MORAINE VALLEY COMMUNITY COLLEGE
3 5029 00383718 2

D1605452

Textbook of Anxiety Disorders

SECOND EDITION

Textbook of Anxiety Disorders

Edited by
Dan J. Stein, M.D., Ph.D.
Eric Hollander, M.D.
Barbara O. Rothbaum, Ph.D., ABPP

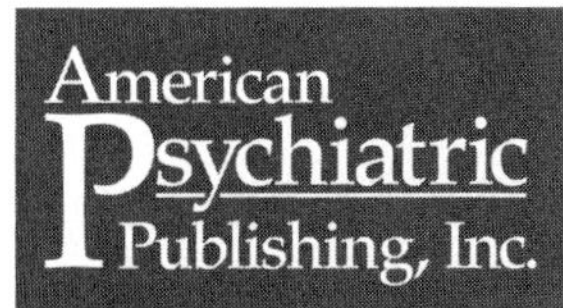

Washington, DC
London, England

Note: The authors have worked to ensure that all information in this book is accurate at the time of publication and consistent with general psychiatric and medical standards, and that information concerning drug dosages, schedules, and routes of administration is accurate at the time of publication and consistent with standards set by the U.S. Food and Drug Administration and the general medical community. As medical research and practice continue to advance, however, therapeutic standards may change. Moreover, specific situations may require a specific therapeutic response not included in this book. For these reasons and because human and mechanical errors sometimes occur, we recommend that readers follow the advice of physicians directly involved in their care or the care of a member of their family.

Books published by American Psychiatric Publishing, Inc., represent the views and opinions of the individual authors and do not necessarily represent the policies and opinions of APPI or the American Psychiatric Association.

Manufactured in the United States of America on acid-free paper
13 12 11 10 09 5 4 3 2 1
Second Edition

Typeset in Adobe's ACaslon and Frutiger

American Psychiatric Publishing, Inc.
1000 Wilson Boulevard
Arlington, VA 22209-3901
www.appi.org

To purchase 25–99 copies of this or any other APPI title at a 20% discount, please contact APPI Customer Service at appi@psych.org or 800-368-5777. If you wish to buy 100 or more copies of the same title, please e-mail bulksales@psych.org for a price quote.

Library of Congress Cataloging-in-Publication Data
Textbook of anxiety disorders / edited by Dan J. Stein, Eric Hollander, Barbara O. Rothbaum. — 2nd ed.
p. ; cm.
Includes bibliographical references and index.
ISBN 978-1-58562-254-2 (alk. paper)
1. Anxiety disorders—Textbooks. I. Stein, Dan J. II. Hollander, Eric, 1957- III. Rothbaum, Barbara Olasov.
[DNLM: 1. Anxiety Disorders. WM 172 T356 2010]
RC531.A525 2010
616.85'22—dc22

2009015495

British Library Cataloguing in Publication Data
A CIP record is available from the British Library.

Contents

PART II
Generalized Anxiety Disorder

PART III

Mixed Anxiety-Depression

PART IV

Obsessive-Compulsive Disorder/Related Disorders

PART V

Panic Disorder/Agoraphobia

PART VI

Social Anxiety Disorder (Social Phobia)

PART VII

Specific Phobia

PART VIII

Posttraumatic Stress Disorder/Acute Stress Disorder

PART IX

Anxiety Disorders in Special Populations

PART X

Social Aspects of Anxiety Disorders

Contributors

Jonathan S. Abramowitz, Ph.D., ABPP
Professor, Department of Psychology, and Director, Anxiety and Stress Disorders Clinic, University of North Carolina at Chapel Hill

Anne Marie Albano, Ph.D., ABPP
Director, Columbia University Clinic for Anxiety and Related Disorders, Columbia University Medical Center, New York, New York

Danielle L. Anderson, M.D.
Assistant Professor, Department of Psychiatry and Behavioral Neuroscience, University of Chicago Hospitals, Chicago, Illinois

Gordon J.G. Asmundson, Ph.D.
Professor and Research Director, Faculty of Kinesiology and Health Studies, University of Regina, Saskatchewan, Canada

Sudie E. Back, Ph.D.
Associate Professor, Clinical Neuroscience Division, Department of Psychiatry and Behavioral Sciences, The Medical University of South Carolina, Charleston, South Carolina

David S. Baldwin, M.D.
Clinical Neuroscience Division, School of Medicine, University of Southampton, Southampton, United Kingdom

Borwin Bandelow, M.D., Ph.D.
Department of Psychiatry and Psychotherapy, University of Göttingen, Göttingen, Germany

Carlos Blanco, M.D., Ph.D.
Associate Professor of Clinical Psychiatry, New York State Psychiatric Institute/Department of Psychiatry, College of Physicians and Surgeons of Columbia University, New York, New York

Kathleen T. Brady, M.D., Ph.D.
Professor and Director, Clinical Neuroscience Division, The Medical University of South Carolina, Charleston, South Carolina

J. Douglas Bremner, M.D.
Professor of Psychiatry and Radiology, Emory University School of Medicine, Atlanta, Georgia; Director of Mental Health Research, Atlanta Veterans Affairs Medical Center, Decatur, Georgia

Timothy A. Brown, Psy.D.
Professor, Center for Anxiety and Related Disorders, Boston University, Boston, Massachusetts

Fredric N. Busch, M.D.
Clinical Associate Professor of Psychiatry, Weill Cornell Medical College; Faculty, Columbia University Center for Psychoanalytic Training and Research, New York, New York

Shawn P. Cahill, Ph.D.
Assistant Professor, Department of Psychology, College of Letters and Science, University of Wisconsin, Milwaukee

Rebecca P. Cameron, Ph.D.
Associate Professor, Department of Psychology, California State University, Sacramento

Raymond Carvajal, M.A.
Doctoral Student, Department of Psychology, Philadelphia College of Osteopathic Medicine, Philadelphia, Pennsylvania

Samuel R. Chamberlain, Ph.D., M.B.B.Ch.
Senior Visiting Clinical Research Fellow, Brain Mapping Unit, Department of Psychiatry, University of Cambridge School of Clinical Medicine, Addenbrooke's Hospital, Cambridge; Clinical Research Associate, Behavioural and Clinical Neuroscience Institute, University of Cambridge, Cambridge, United Kingdom

Dennis S. Charney, M.D.
Dean, Mount Sinai School of Medicine, New York, New York

Denise A. Chavira, Ph.D.
Assistant Professor, Department of Psychiatry, University of California, San Diego

Meredith E. Coles, Ph.D.
Assistant Professor, Department of Psychology, Binghamton University (SUNY), Binghamton, New York

Jeremy D. Coplan, M.D.
Professor of Psychiatry and Director, Division of Neuropsychopharmacology, Department of Psychiatry, State University of New York—Downstate Medical Center, Brooklyn, New York

Bernadette M. Cortese, Ph.D.
Postdoctoral Scholar, Department of Psychiatry and Behavioral Sciences, The Medical University of South Carolina, Charleston, South Carolina

Kevin J. Craig, M.B.B.Ch., M.Phil., MRCPsych
Medical Director, P1vital Limited; University of Oxford Department of Psychiatry, Warneford Hospital, Oxford, United Kingdom

Jonathan R. T. Davidson, M.D.
Professor Emeritus, Department of Psychiatry and Behavioral Sciences, Duke University Medical Center, Durham, North Carolina

Robert A. DiTomasso, Ph.D., ABPP
Professor and Chairman, Department of Psychology, Philadelphia College of Osteopathic Medicine, Philadelphia, Pennsylvania

Darin D. Dougherty, M.D.
Associate Professor of Psychiatry, Harvard Medical School; Director of Medical Education, OCD Institute, Department of Psychiatry, Massachusetts General Hospital, Boston, Massachusetts

Danielle Dufresne, M.A.
Psychology Extern, University of Hartford and The Institute of Living, Hartford, Connecticut

Jane L. Eisen, M.D.
Associate Professor, Psychiatry and Human Behavior, and Associate Dean, Biomedical Faculty, Warren Alpert Medical School of Brown University, Providence, Rhode Island

Jan Fawcett, M.D.
Professor of Psychiatry, University of New Mexico School of Medicine, Albuquerque, New Mexico

Naomi A. Fineberg, M.B.B.S., M.A., MRCPsych
Consultant Psychiatrist and Visiting Professor of the University of Hertfordshire, National OCD Treatment Service, Queen Elizabeth II Hospital, Welwyn, Garden City; Senior Clinical Research Fellow, Department of Psychiatry, University of Cambridge School of Clinical Medicine, Addenbrooke's Hospital, Cambridge, United Kingdom

Edna B. Foa, Ph.D.
Professor and Director of the Center for the Treatment and Study of Anxiety, Department of Psychiatry, School of Medicine, University of Pennsylvania, Philadelphia, Pennsylvania

Arthur Freeman, Ed.D., ABPP
Visiting Professor, Governor's State University, Chicago, Illinois; Clinical Professor, Department of Psychology, Philadelphia College of Osteopathic Medicine, Philadelphia, Pennsylvania

Amanda L. Gamble, Ph.D.
Postdoctoral Research Fellow, Centre for Emotional Health, Department of Psychology, Macquarie University, Sydney, Australia

Maryrose Gerardi, Ph.D.
Assistant Professor, Department of Psychiatry and Behavioral Sciences, Emory University School of Medicine, Atlanta, Georgia

Christina M. Gilliam, Ph.D.
Staff Psychologist, The Institute of Living, Hartford, Connecticut

Andrew W. Goddard, M.D.
Professor of Psychiatry, Department of Psychiatry, Indiana University School of Medicine, Indianapolis, Indiana

Benjamin D. Greenberg, M.D., Ph.D.
Associate Professor of Psychiatry and Human Behavior, Butler Hospital, Warren Alpert Medical School of Brown University, Providence, Rhode Island

Nicola D. Hanson, B.S.
Doctoral candidate, Department of Psychiatry and Behavioral Sciences, Emory University School of Medicine, Atlanta, Georgia

Allison G. Harvey, Ph.D.
Associate Professor, Psychology Department, Sleep and Psychological Disorders Laboratory, University of California, Berkeley

Richard G. Heimberg, Ph.D.
Professor and Distinguished Faculty Fellow in Psychology, Director of the Adult Anxiety Clinic of Temple, Department of Psychology, Temple University, Philadelphia, Pennsylvania

Myron A. Hofer, M.D.
Sackler Professor and Director, Sackler Institute for Developmental Psychobiology, Department of Psychiatry, Columbia University College of Physicians and Surgeons, New York, New York

Stefan G. Hofmann, Ph.D.
Professor of Clinical Psychology, Boston University, Boston, Massachusetts

Elizabeth Hoge, M.D.
Clinical Assistant in Psychiatry, Massachusetts General Hospital; Instructor of Psychiatry, Harvard Medical School, Boston, Massachusetts

Eric Hollander, M.D.
Research Attending Psychiatrist, Montefiore Medical Center, University Hospital of Albert Einstein College of Medicine, New York, New York; formerly Esther and Joseph Klingenstein Professor and Chairman of Psychiatry and Director of the Compulsive, Impulsive and Anxiety Disorders Program, Mount Sinai School of Medicine, New York, New York

Jonathan D. Huppert, Ph.D.
Associate Professor of Psychology, The Hebrew University of Jerusalem, Mt. Scopus, Jerusalem, Israel

Sarah Ketay, Ph.D.
Postdoctoral Fellow, Compulsive and Impulsive Disorder Program, Department of Psychiatry, Mount Sinai School of Medicine, New York, New York

Eric J. Lenze, M.D.
Associate Professor of Psychiatry, Washington University School of Medicine, Department of Psychiatry, St. Louis, Missouri

Ovsanna Leyfer, Ph.D.
Postdoctoral Fellow, Center for Anxiety and Related Disorders, Boston University, Boston, Massachusetts

Michael R. Liebowitz, M.D.
Professor of Clinical Psychiatry, New York State Psychiatric Institute/Department of Psychiatry, College of Physicians and Surgeons of Columbia University, New York, New York

Jeffrey D. Lightfoot, Ph.D.
Clinical Assistant Professor of Psychology in Clinical Psychiatry, Department of Psychiatry, Indiana University School of Medicine, Indianapolis, Indiana

Maria C. Mancebo, Ph.D.
Assistant Professor, Psychiatry and Human Behavior (Research), Brown University, Providence, Rhode Island

Catherine Mancini, M.D., FRCPC
Associate Professor, Department of Psychiatry and Behavioural Neurosciences, McMaster University; Co-director, Anxiety Disorders Clinic, McMaster University Medical Centre—Hamilton Health Sciences, Hamilton, Ontario, Canada

Michael J. Marcangelo, M.D.
Assistant Professor, Department of Psychiatry and Behavioral Neuroscience, University of Chicago Hospitals, Chicago, Illinois

John S. March, M.D., M.P.H.
Professor of Psychiatry and Behavioral Sciences and Director, Division of Neurosciences Medicine, Duke Clinical Research Institute, Duke University Medical Center, Durham, North Carolina

Alexander C. McFarlane, M.D.
Professor, Centre for Military and Veterans' Health Node, University of Adelaide, South Australia

Dean McKay, Ph.D.
Associate Professor, Department of Psychology, Fordham University, Bronx, New York

Barbara L. Milrod, M.D.
Professor of Psychiatry, Weill Cornell Medical College, and Faculty, New York Psychoanalytic Institute, New York, New York

Phoebe S. Moore, Ph.D.
Assistant Consulting Professor, Duke University Medical Center, Durham, North Carolina

Mary Morreale, M.D.
Assistant Professor, Department of Psychiatry, Wayne State University, Detroit, Michigan

Navin Natarajan, M.D.
Resident, Department of Psychiatry, State University of New York—Downstate Medical Center, Brooklyn, New York

Charles B. Nemeroff, M.D., Ph.D.
Reunette W. Harris Professor, Department of Psychiatry and Behavioral Sciences, Emory University School of Medicine, Atlanta, Georgia

Michael W. Otto, Ph.D.
Director, Center for Anxiety and Related Disorders; Professor of Psychology, Boston University, Boston, Massachusetts

Laszlo A. Papp, M.D.
Associate Professor of Clinical Psychiatry, Department of Psychiatry, Columbia University College of Physicians and Surgeons, New York, New York

Beth Patterson, B.Sc.N., B.Ed.
Research Manager, Department of Psychiatry and Behavioural Neurosciences, McMaster University and Anxiety Disorders Clinic, McMaster University Medical Centre—Hamilton Health Sciences, Hamilton, Ontario, Canada

Anthony Pinto, Ph.D.
Adjunct Assistant Professor, Psychiatry and Human Behavior (Research), Brown University, Providence, Rhode Island

Mark H. Pollack, M.D.
Director, Center for Anxiety and Traumatic Stress Disorders, Massachusetts General Hospital; Professor of Psychiatry, Harvard Medical School, Boston, Massachusetts

Kristin E. Pontoski, M.A.
Doctoral Student in Clinical Psychology, Adult Anxiety Clinic of Temple, Department of Psychology, Temple University, Philadelphia, Pennsylvania

Holly J. Ramsawh, Ph.D.
Postdoctoral Fellow, Department of Psychiatry, University of California, San Diego

Ronald M. Rapee, Ph.D.
Professor of Psychology and Director, Centre for Emotional Health, Department of Psychology, Macquarie University, Sydney, Australia

Steven A. Rasmussen, M.D.
Associate Professor, Psychiatry and Human Behavior, Warren Alpert Medical School of Brown University, Providence, Rhode Island

Scott L. Rauch, M.D.
President and Psychiatrist in Chief, McLean Hospital, Belmont, Massachusetts, Chair, Partners Psychiatry and Mental Health, and Professor of Psychiatry, Harvard Medical School, Boston, Massachusetts

Kerry Ressler, M.D., Ph.D.
Associate Professor, Department of Psychiatry and Behavioral Sciences, Yerkes National Primate Center, Emory University School of Medicine, Atlanta, Georgia

Winfried Rief, Ph.D.
Professor of Clinical Psychology, University of Marburg, Marburg, Germany

Jerilyn Ross, M.A., L.I.C.S.W.
President and Chief Executive Officer, Anxiety Disorders Association of America; Director, The Ross Center for Anxiety and Related Disorders, Washington, D.C.

Barbara Olasov Rothbaum, Ph.D., ABPP
Professor, Department of Psychiatry and Behavioral Sciences, and Director, Trauma Anxiety Recovery Program, Emory University School of Medicine, Atlanta, Georgia

William C. Sanderson, Ph.D.
Professor of Psychology, Hofstra University, Hempstead, New York

Casey Sarapas, B.S.
Clinical Research Coordinator, Traumatic Stress Studies Division, Mount Sinai School of Medicine, James J. Peters Veterans Affairs Medical Center, Bronx, New York

Alan F. Schatzberg, M.D.
Professor, Department of Psychiatry and Behavioral Sciences, Stanford University School of Medicine, Stanford, California

Franklin R. Schneier, M.D.
Associate Professor of Clinical Psychiatry, New York State Psychiatric Institute/Department of Psychiatry, College of Physicians and Surgeons of Columbia University, New York, New York

Steven Seay Jr., M.S.
Student, Department of Psychology and Brain Sciences, Indiana University School of Medicine, Bloomington, Indiana

M. Katherine Shear, M.D.
Marion Kenworthy Professor of Psychiatry in Social Work, Columbia University School of Social Work, New York, New York

Ranjeeb Shrestha, M.D.
Resident, Department of Psychiatry, State University of New York—Downstate Medical Center, Brooklyn, New York

Naomi Simon, M.D., M.Sc.
Associate Director, Center for Anxiety and Traumatic Stress Disorders, Massachusetts General Hospital; Associate Professor of Psychiatry, Harvard Medical School, Boston, Massachusetts

William Simpson, B.Sc.
Research Associate, Anxiety Disorders Clinic, McMaster University Medical Centre—Hamilton Health Sciences, Hamilton, Ontario, Canada

Jordan W. Smoller, M.D., Sc.D.
Director, Center for Human Genetic Research, Massachusetts General Hospital; Associate Professor of Psychiatry, Harvard Medical School, Boston, Massachusetts

David A. Spiegel, M.D.
Professor Emeritus, Boston University, Boston, Massachusetts

Dan J. Stein, M.D., Ph.D.
Professor, Department of Psychiatry and Mental Health, University of Cape Town, South Africa

Murray B. Stein, M.D., M.P.H.
Professor, Department of Psychiatry, Department of Family and Preventive Medicine; Director, Anxiety and Traumatic Stress Disorders Program, University of California, San Diego

Michael H. Stone, M.D.
Professor of Clinical Psychiatry, Department of Psychiatry, College of Physicians and Surgeons, Columbia University, New York, New York

Manuel E. Tancer, M.D.
Professor, Department of Psychiatry, Wayne State University, Detroit, Michigan

Steven Taylor, Ph.D., ABPP
Professor, Department of Psychiatry, University of British Columbia, Vancouver, British Columbia, Canada

Margo Thienemann, M.D.
Adjunct Clinical Associate Professor of Psychiatry and Behavioral Sciences, Stanford University Medical Center, Stanford, California

David F. Tolin, Ph.D.
Adjunct Associate Professor of Psychiatry, The Institute of Living and Yale University School of Medicine, Hartford, Connecticut

Christine Truong, B.Sc.
Research Associate, Anxiety Disorders Clinic, McMaster University Medical Centre—Hamilton Health Sciences, Hamilton, Ontario, Canada

Cynthia L. Turk, Ph.D.
Assistant Professor, Department of Psychology, Washburn University, Topeka, Kansas

Thomas W. Uhde, M.D.
Professor and Chair, Department of Psychiatry and Behavioral Sciences, The Medical University of South Carolina, Charleston, South Carolina

Michael Van Ameringen, M.D., FRCPC
Associate Professor, Department of Psychiatry and Behavioural Neurosciences, McMaster University, and Co-Director, Anxiety Disorders Clinic, McMaster University Medical Centre—Hamilton Health Sciences, Hamilton, Ontario, Canada

Oriana Vesga-López, M.D.
Research Scientist, New York State Psychiatric Institute/Department of Psychiatry, College of Physicians and Surgeons of Columbia University, New York, New York

Angela E. Waldrop, Ph.D.
Department of Psychiatry, University of California, San Francisco; Staff Psychologist, PTSD Clinical Team, San Francisco Veterans Affairs Medical Center, San Francisco, California

David Williams, Ph.D.
Florence and Laura Norman Professor of Public Health, Professor of African and African American Studies and of Sociology, and Staff Director, RWJF Commission to Build a Healthier America, Harvard School of Public Health, Department of Society, Human Development and Health, Harvard University, Boston, Massachusetts

Monnica T. Williams, Ph.D.
Assistant Professor of Psychology in Psychiatry, Department of Psychiatry, School of Medicine, University of Pennsylvania, Philadelphia, Pennsylvania

Thomas N. Wise, M.D.
Professor of Psychiatry and Behavioral Sciences, Johns Hopkins University School of Medicine, Baltimore, Maryland; Chairman, Department of Psychiatry, Inova Fairfax Hospital, Fairfax, Virginia

Rachel Yehuda, Ph.D.
Professor of Psychiatry and Director, Traumatic Stress Studies Division, Mount Sinai School of Medicine, James J. Peters Veterans Affairs Medical Center, Bronx, New York

Agustin G. Yip, M.D., Ph.D.
Staff Psychiatrist, Butler Hospital, Providence, Rhode Island

Bruce Zahn, Ed.D., ABPP
Professor, Department of Psychology, Philadelphia College of Osteopathic Medicine, Philadelphia, Pennsylvania

Wei Zhang, M.D., Ph.D.
Director, Anxiety and Traumatic Stress Program, Department of Psychiatry and Behavioral Sciences, Duke University Medical Center, Durham, North Carolina

Disclosure of Interests

The following contributors to this book have indicated a financial interest in or other affiliation with a commercial supporter, a manufacturer of a commercial product, a provider of a commercial service, a nongovernmental organization, and/or a government agency, as listed below:

Anne Marie Albano, Ph.D.—*Grant support:* National Institute of Mental Health (NIMH); *Royalties:* Guilford Press and Oxford University Press.

David S. Baldwin, M.D.—*Research grants* Asahi, AstraZeneca, Cephalon, Eli Lilly, GlaxoSmithKline, Lundbeck, Organon, Pharmacia, Pierre Fabre, Pfizer, Roche, Servier, Sumitomo, and Wyeth; *Consultant:* Asahi, AstraZeneca, Cephalon, Eli Lilly, GlaxoSmithKline, Lundbeck, Organon, Pharmacia, Pierre Fabre, Pfizer, Roche, Servier, Sumitomo, and Wyeth.

Borwin Bandelow, M.D., Ph.D.—*Consultant:* AstraZeneca, Cephalon, Eli Lilly, Lundbeck, Pfizer, Roche, Sanofi-Aventis, and Wyeth; *Speaker's bureau/advisory board:* AstraZeneca, Bristol-Myers Squibb, Dainippon Sumitomo, Janssen-Cilag, Eli Lilly, Lundbeck, Pfizer, Solvay, Wyeth, and Xian-Janssen.

Carlos Blanco, M.D., Ph.D.—*Research support:* GlaxoSmithKline, Pfizer, and Somaxon.

J. Douglas Bremner, M.D.—*Grant support:* National Institutes of Health (NIH): R01 MH56120, T32 MH067547, K24 MH076955; R01 AG026255, R01 HL068630, R01 HL703824, R01 MH068791, P50 MH58922 (as co-investigator), Veterans Affairs: Merit Review, VET-Heal Award, National Alliance for Research on Schizophrenia and Depression (NARSAD) Independent Investigator Award, American Foundation for Suicide Prevention (AFSP), Georgia Research Alliance, GlaxoSmithKline Investigator Initiated Medical Research; *Consultant:* GlaxoSmithKline and Novartis; discussion of off-label medication use: phenytoin.

Dennis S. Charney, M.D.—*Consultant:* AstraZeneca, Bristol-Myers Squibb, Cyberonics, Neurogen, Neuroscience Education Institute, Novartis, Orexigen, and Unilever UK Central Resources Limited; *Patent:* Ketamine.

Jeremy D. Coplan, M.D.—*Grant funding:* GlaxoSmithKline and Pfizer; *Honoraria:* Bristol-Myers Squibb, Forest, and Pfizer.

Kevin J. Craig, M.B.B.Ch., M.Phil.—*Research support:* GlaxoSmithKline; *Consultant:* GlaxoSmithKline.

Jonathan R.T. Davidson, M.D.—*Research and other support:* AstraZeneca, Bristol-Myers Squibb, Cephalon, CME Institute, Forest, GlaxoSmithKline, Janssen, International Psychopharmacology Algorithm Project, Eli Lilly, Pfizer, UCB; *Speaker's bureau:* Duke University Medical Center, GlaxoSmithKline, Forest, Henry Jackson Foundation, Massachusetts Psychiatric Society, North Carolina Psychiatric Association, Pfizer, Psychiatric Society of Virginia, Solvay, Texas Society of Psychiatric Physicians, University of Chicago, University of Hawaii, University of North Carolina, and University of Utah; *Advisor:* Actelion, AstraZeneca, Brain Cells, Epix, Forest, GlaxoSmithKline, Janssen, Jazz Pharmaceuticals, Eli Lilly, MediciNova, Organon, Pfizer, Roche, Sanofi-Aventis, TransOral, and Wyeth; *Royalties:* American Psychiatric Association, Current Medical Science, Guilford Publications, MultiHealth Systems Inc., and Taylor and Francis; *Stock:* Procter and Gamble.

Darin D. Dougherty, M.D.—*Research funding:* Cephalon, Cyberonics, Eli Lilly, Forest, McNeil, Medtronic, and Northstar Neuroscience; *Consultant/advisor:* Jazz, Medtronic, and Trancept Pharmaceuticals; *Honoraria:* Cyberonics, McNeil, Medtronic, and Northstar Neuroscience.

Naomi. A. Fineberg, M.B.B.S., M.A.—*Grant support:* AstraZeneca, Bristol-Myers Squibb, Cephalon, Janssen, and Lundbeck; *Consultant:* GlaxoSmithKline and Lundbeck; *Speaker's bureau:* AstraZeneca and Wyeth.

Andrew W. Goddard, M.D.—*Grant support:* AstraZeneca, Janssen-McNeil, Orexigen, and Pfizer; *Consultant:* Orexigen; *Speaker's bureau:* Astra, Janssen-McNeil, Orexigen, and Pfizer; *Honorarium:* Orexigen.

Benjamin D. Greenberg, M.D., Ph.D.—*Research funding:* Medtronic; *Consultant:* Jazz and Medtronic.

Allison G. Harvey, Ph.D.—*Consultant:* Actelion; *Speaker's bureau:* Sanofi-Aventis and Sleep Medicine Education Institute.

Stefan G. Hoffman, Ph.D.—*Research support:* National Institute of Mental Health; *Consultant:* Organon.

Elizabeth Hoge, M.D.—*Research grants:* AstraZeneca, Bristol-Myers Squibb, Cephalon, Forest Laboratories, GlaxoSmithKline, Janssen, Eli Lilly, NIH, Pfizer, UCB Pharma, and Sepracor.

Eric Hollander, M.D.—*Research grants:* Forest, GlaxoSmithKline, and Solvay; *Consultant:* Jazz Pharmaceuticals.

Eric J. Lenze, M.D.—*Research funding:* Forest and Pfizer.

Michael R. Liebowitz, M.D.—*Clinical trial contracts:* Abbott, AstraZeneca, Avera, Cephalon, Forest, GlaxoSmithKline, Jazz, Johnson & Johnson, Horizon, Eli Lilly, MAP, Novartis, PGX Health, Pherin, Sepracor, Pfizer, Takeda, Tikvah, and Wyeth; *Consultant:* AstraZeneca, Jazz, Lilly, Pherin, Tikvah, and Wyeth; *Speaker's bureau:* AstraZeneca, Bristol-Myers Squibb, Jazz, and Wyeth, *Equity:* ChiMatrix, electronic data capture, and Liebowitz Social Anxiety Scale; *Licensing software or LSAS:* Avera, GlaxoSmithKline, Indevus, Lilly, Pfizer, Servier, and Tikvah.

Catherine Mancini, M.D., FRCPC—*Grant/research support:* AstraZeneca, Canadian Foundation for Innovation (CFI), Cephalon, GlaxoSmithKline, Eli Lilly, Janssen-Ortho, NIH, Novartis, Pfizer, Sanofi-Aventis, Servier, and Wyeth-Ayerst; *Consultant:* Shire; *Speaker's bureau:* GlaxoSmithKline.

John S. March, M.D. M.P.H.—*Research support:* Eli Lilly and Pfizer; *federal:* TADS, CAMS, POTS I, II, and Jr., RUPP-PI, CAPTN, and K24; *foundation:* NARSAD; *Consultant:* GlaxoSmithKline, Lilly, Pfizer, and Wyeth; *Scientific advisor:* Lilly, Pfizer, and Seaside; *DSMB:* AstraZeneca and Johnson & Johnson; *Equity:* MedAvante and Multidimensional Anxiety Scale for Children (MultiHealth Systems),.

Barbara L. Milrod, M.D.—*Lecture/speaker's bureau:* New York Psychoanalytic Institute and Swedish Psychotherapy Association.

Charles B. Nemeroff, M.D., Ph.D.—*Grant support:* AFSP, NARSAD, and NIH; *Scientific advisory board:* AstraZeneca, Forest Laboratories, Johnson & Johnson, NARSAD, Pharma Neuroboost, and Quintiles; *Employed by:* Serves on the Board of Directors of AFSP, APIRE, NovaDel Pharmaceuticals, and the George West Mental Health Foundation. *Equity:* CeNeRx and Reevax. *Stock:* Corcept and NovaDel.

Michael W. Otto, Ph.D.—*Consultant/advisory board:* AstraZeneca, Jazz Pharmaceuticals, and Organon.

Mark H. Pollack, M.D.—*Research grants:* Bristol-Myers Squibb, Cephalon, Forest Laboratories, GlaxoSmithKline, Janssen, Eli Lilly, NARSAD, NIDA, NIMH, Pfizer, Sepracor, UCB Pharma, and Wyeth; *Consultant/advisory board:* AstraZeneca, Brain Cells, Bristol-Myers Squibb, Cephalon, Forest Laboratories, GlaxoSmithKline, Janssen, Jazz, Eli Lilly, Medavante, Neurocrine, Neurogen, Novartis, Otsuka Pharmaceuticals, Pfizer, Predix, Roche Laboratories, Sanofi, Sepracor, Solvay, Tikvah Therapeutics, Transcept, UCB Pharma, and Wyeth; *Speaker's bureau:* Bristol-Myers Squibb, Forest Laboratories, GlaxoSmithKline, Janssen, Lilly, Pfizer, Solvay, and Wyeth; *Equity:* Medavante and Mensante.

Scott L. Rauch, M.D.—*Funded research (through Massachusetts General Hospital):* Cyberonics and Medtronics, Inc.; *Consultant:* Novartis; *Honoraria:* Cyberonics, Medtronics, Neurogen, Novartis, Primedia, and Sepracor.

Kerry Ressler, M.D., Ph.D.—*Grant/funding support:* Burroughs Wellcome Foundation, Lundbeck, NARSAD, National Institute on Drug Abuse (NIDA), NIMH, and Pfizer; *Consultant:* Tikvah Therapeutics.

Barbara O. Rothbaum, Ph.D.—*Research funding:* Janssen, Pfizer, and Wyeth; *Consultant:* Virtually Better; Scientific advisory board: Tikvah Therapeutics; *Equity:* Virtually Better.

Alan F. Schatzberg, M.D.—*Consultant:* Abbott, Aventis, Bristol-Myers Squibb, Corcept, Eli Lilly, Forest Laboratories, GlaxoSmithKline, Innapharma, Janssen, Merck, Novartis, Organon, Pharmacia, Solvay, Somerset, Wyeth; *Grants:* Bristol-Myers Squibb, Eli Lilly, Wyeth; *Equity:* Corcept, Cypress Biosciences, Elan, Merck, Pfizer

M. Katherine Shear, M.D.—*Research funding:* Forest Laboratories; *Consultant/Advisory board:* Forest Laboratories and Pfizer.

Naomi Simon, M.D., M.Sc.—*Grant/research support:* AstraZeneca, Bristol-Myers Squibb, Cephalon, Eli Lilly, Forest Laboratories, GlaxoSmithKline, Janssen, NARSAD, NIMH, Pfizer, Sepracor, and UCB Pharma; *Consultant/advisory board:* Paramount Biosciences and Solvay; *Speaker's bureau:* Forest Laboratories, Janssen, Lilly, Pfizer, Sepracor, and UCB Pharma.

Jordan W. Smoller, M.D., Sc.D.—*Consultant:* Eli Lilly; Advisory board: Roche Diagnostics.

Dan J. Stein, M.D., Ph.D.—*Research grant:* AstraZeneca, Eli Lilly, GlaxoSmithKline, Johnson & Johnson, Lundbeck, Orion, Pfizer, Pharmacia, Roche, Servier, Solvay, Sumitomo, Tikvah, and Wyeth; *Consultant:* AstraZeneca, Eli Lilly, GlaxoSmithKline, Johnson & Johnson, Lundbeck, Orion, Pfizer, Pharmacia, Roche, Servier, Solvay, Sumitomo, Tikvah, and Wyeth.

Murray B. Stein, M.D., M.P.H., FRCPC—*Research support:* Eli Lilly, Forest Laboratories and GlaxoSmithKline; *Consultant:* AstraZeneca, Avera, Bristol-Myers Squibb, Eli Lilly & Company, Forest Laboratories, GlaxoSmithKline, Hoffman-La Roche, Integral Health Decisions, Jazz, Johnson & Johnson, Pfizer, and Virtual Reality Medical Center; *Stock:* Co-owner of NeuroMarkers.

Thomas W. Uhde, M.D.—*Speaker's bureau:* Jazz Pharmaceuticals.

Michael Van Ameringen, M.D.—*Grant/research support:* AstraZeneca, Cephalon, Eli Lilly, GlaxoSmithKline, Janssen-Ortho, National Institutes of Health (NIH), Novartis, Pfizer, Servier, and Wyeth-Ayerst; *Consultant:* Biovail, Cephalon, GlaxoSmithKline, Janssen-Ortho, Novartis, Pfizer, Servier, Shire, and Wyeth-Ayerst; *Speaker's bureau:* GlaxoSmithKline, Janssen-Ortho, Pfizer, and Wyeth-Ayerst.

Angela E. Waldrop, Ph.D.—*Research support:* NIH.

Thomas N. Wise, M.D.—*Speaker's bureau:* Eli Lilly and Pfizer.

The following authors have no competing interests to report:

Jonathan S. Abramowitz, Ph.D.
Danielle L. Anderson, M.D.
Gordon J. G. Asmundson, Ph.D.
Sudie Back, Ph.D.
Kathleen T. Brady, M.D., Ph.D.
Timothy A. Brown, Psy.D.
Fredric N. Busch, M.D.
Shawn P. Cahill, Ph.D.
Rebecca P. Cameron, Ph.D.
Raymond Carvajal, M.A.
Samuel R. Chamberlain, Ph.D., M.B.B.Ch.
Denise A. Chavira, Ph.D.
Meredith E. Coles, Ph.D.
Bernadette M. Cortese, Ph.D.
Robert A. DiTomasso, Ph.D.
Danielle Dufresne, M.A.
Jane L. Eisen, M.D.
Jan Fawcett, M.D.
Edna Foa, Ph.D.
Amanda L. Gamble, Ph.D.
Maryrose Gerardi, Ph.D.
Christina M. Gilliam, Ph.D.
Nicola D. Hanson, B.S.
Richard G. Heimberg, Ph.D.
Myron A. Hofer, M.D.
Jonathan D. Huppert, Ph.D.
Sarah Ketay, Ph.D.
Ovsanna Leyfer, Ph.D.
Jeffrey D. Lightfoot, Ph.D..
Maria C. Mancebo, Ph.D.
Michael J. Marcangelo, M.D.
Alexander C. McFarlane, M.D.
Dean McKay, Ph.D.
Phoebe S. Moore, Ph.D.
Mary Morreale, M.D.
Navin Natarajan, M.D.
Laszlo A. Papp, M.D.
Beth Patterson, B.Sc.N., B.Ed.
Anthony Pinto, Ph.D.
Kristin E. Pontoski, M.A.
Holly J. Ramsawh, Ph.D.
Ronald M. Rapee, Ph.D.
Winfried Rief, Ph.D.
Jerilyn Ross, M.A., L.I.C.S.W.
William C. Sanderson, Ph.D.
Casey Sarapas, B.S.
Franklin R. Schneier, M.D.
Steven J. Seay Jr., M.S.
Ranjeeb Shrestha, M.D.
William Simpson, B.S.
Michael H. Stone, M.D.
Manuel E. Tancer, M.D.
Steven Taylor, Ph.D.
Margo Thienemann, M.D.
David F. Tolin, Ph.D.
Christine Truong, B.Sc.
Cynthia L. Turk, Ph.D.
Oriana Vesga-Lopez, M.D.
David Williams, Ph.D.
Monnica T. Williams, Ph.D.
Rachel Yehuda, Ph.D.
Agustin G. Yip, M.D., Ph.D.
Bruce Zahn, Ed.D.

Foreword

I am delighted, honored, and proud to comment on the second edition of the *Textbook of Anxiety Disorders,* a major and most welcome contribution to the field. I'm delighted that the psychiatric community recognizes the position of anxiety disorders as among the most misdiagnosed and undertreated, yet most prevalent and economically burdensome of all psychiatric syndromes. I'm honored for the opportunity, on behalf of the Anxiety Disorders Association of America (ADAA), to remark on this outstanding collection of contributions by world-renowned experts at the leading edge of research, theory, and clinical knowledge. And I'm proud that the anxiety disorders field is growing at such a rapid pace that an updated edition, designed to reach a broader audience of health care professionals, is warranted.

When the ADAA was established nearly 30 years ago (as the Phobia Society of America), there was no "anxiety disorders field." Not only didn't we have names for the different disorders, we labeled just about everything a phobia. The young man who spent hours each day washing and rewashing his hands was said to have a germ phobia. "Agoraphobia, without avoidance" was how we diagnosed the young mother who had repeated panic attacks but continued to carry out her daily activities. The soldier who returned from the front line who avoided driving for fear of the flashbacks that occurred anytime he heard a loud noise on the road behind him was said to have a "driving phobia caused by shell shock."

In the late 1970s, following a CBS *60 Minutes* program about phobias, thousands of people were relieved to learn that there was a name for what was ailing them—and that they were not alone. Still, they were embarrassed to talk about their irrational fears, thoughts, or behaviors. And when they sought help, they found limited options. When the Phobia Society of America was formed in 1979 by a small group of psychiatrists, psychologists, social workers, patients, and family members, myself included, its purpose was to find answers to these questions: How can we better understand these disorders? What can we do to help those suffering from them?

By 1990, a few years after the *Diagnostic and Statistical Manual of Mental Disorders* (DSM) put forth criteria for differentially diagnosing each distinct anxiety disorder, the organization had changed its name to the Anxiety Disorders Association of America to more accurately reflect the conditions it represents. Although ADAA is not planning to change its name again any time soon, it has participated in the process of the development of the forthcoming DSM-V, and, as a stakeholder, it is eagerly looking forward to that edition's publication in 2012. The information in the new edition of this textbook will help guide that revision, as well as that of the *International Statistical Classification of Diseases and Related Health Problems,* 10th Revision (ICD-10).

During the past few decades, research into the phenomenology, pathophysiology, and neurobiology of anxiety disorders has exploded, offering people with anxiety disorders hope and help. The translation of neuroscience, which looks at what happens in laboratory animals and applies the understanding of how the same mechanisms work in humans, has introduced new insights into the root causes of anxiety, provided us with new and more optimal psychosocial and pharmacological treatments, and led to exciting breakthroughs in the interaction between genes and the environment. But we have a long way to go, especially with regard to understanding the onset of the disorders and their impact on special populations—women, children, adolescents, and the elderly. Posttraumatic stress disorder, common to all populations, presents an ongoing—and growing—global challenge.

The vision of the editors of the second edition of the *Textbook of Anxiety Disorders* to present health professionals in a wide range of disciplines with the translation of neuroscience, as well as a broader understanding of the phenomenology of anxiety disorders, is reflected in the well-considered organization of the book. The beginning chapters focus on the basic mechanisms of anxiety disorders and are followed by a thorough review of each disorder addressed from multiple perspectives. The chapters covering the latest developments in pharmacological and psychosocial interventions for each disorder make the book particularly relevant for clinicians in the medical field as well as psychologists, social workers, counselors, and other mental health professionals involved in the treatment of anxiety disorders. Medical students and those in psychology, social work, and other mental health–related graduate programs preparing for clinical practice will also find this an excellent teaching tool and reference guide. The final section of the book focuses on special populations and the social aspects of anxiety disorders, areas of particular relevance to the efforts of ADAA to overcome stigma, to work toward the prevention, treatment and cure of anxiety disorders, and to improve the lives of all people who suffer from them.

For this invaluable resource we owe a debt of gratitude to the editors: Dan J. Stein, M.D., Ph.D.; Eric Hollander, M.D.; and Barbara Olasov Rothbaum, Ph.D., ABPP. Dr. Stein has made major contributions to the understanding of the psychobiology and management of anxiety disorders, especially in the areas of social anxiety disorder, obsessive-compulsive disorder, and posttraumatic stress disorder. Dr. Hollander has significantly contributed to the knowledge base of OCD and the OCD spectrum disorders through his pioneering research into the understanding of the basic neurobiology of OCD, an expanded notion of repetitive behaviors, and the conceptualization of anxiety disorders.

The addition of Dr. Rothbaum, a clinical psychologist and highly esteemed researcher, as an editor for this edition broadens the book's relevance to both the scientific and clinical communities. Dr. Rothbaum's cutting-edge work in the application of virtual reality to the treatment of anxiety disorders and her use of basic learning mechanisms in exposure therapy have given clinicians new weapons in their arsenal of effective treatments.

Thanks to the contributors to this book, we have a greater understanding of the root causes of anxiety disorders, proven treatments, and new hope for those whose lives have been compromised by persistent, irrational, chronic, or life-altering anxiety. The book will inform and foster discussion. It is poised to influence health professionals in their understanding of anxiety disorders, enhance their clinical skills, and provide them with the background to best communicate with their colleagues, legislators, and the public that anxiety disorders are real, serious, and treatable. It is a major leap forward for the field.

Jerilyn Ross, M.A., L.I.C.S.W.
Director, The Ross Center for Anxiety & Related Disorders
President and CEO, Anxiety Disorders Association of America

Preface

Anxiety is one of the oldest of subjects. The phylogenetic origins of anxiety date back to the origins of the animal kingdom, and philosophers and thinkers have long written about the centrality of anxiety to human life and experience. The experience of anxiety has a ubiquity and a universality that extends across times and across cultures.

At the same time, anxiety is one of the newest of subjects. It is only in the past few decades that scientists and clinicians have been able to develop rigorous diagnostic schemas, to appreciate the prevalence of different anxiety disorders, to understand their underlying psychobiology, and to develop effective pharmacotherapy and psychotherapy interventions.

While the universality of anxiety and its disorders provides this book with its justification, it is these new advances that have often inspired our interest in the anxiety disorders and that provided the immediate impetus to collect a series of contributions at the cutting edge of anxiety disorder research and clinical practice. New advances are also the reason for this second edition of our original volume; we felt that many chapters were in need of updating, and that developments in the field required the text to be supplemented with new chapters.

A number of these advances are particularly worth emphasizing at the outset. First, it is not always appreciated that the anxiety disorders are not only among the most prevalent of the psychiatric disorders, but also among the most disabling. Both the National Comorbidity Survey–Replication and the World Mental Health Survey found that taken together, the anxiety disorders are more common than either mood or substance use disorders.

Furthermore, it has been estimated that one-third of all costs of psychiatric disorders are due to the anxiety disorders; in particular, the anxiety disorders are associated with high indirect costs. Although the high direct costs of disorders such as the psychotic disorders are obvious, the high indirect costs of the anxiety disorders are less so, and therefore require continued emphasis.

Unfortunately, however, the anxiety disorders continue to be misdiagnosed and undertreated. Perhaps the very universality of anxiety makes it more difficult for caregivers to appreciate the morbidity of anxiety disorders, and for patients to seek help. Clinicians and advocacy groups have made important strides in increasing awareness, but much further work remains to be done.

On the other hand, the psychobiology of anxiety disorders is indisputably one of the most interesting and rewarding areas of contemporary medical research. The specific neuroanatomy, neurochemistry, cognitive dysfunctions, and genetic and environmental contributions to each of the anxiety disorders are gradually being outlined. Data from disparate fields are being integrated into powerful and sophisticated models.

Indeed, anxiety disorders provide researchers and clinicians a remarkable locus for integration. Animal models of fear conditioning, for example, provide fascinating parallels with clinical phenomena such as posttraumatic stress. Similarly, functional brain imaging has demonstrated how the pharmacotherapy and psychotherapy of anxiety disorders are both able to normalize underlying functional neuroanatomy, providing a unique opportunity for the integration of brain and mind.

In the remainder of this volume we include subsections on each of the main anxiety disorders (including chapters on their phenomenology, psychobiology, pharmacotherapy, and psychotherapy). The introductory and concluding sections also consider a number of theoretical and clinical issues that cut across the different anxiety disorders.

We would like to express our gratitude to the contributors who have updated their chapters or provided entirely new chapters for this second edition, to our colleagues who have helped support and guide us, to the patients who have taught us about themselves, and to our families for their love and encouragement.

Dan J. Stein, M.D., Ph.D.
Eric Hollander, M.D.
Barbara O. Rothbaum, Ph.D., ABPP

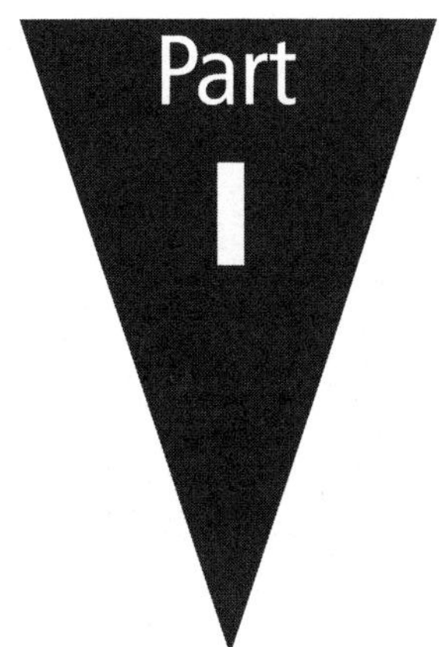

Approaching the Anxiety Disorders

Chapter 1

History of Anxiety Disorders

Michael H. Stone, M.D.

Anxiety goes back to our very beginnings. Perhaps because of the very universality of anxiety as part of the human condition, physicians in ancient times omitted it from their roster of mental illnesses. The Greeks of the classical age had words for mania, melancholia, hysteria, and paranoia. (In fact, those are the Greek words that we still use today.) But they had no word for *anxiety*. In modern Greek, we confront the word *anesuchia*, whose root meaning is "not quiet" or "not calm." The Romans in Cicero's time used the word *anxietas*, which indicated a lasting state of fearfulness, in contrast with *angor*, which signified a momentary state of intense fear, akin to our concept of panic. *Angor* also meant strangling—and derives from the verb *ango*—to press something together, to strangle. The idea of narrowness is another connotation, as in the Latin *angustia* (narrowness), the French *angoisse* (anguish—a more acute, paniclike state), and the German *angst* (fear) and *eng* (narrow). The *angr* root in Indo-European languages also gave rise to our *anger* (akin to Old Norse *angra:* grief) and *angina* (a term also used in Roman times to signify a crushing sensation in the chest and the accompanying dread).

Early Commentaries on Anxiety or Equivalent States

It is easy enough to understand the origins of our modern word because anxiety is often accompanied by a feeling of closeness; a feeling of pressure on the chest, such that one can scarcely breathe; or a feeling of pressure on the abdomen (Littre and Robin 1858).

Berrios and Link (1995) pointed out that, although many references to anxiety-like states are found in older books such as Burton's (1621) *Anatomy of Melancholy*, the term *anxiety* was not used as such in psychiatric parlance until later. Instead, the individual symptoms and manifestations were considered as separate diseases or conditions. That is, the difficulty breathing while in a state of anxiety would be ascribed to some pulmonary abnormality, what we call "butterflies in the stomach" would be understood as some gastric malady, and the dizziness that may accompany intense anxiety might be described as the "condition" of vertigo and seen as a function of a middle-ear problem. Symptoms of this sort would be manifestations of what Berrios and Link (1995) called the *objective* aspects of anxiety. These include what we now call the psychosomatic illnesses that can arise in the context of intense anxiety, such as abdominal pain, palpitations, hot flushes, and breathlessness. The contrasting *subjective* aspects are those that adhere more closely to modern conceptions of anxiety states or disorders, such as feelings of terror; pressing worries; phobias; stage fright; obsessive ruminations about dirt, disease, and death; and experiences of depersonalization or derealization. Burton (1621) hinted that some connection probably existed between the disturbances of the mind and those of the body:

> The Minde most effectually workes upon the Body, producing by his passions and perturbations, miraculous alterations; as Melancholy, despaire, cruell diseases, and sometimes death itselfe. Inso much, that it

> is most true which Plato saith in his *Charmides*: omnia corpora mala ab anima procedere: all the mischiefs of the Body, proceede from the Soule. (p. 78)

But nowhere does Burton mention the term *anxiety* itself.

Anxiety, as we understand it, was often conflated with the concept of melancholia in medieval times and during the Renaissance. Just as contemporary clinicians seldom encounter seriously depressed patients who are not also anxious to a significant degree, "melancholic" persons in bygone times were simultaneously considered pathologically anxious. One common form of this mixed state was (and still is) lovesickness. Presumably, there was something special about lovesickness (or doubting-with-compulsions) that would attract the attention of a physician: persons with these conditions were dysfunctional. The lovesick nephew, for example, was seen as wasting away in bed, lacking appetite and even the will to live. Someone expressing the same worry repeatedly and showing some repetitive behavior (such as hand washing) would strike physicians and laypersons alike as "different" from an ordinary person. What was missing, and what did not become common medical currency until the nineteenth century, was the awareness that anxiety (of this more than "normal" sort) was the red thread that ran through a variety of conditions: lovesickness, obsessive-compulsive symptoms, fainting spells, hypochondriasis, and the like. At the same time, these *anxiety disorders*, as we would call them, usually fell short of necessitating institutional care. Hence, the medical literature from the first printed books (mid-fifteenth century) until this "red thread" was discovered was very sparse in its mention of these disorders.

Among the descriptions of such conditions in the seventeenth century was that of the English moral-tract writer Richard Younge. In his sketches of mental abnormalities (Younge 1638) are some that inspired the characterology of Richard Flecknoe's *Enigmaticall Characters*, written a generation later (Flecknoe 1658). By then, as Hunter and Macalpine (1963) noted, psychiatric labels had come to be attached to these abnormal states. Flecknoe wrote of "anxiety states" in which "one troubles herself with every thing," or the "irresolute person" (the contemporary obsessive-compulsive person), who "hovers in his every choice like an empty Ballance with no weight of Judgment to incline him to either scale...when he begins to deliberate, he never makes an end" (Hunter and Macalpine 1963, p. 116).

A Cross-Cultural Perspective

Attention by the medical community to anxiety disorders was not confined to the West. In many instances, however, the cultural differences that affected how anxiety was understood, experienced, and treated were profound, differing substantially from conceptions familiar to those of a European or American background.

The eleventh-century Persian physician Avicenna ('Ali al-Husayn ibn Sina: 980–1037) wrote an encyclopedic treatise called the *Canons of Medicine*, covering all conditions—including mental conditions such as mania and melancholy. As for anxiety, the story is told (Hajal 1994) of how Avicenna was able to diagnose and cure a case of combined depression and anxiety—known as "lovesickness" (*ishk*)—in a young nobleman who was deeply in love with a woman he thought was "forbidden." He had fallen into a state of intense anxiety and melancholy. Relying on fluctuations in the man's pulse as Avicenna mentioned locales nearer and nearer to where the woman lived, the physician diagnosed that the man was, much to his chagrin, in love with his cousin. His uncle the king considered a union of cousins legitimate, however, and with that blessing the young man quickly recovered.

In ancient China, emphasis was placed on the supposed correspondence between certain emotions and the bodily organs that were deemed especially vulnerable to these emotions. Excess anger, for example, was considered harmful to the liver; excess happiness, to the heart. Fear was deleterious to the kidney; sadness, to the lungs (perhaps because sighing is linked with sadness). As in the case of lovesickness, anxiety and depression often occur together, so it is not surprising that the usual Chinese term for anxiety to this day is *yu-lü*; the first character designates grief, the second character, care or anxiety. Related words express the notion of anticipation (reminiscent of Freud's concept of *anticipatory* anxiety): *lü-huan* (to take precautions against calamity) and *lü-chi* (to anticipate). The main Japanese term for anxiety is the same as in Chinese, using the same characters, though pronounced a bit differently: *yū-ryo,* signifying "anxious-thought."

Traditional Chinese medicine aims to treat anxiety through the kidney, just as it would treat anger through the liver and mania via some intervention involving the heart. Even now, one of the commonest diagnostic terms in psychiatric practice in China is *neurasthenia*—no longer used in the West. Patients so diagnosed are generally rediagnosed with anxiety or depression, or both, when evaluated according to ICD-9 criteria (Zhang 1989). An important variant of neurasthenia in contemporary China is *shenkui* (literally, kidney deficiency), supposedly brought about by excessive masturbation and leading to lassitude and weakness. The anxiety component consists of the worry that this habit may deplete a young man's *yang*, or masculine force (Stone 1997a, p. 419). Still another variety is called *brain neurasthenia*, brought about by excessive studying (*naoshenjing shuai-ruo*), and associated with dizziness, insomnia, and poor concentration. What these examples show is that situations that, worldwide, typically cause anxiety are accompanied by varying somatic and psychic symptoms—shaped by the different cultures within which the situations (exam-fear, love-worries) occur (see Chapter 39, "Cultural and Social Aspects of Anxiety Disorders," in this volume).

In Korea there is an anxiety-related condition to which middle-aged women are particularly prone when troubled by marital unhappiness or domestic violence. They develop *hwa-byung*, in which anxiety, depression, and a sense of burning in the abdomen are combined (the term means fire disease). In bygone times, the condition was often treated by a village shaman, who in effect "exorcised" the offending spirit (which we would identify as the unexpressed anger of the patient). Nowadays, with increasing westernization, treatment is more apt to be antianxiety medication and psychotherapy.

Eighteenth-Century Impressions About Anxiety

At some point in the early eighteenth century, the term *anxiety* began to be used in medical writing about mental illness. We can hardly speak about "psychiatry" yet because this word did not come into medical parlance until Johann Reil coined it in 1808. Use of the term *anxiety* also meant, in effect, that a distinction was being established between the "normal" levels average people experienced after disappointments in love, financial worries, and so on, and the excessive levels noticeable in persons who overreacted grossly to similar life events (as LePois [1618] had commented on a century earlier).

In England, Sir Richard Blackmore (1653–1729), in a treatise on "vapours," advocated "pacifick medicines" for what today we would call anxiety states and other significant psychological disturbances: "If Inquietude be the Distemper, Quiet must be the Cure" (Blackmore 1725). The old term *vapours* was itself analogous in some respects to our concept of anxiety disorders: Aristotle had contended, for example, that the brain condensed vapors that emanated from the heart and that vapors were involved in various "nervous" (especially hysteric) states (Stone 1997a). Blackmore believed that opiates in moderation were helpful in "hypochondriacal and hysteric" cases and did not lead to loss of appetite or mental dullness.

The first psychiatric textbook in English was written by William Battie (1703–1776), director of Bethlem Hospital in London, England, and later (in 1751) the founder of St. Luke's Hospital, also in London.

Although his work concentrated on the more grave (we would say *psychotic*) disorders necessitating hospitalization, he distinguished between "madness" and "anxiety," writing of the latter in this vein:

> It may not be improper to take some notice of those two other disorders...which were excluded from our definition of Madness, viz., praeternatural Anxiety or Sensation too greatly excited by real objects, and its contrary Insensibility or Sensation not sufficiently excited by real objects.... Madness in its proper sense [is] very often preceded by or accompanied with the first and often terminates in the second of these two disorders.... Whatever may be the cause of Anxiety, it chiefly discovers itself by that agonizing impatience observable in some men of black November days, of easterly winds, of heat, cold, damps, etc. (Battie 1758, p. 33)

On the theoretical plane, Battie adhered to the view that anxiety was to be understood mainly in terms of the body, more so than of the mind, insofar as it represented an "excess of sensation." Battie's awareness that many deluded persons (those with "madness") also at times experienced "anxiety," whereas many other persons showed "anxiety" without ever experiencing "madness" confused some of his colleagues, such as James Vere (1700–1779). Vere (1778) was a merchant of London and a governor of the Bethlem Hospital. In his view, nervousness (which we can read as *anxiety*) could be understood as the outcome of an internal war or conflict—between the "lower order of instincts" and the "moral instincts." The lower order of instincts involved the preservation and continuance of existence (which we might read as *sex and aggression*). This strikes the modern ear as very much in keeping with the Freudian tripartite model of the mind, in which the ego is seen as mediating between the impulses stemming from the id and the prohibitions imposed by the superego (Freud 1923/1961). In a similar prelibation of Freudian theory (here, the aspect dealing with the pleasure-pain principle), Vere also spoke of the "two great principles which actuate all animated bodies: appetite and desire [versus] aversion and dislike."

The Scottish neurologist Robert Whytt (1714–1766) focused, as Battie had done, on sensation and the peripheral nervous system in his writings on hysteria, hypochondriasis, and the "nervous disorders" (Whytt 1765). He mentioned that "the coats of the nerves may be obstructed, or inflamed, compressed by hard swellings, or irritated by acrid humours" (p. 85), and viewed abnormalities of this sort (perhaps because of his neurological background) as the root causes of the minor (i.e., nonpsychotic) afflictions he worked with. Whytt also wrote of *nervous exhaustion*—similar to the nineteenth-century concept of *neurasthenia*. Allusions to what we would consider anxiety are found in Whytt's comments on palpitations, in which he states, "In those whose nervous system is easily moved, any sudden and strong passion, but especially fear, will produce palpitations, and an irregular motion of the heart, by rendering it more irritable" (p. 286).

The relationship between anxiety and nightmares was touched on in a treatise on the *incubus* by John Bond in 1753. The idea of an incubus as a causative factor in nightmares stemmed from the belief that some spirit or ghostly person crept in during the night and lay upon the sleeper, so as to constrict the chest and breathing—leading to a sense of suffocation, side by side with a terrifying dream of being either crushed or (in the case of a woman) sexually violated by the (male) incubus or *ephialtes*, as many authors of this period called it. Sleepers thus set upon feel they are about to die—but as Bond (who was himself prone to nightmares) stated, "As soon as they shake off that vast oppression, they are affected with a strong palpitation, great anxiety, languor, and uneasiness—which symptoms gradually abate, and are succeeded by the pleasing reflection of having escaped such imminent danger" (p. 3). Further on, Bond gives examples of women who experienced nightmares in the two or three days before their menses, complaining of anxiety and oppression in the breasts for several days after the menstrual flow began (p. 48). Here, there is an early allusion to "premenstrual tension." But in the more common form of nightmare, Bond pictured the nightmare as causing the anxiety—whereas we would tend to think that certain anxiety-engendering life events from the previous day were the main causative factors. Another way to understand the concept of the incubus is to reflect once again on the root meaning of "anxiety" as referred to above: the (distressing) mental accompaniment of being strangled or suffocated by a weight pressing on the chest.

In France, intense anxiety states were mentioned in the medical text of Boissier de Sauvages (1752), although not yet with the terms *anxiété* or *angoisse*. He spoke, for example, of *panophobia*, a generalized state of anxiety that might express itself by turns as *pavor nocturnus*, intense shaking of the body, insomnia, or feelings of terror arising from the "working of the imagination" (p. 240). The concept of panophobia was echoed a century and a half later in Ribot's term *pantophobia*.

Thus far, as we have seen, the medical practitioners in the field of mental illness (they could be called *alienists* at this stage, but not yet *psychiatrists*) concentrated on patients with delusions and other severe disorders requiring institutional care. The less serious disorders were seen as abnormalities of the nerves, or of the brain to which the nerves were connected. This was a very "biological" view of mental illness. Although there was some awareness of the psychological underpinnings of some of these afflictions, these were seldom placed in the hierarchy of causative factors. One has the impression that ordinary people themselves were less aware of the psychological, interpersonal stresses that underlay their illnesses, and that they tended to somatize—partly *because* they lacked awareness, but also because somatic conditions were the only afflictions that their physicians were equipped to hear about and deal with. Contemporary conditions such *hwa-byung* (burning in the stomach) among Koreans (Stone 1997a, p. 423) seem altogether analogous to the fainting spells of anxious women in the eighteenth and nineteenth centuries, who had little opportunity to escape psychologically intolerable situations except by developing somatic conditions.

This emphasis on the "nerves" is still discernible in the writings of the celebrated Scottish physician William Cullen (1710–1790), who coined the term *neurosis*: "I propose to comprehend, under the title of Neurosis, all those praeternatural affections of sense and motion, which are without pyrexia, and all those which... depend upon a more general affection of the nervous system" (Cullen 1807, p. 387).

The Nineteenth Century: The Early Years

The early years of the nineteenth century witnessed a shift within the mental health field from attention to the somatic causes or accompaniments of mental illness to the possible psychological causes. The German Romantic period was in full swing, having been energized by works such as Goethe's *The Sorrows of Young Werther* (1774). In Goethe's tale of hopeless love for an unavailable woman, the protagonist's suicide precipitated a wave of suicides in Europe, earning the author the contumely of the English vicar Charles Moore (1743–1811), whose magnum opus on suicide (Moore 1790) condemned Goethe for his "lovesick tale."

Nevertheless, during this time (which lasted until about 1840), the first lengthy biographical sketches were written—in the medical literature—about the anxieties, conflicts, and general psychological problems of people in everyday life. Among the earliest of such sketches were those of Christian Spiess (1796) in Germany, John Haslam (1809) in England, and the director of Berlin's Charity Hospital, Karl Ideler (1841).

These influences were not felt in America until sometime later. Cullen's pupil Benjamin Rush (1746–1813), from Philadelphia, Pennsylvania, was writing in his psychiatric text in a still very "somatic" vein about anxiety disorders. "The objects of fear are of two kinds," he remarked: "the reasonable (death and surgical operations) and the Unreasonable (these are, thunder, darkness, ghosts, speaking in public, sailing, riding, certain animals, particularly cats, rats, insects and the like)" (Rush 1812, p. 325). As for the one anxiety disorder that is easily recognizable to us as a type of *social anxiety*, speaking in public, Rush did not elaborate more than to say, "The fear from speaking in public was always obviated by Mr. John Hunter, by taking a dose of laudanum [an opiate] before he met his class every day" (p. 332). The year after Rush's book appeared, Landre-Beauvais (1813) in France used the term *angoisse* to designate anxiety states, defining it as "a certain malaise, restlessness, excessive agitation" that could accompany either acute or chronic conditions and either psychological or somatic expressions of anxiety (Berrios and Link 1995, p. 546). This state of intense fearfulness was still seen as an element in the clinical picture of melancholia (Georget 1820; Pinel 1801). Another label that indicated a condition involving severe anxiety was "monomania with fear." To show the equivalence of this term with our concepts of anxiety disorder, Alexander Morrison (1826) in his lectures on mental diseases appended etchings of typical patients. The caption to Plate VI reads as follows: "This plate is intended to give an idea of partial insanity with fear, what has been termed Panaphobia. The subject is female, although, from her dress, she rather gives the idea of a male. Delusive fear of every object and person keeps her in a state of perpetual distress: it is necessary to watch her closely, to prevent her from committing suicide" (p. 136).

The phrase *anxiety of mind* appeared shortly afterward in a book by the English physician Charles Thackrah (1831). Writing about the tribulations peculiar to each of the five social classes he outlined, he commented that the "health of doctors is impaired particularly by anxiety of mind." Thackrah ascribed this vulnerability to the physician's special need for study and research and (worst of all) for making night calls.

Although, in general, anxiety and "anguish" were by then seen as manifestations of psychiatric disturbances of a severity intermediate between psychosis ("madness," "lunacy," or "insanity") and normalcy, Prichard (1835) nevertheless claimed that care and anxiety, distress, grief, and mental disturbances were the most common causes of insanity.

Jules Angst (1995) mentioned a German physician, Otto Domrich, who wrote in the first half of the nineteenth century about anxiety attacks. These consisted of a combination of anxiety and cardiopulmonary symptoms, such as might be induced (for example, in the present-day description of posttraumatic stress disorder) by the terror of the battlefield.

Implicit in my comment above about German Romanticism is that advances in theory about anxiety did come mostly from German-speaking authors throughout the first half of the nineteenth century. The German school went beyond the empiricism of the British and the French, who were still dwelling on the state of the "nerves" of anxious persons (and on the various anodynes that might soothe those nerves) rather than on the particularities of the individual persons who experienced various forms of anxiety. Friedrich Beneke (1798–1854), for example, argued that certain "ideas" or attitudes of mind could be symbolized within psychosomatic reactions (Beneke 1853). Along similar lines, Baron Ernst von Feuchtersleben (1806–1849) stressed the role of conflict, as Vere had done 50 years earlier, as central to the understanding of mental illness (von Feuchtersleben 1838, 1845). Again, the conflict was seen specifically as the battle between one's "irrational impulses" and one's more reasonable wishes and expectations. As to his "psychosomatic" views, von Feuchtersleben understood that intense anxiety and grief could lead to organic conditions of the heart and the digestive system (Berrios and Link 1995, p. 548). We also must credit the Viennese baron with a thought that may be seen as prefiguring Freud's famous dictum about freeing the psychoanalytic patient from neurotic misery by making the unconscious conscious—in effect, helping the patient to master the anxiety from hidden sources by enabling those sources to reach the level of awareness.

We should also acknowledge the contribution of Jean-Etienne Esquirol (1772–1840), who did not write on the topic of anxiety per se but did provide detailed clinical examples of what we now call obsessive-compulsive disorder (OCD). Esquirol's (1838, p. 62) descriptions served as the inspiration for the even more detailed descriptions of Henri Le Grand du Saulle (1830–1886), one of which I had translated in an earlier communication (Stone 1997b). Here, I give only brief portions taken from the description of one of Esquirol's OCD patients:

> Miss F., age 34, was raised in a merchant household from her earliest days. She feared that she would do wrong to others, and later on, when she handled the payments and receipts, feared that she would make a mistake in giving too little change to a customer.... Back in her parents' shop, she would fear that, in returning change to a customer, she might have retained in her fingers something of value.... She knew her anxiety was "absurd and ridiculous" but could do nothing to control her behavior. She ended up shaking her hands vigorously after touching nothing, to make sure that nothing stuck to her fingers that didn't belong to her. (Esquirol 1838, Vol. 2, pp. 63–64) (my translation)

The Nineteenth Century: The Later Years

By the second half of the nineteenth century, there was more widespread recognition that anxiety, in its more intense or persistent forms, deserved its own place within psychiatric nosology. As was typical of the French school, anxiety was seen as part of a "three-stage process," which began with inquietude, progressed to anxiety, and might end with anguish (*angoisse*) (Littre and Robin 1858). Feelings of "closeness" and "difficulty breathing" were noted in descriptions of both anxiety and anguish.

In Germany, Wilhelm Griesinger (1817–1868) saw mental disease and somatic disease as one; neuropathology and psychiatry were in essence the same field. He realized that not all behavior was consciously determined, and acknowledged the importance of temperament and personality. Although he thought that mental disease must stem from abnormalities of the brain cells (and thus had an "organic" basis), he nevertheless endorsed the idea from his Romanticist predecessors that strong affects could induce mental illness. Such illness might come about, in Griesinger's (1861) view, because of conflicts involving the repression (*Verdraengung*) of sexual urges—a Freudian concept expressed a generation before Freud. Griesinger estimated that one in ten patients who developed a psychosis ("insanity") did so with acute fear as the inciting agent.

A similar theory was espoused by Heinrich Wilhelm Neumann (1814–1884), a contemporary of Griesinger. Neumann (1859) saw mental illness as partaking of a dynamic process in which under normal circumstances a person succeeds in his or her development toward a freedom gained through self-mastery. In pathological circumstances the perturbations of the drives, especially the sexual ones, disturb one's harmony. When the drives cannot be satisfied, anxiety appears. Furthermore, if certain life functions are threatened, the instinctual needs are apt to express themselves in consciousness as "perceptions" (Neumann used the Greek word *aistheses*) or "calls" that make the person aware of impending danger (Beauchesne 1781, p. 51). Neumann's theory anticipated Freud's reworking of his anxiety theory in 1923, wherein he spoke of "signal anxiety."

Psychiatry in the second half of the nineteenth century remained biologically oriented, and this was even more true in France than in Germany. Benedict Morel (1809–1873), to whom we owe the concept of *démence précoce* (Morel 1860) (which gave rise to the later concepts of dementia praecox and schizophrenia), believed that both the psychological and the somatic (subjective and objective) expressions of anxiety could lead to pathological changes in the autonomic nervous system (Berrios and Link 1995, p. 549).

Le Grand du Saulle (1878), a prominent and prolific psychiatrist at the Bicêtre Hospital in Paris, France, wrote a monograph on the *peur des espaces* (fear of spaces) based on Westphal's (1872) article on agoraphobia. Le Grand du Saulle preferred this admittedly more vague designation rather than the term *agoraphobia* that the German school preferred because "although one may see now and again that these patients fear open spaces, they may experience the fear at the theater, at church, on an elevated storey of a building, or while inside near a window giving out to a large courtyard, or on a bus or boat or a bridge" (p. 6, my translation).

In a separate monograph of 1875 entitled *La folie du doute avec délire du toucher* ("doubting mania, with dread of being touched"), Le Grand du Saulle gave clinical descriptions of persons with what we now know as obsessive-compulsive disorder, as well as with related anxiety conditions such as generalized anxiety, or a tormenting conviction of "sinfulness" (in otherwise timid and well-behaved persons) (Le Grand du Saulle 1875). One woman in her mid-20s, for example, became obsessed, as she walked along the streets, that someone might hurl themselves from a window and land in front of her. She would ponder, "Would it be a man or a woman, would the person be killed or just wounded, would there be blood on the sidewalk, should I call for help or run away, would I be held responsible or would people believe my innocence?" In another case, a 30-year-old man was obsessed with colors and numbers. He would ask why trees are green, why brides wear white, why soldiers have red trousers, etc., but he would also find himself counting the objects in a room where he was visiting, telling his host, "You have 44 books on your table, and your vest has seven buttons," then apologizing: "Excuse me, it's involuntary, but I feel I must count things" (p. 12). He felt extremely anxious about this tendency and said he would be willing to do anything to achieve tranquility. In still another case, an 18-year-old orphan girl adopted into a wealthy family was tormented by the memory that she had once laughed in the church where she had her first communion, and by the recollection that she had withheld from the priest at confession one of her "sins." As a penitence for these peccadilloes she decided to starve herself, losing considerable weight in the process. She was also afraid to sleep, lest she die unshriven. The cure that Le Grand du Saulle hit upon was to have her parents provide her with a companion who would sleep in the room with her. This seemed to work, and the girl regained her equanimity. But there is not a hint in any of his vignettes about "dynamics": what may, in a psychological way, have predisposed these patients to manifest the anxious symptoms for which they sought help. Le Grand du Saulle viewed these conditions as exaggerations of *conscience,* as distinct from melancholic or persecutory conditions, in which sadness and suspiciousness are exaggerated. His ideas about etiology were limited to his observations that these anxiety disorders (*névroses*, in his terminology) tended to show up first during puberty. Perhaps a "morbid heredity" played a role (p. 60), given that, in his observations, many such patients had relatives with various forms of mental illness. Also implicated were certain physical diseases: typhoid, cholera, as well as habits, such as "habitual onanism." Yet all of these anxiety disorder patients could give good account of themselves and their symptoms—they were not "psychotic." The only other clue he offered concerning etiology was that women seemed more prone to "doubting folly" than men, and that those in the upper social classes were more vulnerable than those less well off.

Although Le Grand du Saulle (1878) mentioned that psychological causes had been cited by other authors ("too vivid emotions of a person sad by nature, an unexpected fright, the sudden death of a loved one, the good luck to have escaped a great danger, excessive intellectual efforts, insufficient sleep, or sexual excess" [p. 31]), he favored either medical (somatic) rather than psychological factors, or, as previously mentioned, adverse heredity—the latter view endorsed also by Dagonet (1894).

Earlier, Dagonet (1876), a professor of psychiatry in Strasbourg, France, had described several forms of anxiety under the broad heading of *lypemanie* (Esquirol's term for depression, stemming from the Greek *lupeo,* to grieve). He characterized hypochondriasis (*lypemanie hypochondriaque*) as beginning with mild symptoms, which progress in the usual "three stages" customary in all French nineteenth-century psychiatric texts. The patient is "anxious [*inquiet*], preoccupied, and begins to experience fears concerning his health; he inspects his body minutely,...observes scrupulously all the rules of hygiene; he reads books on medicine and is most eager to speak with physicians about his condition" (p. 25, my translation). Dagonet also discussed *lypemanie anxieuse* (anxious depression), also known as *panophobia, angoisse morale* (anguished mood, or in German, *Gemütsbeklemmung*, or *angst*). Dagonet's case descriptions were those of a serious disorder, midway between our concept of generalized anxiety disorder and OCD, bordering on delusion. The clinician encountered as the patient's predominant symptoms "*les angoisses, les inquietudes vagues, les terreurs, des conceptions erronés, et un délire plus ou moins systematisé*" (p. 239) ("feelings of dread, vague anxieties, terror, false ideas, and more or less systematized delusory ideas"). In the lengthier example provided by Dagonet, the patient had a mentally ill grandmother, uncle, and five cousins (all by that uncle), which suggested to Dagonet that heredity was the principal causative agent.

Berrios and Link (1995, p. 551) gave a description of *vertigo*, written by Leroux (1889) for a medical encyclopedia, which could serve well as a defining example of panic attack. In this connection, Berrios credited Le Grand du Saulle with realizing that the patient with "vertigo" did not have an inner-ear malady, as Benedikt was still suggesting in 1870, but was more likely troubled by a *fear* of falling.

The panophobia, or *lypemanie anxieuse*, of which the European psychiatrists of the period were speaking—similar to generalized anxiety disorder—was given the name *neurasthenia* (a weakness of the nerves) by the American neurologist George Miller Beard (1839–1883). Beard enjoyed considerable fame during his lifetime for his application of electrical treatments—"voltaic-galvanic stimulation" or "faradic stimulation"—to the cure of neurasthenia (Beard 1880; Beard and Rockwell 1875). The popularity of Beard's method in the waning years of the century can hardly be overestimated.

The *neurasthenia* concept was so popular that many mental health practitioners placed all types of anxiety-related conditions in this broad category. Sigmund Freud (1856–1939) objected to this tendency: "It can be nothing but a gain to neuropathology if we make an attempt to separate from neurasthenia proper all those neurotic disturbances in which...the symptoms are more firmly linked to one another than to the typical symptoms of neurasthenia (such as intracranial pressure, spinal irritation, and dyspepsia with flatulence and constipation)" (Freud 1895/1962, p. 90). Freud went on to describe *anxiety neurosis,* a term first published in the 1895 paper, although he had used it in letters to Wilhelm Fliess two years earlier. Freud gave credit to Ewald Hecker (1893) for originating the concept (Freud was at first unaware of Hecker's paper), but Hecker had not gone so far as to discriminate between anxiety neurosis and neurasthenia, as Freud was now about to do. The clinical picture was composed, as Freud outlined, of the following elements: 1) general irritability; 2) anxious expectation (Freud gave an example of a woman who fears that her husband has pneumonia every time she hears him cough), which may also take the form of scrupulosity, pedantry, or doubting mania; 3) anxiety that is constantly lurking in the background; 4) rudimentary anxiety attacks; 5) waking up at night in a fright (*pavor nocturnus*); 6) vertigo; 7) phobias (*specific* fears) of snakes, darkness, vermin, and so forth, but also agoraphobia; 8) digestive troubles; 9) paresthesias; and 10) chronic states, such as a constant feeling of lassitude (pp. 92–99).

Freud's description of anxiety neurosis was, as we can see from the list of its defining elements, a fairly broad concept. DSM-IV-TR (American Psychiatric Association 2000), for example, lists 13 anxiety disorders. Of these, panic attack (at least the type represented by *pavor nocturnus*), agoraphobia, specific phobia, and generalized anxiety disorder all would seem to fit within the borders outlined by Freud's "anxiety neurosis." Freud went on to disclose what he believed were the psychological underpinnings of the condition. In fact, all the various character disorders he and the psychoanalytic pioneers described may be seen as resting on a foundation of anxiety—now defined as a common but abnormal state—as distinct from fear, which requires no psychoanalytic uncovering to understand (i.e., fear of the tiger-in-the-room situation, which would be a universal and normal reaction). Still, the predominantly psychological explanation for anxiety neurosis was not universally accepted. The French neurologist Eduard Brissaud (1890), as Berrios and Link (1995) mentioned, could acknowledge that *anxiété* was cerebral in origin, but in his view, *angoisse* (here, to be understood as panic) was a brain stem phenomenon—basically, a physical disorder expressing itself as a sensation of suffocation (in contrast to anxiety, which manifested as a feeling of insecurity).

The Early Twentieth Century

The tendency was still quite strong at the turn of the last century and in the early years of the twentieth century to assume that the main etiological factors behind anxiety were hereditary or strictly biological. Maurice De Fleury (1897), for example, divided the emotions into two groups: "Doubt, humility, sloth, fearfulness, sadness and pity are symptoms—to varying degrees—of cerebral exhaustion. Pride, foolishness, anger, egoism, courage, heroism, and cruelty are the manifestations of exaltation of the spirit" (p. 317, my translation). Freud's original concept of anxiety also shared the notion that energy played a key role: dammed-up libido from ungratified drives led to an excess of energy accumulating in the nervous system, manifested as anxiety. This mechanistic and closed-system model (in keeping with the physics of the last decade of the nineteenth century) gave way two decades later when Freud modified his theory, such that anxiety was no longer measured as so many discrete packets of (ill-distributed) energy but rather as a signal warning (involving very little actual energy) of a threat to one's equilibrium and well-being. This was the so-called *anticipatory anxiety*, as distinct from his term *traumatic anxiety*, in which the psychic apparatus is (understandably) overwhelmed by a psychologically meaningful danger, as in the case of what we now recognize can sometimes lead to panic states or to posttraumatic stress disorder (Busch et al. 1999).

The distinction between fear and anxiety (made, as Pichot [1990] pointed out, in the middle of the nineteenth century by Søren Aabye Kierkegaard [1813–

1855]) was emphasized once again by Karl Jaspers (1913). Several varieties of anxiety disorder that had for many years been neglected began to receive attention. What we now call *social phobia*—the opposite side of the coin of *avoidant personality* (because anxiety is what the avoidant person would experience if forced into social situations)—was alluded to by other terms in earlier writings. Berrios and Link (1995) mentioned Hippocrates and Richard Burton in this connection. Paul Hartenberg (1901) wrote of *timidity*, a concept paralleling that of social phobia. Hartenberg singled out heredity, social or psychological defects, and (maladaptive) learning as contributing factors. Hartenberg was a student of Theodule Ribot (1839–1916), as was the prolific and long-lived Pierre Janet (1859–1947).

Janet was the founder of French dynamic psychiatry. Ribot had been the chairman of the department of experimental psychology at the College de France. Janet, in contrast, was less interested in either experimental methods or statistics, and pursued instead a more clinical path. Janet helped his patients to express the "fixed ideas" that he saw as the source of much of their psychological distress. Feelings, for Janet, were secondary mental states that guided the expression and termination of behaviors. Their effectiveness depended on their "energy" and on one's integrative capacity. Too little energy or too little integrative capacity led to a failure of feelings and to the emergence of primitive behaviors. Anxiety and *angoisse* were the main manifestations of such failure. In his book, Janet (1926) spoke of *tendencies* rather than of drives; also, he described "psychological tension": the capacity of a person to use his or her energy on some more or less elevated level (akin to the psychoanalytic concept of *sublimation*). According to Janet, a person's "dynamism" depended on the quality and quantity of this energy rather than on the conflicts and their respective forces, which Freud placed at the center of his dynamic model.

Janet's case descriptions focused primarily on the here and now: the patient's current situation and feelings; only rare allusions were made to the details of early childhood and to the influence those early events may have had on the shape of the patient's anxious symptoms. In his 1926 book, however, Janet discussed at length the case of "Madelaine," a single 40-year-old woman from a well-to-do family. It is quite possible that Madelaine represents a case of severe anxiety for which the predisposing factors were almost entirely constitutional. In addition to being episodically depressed since adolescence and experiencing obsessions with a delusional force, she was physically handicapped. We could not fault Janet for leaving us in the dark about conflictual or dynamic factors in her early family life—if these were absent or negligible. But Janet's description points out what is so often a tantalizing situation in case histories of anxious patients. Clinicians without a psychoanalytic background too often omit what may be crucial from a family dynamic standpoint. Equally true, psychoanalytic writers too often omit sufficient mention of possible hereditary and constitutional factors. The "complete picture" remains elusive. In any event, just as the experimentalist Ribot influenced the more descriptively oriented Janet, Janet influenced the great psychopharmacologist Jean Delay (1907–1987), whose work (and that of his successors) has brought us closer to an understanding of the neurochemical correlates of anxiety. The work of Delay, Deniker, and Pichot in the 1950s also helped validate the separateness of anxiety and depression and, along the way, helped to develop anxiolytics and antidepressants (Delay and Deniker 1952).

Other notable work in the area of anxiety disorders in the early twentieth century includes that of Ribot (1896, 1911), who made clearer distinctions than were previously available between generalized anxiety disorder ("pantophobia") and the specific phobias of various objects and animals. The major theoretician of behavior therapy, Burrhus Frederick Skinner (1904–1990), explained anxiety as a manifestation of conditioned response to some feared situation (Skinner 1938). The English analyst Wilfred Bion (1897–1979) understood the developing infant as experiencing from birth a series of "psychotic" anxieties in relation to his or her primary caregivers—anxieties that can be reactivated later in various group situations. Bion (1967) had received his inspiration from Melanie Klein (1882–1960), who speculated that infants went through depressive and paranoid "positions" during early development (Klein 1975). The problem with Kleinian theory with regard to anxiety is that it confuses substantive with substance. Infants' reactions are perhaps analogous to certain reactions of adult patients with depressive or paranoid psychosis. But, as has become clearer through contemporary research in psychobiological psychiatry, the "chemistry" of psychotic patients and that of nonpsychotic infants or children is by no means the same. A similar problem confronts us when we examine the theoretical model of Harry Stack Sullivan (1892–1949). Sullivan (1948) saw anxiety as the "basic symptom" underlying all forms of psychopathology; today, we believe this is an overstatement. Most patients with severe psychiatric disorders do report more than their share of anxiety. But at the start of this century, we are beginning to understand the biological correlates of intense anxiety and how certain "harm-avoidant" persons, in Cloninger's (1986) language, are temperamentally (i.e., innately) more prone to experience anxiety than other people (e.g., persons with an "anxious-fearful cluster" personality) (see Chapter 5, "Anxious Traits and Temperaments," this volume). At the other end of the spectrum are persons with antisocial, especially psychopathic, personalities who are less prone to experience anxiety. Perhaps in the twenty-first century, psychiatric advances will allow both the overly anxious and the not-anxious-enough to meet somewhere in a more comfortable middle ground. Likewise, we can hope that the various theories and practices concerning anxiety will be better integrated.

Conclusion

Viewed from the perspective of evolutionary psychiatry, the emotion of fear represents something hard-wired into our genome by virtue of its leading to movements (i.e., behavior) designed to avoid danger (see Chapter 9, "Evolutionary Concepts of Anxiety"). The term *anxiety*, in contrast to *fear*, tends to be reserved for reactions that, albeit understandable, are exaggerated. We *fear* a poisonous snake moving toward us; certain persons become *anxious* when merely looking at a picture of such a snake in a magazine. Before the modern era, physicians focused primarily on the bodily ("objective") manifestations of anxiety, such as palpitations, shortness of breath, and tremulousness. Nightmares were seen as causing anxiety because of their frightening content, whereas we would see the nightmare as being triggered by some antecedent fear- or anxiety-inducing experience. Likewise, treatments were usually directed to relieving the bodily symptoms associated with the anxiety: administering smelling salts for fainting episodes, for example. Another remedy might consist of encouraging a patient to move away from an area where anxiety-inducing "agents" were abundant to places where they were less likely to be encountered. Cultural differences often dictated which bodily organs were considered the culprits in attacks of anxiety; this determined where the somatic treatments would be directed. As late as the latter part of the nineteenth century, the various disorders we now lump together under the heading of anxiety were described as separate entities: agoraphobia, obsessive ruminations ("doubting mania"), compulsive avoidance of touching, panic, and so forth. With the advent of Freud and the psychoanalytic pioneers, the topic was reexamined. Traumatic anxiety was distinguished from anticipatory ("signal") anxiety. In treatment, emphasis shifted from the bodily counterparts to the examination of the *subjective* experiences of the patient (fear of loss of status, fear of losing a love-object, sexual fears that led to diminished contact with one's social milieu or to fear of symbolically connected objects in the real world, such as horses, elevators, or spiders). This change of focus paved the way to a more rational therapy of the anxiety disorders, where both the objective and subjective elements receive appropriate attention.

Key Clinical Points

- Anxiety disorders are a universal phenomenon: exaggerations of evolutionarily hard-wired reactions to dangers to the body or to the psyche.
- Physicians in earlier times focused on the somatic ("objective") manifestations of anxiety, such as palpitations, shortness of breath, and the like.
- Treatment in earlier times was directed primarily to these somatic manifestations.
- Even as recently as the late nineteenth century, the various disorders we subsume under the heading of anxiety were described and considered as separate entities, not yet unified as elements of a particular class of disorders.
- The psychoanalytic pioneers drew attention to the subjective element in anxiety disorders. Professionals associated with general psychiatry began to conceptualize anxiety as the common thread running through a particular group of conditions such as panic disorder, obsessive-compulsive disorder, agoraphobia, and social anxiety. Therapeutic strategies were reshaped so as to take into consideration both the objective and the subjective counterparts to the various anxiety-related disorders.

References

American Psychiatric Association: Diagnostic and Statistical Manual of Mental Disorders, Fourth Edition, Text Revision. Washington, DC, American Psychiatric Association, 2000

Angst J: History and epidemiology of panic. Eur Psychiatry 10:57–59, 1995

Battie W: A Treatise on Madness. London, J Whiston and B White, 1758

Beard GM: A Practical Treatise on Nervous Exhaustion (Neurasthenia). New York, W Wood, 1880

Beard GM, Rockwell AD: A Practical Treatise on the Medical and Surgical Uses of Electricity. New York, W Wood, 1875

Beauchesne EPC: De l'influence des affections de l'âme dans les maladies nerveuses des femmes. Paris, Mequignon, 1781

Benedikt M: Über Platzschwindel. Allgemeine Wiener Medizinische Zeitung 15:488–490, 1870

Beneke FE: Lehrbuch der pragmatischen Psychologie, oder der Seelenlehre in der Anwendung auf das Leben. Berlin, Germany, ES Mittler and Sons, 1853

Berrios G, Link C: Anxiety disorders, in A History of Clinical Psychiatry. Edited by Berrios G, Porter R. New York, New York University Press, 1995, pp 545–562

Bion W: Second Thoughts: Selected Papers on Psychoanalysis. London, Marsfield Reprints, 1967

Blackmore R: A Treatise of the Spleen and Vapours; or Hypochondriacal and Hysterical Affections. London, Pemberton, 1725

Boissier de Sauvages F: Pathologica methodica. Amsterdam, De Tournes, 1752

Bond J: An Essay on the Incubus, or Nightmare. London, Wilson and Durham, 1753

Brissaud E: De l'anxiété paroxystique. Sémaine Medicale 9:410–411, 1890

Burton R [as "Democritus Junior"]: Anatomy of Melancholy. Oxford, England, Lichfield and Short, 1621

Busch FN, Milrod BL, Singer MB: Theory and technique in psychodynamic treatment of panic disorder. J Psychother Pract Res 8:234–242, 1999

Cloninger CR: A unified biosocial theory of personality and its role in the development of anxiety states. Psychiatr Dev 3:167–226, 1986

Cullen W: First Lines on the Practice of Physic. Brookfield, MA, E Merriam, 1807

Dagonet H: Nouveau traité elementaire et pratique des maladies mentales. Paris, J-B Baillière et Fils, 1876

Dagonet H: Traité des maladies mentales. Paris, J-B Baillière et Fils, 1894

De Fleury M: Introduction a la médicine de l'esprit. Paris, Felix Alcan, 1897

Delay J, Deniker P: Trent-huit cas de psychoses traitées par la cure prolongée et continue de 4560RP, in Le Congres des Aliénistes et Neurologues de Langue Français: Contes Rendu du Congres. Paris, Masson, 1952, pp 497–502

Esquirol E: Des maladies mentales considerées sous les rapports médical, hygienique et médico-legal. Paris, J-B Baillière, 1838

Flecknoe R: Enigmaticall Characters, all taken to the life from severall persons, humours, and dispositions. London, 1658

Freud S: On the grounds for detaching a particular syndrome from neurasthenia under the description "anxiety neurosis" (1895), in Standard Edition of the Complete Psychological Works of Sigmund Freud, Vol 3. Edited by Strachey J. London, Hogarth, 1962, pp 90–117

Freud S: The ego and the id (1923), in Standard Edition of the Complete Psychological Works of Sigmund Freud, Vol 19. Edited by Strachey J. London, Hogarth, 1961, pp 12–66

Georget EJ: De la folie: considérations sur cette maladie. Paris, Crevot, 1820

Goethe JW: Die Leiden des jungen Werthers. Leipzig, J Kiermeier-Debre, 1774

Griesinger W: Die Pathologie und Therapie psychischen Krankheiten für Aerzte und Studirende. Braunschweig, Germany, F Wreden, 1861

Hajal F: Diagnosis and treatment of lovesickness: an Islamic medieval case study. Hosp Community Psychiatry 45:647–650, 1994

Hartenberg P: Les timides et la timidité. Paris, Alcan, 1901

Haslam J: Observations on Madness. London, J Callow, 1809

Hecker E: Über larvirte und abortive Angstzustaende bei Neurasthenie. Zentralblatt für Nervenheilkunde 16:565–572, 1893

Hunter R, Macalpine I: Three Hundred Years of Psychiatry: 1535–1860. London, Oxford University Press, 1963

Ideler KW: Biographien Geisteskranken. Berlin, EH Schroeder, 1841

Janet P: De l'angoisse à l'exstase. Paris, Alcan, 1926

Jaspers K: Allgemeine Psychopathologie. Berlin, Springer-Verlag, 1913

Klein M: Love, Guilt and Reparation and Other Works: 1921–1945. New York, Delta, 1975

Landre-Beauvais AJ: Sémiotique ou traité des signes des maladies. Paris, Brosson, 1813

Le Grand du Saulle H: La folie du doute, avec délire du toucher. Paris, V Adrien Delahaye, 1875

Le Grand du Saulle H: Étude clinique sur la peur des espaces (agoraphobie, des allemandes). Paris, V Adrien Delahaye, 1878

LePois C: Selectiorum observatorium. Pont-a-Mousson, France, Carolus Mercator, 1618

Leroux P: Vertige, in Dictionnaire encyclopédique des sciences médicales. Edited by Dechambre A, Lereboullet L. Paris, Masson, 1889, pp 146–188

Littre E, Robin C: Dictionnaire de médicine. Paris, Baillière, 1858

Moore C: A Full Inquiry Into the Subject of Suicide. London, FJ and C Rivington, 1790

Morel B: Traité des maladies mentales. Paris, Masson, 1860

Morrison A: Outlines of Lectures on Mental Diseases. London, Longman, Rees, Orme, Brown and Green, and S Highley, 1826

Neumann H: Lehrbuch der Psychiatrie. Erlangen, F. Enke, 1859

Pichot P: History of the treatment of anxiety, in Handbook of Anxiety, Vol 4: The Treatment of Anxiety. Edited by Noyes R Jr, Roth M, Burrows GD. Amsterdam, Elsevier, 1990, pp 3–25

Pinel P: Traité médico-philosophique sur l'aliénation mentale et la manie. Paris, Richard, Caille and Ravier, 1801

Prichard JC: A Treatise on Insanity and Other Disorders Affecting the Mind. London, Sherwood, Gilbert and Piper, 1835

Reil J: Über den Begriff der Medizin und ihre Verzweigungen, besonders in Beziehung auf die Berichtgung der Topik in der Psychiaterie. In Beyträge zür Beförderung einer Kurmethode auf psychischem Wege. Halle, Curtsche Buchhandlung, 1808

Ribot T: The Psychology of Emotions. London, Walter Scott, 1896

Ribot T: The Psychology of Emotions, 2nd Edition. London, Walter Scott, 1911

Rush B: Medical Inquiries and Observations Upon the Diseases of the Mind. Philadelphia, PA, Kimber and Richardson, 1812

Skinner BF: The Behavior of Organisms: An Experimental Analysis. New York, Appleton-Century, 1938

Spiess CH: Biographien der Wahnsinnigen. Leipzig, 1796

Stone MH: Healing the Mind: A History of Psychiatry From Antiquity to the Present. New York, WW Norton, 1997a

Stone MH: The history of obsessive-compulsive disorder from the early period to the turn of the twentieth century, in Essential Papers on Obsessive-Compulsive Disorder. Edited by Stein D, Stone MH. New York, New York University Press, 1997b, pp 19–29

Sullivan HS: The meaning of anxiety in psychiatry and life. Psychiatry 11:1–13, 1948

Thackrah CT: The Effects of Arts, Trades, and Professions, and of Civic States and Habits of Living, on Health and Longevity. London, Longman, 1831

Vere J: A Physical and Moral Inquiry Into the Causes of That Internal Restlessness and Disorder in Man, Which Has Been the Complaint of All Ages. London, White and Sewell, 1778

von Feuchtersleben E: Zur Diätetik der Seele. Vienna, Carl Armbruster, 1838

von Feuchtersleben E: Lehrbuch aertzlicher Seelenkunde. Vienna, Gerold, 1845

Westphal C: Die Agoraphobie: eine neuropatische Erscheinung. Archiv für Psychiatrie und Nervenkrankheiten 3:138–161, 1872

Whytt R: Observations on the Nature, Causes and Cure of Those Disorders Which Have Commonly Been Called Nervous, Hypochondriac or Hysteric, to Which Are Prefixed Some Remarks on the Sympathy of the Nerves. Edinburgh, Becket and du Hondt, 1765

Younge R: The Drunkard's Character. London, Latham, 1638

Zhang M-Y: Neurasthenia. Cult Med Psychiatry 13:147–161, 1989

Recommended Readings

Berrios G, Porter R: History of Clinical Psychiatry. New York, New York University Press, 1995

Bond MH: Beyond the Chinese Face: Insights from Psychology. New York, Oxford, 1991

Ellenberger H: The Discovery of the Unconscious. New York, Basic Books, 1970

Moore BE, Fine B: Psychoanalysis: The Major Concepts. New Haven, CT, Yale University Press, 1995

Semelaigne R: Les pionniers de la psychiatrie française. Paris, Baillière, 1930

Chapter 2

Classification of Anxiety Disorders

Timothy A. Brown, Psy.D.
Ovsanna Leyfer, Ph.D.

With the publication of DSM-IV (American Psychiatric Association 1994), 12 anxiety disorder categories now exist in the formal nomenclature: panic disorder without agoraphobia, panic disorder with agoraphobia, agoraphobia without history of panic disorder, social phobia, specific phobia, generalized anxiety disorder (GAD), obsessive-compulsive disorder (OCD), posttraumatic stress disorder (PTSD), acute stress disorder, anxiety disorder due to a general medical condition, substance-induced anxiety disorder, and anxiety disorder not otherwise specified. A thirteenth category, mixed anxiety-depressive disorder, was considered for inclusion in DSM-IV but currently resides in the appendix of disorders in need of further study as a possible addition to DSM-V (Zinbarg et al. 1994). In addition to the creation of three new categories (acute stress disorder, anxiety disorder due to a general medical condition, substance-induced anxiety disorder), the definitions of existing categories underwent numerous revisions in DSM-IV. Table 2–1 summarizes these revisions and provides an overview of key diagnostic features for the major anxiety disorder categories.

DSM-IV and its text revision, DSM-IV-TR (American Psychiatric Association 2000), perpetuate the steady increase in the number of categories across its preceding editions and in other major classification systems for mental disorders (e.g., ICD-10; World Health Organization 1992). For instance, DSM-IV includes 12 anxiety disorders, whereas DSM-II (American Psychiatric Association 1968) included only 3 categories. This increase could be viewed as corresponding to expanding cumulative knowledge of the nature of psychopathology and in the classification of disorders. However, many researchers (e.g., Andrews 1996; Tyrer 1989) have expressed concern that the expansion of our nosologies has come at the expense of less empirical consideration of shared or overlapping features of emotional disorders that, relative to unique features of specific disorders, may have far greater significance in the understanding of the prevention, etiology, and course of disorders and in predicting their response to treatment.

Moreover, this expansion has led to questions of compromised discriminant validity; namely, whether our current classification systems are erroneously distinguishing symptoms and disorders that, in reality, are inconsequential variations of broader syndromes. For instance, many anxiety disorders share constituent processes (e.g., apprehension of situations or objects, protective or anxiety-reducing actions) and differ primarily (or solely) at the descriptive level in content or focus of apprehension (e.g., worry about rejection or embarrassment in social phobia, worry about contamination in OCD, worry about several daily matters in GAD) or in the form of protective action (e.g., situational avoidance

TABLE 2–1. Overview of key features and changes to the definitions of major anxiety disorders introduced in DSM-IV

Disorder	Key features	Changes in DSM-IV
Panic disorder	Recurrent, unexpected panic attacks Persistent worry/concern about additional attacks or their consequences	Elimination of panic severity specifiers (mild, moderate, severe) Introduction of a panic typology (unexpected, situationally bound, situationally predisposed) "Recurrent" replaces requirement of history of at least 4 panic attacks in a one-month period Increased emphasis on cognitive features (e.g., worry about panic, cognitive misappraisals) Criterion of "significant change in behavior related to the attacks" for coverage of "nonfearful panic disorder"
Panic disorder with agoraphobia	Meets criteria for panic disorder Agoraphobia: fear/avoidance of situations where panic attacks might occur	See panic disorder Elimination of agoraphobia severity specifiers (mild, moderate, severe)
Social phobia	Marked fear/avoidance of social situations due to possibility of embarrassment or humiliation	Diagnosis permitted in presence of unexpected panic attacks, if attacks confined to social situations (i.e., situationally predisposed attacks)
Specific phobia	Fear/avoidance of circumscribed objects or situations (e.g., heights, enclosed places, receiving injections)	Introduction of phobia types (animal, natural environment, situational, blood-injury-injection, other) Diagnosis permitted in presence of unexpected panic attacks, if attacks confined to phobic situation/object Previously named "simple phobia"
Generalized anxiety disorder	Chronic excessive, uncontrollable worry about a number of events or activities (e.g., job performance, finances)	Criterion of uncontrollable worry "A number of events/activities" replaces requirement of 2 or more worry spheres List of associated symptoms reduced from 18 to 6, primarily via elimination of autonomic symptoms Replaces category of "overanxious disorder" as a child/adolescent diagnosis
Obsessive-compulsive disorder	Recurrent, intrusive thoughts, images, or impulses (e.g., excessive doubting, thoughts of contamination) Repetitive behaviors or mental acts aimed at reducing distress or to "neutralize" an obsession	Recognition of mental/covert compulsions Inclusion of differential diagnostic criterion involving boundary of obsessions and chronic worry Introduction of "with poor insight" specifier for cases in which obsessions and compulsions not recognized as excessive or unreasonable
Posttraumatic stress disorder	Persistent reexperiencing (e.g., dreams, flashbacks), distress, and avoidance of stimuli associated with prior exposure to extreme stress (e.g., rape, combat)	Traumatic event criterion revised to require subjective response (intense fear, horror, helplessness) Introduction of course specifier (acute, chronic) Introduction of a new category, acute stress disorder, for coverage of short-term, extreme stress responses emphasizing dissociative symptoms

in agoraphobia, specific phobia, and social phobia; compulsions in OCD; safety behaviors in all anxiety disorders). Similarly, virtually all current cognitive-behavioral treatments of anxiety disorders contain the elements of exposure (situational, imaginal, and/or interoceptive), cognitive therapy, and between-sessions practice, varying primarily in content and process. Although differentiation may be helpful in conveying information about the nature of the disturbance, the empirical question is whether these manifestations are sufficiently distinct (e.g., beyond variations in content) to warrant separation. Our intent in this chapter is to review issues, extant empirical evidence, and future research directions bearing on the validity of the anxiety disorder categories.

Do the Anxiety Disorders Possess Poor Discriminant Validity?

As noted, the steady rise in the number of anxiety disorder diagnoses has led to questions about the discriminant validity of these categories. Findings of unfavorable diagnostic reliability (interrater agreement) and a high rate of co-occurrence of the anxiety and mood disorders are frequently cited as evidence in support of these concerns. Because most studies to date have approached these issues at the descriptive and diagnostic levels, diagnostic reliability and comorbidity data alone do not allow for firm conclusions regarding the extent or nature of overlap among the anxiety disorders (Brown and Barlow 2005). Nevertheless, although alternative explanations are plausible (see next sections), evidence of unsatisfactory reliability and high comorbidity among diagnoses is consistent with the hypothesis that the anxiety disorders do not represent distinct entities. In addition, data indicating that a wide range of emotional disorders respond similarly to the same psychosocial or medication treatment and evidence that the neurobiological underpinnings of these conditions often overlap have been taken to suggest that the similarities among diagnoses outweigh their differences.

Diagnostic Reliability

Diagnostic reliability refers to the extent to which two (or more) independent raters or interviewers agree on the presence or absence of a given diagnosis. The approach to studying diagnostic reliability of the anxiety disorders has usually taken one of two forms—test-retest or simultaneous—both involving the use of structured clinical interviews such as the Anxiety Disorders Interview Schedule for DSM-IV (ADIS-IV; Di Nardo et al. 1994) and the Structured Clinical Interview for DSM-IV Axis I Disorders (SCID; First et al. 1996). In the test-retest approach, on two separate occasions, the patient is interviewed by different independent evaluators (e.g., Brown et al. 2001b; Di Nardo et al. 1993). In the simultaneous approach, a diagnostic interview is video- or audiotaped and rated by an independent evaluator (e.g., Riskind et al. 1987; Skre et al. 1991). In both approaches, the most widely used index of interrater agreement is the kappa statistic (Fleiss et al. 1979), which ranges in value from 0.0 (poor agreement) to 1.0 (perfect agreement). Clearly, the strategy of interviewing patients on separate occasions is the more stringent approach to estimating diagnostic reliability because it introduces several potential sources of disagreement not found in the single-interview method (e.g., variation in patient report, change in clinical status). Although these issues could be viewed as limitations of this approach, the single-interview method has also been criticized for its potential to provide an overly optimistic estimation of diagnostic reliability (e.g., the independent evaluator's judgments may be strongly influenced by the nature and extent of follow-up questions asked by the initial interviewer; the evaluator may not address the short-term stability in symptoms or in patient report); these factors may bear on confidence in judgments of the presence or absence of a DSM diagnosis (Segal et al. 1994).

Large-scale reliability studies based on DSM-III-R (American Psychiatric Association 1987) and DSM-IV definitions of anxiety and mood disorder categories have indicated that these diagnoses are associated with differential levels of agreement (Brown et al. 2001b; Di Nardo et al. 1993; Mannuzza et al. 1989; Williams et al. 1992). Results of one large-scale study of the DSM-IV anxiety disorders and three of the DSM-III-R anxiety and mood disorders are summarized in Table 2–2 for current diagnoses. All four studies employed the test-retest method, but they differed in the structured interview used; Brown et al. (2001b) used the ADIS-IV–Lifetime Version; Di Nardo et al. (1993) used the ADIS–Revised (Di Nardo and Barlow 1988); Mannuzza et al. (1989) used the Schedule for Affective Disorders and Schizophrenia–Lifetime Anxiety Version (Fyer et al. 1985); and Williams et al. (1992) used the SCID. Following guidelines often used in the interpretation of kappa ($\kappa > 0.75$=excellent agreement; κ between 0.60 and 0.74=good agreement; κ between 0.40 and 0.59=fair agreement; $\kappa < 0.40$=poor agreement; Shrout et al. 1987), results indicated that categories such as panic disorder with agoraphobia, social phobia, specific phobia, OCD, and GAD had good to excellent reliability in the DSM-IV study (Brown et al. 2001b). However, certain categories (e.g., major depressive disorder, dysthymia) were associated with fair agreement at best. The reliability of GAD improved in the DSM-IV study in comparison with the previous studies, which is probably due to the major revision of its criteria in DSM-IV (see Table 2–1). The interrater agreement for dysthymia remained poor across the studies.

Analyses of the sources of diagnostic disagreements indicate that the factors contributing to unreliability are wide-ranging and vary substantially across the anxiety and mood disorders.

For instance, in Brown et al. (2001b), the majority of disagreement involving social phobia, specific phobia, and OCD (62%–67%) stemmed from one interviewer assigning the diagnosis at a clinical level and the other one rating it as subclinical. For GAD, major depression, and dysthymia, this was a relatively rare source of disagreement. The most prevalent reason for disagreements across studies has been "information variance" (patients provide different information to the two interviewers), a source that accounted for 22%–100% of the discrepancies in the Brown et al. (2001b) study.

The sources of unreliability identified by these studies correspond to important issues and problems in the classification of emotional disorders. The fact that clinical severity was significantly associated with unreliability (i.e., disagreements as to whether presenting symptoms are above or below the DSM threshold) speaks to the purely categorical approach of current classification systems. If one assumes that the constituent features of disorders (or the disorder constructs themselves) are dimensional and operate along a continuum (e.g., Brown and Barlow 2005), then a certain degree of measurement error will be inherent to the classification system that imparts a categorical cutoff (i.e., variability in symptom expression is collapsed on either side of the dichotomy). Many researchers have noted difficulties with this approach and have championed alternative systems that incorporate a dimensional component to classification (e.g., Brown and Barlow 2005; Widiger and Samuel 2005).

The frequency with which other disorders were involved in diagnostic disagreements also varied substantially across categories (Brown et al. 2001b). Whereas it was relatively uncommon for social phobia, OCD, and PTSD (8%–13%), it was very frequent for dysthymia, panic disorder with agoraphobia, major depression, and GAD (54%–74%), which are disorders with overlapping definitional features. Moreover, for GAD, 63% of disagreements involving another diagnosis were with mood disorders. This overlap was also evident in disagreements involving anxiety disorder not otherwise specified and depressive disorder not otherwise specified diagnoses. When two or more potential diagnoses are present, the risk for disagreement is heightened by the fact that interviewers may not agree as to whether the features of one disorder should be subsumed under another disorder (e.g., do the symptoms of social anxiety represent a social phobia, or are they better accounted for by panic disorder with agoraphobia—i.e., fear of negative evaluation or of having a panic attack in public?). Indeed, this source of diagnostic disagreement pertains to another major issue concerning the potential poor discriminant validity among emotional disorders—their high rate of co-occurrence.

Diagnostic Comorbidity

Consistent evidence of high comorbidity among anxiety and mood disorders is frequently cited in support of skepticism about the distinguishability of the emotional disorders (Andrews 1990; Tyrer 1989). Comorbidity studies based on DSM-III-R criteria have consistently indicated that at least 50% of patients with a principal anxiety disorder have one or more additional diagnoses at the time of assessment (e.g., Brawman-Mintzer et al. 1993; Brown and Barlow 1992; Sanderson et al. 1990b). Similar findings were obtained in a large-scale study (N=1,127) of the DSM-IV categories with patients presenting to an anxiety disorders specialty clinic (Table 2–3; Brown et al. 2001a). Because of limits in generalizability, such as the nature of inclusion and exclusion criteria used (e.g., active substance use disorders and presence of suicidality were exclusion criteria) and its outpatient setting, this study, like others, probably yielded conservative estimates of diagnostic co-occurrence. Nevertheless, comorbidity rates for many categories were quite high. For instance, consistent with earlier findings, 55% of patients with a principal anxiety or mood disorder had at least one additional anxiety or depressive disorder at the time of the assessment. Although 68% of patients with a principal diagnosis of GAD had at least one additional diagnosis, this comorbidity rate was lower than reported in the Brown and Barlow (1992) study using the DSM-III-R criteria (82%). This finding is important, because the high comorbidity rate associated with GAD (Brown and Barlow 1992) in tandem with evidence that GAD is asso-

TABLE 2–2. Summary of interrater reliability studies for DSM-IV and DSM-III-R anxiety and mood disorders

	Brown et al. (2001b)		Di Nardo et al. (1993)		Mannuzza et al. (1989)		Williams et al. (1992)	
Disorder	*n*	κ	*n*	κ	*n*	κ	*n*	κ
Anxiety disorders								
GAD	113	0.65	108	0.53	11	0.27	8	0.56
OCD	60	0.75	24	0.75	13	0.91	27	0.59
PD	22	0.56	44	0.39	53	0.79	—	—
PDA	102	0.81	53	0.71	34	0.81	35	0.58[a]
PTSD	14	0.59	8	0.55	—	—	—	—
Social phobia	152	0.77	84	0.66	51	0.68	23	0.47
Specific phobia	100	0.71	47	0.63	30	0.29	20	0.52
Mood disorders								
Dysthymia	53	0.31	25	0.35	—	—	23	0.40
MDD	111	0.59	46	0.55	—	—	121	0.64

Note. GAD=generalized anxiety disorder; MDD=major depressive disorder; OCD=obsessive-compulsive disorder; PD=panic disorder; PDA=panic disorder with agoraphobia; PTSD=posttraumatic stress disorder; *n*=number of cases in which diagnosis was assigned by one or both raters; κ=kappa; all kappas pertain to current clinical diagnoses (collapsing across principal and additional diagnoses).

[a]PD and PDA were collapsed under the same category in this study.

ciated with poor to fair diagnostic reliability (e.g., Di Nardo et al. 1993) contributed to the debate during the preparation of DSM-IV regarding whether GAD should be moved to the Appendix of Disorders in Need of Future Study, given uncertainty about its status as a distinct syndrome (see Brown et al. 1994 for a detailed discussion of this issue). However, several other diagnostic categories had levels of comorbidity comparable with or higher than GAD in the DSM-IV study (by Brown et al. 2001a). The most commonly occurring additional diagnoses were social phobia (22%) and major depressive disorder (20%).

However, in part because of their descriptive nature, comorbidity data alone do not have substantial implications for establishing or refuting the discriminant validity of the emotional disorder constructs. The multiple conceptual explanations for diagnostic comorbidity are sufficiently wide-ranging to either support or invalidate current nosologies and conceptualizations of emotional disorders (Andrews 1996; Blashfield 1990; Frances et al. 1990). Accounts for comorbidity that challenge current classification systems include the possibility that disorders co-occur in part because 1) they share overlapping defining criteria or 2) they represent inconsequential variations of a broader underlying syndrome that has been erroneously separated by the classification system. In regard to the first explanation, as currently defined by DSM-IV-TR, the associated symptom criteria for GAD overlap almost entirely with the defining features of major depression and dysthymia (e.g., sleep disturbance, fatigability, concentration difficulties, and restlessness). This overlap could contribute to findings of a differentially high comorbidity rate of GAD and mood disorders (e.g., Brown and Barlow 1992; Sanderson et al. 1990a), although DSM-IV attempts to adjust for this with a hierarchy rule stating that GAD should not be assigned if its features occur exclusively during the course of a mood disorder. The second explanation is akin to arguments that classification systems may have become overly precise to the point of artificial separation from broader disorders (Tyrer 1989).

Explanations for comorbidity that do not suggest problems in the current nosologies include the possibility that disorders co-occur 1) because of artifacts such as their base rates of occurrence in the study setting, 2) because the features of one disorder act as risk factors for another disorder (e.g., severe agoraphobia leads to mood disturbance due to hopelessness, restricted mobility, etc.), and 3) because they emerge from the same diathesis. An illustration of the first explanation is that major depression was the most frequently assigned lifetime additional diagnosis in a study by Brown et al. (2001a). This result may have been more a reflection of the fact that major depression is a prevalent diagnosis in our research setting and in the general population (Kessler et al. 2005), not because it reflects a potential boundary problem with this category. In regard to the second explanation, the results from the Brown et al. (2001a) study indicated that presence of PTSD was associated with a significantly elevated risk of panic disorder with agoraphobia, and that in the majority of the cases, PTSD preceded panic disorder. These findings can be interpreted to suggest that the high autonomic arousability and low perception of personal control associated with PTSD may have served as precipitants to panic disorder. The third explanation is intriguing in terms of its alignment with current theories of emotional disorders, which assert that anxiety and mood disorders emanate from shared genetic, biological, and psychosocial vulnerabilities (e.g., Barlow 2002; Barlow et al. 1996). By these accounts, which are discussed in detail later in this chapter, a certain amount of co-occurrence among disorders would be presumed because of their shared etiological roots.

Nevertheless, other aspects of extant comorbidity findings support questions about the discriminant validity of anxiety and mood disorders. Findings indicate that psychosocial treatment of a given anxiety disorder results in a significant decline in other anxiety or mood diagnoses that are not addressed directly in treatment (Borkovec et al. 1995; Brown et al. 1995a). For instance, Brown et al. (1995a) examined the course of additional diagnoses in a sample of 126 patients who were enrolled in a short-term (11-session) psychosocial treatment program for panic disorder with minimal agoraphobic avoidance. At pretreatment, 26% of the patients had an additional diagnosis of GAD. The rate of comorbid GAD declined significantly at posttreatment to 7%; this rate remained low at 2-year follow-up (9%). Although it might be tempting to attribute this decline to factors such as treatment generalization (e.g., elements of the treatment, such as cognitive restructuring, were powerful enough to reduce symptoms of both panic disorder and GAD), evidence of the resiliency of GAD to current psychosocial and drug treatments mitigates the plausibility of such an explanation (Brown et al. 1994). Instead, other factors such as a lack of independence between disorders, random measurement error (e.g., diagnostic unreliability), and systematic measurement error (e.g., tendency to over-report symptoms at pretreatment or

TABLE 2–3. Percentages of additional diagnoses among patients with anxiety and mood disorders (N=1,127)

	DSM-IV principal diagnosis							
Additional diagnosis	**PD (*n*=36)**	**PDA (*n*=324)**	**SOC (*n*=186)**	**GAD (*n*=120)**	**OCD (*n*=77)**	**SPEC (*n*=110)**	**MDD (*n*=81)**	**Overall[a]**
Any diagnosis	42	62	46	68	57	34	69	57
Anxiety disorders								
PD	—	—	1	3	1	0	4	1
PDA	—	—	3	15	3	5	15	9
SOC	8	15	—	36	26	9	41	22
GAD	19	16	13	—	12	5	5	13
OCD	6	7	8	4	—	3	9	7
SPEC	8	15	8	12	12	—	15	13
Mood disorders								
MDD	8	24	14	26	22	3	—	20
DYS	8	7	13	6	10	4	11	8
MDD or DYS	11	17	20	29	40	4	0	18

Note DYS=dysthymia; GAD=generalized anxiety disorder; MDD=major depressive disorder; OCD=obsessive-compulsive disorder; PD=panic disorder; PDA=panic disorder with agoraphobia; SOC=social phobia; SPEC=specific phobia.

[a]Overall frequency in which category was assigned as an additional current diagnosis.

Source. Adapted from Brown TA, Campbell LA, Lehman CL, Grisham JR, and Mancill RB: "Current and Lifetime Comorbidity of the DSM-IV Anxiety and Mood Disorders in a Large Clinical Sample." *Journal of Abnormal Psychology* 110:585–599, 2001. Copyright © 2001 by the American Psychological Association. Used with permission.

under-report at posttreatment) (Brown and Barlow 1992) might better explain the sharp decline in GAD.

On the other hand, an interesting pattern of results was obtained when overall comorbidity was examined (i.e., collapsing across all additional diagnoses). In this analysis, a significant pre- to posttreatment decline in overall comorbidity (from 40% to 17%) was still evident. At 2-year follow-up, however, the rate of comorbidity had increased to a level (30%) that was no longer significantly different from that of pretreatment. This occurred even though, in the aggregate, patients maintained or improved on gains for panic disorder across the follow-up interval, indicating considerable independence between panic disorder symptoms and overall comorbidity. Although these findings are based on descriptive data and are highly speculative, they could be interpreted in accord with the explanation for comorbidity and theoretical models stating that disorders emerge from the same vulnerabilities. Specifically, although cognitive-behavioral treatment was generally effective in ameliorating the symptoms and the maintaining processes of panic disorder, perhaps the intervention did not substantially reduce the general predispositional features (e.g., trait-negative affect), which left patients vulnerable to the emergence or resilience of other disorders.

Treatment Response Nonspecificity

Although the ability to draw conclusions about the validity of a disorder based on its treatment response is limited, the fact that numerous disorders respond similarly to the same psychosocial or drug treatment has been cited as further evidence of their overlap and poor discriminant validity (e.g., Hudson and Pope 1990; Tyrer et al. 1988). Findings indicating that a wide range of emotional disorders (e.g., major depression, dysthymia, OCD, panic disorder) respond similarly to antidepressant medications have been interpreted as evidence of overlap or a shared pathophysiology among these syndromes (e.g., Hudson and Pope 1990). In one of the largest studies bearing on this issue to date, Tyrer et al. (1988) treated 210 outpatients with GAD, panic disorder, or dysthymia with one of the following five interventions: diazepam, dothiepin, placebo, cognitive-behavioral therapy, or a self-help program. Although some treatment condition differences were noted at posttreatment (e.g., diazepam was less effective than dothiepin, cognitive-behavioral therapy, and self-help), no diagnostic group differences were found. In view of the lack of diagnostic group treatment response differences, Tyrer and colleagues concluded that differential diagnosis of anxiety and mood disorders did not provide a sound basis for treatment prescription. However, these conclusions are limited by several issues, including the absence of long-term outcome data and the fact that the study did not use treatments developed specifically for the key and maintaining features of the disorders in question (e.g., Brown et al. 2001c; Craske and Barlow 2001; Young et al. 2001).

Classification of Emotional Disorders: Limitations of Extant Studies

Although the literature reviewed in this chapter thus far provides clues about boundary issues among disorders and the validity of current nosologies of emotional disorders, most of these studies have design problems that limit their contribution to this subject. Indeed, most studies that bear on the validation of the classification of anxiety and mood disorders have been conducted at the diagnostic level (e.g., family and twin studies; Andrews et al. 1990; Kendler et al. 1992a) or have examined dimensional features within a diagnostic category (e.g., psychometric evaluations of constituent features within a DSM disorder; Marten et al. 1993). As we have discussed at length elsewhere (Brown 1996; Brown and Barlow 2005; Brown and Chorpita 1996), the categorical approach to analysis has many limitations (Costello 1992; Livesley et al. 1994). For instance, studies conducted at the diagnostic level (e.g., comorbidity, genetic or familial aggregation, across-diagnosis comparisons) are restricted by their adherence to the disorders defined by the classification system. (By using diagnoses as the units of analysis, researchers are implicitly accepting or are bound to the nosology they are evaluating.) Moreover, analyses at the diagnostic level rely largely on data that do not reflect the dimensional nature of psychopathological phenomena. Categorization of dimensional variables usually forfeits meaningful information by artificially (and often erroneously) collapsing variability above and below an arbitrary threshold (e.g., presence or absence of a DSM-IV disorder). In addition to reducing statistical power and limiting the ability to detect more complex uni- or multivariate relationships, this categorization often unnecessarily introduces additional measurement error. Brown et al.'s (2001b) diagnostic reliability study, reviewed earlier in this chapter, found that for many diagnostic categories, a common source of unreliability was interviewer disagreements regarding whether the features of a disorder met or surpassed the DSM threshold on the number, duration, or severity of symptoms. Moreover, dimensional ratings of the symptoms of major depression were found to be more reliable than the DSM-IV categorical descriptors (mild, moderate, and severe). Another clear example of this phenomenon can be found in the large-scale study by Di Nardo et al. (1993) on the diagnostic reliability of the DSM-III-R anxiety disorders. Results revealed considerable unreliability for DSM severity specifiers for agoraphobia (i.e., mild, moderate, and severe), a finding that influenced the decision to eliminate these specifiers in DSM-IV. This occurred despite the fact that the zero-order correlation of the first and second interviewers' dimensional ratings of agoraphobic avoidance was quite high (r=0.81). Thus, whereas considerable concordance was observed at the dimensional level, error was inflated when categorization was imposed on these ratings.

Conversely, if assessment were conducted at the dimensional level, the interrelationships among symptoms and syndromes could be examined, as could the extent to which the latent structure of these features corresponds to that specified by major classification systems such as DSM-IV. Methods of structural equation modeling could be used to examine the cross-sectional and longitudinal covariation of these latent factors, adjusting for measurement error and an error theory (e.g., extracting shared method variance from relationships or paths of interest).

Classification studies addressing multiple domains and dimensional features are beginning to appear in the literature on emotional disorders (Brown 2007; Brown et al. 1998; Spence 1997; Zinbarg and Barlow 1996). Spence (1997) examined the structure of anxiety symptoms in 698 children (ages 8–12 years) with confirmatory factor analysis of a questionnaire on the frequency of symptoms from six DSM-IV constructs: panic disorder, separation anxiety disorder, social phobia, specific phobia, OCD, and GAD. Compared with competing models in which disorders were collapsed or factors were constrained to be orthogonal, the six-factor model provided a superior fit to the data. Although factorially distinct, the six disorder factors were highly intercorrelated (r of 0.67–0.88). However, the considerable covariance in these latent factors was satisfactorily accounted for by a higher-order model in which the six disorder factors loaded significantly onto a single second-order factor. This higher-order model is consistent with the underpinnings of the DSM-IV nosology, which asserts that panic disorder, separation anxiety disorder, social phobia, specific phobia, OCD, and GAD, albeit distinct, belong to a common family of disorders. This higher-order model was replicated in a second cohort and was found to be consistent across sexes and age groups. Although this research was limited to some degree by its use of a single self-report measure and a nonclinical sample and by its failure to include a depression factor (since mood disorders may be highly overlapping with some anxiety disorders, such as GAD), the results are nonetheless encouraging with regard to the correspondence of the obtained latent structure with the nosology outlined in DSM-IV.

An example in the area of adult anxiety disorders is a study by Zinbarg and Barlow (1996). In this study, an exploratory factor analysis of various questionnaires on features of anxiety disorders produced a factor structure that was largely consistent with the DSM-III-R nosology (i.e., social anxiety, generalized dysphoria, agoraphobia, fear of fear, obsessions and compulsions, and simple fears). Support for DSM-III-R was also provided by discriminant function analyses indicating that selected diagnostic groups (defined by principal diagnoses established by structured interviews) had characteristic profiles in factor scores generated from a higher-order factor analysis. Although encouraging, as noted by the authors, these findings were limited by factors such as the preponderant use of self-report measures (e.g., method variance could account, in part, for the structure observed) and the fact that mood disorders were poorly represented (i.e., depressive symptoms were assessed by a single measure with a scale under psychometric development). Again, this latter limitation is noteworthy, given evidence that mood disorders (i.e., major depression and dysthymia) may pose greater boundary problems for certain anxiety disorders than do other anxiety disorders (Brown et al. 1995b, 1998; D.A. Clark et al. 1994; Starcevic 1995).

Structure and Pathogenesis of Anxiety/Mood Disorders: Conceptual Models and Evidence

Traditionally, dimensional studies of anxiety and depression have revealed considerable overlap in these constructs. For instance, intercorrelations among widely used self-report measures (e.g., State-Trait Anxiety Inventory and Beck Depression Inventory) and clinical rating scales (e.g., Hamilton Anxiety and Depression Rating Scales) of anxiety and depression have typically exceeded 0.70 (Clark and Watson 1991; Kendall and

Watson 1989). These findings, in tandem with the aforementioned studies conducted at the syndromal level, have led investigators to question whether clinical anxiety and depression are in fact empirically distinct phenomena. Addressing this issue, Clark and Watson (1991) concluded, on the basis of literature review, that although anxiety and depression share a significant nonspecific component encompassing general affective distress and other common symptoms, the two constructs can be distinguished by certain unique features. The investigators proposed a tripartite structure of anxiety and depression consisting of 1) *negative affect*, defined as symptoms of general distress such as worry, irritability, and tension; 2) *positive affect*, defined as the level of pleasurable engagement with the environment and characterized by features such as cheerfulness, sociability, high energy level, and enthusiasm; and 3) *autonomic hyperarousal*, characterized by symptoms such as rapid heart rate, shortness of breath, and trembling. This model illustrates that negative affect is a shared feature of anxiety and mood disorders (i.e., symptoms of tension, worry, irritability, etc., are present in both anxiety and depression). Autonomic hyperarousal is viewed as specific to anxiety. Conversely, an absence of positive affect (anhedonia) is regarded as a feature that differentiates mood disorders from anxiety disorders.

However, the model has several shortcomings. First, it does not account for the diversity of symptoms of anxiety disorders. For example, Brown et al. (1998) found that autonomic hyperarousal was not specific to all anxiety disorders, but instead was a unique component of panic disorder. Additionally, research has demonstrated that absence of positive affect is not specific to depression but is also related to social phobia (e.g., Brown et al. 1998). To address the shortcomings of the tripartite model, Mineka et al. (1998) proposed a reformulation that they termed the "hierarchical model of anxiety and depression." In this model, each disorder consists of both a shared and a unique component. The shared component corresponds to individual differences in general distress and negative affect, representing a higher-order factor common to both anxiety and mood disorders. The unique component for each disorder consists of the specific features that distinguish it from the other disorders. For example, anhedonia, absence of positive affect, and lack of interest are conceptualized as the unique component of depression (Mineka et al. 1998). Unlike in the tripartite model, autonomic hyperarousal is no longer viewed in this model as specific to all anxiety disorders, but rather as the specific component of panic disorder. The size of shared and unique components varies among different disorders. For instance, major depression and GAD include more negative affect and general distress than specific phobia (Watson et al. 2005).

In a related conceptualization, Barlow (2000, 2002) formulated a triple vulnerability model of emotional disorders, which draws from genetics, personality, cognitive science and neuroscience, and emotion and learning theories. The first diathesis, "generalized biological vulnerability," corresponds to the genetically based dimensions of temperament (e.g., neuroticism). Second, the Barlow model posits that certain early life experiences (e.g., overcontrolling parenting style; Chorpita and Barlow 1998) contribute to a perceived sense of uncontrollability, leading to a "generalized psychological vulnerability." This vulnerability is manifested as a propensity for an individual to process failures and perceived deficiencies as an indication of a chronic inability to cope with unpredictable and uncontrollable negative events. Acting together, generalized biological and psychological vulnerabilities may sometimes be sufficient to produce an emotional disorder. However, the Barlow model forwards a third set of vulnerabilities that, in combination with the previous two diatheses, are germane to the development of specific emotional disorders. These "specific psychological vulnerabilities," which also emerge from early learning experiences, reflect a cognitive disposition for anxious apprehension focused on the perceived danger of specific events, thoughts, or objects (e.g., thought-action fusion in OCD, in which individuals learn to equate dangerous thoughts with dangerous actions). For example, "anxiety sensitivity," conceptualized as a specific psychological vulnerability for panic disorder (Taylor 1999), may arise when individuals learn early on from caregivers that unexplained somatic sensations are dangerous and could signal illness or death.

Subsequent research has suggested that these conceptual models of anxiety and depression may have considerable relevance to the understanding of the pathogenesis of these conditions. Extensive evidence indicates that the higher-order dimensions of negative affect and positive affect represent trait vulnerability factors for the development of emotional disorders. For instance, a growing body of literature attests to the heritability of these constructs (e.g., Hettema et al. 2004) and their roles in accounting for the onset, overlap, and maintenance of anxiety and depression (e.g., Brown et al. 1998; Gershuny and Sher 1998; Kasch et al. 2002).

These conceptualizations of the pathogenesis of anxiety and depression may have a strong bearing on issues concerning the classification of emotional disorders. For instance, these models and recent evidence indicate that much of the overlap between anxiety and mood disorders stems from the fact that these disorders emerge from the same biological/genetic and psychosocial diatheses (e.g., Barlow 2002; L.A. Clark et al. 1994). That is, although emotional disorders co-occur in part because they arise from core diatheses, this common vulnerability is manifested heterogeneously (i.e., as different DSM disorders) due to exposure to differing environmental influences, other genetic/biological agents, and so forth (e.g., Barlow 2002; L.A. Clark 2005; Hettema et al. 2005). Genetic evidence is consistent with this position. For example, in a blind study of 1,033 female-female twin pairs, Kendler et al. (1992a) concluded that GAD is a moderately familial disorder, with a heritability estimated at about 30% (the remainder of variance in GAD liability may result from environmental factors not shared by the adult twins). Further research on both all-female (Kendler 1996; Kendler et al. 1992b, 2007) and mixed-sex twin samples (Roy et al. 1995) has indicated that a clear genetic influence exists in GAD, and that the genetic factors in GAD are completely shared with major depression.

Findings and conceptualizations of shared genetic, biological, and psychosocial vulnerability in anxiety and depression could be taken as further indication of the poor boundaries of these conditions. Nevertheless, empirical and conceptual accounts suggest that this may not be the case. For example, Kendler et al. (1992b) found that GAD and major depression share the same genetic factors but their environmental determinants appeared to be mostly distinct. These findings are consistent with conceptual models of emotional disorders (e.g., Barlow 2002) that view the anxiety and mood disorders as sharing vulnerabilities but differing on important dimensions (e.g., specific psychological vulnerability arising from environmental experiences) to the extent that differentiation of these psychopathological phenomena is warranted. Biologically or genetically based traits such as negative affect and behavioral inhibition may underlie social phobia and panic disorder. Whether one or both conditions become manifest from these diatheses could depend on environmental determinants such as direct experiences with social humiliation or scrutiny, vicarious exposure (e.g., parental modeling) to shyness or introversion, and hypochondriacal behavior.

In summary, evidence and predictions emanating from the hierarchical model of anxiety and depression (Mineka et al. 1998), genetic and biological studies (e.g., Kendler 1996; Kendler et al. 1992b, 2007), and comprehensive theories of emotional disorders (e.g., Barlow 2002) align with the position that although most of the constructs underlying the DSM-IV anxiety and mood disorders are relatively distinct (Brown 2007; Brown et al. 1998; Spence 1997; Zinbarg and Barlow 1996), salient overlap exists in these categories. This overlap may include features such as negative affect and behavioral inhibition, which represent expressions of common genetic and biologically or psychosocially based vulnerability dimensions. Of course, alternative explanations also may account to varying degrees for the overlap and high comorbidity among emotional disorders (e.g., erroneous splitting of trivial variations of a broad syndrome into two or more categories and unnecessary overlap in diagnostic criteria). Therefore, extensive research is needed to determine the validity of these positions.

For instance, the debate continues as to whether the DSM-IV diagnosis of GAD represents a distinct syndrome because of high phenotypic overlap (Brown et al. 1994). On the one hand, these findings could be viewed as consistent with the triple vulnerability and hierarchical models of anxiety and depression (Barlow 2002; Mineka et al. 1998), and could suggest the existence of multiple dimensions of risk that have differential relevance to the various emotional disorders (i.e., the vulnerability factors for GAD and depression are neither singular nor entirely overlapping; e.g., L.A. Clark 2005; Mineka et al. 1998). On the other hand, the numerous similarities between GAD and the mood disorders have led some researchers to conclude that GAD represents a variant of or prodrome to depression. As noted earlier, DSM-IV acknowledges this boundary issue with the hierarchy rule, specifying that GAD should not be diagnosed if its features occur exclusively during a mood disorder.

From a classification standpoint, studies are needed that examine the relations and discriminability of the DSM-IV disorder constructs with key vulnerability dimensions. A cross-sectional study of this nature analyzed the structural relations of dimensions of selected emotional disorders and dimensions of negative affect, positive affect, and autonomic arousal (Brown et al. 1998). In a sample of 350 patients with DSM-IV anxiety and mood disorders who were assessed by a variety of questionnaires and clinician ratings, a confirmatory factor analysis of the latent structure of dimensions of key features in selected DSM-IV disorders (i.e., mood disorders, GAD, panic disorder/agoraphobia, OCD, social phobia) supported the discriminant validity of DSM-IV for the five constructs examined. Relative to models that collapsed across all or various disorders, the five-factor model (i.e., mood disorders, GAD, panic disorder/agoraphobia, OCD, social phobia) provided the best fit for the data. Notably, model fit was degraded significantly when indicators of GAD and mood disorders were collapsed into a single factor, thereby lending support for the differentiation of these features. However, the GAD latent factor was most strongly correlated with the mood disorder latent factor (r=0.63), supporting contentions that the features of GAD have the most overlap with the mood disorders.

Also, this study comparatively evaluated several structural models of the relations among the five latent factors for DSM-IV disorder and the three latent factors corresponding to the tripartite model of anxiety and depression (i.e., negative affect, positive affect, autonomic arousal). Superior data fit was associated with a model that 1) specified negative affect and positive affect as higher-order factors, compared with the DSM-IV disorder factors (with significant paths from negative affect to each of the five DSM-IV factors and from positive affect to the mood disorder and social phobia factors only), and 2) specified autonomic arousal as a lower-order factor (with significant paths from panic disorder/agoraphobia and GAD to autonomic arousal). For instance, all paths from negative affect to the DSM-IV disorder factors were statistically significant, in accord with predictions that negative affect is a shared and potentially dispositional feature of emotional disorders that accounts for communality among them (i.e., the considerable zero-order correlations among DSM-IV disorder factors were well accounted for by negative affect, and, for two disorders, by positive affect). Yet the strongest paths from the higher-order factor specified as negative affect to the various DSM-IV factors were to GAD and mood disorder (path coefficients=0.74 and 0.67, respectively)—consistent with arguments and evidence discussed earlier that GAD and depression are associated with the highest levels of negative affect.

Other noteworthy findings from the Brown et al. (1998) study included results involving the structural relations of the DSM-IV disorder factors and the latent factor of autonomic arousal. Counter to prediction and the tripartite model, paths from the DSM-IV disorder factors OCD and social phobia to autonomic arousal were nonsignificant. These results suggest that, although generally unrelated to mood disorders (i.e., results indicated no improvement in model fit with the addition of a path from depression to autonomic arousal), autonomic arousal symptoms may be weakly related to or of less discriminant value for certain anxiety disorders (e.g., discrete social phobias). Accordingly, these findings highlighted a possible refinement of the tripartite model with regard to autonomic arousal. Although autonomic arousal had initially been posited as a discriminating feature for the entire range of anxiety disorders, these data suggest that the relevance of autonomic arousal may be limited primarily to panic disorder/agoraphobia. This interpretation is in accord with the subsequent reconsiderations of the hierarchical model (Mineka et al. 1998), which also now acknowledges the consistent finding of an association between positive affect and social phobia (Brown et al. 1998; Watson et al. 1988). Specifically, the unique relation of social phobia to positive affect relative to the other anxiety disorders has been interpreted as being based on the interpersonal character of low positive affect (e.g., low self-confidence, unassertiveness) (L.A. Clark et al. 1994).

Another interesting finding regarding the construct of autonomic arousal was the statistically significant negative path from GAD to autonomic arousal. In addition to aligning with the results of laboratory studies indicating that the features of GAD (i.e., excessive worry) are associated with autonomic suppression, this finding may point to another distinguishing characteristic of GAD relative to other anxiety disorders (this distinction could be primarily limited to panic disorder, because many other anxiety and mood disorders, although not linked to autonomic suppression, may be characterized by low autonomic arousal).

However, two limitations of this study were that it was a cross-sectional study and thus did not allow for conclusions about directionality of the relation of the disorders and vulnerability constructs, and negative and positive affect were assessed by a single indicator (Positive and Negative Affect Scales). Although developed independently, the constructs of negative affect and positive affect coincide to a considerable degree with trait vulnerability constructs of other leading theories, such as those of Gray (1987), Eysenck (1970), and Barlow et al. (1996). For instance, negative affect is a construct similar to behavioral inhibition, neuroticism, and anxious apprehension in the Gray, Eysenck, and Barlow models, respectively. And the construct of positive affect is similar to behavioral activation and extraversion in the Gray and Eysenck models, respectively.

Brown (2007) expanded on the previous study (Brown et al. 1998), using a sample of 606 patients, with a focus on three disorder constructs: unipolar depression, GAD, and social phobia. Latent factors of neuroticism/behavioral inhibition and behavioral activation/positive affect were assessed using multiple indicators of hypothesized vulnerability dimensions. Confirmatory factor analyses indicated that the latent factors of neuroticism/behavioral inhibition and behavioral activation/positive affect were distinct from GAD, social phobia, and depression. Neuroticism/behavioral inhibition and behavioral activation/positive affect accounted for most of the covariance among the DSM-IV disorder constructs. Although neuroticism/behavioral inhibition was significantly related to all three DSM-IV disorders, it had the strongest relationship with GAD and depression. Behavioral activation/positive affect was more strongly related to depression and social phobia than GAD, a result similar to the findings of Brown et al. (1998).

Brown (2007) also examined the temporal course and temporal structural relationships of dimensions of neuroticism/behavioral inhibition and behavioral activation/positive affect and DSM-IV disorder constructs, reassessing the participants at 1-year and 2-year follow-ups. Because the majority of the study participants (76%) were receiving psychotherapy following their intake, the rate of anxiety and mood disorders decreased significantly between the intake and the 2-year follow-up (100% to 58%). Behavioral activation/positive affect evidenced a very high degree of temporal stability, consistent with its conceptualization as a trait vulnerability construct that is relatively unaffected by treatment. Neuroticism, on the other hand, evidenced the greatest amount of temporal change out of the five constructs examined, which is inconsistent with previous findings (e.g., Kasch et al. 2002). However, it is possible that neuroticism/behavioral inhibition consists of some combination of stable temperament variance with variability due to generalized distress; the latter may be temporally less stable and be more likely to covary with changes in the severity of disorders.

Further examination of the directional effects among temperament and DSM-IV disorder constructs over time revealed that higher initial levels of neuroticism/behavioral inhibition were associated with less change in GAD and social phobia. Initial levels of the DSM-IV disorders, however, did not predict change in temperament over time. Moreover, all the temporal covariance of the DSM-IV disorder constructs was accounted for by change in neuroticism/behavioral inhibition. This finding suggests that either neuroticism may be affected by therapy, or a reduction in disorder severity is associated with reduction in general distress, a feature shared by all emotional disorders and partially reflected in the measurement of neuroticism/behavioral inhibition. Overall, the results of this study demonstrate in a longitudinal context the role of neuroticism/behavioral inhibition as a unifying construct accounting for the covariance among the emotional disorders.

Key Clinical Points and Directions for Future Research

In this chapter, we focused on issues pertaining to the validity of the anxiety disorder categories. The extant literature points to considerable overlap among the various anxiety and mood disorders. This is evident in studies that have demonstrated high rates of current and lifetime comorbidity at the diagnostic level (e.g., Brown et al. 2001a), nonspecificity of treatment response (e.g., Tyrer et al. 1988), and the remission of comorbid conditions following psychosocial treatment of the principal disorder (e.g., Brown et al. 1995a). On the other hand, evidence suggests that the dimensional key features of the DSM anxiety and mood disorders display a high level of discriminant validity, despite a certain degree of overlap (e.g., Brown 2007; Brown et al. 1998). Moreover, most of the shared variance of these emotional disorder constructs can be accounted for by a higher-order dimension of general distress/neuroticism.

The principal position outlined in the preceding section was that overlap in anxiety and mood disorders, although reflective of nosological concerns to varying degrees (perhaps with regard to GAD, in particular), may provide important clues to the understanding of the origins and maintenance of these syndromes. This position is consistent with one potential explanation of comorbidity—that high co-occurrence of disorders at the descriptive level is the result of their common etiological roots. Clearly, these hypotheses await sophisticated, hypothesis-driven research.

Several suggestions have been made throughout this chapter regarding important refinements for future research on the classification of emotional disorders. These suggestions included the following:

1. Increased emphasis on dimensional measures of psychopathological phenomena and disorders to better elucidate the latent structure and interrela-

tionships of these features (which also mitigates the problem of being bound to the existing nosology, if disorders are studied at the diagnostic level)

2. Greater use of latent variable approaches to data analysis (offering the advantages of adjusting for measurement error and an error theory), which foster statistical comparisons of models reflecting competing theories of classification or causality (e.g., models emanating from competing explanations for diagnostic comorbidity; Blashfield 1990; Frances et al. 1990), and evaluating paths or relations only in the context of good model fit (Bollen 1989)
3. Increased within-study focus on a wider range of disorders, given that issues pertaining to overlap and pathogenesis cut across the classes of syndromes outlined in DSM-IV (e.g., although residing in separate chapters in DSM-IV, potential boundary issues exist across the anxiety, mood, somatoform, and personality disorders)
4. Incorporation of multiple measures associated with theoretically salient vulnerability dimensions (e.g., negative affect, behavioral inhibition, perceived control), which fosters examination of issues such as the (differential) prediction of the emergence of diagnostic syndromes and the extent to which the defining features of emotional disorders overlap with these traits (e.g., are the features of GAD best subsumed under these traits, consistent with arguments that GAD simply reflects a nonspecific symptom or trait, or does GAD represent a distinct latent factor that, like other anxiety and mood disorders, is influenced by these higher-order traits?)

   This final focus would also address suggestions made by researchers for increased empirical consideration of the common traits of emotional disorders that may hold strong predictive value for the prevention, etiology, course, and treatment response of emotional disorders.

It is hoped that these methodological refinements will be increasingly applied to two other important avenues of classification and pathogenesis research—genetic and longitudinal studies. Greater emphasis on dimensional assessment of psychopathology (e.g., latent disorder constructs) in twin studies, in tandem with the use of latent variable approaches that are well entrenched in the behavioral genetics literature (Boomsma et al. 1989), could lead to important advances beyond evidence on the heritability and familial aggregation of disorders focused at the diagnostic (categorical) level (e.g., estimates of genetic liability are influenced by heightened measurement error and mitigated statistical power associated with collapsing dimensional variability above and below the DSM threshold). Increasingly, genetic studies of this nature are emerging in the literature (e.g., Kendler et al. 1987).

Important potential avenues for longitudinal research also await exploration. One is the study of at-risk or large nonclinical samples to identify the contribution of dimensions implicated as vulnerability factors (e.g., negative affect) in the prediction of emotional disorders, and whether these higher-order traits are more explanatory than vulnerability constructs suggested to be disorder-specific, such as cognitive vulnerabilities of depression and OCD (Ingram et al. 1998; Salkovskis 1996). In addition, large-scale clinical studies are needed to address issues such as the temporal stability and covariation of disorders and their underlying constructs, the effects of life stress on the relationship between temperament and psychopathology, and the bidirectional influence of temperament and DSM-IV disorders during the course of psychosocial treatment. This methodology is crucial to the better understanding of the direction of the relationships among disorders and potential vulnerability constructs (e.g., theory-driven tests of selected conceptual accounts for comorbidity, such as whether the features of a disorder serve as risk factors to another disorder). For instance, given the evidence that the effects of vulnerability on psychopathology may be affected by stressful life events (Kendler et al. 2004), the Brown (2007) study may have underestimated the influence of neuroticism/behavioral inhibition and behavioral activation/positive affect on the course of the DSM-IV disorder constructs. These questions await longitudinal study in twin, community, at-risk, and clinical samples.

References

American Psychiatric Association: Diagnostic and Statistical Manual of Mental Disorders, 2nd Edition. Washington, DC, American Psychiatric Association, 1968

American Psychiatric Association: Diagnostic and Statistical Manual of Mental Disorders, 3rd Edition, Revised. Washington, DC, American Psychiatric Association, 1987

American Psychiatric Association: Diagnostic and Statistical Manual of Mental Disorders, 4th Edition. Washington, DC, American Psychiatric Association, 1994

American Psychiatric Association: Diagnostic and Statistical Manual of Mental Disorders, 4th Edition, Text Revision.

Washington, DC, American Psychiatric Association, 2000

Andrews G: Classification of neurotic disorders. J R Soc Med 83:606–607, 1990

Andrews G: Comorbidity in neurotic disorders: the similarities are more important than the differences, in Current Controversies in the Anxiety Disorders. Edited by Rapee RM. New York, Guilford, 1996, pp 3–20

Andrews G, Stewart G, Morris-Yates A, et al: Evidence for a general neurotic syndrome. Br J Psychiatry 157:6–12, 1990

Barlow DH: Unraveling the mysteries of anxiety and its disorders from the perspective of emotion theory. Am Psychol 55:1247–1263, 2000

Barlow DH (ed): Anxiety and Its Disorders: The Nature and Treatment of Anxiety and Panic, 2nd Edition. New York, Guilford, 2002

Barlow DH, Chorpita BF, Turovsky J: Fear, panic, anxiety, and disorders of emotion, in Perspectives on Anxiety, Panic, and Fear, Vol 43. Edited by Hope DA. Lincoln, NE, University of Nebraska Press, 1996, pp 251–328

Blashfield RK: Comorbidity and classification, in Comorbidity of Mood and Anxiety Disorders. Edited by Maser JD, Cloninger CR. Washington, DC, American Psychiatric Press, 1990, pp 61–82

Bollen KA: Structural Equations With Latent Variables. New York, Wiley, 1989

Boomsma DI, Martin NG, Neale MC (eds): Genetic analysis of twin and family data: structural equation modeling using LISREL. Behav Genet 19:1–160, 1989

Borkovec TD, Abel JL, Newman H: Effects of psychotherapy on comorbid conditions in generalized anxiety disorder. J Consult Clin Psychol 63:479–483, 1995

Brawman-Mintzer O, Lydiard RB, Emmanuel N, et al: Psychiatric comorbidity in patients with generalized anxiety disorder. Am J Psychiatry 150:1216–1218, 1993

Brown TA: Validity of the DSM-III-R and DSM-IV classification systems for anxiety disorders, in Current Controversies in the Anxiety Disorders. Edited by Rapee RM. New York, Guilford, 1996, pp 21–45

Brown TA: Temporal course and structural relationships among dimensions of temperament and DSM-IV anxiety and mood disorder constructs. J Abnorm Psychol 116:313–328, 2007

Brown TA, Barlow DH: Comorbidity among anxiety disorders: implications for treatment and DSM-IV. J Consult Clin Psychol 60:835–844, 1992

Brown TA, Barlow DH: Dimensional versus categorical classification of mental disorders in the fifth edition of the Diagnostic and Statistical Manual of Mental Disorders and beyond: comment on the special section. J Abnorm Psychol 114:551–556, 2005

Brown TA, Chorpita BF: Reply to Andrews: on the validity and comorbidity of the DSM-III-R and DSM-IV anxiety disorders, in Current Controversies in the Anxiety Disorders. Edited by Rapee RM. New York, Guilford, 1996, pp 48–52

Brown TA, Barlow DH, Liebowitz MR: The empirical basis of generalized anxiety disorder. Am J Psychiatry 151:1272–1280, 1994

Brown TA, Antony MM, Barlow DH: Diagnostic comorbidity in panic disorder: effect on treatment outcome and course of comorbid diagnoses following treatment. J Consult Clin Psychol 63:408–418, 1995a

Brown TA, Marten PA, Barlow DH: Discriminant validity of the symptoms constituting the DSM-III-R and DSM-IV associated symptom criterion of generalized anxiety disorder. J Anxiety Disord 9:317–328, 1995b

Brown TA, Chorpita BF, Barlow DH: Structural relationships among dimensions of the DSM-IV anxiety and mood disorders and dimensions of negative affect, positive affect, and autonomic arousal. J Abnorm Psychol 107:179–192, 1998

Brown TA, Campbell LA, Lehman CL, et al: Current and lifetime comorbidity of the DSM-IV anxiety and mood disorders in a large clinical sample. J Abnorm Psychol 110:585–599, 2001a

Brown TA, Di Nardo PA, Lehman CL, et al: Reliability of DSM-IV anxiety and mood disorders: implications for the classification of emotional disorders. J Abnorm Psychol 110:49–58, 2001b

Brown TA, O'Leary TA, Barlow DH: Generalized anxiety disorder, in Clinical Handbook of Psychological Disorders, 3rd Edition. Edited by Barlow DH. New York, Guilford, 2001c, pp 154–208

Chorpita BF, Barlow DH: The development of anxiety: the role of control in the early environment. Psychol Bull 124:3–21, 1998

Clark DA, Beck AT, Beck JS: Symptom differences in major depression, dysthymia, panic disorder, and generalized anxiety disorder. Am J Psychiatry 151:205–209, 1994

Clark LA: Temperament as a unifying basis for personality and psychopathology. J Abnorm Psychol 114:505–521, 2005

Clark LA, Watson D: Tripartite model of anxiety and depression: psychometric evidence and taxonomic implications. J Abnorm Psychol 100:316–336, 1991

Clark LA, Watson D, Mineka S: Temperament, personality, and the mood and anxiety disorders. J Abnorm Psychol 103:103–116, 1994

Costello CG: Research on symptoms versus research on syndromes: arguments in favour of allocating more research time to the study of symptoms. Br J Psychiatry 60:304–308, 1992

Craske MG, Barlow DH: Panic disorder and agoraphobia, in Clinical Handbook of Psychological Disorders, 3rd Edition. Edited by Barlow DH. New York, Guilford, 2001, pp 1–59

Di Nardo PA, Barlow DH: Anxiety Disorders Interview Schedule-Revised. Albany, NY, Graywind, 1988

Di Nardo PA, Moras K, Barlow DH, et al: Reliability of DSM-III-R anxiety disorder categories using the Anxiety Disorders Interview Schedule-Revised (ADIS-R). Arch Gen Psychiatry 50:251–256, 1993

Di Nardo PA, Brown TA, Barlow DH: Anxiety Disorders Interview Schedule for DSM-IV: Lifetime Version (ADIS-IV-L). San Antonio, TX, Psychological Corporation, 1994

Eysenck HJ: The Structure of Human Personality. London, Methuen, 1970

First MB, Spitzer RL, Gibbon M, et al: Structured Clinical Interview for DSM-IV Axis I Disorders (SCID). Washington, DC, American Psychiatric Press, 1996

Fleiss JL, Nee JCM, Landis JR: Large sample variance of kappa in the case of different sets of raters. Arch Gen Psychiatry 86:974–977, 1979

Frances A, Widiger T, Fyer MR: The influence of classification methods on comorbidity, in Comorbidity of Mood and Anxiety Disorders. Edited by Maser JD, Cloninger CR. Washington, DC, American Psychiatric Press, 1990, pp 41–59

Fyer AJ, Endicott J, Mannuzza S, et al: Schedule for Affective Disorders and Schizophrenia: Lifetime Version (modified for the study of anxiety disorders). New York, Anxiety Disorders Clinic, New York State Psychiatric Institute, 1985

Gershuny BS, Sher KJ: The relation between personality and anxiety: findings from a 3-year prospective study. J Abnorm Psychol 107:252–262, 1998

Gray JS: The Psychology of Fear and Stress, 2nd Edition. New York, Oxford University Press, 1987

Hettema JM, Prescott CA, Kendler KS: Genetic and environmental sources of covariation between generalized anxiety disorder and neuroticism. Am J Psychiatry 161:1581–1587, 2004

Hettema JM, Prescott CA, Myers JM, et al: The structure of genetic and environmental risk factors for anxiety disorders in men and women. Arch Gen Psychiatry 62:182–189, 2005

Hudson JI, Pope HG: Affective spectrum disorder: does antidepressant response identify a family of disorders with a common pathophysiology? Am J Psychiatry 147:552–564, 1990

Ingram RE, Miranda J, Segal ZV: Cognitive Vulnerability to Depression. New York, Guilford, 1998

Kasch KL, Rottenberg J, Arnow BA, et al: Behavioral activation and inhibition systems and the severity and course of depression. J Abnorm Psychol 111:589–597, 2002

Kendall PC, Watson D (eds): Anxiety and Depression: Distinctive and Overlapping Features. San Diego, CA, Academic Press, 1989

Kendler KS: Major depression and generalized anxiety disorder: same genes, (partly) different environments—revisited. Br J Psychiatry 168(suppl):68–75, 1996

Kendler KS, Heath AC, Martin NG, et al: Symptoms of anxiety and symptoms of depression: same genes, different environments? Arch Gen Psychiatry 44:451–457, 1987

Kendler KS, Neale MC, Kessler RC, et al: Generalized anxiety disorder in women: a population-based twin study. Arch Gen Psychiatry 49:267–272, 1992a

Kendler KS, Neale MC, Kessler RC, et al: Major depression and generalized anxiety disorder: same genes, (partly) different environments? Arch Gen Psychiatry 49:716–722, 1992b

Kendler KS, Kuhn J, Prescott CA: The interrelationship of neuroticism, sex, and stressful life events in the prediction of episodes of major depression. Am J Psychiatry 161:631–636, 2004

Kendler KS, Gardner CO, Gatz M, et al: The sources of comorbidity between major depression and generalized anxiety disorder in a Swedish national twin sample. Psychol Med 37:453–462, 2007

Kessler RC, Chiu WT, Demler O, et al: Prevalence, severity, and comorbidity of 12-month DSM-IV disorders in the National Comorbidity Survey Replication. Arch Gen Psychiatry 62:617–627, 2005

Livesley WJ, Schroeder ML, Jackson DN, et al: Categorical distinctions in the study of personality disorder: implications for classification. J Abnorm Psychol 103:6–17, 1994

Mannuzza S, Fyer AJ, Martin LY, et al: Reliability of anxiety assessment, I: diagnostic agreement. Arch Gen Psychiatry 46:1093–1101, 1989

Marten PA, Brown TA, Barlow DH, et al: Evaluation of the ratings comprising the associated symptom criterion of DSM-III-R generalized anxiety disorder. J Nerv Ment Dis 181:676–682, 1993

Mineka S, Watson D, Clark LA: Comorbidity of anxiety and unipolar mood disorders. Annu Rev Psychol 49:377–412, 1998

Riskind JH, Beck AT, Berchick RJ, et al: Reliability of the DSM-III-R diagnoses for major depression and generalized anxiety disorder using the Structured Clinical Interview for DSM-III-R. Arch Gen Psychiatry 44:817–820, 1987

Roy MA, Neale MC, Pedersen NL, et al: A twin study of generalized anxiety disorder and major depression. Psychol Med 25:1037–1040, 1995

Salkovskis PM: Cognitive-behavioral approaches to understanding obsessional problems, in Current Controversies in the Anxiety Disorders. Edited by Rapee RM. New York, Guilford, 1996, pp 103–133

Sanderson WC, Beck AT, Beck J: Syndrome comorbidity in patients with major depression or dysthymia: prevalence and temporal relationships. Am J Psychiatry 147:1025–1028, 1990a

Sanderson WC, Di Nardo PA, Rapee RM, et al: Syndrome comorbidity in patients diagnosed with a DSM-III-R anxiety disorder. J Abnorm Psychol 99:308–312, 1990b

Segal DL, Hersen M, Van Hesselt VB: Reliability of the Structured Interview of DSM-III-R: an evaluative review. Compr Psychiatry 35:316–327, 1994

Shrout PE, Spitzer RL, Fleiss JL: Quantification of agreement in psychiatric diagnosis revisited. Arch Gen Psychiatry 44:172–177, 1987

Skre I, Onstad S, Torgersen S, et al: High interrater reliability for the Structured Clinical Interview for DSM-III-R Axis I (SCID-I). Acta Psychiatr Scand 84:167–173, 1991

Spence J: Structure of anxiety symptoms among children: a confirmatory factor-analytic study. J Abnorm Psychol 106:280–297, 1997

Starcevic V: Pathological worry in major depression: a preliminary report. Behav Res Ther 33:55–56, 1995

Taylor S: Anxiety Sensitivity: Theory, Research, and Treatment of the Fear of Anxiety. New York, Guilford, 1999

Tyrer P: Classification of Neurosis. Chichester, England, Wiley, 1989

Tyrer P, Seivewright N, Murphy S, et al: The Nottingham study of neurotic disorder: comparison of drug and psychological treatments. Lancet 2:235–240, 1988

Watson D, Clark LA, Carey G: Positive and negative affectivity and their relation to the anxiety and depressive disorders. J Abnorm Psychol 97:346–353, 1988

Watson D, Gamez W, Simms L: Basic dimensions of temperament and their relation to anxiety and depression: a symptom-based perspective. J Res Pers 39:46–66, 2005

Widiger TA, Samuel DB: Diagnostic categories or dimensions: a question for DSM-V. J Abnorm Psychol 114:494–504, 2005

Williams JBW, Gibbon M, First MB, et al: The Structured Clinical Interview for DSM-III-R (SCID), II: multisite test-retest reliability. Arch Gen Psychiatry 49:630–636, 1992

World Health Organization: ICD-10 Classification of Mental and Behavior Disorders: Clinical Descriptions and Diagnostic Guidelines. Geneva, Switzerland, World Health Organization, 1992

Young JE, Weinberger A, Beck AT: Cognitive therapy for depression, in Clinical Handbook of Psychological Disorders, 3rd Edition. Edited by Barlow DH. New York, Guilford, 2001, pp 264–308

Zinbarg RE, Barlow DH: Structure of anxiety and anxiety disorders: a hierarchical model. J Abnorm Psychol 105:181–193, 1996

Zinbarg RE, Barlow DH, Liebowitz MR, et al: The DSM-IV field trial for mixed anxiety depression. Am J Psychiatry 151:1153–1162, 1994

Recommended Readings

Barlow DH (ed): Anxiety and Its Disorders: The Nature and Treatment of Anxiety and Panic, 2nd Edition. New York, Guilford, 2002

Barlow DH (ed): Clinical Handbook of Psychological Disorders: A Step-By-Step Treatment Manual, 4th Edition. New York, Guilford, 2007

Brown TA, Barlow DH: Dimensional versus categorical classification of mental disorders in the fifth edition of the Diagnostic and Statistical Manual of Mental Disorders and beyond: comment on the special section. J Abnorm Psychol 114:551–556, 2005

Clark LA: Temperament as a unifying basis for personality and psychopathology. J Abnorm Psychol 114:505–521, 2005

Hettema JM, Neale MC, Kendler KS: A review and meta-analysis of the genetic epidemiology of anxiety disorders. Am J Psychiatry 158:1568–1578, 2001

Chapter 3

Preclinical Models of Anxiety

Nicola D. Hanson, B.S.
Charles B. Nemeroff, M.D., Ph.D.

Animal models of anxiety have been developed for two major purposes: to screen compounds for potential anxiolytic activity and to study the neurobiology of anxiety. One problem that arises from the use of animal models to study anxiety is the diversity of human anxiety disorders. In DSM-IV-TR (American Psychiatric Association 2000), generalized anxiety disorder (GAD), panic disorder, obsessive-compulsive disorder (OCD), specific phobia, social phobia, and posttraumatic stress disorder (PTSD) are considered distinct syndromes; specifying the categories of anxiety disorders into which the various animal models fit is a matter of considerable controversy. There is considerable syndromal and symptom comorbidity, both among the anxiety disorders and between the anxiety disorders and the affective disorders. Both genetic and environmental factors are believed to play a role in the pathophysiology of most anxiety disorders.

One basic criterion a laboratory test for anxiety should fulfill is the ability to discriminate between drugs that are clinically effective in the treatment of anxiety disorders and those that are not. Moreover, a test should ideally also detect agents that are known to be anxiogenic in humans. Indeed, most tests were originally developed on the basis of the effects of benzodiazepines and barbiturates. However, because many tests have failed to detect an anxiolytic action of partial serotonin type 1A (5-HT_{1A}) receptor agonists (i.e., buspirone and the related compounds gepirone, ipsapirone, and tandospirone), investigators have questioned whether these tests are valid models for anxiety or, alternatively, merely screening tests for benzodiazepines and related compounds.

In clinical trials, buspirone shows efficacy equal to that of benzodiazepines in the treatment of GAD. However, the onset of action of buspirone is much slower than that of the benzodiazepines, and the anxiolytic effects of buspirone are not clinically apparent until after several weeks of treatment have elapsed. This suggests that the anxiolytic action of buspirone is mediated through neurochemical changes in brain that develop after repeated administration of the drug, rather than by its acute mechanism of action. Hence, the lack of an anxiolytic action of partial 5-HT_{1A} receptor agonists reported in several anxiety models may result, at least in part, from the fact that most investigators have studied the effects of such drugs only after acute administration. Several antidepressant drugs are also effective in the treatment of certain anxiety disorders, but several weeks of treatment are required before clinical improvement is observed. Thus, in this chapter, only the effects of chronic treatment with 5-HT_{1A} receptor agonists

The authors were supported by National Institutes of Health grants MH42088, MH52899, MH69056, MH77083, and DA015040.

and antidepressant drugs in various anxiety models are reviewed.

In this chapter, we examine conditioned, ethologically based, and genetic models. We also include two models—adversely reared primates and maternal deprivation—that we have designated as etiologically based. Accumulated data from studies that used these models strongly indicate that they constitute valid animal models of anxiety, both on the face (these conditions "seem like" they would produce anxiety in animals) and as constructs (the subjects exhibit many traits that we have come to refer to as "anxiety"). The genetic and etiologically based models probably provide particularly good animal models for the study of the pathophysiology of anxiety because the animals show permanently increased anxiety, which may better reflect the chronic state of human anxiety disorders than the acute anxiety elicited in conditioned or ethologically based models. The paradigms included in this chapter are generally considered to model GAD. Animal models specifically developed to study other anxiety disorders are not discussed here but have been reviewed comprehensively elsewhere (e.g., Joel 2006; Koob et al. 1998; Lister 1990; Stam 2007).

Conditioned Models: Operant Conflict Test

The operant conflict test is one of the most commonly used animal models of anxiety. It was developed by Geller and Seifter (1960) and is therefore often referred to as the *Geller-Seifter test.* It is based on the approach-avoidance test of Masserman and Yum (1946). Approach behavior is induced by stimulating ingestive behavior by food deprivation but is simultaneously reduced by punishment (an aversive event such as electric shock), thus inducing conflict in the animal. The conflict paradigm consists of two components in which freely moving rats are trained to press a lever for food reward. In one component, lever-pressing is reinforced with food after a variable interval of time (i.e., the "unpunished" period). In the second component, a short signal (a tone or light) precedes the delivery of a mild electric shock in conjunction with food reward (i.e., the "punished" period). After several weeks of training, the animal presses the lever much less frequently when the signal is on because it is assumed that the animal is anxious about the impending delivery of the shock. Thus, the anxiety in this model is conditioned. Both benzodiazepines and barbiturates increase the response during the punished period (also called *anticonflict effect*); that is, the animal accepts significantly more electric shocks, which is taken to reflect anxiolytic properties of the drug under study (for reviews, see Iverson 1980; Pollard and Howard 1990). Modification of the Geller-Seifter paradigm by using incremental shock levels beginning at zero has provided a distinct improvement over the original paradigm and is the procedure most often used today. Employment of this paradigm produced drug effects that were qualitatively similar to those reported when the original procedures were used.

A variant of the Geller-Seifter model of anxiety is Vogel's conflict test (Vogel et al. 1971). In this test, water-deprived naïve animals are placed in an experimental chamber with a water tube; they are allowed to drink briefly and then are periodically punished with electric shocks for licking water, thus suppressing licking behavior. Benzodiazepines and barbiturates reverse this suppression. The advantage of this model over the Geller-Seifter test is that it is faster and simpler and does not involve training of animals. However, Vogel's original conflict test used unconditioned suppression of drinking and could not distinguish nonspecific effects such as sedation or ataxia, which confounded the interpretation of the results. Consequently, this model has been further modified by the inclusion of an unpunished responding component and a tone signaling the onset of the shock, as well as training of animals to stable baselines (Ford et al. 1979). This model is often referred to as the *conditioned suppression of drinking* or *conditioned lick-suppression* test. Comparisons with the Geller-Seifter test found that this test is equally sensitive to the antianxiety properties of benzodiazepines and barbiturates. In the remainder of the discussion, the effects of various drug treatments that use the Geller-Seifter test, Vogel's conflict test, or conditioned suppression of drinking test are described together.

Treatment with clinically effective anxiolytic drugs outside of the benzodiazepine or barbiturate class has produced inconsistent results in the operant conflict tests. Chronic treatment with tricyclic antidepressants (TCAs) and monoamine oxidase inhibitors, but not the selective serotonin reuptake inhibitor (SSRI) fluoxetine, which are effective in the treatment of panic disorder and other anxiety disorders, resulted in a gradual increase in punished drinking behavior without affecting water intake (Table 3–1). Remarkably, this effect parallels the slow onset of therapeutic effect observed in panic disorder patients receiving antidepressant treatment. Clearly, additional work with SSRIs and the

TABLE 3–1. Effects of chronic treatment with antidepressant drugs in various animal models of anxiety

Model	Compound	Species	Effect	Reference
Operant conflict	Imipramine	Rats	+	Fontana and Commissaris 1988
	Desipramine	Rats	+	Fontana et al. 1989
	Amitriptyline	Rats	+	Fontana et al. 1989
	Phenelzine	Rats	+	Fontana et al. 1989
	Pargyline	Rats	+	Commissaris et al. 1995
	Fluoxetine	Rats	0	Beaufour et al. 1999
Open field	Imipramine	Rats	–	Dwyer and Roy 1993
	Fluoxetine	Mice	+	Dulawa et al. 2004
	Citalopram	Rats	+	Kugelberg et al. 2002
Elevated plus-maze	Phenelzine	Rats	0	File 1995; Johnston and File 1988
	Imipramine	Rats	0	File and Johnston 1987
	Imipramine	Mice	0	Cole and Rodgers 1995
	Maprotiline	Mice	+/0	Rodgers et al. 1997b
	Mianserin	Rats	+	Rocha et al. 1994
	Cianopramine	Rats	+	Griebel et al. 1994
	Fluvoxamine	Mice	0	Rodgers et al. 1997b
	Paroxetine	Rats	+	Cadogan et al. 1992
	Sertraline	Rats	–	Kurt et al. 2000
	Fluoxetine	Rats	+	Kurt et al. 2000
	Fluoxetine	Rats	0	Silva and Brandão 2000
Defensive burying	Desipramine	Rats	0	Beardslee et al. 1990
	Desipramine	Rats	+	Fernandez-Guasti et al. 1999
	Imipramine	Rats	+	Craft et al. 1988
Social interaction	Clomipramine	Rats	0	File 1985
	Imipramine	Rats	0	Pellow and File 1987
	Phenelzine	Rats	–	Johnston and File 1988
	Maprotiline	Mice	+/0	Cutler et al. 1997b
	Paroxetine	Rats	+	Lightowler et al. 1994
	Fluvoxamine	Mice	0	Cutler et al. 1997b
Isolation-induced ultrasonic vocalizations	Clomipramine	Rats	0	Winslow and Insel 1990
	Fluoxetine	Guinea pigs	+	Kramer et al. 1998
	Substance P receptor antagonists	Guinea pigs	+	Kramer et al. 1998
Maternal deprivation	Paroxetine	Rats	+	Ladd et al. 2000
	Fluoxetine	Rats	+	Ruedi-Bettschen et al. 2004
	Desipramine	Rats	+	MacQueen et al. 2003

Note. + = anxiolytic effect; 0 = no effect; – = anxiogenic effect.

TABLE 3–2. Effects of chronic treatment with partial 5-HT$_{1A}$ receptor agonists in various animal models of anxiety

Model	Compound	Species	Effect	Reference
Operant conflict	Buspirone	Rats	+	Amano et al. 1993
	Buspirone	Rats	+	Schefke et al. 1989
	Buspirone	Rats	+	Yamashita et al. 1995
	Buspirone	Mice	0	Martin et al. 1993
	Gepirone	Rats	+	Yamashita et al. 1995
	Tandospirone	Rats	+	Shimuzu et al. 1987
Elevated plus-maze	Buspirone	Rats	+	Söderpalm et al. 1993
	Buspirone	Rats	–	Moser 1989
	Buspirone	Rats	–	File 1995
	Buspirone	Mice	+	Cole and Rodgers 1994
	Buspirone	Mice	0	Rodgers et al. 1997a
	Gepirone	Rats	+	Motta et al. 1992[a]
	Gepirone	Rats	+	Maisonnette et al. 1993[a]
	Gepirone	Rats	+	Silva and Brandão 2000
	Ipsapirone	Rats	0	Wright et al. 1992
Defensive burying	Buspirone	Rats	+	Treit et al. 1981
	Perospirone	Rats	+	Sakamoto et al. 1998
Social interaction	Buspirone	Mice	+	Cutler 1991
	Buspirone	Mice	+	Gao and Cutler 1992
	Buspirone	Mice	0	Cutler et al. 1997a
Isolation-induced ultrasonic vocalizations	Buspirone	Rats	+	Iijima and Chaki 2005
	Buspirone	Guinea pigs	+	Kramer et al. 1998
Shock-induced ultrasonic vocalizations	Ipsapirone	Rats	+	Baudrie et al. 1993

Note. + =anxiolytic effect; 0=no effect; –=anxiogenic effect; 5-HT$_{1A}$=serotonin type 1A.
[a]Isolated animal.

selective serotonin-norepinephrine reuptake inhibitors, effective in certain anxiety disorders, is warranted. An anxiolytic profile of 5-HT$_{1A}$ receptor agonists has been observed in this test in chronic treatment in rats but not in mice (Table 3–2). Neither acute nor chronic treatment with the β-adrenergic antagonist propranolol, used often to treat fear of public speaking, affected punished responding in the conflict test.

Both compounds that block the γ-aminobutyric acid (GABA) receptor–coupled chloride channel and benzodiazepine inverse agonists were anxiogenic in the conflict tests, as shown by a decrease in punished responding, which is further evidence of the validity of the paradigm. Central administration of corticotropin-releasing factor (CRF), the peptide that coordinates the endocrine, autonomic, immune, and behavioral responses to stress, suppresses both punished and unpunished responding. Both chlordiazepoxide and ethanol reverse the suppressive effects of CRF, as does neuropeptide Y (NPY) (Britton et al. 2000). CRF$_1$ receptor antagonists produce opposite effects to CRF, which is evidence of their anxiolytic properties (see, e.g., Arborelius et al. 1999).

The conflict test has several disadvantages. It is time-consuming to perform, because the animals have to undergo long training periods and need to be deprived of food or water. Drugs that directly affect hunger or thirst confound the interpretation of the results, and drug treatments also may affect motivation for these rewards. Indeed, animals treated with benzodiazepines increase both their intake of rewards and their rate of responding for rewards (for an extensive review on criticisms of this model, see Treit 1985).

Ethologically Based Models

Animal models of anxious behaviors are too numerous to be covered exhaustively here. The seven models detailed in this section were chosen as both the most commonly encountered and the most representative examples of different aspects of anxiety. Those models omitted include the open field and hole-board tests, marble burying, barbering, fear-potentiated startle, and the light-dark transition box (for reviews, see Davis et al. 1993; Bourin and Hascoët 2003; Koob et al. 1998; Lister 1990).

Elevated Plus-Maze Test

The elevated plus-maze (or elevated X- or T-maze) test is one of the most popular of the currently available animal models for anxiety, partly because it is easy and quick to perform, requires only inexpensive equipment, and appears to detect both anxiolytic and anxiogenic effects. The apparatus is a plus-shaped maze, consisting of two open and two enclosed arms, and the whole construction is elevated from the floor. The animal is placed in the center of the maze and observed for a short period (usually 5 minutes). The proportion of entries to the open arms and the time spent in the open arms expressed as percentage of the total time spent in the maze are measured (Handley and Mithani 1984; Pellow et al. 1985). This test was developed as a result of Montgomery's observation that laboratory rats showed a greater fear response, and therefore more avoidance behavior, when exposed to an open maze alley than when exposed to an enclosed alley (1955). Montgomery proposed that exposure to both the open alleys and the enclosed alleys evokes the exploratory drive, but the former evokes greater fear in rodents. Thus, the elevated plus-maze test is considered a conflict test, because it evokes an approach-avoidance conflict (i.e., a conflict between fear and an exploratory drive). If a treatment increases the time spent in the open arms without altering the total number of arm entries, this is interpreted as an *anxiolytic action*. Conversely, if a treatment decreases the animal's preference for open arms without altering the total number of arm entries, this is taken to reflect *anxiogenic action*.

The reluctance of rodents to explore the open arms of the maze reflects their natural aversion to open areas and the elevation of the maze. Physiologically, this was reflected by a greater rise in plasma corticosterone concentrations in animals exposed to open arms when compared to those exposed to enclosed arms (Pellow et al. 1985). Confinement to the open arms was also associated with more anxiety-related behaviors, such as increased freezing and defecation, than confinement in the enclosed arms. Whether it is the novelty, openness, or height that is the predominant anxiogenic stimulus in the elevated plus-maze is unclear. Reducing the height of the plus-maze did not increase exploration of the open arms, and changes in the light level generally did not alter the behavior of the animals in the elevated plus-maze. However, attaching a clear Plexiglas wall along one edge of one of the open arms increased the preference for this arm. Thus, it has been suggested that fear of open spaces is the predominant anxiogenic stimulus in the elevated plus-maze (Treit et al. 1993).

This test has been extensively evaluated pharmacologically and appears to be sensitive to both anxiolytic and anxiogenic drugs in both rats and mice. Thus, both acute and chronic treatment with clinically effective anxiolytics increased the percentage of time spent in open arms and open-arm entries, whereas compounds known to be anxiogenic in both animals and humans reduced the percentage of time spent in and entries to open arms. However, exposure to acute stressors (immobilization or footshock), which normally increases fear in animals, did not increase the preference for the enclosed arms in the elevated plus-maze. In contrast, exposure to social stressors or a more severe stress (i.e., 1-hour restraint) did increase open-arm aversion. The anxiolytic effect of chronic treatment with antidepressants, including SSRIs, has been detected in the elevated plus-maze test in some but not all studies (Table 3–1). Moreover, chronic treatment with clinically effective 5-HT_{1A} receptor agonists produced variable effects in the elevated plus-maze (Table 3–2). Thus, in mice, buspirone produces anxiolytic effects in high but not low doses, and in rats, buspirone or ipsapirone produces anxiolytic, anxiogenic, or no effects.

Indeed, one problem with the elevated plus-maze test is the great interlaboratory variability in pharmacological sensitivity, which has been reported for some compounds (see above), raising serious questions about the validity of the test as a model for anxiety. It has been suggested that the variability of pharmacological responses in this test may be attributed to either different characteristics of the maze, such as the material on the floor of the open arms and the use of transparent or opaque walls on the enclosed arms, or the test procedures used (i.e., prior handling of the animals, single- or group-housed animals, time of the day of testing, and presence of the experimenter during testing). However, adjustments that increase the strength of the test are available, even if they are not widely used. Scoring of risk assessment behaviors, which are more persistent than avoidance behaviors, may increase sensitivity to anxiety-modulating drugs. Additionally, the use of fear potentiation (some stressors being more effective than others, as noted previously in this section) prior to the elevated plus-maze test has been applied to represent an enhanced anxiety state, which may be more representative of certain anxiety disorders (Mechiel Korte and De Boer 2003). For extensive reviews, see Carobrez and Bertoglio 2005, Hogg 1996, and Rodgers and Dalvi 1997.

Defensive Withdrawal Test

Laboratory rats have an innate fear of unfamiliar environments, particularly open areas, but will subsequently start to explore for possible resources (Blanchard et al. 1974). The defensive withdrawal test evolved from so-called timidity tests, in which latency to emerge or move from a sheltered environment is recorded (Archer 1973). The test consists of an illuminated, 1 m^2 open field containing a small enclosed chamber with one open end. The animal is placed in the chamber with the open end facing a corner and is observed for 10 or 15 minutes. The latency to leave the chamber, the number of passages between the chamber and the open field, and the total time spent in the chamber are recorded. An untreated rat spends most of its time withdrawn in the chamber, shows a long latency before leaving the chamber, and makes few entries into the open field. If the same animal is tested a second time, defensive withdrawal behavior is decreased, as shown by a decrease in latency to leave the chamber and a decrease in total time spent in the chamber. CRF appears to be involved in the mediation of defensive behavior and in the adaptation to an unfamiliar environment. Thus, central administration of a CRF receptor antagonist decreases defensive withdrawal in rats and increases exploration of the open field (Gutman et al. 2003; Li et al. 2003); the usual increase in exploration observed when the animal is tested a second time in this model can be blocked by central pretreatment with CRF (Takahashi et al. 1989; Yang et al. 1990). Moreover, local injection of CRF into the locus coeruleus (LC), the origin of the main noradrenergic projections to the forebrain, increases defensive withdrawal, indicating that central noradrenergic systems may also be involved in this behavior. Exposure of rats to acute stressors, such as restraint stress or air-puff startle, markedly increases defensive withdrawal in this test (Engelmann et al. 1996; Yang et al. 1990). Such stress-induced increases in anxiety can be blocked by CRF receptor antagonists.

Few of the clinically used anxiolytics have been tested in this model. The benzodiazepine chlordiazepoxide has anxiolytic effects in this model, as evidenced by a decrease in latency to leave the chamber and in time spent withdrawn in the chamber. β-Adrenergic antagonists (e.g., propranolol), which, as noted above, have some limited anxiolytic effects in humans, decrease defensive withdrawal as well as the anxiogenic effects induced by restraint stress. Conversely, β-adrenergic agonists increase anxiety in this test, providing further support for the involvement of noradrenergic systems in defensive withdrawal behavior.

Defensive Burying Test

The defensive burying test of anxiety was introduced by Pinel and Treit (1978). Following the observation that rats may respond to various types of noxious stimuli by kicking bedding over the offending objects, a standardized shock-prod was used to elicit fear/anxiety behaviors. The most commonly measured parameters are burying latency, duration of burying, prod-directed exploration, freezing, grooming, and ambulation, which can be divided into active and passive avoidance behaviors. There is a sizable variation in behavior among animals, but, typically, an individual's response in this test remains stable over multiple trials. Interestingly, there is no correlation between an animal's behavior in this and the elevated plus-maze test (see section "Elevated Plus-Maze Test" earlier in this chapter), suggesting that the two tests measure either different types of anxiety or different behavioral expressions of anxiety, and that the two depend on independent neural mechanisms (reviewed in De Boer and Koolhaas 2003). The defensive burying test is also sometimes used as a conditioned response test, in which the shock-prod is only electrified at the first contact and subsequent burying behavior reflects fear learning.

During the test, plasma corticosterone concentrations remain low regardless of amount of burying activity, whereas plasma norepinephrine concentrations rise in correlation with time spent burying, which is likely to indicate sympathetic activation associated with increased muscle activity rather than an increase in emotionality. Neurochemical circuits critically involved in burying include the septal region, the dorsal hippocampus, the caudal shell of the accumbens, and the dorsal raphe nuclei but, notably, not the amygdala, bed nucleus of the stria terminalis, and prefrontal cortex. Activation of various regions is greatly dependent on whether the animal adopts an active or passive coping strategy. GABA apparently plays a large role via activation of the $GABA_A$ receptor. Benzodiazepines are very effective anxiolytics in this test, as are the 5-HT_{1A} receptor agonists and some TCAs (see Tables 3–1 and 3–2).

Social Interaction Test

The social interaction test developed by File and colleagues is based on the observation that the time male rat pairs spent in active social interaction (e.g., sniffing and grooming) decreased as the illumination or unfamiliarity of the test arena increased. Because such manipulations have been suggested to be aversive or anxiogenic to rats, File and Hyde (1978) proposed that increased anxiety is also reflected in a decrease in social interaction. In this test, the time spent in active social interaction by a pair of male rats of similar weight (to avoid having one rat be clearly dominant over the other) is measured in four different testing conditions: high-light, unfamiliar; low-light, unfamiliar; high-light, familiar; and low-light, familiar (see, e.g., File and Seth 2003). Drug-naïve rats show the highest level of social interaction when the test area is familiar and has low light. Social interaction is lowest when the test area is brightly lit and unfamiliar. Locomotor activity is also measured during the test, which makes it possible to distinguish between sedative and anxiolytic effects and thus increases the specificity of the test. The test has been validated behaviorally, and it has been shown that the decrease in social interaction is correlated with an increase in more traditional behavioral measures of emotionality (i.e., defecation and freezing) and is not due to an increase in exploratory behavior when animals are tested in an unfamiliar environment. Plasma concentrations of corticosterone were higher in rats placed in unfamiliar environments than in rats placed in familiar environments and were higher in rats tested under high-light conditions than in those tested under low-light conditions in an unfamiliar, but not a familiar, arena.

Some methodological details need special consideration when this model is used. The light level in which the animals are housed should be kept low because rats that are housed in bright light lose their aversion to high-light conditions, and thus changes in illumination no longer influence their social interaction. Interaction is also influenced by prior socialization; therefore, animals are typically housed individually for several days preceding testing in order to maximize their interaction. Moreover, stress decreases social interaction; therefore, repeated handling of the animals before testing, in order to reduce stress during testing, is of great importance.

In the social interaction test, anxiolytic effects of benzodiazepines and barbiturates are observed only after subchronic treatment, when tolerance has developed to the sedative effects of such drugs (File and Seth 2003). Benzodiazepines increase the time spent in social interaction during high-light conditions and unfamiliarity of the test arena, but benzodiazpines have only minimal effects in low-light, familiar conditions, the least anxiety-provoking test condition. Propranolol did not exhibit anxiolytic effects in the social interaction test. Chronic treatment with the antidepressants clomipramine, imipramine, or phenelzine did not produce anxiolytic effects in this test (see Table 3–1). In fact, chronic treatment with phenelzine actually showed anxiogenic activity. In contrast, 3 weeks of treatment with the SSRI paroxetine showed a clear anxiolytic profile, as indicated by a significant increase in social interaction under high-light conditions. Chronic treatment with the 5-HT_{1A} receptor agonist buspirone has been reported to produce anxiolytic or no effects in this test (see Table 3–2). Anxiogenic compounds reduce the time spent in social interaction without concomitant reduction in locomotor activity. Central administration of CRF significantly decreased social interaction, an effect that was prevented by pretreatment with a benzodiazepine. For an exhaustive review of compounds showing positive and negative results in the social interaction test, the reader is directed to File and Seth (2003).

Isolation-Induced Ultrasonic Vocalization in Rat Pups

Following social isolation, rat pups emit vocalizations that probably alert their mothers to retrieve them. The biophysical properties of these sounds (i.e., very high frequency, 35–45 kHz) make them inaudible for most predators as well as for humans. These ultrasonic vocalizations are considered distress calls and have been proposed to reflect anxiety in the pup (for reviews, see Winslow and Insel 1991). Gardner (1985) first observed that ultrasonic vocalizations induced by tail-holding stress in rat pups were decreased by the anxiolytic drugs diazepam and chlordiazepoxide in doses that neither altered locomotion nor had sedative effects. Subsequent studies showed that isolation-induced distress calls were decreased by benzodiazepines, an effect that could be blocked by specific benzodiazepine receptor antagonists, and, conversely, anxiogenic compounds such as benzodiazepine inverse agonists increased the number and the power of such calls, giving further support to the notion that isolation-induced ultrasonic vocalizations in rat pups represent a useful anxiety model. Guinea pig pups may also be used as subjects in this test; anxiolytic results in this species have been obtained from the SSRI fluoxetine and the TCA imipramine as well as the 5-HT_{1A} antagonist buspirone and selective antagonists of the CRF_1 and substance P receptors (Griebel et al. 2002; Kramer et al. 1998).

On the basis of these observations, it has been suggested that the benzodiazepine–$GABA_A$ receptor complex is involved in the physiological mediation of distress calls. Moreover, 25 minutes of isolation resulted in a decrease in benzodiazepine receptor binding in vivo, but not in vitro, in several brain regions, including the neocortex and hippocampus, suggesting the release of an endogenous benzodiazepine during isolation.

Additional evidence that isolation-induced ultrasonic vocalizations in rat pups represent anxiety or increased emotionality comes from studies of inbred rat strains. During isolation, pups from the Maudsley reactive (MR) rat strain, which is considered to be more emotional (see section "Maudsley Reactive and Nonreactive Rat Strains" later in this chapter), emit about five times as many ultrasonic calls as do pups from the less emotional Maudsley nonreactive (MNR) rat strain (Insel and Hill 1987). This finding may also imply that the large variability in the number of isolation-induced distress calls observed across litters could be, at least partly, of genetic origin.

Several variables affect ultrasonic vocalizations in rat pups, including changes in body temperature, locomotion, and coordination. Thus, it is of great importance that the effects on these variables are monitored for each given drug treatment to avoid the confounds of putative anxiolytics in this test. Another confounding factor in this model is change in respiratory rate. The ultrasonic vocalizations are emitted during the expiratory phase of respiration, and consequently, any drug-induced change in respiratory rate would predictably alter vocalizations.

The use of this model for studying drug effects during chronic treatment is limited because ultrasonic vocalizations are evident only in the first 2 weeks after birth. Moreover, chronic drug treatment may alter normal development. Another disadvantage of using infant animals to study drug effects is that changes in receptors, pharmacokinetic factors, and the permeability of the blood-brain barrier may occur during postnatal development. In particular, measures that undergo dramatic shifts during development lead to findings that contradict results in adults, a situation exemplified by the changing expression patterns of CRF receptors in the postnatal brain (Avishai-Eliner et al. 1996). Thus, there are conflicting findings of central administration of CRF or CRF receptor antagonists, both of which have been seen to either increase or decrease ultrasonic distress calls in rat pups in different studies.

Defensive Behavior in Infant Rhesus Monkeys

Kalin and Shelton (1989) have pioneered the study of defensive behavior in infant rhesus monkeys in response to fearful stimuli. They observed that when a young monkey (6–12 months old) was briefly separated from its mother and placed in a cage, it became active and emitted distress calls ("coo" vocalizations). When a human stood outside the cage without making eye contact with the infant monkey, a situation the monkey perceived as frightening, it became silent and froze, remaining completely still in one position. However, if the human stared at the infant, it started to bark and produce so-called threat faces. The cooing is thought to be activated by disruption of the attachment bond and helps the mother locate her infant. The freezing behavior is a common response to threat in many animal species that reduces the likelihood of being attacked, and the aggressive barking serves the purpose of warding off an attack once the infant has been detected by a predator.

On the basis of their observation that freezing is elicited in a threatening situation, Kalin et al. (1998) suggested that this behavior in infant rhesus monkeys is analogous to the responses observed in behaviorally inhibited children who are exposed to unfamiliar environments (Kagan et al. 1988). Because extremely inhibited children are at increased risk for developing anxiety disorders, fear-induced freezing may represent a model for study of behavioral inhibition and the development of anxiety in monkeys. The propensity to freeze shows marked interindividual differences in infant rhesus monkeys, and these differences appear to be stable over time (Kalin and Shelton 1989). In one study (Kalin et al. 1998), basal plasma cortisol levels were positively correlated with freezing duration. It is noteworthy that elevated levels of salivary cortisol have also been reported in behaviorally inhibited children. Additionally, fearful monkeys have been reported to have elevated levels of cerebrospinal CRF (Kalin et al. 2000). Benzodiazepines have been shown to reduce freezing behavior in infant monkeys in response to a human intruder not engaged in eye contact with the solitary infant. But, an inverse benzodiazepine agonist increases freezing in this situation, which is consistent with the anxiogenic effects of such drugs. These findings give further support to the notion that freezing may reflect anxiety in infant rhesus monkeys.

Quinpirole-Induced Compulsive Checking

Szechtman et al. (1998) developed the compulsive checking model based on rituals described by patients with OCD, in which they feel compelled to repeat routine behaviors. In this model, rats are tested in an open field containing several small objects for measures of locomotion and exploration of the objects. Checking behavior is distinguished by an excessive number of returns to a particular object, excessive rapid return time to the object, few visits to other places, and motor rituals (a few types of motor acts repeated to the exclusion of other types of acts). It was found that chronic treatment with the D_2/D_3 agonist quinpirole produces compulsive checking behavior in rats, and that treatment with the TCA clomipramine, which is often used clinically to treat OCD, could partially block this effect of quinpirole. Beyond this, there have been no tests conducted on the effects of drugs used to treat OCD in this model, although the monoamine oxidase inhibitors clorgyline and pargyline produce an interesting redirection into a compulsive mouthing behavior. Recent research into the quinpirole model has largely focused on exploring the dopaminergic circuitry involved (Eilam and Szechtman 2005).

Genetic Models

The genetic models of anxiety fall into three categories: the selectively bred (discussed here, Maudsley reactive and nonreactive and Roman high-avoidance and low-avoidance strains), the natural variants ("uptight" and "laid-back" rhesus monkeys), and the genetically engineered (5-HT_{1A} knockout and DICT-7 line transgenic mice). The final category especially contains many more examples than the ones included in this chapter (for a useful review, see Finn et al. 2003).

Maudsley Reactive and Nonreactive Rat Strains

The MR and MNR rats were selectively bred in London, England, in the 1960s from Wistar rats on the basis of their high or low rates of defecation in the open field, respectively (Blizard and Adams 2002; Broadhurst 1975). Defecation rate in the open-field test has been suggested to indicate the level of emotionality of the animal, with the MR rats showing high levels of emotionality and the MNR rats showing low levels of emotionality. In a wide range of tests designed to measure anxiety or fear, or under stressful conditions, the MR rats showed greater levels of anxiety than did MNR rats, but not under basal conditions. Because results from early studies examining the differences between the strains are comprehensively reviewed elsewhere (Blizard and Adams 2002; Broadhurst 1975), we mainly review recent research on Maudsley rat colonies established in the United States in the 1960s.

The MR rats show less activity in the open field test and accept less shock in conditioned suppression of drinking or feeding paradigms than do MNR rats. Moreover, MR rats spend less time in the open arms of the elevated plus-maze and show less exploratory "rearing" behavior in the staircase test than do MNR rats. In the infant separation test, MR rat pups show greater distress, manifested as an increased number of ultrasonic calls, compared with MNR rat pups. Interestingly, the latter study result suggests that increased anxiety in the MR rats is already apparent early in development. However, the Maudsley rat strains do not differ in all animal models of anxiety or emotionality. In defensive burying behavior and active avoidance performance, no differences were seen between MR and MNR rats. Thus, the MR rat strain clearly differs from other emotional rat strains (i.e., the Roman low-avoidance rats, which were selectively bred for their poor performance in active avoidance) (see the section "Roman High-Avoidance and Low-Avoidance Rats" later in this chapter). In the forced swim test, the MR rats are more immobile than their less reactive counterparts, suggesting that the MR rats also may exhibit depressive-like behaviors. Taken together, most studies support the view that the MR rats have an increased level of emotionality and, thus, provide a valid animal model for studying genetically based anxiety. The increased anxiety in the MR rats does not appear to be linked to a learning deficit, because they do equally as well as or even better than MNR rats in most learning tasks. However, the MR rats do display a deficit in the 12-arm radial maze, a task that emphasizes working memory, which appears to be correlated with lower muscarinic receptor binding in the central nervous system.

The Maudsley rat strains provide an excellent model for characterizing the physiological, neuroendocrine, and neurochemical basis for anxiety. However, no difference in basal or stress-induced plasma levels of corticosterone has been found between MR and MNR rats, which indicates that the two rat strains also do not differ in hypothalamic-pituitary-adrenal (HPA) axis activity. In contrast, a higher sympathetic tone is observed in the less emotional MNR rats (for review, see Blizard 1988). Thus, the MNR rats show higher tissue levels of norepinephrine in several peripheral organs, including the heart, adrenals, small intestine, and colon. However, in response to various stressors, the MR, but not the MNR, rats show an increase in plasma norepinephrine, which largely reflects norepinephrine release from peripheral nerve endings; plasma epinephrine concentrations increase in both strains in response to moderate stress. Central noradrenergic systems have also been extensively studied in the Maudsley rat strains. Although some results appear contradictory, the differences in central noradrenergic neuronal reactivity in MR rats compared with MNR rats are noteworthy, in that the noradrenergic systems, especially the LC, have been implicated in mediating fear and anxiety in animals and in humans. However, this model has been called into question by the fact that chlordiazepoxide administration produces similar effects in both strains (Paterson et al. 2001). In addition, it is possible that the MNR rats are the "pathologic" strain in that they are unusually nonresponsive to stressful stimuli.

Roman High-Avoidance and Low-Avoidance Rats

The Roman rat lines were derived from Wistar rats and were psychogenetically selected on the basis of their performance in active avoidance. The Roman high-avoidance (RHA) rats show unusually rapid acquisition of active avoidance on shock presentation in a shuttle box (a box divided into two equal-sized compartments connected by one opening), whereas the Roman low-avoidance (RLA) rats fail to acquire this behavior but show escape or freezing behavior in this test (for reviews, see Castanon and Moremède 1994; Driscoll and Bättig 1982). Numerous behavioral studies have suggested that RLA rats are more anxious and emotionally reactive than are RHA rats. Thus, RLA rats placed in an open field show signs of increased anxiety, such as decreased locomotion, decreased rearing, and increased grooming behavior and defecation, compared with RHA rats. The RLA rats also show increased anxiety in several other tests involving exposure to a novel environment, such as decreased feeding in the so-called hyponeophagia test; decreased head-dipping, which is a measure of exploratory behavior; and less frequent entering of the brightly illuminated center of a hexagonal tunnel maze than their RHA counterparts.

Physiologically, RLA rats have a greater increase in heart rate in unconditioned stressful situations than do RHA rats and a pronounced bradycardia in response to conditioned emotional stressors. The release of renin, which can be used as an indirect index of sympathetic reactivity, has also been reported to be higher in RLA rats than in RHA rats, when tested in the open field (Castanon and Moremède 1994). Neuroendocrine activation during stress is another important measure of emotional state, and indeed, differences in activation of the HPA axis after stress have been described between the two rat lines. Thus, RLA rats have greater adrenocorticotropic hormone (ACTH), corticosterone, and prolactin responses to various stressors than do RHA rats. No differences in basal or stress-induced increases in CRF messenger ribonucleic acid (mRNA) expression have been observed between the two rat lines. CRF infused into the central nucleus of amygdala increased heart rate and behavioral activity in RHA rats, but not RLA rats, and caused a differential local decrease in fos-positive cells in RHA rats but an increase in RLA rats (Wiersma et al. 1998). Additionally, increased basal vasopressin mRNA expression was found in RLA rats.

Several neurochemical studies of the central nervous system (CNS) of the two Roman rat strains have been conducted. Because impaired GABAergic transmission has been implicated in anxiety disorders and increasing GABAergic transmission produces anxiolytic effects, whereas drugs that decrease GABAergic transmission increase anxiety, GABA systems have been the focus of some studies. One study revealed lower [^{3}H]diazepam binding in several brain areas, including cortex, striatum, hippocampus, thalamic regions, and pons medulla in RLA rats compared with RHA rats. Other studies have shown a decrease in GABA receptor–effector coupling, but not in GABA or benzodiazepine receptor binding, in the cortex of RLA rats compared with RHA rats. Thus, a decrease in benzodiazepine binding sites and/or a decrease in GABA receptor function in RLA rats may, at least partly, account for their increased anxiety.

Diazepam or propranolol treatment reduced anxiety in the hyponeophagia test in both rat strains, but RLA rats were more sensitive to both drugs. Several different treatment paradigms have been found to increase the performance of RLA rats in the active avoidance test, such as an acute dose of pentobarbital, prenatal diazepam or perinatal flumazenil, neonatal handling, and extensive training. Neonatal handling also decreased anxiety and increased exploratory behavior in RLA rats.

RLA rats that have previously been exposed to an experimental stressor (i.e., the shuttle box) showed a marked decrease in locomotor activity and an increased ACTH response when subsequently tested in the open field. In contrast, RHA rats showed no difference in performance in the open field with or without previous testing in the shuttle box. Thus, RLA rats appear to be particularly vulnerable to stressors, and this rat strain may therefore serve as a good model for identifying individuals with a genetic risk of developing anxiety disorders. RLA rats have also come to be used as models for studying addictive behavior, because they show markedly dimorphic behavioral and neurochemical response patterns to drugs of abuse (e.g., Giménez-Llort et al. 2005; Giorgi et al. 2005).

Uptight and Laid-Back Rhesus Monkeys

From extensive studies of individual behavior of rhesus monkeys, Suomi (1991) obtained strong evidence for a hereditary anxiety trait present in approximately 20% of the monkeys found in both a self-sufficient breeding colony and in the wild. These monkeys showed nervous, fearful, and anxiety-like behaviors when faced with challenge or novelty, which elicited interest and exploration from the other monkeys in the colony. Suomi and colleagues used the term *uptight* to describe the behavioral characteristics of the fearful animals, as opposed to the other animals that are more *laid back*. These differences in response to novelty or challenge appear very early in life and are apparently stable over the life span. Physiologically, the uptight monkeys had a greater increase in heart rate when exposed to novelty than the less reactive, laid-back monkeys. After some time in the novel environment, the heart rate of the less reactive subjects decreased, whereas the heart rate of the behaviorally reactive monkeys showed little change. In addition, when subjected to novelty, uptight monkeys not only had a greater increase in plasma ACTH and cortisol concentrations, but these stress hormones remained elevated for longer than in the laid-back monkeys. In contrast, during familiar, unchallenging conditions, no obvious differences in behavior or physiological reactions were evident between the uptight and laid-back monkeys. Moreover, if the behaviorally reactive monkeys stayed in the novel environment for several hours or were repeatedly reintroduced to it, both their cardiac and neuroendocrine functions normalized, and the behavioral distinction between the reactive subjects and the laid-back subjects diminished. Taken together, the characteristic behavioral and physiological responses to environmental challenge and novelty observed in the reactive uptight rhesus monkeys resemble the human infants and children described by Kagan et al. (1988) as "behaviorally inhibited to the unfamiliar" (see section "Defensive Behavior in Infant Rhesus Monkeys" earlier in this chapter). Behaviorally inhibited children are believed to be at increased risk for developing anxiety disorders in adulthood.

When subjected to short-term separation from either parents or peers, the uptight monkeys showed depressive-like behaviors and a greater activation of the HPA axis, decreased cerebrospinal fluid (CSF) norepinephrine concentrations, and increased CSF concentrations of the major norepinephrine metabolite, MHPG (3-methoxy-4-hydroxyphenylglycol). In contrast, their more laid-back counterparts showed rapid adjustment to such separations. The behavioral, physiological, and biochemical changes observed in reactive individuals in response to separation can be reversed by treatment with TCAs or SSRIs. The observations that the more anxious and fearful monkeys are also more prone to develop depressive-like symptoms parallel findings that show the close relation between anxiety disorders and depression in humans.

5-HT_{1A} Knockout Mice

Accumulated pharmacological and neurobiological evidence of the involvement of the 5-HT_{1A} receptor in anxiety has made it a natural target for creation of a genetic knockout. In 1998, three independent groups reported development of 5-HT_{1A} knockout mice (Heisler et al. 1998; Parks et al. 1998; Ramboz et al. 1998). These lines demonstrate a clearly anxious phenotype, showing reduced numbers of open-arm entries into the elevated plus-maze and reduced time spent inside the open arms; reduced time spent in the center area of an open field; reduced exploration of a novel object or in a novel environment; and increased freezing when stressed. These lines also show greater increases in heart rate and blood pressure when exposed to novel or stressful conditions, although their baseline levels do not differ from wild-type mice, indicating a greater autonomic expression of anxiety. In Vogel's lick-suppression test, knockouts and wild-types display an equal threshold for behavioral inhibition. They behave identically in contextual fear conditioning to environment and in extinction of the conditioning, which reveals that both types of mice are not impaired in associating aversive stimuli to contextual cues. However, when the testing environment is similar but not identical to the training environment, knockouts express greater fear behavior than wild-types, suggesting a hypervigilance or overgeneralization of threat such as that seen in PTSD patients (Klemenhagen et al. 2006).

Gross et al. (2002) demonstrated, using a conditional rescue model, that expression of the 5-HT_{1A} receptor in the forebrain but not the raphe nucleus is sufficient to restore normal anxiety behavior in the knockouts. Additionally, the researchers established that there is a critical period during postnatal development when the 5-HT_{1A} receptor is necessary for the production of a normal adult behavioral phenotype. Turning off receptor expression in adulthood had no effect on anxiety behavior.

Baseline corticosterone levels remain normal under these conditions, but the stress-induced increase in corticosterone is blunted in knockout mice. In two of the mouse lines in which 5-HT_{1A} knockouts have been studied (Swiss-Webster and 129/sv), extracellular levels of serotonin are unchanged, which may be the result of a compensatory increase in 5-HT_{1B} autoreceptor activity. A third mouse line (C57B/6) with a 5-HT_{1A} knockout shows increased serotonin concentrations in the frontal cortex and hippocampus. This may be due to the greater general anxiety level of C57B/6 mice, given that serotonin release increases under stressful conditions such as those used in the experiments. Electrophysiological studies on mice of the 129/sv knockout line also found abnormalities in paired-pulse inhibition and facilitation in hippocampal areas, although serotonin release in these areas was unchanged.

An unexpected feature of this model is the insensitivity of the Swiss-Webster knockout line to diazepam and other benzodiazepines, although the two other lines display normal anxiolytic and sedative responses to these drugs. This benzodiazepine resistance is associated with decreased cortical expression of $GABA_A$ subunits, whereas knockout animals of the C57B/6 strain show normal $GABA_A$ expression (Bailey and Toth 2004). Also unexpectedly, the ability of fluoxetine to reduce immobility in the tail suspension test is abolished in the 5-HT_{1A} knockout mice, whereas the similar effect of desipramine, a norepinephrine reuptake inhibitor, is retained. Fluoxetine administration results in a much greater increase in extracellular serotonin concentrations in the 5-HT_{1A} knockouts than in wild-type animals. Thus, it appears that 5-HT_{1A} receptors play an essential role in the therapeutic action of SSRIs. (For review, see Olivier et al. 2001 and Toth 2003.)

DICT-7 Transgenic Mice

The DICT-7 transgenic mouse model was engineered to express a neuropotentiating protein (cholera toxin A1 subunit) within a cortical-limbic subset of dopamine D_1 receptor–expressing (D_1^+) neurons (Campbell et al. 1999a, 1999b; McGrath et al. 1999b). It was found that these mice displayed characteristics similar to obsessive-compulsive disorder, including behavioral perseveration and repetitive nonaggressive biting, and a higher basal level of anxiety than wild-type mice. These behaviors differ qualitatively from the stereotypy that results from limbic seizures or cocaine administration. Stereotypical behavior can be exacerbated in these mice by a stressful experience (exposure to predator odor) (McGrath et al. 1999a). Expression of the transgene is mainly confined to the amygdala and limbic cortex, areas that have been linked to compulsive behaviors in humans, which is further evidence that these transgenic mice may represent a valid model of OCD. No anxiolytic or antidepressant drugs have yet been tested in this model.

Etiologically Based Models

Exposure to repeated early life stress has been proposed to constitute a model of anxiety primarily based on the relation between stress and the development of anxiety disorders. Although stress has generally been associated with the development of affective disorders, several studies have shown that adverse early life experiences, such as childhood abuse and neglect, are also associated with an increased risk for anxiety disorders in adulthood, including social anxiety disorder and PTSD (see, e.g., Arborelius et al. 1999). Moreover, anxiety disorders, like mood disorders, are likely to develop from dysfunction of certain neuronal systems in the brain. Thus, a growing body of evidence now suggests that both hereditary factors and stressful early life events exert significantly long-lasting effects on neuronal pathways.

Adversely Reared Primates

Coplan and colleagues (1995) developed a primate model for early life experiences in which one of the conditions may resemble the adverse events hypothesized to predispose humans to anxiety disorders. In this model, bonnet macaque infants are raised under different rearing conditions in which the mothers are confronted with different foraging demands. Mothers that have low foraging demands (LFD) can easily find food, whereas mothers that have consistently high (but predictable) foraging demands (HFD) must work to find food. A third group of mothers are exposed to variable (unpredictable) foraging demands (VFD). The VFD paradigm appears to be the most stressful for the mother-infant dyad. These mothers appear to be more anxious, presumably because of the uncertainty of the environment, and they are more neglectful of their infants. Infant monkeys raised by VFD mothers show several signs of increased anxiety; for example, they are more timid, less social, and more frightened by novelty than are LFD and HFD offspring (Coplan et al. 1995). The behaviors seen in VFD offspring have several similarities to those observed in young children identified as behaviorally inhibited, who are at increased risk for the development of anxiety disorders in adulthood (see section "Defensive Behavior in Infant Rhesus Monkeys" earlier in this chapter). It is also interesting that, although VFD-reared infants achieve an equal rate of growth compared with their LFD counterparts, at puberty they show an increased level of glucagon-like peptide-1, as well as an increased tendency toward obesity, metabolic syndrome, and insulin resistance (Kaufman et al. 2007).

Several biochemical differences that indicate dysfunction of central neuronal systems have been observed in young adult monkeys raised by VFD mothers. The CSF concentrations of the dopamine metabolite homovanillic acid and the serotonin metabolite 5-hydroxyindoleacetic acid were significantly elevated, whereas cortisol was decreased in VFD-reared monkeys compared with LFD- and HFD-reared subjects (Coplan et al. 1996; Mathew et al. 2002). The timing of the period of foraging demand seems to be critical, resulting in either lower or higher CSF CRF concentrations in VFD-reared monkeys when compared with nonadversely reared peers (Coplan et al. 2006). The results are concordant with the rodent and human data, which support the idea that stress early in life results in persistent elevations in CSF CRF concentrations. Moreover, VFD-reared subjects showed a behavioral hyperresponsiveness after administration of yohimbine, an α_2-adrenoceptor antagonist that stimulates central noradrenergic activity. Interestingly, in humans, patients with panic disorder and PTSD experienced larger biochemical and cardiovascular effects after yohimbine administration than did healthy subjects, as well as an increase in panic attacks and flashbacks. A reduced growth-hormone response to the α_2-adrenoceptor agonist clonidine, a biological marker found in several anxiety disorders, has been found in VFD-reared monkeys (Coplan et al. 2000). In contrast, VFD-reared monkeys showed hyporesponsiveness to the behavioral effects of the serotonergic agonist *m*-chlorophenylpiperazine, which has been shown to exacerbate the symptoms in patients with anxiety disorders, including panic disorder, OCD, and PTSD (Rosenblum et al. 1994).

Another model of early life stress in primates, developed to mirror the success of the rat maternal deprivation model (see next section, "Maternal Deprivation in Rats"), involves rhesus macaques that underwent repeated brief periods of maternal separation between the ages of 3 and 6 months (Sánchez et al. 2005). When studied later in life, these animals display an increased acoustic startle response, sleep disturbances, and flattened diurnal cortisol rhythms (although this last effect appears to lessen with age). The macaques also exhibit reduced serotonin transporter binding, as assessed with micro positron emission tomography (PET) imaging methods.

Taken together, these studies in nonhuman primates support the notion that early life stress permanently alters central noradrenergic, serotonergic, and CRFergic systems in the CNS. Results of the above-cited studies on early life stress in nonhuman primates strongly parallel many clinical research findings on humans and may therefore constitute a valid animal model of anxiety. However, information on the effects of anxiolytic compounds in this model is still lacking.

Maternal Deprivation in Rats

The rat maternal deprivation model has been suggested to constitute a valid model of early life stress in humans. In different separation paradigms, rat pups are subjected to various intervals of separation from their mothers during the first 2–3 weeks after birth. Maternally deprived rats may be compared with so-called handled rats, which are subjected to daily handling during the same period, or with facility-reared animals. As adults, maternally deprived rats show several signs of increased anxiety, including decreased exploration in a novel open field, increased defensive withdrawal behavior, increased novelty-induced suppression of feeding, increased startle response, and a distinct preference for alcohol, cocaine, and morphine, compared with handled rats (Caldji et al. 2000; Moffett et al. 2007). Maternally deprived rats also show an enhanced neuroendocrine response to an acute psychological, but not somatic, stressor, as evidenced by a larger rise in plasma ACTH and corticosterone concentrations than in nondeprived rats (Ladd et al. 2000).

The hyperresponsiveness to stress may be related to the observed hypersecretion of hypothalamic CRF, coupled with the decrease in glucocorticoid receptor binding and expression in the hippocampus and medial prefrontal cortex, in maternally deprived rats. Moreover, changes in extrahypothalamic CRF systems have been observed in maternally deprived rats. Notably, CRF binding sites are increased in both the dorsal raphe nucleus, the major site of origin of the widespread serotonergic innervation of the forebrain, and the LC, the origin of the noradrenergic innervation. In addition, maternally deprived rats show an increased release of hypothalamic norepinephrine in response to restraint stress and decreased α_2-adrenoceptor binding in the LC, compared with handled rats. These findings are of particular interest in view of the possible involvement of these monoaminergic pathways in the pathogenesis of human anxiety. Decreased binding of $GABA_A$ receptors and reduced benzodiazepine binding sites also have been found in several different brain regions, including the LC, in maternally deprived rats, which may contribute to the increased anxiety observed in such animals. In the central nucleus of the amygdala, a brain region presumably involved in fear and anxiety, benzodiazepine binding sites are decreased and CRF mRNA expression is increased in maternally deprived rats (Caldji et al. 2000; Ladd et al. 2000). The effects of benzodiazepines have not yet been studied in maternally deprived rats. However, chronic treatment with the SSRI paroxetine, effective in the treatment of several anxiety disorders, almost completely normalizes stress-induced neuroendocrine hyperresponsiveness, reduces anxiety behaviors in the elevated plus-maze test and the defensive withdrawal test, and reduces alcohol preference in such animals (Ladd et al. 2000; Moffett et al. 2007; Plotsky et al. 2005).

Although study of negative early life experiences is much more widespread, good maternal care has also been shown to have a profound and long-lasting effect on anxiety state. As would be expected, many of the characteristics of maternally deprived animals are reversed in animals exposed to an exceptionally high level of maternal attention (e.g., decreased stress responsivity and increased negative feedback of the HPA axis [Champagne and Meaney 2001]).

Conclusion

Our purpose in this chapter was to present a selection of different types of animal models of anxiety (i.e., conditioned models, ethologically based models, genetic models, and etiologically based models). Overall, it is clear that the different types of animal models can serve various purposes to increase our understanding of anxiety disorders. Because human anxiety disorders are believed to result from genetic and environmental factors (one such factor being adverse early life experiences), and such disorders are often chronic in nature, the genetically and etiologically based models in which the animals showed permanently increased anxiety may serve as better models to study the pathophysiology of anxiety disorders than the conditioned and ethologically based models. However, a more complete pharmacological validation is needed for the genetic and etiologically based models, because the effects of only a few of the clinically effective anxiolytic drugs have been studied. Further, the conditioned and ethologically based models are important tools for studying "state" anxiety, and these paradigms are necessary to evaluate the level of anxiety of animals in the genetic and etiologically based models. Whether the inconsistent results of chronic treatment with partial 5-HT_{1A} receptor agonists and various antidepressants in these anxiety models are due to pharmacological factors, confounding factors, species differences, or the fact that the models do not really model human anxiety remains to be elucidated.

Interestingly, in the genetic models of anxiety, the animals showing high levels of anxiety respond with helpless behavior in certain situations, suggesting that these animals may also be at increased risk to develop depression. Moreover, because adverse early life experience is associated with increased risk for developing depression in humans, the etiologically based animal models have also been used to study the pathophysiology of depression. The results parallel observations made in studies of humans, in whom comorbid anxiety disorders and depression are common. The findings suggest that the genetic and etiologically based models may also be valid models for studying mixed anxiety-depression in animals.

◀ Key Clinical Points ▶

- When considering the clinical impact of the information presented in this chapter, it is important to first note that animal models must be considered to merely mimic many behaviors associated with anxiety, rather than to present a true anxiety syndrome. The key characteristic of generalized anxiety disorder—excessive worry—is something that cannot be measured in a nonhuman, even if one were to argue for its existence.
- Most animal models of anxiety were developed (and are currently utilized) as screening tests for anxiolytic properties of drugs.

  Implications for pharmacotherapy: Drugs that decrease what we call "anxious characteristics" in animals are likely to decrease the severity of anxiety disorders in patients.
- Models derived from genetic manipulations and models derived from environmental manipulations can display very similar behavioral phenotypes, suggesting that the pathogenesis of clinical anxiety disorders may likewise be either genetic or environmental (or, more likely, a combination of both).

  Implications for genetics-based interventions: As new anxiety-related genes are identified, new treatments can be developed to target the specific products of these genes in preclinical models. Likewise, polymorphisms identified in clinical populations can be explored by using transgenic mouse models.

  Implications for environment-based interventions: The prevalence of early life stress in anxiety models suggests that a clinical emphasis on preventative measures in children at risk for developing anxiety would be appropriate.

References

Amano M, Goto A, Sakai A, et al: Comparison of the anticonflict effect of buspirone and its major metabolite 1-(2-pyrimidinyl)-piperazine (1-PP) in rats. Jpn J Pharmacol 61:311–317, 1993

American Psychiatric Association: Diagnostic and Statistical Manual of Mental Disorders, 4th Edition, Text Revision. Washington, DC, American Psychiatric Association, 2000

Arborelius L, Owens MJ, Plotsky PM, et al: The role of corticotropin-releasing factor in depression and anxiety disorders. J Endocrinol 160:1–12, 1999

Archer J: Tests for emotionality in rats and mice: a review. Anim Behav 21:205–235, 1973

Avishai-Eliner S, Yi S-J, Baram TZ: Developmental profile of messenger RNA for the corticotropin-releasing hormone receptor in the rat limbic system. Brain Res Dev Brain Res 91:159–163, 1996

Bailey SJ, Toth M: Variability in the benzodiazepine response of serotonin 5-HT1A receptor null mice displaying anxiety-like phenotype: evidence for genetic modifiers in the 5-HT-mediated regulation of GABAA receptors. J Neurosci 24:6343–6351, 2004

Baudrie V, De Vry J, Broqua P, et al: Subchronic treatment with the anxiolytic doses of the 5-HT1A receptor agonist ipsapirone does not affect 5-HT2 receptor sensitivity in the rat. Eur J Pharmacol 231:395–406, 1993

Beardslee SL, Papadakis E, Fontana DJ, et al: Antipanic drug treatments: failure to exhibit anxiolytic-like effects on defensive burying behavior. Pharmacol Biochem Behav 35:451–455, 1990

Beaufour CC, Ballon N, Le Bihan C, et al: Effects of chronic antidepressants in an operant conflict procedure of anxiety in the rat. Pharmacol Biochem Behav 62:591–599, 1999

Blanchard RJ, Kelley MJ, Blanchard DC: Defensive reactions and exploratory behavior in rats. J Comp Physiol Psychol 87:1129–1133, 1974

Blizard DA: The locus coeruleus: a possible neural focus for genetic differences in emotionality. Experientia 44:491–495, 1988

Blizard DA, Adams N: The Maudsley Reactive and Nonreactive strains: a new perspective. Behav Genet 32:277–299, 2002

Bourin M, Hascoët M: The mouse light/dark box test. Eur J Pharmacol 463:55–65, 2003

Britton KT, Akwa Y, Spina MG, et al: Neuropeptide Y blocks anxiogenic-like behavioral action of corticotropin-releasing factor in an operant conflict test and elevated plus maze. Peptides 21:37–44, 2000

Broadhurst PL: The Maudsley reactive and nonreactive strains of rats: a survey. Behav Genet 5:299–319, 1975

Cadogan A-K, Wright IK, Coombs CA, et al: Repeated paroxetine administration in the rat produces an anxiolytic profile in the elevated X-maze and a decreased 3H-ketanserin binding. Neurosci Lett 42(suppl):S8, 1992

Caldji C, Francis D, Sharma S, et al: The effects of early rearing environment on the development of GABAA and central benzodiazepine receptor levels and novelty-induced fearfulness in the rat. Neuropsychopharmacology 22:219–229, 2000

Campbell KM, de Lecea L, Severynse DM, et al: OCD-Like behaviors caused by a neuropotentiating transgene targeted to cortical and limbic D1+ neurons. J Neurosci 19:5044–5053, 1999a

Campbell KM, McGrath MJ, Burton FH: Differential response of cortical-limbic neuropotentiated compulsive mice to dopamine D1 and D2 receptor antagonists. Eur J Pharmacol 371:103–111, 1999b

Carobrez AP, Bertoglio LJ: Ethological and temporal analyses of anxiety-like behavior: the elevated plus-maze model 20 years on. Neurosci Biobehav Rev 29:1193–1205, 2005

Castanon N, Morméde P: Psychobiogenetics: adapted tools for the study of the coupling between behavioral and neuroendocrine traits of emotional reactivity. Psychoneuroendocrinology 19:257–282, 1994

Champagne F, Meaney MJ: Like mother, like daughter: evidence for non-genomic transmission of parental behavior and stress responsivity. Prog Brain Res 133:287–302, 2001

Cole JC, Rodgers RJ: Ethological evaluation of the effects of acute and chronic buspirone treatment in the murine elevated plus-maze test: comparison with haloperidol. Psychopharmacology 114:288–296, 1994

Cole JC, Rodgers RJ: Ethological comparison of the effects of diazepam and acute/chronic imipramine on behavior of mice in the elevated plus-maze. Pharmacol Biochem Behav 52:473–478, 1995

Commissaris RL, Humrich J, Johns J, et al: The effects of selective and non-selective monoamine oxidase (MAO) inhibitors on conflict behavior in the rat. Behav Pharmacol 6:195–202, 1995

Coplan JD, Rosenblum LA, Gorman JM: Primate models of anxiety: longitudinal perspectives. Psychiatr Clin North Am 18:727–743, 1995

Coplan JD, Andrews MW, Rosenblum LA, et al: Persistent elevations of cerebrospinal fluid concentrations of corticotrophin-releasing factor in adult nonhuman primates exposed to early life stressors: implications for the pathophysiology of mood and anxiety. Proc Natl Acad Sci USA 93:1619–1623, 1996

Coplan JD, Trost RC, Owens MJ, et al: Cerebrospinal fluid concentrations of somatostatin and biogenic amines in grown primates reared by mothers exposed to manipulated foraging conditions. Arch Gen Psychiatry 55:473–477, 1998

Coplan JD, Smith ELP, Trost RC, et al: Growth hormone response to clonidine in adversely reared young adult primates: relationship to serial cerebrospinal fluid corticotropin-releasing factor concentrations. Psychiatry Res 95:93–102, 2000

Coplan JD, Smith EL, Altemus M, et al: Maternal-infant response to variable foraging demand in nonhuman primates: effects of timing of stressor on cerebrospinal fluid corticotropin-releasing factor and circulating glucocorticoid concentrations. Ann N Y Acad Sci 1071:525–533, 2006

Craft RM, Howard JL, Pollard GT: Conditioned defensive burying as a model for identifying anxiolytics. Pharmacol Biochem Behav 30:775–780, 1988

Cryan JF, Holmes A: The ascent of mouse: advances in modeling human depression and anxiety. Nat Rev Drug Discov 4:775–790, 2005

Cutler MG: An ethological study of the effects of buspirone and the 5-HT3 receptor antagonist BRL 43694 (granisetron) on behavior during social interactions in female and male mice. Neuropharmacology 30:299–306, 1991

Cutler MG, Rodgers RJ, Jackson JE: Behavioral effects in mice of subchronic buspirone, ondansetron and tianeptine, I: social interactions. Pharmacol Biochem Behav 56:287–293, 1997a

Cutler MG, Rodgers RJ, Jackson JE: Behavioral effects in mice of subchronic chlordiazepoxide, maprotiline, and fluvoxamine, I: social interactions. Pharmacol Biochem Behav 57:119–125, 1997b

Davis M, Falls WA, Campeau S, et al: Fear-potentiated startle: a neural and pharmacological analysis. Behav Brain Res 58:175–198, 1993

De Boer SF, Koolhaas KM: Defensive burying in rodents: ethology, neurobiology and psychopharmacology. Eur J Pharmacol 463:145–161, 2003

Driscoll P, Bättig K: Behavioral, emotional and neurochemical profiles of rats selected for extreme differences in active, two-way avoidance performance, in Genetics of the Brain. Edited by Lieblich I. Amsterdam, The Netherlands, Elsevier, 1982, pp 95–123

Dulawa SC, Holick KA, Gundersen B, et al: Effects of chronic fluoxetine in animal models of anxiety and depression. Neuropsychopharmacology 29:1321–1330, 2004

Dwyer KD, Roy EJ: Juvenile desipramine reduces adult sensitivity to imipramine in two behavioral tests. Pharmacol Biochem Behav 45:201–207, 1993

Eilam D, Szechtman H: Psychostimulant-induced behavior as an animal model of obsessive-compulsive disorder: an ethological approach to the form of compulsive rituals. CNS Spectr 10:191–202, 2005

Engelmann M, Thrivikraman KV, Su Y, et al: Endocrine and behavioral effects of airpuff-startle in rats. Psychoneuroendocrinology 21:391–400, 1996

Fernandez-Guasti A, Martinez-Mota L, Estrada-Camarena E, et al: Chronic treatment with desipramine induces an

estrous cycle-dependent anxiolytic-like action in the burying behavior, but not in the elevated plus-maze test. Pharmacol Biochem Behav 63:13–20, 1999
File SE: Animal models for predicting clinical efficacy of anxiolytic drugs: social behavior. Neuropsychobiology 13:55–62, 1985
File SE: Animal models of different anxiety states. Adv Biochem Psychopharmacol 48:93–113, 1995
File SE, Hyde JR: Can social interaction be used to measure anxiety? Br J Pharmacol 62:19–24, 1978
File SE, Johnston AL: Chronic treatment with imipramine does not reverse the effects of 3 anxiogenic compounds in a test of anxiety in the rat. Neuropsychobiology 17:187–192, 1987
File SP, Seth P: A review of 25 years of the social interaction test. Eur J Pharmacol 463:35–53, 2003
Finn DA, Rutledge-Gorman MT, Crabbe JC: Genetic animal models of anxiety. Neurogenetics 4:109–135, 2003
Fontana DJ, Commissaris RL: Effects of acute and chronic imipramine administration on conflict behavior in the rat: a potential "animal model" for the study of panic disorder? Psychopharmacology 95:147–150, 1988
Fontana DJ, Carbary TJ, Commissaris RL: Effects of acute and chronic anti-panic drug administration on conflict behavior in the rat. Psychopharmacology 98:158–162, 1989
Ford RD, Rech RH, Commissaris RL, et al: Effects of acute and chronic interactions of diazepam and D-amphetamine on punished behavior of rats. Psychopharmacology 65:197–204, 1979
Gao B, Cutler MG: Effects of sub-chronic treatment with chlordiazepoxide, buspirone and the 5-HT3 receptor antagonist, BRL 46470, on the social behavior of mice. Neuropharmacology 31:207–213, 1992
Gardner CR: Distress vocalizations in rat pups: a simple screening method for anxiolytic drugs. J Pharmacol Methods 14:181–187, 1985
Geller I, Seifter J: The effect of meprobamate, barbiturates, d-amphetamine and promazine on experimentally induced conflict in the rat. Psychopharmacologia 1:482–491, 1960
Giménez-Llort L, Canete T, Guitart-Masip M, et al: Two distinctive apomorphine-induced phenotypes in the Roman high- and low-avoidance rats. Physiol Behav 86:458–466, 2005
Giorgi O, Piras G, Lecca D, et al: Differential activation of dopamine release in the nucleus accumbens core and shell after acute or repeated amphetamine injections: a comparative study in the Roman high- and low-avoidance rat lines. Neuroscience 135:987–988, 2005
Griebel G, Moreau JL, Jenck F, et al: Acute and chronic treatment with 5-HT reuptake inhibitors differentially modulate emotional responses in anxiety models in rodents. Psychopharmacology 113:463–470, 1994
Griebel G, Simiand J, Steinberg R, et al: 4-(2-Chloro-4-methoxy-5-methylphenyl)-N-[(1S)-2-cyclopropyl-1-(3-fluoro-4-methylphenyl)ethyl]5-methyl-N-(2-propynyl)-1,3-thiazol-2-amine hydrochloride (SSR125543A): a potent and selective corticotrophin-releasing factor 1 receptor antagonist, II: characterization in rodent models of stress-related disorders. J Pharmacol Exp Ther 301:333–345, 2002
Gross C, Zhuang X, Stark K, et al: Serotonin-1A receptor acts during development to establish normal anxiety-like behaviour in the adult. Nature 416:396–400, 2002
Gutman DA, Owens MJ, Skelton KH, et al: The corticotropin-releasing factor 1 receptor antagonist R121919 attenuates the behavioral and endocrine responses to stress. J Pharmacol Exp Ther 304:874–880, 2003
Handley SL, Mithani S: Effects of alpha-adrenoceptor agonists and antagonists in a maze-exploration model of "fear"-motivated behaviour. Naunyn Schmiedebergs Arch Pharmacol 327:1–5, 1984
Heisler LK, Chu HM, Brennan TJ, et al: Elevated anxiety and antidepressant-like responses in serotonin 5-HT1A receptor mutant mice. Proc Natl Acad Sci USA 95:15049–15054, 1998
Hogg S: A review of the validity and variability of the elevated plus-maze as an animal model of anxiety. Pharmacol Biochem Behav 54:21–30, 1996
Iijima M, Chaki S: Separation-induced ultrasonic vocalization in rat pups: further pharmacological characterization. Pharmacol Biochem Behav 82:652–657, 2005
Insel TR, Hill JL: Infant separation distress in genetically fearful rats. Biol Psychiatry 22:783–786, 1987
Iverson SD: Animal models of anxiety and benzodiazepine actions. Arzneimittelforschung 30:862–868, 1980
Joel D: The signal attenuation rat model of obsessive-compulsive disorder: a review. Psychopharmacology 186:487–503, 2006
Johnston AL, File SE: Profiles of the antipanic compounds, triazolobenzodiazepines and phenelzine, in two animal tests of anxiety. Psychiatry Res 25:81–90, 1988
Kagan J, Reznick JS, Snidman N: Biological bases of childhood shyness. Science 240:161–171, 1988
Kalin NH, Shelton SE: Defensive behavior in infant rhesus monkeys: environmental cues and neurochemical regulation. Science 243:1718–1721, 1989
Kalin NH, Shelton SE, Rickman M, et al: Individual differences in freezing and cortical in infant and mother rhesus monkeys. Behav Neurosci 112:251–254, 1998
Kalin NH, Shelton SE, Davidson RJ: Cerebrospinal fluid corticotropin-releasing hormone levels are elevated in monkeys with patterns of brain activity associated with fearful temperament. Biol Psychiatry 47:579–585, 2000
Kaufman D, Banerji MA, Shorman I, et al: Early life stress and the development of obesity and insulin resistance in juvenile bonnet macaques. Diabetes 56:1382–1386, 2007

Klemenhagen KC, Gordon JA, David DJ, et al: Increased fear response to contextual cues in mice lacking the 5-HT1A receptor. Neuropsychopharmacology 31:101–111, 2006

Koob GF, Heinrichs S, Britton K: Animal models of anxiety disorders, in The American Psychiatric Press Textbook of Psychopharmacology, 2nd Edition. Edited by Schatzberg AF, Nemeroff CB. Washington, DC, American Psychiatric Press 1998, pp 141–152

Kramer MS, Cutler N, Feighner J, et al: Distinct mechanism for antidepressant activity by blockade of central substance P receptors. Science 281:1640–1645, 1998

Kugelberg FC, Apelqvist G, Bengtsson F: Effects of chronic citalopram treatment on central and peripheral spontaneous open-field behaviours in rats. Pharmacol Toxicol 90:303–310, 2002

Kurt M, Arik AC, Celik S: The effects of sertraline and fluoxetine on anxiety in the elevated plus-maze test in mice. J Basic Clin Physiol Pharmacol 11:173–180, 2000

Ladd CO, Huot RL, Thrivikraman KV, et al: Long-term behavioral and neuroendocrine adaptations to adverse early experience, in The Biological Basis of Mind Body Interaction (Progress in Brain Research, Vol 122). Edited by Mayer EA, Saper CB. Amsterdam, The Netherlands, Elsevier Science, 2000, pp 81–103

Li Y-W, Hill G, Wong H, et al: Receptor occupancy of nonpeptide corticotropin-releasing factor 1 antagonist DMP696: correlation with drug exposure and anxiolytic efficacy. J Pharmacol Exp Ther 305:86–96, 2003

Lightowler S, Kennett GA, Williamson IJR, et al: Anxiolytic-like effect of paroxetine in a rat social interaction test. Pharmacol Biochem Behav 49:281–285, 1994

Lister RG: Ethologically based animal models of anxiety disorders. Pharmacol Ther 46:321–340, 1990

MacQueen GM, Ramakrishnan K, Ratnasingan R: Desipramine treatment reduces the long-term behavioural and neurochemical sequelae of early life maternal separation. Int J Neuropsychopharmacol 6:391–396, 2003

Martin JR, Moreau JL, Jenck F, et al: Acute and chronic administration of buspirone fails to yield anxiolytic-like effects in a mouse operant punishment paradigm. Pharmacol Biochem Behav 46:905–910, 1993

Masisonnette S, Morato S, Brandao ML: Role of resocialization and of 5-HT1A receptor activation on the anxiogenic effects induced by isolation in the elevated plus-maze test. Physiol Behav 54:753–758, 1993

Masserman JH, Yum KS: An analysis of the influence of alcoholism: experimental neuroses in cats. Psychosom Med 8:36–52, 1946

Mathew SJ, Coplan JD, Smith EL, et al: Cerebrospinal fluid concentrations of biogenic amines and corticotropin-releasing factor in adolescent non-human primates as a function of the timing of adverse early rearing. Stress 5:185–193, 2002

McGrath MJ, Campbell KM, Burton FH: The role of cognitive and affective processing in a transgenic mouse model of cortical-limbic neuropotentiated compulsive behavior. Behav Neurosci 113:1249–1256, 1999a

McGrath MJ, Campbell KM, Veldman MB, et al: Anxiety in a transgenic mouse model of cortical-limbic neuropotentiated compulsive behavior. Behav Pharmacol 10:435–443, 1999b

Mechiel Korte S, De Boer SF: A robust animal model of state anxiety: fear-potentiated behaviour in the elevated plus-maze. Eur J Pharmacol 463:163–175, 2003

Moffett MC, Vicentic A, Kozel M: Maternal separation alters drug intake patterns in adulthood in rats. Biochem Pharmacol 73:321–330, 2007

Montgomery KC: The relationship between fear induced by novel stimulation and exploratory behavior. J Comp Physiol Psychol 48:254–260, 1955

Moser PC: An evaluation of the elevated plus-maze test using the novel anxiolytic buspirone. Psychopharmacology 99:48–53, 1989

Motta V, Maisonnette S, Morato S, et al: Effects of blockade of 5-HT2 receptors and activation of 5-HT1A receptors on the exploratory activity of rats in the elevated plus-maze. Psychopharmacology 17:135–139, 1992

Olivier B, Pattij T, Wood SJ, et al: The 5-HT(1A) receptor knockout mouse and anxiety. Behav Pharmacol 12:439–450, 2001

Parks CL, Robinson PS, Sibille E, et al: Increased anxiety of mice lacking the serotonin 1A receptor. Proc Natl Acad Sci USA 95:10734–10739, 1998

Paterson A, Whiting PJ, Gray JA: Lack of consistent behavioural effects of Maudsley reactive and non-reactive rats in a number of animal tests of anxiety and activity. Psychopharmacology 154:336–342, 2001

Pellow S, File SE: Can anti-panic drugs antagonize the anxiety produced in the rat by drugs acting at the GABA-benzodiazepine receptor complex? Neuropsychobiology 17:60–65, 1987

Pellow S, Chopin P, File SE, et al: Validation of open:closed arm entries in an elevated plus-maze as a measure of anxiety in the rat. J Neurosci Methods 14:149–167, 1985

Pinel JPJ, Treit D: Burying as a defensive response in rats. J Comp Physiol Psychol 92:708–712, 1978

Plotsky PM, Thrivikraman KV, Nemeroff CB, et al: Long-term consequences of neonatal rearing on central corticotropin-releasing factor systems in adult male rat offspring. Neuropsychopharmacology 30:2192–2204, 2005

Pollard GT, Howard JL: Effects of drugs on punished behavior: pre-clinical test for anxiolytics. Pharmacol Ther 45:403–424, 1990

Ramboz S, Oosting R, Amara DA, et al: Serotonin receptor 1A knockout: an animal model of anxiety-related disorder. Proc Natl Acad Sci USA 95:14476–14481, 1998

Rocha B, Rigo M, Di Scala G, et al: Chronic mianserin or eltoprazine treatment in rats: effects on the elevated plus-maze test and on limbic 5-HT2C receptor levels. Eur J Pharmacol 262:125–131, 1994

Rodgers RJ, Dalvi A: Anxiety, defence and the elevated plus-maze. Neurosci Biobehav Rev 21:901–810, 1997

Rodgers RJ, Cutler MG, Jackson JE: Behavioral effects in mice of subchronic buspirone, ondansetron and tianeptine, II: the elevated plus-maze. Pharmacol Biochem Behav 56:295–303, 1997a

Rodgers RJ, Cutler MG, Jackson JE: Behavioral effects in mice of subchronic chlordiazepoxide, maprotiline and fluvoxamine, II: the elevated plus-maze. Pharmacol Biochem Behav 57:127–136, 1997b

Rosenblum LA, Coplan JD, Friedman S, et al: Adverse early experiences affect noradrenergic and serotonergic functioning in adult primates. Biol Psychiatry 35:221–227, 1994

Rüedi-Bettschen D, Feldon J, Pryce CR: The impaired coping induced by early deprivation is reversed by chronic fluoxetine treatment in adult Fischer rats. Behav Pharmacol 15:413–421, 2004

Sakamoto H, Matsumoto K, Ohno Y, et al: Anxiolytic-like effects of perospirone, a novel serotonin-2 and dopamine-2 antagonist (SDA)-type antipsychotic agent. Pharmacol Biochem Behav 60:873–878, 1998

Sánchez MM, Noble PM, Lyon CK, et al: Alterations in diurnal cortisol rhythm and acoustic startle response in nonhuman primates with adverse rearing. Biol Psychiatry 57:373–381, 2005

Schefke DM, Fontana DJ, Commissaris RL: Anti-conflict efficacy of buspirone following acute versus chronic treatment. Psychopharmacology 99:427–429, 1989

Shimuzu H, Hirose A, Tatsuno T, et al: Pharmacological properties of SM-3997: a new anxioselective anxiolytic candidate. Jpn J Pharmacol 45:493–500, 1987

Silva RC, Brandão ML: Acute and chronic effects of gepirone and fluoxetine in rats tested in the elevated plus-maze: an ethological analysis. Pharmacol Biochem Behav 65:209–216, 2000

Söderpalm B, Lundin B, Hjorth S: Sustained 5-hydoxytryptamine release-inhibitory and anxiolytic-like action of the partial 5-HT1A receptor agonist, buspirone, after prolonged chronic administration. Eur J Pharmacol 239:69–73, 1993

Stam R: PTSD and stress sensitization: a tale of brain and body: part 2. Neurosci Biobehav Rev 31:558–584, 2007

Suomi SJ: Uptight and laid-back monkeys: individual differences in the response to social challenges, in Plasticity of Development. Edited by Branch S, Hall W, Dooling E. Cambridge, MA, MIT Press, 1991, pp 27–55

Szechtman H, Sulis W, Eilam D: Quinpirole induces compulsive checking behavior in rats: a potential animal model of obsessive-compulsive disorder (OCD). Behav Neurosci 12:1475–1485, 1998

Takahashi LK, Kalin NH, Vanden Burgt JA, et al: Corticotropin-releasing factor modulates defensive-withdrawal and exploratory behavior in rats. Behav Neurosci 103:648–654, 1989

Toth M: 5-HT1A receptor knockout mouse as a genetic model of anxiety. Eur J Pharmacol 463:177–184, 2003

Treit D: Animal models for the study of anti-anxiety agents: a review. Neurosci Biobehav Rev 9:203–222, 1985

Treit D, Pinel JP, Fibiger HC: Conditioned defensive burying: a new paradigm for the study of anxiolytic agents. Pharmacol Biochem Behav 15:619–626, 1981

Treit D, Meynard J, Royan C: Anxiogenic stimuli in the elevated plus-maze. Pharmacol Biochem Behav 44:463–469, 1993

Vogel JR, Beer B, Clody DE: A simple and reliable conflict procedure for testing anti-anxiety agents. Psychopharmacologia 21:1–7, 1971

Wiersma A, Konsman JP, Knollema S, et al: Differential effects of CRH infusion into the central nucleus of the amygdala in the Roman high-avoidance and low-avoidance rats. Psychoneuroendocrinology 23:261–274, 1998

Winslow JT, Insel TR: Serotonergic and catecholaminergic reuptake inhibitors have opposite effects on the ultrasonic isolation calls of rats pups. Neuropsychopharmacology 3:51–59, 1990

Winslow JT, Insel TR: The infant rat separation paradigm: a novel test for novel anxiolytics. Trends Pharmacol Sci 12:402–404, 1991

Wright IK, Heaton M, Upton N, et al: Comparison of acute and chronic treatment of various serotonergic agents with those of diazepam and idazoxan in the rat elevated X-maze. Psychopharmacology 107:405–414, 1992

Yamashita S, Oishi R, Gomita Y: Anticonflict effects of acute and chronic treatments with buspirone and gepirone in rats. Pharmacol Biochem Behav 50:477–479, 1995

Yang X-M, Gorman AL, Dunn AJ: The involvement of central noradrenergic systems and corticotropin-releasing factor in defensive-withdrawal behavior in rats. J Pharmacol Exp Ther 255:1064–1070, 1990

Recommended Readings

The chapter by Koob et al. provides the broadest coverage for further reading on this topic. The reader may also consult the specific reviews listed below for primate models (Coplan et al.), rodent models (File, Lister), and models for distinguishing between characteristics of depression and anxiety (Cryan and Holmes).

Coplan JD, Rosenblum LA, Gorman JM: Primate models of anxiety: longitudinal perspectives. Psychiatr Clin North Am 18:727–743, 1995

Cryan JF, Holmes A: The ascent of mouse: advances in modeling human depression and anxiety. Nat Rev Drug Discov 4:775–790, 2005

File SE: Animal models of different anxiety states. Adv Biochem Psychopharmacol 48:93–113, 1995

Koob GF, Heinrichs S, Britton K: Animal models of anxiety disorders, in The American Psychiatric Press Textbook of Psychopharmacology, 2nd Edition. Edited by Schatzberg AF, Nemeroff CB. Washington, DC, American Psychiatric Press 1998, pp 141–152

Lister RG: Ethologically based animal models of anxiety disorders. Pharmacol Ther 46:321–340, 1990

Chapter 4

Neural Circuits in Fear and Anxiety

J. Douglas Bremner, M.D.
Dennis S. Charney, M.D.

In this chapter, we review neural correlates of fear and anxiety and the clinical neuroscience of human anxiety disorders built on basic research. We make connections between neurobiology and functional neuroanatomy and the clinical and symptomatic presentation of patients with anxiety disorders. This work is ongoing, and many of the models proposed may be subject to modification and revision as our knowledge base in this exciting area continues to expand.

Development of a Model for the Neural Circuitry of Fear and Anxiety

History of Biological Models for Anxiety

There has been a long history of hypotheses related to the neurobiology of human anxiety. Early neuroanatomical studies showed that removal of the cerebral cortex of the cat—which left only subcortical regions including the amygdala, thalamus, hippocampus, and hypothalamus—resulted in accentuated fearful responses to potentially threatening or novel stimuli, accompanied by signs of diffuse sympathetic activation such as increased blood pressure, sweating, piloerection, and increased secretion of epinephrine from the adrenal medulla (Cannon 1927). This behavioral response came to be referred to as *sham rage* and led to the original hypothesis that subcortical brain structures above the level of the midbrain, such as the hypothalamus, hippocampus, cingulate, entorhinal cortex, and thalamus, mediate human anxiety responses (Papez 1937; reviewed in LeDoux 1996). MacLean later added the amygdala to the "Papez circuit" of "limbic" brain structures, so called because of their evolutionary relationship to olfaction, which was hypothesized to play a role in fear and anxiety (reviewed in LeDoux 1996). More recent work by LeDoux (1993) and Davis (1992) has confirmed the important role of the amygdala in animal models of anxiety. Neuroanatomical hypotheses have subsequently been developed related to specific anxiety disorders, including panic disorder (Gorman et al. 1989) and posttraumatic stress disorder (PTSD) (Pitman 1989). Alterations in neurochemical and neurotransmitter systems—including norepinephrine, cortisol, benzodiazepines, and other neurochemical systems that mediate the stress response—have been hypothesized to play a role in anxiety (Charney and Bremner 1999).

A Working Model for Fear and Anxiety

Based on studies of the effects of stress on animals and emerging work in the clinical neuroscience of anxiety disorders, we have developed a working model for the neural circuitry of fear and anxiety (Bremner et al.

1999a; Charney and Deutch 1996). The model must explain how information related to a threatening stimulus (e.g., someone approaches you with a gun in a dark alley) enters the primary senses (smell, sight, touch, hearing), is integrated into a coherent image that is grounded in space and time, activates memory traces of prior similar experiences with the appropriate emotional valence (necessary to evaluate the true threat potential of the stimulus), and triggers an appropriate motor response. Specific brain circuits that mediate these responses make up the neural circuitry of fear and anxiety.

In the development of human fear and anxiety, afferent sensory input enters through the senses of smell, sight, touch, and hearing and the body's own visceral information, or through any combination of these. These sensory inputs are relayed through the dorsal thalamus to cortical brain areas, such as primary visual (occipital), auditory (temporal), or tactile (postcentral gyrus) cortical areas. Olfactory sensory input, however, has direct inputs to the amygdala and entorhinal cortex. Input from peripheral visceral organs is relayed through the nucleus paragigantocellularis and nucleus tractus solitarii in the brain stem to the locus coeruleus, site of most of the brain's noradrenergic neurons, and from there to central brain areas.

Information that reaches primary sensory areas is then processed by secondary cortical association areas (Jones and Powell 1970). These secondary areas are often physically adjacent to the primary sensory areas from which they receive information. For instance, the primary sensory area for vision is in the medial portion of the occipital lobe (Brodmann area 17), which is in the posterior portion of the brain. Just lateral to this area is the visual association cortex (Brodmann areas 18 and 19). Thus, the primary occipital cortex is responsible for determining an object's color, for example, whereas the visual association cortex is responsible for forming a visual image of the object. More complex visual processing involves recognition of faces, which is mediated by the lingual gyrus (posterior parahippocampal region), fusiform gyrus, and inferior temporal gyrus. These brain areas have projections to multiple areas, including the amygdala, hippocampus, entorhinal cortex, orbitofrontal cortex, and cingulate, that are involved in mediating memory and emotion.

Prefrontal and Parietal Cortex

Cognitive appraisal of potential threat is also an important aspect of the stress response. The cognitive response to threat involves placing the threatening object in space and time. Specific brain areas are involved in these functions. For example, the parietal cortex is involved in determining where an object is located in space. Posterior portions of the cingulate have connections to the parietal cortex, hippocampus, and adjacent cortex. This region plays an important role in visuospatial processing (Vogt et al. 1992). The prefrontal cortex also is involved in memory and cognition and, with the parietal cortex, has important dual reciprocal connections with all of the subcortical areas mentioned above (Selemon and Goldman-Rakic 1988). The dorsolateral prefrontal cortex has a range of functions, including declarative and working memory and planning of action, whereas the parietal cortex, as mentioned, plays an important role in spatial memory (Goldman-Rakic 1988). The prefrontal cortex and parietal cortex work in concert in the alerting and planning aspects of the stress response that is critical for survival. Anterior cingulate (Brodmann area 32) is involved in selection of responses for action as well as emotion (Devinsky et al. 1995). This area and other medial portions of the prefrontal cortex, including subgenual area (Brodmann area 25) and orbitofrontal cortex, modulate emotional and physiological responses to stress. These parts of the prefrontal cortex are discussed in more detail below.

Another important aspect of the stress response is incorporation of a person's prior experience (memory) into the cognitive appraisal of stimuli. For example, if one is approached by another person in a potentially threatening situation, it is important to determine whether the person is someone familiar or is a stranger who may be more threatening. In addition, it is important to place the situation in time and place. Entering a dark alley may trigger memories of being robbed, with associated negative emotions and physiological arousal. These memories may have survival value, in that the individual will avoid the situation in which the previous negative event took place. Finally, it is critical to effectively lay down memory traces related to a potential threat so as to avoid this type of threat in the future. Specific brain areas are involved in retrieval of memory.

Hippocampus

The hippocampus, which is particularly vulnerable to stress, plays an important role in memory. The hippocampus and adjacent cortex mediate declarative memory function (e.g., recall of facts and lists) and play an important role in integration of memory elements at the time of retrieval, as well as in assigning significance to events within space and time (Squire and Zola-Morgan

1991). The hippocampus also plays an important role in mediating emotional responses to the context of a stressor; for example, in animal studies, lesions of the hippocampus disrupted the formation of emotional memories of the context (e.g., the box) in which the stressor (e.g., electric footshock) took place. High levels of glucocorticoids released during stress were also associated with damage to the CA3 region of the hippocampus (Sapolsky 1996) and related memory deficits (McEwen et al. 1992). Other factors implicated in the effects of stress on the hippocampus include stress-induced decreases in brain-derived neurotrophic factor (Nibuya et al. 1995) and increased glutamate (Moghaddam et al. 1997). Stress also decreases neurogenesis (new neuron formation) (Gould et al 1997); these effects are reversed by antidepressants (Duman et al. 2001; Santarelli et al. 2003). These findings may be applicable to patients with PTSD and other anxiety disorder (see section "A Working Model for the Neural Circuitry of Anxiety Disorders," later in this chapter).

With long-term storage, memories shift from the hippocampus to the neocortical areas (Squire and Zola-Morgan 1991). The shift in memory storage to the cortex may represent a shift from conscious representational memory to unconscious memory processes that indirectly affect behavior. *Traumatic cues*, such as a particular sight or sound reminiscent of the original traumatic event, will trigger a cascade of anxiety- and fear-related symptoms, often without conscious recall of the original traumatic event. In patients with PTSD, however, the traumatic stimulus is always potentially identifiable. Symptoms of anxiety in patients with panic or phobic disorder, however, may be related to fear responses to a traumatic cue (in individuals who are vulnerable to increased fear responsiveness, through either constitution or previous experience) when there is no possibility that the original fear-inducing stimulus will ever be identified.

Amygdala

The amygdala is involved in memory for the emotional valence of events. The paradigm of conditioned fear has been used as an animal model for stress-induced abnormalities of emotional memory (Davis 1992; LeDoux 1993). Conditioned fear, in which pairing of a neutral (conditioned) stimulus to a fear-inducing (unconditioned) stimulus results in fear responses to the neutral (conditioned) stimulus alone, has been used as a probe of amygdala function (Davis 1992; LeDoux et al. 1990). Lesions of the central nucleus of the amygdala have been shown to completely block fear conditioning, whereas electrical stimulation of the central nucleus increases acoustic startle. The central nucleus of the amygdala projects to a variety of brain structures via the stria terminalis and the ventral amygdalofugal pathway. One pathway is from the central nucleus to the brain stem–startle-reflex circuit (nucleus reticularis pontis caudalis) (Davis 1992). Pathways from the amygdala to the lateral hypothalamus effect peripheral sympathetic responses to stress (Iwata et al. 1986). Electrical stimulation of the amygdala in cats resulted in peripheral signs of autonomic hyperactivity and fear-related behaviors seen in the wild when the animal is being attacked or is attacking, including alerting, chewing, salivation, piloerection, turning, facial twitching, arching of the back, hissing, and snarling, associated with an increase in catecholamine turnover (Hilton and Zbrozyna 1963). Electrical stimulation of the amygdala in human subjects resulted in signs and symptoms of fear and anxiety, including an increase in heart rate and blood pressure, increased muscle tension, subjective sensations of fear or anxiety (Chapman et al. 1954), and increases in peripheral catecholamines (Gunne and Reis 1963). These findings show that the amygdala plays an important role in conditioned fear and emotional responding and modulates peripheral stress responses. Also, connections between cortical association areas, thalamus, and amygdala are important in shaping the emotional valence of the cognitive response to stressful stimuli. In addition to thalamic-cortical-amygdalar connections, there are direct pathways from thalamus to amygdala, which could account for fear-responding below the level of conscious awareness (LeDoux et al. 1989; Romanski and LeDoux 1993).

Frontal cortical areas modulate emotional responsiveness through inhibition of amygdala function, and we have hypothesized that dysfunction in these regions may underlie pathological emotional responses in patients with anxiety disorders (Charney and Bremner 1999). The medial prefrontal cortex has projections to the amygdala that are involved in the modulation of amygdalar responsiveness to fearful cues. Dysfunction of this area may be responsible for the failure of extinction to fearful cues, which is an important part of the anxiety response (Morgan and LeDoux 1995; Morgan et al. 1993; Quirk et al. 2006). This area is involved in regulation of peripheral responses to stress, including heart rate, blood pressure, and cortisol response (Roth et al. 1988). Finally, case studies of humans with brain lesions have implicated the medial prefrontal cortex (including orbitofrontal cortex [Brodmann area 25] and anterior cingulate [Brodmann area 32]) in "emotion" and socially appropriate interactions (Damasio et al. 1994). The most replicated finding from brain imaging studies of PTSD is decreased function of medial prefrontal cortex with traumatic reminders.

Neocortex

A final component of the stress response involves preparation for a response to potential threat. Preparation for responding to threat requires an integration between brain areas involved in assessing and interpreting the potentially threatening stimulus and brain areas involved in responding. For instance, the prefrontal cortex and anterior cingulate play an important role in the planning of action and in holding multiple pieces of information in working memory during the execution of a response (Goldman-Rakic 1988). The parietal cortex and posterior cingulate are involved in visuospatial processing, which is an important component of the stress response. The motor cortex represents the neural substrate of planning for action. The cerebellum has a well-known role in motor movement and is involved in planning for action; however, studies are consistent with a role in cognition as well. Connections between parietal and prefrontal cortex are required to permit the organism to rapidly and efficiently execute motor responses to threat. It is therefore not surprising that these areas have important innervations to precentral (motor) cortex, which is responsible for skeletal motor responses to threat that facilitate survival. The striatum (caudate and putamen) modulates motor responses to stress. The dense innervation of the striatum and prefrontal cortex by the amygdala indicates that the amygdala can regulate both of these systems. These interactions between the amygdala and the extrapyramidal motor system may be very important for generating motor responses to threatening stimuli, especially those related to prior adverse experiences (McDonald 1991a, 1991b).

Neurohormonal Responses

The organism must rapidly effect peripheral responses to threat, which are mediated by the stress hormone cortisol and the sympathetic and parasympathetic systems. Stimulation of the lateral hypothalamus results in sympathetic system activation, producing increases in blood pressure and heart rate, sweating, piloerection, and pupil dilatation. Stress stimulates release of corticotropin-releasing factor (CRF) from the paraventricular nucleus (PVN) of the hypothalamus, which increases peripheral adrenocorticotropic hormone (ACTH) and cortisol levels. The medial prefrontal cortex, as mentioned earlier in the chapter, also mediates increased blood pressure and pulse rate as well as elevated cortisol levels in response to stress. Striatum, amygdala, and bed nucleus of the stria terminalis also effect peripheral responses to threat through the lateral nucleus of the hypothalamus (Sawchenko and Swanson 1983a, 1983b).

The vagus and splanchnic nerves are major projections of the parasympathetic nervous system. Afferents to the vagus include the lateral hypothalamus, PVN, locus coeruleus, and amygdala. There are afferent connections to the splanchnic nerves from the locus coeruleus (Clark and Proudfit 1991). This innervation of the parasympathetic nervous system is important for visceral symptoms commonly associated with anxiety, such as gastrointestinal and genitourinary disturbances (Mayer et al. 2001).

Function of these brain areas is mediated by specific neurochemical systems that mediate the stress response. Increased release of glucocorticoids, catecholamines (norepinephrine, epinephrine, and dopamine), serotonin, benzodiazepines, and endogenous opiates is associated with acute stress exposure. We have hypothesized that long-term dysregulation of these systems, acting on brain areas outlined earlier in this chapter, mediates the symptoms of pathological anxiety (Bremner et al. 1999a).

HPA Axis

The hypothalamic-pituitary-adrenal (HPA) axis is an important component of the stress response system. This axis is involved in a negative feedback loop that regulates cortisol release (as well as regulatory feedback with the noradrenergic system, which is discussed in more detail later in this chapter). Cortisol has a variety of functions in the body, regulating primarily energy use but also bone resorption, reproduction, and immunity. The purpose of the functions of cortisol is to help the organism rapidly adapt to cope with stressors. In addition to the PVN of the hypothalamus, binding sites for cortisol and CRF are located in multiple central brain areas involved in fear and the stress response. Binding sites for glucocorticoids include the type I and type II receptors, which have varying affinities for cortisol and the other glucocorticoids (such as dexamethasone). There are at least three CRF receptors—the corticotropin-releasing hormone (CRH) type 1, 2A, and 2B receptors—each constituting seven putative spanning domains characteristic of G_s protein–coupled receptors (Chalmers et al. 1996). CRH_1 receptors are most abundant in neocortical, cerebellar, and sensory relay structures. CRH_2 receptors are generally localized to specific subcortical structures, most notably, lateral septal nuclei, choroid plexus, olfactory bulb, specific amygdaloid nuclei, and various hypothalamic areas. Within the pituitary, CRH_1 expression predominates over CRH_2 expression, suggesting that CRH_1 receptors may mediate CRH-induced changes in ACTH release. CRF has direct behavioral effects in the brain that lead to anxiety. As described later in this chapter, CRF can also exert behavioral effects during stress by stimulating other systems, such as norepinephrine.

Acute stress of many types results in release of CRF, ACTH, and cortisol. The mechanism responsible for transient stress-induced hyperadrenocorticism and feedback resistance may involve a downregulation of glucocorticoid receptors. High glucocorticoid levels (such as those elicited by acute stress) decrease the number of hippocampal glucocorticoid receptors, resulting in increased corticosterone secretion and feedback resistance. Following stress termination, when glucocorticoid levels decrease, receptor numbers increase and feedback sensitivity normalizes (Sapolsky et al. 1984).

The effects of chronic stress on ACTH and corticosterone secretion vary depending on the experimental paradigm. It has been reported that an adaptation to chronic stress may occur, resulting in decreased plasma ACTH and corticosterone levels compared with levels following a single stressor. However, other investigations have reported enhanced corticosterone secretion after chronic stressor regimens. Evidence also indicates that the experience of prior stress may result in augmented corticosterone responses to a subsequent stress exposure (Caggiula et al. 1989; Dallman and Jones 1973). It is not known which factors determine whether adaptation or sensitization of glucocorticoid activity will occur following chronic stress (Yehuda et al. 1991).

The HPA axis has important functional interactions with the norepinephrine system that facilitate a sophisticated range of responses to stress. Glucocorticoids inhibit stress-induced activation of catecholamine synthesis in the PVN. CRF increases activity of the locus coeruleus, and CRF injected into the locus coeruleus intensifies anxiety-related responses. These findings support the notion that CRF serves as an excitatory neurotransmitter in the locus coeruleus, which may represent the pathway for the behavioral effects of CRF.

Stressors early in life have long-term effects on the HPA axis. Both prenatal (light and noise) (Fride et al. 1986) and early maternal deprivation stress (Levine et al. 1993; Stanton et al. 1988) and early-manipulation stress (Levine 1962) resulted in increased glucocorticoid response to subsequent stressors. Prenatal stress was associated with a failure of habituation of glucocorticoid responsiveness to novel stimuli (Fride et al. 1986). Increased glucocorticoid responsivity to ACTH challenge in maternal deprivation stress suggested an increase in adrenocortical responsivity with early stress (Stanton et al. 1988).

Early postnatal adverse experiences altered hypothalamic CRF messenger ribonucleic acid (mRNA), median eminence CRF content, and stress-induced CRF release (Plotsky and Meaney 1993) and ACTH release (Ladd et al. 1996) in male rats. Maternally deprived rats had decreased numbers of glucocorticoid receptors, as measured by dexamethasone binding in the hippocampus, hypothalamus, and frontal cortex. They also had increased norepinephrine levels in the PVN, as determined by microdialysis. In nonhuman primates, early adverse experiences induced by variable maternal foraging requirements resulted in profound behavioral disturbances (more timid, less social, and more subordinate) years later. Adult monkeys raised in the variable maternal foraging environment were also hyperresponsive to yohimbine and had elevated levels of cerebrospinal fluid and decreased CSF cortisol levels in adulthood, a picture that is closer to PTSD than depression (Coplan et al. 1996). These observations suggest that early adverse experience permanently affects the HPA axis.

Positive early-life experiences during critical periods of development may have long-term beneficial consequences on an animal's ability to mount adaptive responses to stress or threat. An animal model that appears to be of use in studying this phenomenon is postnatal handling. Postnatal handling has important effects on the development of behavioral and endocrine responses to stress. For example, daily handling within the first few weeks of life (picking up rat pups and then returning them to their mother) resulted in increased type II glucocorticoid receptor binding, which persisted throughout life. This was associated with increased feedback sensitivity to glucocorticoids and reduced glucocorticoid-mediated hippocampal damage in later life (Meaney et al. 1988, 1989). These effects appear to be the result of a type of "stress inoculation" from the mother's repeated licking of the handled pups. Considered together, these findings suggest that early in the postnatal period, the naturally occurring brain plasticity in key neural systems may "program" an organism's biological response to threatening stimuli.

Coordinated functional interactions between the HPA axis and noradrenergic neuronal systems may be critical in promoting adaptive responses to stress, anxiety, or fear. CRF increases locus coeruleus firing, resulting in enhanced norepinephrine release in cortical and subcortical areas throughout the brain. The PVN of the hypothalamus, site of most CRF-containing neurons in the hypothalamus, is an important site in effecting cardiovascular and neuroendocrine responses to stress. Norepinephrine increases CRF in the PVN of the hypothalamus. In chronically stressed animals, the locus coeruleus (as opposed to other norepinephrine neurons in the medulla) may be preferentially responsible for norepinephrine release in the PVN. High levels of circulating cortisol act through a negative feedback pathway to decrease both CRF and norepinephrine synthesis at the level of the PVN. Glucocorticoid inhibition of norepinephrine-induced CRF stimulation may be evident primarily during stressor-induced cortisol release, and not under resting conditions. High levels of cortisol likely inhibit the effects of norepinephrine on CRF release from the PVN, serving to restrain the stress-induced neuroendocrine and cardiovascular effects mediated by the PVN. Norepinephrine, cortisol, and CRF thus appear to be tightly linked in a functional system that provides a broad homeostatic mechanism for coping with stress.

Norepinephrine

Norepinephrine release in the brain is an important part of the stress response (reviewed in Bremner et al. 1996a, 1996b). Most noradrenergic cell bodies are located in the brain stem, in the locus coeruleus region of the pons, with axons that extend throughout the cerebral cortex and to multiple subcortical areas. Neurons in the locus coeruleus are activated in association with fear and anxiety states (Abercrombie and Jacobs 1987; Redmond 1987), and the limbic and cortical regions innervated by the locus coeruleus are those involved in the elaboration of adaptive responses to stress. Stressors such as a cat seeing a dog result in an increase in firing of neurons in the locus coeruleus and enhanced norepinephrine release in the hippocampus and medial prefrontal cortex. Exposure to chronic stress also results in a potentiation of norepinephrine release with subsequent stressors (reviewed in Bremner et al. 1996a, 1996b). Consistent with these findings, noradrenergic stimulation resulted in decreased metabolism in the hippocampus (consistent with high levels of norepinephrine release) and relative failure of activation in the medial prefrontal cortex in PTSD patients, but not in subjects without PTSD. A relation between this metabolic response and increased panic or anxiety was also found (Bremner et al. 1997a).

Dopamine

Acute stress increases dopamine release and metabolism in several specific brain areas (reviewed in Thierry et al. 1998). However, the dopamine innervation of the medial prefrontal cortex appears to be particularly vulnerable to stress. Sufficiently low-intensity stress (such as that associated with conditioned fear) or brief exposure to stress increases dopamine release and metabolism in the prefrontal cortex in the absence of overt changes in other mesotelencephalic dopamine regions (Deutch and Roth 1990). Low-intensity electric footshock increases in vivo tyrosine hydroxylase and dopamine turnover in the medial prefrontal cortex, but not in the nucleus accumbens or striatum. Stress can enhance dopamine release and metabolism in other areas receiving dopamine innervation, provided that stress is of greater intensity or longer duration. Thus, the medial prefrontal cortex dopamine innervation is preferentially activated by stress, compared with mesolimbic and nigrostriatal systems, and the mesolimbic dopamine innervation appears to be more sensitive to stress than the striatal dopamine innervation (Deutch and Roth 1990).

Serotonin

The effects of stress on serotonin systems have been studied less thoroughly than the effects on noradrenergic systems. Animals exposed to a variety of stressors, including footshock, tail shock, tail pinch, and restraint stress, all produced an increase in serotonin turnover in the medial prefrontal cortex, nucleus accumbens, amygdala, and lateral hypothalamus, with preferential release during conditioned fear in the medial prefrontal cortex. Chronic electric shock, producing learned helplessness behavioral deficits, was associated with reduced in vivo serotonin release in the frontal cortex (Petty et al. 1992), probably reflecting a situation in which synthesis cannot keep pace with demand. Serotonin antagonists produce behavioral deficits resembling those seen following inescapable shock. Drugs that enhance serotonin neurotransmission (selective serotonin reuptake inhibitors [SSRIs}) are effective in reversing learned helplessness (Petty and Sherman 1980). Preadministration of benzodiazepines or tricyclic antidepressants prevents stress-induced decreases in serotonin and the acquisition of behavioral deficits, whereas injection of serotonin into the frontal cortex after stress exposure reverses behavioral deficits. Chronic restraint stress results in a decrease in serotonin type 1A (5-HT_{1A}) receptor binding in the hippocampus. Animals exposed to social stress had decreased 5-HT_{1A} receptor binding in the hippocampus and dentate gyrus and decreased serotonin type 2 (5-HT_2) receptor binding in the parietal cortex. Administration of 5-HT_{1A} agonists such as buspirone results in a reversal of stress-induced behavioral deficits.

Stress-induced activation of serotonin turnover stimulates a system that has both anxiogenic and anxiolytic pathways within the forebrain (Graeff 1993). A primary distinction in the qualitative effects of serotonin may be between the dorsal and the median raphe nuclei, the two midbrain nuclei that produce most of the forebrain serotonin. The serotonergic innervation of the amygdala and the hippocampus by the dorsal raphe is believed to mediate anxiogenic effects via 5-HT_2 receptors. In contrast, the median raphe innervation of hippocampal 5-HT_{1A} receptors has been hypothesized to facilitate the disconnection of previously learned associations with aversive events or to suppress formation of new associations, thus providing a resilience to aversive events (Graeff 1993). Chronic stress increases cortical binding at 5-HT_2 receptors and reduces it at hippocampal 5-HT_{1A} receptors (Mendelson and McEwen 1991).

Benzodiazepine Systems

Endogenous benzodiazepines also play an important role in the stress response and anxiety. Benzodiazepine receptors are present throughout the brain, with the highest concentration in cortical gray matter. Benzodiazepines potentiate and prolong the synaptic actions of the inhibitory neurotransmitter γ-aminobutyric acid (GABA). Central benzodiazepine receptors and $GABA_A$ receptors are part of the same macromolecular complex. These receptors have distinct binding sites, but they are functionally coupled and regulate one another in an allosteric manner. Administration of inverse agonists of benzodiazepine receptors, such as β-carboline-3-carboxylic acid ethyl ester (β-CCE), results in behavioral and biological effects similar to those seen in anxiety and stress, including increases in heart rate, blood pressure, plasma cortisol, and catecholamines. These effects are blocked by administration of benzodiazepines or pretreatment with the benzodiazepine antagonist flumazenil. Animals exposed to acute, inescapable stress in the form of cold swim or footshock developed a decrease in benzodiazepine receptor binding (density [B_{max}] but not typically affinity [K_D]) in the frontal cortex, with mixed results for the cerebral cortex, hippocampus, and hypothalamus and no change in the occipital cortex, striatum, midbrain, thalamus, cerebellum, and pons. Chronic stress in the form of footshock or cold swim resulted in decreases in benzodiazepine receptor binding in the cerebral cortex, frontal cortex, hippocampus, and hypothalamus, with mixed results for the cerebellum, midbrain, and striatum, and no change in the occipital cortex or pons. Decreases in benzodiazepine receptor binding are associated with alterations in memory manifested by deficits in maze escape behaviors. Changes in benzodiazepine receptor function appear to be specific to uncontrollable stress, as opposed to controllable stress, and are prevented by preadministration of benzodiazepines. A decrease in benzodiazepine receptor binding has been found in the so-called Maudsley genetically fearful (reactive) strain of rat, in comparison to nonfearful (nonreactive) rats, in several brain structures including the hippocampus.

Neuropeptides

Several neuropeptides also mediate the response to stress. Cholecystokinin (CCK), an anxiogenic neuropeptide present in the gastrointestinal tract and the brain, has been suggested as a neural substrate for human anxiety. CCK-containing neurons are found in high density in the cerebral cortex, amygdala, and hippocampus. They are also found in the midbrain, including the periaqueductal gray, substantia nigra, and raphe nuclei. Iontophoretic administration of CCK has depolarizing effects on pyramidal neurons, which suggests that it may serve as an excitatory neurotransmitter. CCK_{4-8} have stimulatory effects on action potentials in the dentate gyrus of the hippocampus. Activation of hippocampal neurons is suppressed by low-dose benzodiazepines. CCK agonists are anxiogenic in a variety of animal models of anxiety, whereas CCK antagonists have anxiolytic effects in these tests. Stress is associated with an increase in endogenous opiate release, with a decreased density of μ opiate receptors, which may mediate the analgesia associated with stress. Other neuropeptides under investigation that appear to play a role in the stress response are neuropeptide Y, somatostatin, and thyrotropin. Stress also has important effects on the immune system that are not reviewed here in detail.

Application of the Neural Circuitry Model of Anxiety and Fear to Anxiety Disorders

The primary goal in research related to the clinical neuroscience of anxiety disorders is to apply findings related to the effects of stress on the brain in animals (which are used as models of anxiety) to patients with anxiety disorders. Ideally, animal studies are used to measure the effects of chronic stress on neurochemical systems and brain areas that are particularly sensitive to stress. This approach assumes that animal models of the anxiety disorders are directly applicable to human anxiety disorders. However, it can immediately be seen that this is not possible because different anxiety disorders are expressed in different ways (e.g., panic disorder has important symptomatic differences from PTSD). Animal models used for anxiety disorders (e.g., chronic stress) are also used as models for depression. If there is any validity to our differentiation of unique disorders of anxiety and depression, then it is not possible that, when it comes to animal models, "one size fits all."

However, given these limitations, animal models can be very useful in guiding research in the anxiety disorders. The animal model of chronic stress can go a long way in explaining many of the neurobiological changes associated with anxiety disorders (and possibly depression) (see Chapter 3, "Classification of Anxiety Disorders," in this volume). We have posited that PTSD, panic disorder, and phobic disorders share many neurobiological and phenomenological characteristics and can benefit from the application of animal models of stress (Charney and Bremner 1999). Obsessive-compulsive disorder does not fit as easily with these disorders (and, therefore, is not discussed in depth in this chapter).

Neural circuits mediating symptoms of anxiety disorders can be studied by measuring neurotransmitter and hormone levels in blood, urine, and saliva; assessing behavioral and biochemical responses to pharmacological challenge to specific neurochemical systems; measuring brain structures with structural neuroimaging; provoking disease-specific symptoms in conjunction with functional neuroimaging; or using imaging to measure neuroreceptors.

Brain Imaging Studies in Posttraumatic Stress Disorder

Several replicated studies showed hippocampal atrophy with associated verbal memory deficits in PTSD (Bremner et al. 1995; Kitayama et al. 2005; Smith 2005). Studies have also shown a reduction in *N*-acetyl aspartate, a marker of neuronal activity, in the hippocampus, as well as a failure of hippocampal activation during memory task as measured with functional neuroimaging (Bremner 2006). One study showed a genetic contribution to smaller hippocampal volume in PTSD (Gilbertson et al. 2002). Treatment with the SSRI paroxetine resulted in an increase in hippocampal volume in PTSD patients (Vermetten et al. 2003). Considering the role played by the hippocampus in the integration of memory elements that have been stored in primary sensory and secondary association cortical areas at the time of retrieval, the findings suggest a possible neural correlate for symptoms of memory fragmentation and dysfunction in PTSD (Bremner 2006).

The anterior cingulate/medial prefrontal cortex is also implicated in PTSD. Studies in animals showed that early stress results in a decrease in neuronal branching in the medial prefrontal cortex (Radley et al. 2004). Researchers have used magnetic resonance imaging (MRI) to show smaller volume of the anterior cingulate in PTSD (Kitayama et al. 2006; Rauch et al. 2003; Woodward et al. 2006).

Researchers have used functional imaging, including functional magnetic resonance imaging (fMRI) and positron emission tomography (PET), during provocation of PTSD symptom states to identify neural correlates of PTSD symptomatology and of traumatic remembrance in PTSD (Bremner 2007). For example, stimulation of the noradrenergic systems with yohimbine resulted in an increase in PTSD symptoms and a decrease in prefrontal function in PTSD (Bremner et al. 1997a). Norepinephrine has a U-shaped curve type of effect on brain function—lower levels of release cause an increase in metabolism, and very high levels of release actually cause a decrease in metabolism. Therefore, these findings are consistent with an increased release of norepinephrine in the brain after yohimbine administration in PTSD patients. The findings are also consistent with PET metabolism studies showing an inverse-U relationship between anxiety and cortical function (similar to the Yerkes-Dodson law), with low levels of anxiety causing an increase in cortical metabolism and high levels causing a decrease in cortical metabolism (Gur et al. 1987; Rodriguez et al. 1989).

A number of functional imaging studies have measured neural correlates of exposure to traumatic reminders in the form of traumatic slides and sounds or traumatic scripts (Bremner 2007; Liberzon and Phan 2003; Pitman 2001; Rauch et al. 2006). The most consistent finding from these studies is a decrease in medial prefrontal function (Bremner et al. 1999b; Shin et al. 2004), with some studies showing decreased hippocampal and parietal function and increased posterior cingulate function. Exposure to external threatening stimuli, such as exposure to fearful faces (Rauch et al. 2000) or fear conditioning (Bremner et al. 2005), was associated with increased amygdala function.

Several studies showed alterations in hippocampus and adjacent cortex (parahippocampus) function in panic disorder, with no change in hippocampal volume. Individuals with social phobia show increased amygdala response to contemptuous faces (Stein et al. 2002). In simple phobias, altered amygdala function has not been consistently shown; instead a circuit including increased visual association and decreased dorsolateral and hippocampal function has been associated with induction of phobic symptoms (Bremner 2005).

These findings point to a network of related regions as mediating symptoms of anxiety disorders. The anterior cingulate/medial prefrontal cortex, as reviewed here, plays an important role in modulation of emotion and extinction of fear through inhibition of amygdala function. The amygdala is responsible for execution of the fear response. The posterior cingulate plays an important role in visuospatial processing (Devinsky et al. 1995; Vogt et al. 1992) and is therefore an important component of preparation for coping with a physical threat. The posterior cingulate has functional connections with the hippocampus and adjacent cortex, which led to its original classification as part of the "limbic brain" (Gray 1982). The hippocampus is involved in declarative memory as well as contextual fear.

Findings from imaging studies may also be relevant to the failure of extinction to fear responding that is characteristic of PTSD and other anxiety disorders. Following the development of conditioned fear, as in the pairing of a neutral stimulus (bright light, the conditioned stimulus) with a fear-inducing stimulus (electric shock, the unconditioned stimulus), repeated exposure to the conditioned stimulus alone usually results in the gradual loss of fear responding. The phenomenon, known as *extinction to conditioned fear*, has been hypothesized to be secondary to the formation of new memories that mask the original conditioned fear memory. The extinguished memory is rapidly reversible after reexposure to the conditioned-unconditioned stimulus pairing, even up to 1 year after the original period of fear conditioning, suggesting that the fear response did not disappear but was merely inhibited. Recent evidence, in fact, suggests that extinction is mediated by cortical inhibition of amygdala responsiveness. The medial prefrontal cortex (anterior cingulate—Brodmann areas 24, 25, and 32) has inhibitory connections to the amygdala that play a role in extinction of fear responding, an important component of the symptom profile of PTSD. PET studies in PTSD reviewed earlier in this chapter showed decreased blood flow of the medial prefrontal cortex/anterior cingulate region. On the basis of these findings, we previously argued that anterior cingulate/medial prefrontal activation represents a "normal" brain response to traumatic stimuli that serves to inhibit feelings of fearfulness when no true threat is present. Failure of activation in this area and/or decreased blood flow in this region in individuals with PTSD may lead to increased fearfulness that is not appropriate for the context, a behavioral response that is highly characteristic of patients with PTSD.

Fear conditioning has been used as a model for the occurrence of pathological anxiety responses to seemingly neutral stimuli. According to this model, the neutral stimulus was originally paired with a truly fearful stimulus, which may subsequently be forgotten. Patients then begin to avoid these stimuli in their everyday life. These subcortical memory traces may be indelible and account for repetitive memories specific to PTSD that are often resistant to cognitively based therapies. Patients with anxiety disorders also have symptoms that reflect a continuous perception of threat. The inability to distinguish true threat from perceived threat in innocuous situations is in fact highly characteristic of the anxiety disorders. The animal model of contextual fear conditioning may represent a good model for these symptoms. Preclinical data suggest that the hippocampus (as well as the bed nucleus of the stria terminalis and the periaqueductal gray; see previous section) plays an important role in the mediation of contextual fear and that increased responding to a conditioned stimulus is due to hippocampal dysfunction. Hippocampal atrophy in PTSD, as described earlier in this chapter, therefore provides a possible neuroanatomical substrate for abnormal contextual fear conditioning and chronic feelings of threat and anxiety in PTSD. Interestingly, in light of studies showing abnormal noradrenergic function in PTSD, the bed nucleus of the stria terminalis has some of the densest noradrenergic innervation of any area in the brain.

Alterations in Neurochemical Stress Response Systems in Patients With Anxiety Disorders

Patients with anxiety disorders have long-term alterations in neurochemical systems that mediate the stress response and that have been shown to be sensitive to chronic stress (Tables 4–1, 4–2, 4–3).

HPA Axis Function in Posttraumatic Stress Disorder

Studies on the effects of stress on neurohormonal systems in animals have been applied to PTSD, with a number of studies reporting alterations in HPA axis function in PTSD (reviewed in Yehuda 2006). In 1986, Mason and colleagues reported that although combat veterans with PTSD demonstrated sustained elevations in urinary catecholamine levels, cortisol levels were significantly lower in veterans with PTSD than among those with other psychiatric disorders (Mason et al. 1986). These observations were later confirmed by carefully controlled studies of plasma cortisol release over the diurnal cycle (Bremner et al. 2007; Yehuda et al. 1996). Studies using 24-hour urinary collections or plasma or salivary samples chosen from less frequent sampling over the diurnal cycle showed cortisol to be either reduced or unchanged (Yehuda 2006). Other findings in PTSD include enhanced cortisol negative feedback inhibition that seems to result from increased responsiveness of glucocorticoid receptors (Yehuda et al. 1993). Exposure to a traumatic reminder was associated with a potentiated release of cortisol in PTSD (Elzinga et al. 2003). In PTSD patients, cerebrospinal fluid CRF levels were found to be increased with single lumbar-puncture sampling (Bremner et al. 1997b) as well as throughout a 24-hour period (Baker et al. 2005). The neuroendocrine alterations observed in PTSD suggest an increased sympathetic and central CRF activation in the face of reduced cortisol signaling.

Norepinephrine in Posttraumatic Stress Disorder

Studies have documented alterations in other stress-responsive neurochemical systems in PTSD. Patients with PTSD have increased norepinephrine in blood and urine, increased norepinephrine response to traumatic reminders, and increased behavioral and biochemical response (Bremner et al. 1996a, 1996b; Southwick et al. 1993) as well as brain response (Bremner et al. 1997a) to yohimbine (which stimulates the norepinephrine system). Psychophysiology studies are also consistent with increased noradrenergic function. For example, PTSD is characterized by increased heart rate and blood pressure response to reminders of trauma; these physiological indicators are controlled by noradrenergic function, and they increase the risk of cardiac morbidity.

TABLE 4–1. Evidence for alterations in catecholaminergic function in anxiety disorders

Finding	PTSD	Panic disorder
Increased resting heart rate and blood pressure	±	±
Increased heart rate and blood pressure response to traumatic reminders/panic attacks	+++	++
Increased resting urinary NE and epinephrine	+	+±
Increased resting plasma NE or MHPG	–	–
Increased plasma NE with traumatic reminders/panic attacks	+	±
Increased orthostatic heart rate response to exercise	+	+
Decreased binding to platelet α_2 receptors	+	±
Decrease in basal and stimulated activity of cAMP	±	+
Decrease in platelet monoamine oxidase activity	+	?
Increased symptoms, heart rate, and plasma MHPG with yohimbine noradrenergic challenge	+	+++
Differential brain metabolic response to yohimbine	+	+

Note. – = one or more studies did not support this finding (with no positive studies), or the majority of studies did not support this finding; ± = an equal number of studies supported this finding as studies that did not support this finding; + = at least one study supported this finding, with no studies not supporting the finding, or the majority of studies supported the finding; ++ = two or more studies supported this finding, with no studies not supporting the finding; +++ = three or more studies supported this finding, with no studies not supporting the finding. cAMP = cyclic adenosine monophosphate; MHPG = 3-methoxy-4-hydroxyphenylglycol; NE = norepinephrine; PTSD = posttraumatic stress disorder.

TABLE 4–2. Evidence for alterations in CRF/HPA axis function in anxiety disorders

Finding	PTSD	Panic disorder
Alterations in urinary cortisol	±[a]	±
Altered plasma cortisol with 24-hour sampling	++	+ (increased)
Supersuppression with DST	+++	–
Blunted ACTH response to CRF	±	±
Elevated CRF in CSF	+++	+
Increased lymphocyte glucocorticoid receptors	++	NT

Note. –=one or more studies did not support this finding (with no positive studies), or the majority of studies did not support this finding; ±=an equal number of studies supported this finding as studies that did not support this finding; +=at least one study supported this finding, with no studies not supporting the finding, or the majority of studies supported the finding; ++=two or more studies supported this finding, with no studies not supporting the finding; +++=three or more studies supported this finding, with no studies not supporting the finding. ACTH=adrenocorticotropic hormone; CRF=corticotropin-releasing factor; CSF=cerebrospinal fluid; DST=dexamethasone suppression test; HPA=hypothalamic-pituitary-adrenal; NT=not tested (to our knowledge); PTSD=posttraumatic stress disorder.

[a]Findings of decreased urinary cortisol in older male combat veterans and Holocaust survivors and increased cortisol in younger female abuse survivors may be explainable by differences in sex, age, trauma type, or developmental epoch at the time of the trauma.

Neurohormonal Function in Panic Disorder

In patients with panic disorder, the responsiveness of the HPA system to a combined dexamethasone-CRF challenge test was higher than in psychiatrically healthy control subjects but lower than in depressed patients. The difference in responsiveness between patients with panic disorder and those with depression may be due to overexpression of vasopressin in major depression, which is known to synergize the effect of CRF at corticotropes. The results of the combined dexamethasone-CRH test indicate that a substantial portion of patients with panic disorder have disturbed HPA system regulation. If sensitization by repetitive panic attacks is indeed responsible for progressive HPA dysregulation, and if progressive HPA dysregulation is indeed of decisive importance for the pathogenesis of panic disorder, then therapeutic strategies capable of dampening the hyperactivity of the HPA–locus coeruleus "alarm system" are indicated. Patients with panic disorder have also been shown to have increased noradrenergic function as measured by increased responsiveness to yohimbine and other measures.

Release of glucocorticoids and/or catecholamines with stress may modulate the encoding of memories of the stressful event. Among the most characteristic features of anxiety disorders such as PTSD and panic disorder is that memories of the traumatic experience or original panic attack remain indelible for decades and are easily reawakened by all sorts of stimuli and stressors. The strength of traumatic memories relates, in part, to the degree to which certain neuromodulatory systems, particularly catecholamines and glucocorticoids, are activated by the traumatic experience. Evidence from experimental and clinical investigations suggests that memory processes remain susceptible to modulating influences after information has been acquired. Long-term alterations in these catecholaminergic and glucocorticoid systems may also be responsible for fragmentation of memories, hyperamnesia, amnesia, deficits in declarative memory, delayed recall of abuse, and other aspects of the wide range of memory distortions in PTSD.

Effects of Pharmacotherapy on Brain Circuits Mediating Anxiety

Pharmacotherapy of anxiety is associated with a modulation of neurohormonal systems mediating symptoms of anxiety. Administration of benzodiazepine medications acts directly on the GABA/benzodiazepine complex to promote release of the inhibitory neurotransmitter GABA. The SSRIs increase serotonin concentrations, which has secondary effects on glucocorticoid and noradrenergic systems. SSRIs have been shown to decrease cortisol response and autonomic response to stress in PTSD patients (Vermetten et al. 2006). Antidepressants also promote nerve growth in the hippocampus, an effect that has been hypothesized to underlie the mechanism by which antidepressants are efficacious for anxiety and depression (Santarelli et al. 2003).

For the clinician, some reference to how pharmacotherapy acts to normalize these systems might be useful. It may also be helpful to reference some of the recent

TABLE 4–3. Evidence for alterations in other neurotransmitter systems in anxiety disorders

Finding	PTSD	Panic disorder
Benzodiazepine		
Increased symptomatology with benzodiazepine antagonist	–	++
Opiate		
Naloxone-reversible analgesia	+	
Increased plasma β-endorphin response to exercise	+	
Increased endogenous opiates in CSF	+	
Serotonin		
Decreased serotonin reuptake site binding in platelets	++	
Decreased serotonin transmitter in platelets	–	
Blunted prolactin response to buspirone (5-HT_{1A} probe)	–	
Altered serotonin effect on cAMP in platelets (5-HT_{1A} probe)	–	
Thyroid		
Increased baseline thyroxine	+	
Increased TSH response to TRH	+	
Somatostatin		
Increased somatostatin levels at baseline in CSF	+	
Cholecystokinin (CCK)		
Increased anxiety symptoms with CCK administration	NT	++

Note. – = one or more studies did not support this finding (with no positive studies), or the majority of studies did not support this finding; + = at least one study supported this finding, with no studies not supporting the finding, or the majority of studies supported the finding; ++ = two or more studies supported this finding, with no studies not supporting the finding. cAMP = cyclic adenosine monophosphate; CSF = cerebrospinal fluid; 5-HT_{1A} = serotonin type 1A; NT = not tested (to our knowledge); PTSD = posttraumatic stress disorder; TRH = thyrotropin-releasing hormone; TSH = thyroid-stimulating hormone.

reviews of the concept of neuroplasticity, insofar as this is relevant to understanding anxiety.

A Working Model for the Neural Circuitry of Anxiety Disorders

Findings of the studies reviewed in this chapter are consistent with dysfunction of an interrelated neurochemical and neuroanatomical system in human anxiety disorders. PTSD and panic disorder have several biological and phenomenological similarities that allow them to be considered in relation to each other. Investigation of phobic disorders and generalized anxiety disorder is still in the early stages; although they have some phenomenological similarities to PTSD and panic disorder, it is premature to include them in a model for human anxiety disorders. Obsessive-compulsive disorder is different in many ways from these other disorders and therefore has not been reviewed in this chapter. Of the two anxiety disorders that are the focus of subsequent discussion—PTSD and panic disorder—PTSD is related more to the deleterious effects of environmental stress, whereas panic disorder is not as clearly related to stress and may be related more to genetic variability in anxiety. Therefore, a model can be created that incorporates information from animal and clinical research relevant to these disorders, keeping in mind that working models are subject to modification with new information, and that generalizations involving causality should be seen as merely speculative when derived from clinical studies that are, by their very nature, cross-sectional.

A biological model to explain pathological human anxiety should include both brain stem circuits and cortical and subcortical regions involved in memory and modulation of emotion. The evidence reviewed in this chapter is consistent with chronically increased function of neurochemical systems (CRF and norepinephrine) that mediate the stress response in anxiety disorders. Although activity at the central portion of the HPA axis is increased, responses at other portions of the HPA axis, including the pituitary and adrenal, and long-term effects on the hormonal final product, cortisol, do not show increased concentrations of the hormone; instead, levels are normal or low. Increased norepinephrine and CRF released in the brain act on specific brain areas (including the hippocampus; medial prefrontal, temporal, and parietal cortex; and cingulate) that are dysfunctional in human anxiety disorders. Other neurochemical systems, including benzodiazepines, opiates, dopamine, CCK, and neuropeptide Y, also play a role.

Hippocampal dysfunction may play a role in the pathological symptoms of anxiety. In stress-related anxiety disorders (i.e., PTSD), symptoms and cognitive dysfunction associated with PTSD may be linked to hippocampal dysfunction. Release of glucocorticoids or other stress-related factors (e.g., stress-induced decreases in brain-derived neurotrophic factor) may result in hippocampal damage, with lasting deficits in verbal declarative memory dysfunction in PTSD. Although hippocampal volume reduction appears to be specific to stress-related anxiety disorders, patients with panic disorder have had alterations of parahippocampal gyrus and other portions of extrahippocampal temporal lobe that may underlie declarative memory deficits also seen in panic disorder. Increased cortisol release with stress in both PTSD and panic disorder may result in amnesia and cognitive dysfunction associated with these disorders. Excessive release of norepinephrine with stressors in anxiety disorder patients will be predicted to result in decreased function of neurons, which may be related to both cognitive dysfunction and increased anxiety with stress. In addition, given the known role of the hippocampus in contextual fear, lasting damage to the hippocampus may contribute to excessive anxiety and fear responding in anxiety disorders. Finally, because the hippocampus is involved in integration of individual aspects of memory at the time of memory retrieval, hippocampal dysfunction may lead to memory fragmentation and amnesia in anxiety disorders.

The medial prefrontal cortex also plays a prominent role in anxiety. Moving up in terms of species complexity, the most salient change in brain architecture is the massive increase in cortical gray matter, especially frontal cortex. It is therefore not surprising that the frontal lobe plays a role in the phenomenon uniquely associated with our species—that is, emotion. The medial portion of the prefrontal cortex seems to have an important role in human emotion and anxiety. The medial prefrontal cortex (subcallosal gyrus [Brodmann area 25] and anterior cingulate [Brodmann area 32]) has inhibitory inputs that decrease amygdala responsiveness and has been hypothesized to mediate extinction of fear responding. Brodmann area 25 also stimulates the peripheral cortisol and sympathetic response to stress. Activation of this area has been shown to be a normal response to stress or increased emotionality. We have hypothesized that dysfunction in this area may mediate increased emotionality and failure of extinction to fear-inducing cues in anxiety disorders. Evidence to support this idea includes failure of normal activation in this area with yohimbine-induced provocation of anxiety in both PTSD and panic disorder and failure of activation/decreased blood flow with traumatic cue exposure in PTSD. Again, potentiated release of norepinephrine with stressors in PTSD and panic disorder is expected to be associated with a relative decrease in function of neurons in this area. Findings in anxiety disorder research are consistent, with a long history of literature, mostly from studies of lesions in human subjects, supporting a role for medial prefrontal cortex in emotionality.

◀ Key Clinical Points ▶

- Underlying the symptoms of anxiety disorders are alterations in the function and structure of brain areas involved in stress and memory. These alterations involve neurotransmitters and neural circuits that play a critical role in the stress response.
- Specific alterations include increased function of neurochemical systems (corticotropin-releasing factor and norepinephrine) that mediate the stress response, as well as dysregulation of the hypothalamic-pituitary-adrenal axis.
- The affected neurotransmitters and neurohormones are released in specific brain areas (including the hippocampus; medial prefrontal, temporal, and parietal cortex; and cingulate) that are dysfunctional in human anxiety disorders.
- Other neurochemical systems, including benzodiazepines, opiates, dopamine, cholecystokinin, and neuropeptide Y, also play a role in the maintenance of anxiety symptoms.
- Studies performed to date are encouraging, in that many findings from animal studies have been successfully applied to human anxiety disorders.
- The past decade has seen an exciting expansion of research in human anxiety disorders. Future research must continue to apply findings from the revolution in neuroscience to increase understanding of human anxiety disorders.

References

Abercrombie ED, Jacobs BL: Single-unit response of noradrenergic neurons in the locus coeruleus of freely moving cats, I: acutely presented stressful and nonstressful stimuli. J Neurosci 7:2837–2843, 1987

Baker DG, Ekhator NN, Kasckow JW, et al: Higher levels of basal serial CSF cortisol in combat veterans with posttraumatic stress disorder. Am J Psychiatry 162:992–994, 2005

Bremner JD: Brain Imaging Handbook. New York, WW Norton, 2005

Bremner JD: Traumatic stress: effects on the brain. Dialogues Clin Neurosci 8:445–461, 2006

Bremner JD: Functional neuroimaging in posttraumatic stress disorder. Exp Rev Neurotherapeutics 7:393–405, 2007

Bremner JD, Randall PR, Scott TM, et al: MRI-based measurement of hippocampal volume in patients with combat-related posttraumatic stress disorder. Am J Psychiatry 152:973–981, 1995

Bremner JD, Krystal JH, Southwick SM, et al: Noradrenergic mechanisms in stress and anxiety, I: preclinical studies. Synapse 23:28–38, 1996a

Bremner JD, Krystal JH, Southwick SM, et al: Noradrenergic mechanisms in stress and anxiety, II: clinical studies. Synapse 23:39–51, 1996b

Bremner JD, Innis RB, Ng CK, et al: Positron emission tomography measurement of cerebral metabolic correlates of yohimbine administration in combat-related posttraumatic stress disorder. Arch Gen Psychiatry 54:246–254, 1997a

Bremner JD, Licinio J, Darnell A, et al: Elevated CSF corticotropin-releasing factor concentrations in posttraumatic stress disorder. Am J Psychiatry 154:624–629, 1997b

Bremner JD, Southwick SM, Charney DS: The neurobiology of posttraumatic stress disorder: an integration of animal and human research, in Posttraumatic Stress Disorder: A Comprehensive Text. Edited by Saigh P, Bremner JD. New York, Allyn and Bacon, 1999a, pp 103–143

Bremner JD, Staib L, Kaloupek D, et al: Neural correlates of exposure to traumatic pictures and sound in Vietnam combat veterans with and without posttraumatic stress disorder: a positron emission tomography study. Biological Psychiatry 45:806–816, 1999b

Bremner JD, Vermetten E, Schmahl C, et al: Positron emission tomographic imaging of neural correlates of a fear acquisition and extinction paradigm in women with childhood sexual abuse-related posttraumatic stress disorder. Psychol Med 35:791–806, 2005

Bremner JD, Vermetten E, Kelley ME: Cortisol, dehydroepiandrosterone, and estradiol measured over 24 hours in women with childhood sexual abuse-related posttraumatic stress disorder. J Nerv Ment Dis 195:919–927, 2007

Caggiula AR, Antelman SM, Aul E, et al: Prior stress attenuates the analgesic response but sensitizes the corticosterone and cortical dopamine responses to stress 10 days later. Psychopharmacology 999:233–237, 1989

Cannon WB: The James-Lange theory of emotions: a critical examination and an alternative theory. Am J Psychol 39:106–124, 1927

Chalmers DT, Lovenberg TW, Grigoriadis DE, et al: Corticotropin-releasing factor receptors: from molecular biology to drug design. Trends Pharmacol Sci 17:166–172, 1996

Chapman WP, Schroeder HR, Guyer G, et al: Physiological evidence concerning the importance of the amygdaloid nuclear region in the integration of circulating functions and emotion in man. Science 129:949–950, 1954

Charney DS, Bremner JD: The neurobiology of anxiety disorders, in Neurobiology of Mental Illness. Edited by Charney DS, Nestler EJ, Bunney SS. Oxford, UK, Oxford University Press, 1999, pp 494–517

Charney DS, Deutch A: A functional neuroanatomy of anxiety and fear: implications for the pathophysiology and treatment of anxiety disorders. Crit Rev Neurobiol 10:419–446, 1996

Clark FM, Proudfit HK: The projection of locus coeruleus neurons to the spinal cord in the rat determined by anterograde tracing combined with immunocytochemistry. Brain Res 538:231–245, 1991

Coplan JD, Andrews MW, Rosenblum LA, et al: Persistent elevations of cerebrospinal fluid concentrations of corticotropin-releasing factor in adult nonhuman primates exposed to early-life stressors: implications for the pathophysiology of mood and anxiety disorders. Proc Natl Acad Sci USA 93:1619–1623, 1996

Dallman MF, Jones MT: Corticosteroid feedback control of ACTH secretion: effect of stress-induced corticosterone secretion on subsequent stress responses in the rat. Endocrinology 92:1367–1375, 1973

Damasio H, Grabowski T, Frank R, et al: The return of Phineas Gage: clues about the brain from the skull of a famous patient. Science 264:1102–1105, 1994

Davis M: The role of the amygdala in fear and anxiety. Annu Rev Neurosci 15:353–375, 1992

Deutch AY, Roth RH: The determinants of stress-induced activation of the prefrontal cortical dopamine system. Prog Brain Res 85:367–402, 1990

Devinsky O, Morrell MJ, Vogt BA: Contributions of anterior cingulate to behavior. Brain 118:279–306, 1995

Duman RS, Malberg JE, Nakagawa S: Regulation of adult neurogenesis by psychotropic drugs and stress. J Pharmacol Exp Ther 299:401–407, 2001

Elzinga BM, Schmahl CS, Vermetten E, et al: Higher cortisol levels following exposure to traumatic reminders in abuse-related PTSD. Neuropsychopharmacology 28:1656–1665, 2003

Fride E, Dan Y, Feldon J, et al: Effects of prenatal stress on vulnerability to stress in prepubertal and adult rats. Physiol Behav 37:681–687, 1986

Gilbertson MW, Shenton ME, Ciszewski A, et al: Smaller hippocampal volume predicts pathologic vulnerability to psychological trauma. Nat Neurosci 5:1242–1247, 2002

Goldman-Rakic PS: Topography of cognition: parallel distributed networks in primate association cortex. Annu Rev Neurosci 11:137–156, 1988

Gorman JM, Liebowitz MR, Fyer AJ, et al: A neuroanatomical hypothesis for panic disorder. Am J Psychiatry 146:148–161, 1989

Gould E, McEwen BS, Tanapat P, et al: Neurogenesis in the dentate gyrus of the adult tree shrew is regulated by psychosocial stress and NMDA receptor activation. J Neurosci 17:2492–2498, 1997

Graeff F: Role of 5HT in defensive behavior and anxiety. Rev Neurosci 4:181–211, 1993

Gray JA: The Neuropsychology of Anxiety. New York, Oxford University Press, 1982

Gunne LM, Reis DJ: Changes in brain catecholamines associated with electrical stimulation of amygdaloid nucleus. Life Sci 11:804–809, 1963

Gur RC, Gur RE, Resnick SM, et al: The effect of anxiety on cortical cerebral blood flow and metabolism. J Cereb Blood Flow Metab 7:173–177, 1987

Hilton SM, Zbrozyna AW: Amygdaloid region for defense reactions and its efferent pathway to the brain stem. J Physiol 165:160–173, 1963

Iwata J, LeDoux JE, Meeley MP, et al: Intrinsic neurons in the amygdaloid field projected to by the medial geniculate body mediate emotional responses conditioned to acoustic stimuli. Brain Res 383:195–214, 1986

Jones EG, Powell TP: An anatomical study of converging sensory pathways within the cerebral cortex of the monkey. Brain 93:793–820, 1970

Kitayama N, Vaccarino V, Kutner M, et al: Magnetic resonance imaging (MRI) measurement of hippocampal volume in posttraumatic stress disorder: a meta-analysis. J Affect Disord 88:79–86, 2005

Kitayama N, Quinn S, Bremner JD: Smaller volume of anterior cingulate cortex in abuse-related posttraumatic stress disorder. J Affect Disord 90:171–174, 2006

Ladd CO, Owens MJ, Nemeroff CB: Persistent changes in CRF neuronal systems produced by maternal separation. Endocrinology 137:1212–1218, 1996

LeDoux JE: Emotional memory systems in the brain. Behav Brain Res 58:69–79, 1993

LeDoux JE: The Emotional Brain: The Mysterious Underpinnings of Emotional Life. New York, Simon & Schuster, 1996

LeDoux JE, Romanski L, Xagoraris A: Indelibility of subcortical emotional memories. J Cogn Neurosci 1:238–243, 1989

LeDoux JE, Cicchetti P, Xagoraris A, et al: The lateral amygdaloid nucleus: sensory interface of the amygdala in fear conditioning. J Neurosci 10:1062–1069, 1990

Levine S: Plasma-free corticosteroid response to electric shock in rats stimulated in infancy. Science 135:795–796, 1962

Levine S, Weiner SG, Coe CL: Temporal and social factors influencing behavioral and hormonal responses to separation in mother and infant squirrel monkeys. Psychoneuroendocrinology 4:297–306, 1993

Liberzon I, Phan KL: Brain-imaging studies of posttraumatic stress disorder. CNS Spectr 8:641–650, 2003

Mason JW, Giller EL, Kosten TR, et al: Urinary free cortisol levels in post-traumatic stress disorder patients. J Nerv Ment Dis 174:145–149, 1986

Mayer EA, Naliboff BD, Chang L, Coutinho SV: Stress and the gastrointestinal tract, V: stress and irritable bowel syndrome. Am J Gastrointest Liver Physiol 280:G519-G524, 2001

McDonald AJ: Organization of amygdaloid projections to prefrontal cortex and associated striatum in the rat. Neuroscience 44:1–14, 1991a

McDonald AJ: Topographical organization of amygdaloid projections to the caudatoputamen nucleus accumbens, and related striatal-like areas of the rat brain. Neuroscience 44:15–33, 1991b

McEwen BS, Angulo J, Cameron H, et al: Paradoxical effects of adrenal steroids on the brain: protection versus degeneration. Biol Psychiatry 31:177–199, 1992

Meaney MJ, Aitken DH, van Berkel C, et al: Effect of neonatal handling on age-related impairments associated with the hippocampus. Science 239:766–768, 1988

Meaney MJ, Aitken DH, Sharma S, et al: Neonatal handling alters adrenocortical negative feedback sensitivity and hippocampal type II glucocorticoid receptor binding in the rat. Neuroendocrinology 50:597–604, 1989

Mendelson S, McEwen BS: Autoradiographic analyses of the effects of restraint-induced stress on 5-HT1A, 5-HT1C and 5-HT2 receptors in the dorsal hippocampus of male and female rats. Neuroendocrinology 54:454–461, 1991

Moghaddam B, Adams B, Verma A, et al: Activation of glutamatergic neurotransmission by ketamine: a novel step in the pathway from NMDA receptor blockade to dopaminergic and cognitive disruptions associated with the prefrontal cortex. J Neurosci 17:2912–2127, 1997

Morgan MA, LeDoux JE: Differential contribution of dorsal and ventral medial prefrontal cortex to the acquisition and extinction of conditioned fear in rats. Behav Neurosci 109:681–688, 1995

Morgan MA, Romanski LM, LeDoux JE: Extinction of emotional learning: contribution of medial prefrontal cortex. Neurosci Lett 163:109–113, 1993

Nibuya M, Morinobu S, Duman RS: Regulation of BDNF and trkB mRNA in rat brain by chronic electroconvulsive seizure and antidepressant drug treatments. J Neurosci 15:7539–7547, 1995

Papez JW: A proposed mechanism of emotion. AMA Archives of Neurology and Psychiatry 38:725–743, 1937

Petty F, Sherman AD: Regional aspects of the prevention of learned helplessness by desipramine. Life Sci 26:1447–1452, 1980

Petty F, Kramer G, Wilson L: Prevention of learned helplessness: in vivo correlation with cortical serotonin. Pharmacol Biochem Behav 43:361–367, 1992

Pitman RK: Posttraumatic stress disorder, hormones, and memory (editorial). Biol Psychiatry 26:221–223, 1989

Pitman RK: Investigating the pathogenesis of posttraumatic stress disorder with neuroimaging. J Clin Psychiatry 62:47–54, 2001

Plotsky PM, Meaney MJ: Early, postnatal experience alters hypothalamic corticotropin-releasing factor (CRF) mRNA, median eminence CRF content and stress-induced release in adult rats. Brain Res Mol Brain Res 18:195–200, 1993

Quirk GJ, Garcia R, Gonzalez-Lima F: Prefrontal mechanisms in extinction of conditioned fear. Biol Psychiatry 60:337–343, 2006

Radley JJ, Sisti HM, Hao J, et al: Chronic behavioral stress induces apical dendritic reorganization in pyramidal neurons of the medial prefrontal cortex. Neuroscience 125:1–6, 2004

Rauch SL, Whalen PJ, Shin LM, et al: Exaggerated amygdala response to masked facial stimuli in posttraumatic stress disorder: a functional MRI study. Biological Psychiatry 47:769–776, 2000

Rauch SL, Shin LM, Segal E, et al: Selectively reduced regional cortical volumes in post-traumatic stress disorder. Neuroreport 14:913–916, 2003

Rauch SL, Shin LM, Phelps EA: Neurocircuitry models of posttraumatic stress disorder and extinction: human neuroimaging research—past, present, and future. Biol Psychiatry 60:376–382, 2006

Redmond DE: Studies of the nucleus locus coeruleus in monkeys and hypotheses for neuropsychopharmacology, in Psychopharmacology: The Third Generation of Progress. Edited by Meltzer HY. New York, Raven, 1987, pp 967–975

Rodriguez G, Cogorno P, Gris A, et al: Regional cerebral blood flow and anxiety: a correlation study in neurologically normal patients. J Cereb Blood Flow Metab 9:410–416, 1989

Romanski LM, LeDoux JE: Information cascade from primary auditory cortex to the amygdala: corticocortical and corticoamygdaloid projections of temporal cortex in the rat. Cereb Cortex 3:515–532, 1993

Roth RH, Tam SY, Ida Y, et al: Stress and the mesocorticolimbic dopamine systems. Ann N Y Acad Sci 537:138–147, 1988

Santarelli L, Saxe M, Gross C, et al: Requirement of hippocampal neurogenesis for the behavioral effects of antidepressants. Science 301:805–809, 2003

Sapolsky RM: Why stress is bad for your brain. Science 273:749–750, 1996

Sapolsky RM, Krey LC, McEwen BS: Glucocorticoid-sensitive hippocampal neurons are involved in terminating the adrenocortical stress response. Proc Natl Acad Sci USA 81:6174–6178, 1984

Sawchenko PE, Swanson LW: Central noradrenergic pathways for the integration of hypothalamic neuroendocrine and autonomic responses. Science 214:685–687, 1983a

Sawchenko PE, Swanson LW: The organization of forebrain afferents to the paraventricular and supraoptic nuclei of the rat. J Comp Neurol 218:121–144, 1983b

Selemon LD, Goldman-Rakic PS: Common cortical and subcortical targets of the dorsolateral prefrontal and posterior parietal cortices in the rhesus monkey: evidence for a distributed neural network subserving spatially guided behavior. J Neurosci 8:4049–4068, 1988

Shin LM, Orr SP, Carson MA: Regional cerebral blood flow in the amygdala and medial prefrontal cortex during traumatic imagery in male and female Vietnam veterans with PTSD. Arch Gen Psychiatry 61:168–176, 2004

Smith ME: Bilateral hippocampal volume reduction in adults with post-traumatic stress disorder: a meta-analysis of structural MRI studies. Hippocampus 15:798–807, 2005

Southwick SM, Krystal JH, Morgan CA, et al: Abnormal noradrenergic function in posttraumatic stress disorder. Arch Gen Psychiatry 50:295–305, 1993

Squire LR, Zola-Morgan S: The medial temporal lobe memory system. Science 253:2380–2386, 1991

Stanton ME, Gutierrez YR, Levine S: Maternal deprivation potentiates pituitary-adrenal stress responses in infant rats. Behav Neurosci 102:692–700, 1988

Stein MB, Goldin PR, Sareen J, et al: Increased amygdala activation to angry and contemptuous faces in generalized social phobia. Arch Gen Psychiatry 59:1027–1034, 2002

Thierry AM, Pirot S, Gioanni Y, et al: Dopamine function in the prefrontal cortex. Adv Pharmacol 42:717–720, 1998

Vermetten E, Vythilingam M, Southwick SM, et al: Long-term treatment with paroxetine increases verbal declarative memory and hippocampal volume in posttraumatic stress disorder. Biol Psychiatry 54:693–702, 2003

Vermetten E, Vythilingam M, Schmahl C, et al: Alterations in stress reactivity after long-term treatment with paroxetine in women with posttraumatic stress disorder. Ann NY Acad Sci 1071:184–202, 2006

Vogt BA, Finch DM, Olson CR: Functional heterogeneity in cingulate cortex: the anterior executive and posterior evaluative regions. Cereb Cortex 2:435–443, 1992

Woodward SH, Kaloupek DG, Streeter CC, et al: Decreased anterior cingulate volume in combat-related PTSD. Biol Psychiatry 59:582–587, 2006

Yehuda R: Advances in understanding neuroendocrine alterations in PTSD and their therapeutic implications. Ann NY Acad Sci 1071:137–166, 2006

Yehuda R, Lowy MT, Southwick SM, et al: Lymphocyte glucocorticoid receptor number in posttraumatic stress disorder. Am J Psychiatry 149:499–504, 1991

Yehuda R, Southwick SM, Krystal JH, et al: Enhanced suppression of cortisol with low dose dexamethasone in posttraumatic stress disorder. Am J Psychiatry 150:83–86, 1993

Yehuda R, Teicher MH, Trestman RL, et al: Cortisol regulation in posttraumatic stress disorder and major depression: a chronobiological analysis. Biol Psychiatry 40:79–88, 1996

Recommended Readings

Bremner JD: Does Stress Damage the Brain? Understanding Trauma-Related Disorders From a Mind-Body Perspective. New York, WW Norton, 2002

Bremner JD: Functional neuroimaging in posttraumatic stress disorder. Expert Rev Neurother 7:393–405, 2007

Bremner JD, Elzinga B, Schmahl C, et al: Structural and functional plasticity of the human brain in posttraumatic stress disorder. Prog Brain Res 167:171–186, 2008

Charney DS: Psychobiological mechanisms of resilience and vulnerability: implications for successful adaptation to extreme stress. Am J Psychiatry 161:195–216, 2004

Charney DS, Bremner JD: The neurobiology of anxiety disorders, in Neurobiology of Mental Illness. Edited by Charney DS, Nestler EJ, Bunney SS. Oxford, UK, Oxford University Press, 1999, pp 494–517

Nemeroff CB, Bremner JD, Foa EB, et al: Posttraumatic stress disorder: a state-of-the-science review. J Psychiatr Res 40:1–21, 2006

Pitman RK: Investigating the pathogenesis of posttraumatic stress disorder with neuroimaging. J Clin Psychiatry 62:47–54, 2001

Trauma Links. Available at http://www.dougbremner.com/traumalinks.html. Accessed December 3, 2008.

Chapter 5

Anxious Traits and Temperaments

Steven Taylor, Ph.D., ABPP
Jonathan S. Abramowitz, Ph.D., ABPP
Dean McKay, Ph.D.
Gordon J.G. Asmundson, Ph.D.

Traits are dispositions that pervasively influence a person's behavior across many situations and thereby lead to consistency in behavior (Guilford 1959; Mischel 1973). Trait concepts refer, as a rule, to relatively enduring characteristics that have some value in predicting behavior and differentiating one person from another (Anastasi 1948). Thus, traits tend to be stable for years, although they may change over time, for example, as a result of maturation or other developmental factors. Most traits are probably dimensional variables, although some are categorical (present vs. absent) (Waller and Meehl 1998). Traits include narrow variables, such as trait anxiety (anxiety proneness), and broader factors, such as negative affectivity (also called neuroticism), that subsume many narrow traits. Negative affectivity, for example, subsumes trait anxiety as well as proneness to experience other aversive emotional states, such as irritability or depressed mood (Costa and McCrae 1995). The severity of a person's level of negative affectivity corresponds to his or her risk of developing emotional problems; people with high scores on this trait, compared to people with low scores, are at greater risk for developing anxiety disorders and other emotional problems (Krueger and Tackett 2006).

Temperamental variables are particular types of traits, which appear early in child development (e.g., by 18 months of age), are influenced by genetic factors, and are at least moderately stable over time (Rettew and McKee 2005). The boundaries between temperament and personality are not entirely clear. Negative affectivity, for example, can be regarded as a personality dimension or as a temperamental trait. Similarly, extraversion or positive affectivity can be regarded as both a personality dimension and a temperament. One way of distinguishing personality from temperament is to reserve the latter for early-appearing and more constitutionally based predispositions onto which personality traits are built and modified over the life span (Cloninger and Svrakic 1997; Rettew and McKee 2005; Rothbart and Ahadi 1994). From this perspective, temperaments are the building blocks on which more complex personality traits are formed as a function of experience (e.g., social learning) and cognitive development. Personality, unlike temperament, is characterized by complex patterns of evaluating the self and others, goals, beliefs, and values, and behavioral repertoires acquired over the life span. Given the assumption that temperament and the environment interact to produce personality, researchers have typically used the term *temperament* in describing children and infants, whereas personality is generally applied to adults and adolescents, even if the specific dimensions being measured appear to be quite similar (Kagan 1997). In this chapter we follow the convention in the literature by referring to temperament variables as those assessed in children and infants, and personality variables as those assessed in adults and adolescents, regardless of the overlap in those constructs. Throughout this chapter, we use the term *trait* as shorthand for personality trait. When we specifically refer to temperamental traits, the term *temperament* is used, even though the distinction between personality and temperament is to a large degree arbitrary.

There are three main reasons why personality and temperament are important for understanding anxiety disorders. First, specific, narrow traits (e.g., anxiety sensitivity, intolerance of uncertainty) may be vulnerability factors for particular anxiety disorders (e.g., panic disorder) or specific features or subtypes of disorders (e.g., compulsive checking). Second, broad traits (e.g., negative affectivity) may be vulnerability factors that influence a person's risk for several kinds of disorders, such as one or more anxiety or mood disorders. Such broad traits could explain why anxiety and mood disorders (and other disorders) are so commonly comorbid with one another; they are all purportedly influenced by common traits. The combined influences of narrow and broad traits may explain why some people develop a particular disorder (e.g., panic disorder), whereas other people develop multiple disorders (e.g., comorbid panic disorder, social phobia, and major depressive disorder). This is a diathesis-stress model of anxiety disorders; the diathesis (i.e., the trait or the etiologic factors that shape the trait) interacts with particular stressors (e.g., events that evoke a high degree of anxiety, such as a bank holdup) to give rise to a particular disorder (e.g., posttraumatic stress disorder).

The third reason for the importance of traits and temperaments is that some of them may be endophenotypes, that is, trait-like variables that are correlated with a given disorder and are assumed to lie somewhere in the causal chain between genes and psychiatric symptoms or disorders (Gottesman and Gould 2003). To meet the criteria for an endophenotype, a marker must be present in affected individuals, it should be heritable and cosegregate with the disorder, it should be state independent (i.e., manifested in an individual, whether or not the disorder is active), and it must be found among unaffected relatives of patients at a higher rate than in the general population (Delorme et al. 2005). The endophenotype concept is broad; it potentially includes any trait-like variable or stable marker that lies anywhere in the causal chain between genes and disorders. In addition to personality and temperament, candidate endophenotypes may include neurophysiological, biochemical, endocrinological, neuroanatomical, cognitive, or neuropsychological variables and physiological traits or markers, such as the ease by which conditioned fears are acquired (*conditionability*) (Cannon and Keller 2006; Gottesman and Gould 2003). Endophenotypes do not include phenotypes (i.e., symptoms or disorders).

Why study endophenotypes? Given the phenotypic and etiologic complexity of anxiety disorders, it appears likely that many different types of genetic and environmental factors (e.g., learning experiences) play a role in the generation of anxiety disorders, with each of these factors having a small, cumulative effect on a person's risk for developing anxiety problems (Cannon and Keller 2006). To add to the complexity, genes and the environment are likely to interact with one another. Several candidate genes have been identified, as reviewed elsewhere in this volume (see chapters on pathogenesis of specific disorders). However, the process of gene hunting has been slow and laborious, with many false starts, including failures to replicate earlier results. Accordingly, researchers have focused their attention on endophenotypes in an effort to identify traits or markers associated with particular brain systems or circuits that may be involved in a given disorder. Endophenotypes are thought to be important because, in terms of the causal chain, they are closer to the genes influencing these disorders than are complex phenotypes such as anxiety disorders. Moreover, the study of endophenotypes enables researchers to simplify the study of anxiety disorders; if an endophenotype is associated with a particular brain circuit (out of the many circuits involved in a given disorder), then the study of endophenotypes can help researchers identify the genetic and environmental factors that shape the function or malfunction of the circuit (Cannon and Keller 2006).

In the remainder of this chapter, we review the major traits and temperaments that are relevant for understanding the etiology of anxiety disorders. First, we review the role of temperament in anxiety disorders, including an examination of the way in which early temperamental factors may be related to later emergence of anxiety disorders. Second, we review the narrow and broad personality traits and place them in the context of a proposed hierarchical structure of personality in which narrow traits are structured to form broad traits. Third, we review major findings from behavioral-genetic research, providing clues about the broad and narrow genetic traits that play a role in anxiety disorders. Some of these factors may represent the genetic elements shaping the major temperaments and personality dimensions. Fourth, we provide a review of endophenotypes that are not covered in the review of personality or temperament traits (e.g., conditionability). We conclude the chapter with a discussion of the clinical implications of the current state of knowledge of traits and temperaments for treating anxiety disorders and for reducing the risk that vulnerable individuals will develop these disorders in the first place.

Temperament

Various dimensional systems of temperament have been proposed, many of which are hierarchically organized; that is, narrow temperament traits form broader, high-order temperament traits. Three higher-order traits are common to most models of temperament (Rettew and McKee 2005): the first is the degree of sensitivity to signals of punishment and the propensity to experience negative emotions. This trait is variously known as *negative affectivity*, *neuroticism*, or *harm avoidance*. The second is the tendency toward novelty- or sensation-seeking, along with high energy, impulsivity, and the propensity to experience positive emotions. This trait is variously labeled as *novelty-seeking*, *sensation-seeking*, or *extraversion*. The third is the extent to which the person is able to engage in emotional regulation that involves an ability to persist, pay attention, delay gratification, plan, and modulate emotional responses. This trait, variously called *effortful control* or *persistence*, can serve to modify or override the outward expression of the first two broad dimensions.

Studies of children, including longitudinal research, indicate that high risk of developing an anxiety or mood disorder is associated with particular patterns of temperament, especially high levels of negative affectivity, low levels of extraversion, and low levels of effort control (Lohr et al. 2004; Rettew and McKee 2005). A related finding is that high levels of behavioral inhibition (BI) in children are associated with a heightened risk of developing anxiety or mood disorders in adolescence or adulthood (Biederman et al. 1993; Schwartz et al. 1999). BI, which contains elements of high negative affectivity and low extraversion, is characterized by the tendency to be highly physiologically reactive, fearful, and reticent in novel social and nonsocial situations (Kagan 1994). BI is one of the most stable temperamental characteristics in childhood, although there is evidence BI can become less severe over time. BI may be more likely to abate over time if the child also has a high degree of another temperamental trait—effortful control. In such cases, the child would probably be strongly motivated to overcome his or her fears, which would thereby facilitate the development of emotion coping skills. BI may also diminish as a result of supportive caregivers who encourage the child to enter fearful situations and reinforce the child's efforts to develop coping skills (Degnan and Fox 2007).

Various attempts have been made to explain the association between temperament and psychopathology. Among the most promising is the diathesis-stress model (Lohr et al. 2004; Rettew and McKee 2005). In this model, temperament traits, alone or in combination, predispose the child to develop later psychopathology; however, extreme temperaments do not inevitably lead to emotional disorders. Temperaments that are at odds with the demands of the surroundings put the person at risk for psychopathology, whereas a good match between the person's disposition and the supports and demands of various contexts (family, school, and peer group) promotes positive adjustment (Lohr et al. 2004).

The diathesis-stress model predicts that the development of specific disorders is a result of an interaction between particular types of stressors and particular temperaments. Consistent with this model, evidence suggests that among children who are exposed to recurrent teasing by peers, the risk for developing social anxiety disorder later in life is greater for children with high levels of BI, in contrast to children with low BI (Lerman 2004). Similarly, children with high levels of BI, in contrast to those with low BI, are at greater risk of developing posttraumatic stress disorder after being exposed to a traumatic event (Podniesinski 2004).

Temperament may also have indirect effects on psychological adjustment, because it influences the selection of environments, activities, and people (Strelau 1983). A child with severe BI, for example, would tend to avoid novel or unfamiliar situations, thereby constraining his or her life experiences (Sroufe 1997). This could lead to failure to develop adequate social skills (Henderson and Fox 1998). As a result, peers may perceive the person as socially inept or odd and therefore may shun, ridicule, or reject him or her. In turn, this could lead to further avoidance and intensified social anxiety.

To add to the complexity of the temperament-psychopathology relationship, it is also possible that psychopathology influences temperament (Lohr et al. 2004; Rettew and McKee 2005). This is known as the *scar hypothesis*. To illustrate, posttraumatic stress disorder could lead the individual to become pervasively hypervigilant for threat, and therefore the person would become physiologically aroused and fearful in unfamiliar situations. In other words, posttraumatic stress disorder could increase the severity of BI.

Although evidence supports the role of temperaments in shaping the child's risk of developing later psychopathology, it is quite likely that a given disorder can arise from various developmental pathways (Rettew and McKee 2005). To illustrate, the risk of developing obsessive-compulsive disorder (OCD) may be shaped by particular temperaments (e.g., negative affectivity) in some children and may arise from autoimmune mechanisms in others (Swedo 2002).

Broad Personality Traits

Negative Affectivity

Negative affectivity may serve as the most general of the personality factors that have been found to be predictive of later anxiety problems (Craske 2003; Watson and Clark 1984). Contemporary models of personality regard negative affectivity as a trait of major importance. It is one of the "Big Five" personality factors (Costa and McCrae 1995) and is also one of the three dimensions of the tripartite model of personality (Clark and Watson 1991).

Negative affectivity has been implicated in several general models of anxiety disorder risk, whereby the narrow traits subsumed under negative affectivity each contribute to particular symptoms (Zinbarg and Barlow 1996). This association is illustrated in Table 5–1. If the categories of anxiety disorders described in DSM-IV-TR (American Psychiatric Association 2000) are to be considered valid, then it is essential that vulnerability factors specific to each one be identified. Preliminary research supports this contention (Zinbarg and Barlow 1996). For example, anxiety sensitivity (a lower-order trait) predicts the occurrence of panic attacks (Zinbarg and Barlow 1996).

Tripartite Model of Anxiety and Depression

A model of general vulnerability that has gained considerable attention is the tripartite model of anxiety and depression (Clark and Watson 1991; Clark et al. 1994). The three factors specified by the model are negative affectivity, positive affectivity (i.e., the tendency to experience positive emotions), and physiological arousal (the tendency to become physiologically aroused). The model proposes that anxiety disorders (and depression) arise from proneness to negative affectivity, with (low) positive affectivity associated with depression proneness, and elevated physiological arousal accounting for anxiety disorders generally. The model also allows for the possibility that narrow personality factors contribute to vulnerability to specific anxiety diagnoses.

The tripartite model has received substantial empirical scrutiny. Research findings support the assumption that negative affectivity and physiological hyperarousal are related to anxiety symptoms (e.g., Watson et al. 1995a, 1995b). Physiological hyperarousal is especially predictive of panic attacks (Joiner et al. 1999). Low positive affectivity was found to be associated with depression in the aforementioned studies. However, other research evidence suggests that low positive affectivity is also associated with social anxiety disorder (Hughes et al. 2006; Kotov et al. 2007). This result challenges the model's assumption that low positive affectivity is specifically linked to depression.

Two-Factor Model

In order to examine how various psychiatric disorders tend to co-occur, Krueger (1999) conducted a factor analysis using data from a large multisite epidemiological study of psychiatric comorbidity (Kessler et al. 1994). Two factors were identified: externalizing (representing substance use disorders) and internalizing (representing anxiety and depressive disorders). The internalizing factor, which resembles the broad trait of negative affectivity, was composed of two narrower factors labeled anxious-misery and fear (see Table 5–1). This model has since been replicated, and the factors have been shown to be stable at approximately one month follow-up (Vollebergh et al. 2001).

Although the research literature on this model is still in early development, there are indications that it will result in more precise prediction than either negative affectivity or the tripartite model. For example, Cox et al. (2002) showed that the anxious-misery factor predicted posttraumatic stress disorder but the fear factor did not. This model may also be promising for use in making predictions regarding the role of depression in anxiety, and for clearer conceptualizations of the relation between depression and anxiety. This application would be particularly relevant given the high rate of comorbidity of depression with anxiety disorders (Craske 1999).

TABLE 5–1. Broad and narrow traits related to anxiety disorders

Anxiety-related broad traits	Anxiety-related narrow traits subsumed within broad traits	Symptoms correlated with elevated scores on traits
Traits from tripartite model		
Negative affectivity		All anxiety and depressive symptoms associated with elevated negative affectivity
	Trait anxiety	All anxiety symptoms associated with elevated trait anxiety
	Anxiety sensitivity	Anxiety in general and panic attacks in particular
	Intolerance of uncertainty	Related to all anxiety symptoms, but particularly to worry, obsessions, and compulsions
Physiological arousal		All anxiety symptoms are associated with elevated physiological arousal. Panic attacks are especially strongly related to high physiological arousal.
Traits from two-factor model		
Internalizing		Linked to symptoms of all anxiety and depressive disorders
	Anxious-misery	Depression, worry, and symptoms of posttraumatic stress disorder
	Fear proneness	Symptoms of social and specific phobias, agoraphobia, and panic attacks

Broad Traits in Perspective

To summarize, broad trait models of anxiety risk have been refined in recent years to include a three-factor model (tripartite model) and a two-factor model that are part of a larger model describing all psychiatric disorders. At present, these models are useful for making predictions about constellations of anxiety disorders. However, these conceptualizations do not stand alone; instead, they are the basis for hierarchical models that include narrow traits that have greater specificity for individual disorders. Components of the tripartite model (e.g., physiological arousal) and the two-factor model (e.g., anxious-misery) show promise for describing anxious conditions beyond that offered by a single-factor model such as negative affectivity. In order to adequately describe treatment models, refinement of the broad trait models necessarily requires the inclusion of narrow traits.

Narrow Personality Traits

Narrow traits are concrete personality variables with clear behavioral connotations. This is in contrast to the broad personality traits, which are more general or abstract. In this section, we describe the narrow traits with the strongest empirical support for linkage to anxiety symptoms and disorders.

Trait Anxiety

Trait anxiety is defined as proneness to respond with tension, apprehension, and heightened autonomic nervous system activity (Spielberger et al. 1970). From an evolutionary perspective, trait anxiety is adaptive because it activates the body's natural defense mechanisms (e.g., sympathetic arousal, urges to escape) under threatening situations and thereby increases the chances of survival. Although trait anxiety varies widely among people, those with anxiety disorders reliably evidence the highest levels (Zinbarg and Barlow 1996).

Two types of models of trait anxiety have been advanced. Neurophysiological models propose that individuals susceptible to anxiety disorders have greater reactivity of the brain's BI system (i.e., the septohippocampal circuits), which makes the person highly sensitive to signals of punishment, nonreward, and novelty (Gray and McNaughton 1996). Norepinephrine, serotonin, and gamma-aminobutyric acid have been cited as neurotransmitters that might mediate such sensitivities (e.g., Zuckerman 1995). Although neurophysiological models garner some empirical support from animal research, the wealth of research with humans has produced findings inconsistent with this approach and implicates the importance of cognitive variables.

Cognitive models of trait anxiety posit that anxiety arises from systematic biases in information processing involving the tendency to closely attend to threat-relevant stimuli and to interpret such stimuli in ways that magnify the perceived probability and severity of threat (e.g., Williams et al. 1997). These models predict that highly trait-anxious individuals are characterized by 1) hypervigilance to threat and 2) the tendency to interpret ambiguous stimuli in threatening ways. There is considerable experimental evidence directly supporting cognitive models of trait anxiety in nonclinical and clinical populations (e.g., Calvo and Castillo 1997). Moreover, studies that have directly tested both the cognitive and neurophysiological models have found evidence favoring the former over the latter (e.g., Calvo and Cano-Vindel 1997).

Anxiety Sensitivity

Anxiety sensitivity (AS) is the fear of arousal-related body sensations based on beliefs that these sensations have harmful physical, psychological, or social consequences (Reiss and McNally 1985). AS is conceptualized as a contributor to individual differences in general fearfulness and as a diathesis for various types of anxiety disorders (Reiss and McNally 1985; Taylor 1999). This is because AS is an anxiety amplifier; when highly anxiety-sensitive people become anxious, they become alarmed about their arousal-related sensations, which further intensifies their anxiety. Consistent with this formulation, evidence shows that AS is elevated in people with various types of anxiety disorders, compared with control subjects, and that a person's current level of AS predicts the risk of future anxiety symptoms, particularly the risk for panic attacks (Cox et al. 1999; Schmidt et al. 1997, 1999).

Although AS is moderately correlated with trait anxiety, the two can be distinguished on empirical and conceptual grounds. Conceptually, trait anxiety is the proneness to experience anxiety (i.e., the frequency and intensity with which a person experiences anxiety), whereas AS is the *fear of* arousal-related sensations. Empirically, AS, compared with trait anxiety, is a stronger predictor of panic attacks (Taylor 1999).

Empirical studies suggest that AS comprises three dimensions: physical concerns (e.g., "when I feel pain in my chest, I worry I might be having a heart attack"), social concerns (e.g., "I worry that other people will notice my anxiety"), and cognitive concerns (e.g., "when my thoughts seem to speed up, I worry that I might be going crazy") (Taylor et al. 2007). Particular relationships between these components of AS and various forms of anxiety psychopathology have been found. The most robust findings link panic disorder and health anxiety to high levels of physical concerns, posttraumatic stress disorder to psychological concerns (Asmundson and Stapleton 2008; Feldner et al. 2006; Lang et al. 2002), and social phobia to the social concerns dimension (e.g., Deacon and Abramowitz 2006; Taylor et al. 2007). Relationships between AS dimensions and OCD, generalized anxiety disorder, and specific phobias have not been consistently reported and thus require further study.

Intolerance of Uncertainty

Intolerance of uncertainty (IU) has been defined in various ways. Sookman and Pinard (1995) characterized IU as a difficulty with ambiguity, newness, and unpredictable change. Kruglansky (1990) related IU to the need for cognitive closure and desire for an answer (any answer—regardless of accuracy) on a given topic. Freeston et al. (1994) defined the construct as emotional, cognitive, and behavioral reactions to 1) ambiguous situations, 2) implications of being uncertain, and 3) attempts to control the future. Another definition by Ladouceur et al. (2000) emphasized a negative appraisal of uncertainty and posited IU to be a "predisposition to react negatively to an uncertain event or situation, independent of its probability of occurrence and of its associated consequences" (p. 934). Finally, Dugas et al. (2001) proposed that IU is an excessive tendency to consider it unacceptable that a negative event may occur, however small the likelihood of its occurrence.

Defined broadly, IU has been associated with OCD (Obsessive Compulsive Cognitions Working Group 1997), based on the assertion that IU underlies anxiety evoked by obsessional doubts. Kozak et al. (1988) proposed that whereas individuals without OCD generally perceive situations as safe unless there is a reliable sign of danger, those with the disorder view situations related to their obsessive fears as uncertain and therefore "dangerous" unless they are assured of safety. Accordingly, research has uncovered associations between IU and OCD, with the strongest associations involving doubting-obsessions and checking rituals (Tolin et al. 2003).

IU has also been specifically linked with pathological worry and generalized anxiety disorder (e.g., Dugas et al. 2005; Freeston et al. 1994). The basis for this association is the assertion that IU leads to overestimation of the probability and severity of danger and is associated with the belief that it is unacceptable not to know for sure whether a negative event has occurred or will occur. Moreover, IU prevents a more adaptive focus on trying to solve the problem at hand.

Although the IU construct is most strongly associated with generalized anxiety disorder and OCD, patients with panic disorder and social anxiety show elevated levels of IU relative to healthy individuals (Deacon et al., submitted). Carleton et al. (2007) found evidence to suggest that IU may be associated with all anxiety disorders.

Even though IU is correlated with AS (Carleton et al. 2007), the two can be conceptually distinguished. IU refers to the uncertainty about all kinds of outcomes, including outcomes about external events (e.g., about whether a loved one will have a safe flight). In comparison, AS refers to fears of internal events and can occur even if the person has no uncertainty about the meaning of these events (e.g., "When my heart beats rapidly, I *know* I'm going to have a heart attack if I don't find some way of slowing it down.").

Traits Identified in Behavioral-Genetic Studies

Multivariate behavioral-genetic studies have been conducted to determine the extent to which anxiety symptoms and disorders arise from disorder-nonspecific (common) and disorder-specific etiologic factors. The largest, most sophisticated, and most comprehensive research program consisted of a series of investigations by Kendler and colleagues (see Kendler and Prescott 2006). Several thousand twins were enrolled in the studies, in which they completed structured clinical interviews and other measures to assess a range of psychopathology, including anxiety disorders, mood disorders, and substance use disorders. In this section, we will review those findings as they apply to the identification of genetic traits for anxiety disorders. Environmental factors, although important, will be reviewed in less detail because of our focus on intrapersonal factors (traits).

Kendler and colleagues found that genetic factors made "significant but not overwhelming contributions to individual differences in risk for the common mood and anxiety disorders" (Kendler and Prescott 2006, p. 74). Although the importance of genetic factors varied to some extent across disorders, genes accounted for approximately 30% of variance. Similar findings have been reported in other studies of anxiety disorders (Jang 2005). Evidence also indicated that nonshared environment (i.e., environment that was not shared by each member of a twin pair) was more important than shared environment. The latter included family experiences common to both members of a twin pair. Results further suggested that the risk for adult psychiatric disorders (including anxiety disorders) was associated with childhood abuse, including sexual abuse. These risk factors were generally nonspecific (i.e., applied equally across disorders).

Kendler's research revealed that anxiety disorders are influenced by a mix of disorder-specific genetic factors and a nonspecific genetic factor. The latter influenced anxiety disorders and major depressive disorder, but not substance use disorders. The nonspecific genetic factor has a greater impact on some disorders than others. To illustrate, for phobic disorders (i.e., specific phobias, social phobia, and agoraphobia), the disorder-specific genetic factors accounted for 7%–15% of variance, whereas the nonspecific genetic factor accounted for 5%–22% of variance across the phobic disorders. Specific phobias (i.e., animal, situation, and blood-injury injection phobias) were much more strongly influenced by this nonspecific factor (15%–22% variance) than agoraphobia (11%) and social phobia (5%).

A shortcoming of Kendler's research is that the assessment of anxiety disorders was limited to phobic disorders, panic disorder, and generalized anxiety disorder. It remains to be determined whether these disorders have genetic traits in common with other anxiety disorders, such as posttraumatic stress disorder and obsessive-compulsive disorder.

Further research is needed to determine how the specific and nonspecific genetic factors are related to personality and temperament. It may be that the disorder-specific genetic factors may form part of the etiologic underpinnings for narrow personality traits. For example, the genetic factors specific to panic disorder may be the same as the genetic factors underlying the physical concerns dimension of AS. The nonspecific genetic factors may represent the genetic component of broad personality or temperament traits, such as negative affectivity. The particular genes involved in these genetic factors also remained to be determined. The genes involved in the regulation of serotonin may play a role in determining symptoms of anxiety and depression (Hariri et al. 2006; Pezawas et al. 2005), and therefore may play a role in shaping the disorder-nonspecific genetic factor.

A growing body of research suggests that it is not genes per se that are most important in shaping the risk for psychopathology, but rather the interaction of particular genes with particular types of environmental events (Moffitt et al. 2006). For example, people possessing one or more copies of the short allele of the serotonin transporter gene, compared with people with two copies of the long allele, are more likely to develop symptoms of anxiety and depression in response to stressful life events (Leonardo and Hen 2006; Moffitt et al. 2006). Research is needed to investigate the possible role of interactions between genetic traits and environmental events in shaping the risk for developing anxiety disorders.

Endophenotypes

Endophenotypes are trait-like variables that lie somewhere in the causal link between genes and psychiatric disorders. For some anxiety disorders there has been very little research on endophenotypes, whereas for other disorders much more is known. In addition, some endophenotypes have been identified that are associated with more than one anxiety disorder. These general endophenotypes may be markers for the brain systems that are involved in many anxiety disorders, or perhaps emotional disorders in general, and may shed light on the causes of comorbidity among various disorders.

General Endophenotypes

The enhanced tendency to acquire conditioned fear responses and resistance to fear extinction may be a vulnerability factor for anxiety disorders. This enhanced conditionability may reflect hypersensitivity of fear-related brain circuits, such as circuits involving the amygdala, orbitofrontal cortex, hippocampus, and other brain structures. A small number of studies have examined this endophenotype. The results have been inconsistent. Compared with nonclinical control subjects, people with posttraumatic stress disorder have shown enhanced fear conditioning in some studies (Orr et al. 2000; Rothbaum et al. 2001), but not in others (Orr et al. 2006). Preliminary evidence suggests that people with panic disorder and people with generalized social anxiety disorder, compared with control subjects, do not have enhanced fear acquisition but may have greater resistance to fear extinction (Hermann et al. 2002; Michael et al. 2007). In summary, there is currently insufficient evidence to determine whether conditionability is a reliable endophenotype for anxiety disorders. The available evidence has provided mixed or inconsistent support.

Investigators have conducted several studies to determine whether exaggerated startle response, as measured by physiological indices, is an endophenotype for anxiety disorders. In the case of posttraumatic stress disorder, this variable is not, strictly speaking, an endophenotype, because exaggerated startle response is one of the symptoms used to diagnose the disorder (American Psychiatric Association 2000). Most people with posttraumatic stress disorder display exaggerated startle response (Broekman et al. 2007). Although this variable is a phenotype, rather than an endophenotype, it remains possible that the study of physiological indices and determinants of exaggerated startle response may enhance our understanding of the brain mechanisms involved in posttraumatic stress disorder.

Exaggerated startle response, as assessed by physiologic measures (e.g., eyeblink response or changes in skin conductance), has been investigated in several other anxiety disorders. Here, one can distinguish between context-specific startle response (i.e., fear-potentiated startle, such as when a person with a dog phobia is exposed to a dog) and context-nonspecific startle response (e.g., exaggerated startle response regardless of context) (Grillon 2002). Posttraumatic stress disorder, by definition, is associated with the latter (American Psychiatric Association 2000), although it is unclear whether this applies to other anxiety disorders. There is some evidence, however, that anxiety disorders are associated with exaggerated startle response in the context of fear-evoking stimuli (Grillon 2002). For example, people with social anxiety disorder display exaggerated startle response when exposed to fear-evoking social cues (Cornwell et al. 2006). The startle response is sensitive to genetic variation of serotonergic function and thus serves as an endophenotype of fear processing and underlying serotonergic influences (Brocke et al. 2006). Accordingly, further research on the startle-response endophenotype may lead to advances in understanding the role of serotonergic systems in the anxiety disorders.

Panic Disorder

Endophenotypes associated with panic disorder include the tendency for people with panic disorder, compared with control subjects, to be more likely to experience panic attacks when they are exposed to various biological agents, such as by caffeine ingestion, carbon dioxide inhalation, or infusions of yohimbine, sodium lactate, or cholecystokinin tetrapeptide (Leonardo and Hen 2006;

McNally 1994). Such findings raise the question of whether panic disorder can arise from dysregulations in various neurotransmitter systems, particularly serotonergic and noradrenergic systems (McNally 1994). On the other hand, the panicogenic effects of these agents could simply be due to elevated AS as discussed earlier, without necessarily involving dysregulated neurotransmitter systems (Taylor 2000).

Obsessive-Compulsive Disorder

Very little is known about the endophenotypes associated with OCD (Miguel et al. 2005). Preliminary evidence suggests peripheral serotonergic (5-HT) abnormalities in people with OCD and their unaffected relatives, compared with nonclinical controls and their relatives. Such abnormalities include lower whole blood 5-HT concentration and fewer platelet 5-HT binding sites (Delorme et al. 2005). If such results prove to be stable within individuals and replicable across individuals, then these abnormalities may be endophenotypes of OCD, and the study of such endophenotypes may facilitate the study of brain serotonergic functioning in OCD. However, such endophenotypes may not be specific to this disorder, as serotonergic abnormalities have been implicated in several anxiety and mood disorders and in other disorders.

Some evidence suggests that OCD is associated with particular neuropsychological deficits, such as problems in executive functioning (e.g., planning, organization, response inhibition) (Chamberlain et al. 2005; Greisberg and McKay 2003). The findings suggest that dysregulations in orbitofrontal brain circuits may be implicated. Available evidence is inconsistent with regard to memory deficits in OCD, although memory problems tend to be most apparent for tasks requiring an implicit organizational strategy (such as the need to organize or chunk material to facilitate encoding and recollection) (Greisberg and McKay 2003). Such deficits may contribute to obsessional doubting and compulsive checking.

One problem encountered in identifying endophenotypes associated with OCD, which may partly account for inconsistent findings, is that this disorder is clinically heterogeneous and is likely to be etiologically heterogeneous as well (Abramowitz et al. 2008; Delorme et al. 2005). To identify robust endophenotypes, it may be necessary for researchers to focus on specific subtypes or dimensions of the disorder, such as obsessions and compulsions associated with particular symptom domains (e.g., contamination, checking, aggression, sexuality, hoarding).

Posttraumatic Stress Disorder

There is preliminary evidence that posttraumatic stress disorder is associated with particular memory problems, such as difficulty recalling specific details of everyday events (i.e., vague or overgeneralized autobiographic memories; Taylor 2006). There is some evidence that posttraumatic stress disorder is associated with elevated autonomic arousal, although it is not clear whether it is a feature that distinguishes this disorder from other anxiety disorders. It is also not clear whether this finding can be generalized to all forms of posttraumatic stress disorder, because most of the research has focused on male combat veterans (Pole 2007). There is some evidence that the disorder is associated with dysregulation of the hypothalamic-pituitary-adrenal axis (HPA) (Broekman et al. 2007), although there have been many failures to replicate this research (Yehuda 2006). It is possible that variables associated with HPA axis dysregulation are endophenotypes for only particular subtypes of posttraumatic stress disorder (Yehuda 2006).

Other Anxiety Disorders

Little is known about the endophenotypes that are specific to other anxiety disorders, such as specific phobia, social anxiety disorder, and generalized anxiety disorder. Further research is required.

Implications for Treatment

How can an understanding of traits and temperament influence treatment? Responsible selection from among the empirically supported options for treating the anxiety disorders involves comprehensive assessment and consideration of the person's treatment preferences. Assessment is, in large part, a conceptually driven process; that is, theory is at the foundation of any decisions made regarding what is important to assess in any given case. The information gleaned from assessment is then used to develop the case formulation and, on this basis, the treatment plan. Although practitioners are fortunate in that they have fairly well-developed theories regarding a large number of psychopathologies, it is often challenging to find a starting point when a person presents with multiple or comorbid complaints. This is often the case for people presenting for treatment of anxiety disorders; it is thereby difficult to identify which of the presenting problems to focus on in treatment. The theoretical and empirical literature regarding broad traits and temperament, as discussed above, provides practitioners with a starting point that is ostensibly rooted in nonspecific vulnerability factors for the anxiety disorders. Consequently, even in cases in which the person presents with more than one anxiety disorder, or with some other co-occurring psychopathology (e.g., major depression), intervening at the level of the vulnerability factor may effectively alleviate anxiety-related and other pathology. Moreover, this approach may prove useful as a primary prevention strategy to reduce psychopathology.

With regard to narrow traits, Smits et al. (2004) found that changes in AS mediate the relationship between cognitive-behavioral therapy and treatment outcome in patients with panic disorder; that is, changes in AS were important in determining response to treatment. This finding suggests that interventions that target the narrow trait of AS may be important in reducing a person's risk of developing panic attacks and panic disorder. AS is typically reduced through some combination of psychoeducation, interoceptive exposure (i.e., exposure to feared arousal-related sensations), and cognitive restructuring (see Taylor 2000).

To investigate the prophylactic effects of reducing AS, Schmidt et al. (2007) randomly assigned 404 people with high AS to either a brief intervention designed to reduce AS (i.e., Anxiety Sensitivity Amelioration Training [ASAT]) or to a control condition. ASAT comprised psychoeducation and interoceptive exposure. Those participants receiving ASAT had greater reductions in AS than did those in the control condition. Data collected at 24 months postintervention indicated that the treatment group had a lower but statistically insignificant incidence of anxiety disorder diagnoses (4%) compared with the control group (8%). Further research, using larger samples and perhaps longer follow-up intervals, may be needed to fully evaluate the benefits of ASAT.

Research on interventions designed to reduce BI in children has yielded evidence of preventive efficacy. Dadds and colleagues (Dadds et al. 1997, 1999), for example, identified 128 anxious and inhibited children, ages 7–14 years, who were deemed at risk for developing clinically significant anxiety. The schools these children attended were randomly assigned to either an intervention or a control (i.e., monitoring only) condition. The intervention comprised relaxation training, cognitive restructuring, attentional training, parent-assisted in vivo exposure, family/peer support, and parent training. At both 6 and 24 months postintervention, reduced rates of anxiety disorders, as well as some significant behavioral differences, were observed in the intervention group, compared with a monitoring group. However, temperament per se was not used to define the at-risk group, and some of the participants met criteria for diagnosis of an anxiety disorder at the outset of the study.

These findings collectively suggest that early identification of trait and temperamental risk factors may be fruitful in efforts at early intervention, potentially shifting vulnerable adults and children away from pathological trajectories. In future efforts, researchers might seek to determine whether it is possible to match a particular intervention modality to a person's trait or temperamental strengths. For example, one could attempt to enhance the trait of effortful control, thereby maximizing its moderating effect on other temperament dimensions, such as negative affectivity. A child with high negative affectivity but good effortful control may be better suited to take advantage of coping strategies, such as distraction or cognitive restructuring, than a child with lower levels of this trait. Conversely, children with poor effortful control may need proportionally more effort, at least initially, devoted to reducing the effect of environmental stressors or their physiological manifestations. Given that a number of traits, both narrow and broad, and temperaments have been associated with anxiety-related psychopathology, there are innumerable possibilities for developing and empirically scrutinizing interventions tailored to maximize trait and temperamental strengths and bolster strategies to minimize vulnerabilities.

Conclusion

Research into traits and temperaments can shed light into the etiology of anxiety disorders and may have important implications for treating or preventing these disorders. In this chapter, we reviewed 1) temperaments associated with the anxiety disorders, 2) narrow and broad personality traits, placing them in the context of empirically supported models that hierarchically structure the former as lower-order components of the latter, 3) relevant behavioral-genetics studies, and 4) important trait-like variables—endophenotypes—that are correlated with a given disorder and assumed to lie somewhere in the causal link between genes and psychiatric symptoms or disorders. Finally, we provided a selective review of relevant treatment and preventive intervention studies that capitalize on maximizing a person's ability to cope with trait and temperamental vulnerabilities for anxiety-related psychopathology.

Although there is a considerable degree of general knowledge regarding traits and temperaments and their association with the anxiety disorders, much remains to be learned. There are a number of avenues for future research, both basic and applied, stemming from the current state of the art regarding anxious traits and temperaments. For example, although the association of some of the narrow personality traits with specific anxiety disorders is well understood, such as in the case of the relationship between AS and panic disorder, many unanswered questions remain about the roles that each of these traits play in each of the anxiety disorders. Likewise, there is need for additional longitudinal studies to answer the question of which traits and temperaments are causes of which anxiety disorders, and which are consequences and correlates. Further behavioral-genetic research is needed to determine how specific and nonspecific genetic factors are related to personality and temperament. Although this area of inquiry is in its infancy, it offers considerable potential for improving our understanding of the way in which genes and environment interact to increase risk for developing anxiety-related psychopathology. Likewise, additional research of endophenotypes is needed to clarify inconsistent findings in the research on some of the anxiety disorders (e.g., posttraumatic stress disorder) in order to provide initial insights for specific phobia, social anxiety disorder, and generalized anxiety disorder, and to establish how knowledge of endophenotypes can be practically applied. With regard to applied research, available studies provide a sound foundation on which treatment tailoring and primary prevention efforts incorporating traits and temperament can build. Applied efforts such as these have considerable potential to alleviate the suffering and disability that are characteristic of the anxiety disorders and to thereby improve the quality of life for many.

◀ Key Clinical Points ▶

- An understanding of traits and temperaments can provide the practitioner with a conceptual framework on which to base assessment, case formulation, and treatment planning for people presenting with anxiety disorders.
- This approach may be of particular benefit in complex cases in which there are multiple presenting problems, including comorbid disorders.
- People with high test scores on particular traits and temperaments (e.g., negative affectivity) are at heightened risk for developing anxiety and other disorders. Accordingly, these disorders may be prevented by identifying at-risk individuals and initiating primary prevention programs to target the relevant traits and temperaments. These programs, such as Anxiety Sensitivity Amelioration Training, are promising, but more research is needed.

References

Abramowitz JS, Taylor S, McKay D: Obsessive-Compulsive Disorder: Subtypes and Spectrum Conditions. New York, Elsevier, 2008

American Psychiatric Association: Diagnostic and Statistical Manual of Mental Disorders, 4th Edition, Text Revision. Washington, DC, American Psychiatric Association, 2000

Anastasi A: The nature of psychological "traits." Psychol Rev 55:127–138, 1948

Asmundson GJ, Stapleton JA: Associations between dimensions of anxiety sensitivity and PTSD symptom clusters in active-duty police officers. Cogn Behav Ther 37:66–75, 2008

Biederman J, Rosenbaum JF, Bolduc-Murphy EA, et al: A 3-year follow-up of children with and without behavioral inhibition. J Am Acad Child Adolesc Psychiatry 32:814–821, 1993

Brocke B, Armbruster D, Muller J, et al: Serotonin transporter gene variation impacts innate fear processing: acoustic startle response and emotional startle. Mol Psychiatry 11:1106–1112, 2006

Broekman BFP, Olff M, Boer F: The genetic background to PTSD. Neurosci Biobehav Rev 31:348–362, 2007

Calvo MG, Cano-Videl A: The nature of trait anxiety: cognitive and biological vulnerability. Eur Psychol 2:301–312, 1997

Calvo MG, Castillo MD: Mood-congruent bias in interpretation of ambiguity: strategic processes and temporary activation. QJ Exp Psychol 50:163–182, 1997

Cannon TD, Keller MC: Endophenotypes in the genetic analyses of mental disorders. Annu Rev Clin Psychol 2:267–290, 2006

Carleton RN, Sharpe D, Asmundson GJG: Anxiety sensitivity and intolerance of uncertainty: requisites of the fundamental fears? Behav Res Ther 45:2307–2316, 2007

Chamberlain SR, Blackwell AD, Fineberg NA, et al: The neuropsychology of obsessive compulsive disorder: the importance of failures in cognitive and behavioural inhibition as candidate endophenotypic markers. Neurosci Biobehav Rev 29:399–419, 2005

Clark LA, Watson D: Tripartite model of anxiety and depression: psychometric evidence and taxonomic implications. J Abnorm Psychol 100:316–336, 1991

Clark LA, Watson D, Mineka S: Temperament, personality, and the mood disorders. J Abnorm Psychol 103:103–116, 1994

Cloninger CR, Svrakic DM: Integrative psychobiological approach to psychiatric assessment and treatment. Psychiatry 60:120–141, 1997

Cornwell BR, Johnson L, Berardi L, et al: Anticipation of public speaking in virtual reality reveals a relationship between trait social anxiety and startle reactivity. Biol Psychiatry 59:664–666, 2006

Costa PT, McCrae RR: Domains and facets: Hierarchical personality assessment using the Revised NEO Personality Inventory. J Pers Assess 64:21–50, 1995

Cox BJ, Borger SC, Enns MW: Anxiety sensitivity and emotional disorders: psychometric studies and their theoretical implications, in Anxiety Sensitivity: Theory, Research, and Treatment of the Fear of Anxiety. Edited by Taylor S. Mahwah, NJ, Erlbaum, 1999, pp 115–148

Cox BJ, Clara IP, Enns MW: Posttraumatic stress disorder and the structure of common mental disorders. Depress Anxiety 15:168–171, 2002

Craske MG: Anxiety Disorders: Psychological Approaches to Theory and Treatment. Boulder, CO, Westview Press, 1999

Craske MG: Origins of Phobias and Anxiety Disorders: Why More Women Than Men? Amsterdam, The Netherlands, Elsevier, 2003

Dadds MR, Spence SH, Holland D, et al: Prevention and early intervention of anxiety disorders: a controlled trial. J Consult Clin Psychol 65:627–635, 1997

Dadds MR, Holland DE, Laurens KR, et al: Early intervention and prevention of anxiety disorders in children: results at 2-year follow-up. J Consult Clin Psychol 67:145–150, 1999

Deacon BJ, Abramowitz JS: Anxiety sensitivity and its dimensions across the anxiety disorders. J Anxiety Disord 20:837–857, 2006

Deacon BJ, Abramowitz JS, Maak DJ: Intolerance of uncertainty and the anxiety disorders. Manuscript submitted for publication

Degnan KA, Fox NA: Behavioral inhibition and anxiety disorders: multiple levels of a resilience process. Dev Psychopathol 19:729–746, 2007

Delorme R, Betancur C, Callebert J, et al: Platelet serotonergic markers as endophenotypes for obsessive-compulsive disorder. Neuropsychopharmacology 30:1539–1547, 2005

Dugas M, Gosselin M, Ladouceur R: Intolerance of uncertainty and worry: Investigating narrow specificity in a nonclinical sample. Cognit Ther Res 25:551–558, 2001

Dugas M, Marchand A, Ladouceur R: Further validation of a cognitive-behavioral model of generalized anxiety disorder: diagnostic and symptom specificity. J Anxiety Disord 19:329–343, 2005

Feldner MT, Lewis SF, Leen-Feldner EW, et al: Anxiety sensitivity as a moderator of the relation between trauma exposure frequency and posttraumatic stress symptomatology. J Cognit Psychother 20:201–213, 2006

Freeston MH, Rhéaume J, Letarte H, et al: Why do people worry? Pers Individ Dif 17:791–802, 1994

Gottesman II, Gould TD: The endophenotype concept in psychiatry: etymology and strategic intentions. Am J Psychiatry 160:636–645, 2003

Gray JA, McNaughton N: The neuropsychology of anxiety: reprise, in Perspectives on Anxiety, Panic, and Fear: Nebraska Symposium on Motivation, Vol 13. Edited by Hope DA. Lincoln, University of Nebraska Press, 1996, pp 61–134

Greisberg S, McKay D: Neuropsychology of obsessive-compulsive disorder: a review and treatment implications. Clin Psychol Rev 23:95–117, 2003

Grillon C: Startle reactivity anxiety disorders: aversive conditioning, context, and neurobiology. Biol Psychiatry 52:958–975, 2002

Guilford JP: Personality. New York, McGraw-Hill, 1959

Hariri AR, Brown SM, Tamminga CA: Images in neuroscience: serotonin. Am J Psychiatry 163:12, 2006

Henderson HA, Fox NA: Inhibited and uninhibited children: challenges in school settings. School Psych Rev 27:492–505, 1998

Hermann C, Ziegler S, Birbaumer N, et al: Psychophysiological and subjective indicators of aversive Pavlovian conditioning in generalized social phobia. Biol Psychiatry 52:328–337, 2002

Hughes AA, Heimberg RG, Coles ME, et al: Relations of the factors of the tripartite model of anxiety and depression to types of social anxiety. Behav Res Ther 44:1629–1641, 2006

Jang KL: The Behavioral Genetics of Psychopathology: A Clinical Guide. Mahwah, NJ, Erlbaum, 2005

Joiner TE, Steer RA, Beck AT, et al: Physiological hyperarousal: construct validity of a central aspect of the tripartite model of depression and anxiety. J Abnorm Psychol 108:290–298, 1999

Kagan J: Galen's Prophecy: Temperament in Human Nature. New York, Basic Books, 1994

Kagan J: In the beginning: the contribution of temperament to personality development. Modern Psychoanalysis 22:145–155, 1997

Kendler KS, Prescott CA: Genes, Environment, and Psychopathology: Understanding the Causes of Psychiatric and Substance Use Disorders. New York, Guilford, 2006

Kessler RC, McGonagle KA, Zhao S, et al: Lifetime and 12-month prevalence of DSM-III-R psychiatric disorders in the United States: results from the National Comorbidity Survey. Arch Gen Psychiatry 51:8–19, 1994

Kotov R, Watson D, Robles JP, et al: Personality traits and anxiety symptoms: the multilevel trait predictor model. Behav Res Ther 45:1485–1503, 2007

Kozak MJ, Foa EB, McCarthy PR: Obsessive-compulsive disorder, in Handbook of Anxiety Disorders. Edited by Last CG, Hersen M. New York, Pergamon, 1988, pp 87–108

Krueger RF: The structure of common mental disorders. Arch Gen Psychiatry 56:921–926, 1999

Krueger RF, Tackett JL: Personality and Psychopathology. New York, Guilford, 2006

Kruglansky A: Motivations for judging and knowing: implications for causal attribution, in The Handbook of Motivation and Cognition: Foundations of Social Behavior, Vol 2. Edited by Higgins ET, Sorrento R. New York, Guilford, 1990, pp 333–368

Ladouceur R, Gosselin P, Dugas MJ: Experimental manipulation of intolerance of uncertainty: a study of a theoretical model of worry. Behav Res Ther 38:933–941, 2000

Lang AJ, Kennedy CM, Stein MB: Anxiety sensitivity and PTSD among female victims of intimate partner violence. Depress Anxiety 16:77–83, 2002

Leonardo ED, Hen R: Genetics of affective and anxiety disorders. Annu Rev Psychol 57:117–137, 2006

Lerman A: Predictors of Social Anxiety Disorder and Contingent Self-Worth: Behavioral Inhibition and Relationships With Parents and Peers During Childhood. Unpublished doctoral dissertation, Department of Psychology, Illinois Institute of Technology, 2004

Lohr LB, Teglasi H, French M: Schemas and temperament as risk factors for emotional disability. Pers Individ Dif 36:1637–1654, 2004

McNally RJ: Panic Disorder: A Critical Analysis. New York, Guilford, 1994

Michael T, Blechert J, Vriends N, et al: Fear conditioning in panic disorder: enhanced resistance to extinction. J Abnorm Psychol 116:612–617, 2007

Miguel EC, Leckman JF, Rauch S, et al: Obsessive-compulsive disorder phenotypes: implications for genetic studies. Mol Psychiatry 10:258–275, 2005

Mischel W: Towards a cognitive social learning reconceptualization of personality. Psychol Rev 80:252–283, 1973

Moffitt TE, Caspi A, Rutter M: Measured gene-environment interactions in psychopathology. Perspect Psychol Sci 1:5–27, 2006

Obsessive Compulsive Cognitions Working Group: Cognitive assessment of obsessive-compulsive disorder. Behav Res Ther 35:667–681, 1997

Orr SP, Metzger LJ, Lasko NB, et al: De novo conditioning in trauma-exposed individuals with and without posttraumatic stress disorder. J Abnorm Psychol 109:290–298, 2000

Orr SP, Milad MR, Metzger LJ, et al: Effects of beta blockade, PTSD diagnosis, and explicit threat on the extinction and retention of an aversively conditioned response. Biol Psychol 73:262–271, 2006

Pezawas L, Meyer-Lindenberg A, Drabant EM, et al: 5-HTTLPR polymorphism impacts human cingulate-amygdala interactions. Nat Neurosci 8:828–834, 2005

Podniesinski EM: Posttraumatic Stress Symptoms in Children After the World Trade Center Attack: Investigating the Triple Vulnerability Model of Etiology. Unpublished doctoral dissertation, Department of Psychology, Boston University, 2004

Pole N: The psychophysiology of posttraumatic stress disorder: a meta-analysis. Psychol Bull 133:725–747, 2007

Reiss S, McNally RJ: Expectancy model of fear, in Theoretical Issues in Behavior Therapy. Edited by Reiss S, Bootzin RR. San Diego, CA, Academic Press, 1985, pp 107–121

Rettew DC, McKee L: Temperament and its role in developmental psychopathology. Harv Rev Psychiatry 13:14–27, 2005

Rothbart MK, Ahadi SA: Temperament and the development of personality. J Abnorm Psychol 103:55–66, 1994

Rothbaum BO, Kozak MJ, Foa EB, et al: Posttraumatic stress disorder in rape victims: autonomic habituation to auditory stimuli. J Trauma Stress 14:283–293, 2001

Schmidt NB, Lerew DR, Jackson RJ: The role of anxiety sensitivity in the pathogenesis of panic: prospective evaluation of spontaneous panic attacks during acute stress. J Abnorm Psychol 106:355–364, 1997

Schmidt NB, Lerew DR, Jackson RJ: Prospective evaluation of anxiety sensitivity in the pathogenesis of panic: replication and extension. J Abnorm Psychol 108:532–537, 1999

Schmidt NB, Eggleston ME, Woolaway-Bickel K, et al: Anxiety Sensitivity Amelioration Training (ASAT): a longitudinal primary prevention program targeting cognitive vulnerability. J Anxiety Disord 21:302–319, 2007

Schwartz CE, Snidman N, Kagan J: Adolescent social anxiety as an outcome of inhibited temperament in childhood. J Am Acad Child Adolesc Psychiatry 38:1008–1015, 1999

Smits JA, Powers MB, Cho Y, et al: Mechanism of change in cognitive-behavioral treatment of panic disorder: evidence for the fear of fear mediational hypothesis. J Consult Clin Psychol 72:646–652, 2004

Sookman D, Pinard G: The Cognitive Schemata Scale: a multidimensional measure of cognitive schemas in obsessive-compulsive disorder. Paper presented at the World Congress of Behavioral and Cognitive Therapies, Copenhagen, Denmark, July 1995

Spielberger CD, Gorsuch RC, Lushene RE: Manual for the State Trait Anxiety Inventory. Palo Alto, CA, Consulting Psychologists Press, 1970

Sroufe LA: Psychopathology as an outcome of development. Dev Psychopathol 9:251–268, 1997

Strelau J: A regulative theory of temperament. Aust J Psychol 35:305–317, 1983

Swedo SE: Pediatric autoimmune neuropsychiatric disorders associated with streptococcal infections (PANDAS). Mol Psychiatry 7(suppl):S24–S25, 2002

Taylor S: Anxiety Sensitivity: Theory, Research, and Treatment of the Fear of Anxiety. Mahwah, NJ, Lawrence Erlbaum, 1999

Taylor S: Understanding and Treating Panic Disorder. New York, Wiley, 2000

Taylor S: Clinician's Guide to PTSD. New York, Guilford, 2006

Taylor S, Zvolensky M, Cox B, et al: Robust dimensions of anxiety sensitivity: development and initial validation of the Anxiety Sensitivity Index-3 (ASI-3). Psychol Assess 19:176–188, 2007

Tolin DF, Abramowitz JS, Brigidi B, et al: Intolerance of uncertainty in obsessive-compulsive disorder. J Anxiety Disord 17:233–242, 2003

Vollebergh WAM, Iedema J, Bijl RV, et al: The structure and stability of common mental disorders: the NEMESIS study. Arch Gen Psychiatry 58:597–603, 2001

Waller NG, Meehl PE: Multivariate Taxometric Procedures: Distinguishing Types From Continua. Thousand Oaks, CA, Sage, 1998

Watson D, Clark LA: Negative affectivity: the disposition to experience negative emotional states. Psychol Bull 96:465–490, 1984

Watson D, Clark LA, Weber K, et al: Testing a tripartite model, II: exploring the symptom structure of anxiety and depression in student, adult, and patient samples. J Abnorm Psychol 104:15–25, 1995a

Watson D, Weber K, Assenheimer JS, et al: Testing a tripartite model, I: evaluating the convergent and discriminant validity of anxiety and depression symptom scales. J Abnorm Psychol 104:3–14, 1995b

Williams JM, Watts FN, MacLeod C, et al: Cognitive Psychology and Emotional Disorders, 2nd Edition. Chichester, UK, Wiley, 1997

Yehuda R: Psychobiology of Posttraumatic Stress Disorder: A Decade of Progress. Malden, MA, Blackwell, 2006

Zinbarg R, Barlow DH: Structure of anxiety and the anxiety disorders: a hierarchical model. J Abnorm Psychol 106:181–193, 1996

Zuckerman H: Good and bad humors: biochemical bases of personality and its disorders. Psychol Sci 6:325–332, 1995

Recommended Readings

Barlow DH: Anxiety and Its Disorders: The Nature and Treatment of Anxiety and Panic, 2nd Edition. New York, Guilford, 2002

Cannon TD, Keller MC: Endophenotypes in the genetic analyses of mental disorders. Annu Rev Clin Psychol 2:267–290, 2006

Kagan J: Galen's Prophecy: Temperament in Human Nature. New York, Basic Books, 1994

Kendler KS, Prescott CA: Genes, Environment, and Psychopathology: Understanding the Causes of Psychiatric and Substance Use Disorders. New York, Guilford, 2006

Krueger RF, Tackett JL: Personality and Psychopathology. New York, Guilford, 2006

Rettew DC, McKee L: Temperament and its role in developmental psychopathology. Harv Rev Psychiatry 13:14–27, 2005

Chapter 6

The Neuropsychology of Anxiety Disorders

Kevin J. Craig, M.B.B.Ch., M.Phil., MRCPsych
Samuel R. Chamberlain, Ph.D., M.B.B.Ch.

The neuropsychology of anxiety has been studied for more than a century and has given rise to a large corpus of literature. Broadly speaking, studies have addressed two main themes. First, there is a long history of attempts to model the etiology of anxiety, such as through fear conditioning (Watson and Rayner 1920). Second, experiments have focused on the pathophysiology and maintenance of these disorders by examining cognitive domains germane to anxiety, such as executive function, attention, and memory.

Anxiety is a common human state that can facilitate performance and inform learning about outcomes. As such, it is adaptive within certain limits. Under non-challenging conditions of low cognitive load, mild anxiety may enhance emotional processing and attentional control (Wood et al. 2001). High levels of anxiety, on the other hand, lead to decrements in cognitive performance, especially in domains such as attention and executive function. There has been extensive research on the impact of anxious states.

In recent years, neuropsychological tests have been combined with and augmented by advances in pharmacological dissection, neuroanatomical staining, and functional imaging to broaden our understanding of understanding of the neural substrates that give rise to the symptoms of anxiety. This advancement has been greatly aided by the fact that the neural mechanisms of fear and anxiety are highly conserved across species, which has allowed inferences to be made regarding the neurobiology of fear and anxiety in humans (LeDoux 1995) (see Chapter 4, "Neural Circuits in Fear and Anxiety," in this volume).

Studies on anxiety in humans can generally be divided into three types: 1) studies in which anxiety levels are manipulated in healthy control subjects and cognitive performance is measured as a function of anxiety; 2) studies that compare high and low trait anxiety in community samples on measures of cognitive performance; and 3) studies of clinical groups with anxiety disorders; in these cases, a categorical diagnosis is made, based on criteria from DSM-IV-TR (American Psychiatric Association 2000) or ICD-10 (World Health Organization 1993).

It is assumed that these groups represent a continuum of anxiety, from low trait-anxious individuals, through more anxious nonclinical groups, to those with diagnos-

The Behavioural and Clinical Neuroscience Institute is supported by a joint award from the Medical Research Council and the Wellcome Trust. The authors wish to thank Professor Trevor Robbins for comments about the substance and style of this article and the intellectual environment in which these thoughts were conceived.

able anxiety disorders. Although this is a common assumption, few studies have examined this hypothesis systematically. In particular, the diagnostic group of anxiety disorders represents a number of discrete diagnostic entities, and it is unclear whether high trait anxiety represents a common factor within this group or lies on a continuum with one or another individual anxiety disorder, such as generalized anxiety disorder (GAD) (see Chapter 5, "Anxious Traits and Temperaments").

Our aim in this chapter is to outline current understanding about the role of anxiety and fear in normal cognitive functioning, before going on to describe psychopathology arising from these processes in various anxiety disorders.

Fear Versus Anxiety

As noted elsewhere, anxiety disorders represent a large group of syndromes in which an important distinction can be made between fear and anxiety. From a phenomenological perspective, fear has a clear object and is usually elicited by an imminent threat. Anxiety tends to be more generalized, has no object (Marks 1987), and represents the expectation of negative events or outcomes at some time in the future. Anxiety is thus more future-oriented and is not linked to a specific cue. Fear, however, develops once an association has been learned between an object or event and an aversive outcome. In this way, for example, the experimental animal learns to fear the tone that predicts the shock, and the patient with posttraumatic stress disorder (PTSD) develops an excessive fear of events or objects that have become associated with their attendant trauma.

Clinically, phobia is conceptualized as a syndrome of pathological fear. Similarly, GAD and the future-oriented worries of obsessive-compulsive disorder (OCD) are prototypical of anxiety. Although both phobic disorders and anxiety disorders are thought to represent inappropriate activation of normally adaptive defense mechanisms, there is significant empirical evidence for differentiating the two. For example, anxiolytic drugs, such as benzodiazepines, are relatively ineffective in the treatment of fear-related disorders, such as phobia, but remain effective for the treatment of generalized anxiety (Marks 1987).

Psychometric Measures of Anxiety

In most studies, it is assumed that anxiety lies on a continuum. Some individuals have a more anxious disposition than others, and anxiety disorders are thought to represent the most extreme end of this continuous range. In this way, studies divide community populations into high- and low-anxiety groups based on self-report measures. The insights gained are assumed to shed light on clinical populations, which are considered to be different only in degree of anxiety. Another view, which holds that anxiety disorders are qualitatively different from normal anxiety, is less in favor at present, although it is an interpretation that has been the subject of intense debate in the past.

Examples of Nonclinical Measures

State-Trait Anxiety Inventory

In 1966, Spielberger made a conceptual distinction between state and trait anxiety. He defined trait anxiety as an individual's predisposition to respond to a given anxiogenic event and state anxiety as a transitory emotion, characterized by cognitive, behavioral, and physiological changes. The State-Trait Anxiety Inventory (Spielberger 1983) is a self-report scale that measures both aspects of anxiety in a dimensional fashion. It has good reliability and validity and has been used extensively in clinical and nonclinical populations, although it is not a diagnostic questionnaire.

Behavioral Inhibition System and Behavioral Activation System

Gray (1987) described two opposing neurological constructs called the behavioral inhibition system (BIS) and the behavioral activation [or approach] system (BAS). The BAS regulates appetitive motives, in which the organism must move toward something in order to attain its goal. BIS is responsible for stopping behavior that is expected to lead to punishment or the loss of reward. It is involved in reallocation of attentional resources and increased arousal in response to conditioned fear and novel stimuli. It can also motivate risk assessment behavior or behavioral caution (see Figure 6–1). BIS activity is thus closely related to trait anxiety (Gray 1987; Gray and McNaughton 2000) and vulnerability to anxiety.

Carver and White (1994) operationalized Gray's BIS/BAS theory by creating a self-report scale to assess differential BIS and BAS sensitivities. The scale has good reliability and validity and is one of the more widely used measures in the field, although it has been criticized for focusing mainly on the consequences of BIS/BAS activity and not on the BIS/BAS activity itself. The questionnaire comprises one BIS scale and

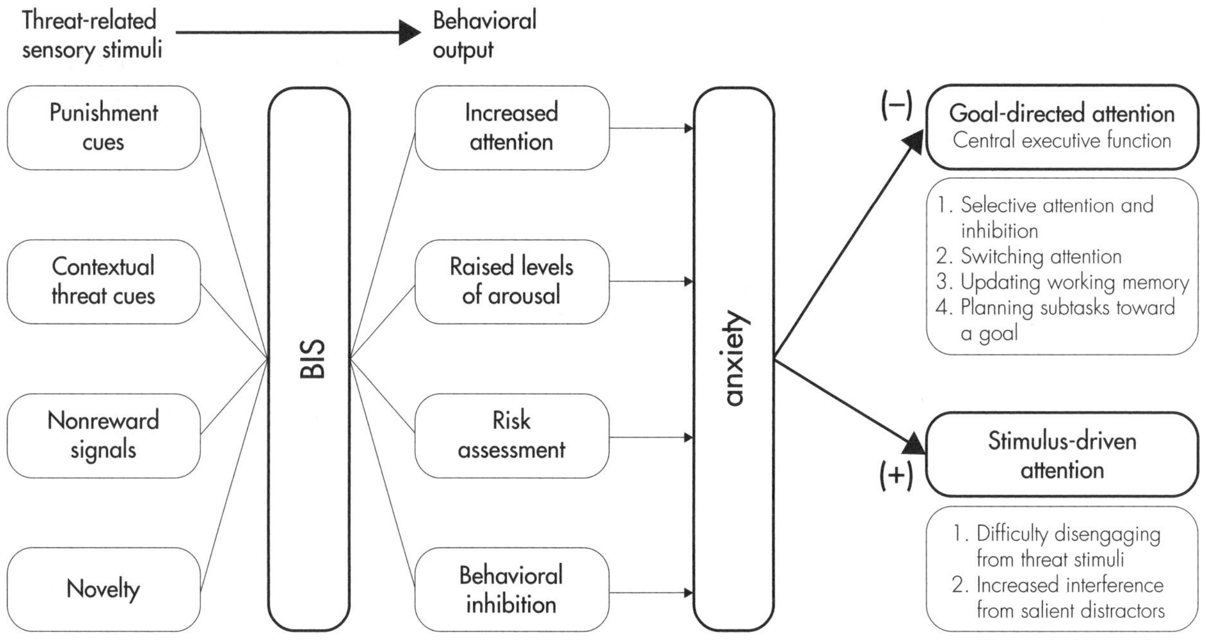

FIGURE 6–1. Behavioral inhibition system (BIS) described by Gray and McNaughton (2000) is linked to trait anxiety and is the putative substrate for anxiolytic drugs.

The construct is thought to operate when threat-related stimuli are linked to the attainment of goals, requiring approach where avoidance would normally occur. The BIS is thus a mechanism for conflict resolution. Sensory inputs relevant to threat generate anxiety-like behaviors aimed at resolving the conflict. The balance between reactivity and control is an important basis for the emotional modulation of attention. Competition among stimuli for limited attentional resources may be influenced by both bottom-up, sensory-driven mechanisms and top-down, goal-driven control. Anxiety disrupts the bidirectional influences of these two attentional systems. It is associated with an increased sensitivity to stimulus-driven threat cues via automatic processing of threat-related stimuli and to a decrease in the efficacy of top-down cognitive control.

three BAS scales. The BIS scale attempts to measure beliefs about the possible occurrence of negative events and sensitivity to such events when they do occur. The BAS part of the questionnaire is divided into three subscales: reward responsiveness, drive, and sensation-seeking. The results of large epidemiological studies have indicated that high BIS scores are most highly correlated with personality traits such as neuroticism (Campbell-Sills et al. 2004), but high scorers are also more vulnerable to depression and anxiety (Johnson et al. 2003). Individuals who show BIS sensitivity are thought to demonstrate attention biases, particularly toward threat- and fear-related stimuli (Bishop et al. 2004; Gray and McNaughton 2000; Mathews and MacKintosh 1998).

Psychophysiology

Psychophysiology is concerned with the physiological changes related to psychological processes. In contrast to the measures mentioned above, indices relating to physiology are generally used experimentally to assess short-term (second to minute) changes in emotional response. There is a long tradition of psychophysiological experiments in anxiety, mostly relating to physiological responses and organ systems innervated by the autonomic nervous system. Cardiovascular changes accompanying anxiety (such as heart rate, heart rate variability, and blood pressure changes) have been central to the concept of anxiety for more than a century and are still commonly measured. More modern psychophysiological measures utilize event-related potentials, electroencephalography, and functional magnetic resonance imaging.

Skin Conductance Response

One method of measuring the relationship between sympathetic activity and emotional arousal is the skin conductance response (SCR), which measures the electrical resistance of the skin. The SCR is highly sensitive to emotions, but it does not identify which emotion is being experienced, because considerable similarity exists in the SCR response to differing emotions. Fear, anger, startle response, and orienting response are among the emotions that may produce changes in SCR.

Fear-Potentiated Startle

The fear-potentiated startle response is another measure that has been used in animals and is being used increasingly in human studies (Grillon 2002b; Grillon and Davis 1997). A startle reflex is elicited by sudden, intense stimuli (such as a loud noise) and involves a stereotypical set of involuntary behaviors. In humans, the magnitude of orbicularis oculi muscle contraction (eyeblink) has been used to quantify the startle reflex reaction. In learning paradigms, anticipation of an aversive stimulus increases the startle response, called *fear-potentiated startle*. The fact that fear-potentiated startle is well preserved across species has made it an increasingly popular measure for translational research in the field of anxiety (see Filion et al. 1998, for a review).

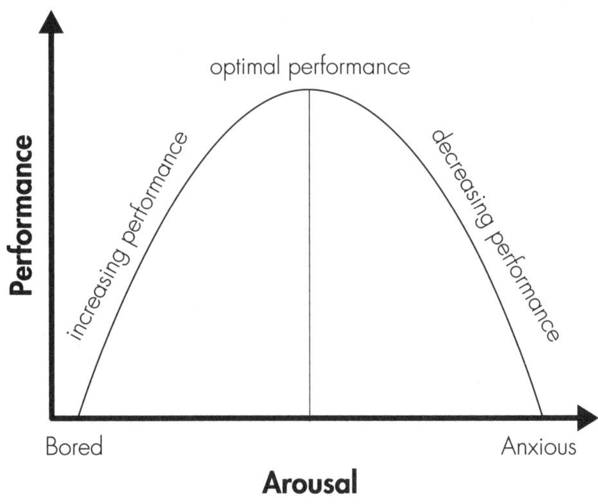

FIGURE 6–2. The Yerkes-Dodson law, which predicts a U-shaped function between arousal and performance.

Across a broad range of experimental settings, it has been shown that optimal performance is attained with moderate levels of arousal that allow for the establishment of task goals, feedback monitoring of task performance, and appropriate resource allocation. The principle indicates that performance increases with cognitive arousal, but only to a certain point. Higher levels of arousal (or stress) may be detrimental to performance because of poor efficacy of allocation.

Cognitive Functioning

Attention

One of the most important findings with respect to cognitive efficiency is the so-called Yerkes-Dodson law (Yerkes and Dodson 1908), which predicts a U-shaped functional relationship between arousal and performance (see Figure 6–2). Across a broad range of experimental settings, it has been shown that optimal performance is attained with moderate levels of arousal that allow for the establishment of task goals, feedback monitoring of task performance, and appropriate resource allocation. The principle suggests that performance increases with cognitive arousal, but only to a certain point.

Anxiety is thus important within the field of cognition and performance because it is often associated with adverse effects on the performance of cognitive tasks. Cognitive resources, of which attention is one example, are limited in their capacity. Therefore, actors that compete for attention will limit the extent to which cognitive resources can be marshaled in the attainment of goals. Higher levels of arousal (or stress) may be detrimental to performance because of poor efficacy of attentional allocation.

Processing-efficiency theory is based on the tripartite working-memory model described by Baddeley (1986, 2001). According to the original model, the limited-capacity working-memory system consists of 1) a modality-free central executive, involved in the processing of information and self-regulatory functions (e.g., performance monitoring, planning, and strategy selection); 2) a phonological loop for the rehearsal and short-term storage of verbal information; and 3) a visuospatial sketchpad for the processing and short-term storage of visual and spatial information.

Converging evidence suggests that it is the central executive that is most affected by anxiety (for a review, see Eysenck et al. 2007). Miyake et al. (2000) further subdivided the functions of the central executive into the following categories:

1. Updating and monitoring working-memory representations. Worrisome thoughts interfere predominantly with this processing and storage function.
2. Shifting back and forth between multiple tasks, operations, or mental sets, involving adaptive changes in attentional control, based on task demands.
3. Inhibiting disruptive responses. Inhibition is "one's ability to deliberately inhibit dominant, automatic, or prepotent responses when necessary." Inhibition involves using attentional control to resist disruption or interference from task-irrelevant stimuli or responses. (Miyake et al. 2000)

The effects of extreme anxiety states on cognitive performance are twofold. First, anxiety increases the extent to which threat-related stimuli (such as fearful faces or salient words) capture attention, which in turn leads to impaired cognitive control. Second, anxiety impairs attentional control, even when no threat-related stimuli are present. Worrisome thoughts consume some of the limited attentional resources of working memory, which are therefore less available for concurrent task processing. Anxiety leads to cognitive interference, limiting the processing and temporary storage capacity of working memory. In this sense, anxiety has a more general effect on cognitive performance and does not require the presentation of anxiety-provoking stimuli to elicit demonstrated cognitive deficits. Studies have addressed this more general effect of anxiety on cognitive performance by looking at the effects of trait anxiety or anxiety disorders, manipulating anxiety levels, and ascertaining the effects on standard measures of working memory and executive function. The detrimental effects of anxiety have been shown in numerous tasks assessing the response-inhibitory functions of the central executive, although many individuals manage to compensate with increased cognitive effort.

Anxiety also has an impact on the inhibiting function of the central executive due to resource allocation costs. The adverse effects of anxiety on the inhibition function mean that anxious individuals are more distracted than nonanxious individuals by external task-irrelevant stimuli (presented by the experimenter) and by internal task-irrelevant stimuli (e.g., worrying thoughts; self-preoccupation). Studies using the Stroop color-word task with low- and high-anxious individuals have shown that anxiety adversely affected performance speed only in the condition requiring inhibition of prepotent responses (i.e., color naming of other color words) (Hochman 1967; Pallak et al. 1975). In both studies, individuals in the high-stress condition performed significantly worse than participants in the low-stress condition when the color name and the color word conflicted. Anxiety has been shown to consistently impair the inhibition function of attention in more than 30 studies on the performance of the "emotional" Stroop task (described in the "Attentional Systems" subsection of this chapter; for review, see Eysenck et al. 2007).

Attentional Bias

Anxiety increases the extent to which threat-related stimuli capture attention, which in turn leads to impaired cognitive control. It is not advantageous for an individual under threat and experiencing anxiety to maintain high attentional focus on a specific stimulus or location. Instead, the optimal strategy is to allocate attentional resources widely, thereby reducing attentional focus with respect to any given task. Attentional bias paradigms such as the emotional Stroop task and the dot-probe task are designed to address this interaction of anxiety with cognitive control.

Relative to healthy participants, anxious patients allocate more attention to threatening information than to neutral information. Evolution has enabled the brain to prioritize attentional resources to threat-related stimuli, even when those stimuli are not fully perceived via preconscious, fast neural pathways (LeDoux 1996). Certain stimuli, such as snakes, spiders, and facial expressions, as well as blood and mutilations, have emotional relevance and have had "privileged" access to attention evolution. These evolutionary "prepared" stimuli (Ohman and Mineka 2001) activate emotional processing modes, even at weak strength or in short duration.

Evidence supporting the notion that threat-related material captures attention preferentially has come from studies of attentional bias (see Eysenck 1992, for review). Attentional bias is the tendency to concentrate on threat-related stimuli (or, more often, to show slow attentional disengagement from such stimuli) when presented concurrently with neutral stimuli. The automatic attentional bias is considered an example of information processing modes activated by specific privileged stimuli. The attentional bias hypothesis is embedded in general emotion theory and would be expected to apply to both clinical and nonclinical individuals showing elevated levels of anxiety.

Attentional Systems

Corbetta and Shulman (2002) distinguish between a *goal-directed* attentional system, which is influenced by expectation, knowledge, and current goals, and a *stimulus-driven* attentional system, which responds maximally to salient threat-related stimuli. The stimulus-driven attentional system, instantiated in the temporoparietal and ventral frontal cortex, is involved in the bottom-up control of attention and "is recruited during the detection of behaviorally relevant sensory events, particularly when they are salient and unattended" (Corbetta and Shulman 2002). The balance between reactivity and control is an important basis for the emotional modulation of attention (see Pashler et al. 2001 for a review). Competition among stimuli for limited attentional resources may be influenced by both bottom-up, sensory-driven mechanisms and top-down, goal-driven control.

According to attentional control theory, anxiety disrupts the bidirectional influences of these two attentional systems (see Figure 6–1). It is associated with an increased sensitivity to stimulus-driven threat cues (Mathews and MacKintosh 1998) via automatic processing of threat-related stimuli (Fox et al. 2005) or with a decreased efficacy of top-down cognitive control in areas such as the anterior cingulate and prefrontal cortex (Bishop et al. 2004). Common tasks that measure attentional bias include the dot-probe task and the emotional Stroop.

In more than two decades of research, the dot-probe task has been used to measure selective visual attention to threat and reward stimuli as a function of individual differences in anxiety. In this paradigm, two stimuli are simultaneously presented and occasionally a small dot appears in one of the two locations previously occupied by one of the stimuli. Participants are required to detect the dot as quickly as possible and to respond by pressing a button. Visual attention to particular stimuli results in quick detection of dots appearing in the same region and slow detection of dots appearing in a different region (see Figure 6–3). Attentional bias in anxious patients is inferred from relatively faster detection of dots that replace anxiety-related stimuli than of dots that replace neutral stimuli (Mogg et al. 2000; Pishyar et al. 2004).

Findings on attentional bias support the assumption that the stimulus-driven attentional system is more affected by threat-related stimuli in anxious individuals than in nonanxious individuals. A number of studies have shown that attentional bias depends mainly on the difficulty individuals have in disengaging from threat-related stimuli, rather than on faster orientation toward stimuli (Fox et al. 2002; Salemink et al. 2007). In general, high-trait-anxious individuals, in contrast to low-trait-anxious individuals, demonstrate a specific tendency to dwell on fear-relevant stimuli, as opposed to negative information. It is possible that delayed disengagement from threat is important in the maintenance of anxiety states.

The emotional Stroop task is another measure of the extent to which adverse effects of anxiety on task performance are caused by task-irrelevant stimuli; these effects are greater when the stimuli are threat-related rather than neutral (see Williams et al. 1996, for a review). In the emotional Stroop task, neutral or threat-related words are presented in color and participants name the color as rapidly as possible. The prediction is that the effect of anxiety in slowing the pace of color-naming performance should be greater when the words are threat-related; that effect is called the *emotional Stroop interference effect*. The slowing of color naming by fear words in high-anxious groups is traditionally accounted for by an automatic bias directing attention toward the emotional meaning of the words, which leads to interference in color naming (Fox 1996; Mathews and MacLeod 2002; Mogg and Bradley 2005; Williams et al. 1996). Other authors have suggested that the effect is more likely to be caused by a slow disengagement process than by a fast orienting bias (Phaf and Kan 2007), and that inhibition of color processing/naming is task-relevant; therefore, slowed responses imply that there is insufficient inhibition.

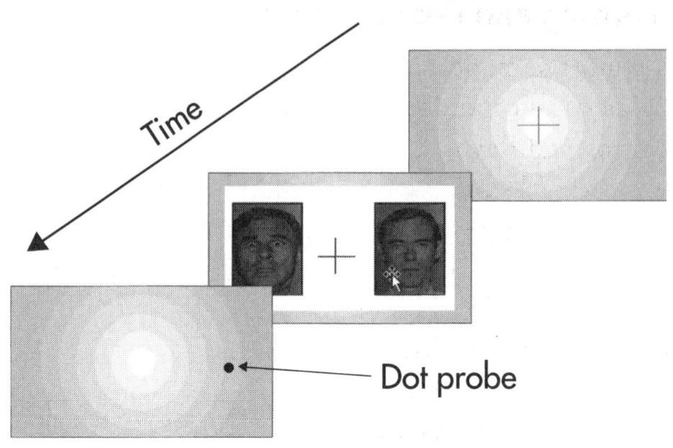

FIGURE 6–3. The dot-probe task.

In this case, two pictures are simultaneously presented and occasionally a small dot appears in one of the two locations previously occupied by one of the stimuli. Participants are required to detect the dot as quickly as possible and to respond by pressing a button. Visual attention to particular stimuli results in quick detection of dots appearing in a same region and slow detection of dots appearing in a different region. Attentional bias in anxious patients is inferred from relatively faster detection of dots replacing fearful faces than neutral faces. Anxious individuals are more likely to have difficulty disengaging from the fearful face once their attention has been oriented toward it.

In a meta-analysis by Phaf and Kan (2007), the largest Stroop effect was obtained for anxious patients, and the second-largest (more modest) effect was for high-anxious nonclinical participants, implying a graded response depending on severity of anxiety.

Learning and Conditioning

Attempts to model anxiety disorders in humans by using classical conditioning go back to the 1920s, when Watson and Rayner (1920) reported their experiments on "Little Albert" (see boxed text). Pavlovian aversive-conditioning paradigms remain key to theories of pathogenesis for both fear and anxiety (Ohman and Mineka 2001). During conditioning, an aversive *unconditioned stimulus* (US) (e.g., a footshock) is paired repeatedly with a neutral *conditioned stimulus* (CS) (e.g., a sound). Once the association is learned, the CS signals the imminent onset of the aversive stimulus. Symptoms of fear are thus elicited when the CS is presented.

If the conditioned stimulus is repeatedly presented without the neutral unconditioned stimulus, the CS usually loses its ability to produce a response, through the process of *extinction*. In contrast, the attenuation of the fear response does not seem to occur in many anxiety disorders—in which operant learning may perpetuate the behavior. In operant theory, the individual will make every attempt to avoid the fear of anxiety associated with the feared object. By avoiding the anxiety-provoking stimulus, the individual experiences an accompanying reduction in fear, and thus feels better. The behavior is thus reinforced and the disorder may remain without any external reinforcement for many years. The result is that the individual does not receive an opportunity to test his or her fears, which would allow extinction of the phobia to occur.

Mowrer's (1947) two-factor model of phobias integrates contributions from classical conditioning and operant conditioning to explain how phobias are acquired and maintained. The combined classical-operant conditioning model is the basis for behavioral treatment strategies such as exposure and desensitization. These therapies are based on the idea that exposure will allow extinguishment of the learned association between the anxiety-provoking situation and fear. They have proved to be successful in the management of phobias, posttraumatic stress disorder, and obsessive-compulsive disorder.

The study of fear conditioning as it relates to anxiety disorders has made significant progress in the past decade, as researchers conducted animal studies in which they identified temporoamygdalolimbic circuits integral to fear conditioning (Blair et al. 2001; Schafe et al. 2001). Human imaging studies have suggested similar neural substrates (LaBar et al. 1998). It has become clear that fear circuitry is highly conserved across species, offering a significant opportunity for translational work in the field.

Watson and Rayner's "Conditioned Emotional Reactions"

In 1920, Watson and Rayner wrote a paper called "Conditioned Emotional Reactions." In this article, they described the experiences of Little Albert, an 11-month-old child with an acquired fear of rabbits and rodents. Unlike Little Hans, a child described by Freud, who presented with phobia that arose in the natural course of his development, Little Albert's phobias were the direct result of the experimental intervention conducted by the two scientists.

Watson and Rayner were attempting to replicate studies of conditioned fear in animals. They theorized that phobias arose due to the conditioned pairing of a fear-inducing stimulus, such as a loud noise (unconditioned stimulus), with a neutral stimulus (conditioned stimulus). Over successive pairings, the neutral stimulus (or conditioned stimulus) becomes associated with the anxiety provoked by the unconditioned stimulus through Pavlovian conditioning. Eventually, the presentation of the conditioned stimulus alone will provoke a fear response. The investigators established this effect by presenting Albert with a rat (conditioned stimulus) and a simultaneous loud noise (unconditioned stimulus), produced by striking an iron bar. After a number of pairings, the boy began to cry whenever a rat was brought into the room. The paradigm was suggested as a possible model for the etiology of phobias.

In a cued fear conditioning experiment, the CS represents a clear threat signal that predicts the onset of an aversive event. Once the association is learned, the presentation of the CS induces acute fear, which subsides after a short period of time. In animal studies, however, startle responses gradually increase over the course of aversive conditioning (Gewirtz et al. 1998), possibly reflecting growing anxiety or distress. This gradual rise in startle responses is not linked to specific fear cues in the classical sense. Instead, the testing environment is more generally linked to a sense that aversive events are likely to occur in the future. Humans too show increased baseline startle responses to numerous contextual cues, including being told that shocks will be administered

(Bocker et al. 2001), the sight of shock electrodes, and darkness (Grillon and Ameli 1998). The experimental paradigm, therefore, leads to fear that is associated with the context in which conditioning takes place. *Context conditioning* induces a state of hypervigilance and distress, similar to anxiety, which is not linked to a specific cue but rather to a more diffuse potential threat. Context conditioning can be thought of as an experimental model for anxiety in the same way that cued fear conditioning is a model for fear.

Animal research has demonstrated dissociable anatomical correlates of contextual versus cued fear conditioning. For example, a study by Selden et al. (1991) showed that lesions of the amygdala impaired aversive conditioning to an explicit auditory cue but did not affect contextual conditioning. In contrast, lesions of the hippocampus prevented contextual conditioning but did not affect aversive conditioning to explicit cues (CS). Although controversial, these findings have been replicated in other studies, suggesting that the nuclei of the amygdala are important in cued fear conditioning (Davis 1998; LeDoux 1998), whereas the dorsal hippocampus and the amygdala are important in context conditioning (Phillips and LeDoux 1992).

Animal studies reveal that the central nucleus of the amygdala is involved in the expression of reflexive fear responses, whereas the basolateral amygdala is part of a system responsible for instrumental choice based on emotional events such as fear (Killcross et al. 1997). This information suggests that anxiety states may result from the interaction between different substrates involved in voluntary avoidance behavior and the behavioral expression of fear.

Patients with anxiety disorders show increased baseline startle responses, compared with control subjects, in experiments in which they are expecting an aversive stimulus (e.g., threat of shock), although baseline responses of the two groups did not differ in nonthreatening experiments (see Figure 6–4) (Grillon 2002b; Grillon et al. 1998b). This result suggests that anxious patients are overly sensitive to threatening contexts. Unlike phobic patients, however, anxious patients do not exhibit an increased fear response in cued fear experiments (de Jong et al. 1996; Vrana et al. 1992).

Uncertainty and Associative Learning

Cognitive theorists have suggested that abnormalities in appraisal or information processing are potential causes of anxiety. Intolerance of uncertainty is an important concept that has been associated with generalized anxiety disorder (Dugas and Ladouceur 2000; Dugas et al. 1998, 2005) and symptom severity in OCD (Steketee et al. 1998). It has been defined as a "difficulty with ambiguity, newness, and unpredictable change" (Sookman and Pinard 1995); other definitions also emphasize the negative appraisal of uncertainty by anxious individuals (Starcevic et al. 2006) (see Chapter 5, "Anxious Traits and Temperaments," this volume). Learning decreases uncertainty, and an effective fear conditioning system would allow the organism to predict aversive events by linking them to specific stimuli. Fear conditioning and associative learning may thus decrease anxiety by allowing the subject to focus on stimuli that predict aversive outcomes.

When shocks are signaled by a tone (and thus are predictable), cued fear results. If stimuli are unpredictable or paired associations are not yet learned, then the entire environment remains linked to aversive events and contextual fear, and the result is anxiety. The lack of predictable signals means that there is no implied safety, and the organism remains in a state of ongoing anxiety. Seligman and Binik (1977) suggested that when an organism can predict an aversive event via a signal, then the absence of that signal also predicts the absence of danger: a so-called *safety signal*. As conditioning continues in a new context, there is a reduction in the number of stimuli that elicit fear as the fear response becomes specific to certain stimuli. Conditioning therefore allows subjects to reduce uncertainty and make predictions about aversive outcomes in the environment.

The safety signal theory has been tested experimentally by presenting two or more different stimuli, one being paired with an aversive stimulus (CS+) while another is not (CS–). CS– conditions therefore function as a safety signal in aversive learning paradigms. Seligman and Binik's results have been confirmed by others, supporting the notion that uncertainty about cue-outcome association leads to anxiety—for example, by showing increased fear responses to CS– in anxious populations relative to low-anxious individuals (Grillon and Ameli 2001; Grillon and Morgan 1999; Orr et al. 2000; Peri et al. 2000). An increase in reported anticipatory anxiety following CS– presentation has also been reported in patients with anxiety, relative to control subjects with normal trait anxiety (Hermann et al. 2002).

Explicit knowledge about CS–US pairings, termed *contingency awareness* (Lovibond and Shanks 2002), can be ascertained in human conditioning experiments by asking subjects whether aversive events were linked to cues. There is significant variability in contingency

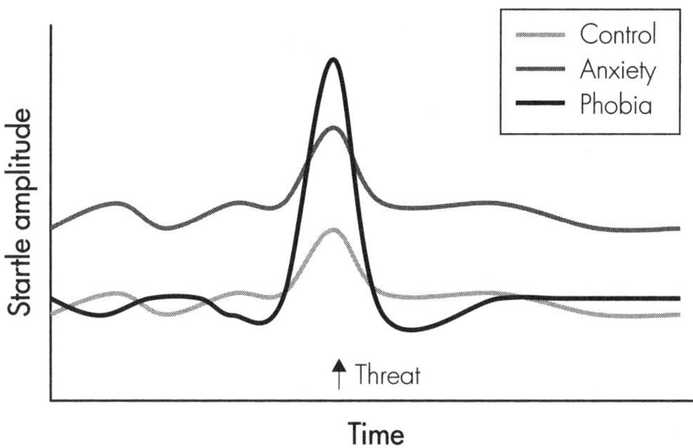

FIGURE 6–4. Differing profiles of startle response in anxious patients and phobic patients versus control subjects.

Anxious patients show a generalized increase in baseline startle during an aversive task (e.g., threat of shock). In contrast, fear-related disorders such as phobia show normal baseline but an exaggerated fear response when patients are presented with the object of their fear (e.g., a picture of a spider).

awareness among humans, with 30%–40% of subjects in some studies characterized as unable to verbalize the CS–US pairings (Chan and Lovibond 1996; Hamm and Vaitl 1996). Studies have shown that those who did not learn the response contingencies (and therefore perceived shocks as unpredictable) showed increased contextual fear and subjective anxiety on subsequent testing days (Grillon 2002a).

Contingency awareness is likely to be a higher cognitive process, and there is some evidence that subjects do learn the contingencies via preconscious, subcortical fast pathways, as indexed by psychophysiological recordings (Hamm and Weike 2005). A similar theory has been put forward by Davis et al. (2000), who suggested that anxiety results from failure to inhibit the fear response in the presence of safety signals. The idea that nonsalient cues generate an increased fear response is compatible with the idea of uncertainty and may speak to the mechanisms underlying deficits in cue-outcome associations underlying uncertainty.

Trait anxiety is strongly correlated with associative learning deficits in aversive conditioning experiments (Chan and Lovibond 1996), although whether it is a cause or effect remains unclear. It is possible that attention deficits associated with trait anxiety may lead to difficulty in learning CS–US associations. Measures of SCR provide some evidence in support of this explanation. The orienting response (OR), a measure of attention, is important in CS–US association. Deficits in OR are associated with poor contingency awareness. Like trait anxiety, variability in OR appears very early in development. Differences in OR relating to autonomic conditioning have been demonstrated among 3-month-old infants (Ingram and Fitzgerald 1974). Attentional and associative learning deficits may cause the world to seem unpredictable, and thus lead to higher levels of anxiety.

In summary, the conditioned fear model has remained one of the major theories for the acquisition of phobias for nearly a century. It has good face validity and is highly conserved across species, making it useful for translational research (see Chapter 3, "Preclinical Models of Anxiety," this volume). Despite criticism of the model, it has been validated by numerous findings, including 1) the increased rates of anxiety disorders among individuals who experienced trauma (Green et al. 1990b) or combat (Green et al. 1990a), 2) the effectiveness of exposure therapy for many anxiety disorders, and, more recently, 3) the observation that D-cycloserine, which improves extinction of the fear conditioned response, improves outcomes in exposure therapy (Ressler et al. 2004) (see also Chapter 10, "Combined Treatment of Anxiety Disorders," this volume).

Anxiety Disorders

In the previous sections, we reviewed the general neurocognitive effects of anxiety. The following section highlights some of the cognitive deficits that have been reported in specific anxiety disorders. The individual differences in cognitive profiles are summarized in Table 6–1.

TABLE 6–1. Cognitive deficits in anxiety disorders

Cognitive domain	GAD	PD	SAD	Simple phobia	OCD	PTSD
Working memory	+++	–	++	–	++	+++
Attention bias (e.g., emotional Stroop and dot-probe)	+++	+++	+++	+++	+++	+++
Cognitive flexibility (e.g., WCST and ID/ED)	–	–	+*	–	+++	–
Response inhibition (e.g., go/no-go and SSRT)	–	–	–	–	+++	–
FPS	–	–	–	?	–	–
Increased baseline startle	++	+++	+++	?	+++	+++
Disgust sensitivity	–	–	–	++	–	–

Note. +=limited effect; ++=moderate effect; +++=strong effect; –=evidence of no effect; ?=no evidence.
FPS=fear-potentiated startle; GAD=generalized anxiety disorder; ID/ED=Intradimensional/Extradimensional Set Shifting task; OCD=obsessive-compulsive disorder; PD=panic disorder; PTSD=posttraumatic stress disorder; SAD=social anxiety disorder; SSRT=stop signal reaction time; WCST=Wisconsin Card Sorting Test.

*When tested in stressful situations.

Generalized Anxiety Disorder

Pathological worry is conceptualized in DSM-IV-TR as excessive, out of proportion to the actual problem, pervasive, present most of the time, focused on several themes or topics (typically, those that pertain to "everyday, routine, life circumstances" and/or "minor matters"), uncontrollable, having a tendency to interfere with functioning, and causing high levels of distress and impairment.

There is evidence that individuals with GAD have an interpretive bias, in which they tend to interpret threatening meanings of emotionally ambiguous events or information. Attentional bias may be a state marker for anxiety. It is perhaps possible to train highly anxious individuals to adopt more benign attentional and interpretive biases. For example, a study by Mogg et al. (1995) showed that attentional bias, as measured by the emotional Stroop task, improved alongside anxiety symptoms following cognitive-behavioral therapy.

Panic Disorder

In contrast to most other anxiety disorders, panic disorder has few associated neurocognitive impairments, apart from deficits in aspects of attention (Lautenbacher et al. 2002). Attention bias has also been well replicated in studies. Indeed, panic patients may have attention bias toward their own somatic symptoms; studies have shown, for example, that panic symptoms themselves increase anxiety sensitivity (Schmidt et al. 2000). Learning theories indicate that panic symptoms are maintained by interoceptive conditioning (conditioned fear of internal somatic cues). Preconscious somatic cues (e.g., increased heart rate) elicit a conditioned fear response as a result of previous associative pairings with anxiety and panic.

Social Anxiety Disorder

Social anxiety disorder (SAD, also called social phobia, involves persistent anxiety about negative evaluation by others, and is associated with significant functional impairment. Milder forms of performance anxiety are more common and have been studied by placing individuals in socially stressful situations (e.g., public speaking) and then measuring cognitive performance. There is general support for the notion of attention bias in SAD. Individuals with SAD exhibit increased attention to potentially threatening social information. They tend to interpret ambiguous social information as negative and fail to generate positive interpretations of social information.

Compared with control subjects, under conditions of stress, individuals with SAD show more generalized cognitive dysfunction, including failures in working memory and set-shifting (Graver and White 2007). There is also some evidence of memory bias: patients with SAD exhibit increased memory for information that is related to negative evaluation from others and to negative self-referential memories.

Obsessive-Compulsive Disorder

People with obsessive-compulsive disorder (OCD) manifest some distinct cognitive deficits that differentiate the condition from other anxiety disorders. In addition to explicit attentional biases to OCD-relevant stimuli, OCD patients show impairment in cognitive and behavioral inhibitory processes that are thought to underlie many of the symptoms and neurocognitive findings of the condition (for a review, see Chamberlain et al. 2005). Specifically, deficits in set-shifting and response inhibition are widely reported in research on OCD, but not in investigations on other anxiety disorders.

Response inhibition (RI) refers to cognitive processes directing executive control over prepotent motor responses (Aron et al. 2003; Logan et al. 1984). In go/no-go tasks, subjects have to perform a simple motor response (such as pressing a button) as quickly as possible when target stimuli are presented, and withhold the motor response when nontarget stimuli are presented. Many studies have revealed that OCD patients show deficits in response inhibition versus healthy control subjects. These deficits are manifested in terms of increased numbers of commission errors (inappropriate responses to no-go stimuli) and longer stop-signal reaction times (an index of the time it takes for the brain to suppress a prepotent response).

Set-shifting represents the ability to switch attention from one aspect of a stimulus to another in an ongoing task, in accordance with changing reinforcement contingencies. Deficits have been reported using a number of different tests, including the Wisconsin Card Sorting Test (WCST; Berg 1948), the Object Alternation Test (OAT; Freedman 1990) and Delayed Alternation Test (DAT; Freedman and Oscar-Berman 1986), the Intradimensional/Extradimensional Set Shift task (ID/ED; Roberts et al. 1988), and the Cambridge Neuropsychological Test Automated Battery (CANTAB; Cambridge Cognition 2006).

Although anxiety remains a key feature of OCD, structural and functional abnormalities in the orbitofrontal cortex, anterior cingulate gyrus, and basal ganglia (Saxena and Rauch 2000; Saxena et al. 1999) indicate orbitofrontal loop dysfunction rather than primary amygdala or septohippocampal differences.

Posttraumatic Stress Disorder

Unlike many anxiety disorders, posttraumatic stress disorder (PTSD) is understood to have a clear causal event, although why some individuals are vulnerable to developing symptoms following trauma is still unclear. Classical fear conditioning has long been seen as a paradigm for PTSD, in which strong cue-response associations are learned at the time of the trauma. Subsequent presentation of environmental cues leads to feelings of panic and fear. Recently, it has been suggested that individuals with PTSD may have a greater sensitivity to contextual fear conditioning, which would explain the sustained hyperarousal and vigilance associated with the disorder (Grillon and Morgan 1999; Grillon et al. 1998a). For example, aversive anticipation, measured by baseline startle response in the face of perceived threats, may be augmented by contextual cues, such as darkness and information, about expected fear stimuli.

The basolateral amygdala is an important locus for memory of aversive CS–US associations. Animal studies have shown that previously formed fear memories can be reactivated by representation of the CS. Once the fear memory is reactivated, reconsolidation is thought to be necessary to maintain, strengthen, or modify the memory, and this reconsolidation process can be disrupted (Nader 2003) through *N*-methyl-D-aspartate receptor manipulations (Lee et al. 2006), noradrenergic blockade, or disruption of protein synthesis within the basolateral amygdala (Tronson and Taylor 2007). Although these study findings suggest an intriguing therapeutic mechanism for disorders such as PTSD, few human studies have been carried out to date.

Simple Phobia

In contrast to anxiety disorders, phobia is considered a disorder of fear, in that there is a specific object (e.g., spiders) or environment (e.g., heights) that is feared. Phobia is generally associated with the expectation that aversive, harm-related consequences will follow exposure to the phobic cue. One of the first models for the pathogenesis of phobia involved classical fear conditioning (see boxed text, p. 93). Phobia is believed to be perpetuated by avoidance of phobic stimuli through operant learning. Avoidance, in turn, means that the object of the phobia is not confronted and extinction does not occur. As predicted by this model, exposure therapy is an effective treatment for phobia.

Critics of the learning model argue that phobias should develop with any pairing of fear with an unconditioned stimulus. The model should reliably predict a more varied array of phobias; but, in fact, most phobias are stereotyped and fall into a few categories. In practice, fear conditioning for stimuli that are common in phobias (e.g., spiders, snakes) is fairly easy to achieve. In contrast, it is more difficult to achieve fear conditioning for stimuli that are dangerous but do not commonly elicit phobias (guns, for example). Other limitations to the application of learning theory to phobias include the fact that many people with phobias do not recall a traumatic event linked to the onset of their phobia. This limitation is particularly apparent in the case of environmental phobias (such as phobia of heights or water) and in phobias of spiders and snakes; indeed, many people have limited previous exposure to the feared stimuli. There are also many instances in which people experience trauma in association with a particular object and do not develop phobias. For instance, most people receive numerous painful injections as children without developing needle phobia.

There is a body of evidence suggesting that abnormal *disgust sensitivity* is present in small-animal phobias (de Jong et al. 2002). For example, compared with nonphobic individuals, those who are spider-phobic report experiencing elevated fear and disgust (independent of fear) when viewing pictures of spiders (Sawchuk et al. 2002). Studies have also shown that spider-phobic individuals score significantly higher than nonphobic individuals on general measures of disgust. In fact, disgust sensitivity is a better predictor of avoidance of small animals such as spiders than is fear. Evolutionary theories propose that disgust evolved to prevent the spread of disease. Common phobias, such as rat and cockroach phobias, may be historically associated with the spread of disease.

Conclusion

There are many areas of overlap in the cognitive profile of anxiety disorders. Perhaps the hallmark of this group of disorders is the privileged access that salient stimuli have to limited attentional resources. Although the content is particular to specific disorders in some circumstances, anxiety disorders as a whole are associated with some degree of attention bias. In addition, individuals with disorders that are characterized by chronic worry and anxiety tend to display limitations in the allocation of limited cognitive resources. People with disorders such as GAD, OCD, and PTSD show decrements in working memory and other functions of the central executive. Those with anxiety disorders, as a whole, are more prone to experience anxiety when provoked (e.g., by public speaking for SAD, or by spiders for spider phobia). In these circumstances there is a general trend toward greater cognitive impairment in patients with anxiety disorders compared with control subjects. At present, it is not possible to comment on the direction of causality in terms of cognitive failures and anxiety, but there is some evidence that clinical improvement is associated with improvement in cognitive measures (e.g., improved attention bias [Mogg et al. 1995]).

Animal models of aversive learning have been invaluable in the attempt to understand how pathological anxiety might arise. Recent advances in neuroscientific techniques have led to a renewed interest in this area. In addition, neural mechanisms of fear and anxiety are conserved across species, although many of the animal models (e.g., fear-potentiated startle) have only recently been used in human research.

There is significant conflicting evidence for links between anxiety and general deficits in higher cognitive functions such as planning, strategy, and memory. The effects of anxiety on attention and on the central executive present a potential confound that makes this aspect difficult to address. Nonetheless, considerable progress has been made in differentiating anxiety disorders according to their neuropsychological endophenotype.

Key Clinical Points

- There are both overlapping and distinct cognitive deficits in anxiety disorders.
- Anxiety is a common human condition that can facilitate performance and inform learning about outcomes. Higher levels of anxiety lead to cognitive impairment and poor performance, particularly in terms of working memory.
- Anxiety-provoking stimuli have privileged access to limited cognitive resources. Salient stimuli capture attention, leading to a predisposition toward stimulus-driven attention biases that interfere with goal-directed cognitive processes.
- Fear conditioning has been suggested as a potential model for disorders of fear.
- Learning theory has led to effective behavioral therapies for anxiety disorders.
- Abnormalities in the learning of stimulus-outcome associations can lead to difficulties in recognizing when an environment is safe and when to expect danger. Thus, uncertainty may be an important factor leading to anxiety.

References

American Psychiatric Association: Diagnostic and Statistical Manual of Mental Disorders, 4th Edition, Text Revision. Washington, DC, American Psychiatric Association, 2000

Aron AR, Fletcher PC, Bullmore ET, et al: Stop-signal inhibition disrupted by damage to right inferior frontal gyrus in humans. Nat Neurosci 6:115–116, 2003

Baddeley AD: Working Memory. Oxford, England, Clarendon, 1986

Baddeley AD: Is working memory still working? Am Psychol 56:851–864, 2001

Berg E: A simple objective technique for measuring flexibility in thinking. J Gen Psychol 39:15–22, 1948

Bishop S, Duncan J, Brett M, et al: Prefrontal cortical function and anxiety: controlling attention to threat-related stimuli. Nat Neurosci 7:184–188, 2004

Blair HT, Schafe GE, Bauer EP, et al: Synaptic plasticity in the lateral amygdala: a cellular hypothesis of fear conditioning. Learn Mem 8:229–242, 2001

Bocker KB, Baas JM, Kenemans JL, et al: Stimulus-preceding negativity induced by fear: a manifestation of affective anticipation. Int J Psychophysiol 43:77–90, 2001

Cambridge Cognition: Cambridge Neuropsychological Test Automated Battery (CANTAB). Cambridge, UK, Cambridge Cognition, 2006. Available at http://www.camcog.com. Accessed March 31, 2009.

Campbell-Sills L, Liverant GI, Brown TA: Psychometric evaluation of the behavioral inhibition/behavioral activation scales in a large sample of outpatients with anxiety and mood disorders. Psychol Assess 16:244–254, 2004

Carver CS, White TL: Behavioral inhibition, behavioral activation, and affective responses to impending reward and punishment: the BIS/BAS scales. J Pers Soc Psychol 67:319–333, 1994

Chamberlain SR, Blackwell AD, Fineberg NA, et al: The neuropsychology of obsessive compulsive disorder: the importance of failures in cognitive and behavioural inhibition as candidate endophenotypic markers. Neurosci Biobehav Rev 29:399–419, 2005

Chan CK, Lovibond PF: Expectancy bias in trait anxiety. J Abnorm Psychol 105:637–647, 1996

Corbetta M, Shulman GL: Control of goal-directed and stimulus-driven attention in the brain. Nat Rev Neurosci 3:201–215, 2002

Davis M: Are different parts of the extended amygdala involved in fear versus anxiety? Biol Psychiatry 44:1239–1247, 1998

Davis M, Falls WA, Gewirtz JC: Neural systems involved in fear inhibition: extinction and conditioned inhibition, in Contemporary Issues in Modeling Psychopathology. Edited by Myslobodsky M, Weiner I. New York, Kluwer Academic, 2000, pp 113–142

de Jong P, Visser S, Merckelback H: Startle and spider phobia: unilateral probes and the prediction of treatment response. J Psychophysiol 10:150–160, 1996

de Jong PJ, Peters M, Vanderhallen I: Disgust and disgust sensitivity in spider phobia: facial EMG in response to spider and oral disgust imagery. J Anxiety Disord 16:477–493, 2002

Dugas MJ, Ladouceur R: Treatment of GAD: targeting intolerance of uncertainty in two types of worry. Behav Modif 24:635–657, 2000

Dugas MJ, Freeston MH, Ladouceur R, et al: Worry themes in primary GAD, secondary GAD, and other anxiety disorders. J Anxiety Disord 12:253–261, 1998

Dugas MJ, Marchand A, Ladouceur R: Further validation of a cognitive-behavioral model of generalized anxiety disorder: diagnostic and symptom specificity. J Anxiety Disord 19:329–343, 2005

Eysenck MW: Anxiety: The Cognitive Perspective. Hove, England, Erlbaum, 1992

Eysenck MW, Derakshan N, Santos R, et al: Anxiety and cognitive performance: attentional control theory. Emotion 7:336–353, 2007

Filion DL, Dawson ME, Schell AM: The psychological significance of human startle eyeblink modification: a review. Biol Psychol 47:1–43, 1998

Fox E: Selective processing of threatening words in anxiety: the role of awareness. Cogn Emot 10:449–480, 1996

Fox E, Russo R, Dutton K: Attentional bias for threat: evidence for delayed disengagement from emotional faces. Cogn Emot 16:355–379, 2002

Fox E, Russo R, Georgiou GA: Anxiety modulates the degree of attentive resources required to process emotional faces. Cogn Affect Behav Neurosci 5:396–404, 2005

Freedman M: Object alternation and orbitofrontal system dysfunction in Alzheimer's and Parkinson's disease. Brain Cogn 14:134–143, 1990

Freedman M, Oscar-Berman M: Comparative neuropsychology of cortical and subcortical dementia. Can J Neurol Sci 13:410–414, 1986

Gewirtz JC, McNish KA, Davis M: Lesions of the bed nucleus of the stria terminalis block sensitization of acoustic startle reflex produced by repeated stress, but not fear potentiated startle. Prog Neuropsychopharmacol Biol Psychiatry 22:625–648, 1998

Graver CJ, White PM: Neuropsychological effects of stress on social phobia with and without comorbid depression. Behav Res Ther 45:1193–1206, 2007

Gray JA: The Psychology of Fear and Stress. Cambridge, UK, Cambridge University Press, 1987

Gray JA, McNaughton N: The Neuropsychology of Anxiety (Oxford Psychology Series). New York, Oxford University Press, 2000

Green BL, Grace MC, Lindy JD, et al: Risk factors for PTSD and other diagnoses in a general sample of Vietnam veterans. Am J Psychiatry 147:729–733, 1990a

Green BL, Lindy JD, Grace MC, et al: Buffalo Creek survivors in the second decade: stability of stress symptoms. Am J Orthopsychiatry 60:43–54, 1990b

Grillon C: Associative learning deficits increase symptoms of anxiety in humans. Biol Psychiatry 51:851–858, 2002a

Grillon C: Startle reactivity and anxiety disorders: aversive conditioning, context, and neurobiology. Biol Psychiatry 52:958–975, 2002b

Grillon C, Ameli R: Effects of threat of shock, shock electrode placement and darkness on startle. Int J Psychophysiol 28:223–231, 1998

Grillon C, Ameli R: Conditioned inhibition of fear-potentiated startle and skin conductance in humans. Psychophysiology 38:807–815, 2001

Grillon C, Davis M: Fear-potentiated startle conditioning in humans: explicit and contextual cue conditioning following paired versus unpaired training. Psychophysiology 34:451–458, 1997

Grillon C, Morgan CA 3rd: Fear-potentiated startle conditioning to explicit and contextual cues in Gulf War veterans with posttraumatic stress disorder. J Abnorm Psychol 108:134–142, 1999

Grillon C, Morgan CA 3rd, Davis M, et al: Effect of darkness on acoustic startle in Vietnam veterans with PTSD. Am J Psychiatry 155:812–817, 1998a

Grillon C, Morgan CA 3rd, Davis M, et al: Effects of experimental context and explicit threat cues on acoustic startle in Vietnam veterans with posttraumatic stress disorder. Biol Psychiatry 44:1027–1036, 1998b

Hamm AO, Vaitl D: Affective learning: awareness and aversion. Psychophysiology 33:698–710, 1996

Hamm AO, Weike AI: The neuropsychology of fear learning and fear regulation. Int J Psychophysiol 57:5–14, 2005

Hermann C, Ziegler S, Birbaumer N, et al: Psychophysiological and subjective indicators of aversive pavlovian conditioning in generalized social phobia. Biol Psychiatry 52:328–337, 2002

Hochman SH: The effects of stress on Stroop color-word performance. Psychon Sci 9:475–476, 1967

Ingram E, Fitzgerald HE: Individual differences in infant orienting and autonomic conditioning. Dev Psychobiol 7:359–367, 1974

Johnson SL, Turner RJ, Iwata N: BIS/BAS Levels and Psychiatric Disorder: an epidemiological study. J Psychopathol Behav Assess 25:25–36, 2003

Killcross S, Robbins TW, Everitt BJ: Different types of fear-conditioned behaviour mediated by separate nuclei within amygdala. Nature 388:377–380, 1997

LaBar KS, Gatenby JC, Gore JC, et al: Human amygdala activation during conditioned fear acquisition and extinction: a mixed-trial fMRI study. Neuron 20:937–945, 1998

Lautenbacher S, Spernal J, Krieg JC: Divided and selective attention in panic disorder: a comparative study of patients with panic disorder, major depression and healthy controls. Eur Arch Psychiatry Clin Neurosci 252:210–213, 2002

LeDoux J: Emotion: clues from the brain. Annu Rev Psychol 46:209–235, 1995

LeDoux J: The Emotional Brain. New York, Simon and Schuster, 1996

LeDoux J: Fear and the brain: where have we been, and where are we going? Biol Psychiatry 44:1229–1238, 1998

Lee JL, Milton AL, Everitt BJ: Reconsolidation and extinction of conditioned fear: inhibition and potentiation. J Neurosci 26:10051–10056, 2006

Logan GD, Cowan WB, Davis KA: On the ability to inhibit simple and choice reaction time responses: a model and a method. J Exp Psychol Hum Percept Perform 10:276–291, 1984

Lovibond PF, Shanks DR: The role of awareness in pavlovian conditioning: empirical evidence and theoretical implications. J Exp Psychol Anim Behav Process 28:3–26, 2002

Marks I: Fears, Phobias and Rituals: Panic, Anxiety and Their Disorders. New York, Oxford University Press, 1987

Mathews A, MacKintosh BA: A cognitive model of selective processing in anxiety. Cogn Ther Res 22:539–560, 1998

Mathews AM, MacLeod C: Induced processing biases have causal effects on anxiety. Cogn Emot 16:331–354, 2002

Miyake A, Friedman NP, Emerson MJ, et al: The unity and diversity of executive functions and their contributions to complex "frontal lobe" tasks: a latent variable analysis. Cognit Psychol 41:49–100, 2000

Mogg K, Bradley BP: Attentional bias in generalized anxiety disorder versus depressive disorder. Cogn Ther Res 29:29–45, 2005

Mogg K, Bradley BP, Millar N, et al: A follow-up study of cognitive bias in generalized anxiety disorder. Behav Res Ther 33:927–935, 1995

Mogg K, Bradley BP, Dixon C, et al: Trait anxiety, defensiveness and selective processing of threat: an investigation using two measures of attentional bias. Pers Individ Dif 28:1063–1077, 2000

Mowrer OH: On the dual nature of learning: a reinterpretation of "conditioning" and "problem-solving." Harv Educ Rev 17:102–148, 1947

Nader K: Neuroscience: re-recording human memories. Nature 425:571–572, 2003

Ohman A, Mineka S: Fears, phobias, and preparedness: toward an evolved module of fear and fear learning. Psychol Rev 108:483–522, 2001

Orr SP, Metzger LJ, Lasko NB, et al: De novo conditioning in trauma-exposed individuals with and without posttraumatic stress disorder. J Abnorm Psychol 109:290–298, 2000

Pallak MS, Pittman TS, Heller JF, et al: The effect of arousal on Stroop colour-word task performance. Bull Psychon Soc 6:248–250, 1975

Pashler H, Johnston JC, Ruthruff E: Attention and performance. Annu Rev Psychol 52:629–651, 2001

Peri T, Ben-Shakhar G, Orr SP, et al: Psychophysiologic assessment of aversive conditioning in posttraumatic stress disorder. Biol Psychiatry 47:512–519, 2000

Phaf RH, Kan KJ: The automaticity of emotional Stroop: a meta-analysis. J Behav Ther Exp Psychiatry 38:184–199, 2007

Phillips RG, LeDoux JE: Differential contribution of amygdala and hippocampus to cued and contextual fear conditioning. Behav Neurosci 106:274–285, 1992

Pishyar R, Harris LM, Menzies RG: Attentional bias for words and faces in social anxiety. Anxiety Stress Coping 17:23–36, 2004

Ressler KJ, Rothbaum BO, Tannenbaum L, et al: Cognitive enhancers as adjuncts to psychotherapy: use of D-cycloserine in phobic individuals to facilitate extinction of fear. Arch Gen Psychiatry 61:1136–1144, 2004

Roberts AC, Robbins TW, Everitt BJ: The effects of intradimensional and extradimensional shifts on visual discrimination learning in humans and non-human primates. Q J Exp Psychol B 40:321–341, 1988

Salemink E, van den Hout MA, Kindt M: Selective attention and threat: quick orienting versus slow disengagement and two versions of the dot probe task. Behav Res Ther 45:607–615, 2007

Sawchuk CN, Lohr JM, Westendorf DH, et al: Emotional responding to fearful and disgusting stimuli in specific phobics. Behav Res Ther 40:1031–1046, 2002

Saxena S, Rauch SL: Functional neuroimaging and the neuroanatomy of obsessive-compulsive disorder. Psychiatr Clin North Am 23:563–586, 2000

Saxena S, Brody AL, Maidment KM, et al: Localized orbitofrontal and subcortical metabolic changes and predictors of response to paroxetine treatment in obsessive-compulsive disorder. Neuropsychopharmacology 21:683–693, 1999

Schafe GE, Nader K, Blair HT, et al: Memory consolidation of pavlovian fear conditioning: a cellular and molecular perspective. Trends Neurosci 24:540–546, 2001

Schmidt NB, Lerew DR, Joiner TE Jr: Prospective evaluation of the etiology of anxiety sensitivity: test of a scar model. Behav Res Ther 38:1083–1095, 2000

Selden NR, Everitt BJ, Jarrard LE, et al: Complementary roles for the amygdala and hippocampus in aversive conditioning to explicit and contextual cues. Neuroscience 42:335–350, 1991

Seligman MEP, Binik YM: The safety signal hypothesis, in Operant Pavlovian Interactions. Edited by Davis H, Hurwitz HMB. New York, Hillsdale, 1977, pp 165–187

Sookman D, Pinard G: The Cognitive Schemata Scale: a multidimensional measure of cognitive schemas in obsessive-compulsive disorder. Presented at the World Congress of Behavioural and Cognitive Therapies, Copenhagen, Denmark, May 1995

Spielberger CD: The effects of anxiety on complex learning and academic achievement, in Anxiety and Behavior. Edited by Spielberger CD. New York, Academic Press, 1966, pp 361–398

Spielberger CD: Manual for the State-Trait Anxiety Inventory (Form V). Palo Alto, CA, Consulting Psychologists Press, 1983

Starcevic V, Berle D: Cognitive specificity of anxiety disorders: a review of selected key constructs. Depress Anxiety 23:51–61, 2006

Steketee G, Frost RO, Cohen I: Beliefs in obsessive-compulsive disorder. J Anxiety Disord 12:525–537, 1998

Tronson NC, Taylor JR: Molecular mechanisms of memory reconsolidation. Nat Rev Neurosci 8:262–275, 2007

Vrana SR, Constantine JA, Westman JS: Startle reflex modification as an outcome measure in the treatment of phobia: two case studies. Behav Assess 14:279–291, 1992

Watson JB, Rayner R: Conditioned emotional reactions. J Exp Psychol 3:1–14, 1920

Williams JMG, Mathews A, McLeod C: The emotional Stroop task and psychopathology. Psychol Bull 120:3–24, 1996

Wood J, Mathews A, Dalgleish T: Anxiety and cognitive inhibition. Emotion 1:166–181, 2001

World Health Organization: The ICD-10 Classification of Mental and Behavioural Disorders: Diagnostic Criteria for Research. Geneva, Switzerland, World Health Organization, 1993

Yerkes RM, Dodson JD: The relation of strength of stimulus to rapidity of habit-formation. Journal of Comparative Neurology and Psychology 18:459–482, 1908

Recommended Readings

Chamberlain SR, Blackwell AD, Fineberg NA, et al: The neuropsychology of obsessive compulsive disorder: the importance of failures in cognitive and behavioural inhibition as candidate endophenotypic markers. Neurosci Biobehav Rev 29:399–419, 2005

Eysenck MW, Derakshan N, Santos R, et al: Anxiety and cognitive performance: attentional control theory. Emotion 7:336–353, 2007

Gray JA, McNaughton N: The Neuropsychology of Anxiety (Oxford Psychology Series). New York, Oxford University Press, 2000

Grillon C: Startle reactivity and anxiety disorders: aversive conditioning, context, and neurobiology. Biol Psychiatry 52:958–975, 2002

Kim JJ, Jung MW: Neural circuits and mechanisms involved in pavlovian fear conditioning: a critical review. Neurosci Biobehav Rev 30:188–202, 2006

Lissek S, Powers AS, McClure EB, et al: Classical fear conditioning in the anxiety disorders: a meta-analysis. Behav Res Ther 43:1391–1424, 2005

Starcevic V, Berle D: Cognitive specificity of anxiety disorders: a review of selected key constructs. Depress Anxiety 23:51–61, 2006

Chapter 7

Cognitive-Behavioral Concepts of Anxiety

Robert A. DiTomasso, Ph.D., ABPP
Arthur Freeman, Ed.D., ABPP
Raymond Carvajal, M.A.
Bruce Zahn, Ed.D., ABPP

It would be virtually impossible to conceive of living without experiencing concerns for safety, well-being, or security at some point during the life cycle. These concepts derive from a common concern for anticipated adverse consequences embodied in the cognitive issue of what has been termed the "What if..." phenomenon. In the biological realm, an important matter for any organism is the extent to which the nutrients on which survival hinges can be obtained. In the emotional realm, being free from assault or harm to one's physical well-being or sense of self-esteem is critical. Thus, perception of safety plays a crucial role, because without it, the organism would be in a constant state of anxiety or arousal and prepared for fight-or-flight responses. The cognitive realm encompasses the thoughts, attitudes, beliefs, assumptions, and images that guide feelings and behaviors. In theorizing and attempting to understand the human condition, including the experience of anxiety, the cognitive realm, which was traditionally largely ignored, has gained more attention through its inclusion as part of a model for understanding anxiety (Barlow 2002; Foa and Kozak 1986; Lang and McNeil 2006; Nemeroff et al. 2006; Shafran and Rachman 2004).

Over the past three decades, the field of psychology has undergone a cognitive revolution (Beck 1991, 2005; Mahoney 1974; Meichenbaum 1977). This cognitive or, more aptly termed, cognitive-behavioral revolution has been energized by the interaction among several factors, including the needs of clinical practice, the experimental tradition of behavioral psychology, accountability, and the demand for evidenced-based interventions. This vital interaction has yielded a theoretical model that has produced several empirically supported treatments, a major part of which has been the development and refinement of cognitive-behavioral strategies and techniques (Leahy 2003). Although some debate remains about the relative primacy of behavioral or cognitive approaches (Beck 1991; Simon and Fleming 1985), the therapeutic mix is arguably dependent on the specific goals of therapy, the skills of the patient, and the skills of the therapist (Freeman et al. 1990). To date, cognitive-behavioral therapy (CBT) has been demonstrated to be effective in treating such anxiety conditions as generalized anxiety disorder, posttraumatic stress disorder, social phobia, and childhood anxiety disorders (A.C. Butler et al. 2006). It has also been indicated in the treatment of panic disorder with or without agoraphobia (Friedman et al. 2006), late-life generalized anxiety disorder (Stanley et al. 2003), and comorbid generalized anxiety disorder and panic disorder with agoraphobia (Labrecque et al. 2006). Moreover, treatment gains with CBT for anxiety tend to endure following treatment termination (Hollon et al. 2006), and evidence-based treatments for anxiety disorders, featuring CBT, are to found to be more cost-effective (Myhr and Payne 2006).

The earliest roots of the role and importance of cognition in human behavior can be traced to Eastern, Greek, and Roman philosophers (Beck and Weishaar 1989) and the early work of George Kelly (1955). There is little doubt, however, that the theories of Albert Ellis (1962) and Aaron T. Beck (1967) have been the most influential sources in creating, guiding, and nurturing the cognitive movement. The so-called Third Wave cognitive-behavioral therapies, including Acceptance and Commitment Therapy (ACT; Hayes and Pierson 2005) and Mindfulness-Based Cognitive Therapy (MBCT; Baer 2003), are rapidly gaining in popularity.

In this chapter, we outline and discuss the cognitive-behavioral theory and model of anxiety and anxiety disorders. We address the definition of anxiety and anxiety disorders; basic assumptions of the cognitive-behavioral theory of anxiety; the role of predisposing and precipitation factors; a cognitive-behavioral case conceptualization; and common misconceptions about cognitive theory. Where relevant, we use clinical research and case examples to illustrate our conceptual points.

Definition of Anxiety

Anxiety may be defined as a diffuse state (Barlow and Cerney 1988) "characterized by an unpleasant affective experience marked by a significant degree of apprehensiveness about the potential appearance of future aversive or harmful events" (DiTomasso and Gosch 2002, p. 1). The common elements of the anxiety experience include the following descriptions: a tense emotional state characterized by a variety of sympathomimetic symptoms such as chest pain, palpitations, and shortness of breath; painful uneasiness of mind over an anticipated ill; abnormal apprehension; self-doubt as to the nature of a threat; belief about the reality of the threat; and lapses or weaknesses of coping potential. The human nervous system is designed to prepare and mobilize the individual to respond in one of three ways to an *objective* and physically dangerous threat. We can fight (attack or defend against the force); flee (escape or avoid); or freeze (become paralyzed). The hallmark of the anxious patient, however, is the presence of a powerful perceived threat and the activation of the physical concomitants in the absence of an objective real threat (DiTomasso and Gosch 2002). In other words, the anxious person sees threat and reacts accordingly when no real threat exists. As a way of highlighting this point, we differentiate between fear, which we define as a response to a stimulus that is consensually validated to be scary, and anxiety, a more idiosyncratic response. For example, some individuals can be anxious about flying in an airliner, whereas others may absolutely refuse to fly because of similar concerns. Refusal to fly would be considered an anxiety response, inasmuch as many people do fly with greater or less difficulty. Although some have made this distinction in behavioral terms, others have referred to fear as an unconditioned response and to anxiety as a conditioned response (Barlow 2002).

Basic Assumptions

The cognitive model of anxiety—an information-processing model—makes several basic assumptions about anxiety, its evocation, its mediation, and its significance (Beck 2005; Beck et al. 1985; Wells 1997). These assumptions are crucial to understanding the phenomenon of anxiety and the nature of anxiety disorders from a cognitive perspective.

Beck (2005) proposes that anxiety is a product of biased information processing of stimuli that occur either within or outside the person as *threatening*, which results in the systematic distortion of the person's thinking and construction of his or her experiences, as evidenced in thinking errors called *cognitive distortions* (Yurica and DiTomasso 2005). Underlying these cognitive errors are more lasting dysfunctional beliefs, or *cognitive content*, contained within cognitive structures known as *schemas*. More specifically, the cognitive model of anxiety "stipulates that danger-oriented beliefs (embedded in cognitive schemas) predispose individuals to narrow their attention to threat, engage in dysfunctional *safety behaviors*, and make catastrophic interpretations of ambiguous stimuli" (Beck 2005, p. 955). This threat-based bias, seen in each of the disorders of anxiety, is found in all aspects of information processing, including an individual's perception of a stimulus, his or her interpretation of it, and even the recall of the stimulus and related information (Beck 2005). The assumptions contained in the cognitive-behavioral model of anxiety are presented below.

1. Fear, an emotional response with adaptive significance for humans, is evoked in response to objective danger and is a survival mechanism (Beck et al. 1985; Emery and Tracy 1987; Freeman and Simon 1989; Izard and Blumberg 1985; Lindsley 1952, 1957, 1960; Plutchik 1980; Wells 1997).
2. The evocation of anxiety reactions in response to misperceived or exaggerated perceptions of danger when there truly is no danger, or, if there is any danger at all, it is actually quite remote, is by definition maladaptive (Beck and Greenberg 1988; Beck et al. 1985; DiTomasso and Gosch 2002; Foa and Kozak 1986; Freeman and Simon 1989; Wells 1997).
3. Individuals with anxiety disorder are prone to precipitate false alarms that create a relatively constant state of emotional arousal, tension, and subjective distress. These "fire drills" keep an individual in a relatively constant state of readiness, in which he or she is prepared to confront an anticipated threatening stimulus or situation that never truly materializes (Barlow and Cerney 1988; Beck and Greenberg 1988; Beck et al. 1985; Freeman and Simon 1989; Wells 1997).
4. The cognitive, physiological, motivational, affective, and behavioral systems are all involved and interrelated during anxiety states (Freeman and Simon 1989; Persons 1989; Taylor 1988; Wells 1997).
5. The cognitive system plays a primary, vital, and essential role in appraising danger and resources and activating the physiological, motivational, affective, and behavioral systems, each of which alone and in concert serve important functions (Beck et al. 1985; Foa and Kozak 1986; Freeman and Simon 1989; Lazarus 1991; Wells 1997).
6. The cognitive system mediates its influence through repetitive, unpremeditated, and rapid involuntary thoughts and/or images related to threat or danger of which the individual is unaware (unless attention is called to them), and which the individual accepts as valid without question or challenge (Beck 2005; Beck and Greenberg 1988; Beck et al. 1985; Emery and Tracy 1987; Freeman and Simon 1989; Wells 1997).
7. Automatic thoughts are derived from underlying deeper cognitive structures called schemas, which contain underlying threatening beliefs or assumptions (Beck 2005; Emery and Tracy 1987; Foa and Kozak 1986; Freeman and Simon 1989; Kendall and Ingram 1987; Persons 1989; Wells 1997).
8. Automatic thoughts and schemas are disorder-specific and, in the case of anxiety, reflect themes of danger and threat, as opposed to the themes of loss typically seen in depressed individuals (Beck 2005; Beck and Rush 1975; Beck and Weishaar 1989; Beck et al. 1985; Foa and Kozak 1986; Freeman and Simon 1989; Hilbert 1984; Wells 1997).
9. Anxiety reactions and disorders may be understood by elucidating the individual's automatic thoughts, cognitive distortions, and underlying assumptions (Beck 1976; G. Butler and Matthews 1983; Deffenbacher et al. 1986; DiTomasso and Gilman 2005; Freeman and Simon 1989; Freeman et al. 1990; Merluzzi and Boltwood 1989; Wells 1997).
10. In anxiety-provoking trigger situations, individuals with anxiety disorders tend to activate danger or threat schema, by which they selectively screen-in stimuli and information that indicate danger, and screen-out data that are incompatible with danger or threat (Beck 1976, 2005; Beck et al. 1985; Freeman and Simon 1989; Freeman et al. 1990; Wells 1997).
11. Individuals with anxiety problems have impaired objectivity and ability to evaluate their threat-bound cognitions in a rational and realistic manner (Beck et al. 1985; Wells 1997).
12. Individuals with anxiety disorders show systematic errors in processing information by, for example, overestimating the likelihood of adverse events (Barlow 2002), catastrophizing, selectively abstracting, thinking dichotomously, and jumping to arbitrary conclusions (Beck 2005; Beck et al. 1985; Freeman and Simon 1989; Wells 1997).
13. Conceived from Barlow's triple vulnerability model (Barlow 2002) of the etiology of anxiety disorders, an integrated set of three vulnerabilities is relevant to the development of anxiety and related emotional disorders: a) *generalized biological vulnerability,* which refers to the genetic contributions to the development of anxiety and negative affect (estimated to account for approximately 30% to 50% of the variance), b) *generalized psychological vulnerability,* which refers to the development of a lack of a sense of control over salient events in one's life, based on early life experiences (e.g., early parenting), and c) *specific psychological vulnerability,* in which one learns, based on early life experiences, to focus anxiety on specific objects or events (e.g., somatic symptoms related to panic or to social evaluation), which in turn become associated

with threat and danger. The synergism of these three vulnerabilities is believed to contribute to the development of anxiety.

More recent cognitive-behavioral treatments share commonalities with traditional CBT but also include very distinctive features. Traditional cognitive-behavioral approaches primarily emphasize the importance of altering and restructuring dysfunctional thoughts. As mentioned previously, Acceptance and Commitment Therapy is one of the so-called Third Wave therapies within the cognitive-behavioral realm, with strong roots in behavior therapy and functional contextualism. ACT has gained in popularity and credibility in recent years and stands as an alternative to traditional cognitive therapy, which seeks to change distorted cognitions and related affect, as well as to more purely behaviorally based approaches that seek to alter contingencies that reinforce avoidance behaviors. ACT is grounded in Relational Frame Theory and considers symbolic language to be the primary source of painful affect because of its use of experiential avoidance and cognitive fusion (Hayes and Pierson 2005).

In treating anxiety disorders with ACT, the therapist focuses on refraining from evaluation through the use of defusion and distancing techniques, while teaching methods for refocusing on the experience in the here and now. In ACT, patients with anxiety are taught to observe their thoughts and images as inner language as they separate the words of private dialogue from the actual experience of threat. Patients are taught to accept negative and painful experiences as paradoxically vital components of living a full life, rather than continue trying to restrict their experience through the use of escape and avoidance in order to reassure themselves of relief from suffering. Techniques typically used in ACT include meditation and mindfulness, paradoxical acceptance, and nonjudgmental cognitive defusion. In the final phases of ACT, patients are taught to reassess their values about meaning-making in life. They are asked to commit to living life on life's terms in the present and not trying to control experience by anticipating potential threats to safety and potential ways to avoid them.

Mindfulness-Based Cognitive Therapy (Baer 2003) is based on the work of John Cabot-Zinn. In this type of therapy, patients are taught to identify and accept feelings and thoughts on a transitory basis, to increase their awareness, and to decide to respond instead of reacting automatically to thoughts, feelings, and situations. MBCT assists patients in overcoming the habitual tendency to react automatically. Specifically, mindfulness-based interventions have been found to improve symptoms related to generalized anxiety and panic, among other problems (Baer 2003).

Critical to the general cognitive-behavioral model is the cognitive appraisal of the individual about stressor events. This model of anxiety also makes explicit assumptions about the predisposing and precipitating factors that are associated with the onset of anxiety disorders. In the sections that follow, we discuss several predisposing and precipitating variables related to anxiety disorders. It is important to bear in mind that any combination of these factors may set the stage and provide the impetus for the development, onset, maintenance, and exacerbation of anxiety problems.

Predisposing Factors

According to the cognitive model of anxiety (Beck et al. 1985), five possible factors may predispose or make an individual vulnerable and thus more prone to anxiety and anxiety disorders: 1) genetic heritability; 2) physical disease states; 3) psychological trauma; 4) absence of coping mechanisms; and 5) dysfunctional thoughts, beliefs, assumptions, and cognitive processing. We discuss each of these factors in detail. As a result of individual differences, an anxiety disorder may result from a unique combination of predisposing and precipitating variables (Beck et al. 1985).

Genetics

In recent years, the possibility that genetic factors play a role in certain psychopathological disorders has assumed more importance. Anxiety disorders are no exception. Panic disorder, specific phobia, and obsessive-compulsive disorder are more common among first-degree biological relatives of patients with these disorders. Nonetheless, the question of *how* heredity exerts an influence in anxiety disorders is important to consider in the conceptualization of anxiety. Heredity may manifest its influence by the existence of an easily aroused or labile autonomic nervous system (Barlow 2002; Barlow and Cerney 1988). In other words, in certain anxiety conditions, a family history of the disorder may make it more likely that a patient will have anxiety symptoms under the right set of conditions. Thus, the role of genetic vulnerability cannot be fully appreciated without considering the interactive role of environmental, psychological, and social factors (Barlow 2002; Barlow and Cerney 1988).

Physical Disease

The cognitive-behavioral model also considers the possible role of physical factors in making an individual vulnerable to an anxiety disorder. Two issues must be considered here. First, possible physical causes that can mimic anxiety must be ruled out in assessing anxiety disorders. In many instances, treating the physical problem alone may resolve the symptoms. Second, the existence of a physical problem does not necessarily preclude the existence of an anxiety problem. A physical problem can coexist with an anxiety disorder, and both problems may require treatment. Studies focused on the treatment of anxiety disorders in the primary care setting, where the majority of patients with anxiety disorders seek treatment—and where anxiety often masquerades as a physical disease—have demonstrated that CBT is effective in treating anxiety in the primary care context, as it is in more controlled research settings (Craske et al. 2006; Roy-Byrne et al. 2005).

Psychological Trauma

Mental trauma experienced during development (Beck et al. 1985) may render an individual more vulnerable to feeling anxiety in situations that are similar to the experience of the trauma. This may have been a single event or, more likely, a series of traumatic experiences. Developmental traumas occurring in the context of high emotional arousal can result in the individual's formulating specific schemas about threat ("that situation is dangerous") or broader threat scripts. This latter concept refers to a series of schemas that meet two conditions: they occur in a designated sequence, and they are predictable. For example, the script might be as follows: "That is dangerous." "I can't cope." "Given my inability to cope, I will be hurt." "If I am hurt, I may be damaged beyond repair." "If I run, I may be saved." Such schemas presumably would be related to themes of danger in anxious persons and could be expected to become active in situations resembling the circumstances in which the schema was originally learned. As Foa and Kozak (1986) noted, "A fear memory is accessed when a fearful individual is presented with fear information that matches some of the information structure in memory" (p. 23). According to the emotional processing model described by Foa and Kozak, fear is expressed as a memory network that incorporates information about the stimulus situations and responses and the meaning of the stimuli and responses. Fear structures, by definition, involve themes of danger.

Absence of Coping Mechanisms

Another predisposing factor in the development of anxiety disorders is an individual's deficit in coping response, coupled with a negatively distorted view of ability to cope. Not only are the primary appraisals of situations more likely to result in perceptions of threat when no threat exists in anxiety-prone individuals, but their secondary appraisals of their resources to cope with threat more often reveal inability to cope. Patients with anxiety may have learned to use responses such as avoidance, which have served to strengthen their anxiety and preclude effective coping. As a result, they may find themselves more vulnerable to experiencing anxiety in the presence of life events or other daily stressors. The anxious individual makes primary, secondary, and tertiary evaluations and converts them into a rough ratio equation. This risk-to-resources ratio involves the perception of risk and the perception of resources available to cope effectively with the perceived risk. If the resources are greater than the risk, no anxiety occurs. If the risk is viewed as outweighing the resources, then anxiety occurs.

Instilling effective coping mechanisms in patients with anxiety will increase their resources and is therefore an integral part of CBT. Preliminary evidence suggests that relaxation training by itself has the capability of producing treatment effects similar to CBT (Norton and Price 2007). Enhancement of coping techniques through methods such as relaxation training therefore serves to facilitate, if not produce, positive treatment outcomes for anxiety.

Irrational Thoughts, Assumptions, and Cognitive Processing Errors

The cognitive model of anxiety places primary emphasis on the role of cognitive factors in predisposing individuals to anxiety disorders. In individuals with anxiety disorders, underlying unrealistic beliefs about threat or danger are presumed to be activated by trigger-events or situations that the individual believes are similar to conditions during which these schemas were learned. When these schemas are activated, they fuel the patient's thinking, behavior, and emotion, all of which can serve to reciprocally reinforce one another and the underlying schema. When the anxiety is stimulated, the individual moves to a response that is egocentric, global, and involuntary. The effort is geared to survival, devoid of objectively threatening stimuli. CBT has been shown to alter these dysfunctional cognitions fueling anxiety disorders. The maladaptive beliefs associated with generalized anxiety disorder and panic disorder with agoraphobia, for example, have been modified with CBT, and this has contributed to the recovery of patients with these disorders (Labrecque et al. 2006).

Precipitating Factors

The cognitive model of anxiety (Beck et al. 1985) posits several possible factors that may precipitate anxiety: physical disease or toxic substances, severe external stressors, long-term stressors, and stressors affecting a specific emotional vulnerability or threshold of an individual.

Physical Problems or Toxic Substances

Anxiety can be precipitated by the onset of a physical problem that does or does not mimic anxiety. For example, during an individual's attempt to adjust to illness, it is not an uncommon reaction to develop anxiety after the onset of a physical problem. Physical problems may cause symptoms, such as fatigue or depression, which could compromise or overtax the individual's ability to tolerate or manage even normal, everyday stressors. As a result, previously handled stressors may overburden the individual's resources. In addition, a physical problem may present an individual with an array of symptoms that are viewed as signs of a serious problem—when the problem is actually relatively benign. Some anxious patients seem to be hypervigilant about normal bodily reactions that they interpret in a threatening manner.

Respiratory difficulties may lead to a disruption of the oxygen and carbon dioxide balance. This may manifest as anxiety-like symptoms. In some instances, individuals ingest a psychoactive substance that produces some physical affect that is interpreted as threatening. Everly (1983) discussed the notion of biogenic stressors or substances, such as caffeine and amphetamine, which are capable of precipitating a stress response by circumventing the cognitive appraisal mechanism. Of course, cognitive appraisal of the stress response can serve to exacerbate the response. Another pharmacological source of anxiety-like symptoms involves the use of prescription drugs that are stimulants. Certain decongestants or bronchodilators have the effect of increasing the heart rate and causing lightheadedness. These symptoms may also be interpreted as threatening and cause anxiety, creating a vicious cycle.

In summary, many substances can be classified as biogenic stressors that circumvent the cognitive appraisal system and act directly on the nervous system (Everly 1983). However, cognitive appraisal may exacerbate even those symptoms precipitated by the biogenic stressor.

Patients with panic disorder, for example, tend to make catastrophic interpretations of bodily sensations (Beck 2005). In primary care settings, where these patients often present, the combination of CBT and medication has been shown to produce great initial and long-term benefits (Craske et al. 2005). The degree of improvement experienced by patients who present with panic disorder in primary care settings increases relative to the number of CBT sessions attended and follow-up telephone contacts completed by the patients (Craske et al. 2006).

Severe External Stressors

The occurrence of a severe stressor or life event, such as loss of a job or loved one, is another possible precipitant of anxiety. The role of life events in precipitating anxiety reactions is well known (Last et al. 1984). The traumatic experiences and associated reactions of patients with posttraumatic stress disorder clearly illustrate this process. Patients with posttraumatic stress disorder typically endorse negative appraisals of their traumatic experiences and poorly integrate their traumatic experiences into their autobiographical memories (Beck 2005). This leads to strong anxiety reactions in anticipation of or when faced with stimuli associated with their traumatic experiences.

Long-Term Stressors

Stressors may accumulate over time and may piggyback on each other, overtaxing an individual. The result may be a situation in which a person's coping resources are exhausted and overwhelmed. McEwen (2005) described this process in presenting his theory of *allostasis* and *allostatic overload.* Based on his reconceptualization of Selye's general adaptation syndrome, McEwen defines allostasis as the adaptive processes that maintain homeostasis (i.e., the stability of the physiological systems that maintain life) through the production of physiological mediators, such as hormones of the hypothalamic-pituitary-adrenal axis, catecholamines, and cytokines. When the set-points of the physiological variables that maintain homeostasis (pH, body temperature, glucose levels, oxygen tension) vary beyond the limits of these homeostatic mechanisms, an allostatic state occurs. The result is an imbalance of the previously mentioned primary mediators of allostasis, and wear on the regulatory systems in the brain and body through their repeated exposure to elevated levels of these mediators (from being "stressed out"). The cumulative effect of an allostatic state is termed allostatic overload, which predisposes a person to disease (e.g., atherosclerosis, heart disease). Thus, although the body responds adaptively to acute stress through allostasis, allostatic overload results when these acute responses are overused or poorly managed in times of chronic stress. In current research efforts, attention is focused on how to improve the efficiency of the allostatic response to stress while preventing overactivity of its mechanisms.

Stressors Affecting Vulnerability and Threshold

Circumstances, situations, or areas of deficit may have the effect of decreasing an individual's ability to cope effectively with life stressors. Whether because of a single factor or the cumulative effect of several factors combined, the individual may either lose possible options or fails to see available options for thoughts, feelings, or actions, and becomes threatened as a result. The normal exigencies of life may be such that an individual's coping capacity is sufficient. Trouble arises when an individual's threshold for coping is exceeded. Vulnerability factors serve to lower the patient's threshold or tolerance for handling stressful life situations. Consequently, circumstances that were more easily handled previously now become overwhelming. This increased level of vulnerability may serve to increase the patient's difficulty in several areas of life. Vulnerability factors may have contributed to the current difficulty, may exacerbate it, or may contribute to future difficulty. Fortunately, the cognitive processes associated with many of these difficulties have been accounted for by the cognitive model (Beck 2005), and moderate to large treatment effects with CBT have been found for depression, generalized anxiety disorder, social phobia, marital distress, and chronic pain (A.C. Butler et al. 2006). Notably, however, symptoms associated with generalized anxiety disorder tend to persist in the long term despite treatment with CBT, which highlights the chronic nature of generalized anxiety disorder and the need to refine treatment methods for this particular condition (Durham et al. 2003; Stanley et al. 2003).

Other Precipitating Factors

Various other factors can precipitate anxiety reactions, including health status changes, aging, and changes in life circumstances. Acute health impairment may range from transient illness, such as headaches, viral infections, or colds, to more severe and debilitating health issues that require medical intervention or even hospitalization. Chronic health problems may decrease one's ability to confront stressors and lead to feelings of overwhelming anxiety. Aging, in and of itself, may result in the inability to perform up to expectations appropriate at other times in one's life. Fatigue may adversely influence problem-solving ability and the energy needed to handle events. Changes in one or more areas of one's life, especially changes in health, may also precipitate anxiety problems. Cognitive therapy has been effectively used as an adjunctive treatment for a variety of medical conditions, such as heart disease, hypertension, cancer, and chronic pain (Beck 2005) and thus likely helps to preserve adequate functioning in the face of these conditions.

It is worth noting that stressors may strike at an individual's particular vulnerability; what may precipitate anxiety in one person may not do so in another. Understanding an individual's vulnerability points may be very helpful in predicting the onset of anxiety problems. For example, an individual who believes that to be secure, one must be loved by everyone may be expected to become symptomatic at times of rejection. In the next sections, we present a case that elucidates the basic facets of the cognitive model.

Cognitive-Behavioral Case Conceptualization

Mr. G, a 49-year-old self-employed businessman in the furniture trade, had a history of generalized anxiety disorder during most of his adult life. By use of the cognitive model and the Persons (1989) formulation model, the following areas were identified: problem list, behavioral factors, cognitive factors, hypothesized mechanisms, relation between mechanisms and problem, current precipitants, and predicted obstacles to treatment. This conceptualization emphasizes the interaction between the predisposing and the precipitating factors.

I. Problem List

A. Feelings. *1) Generalized anxiety:* Mr. G had a chronic sense of anxiety and anticipated personal and financial doom related to the uncertainty of the outcome of his business decisions and the unpredictability of his personal investments. He lived with a constant sense of anxiety related to anticipated negative outcomes, which had direct bearing on his sense of self-efficacy, self-esteem, and general well-being. He also had strong feelings of guilt and shame, and believed that he had disappointed everyone who was important to him, including his wife and children. *2) Panic attacks:* Mr. G experienced panic attacks at a frequency of about once a month when he had an "off day" and trade was slow in his furniture business. He had been in the business for almost 25 years, and he knew intellectually that often things evened out and business would pick up. However, at certain times he became flooded with self-doubt and began to suffer from symptoms of lightheadedness associated with hyperventilation, out-of-body sensations, tingling in his extremities, tightness in his chest, and a sense of impending doom. *3) Depressed mood:* From time to time, Mr. G reported increases in depressive feelings related to events and momentary negative outcomes, which he believed confirmed his underlying fears of inadequacy and sense of failure. During these times, he had fleeting thoughts that he would be better off dead, although these typically passed within several hours to a day. He had never made a suicide attempt, nor did he have any immediate intent or plan to kill himself.

B. Behavior. *1) Irritability and restlessness:* Mr. G was generally pleasant in his interactions with others when he was not feeling anxious, but people observed him to be short-tempered and snappy when he was anxious. In addition, he had difficulty sleeping at night and would often stay up into the early morning hours worrying about his business. When he would finally fall asleep, it would only be for a few hours before he would awaken around 5:00 A.M., and begin worrying again about the day ahead of him. *2) Social isolation:* Mr. G demonstrated no social avoidance, but when he became flooded with anxiety, he would isolate himself from others, especially those who might be supportive to him. He would turn over his business to an associate, and walk up and down the street with his head hung down, like a "prisoner marching to the gallows." During this time, he would ruminate about how alone he was and fantasize about his utter demise, imagining that everyone else on the street was enjoying the spoils of victory while casting negative and disapproving glances his way. *3) Impaired marital and family relationships:* Mr. G would typically seek an outlet for his anxiety by attempting to engage his wife in conversation about his worries. When he would do so, she would usually become very angry with him. She felt threatened by his worries that they would lose their house and lifestyle as well as close friendships that had been forged in the community over the years. Most recently, she intimated that if his attitude did not change, she and her daughters might be better off without him. Mr. G had two teenage daughters attending high school and college who had "complicated social lives." Mr. G typically did not become too involved in dialogue with his daughters, and he avoided discussions with them about their social lives and responsibilities that might be potentially conflict-laden. As a result, he insulated himself from their world, which only served to reinforce his feelings of being "shut out" from experiences involving the people who were most important to him.

C. Cognitive. *1) Cognitive distortions:* Mr. G was often engulfed in a variety of cognitive distortions, including arbitrary inference, all-or-nothing thinking, catastrophizing and fortune telling, overgeneralization, magnification, and emotional reasoning. He tended to react to short-term business downturns as signals of impending financial crisis and ruin, and he became quickly absorbed in his own hopeless and panicky feelings. He perceived these feelings as further evidence of the urgency of his dire condition. Furthermore, Mr. G tended to engage in mental imagery about the future, picturing himself having to sell his dream house and move into shabby living quarters by himself. In his fantasy, his wife and daughters left him to live out the rest of his years in abject despair and squalor, while they fended for themselves and carved out a life that was ultimately more rewarding and financially stable without him. *2) Intolerance of uncertainty:* Mr. G consistently engaged in negative thoughts about the future, especially distinguished by "what if" thinking. He found it extremely difficult to tolerate ambiguity, and he frequently sought reassurance from his wife and business associates that everything would be all right. However, it was difficult to satisfy his nagging doubts in the absence of absolute and tangible proof that his financial picture would immediately improve. He frequently contradicted the very reassurance that he sought by sparring with his counterpart in a devil's advocate exercise, as if he was trying to refute positive encouragement with depressive reality. Mr. G quickly discarded the efforts of others at positive thinking and encouragement as superficial, and he embraced temporary setbacks as harbingers of permanent disaster. *3) Impaired problem-solving:* When Mr. G became engulfed in anxiety and panic, he was unable to use rational problem solving to think through his situation in realistic terms. At times, he found that his brain became "frozen" and that he was not able to think straight. He imagined that he looked like a zombie to others, and when he left the office, he walked around the business district with a "deer in the headlights" look about him. He even found it difficult to speak to others at these times, and he reported feeling shell-shocked and extremely challenged to process information.

II. Hypothesized Mechanisms

A. Cognitive: Mr. G had a number of underlying schemas that were the underpinnings of his distorted thoughts and related feelings and behaviors. Some examples of his core schema were as follows: *1) Need for certainty/intolerance of ambiguity:* "I must know the outcomes before they occur, since I cannot tolerate uncertainty or the possibility of a negative outcome. I am weak and unable to contain uncomfortable feelings related to not knowing." Interestingly, several years ago Mr. G was diagnosed with prostate cancer for which he was successfully treated with surgery and radiation. He reported feeling significantly less anxious then than he did during his current episode. Although he admitted to some initial feelings of anxiety when he was first diagnosed, he indicated that once he saw the handwriting on the wall, he "bucked up and faced the music." It helped him to believe that if treatment was successful, he would recover and resume his life, and if it was not successful, he would likely die and end his suffering. These stark choices offered some comfort to him, and allowed him to compartmentalize his feelings in ways that diminished his anxiety. *2) Vulnerability:* "I need other people to tell me that I'll be OK, or else I'll go crazy. I require reassurance from others, even though I understand that it does not reduce anxiety, and it only serves to push others away. I am a helpless victim, just as my father was, and there doesn't seem to be much I can do about it." *3) Failure:* "No matter what I try, I am doomed to failure. My father was a failure, and I am cut from the same cloth. It must be genetic. No matter how successful I am, my success is not likely to last. I'm like the donkey character, Eeyore, in Winnie the Pooh. There is a dark cloud over my head that follows me, no matter where I go or what I do." *4) Negative view of self, environment, and future:* "I am inept at the core. The world is a stage that serves to confirm my inadequacy, and this is not likely to change in the future. Some people are winners and others are losers. I was raised in a joyless family in which we were always waiting for the other shoe to drop, thereby confirming our miserable heritage."

B. Social: Although Mr. G had acquired many of the symbols of a secure and comfortable life in the suburbs, including a large house, three fine cars, a lovely wife, two daughters, and several close friends who had stood with him through thick and thin for nearly 30 years, he frequently felt alone in his suffering. He was concerned that if he kept requesting reassurance from his wife and friends, they would distance themselves from him more and more, which would confirm and validate his prediction of living out the remaining years of his life in total isolation. Mr. G felt trapped by his anxiety, and he struggled mightily to contain his catastrophic thoughts without having them boil over into desperate pleas for reassurance. He felt alienated from the very people who were close to him and upon whom he relied, yet he felt that he had to put up a false front for them lest he drive them away. Consequently, he also felt alienated from himself and estranged from others, and he often engaged in ruminative existential self-doubt.

C. Biological: Mr. G reported that his mother frequently suffered from "nerves" and appeared to have had at least two panic attacks during his early years. His father suffered from alcohol dependence and chronic depression, and he was occupationally disabled by his mid-40s. Mr. G's eldest daughter had experienced several panic attacks since the onset of adolescence, and was seeing a psychiatrist and therapist for this problem. These findings suggest the possibility of genetic vulnerability to anxiety when triggered by stressors as well as an underlying genetic vulnerability to depression and dysthymia.

III. Relation Between Mechanisms and Problem

Mr. G's anxiety symptoms seemed to be related to several precipitants, including recent stressful life events, a possible biological predisposition to anxiety and depression, and the activation of previously dormant schema, or core vulnerabilities, related to perceived threat, vulnerability, and uncertainty. Although he was a person who enjoyed his independence in the business world by being self-employed, Mr. G felt extremely threatened by the associated risks of independence when business trends appeared to be on the downturn. Where others saw opportunity in crises, he forecasted doom and gloom. For example, Mr. G would typically listen to the stock market results on a small TV that played in his office all day long, which would either confirm that his investments were "winners" or "losers." When he lost money on his investments or when business was slow, he would typically berate himself, much in the same manner that he recalled his father doing, and he would then predict that such a bad day was a signal for his eventual financial collapse and personal ruin. He evaluated his self-worth on tangible variables that were external to him and often beyond his immediate control, rather than basing it on stable internal qualities. When his life looked bright, he dismissed his successes as being lucky, but when things looked dark, he heaped full responsibility on himself for his perceived failures.

Mr. G's anxiety was typically sparked by events that signaled a threat to his security, which was relatively brittle. His need for reassurance that everything would be "all right" could be traced to his childhood, as he remembered how he would desperately wish for his father's validation when he did well in school or sports, only to be knocked back down with pessimistic or negative comments about how he was a burdensome nuisance. Mr. G's mother was recalled as a meek "silent partner" who always seemed to be nervous and easily startled by her husband's boisterous tirades once he started drinking. Mr. G's intolerance of uncertainty was linked to his recollections of coming home from school, nervously counting the minutes until his father would explode in bitter fury about the unfairness of the world and, more specifically, about how Mr. G was a stupid and naïve troublemaker who was responsible for saddling his family with the misfortune of his mere existence. He learned to always anticipate the worst outcome, given that more often than not, it was confirmed for him on a daily basis. As he stated in therapy, "I'm always waiting for the other shoe to drop, and I can't stand not knowing when it will."

Mr. G's problem-solving skills in concrete and tangible events were as effective as anyone else's, but when his perceived personal safety and security were at stake, he quickly became flooded with catastrophic and immobilizing thoughts. Not surprisingly, his anxiety did not signal a call to arms or help him to mobilize his psychological resources in order to protect his vulnerabilities. Rather, it served to signal him to "duck and cover" until he was given the "all clear" signal. During these times, he retreated into his office or his den at home, where he replayed in his head old movies of financial ruin and lonely despair. These images became self-reinforcing by serving to confirm for him that despite his periodic times of seeming success, he was back at "home" where he belonged, taking his place among his family legacy of failures.

Mr. G had sought therapy for several years, beginning approximately 12 years ago, but he found that understanding his family dynamics did little to relieve his anxiety or break the vicious cycle of generalized anxiety, panic, and depression. He had been prescribed an antidepressant with antianxiety benefits for the previous 10 years or so by his primary care physician. Although the medication seemed to reduce the intensity of his depression somewhat, it did little to mitigate his anxiety. He once took a trial of benzodiazepine medication for anxiety, but he did not like the dulling feeling it provided, which seemed to exacerbate his dysthymic mood.

IV. Precipitants

The historic precipitants of Mr. G's anxiety related to family situations in which his father would unpredictably explode into negative, condemning tirades that were especially painful to Mr. G as a young boy. He learned that at any given time, failure and demoralizing repudiation were just around the corner, and he lived in constant anticipation of their damaging consequences, even though he never seemed to learn self-protective strategies. The current precipitant of his anxiety was related to Mr. G's worsening business, investment losses, and marital communication difficulties, as his wife grew tired of hearing his dreadful prophecies and made vague allusions to leaving him unless things changed.

V. Predicted Obstacles to Treatment

Several factors were hypothesized to potentially interfere with treatment. First, Mr. G seemed to externalize responsibility for his mood states, and saw himself as a passive and tragic victim of his family legacy of failure and current business woes. Second, he seemed to enjoy intellectualizing his problems, but had not yet resolved to take action on learning how to change his perceptions about himself, the world, and the future so that he might feel different.

The above-described case provides a typical cognitive conceptualization of a patient suffering from an anxiety disorder. In the next section, we discuss common myths about the cognitive model.

Misconceptions About the Cognitive Model of Anxiety

Many misconceptions exist about the cognitive model of psychiatric disorders (Freeman et al. 1990) and anxiety in general. In this section, we state each of these misconceptions and then provide an accurate description of what the cognitive model implies.

- *Faulty cognitions cause anxiety disorders.* This misconception is perhaps the most commonly cited, unjustified criticism of the cognitive model. The cognitive model does not assume that thoughts cause anxiety disorders. Rather, a variety of predisposing and precipitating factors, including cognitive patterns, may coexist with and relate to the development of anxiety disorders. Cognitions and cognitive processing are not the only important elements, but they do represent a useful focus for intervening.
- *The cognitive model is simply a variant of Norman Vincent Peale's Power of Positive Thinking.* The cognitive model of anxiety assumes that individuals with anxiety disorders perceive and appraise threat when no real danger exists. Actually, anxiety patients have unrealistic thinking and are unlikely to respond to positive, reassuring thoughts in the long run. Numerous individuals, including family members, friends, and physicians, have encouraged positive thinking in these individuals to no avail. The model proposes that patients must learn to evaluate the triggers for anxiety in a realistic, valid manner.
- *The cognitive model denies the importance of behavioral principles, such as exposure, in overcoming anxiety and associated avoidance.* Although this model places primary importance on the cognitive apparatus of the individual, it is simply untrue that the importance of behavioral principles is overlooked. The model may more aptly be described as the cognitive-behavioral-emotive model (Freeman and Simon 1989). Cognitive therapists freely use techniques that are designed to modify behavior (e.g., assertiveness training) and emotions (e.g., relaxation training). These techniques

are found to be effective in treating anxiety. In a recent meta-analysis, for example, cognitive therapy and exposure therapy alone, in combination, or combined with relaxation training resulted in positive treatment outcomes in patients with a variety of anxiety disorders (Norton and Price 2007). Treatment effect sizes did not differ with various combinations of CBT components for any specific diagnosis.

- *Applying the cognitive model is simply a matter of talking patients out of their fears.* The cognitive approach actively relies on the principles of collaborative empiricism and guided discovery. The model assumes the Socratic approach by having the therapist lead patients through questioning to examine and alter faulty cognitions and underlying beliefs; the cognitive therapist actively teaches the patient a process he or she can take away and use. Cognitive therapists do not talk patients out of their problems by persuading them or cajoling them to adopt a new perspective. Rather, they talk to patients in ways that help them guide their patients to think, act, and feel more realistically and adaptively. These techniques are found to be effective in treating anxiety.

Conclusion

The cognitive-behavioral model of anxiety appears to be both a viable and a useful vehicle for furthering our understanding of the complex phenomenon of anxiety and the onset, development, exacerbation, and treatment of anxiety disorders. Recent clinical applications of the cognitive model of anxiety include the use of self-help manuals in primary care settings (van Boeijen et al. 2005) and brief, intensive CBT (Deacon and Abramowitz 2006). Although more research is needed, clinical research supports the efficacy of the cognitive-behavioral model of psychotherapy for specific phobias (Beck 2005), panic disorder with and without agoraphobia (Friedman et al. 2006), social anxiety (Heimberg 2002; Rodebaugh et al. 2004), posttraumatic stress disorder (Ehlers et al. 2005), obsessive-compulsive disorder (Clark 2005), and generalized anxiety disorder (Lang 2004). Continued clinical research designed both to refine the hypotheses of the cognitive theory of anxiety and to develop the optimal delivery of cognitive-behavioral treatment by specific disorders and contexts are warranted.

◀ Key Clinical Points ▶

The treatment of anxiety disorders from a cognitive-behavioral perspective incorporates some of the following clinical points that are directly derived from the model:

- Given the nature of the treatment, which ultimately incorporates confronting and addressing uncomfortable stimuli, the establishment of a sound therapeutic alliance is critical.
- The patient should be "psychoeducated" about a number of fundamentals, including the model, the therapy process, an explanation of symptoms, the identification of patterns of escape/avoidance, and the development of a case formulation that integrates the patient's thoughts, feelings, behaviors, beliefs, assumptions, and triggers. Psychoeducation may be viewed as a means of justifying the elements of the treatment package, and it provides a comprehensive framework allowing the patient to assimilate the treatment.
- The monitoring of symptoms, arousal level, situational triggers, thoughts, feelings, and behaviors is important in establishment of baseline levels, ongoing monitoring of progress, and ultimate outcome.
- Some form of relaxation training and breathing retraining may be employed as a means of reducing arousal.
- Cognitive interventions are often employed to reduce catastrophizing and the overestimation of negative outcomes.
- Exposing the patient to anxiety-related situations, thoughts, feelings, and behavior is critical.
- Mutually developed homework exercises designed to bridge the gap between the session and the in vivo environment is essential. Homework provides significant opportunities to test out unrealistic beliefs, practice new behaviors, expose oneself to feared stimuli and extinguish anxiety responses, develop more adaptive behavior patterns, and enhance self-efficacy.

References

Baer RA: Mindfulness training as a clinical intervention: a conceptual and empirical review. Clin Psychol Sci Pract 10:125–143, 2003

Barlow DH: Anxiety and Its Disorders, 2nd Edition. New York, Guilford, 2002

Barlow DH, Cerney JA: Psychological Treatment of Panic. New York, Guilford, 1988

Beck AT: Depression: Causes and Treatment. Philadelphia, University of Pennsylvania, 1967

Beck AT: Cognitive Therapy and the Emotional Disorders. New York, International Universities Press, 1976

Beck AT: Cognitive therapy: a 30-year retrospective. Am Psychol 46:368–375, 1991

Beck AT: The current state of cognitive therapy: a 40-year retrospective. Arch Gen Psychiatry 62:953–959, 2005

Beck AT, Greenberg RL: Cognitive therapy of panic disorders, in American Psychiatric Press Review of Psychiatry, Vol 7. Edited by Frances AJ, Hales RE. Washington, DC, American Psychiatric Press, 1988, pp 571–583

Beck AT, Rush AJ: A cognitive model of anxiety formation and anxiety resolution, in Stress and Anxiety. Edited by Saranson JD, Spielberger CD. Washington, DC, Hemisphere Publishing, 1975, pp 69–80

Beck AT, Weishaar M: Cognitive therapy, in Comprehensive Handbook of Cognitive Therapy. Edited by Freeman A, Simon KM, Butler LE, et al. New York, Plenum, 1989, pp 21–36

Beck AT, Emery G, Greenberg RL: Anxiety Disorders and Phobias: A Cognitive Perspective. New York, Basic Books, 1985

Butler AC, Chapman JE, Forman EM, et al: The empirical status of cognitive-behavioral therapy: a review of meta-analyses. Clin Psychol Rev 26:17–31, 2006

Butler G, Matthews A: Cognitive processes in anxiety. Advances in Behavior Research and Therapy 5:51–62, 1983

Clark DA: Focus on "cognition" in cognitive behavior therapy for OCD: is it really necessary? Cogn Behav Ther 34:131–139, 2005

Craske MG, Golinelli D, Stein MB, et al: Does the addition of cognitive behavioral therapy improve panic disorder

treatment outcome relative to medication alone in the primary care setting? Psychol Med 35:1645–1654, 2005
Craske MG, Stein MB, Hazlett-Stevens H, et al: CBT intensity and outcome for panic disorder in a primary care setting. Behav Ther 37:112–119, 2006
Deacon B, Abramowitz J: A pilot study of two-day cognitive-behavioral therapy for panic disorder. Behav Res Ther 44:807–817, 2006
Deffenbacher JL, Zwemer WA, Whisman MA, et al: Irrational beliefs and anxiety. Cognit Ther Res 10:281–292, 1986
DiTomasso RA, Gilman R: Behavioral assessment, in Encyclopedia of Cognitive and Behavioral Therapy. Edited by Freeman A, Felgoise SH, Nezu A, et al. New York, Kluwer, 2005, pp 61–65
DiTomasso RA, Gosch EA (eds): Anxiety Disorders: A Practitioner's Guide to Comparative Treatment. New York, Springer, 2002
Durham RC, Chambers JA, MacDonald RR, et al: Does cognitive-behavioural therapy influence the long-term outcome of generalized anxiety disorder? An 8–14 year follow-up of two clinical trials. Psychol Med 33:499–509, 2003
Ehlers A, Clark DM, Hackman A, et al: Cognitive therapy for post-traumatic stress disorder: development and evaluation. Behav Res Ther 43:413–431, 2005
Ellis A: Reason and Emotion in Psychotherapy. New York, Lyle Stuart, 1962
Emery G, Tracy NL: Theoretical issues in the cognitive-behavioral treatment of anxiety disorders, in Anxiety and Stress Disorders: Cognitive-Behavioral Assessment and Treatment. Edited by Michaelson L, Ascher LM. New York, Guilford, 1987, pp 3–38
Everly GS: A Clinical Guide to the Treatment of the Human Stress Response. New York, Plenum, 1983
Foa EB, Kozak MJ: Emotional processing of fear: Exposure of corrective information. Psychol Bull 99:10–35, 1986
Freeman A, Simon KM: Cognitive therapy of anxiety, in Comprehensive Handbook of Cognitive Therapy. Edited by Freeman A, Simon KM, Beutler LE, et al. New York, Plenum, 1989, pp 347–365
Freeman A, Pretzer J, Fleming B, et al: Clinical Applications of Cognitive Therapy. New York, Plenum, 1990
Friedman S, Braunstein JW, Halpern B: Cognitive behavioral treatment of panic disorder and agoraphobia in a multiethnic urban outpatient clinic: Initial presentation and treatment outcome. Cogn Behav Pract 13:282–292, 2006
Hayes S, Pierson H: Acceptance and commitment therapy, in Encyclopedia of Cognitive and Behavioral Therapy. Edited by Freeman A, Felgoise SH, Nezu A, et al. New York, Kluwer, 2005, pp 1–4
Heimberg RG: Cognitive-behavioral therapy for social anxiety disorder: current status and future directions. Biol Psychiatry 51:101–108, 2002
Hilbert GN: Ideational components of anxiety: their origin and content. Br J Psychiatry 144:618–624, 1984
Hollon SD, Stewart MO, Strunk D: Enduring effects for cognitive behavior therapy in the treatment of depression and anxiety. Annu Rev Psychol 57:285–315, 2006
Izard EE, Blumberg SH: Emotion theory and the role of emotions in children and adults, in Anxiety and the Anxiety Disorders. Edited by Tuma AH, Maser J. Hillsdale, NJ, Erlbaum, 1985, pp 109–125
Kelly G: The Psychology of Personal Constructs. New York, WW Norton, 1955
Kendall PC, Ingram R: The future for cognitive assessment of anxiety: let's get specific, in Anxiety and Stress Disorders: Cognitive-Behavioral Assessment and Treatment. Edited by Michaelson L, Ascher LM. New York, Guilford, 1987, pp 89–104
Labrecque J, Dugas MJ, Marchand A, et al: Cognitive-behavioral therapy for comorbid generalized anxiety disorder and panic disorder with agoraphobia. Behav Modif 30:383–410, 2006
Lang AJ: Treating generalized anxiety disorder with cognitive-behavioral therapy. J Clin Psychiatry 65(suppl):14–19, 2004
Lang AJ, McNeil DE: Use of the anxiety control questionnaire in psychiatric inpatients. Depress Anxiety 23:107–112, 2006
Last CG, Barlow DH, O'Brien GT: Cognitive change during behavioral and cognitive-behavioral treatment of agoraphobia. Behav Modif 8:181–210, 1984
Lazarus RL: Progress on a cognitive-motivational-relations theory of emotion. Am Psychol 46:819–834, 1991
Leahy RL: Cognitive Therapy Techniques: A Practitioner's Guide. New York, Guilford, 2003
Lindsley DB: Psychological phenomena and the electroencephalogram. Electroencephalogr Clin Neurophysiol 4:443–456, 1952
Lindsley DB: Psychophysiology and motivation, in Nebraska Symposium on Motivation. Edited by Jones MR. Lincoln, University of Nebraska Press, 1957, pp 45–105
Lindsley DB: Attention, consciousness, sleep, and wakefulness, in Handbook of Physiology, Vol 3. Edited by Freld J, Magoan HW. Washington, DC, Harper and Row, 1960, pp 1553–1593
Mahoney MJ: Cognition and Behavior Modification. Cambridge, MA, Ballinger, 1974
McEwen BS: Stressed or stressed out: what is the difference? J Psychiatry Neurosci 30:315–318, 2005
Meichenbaum D: Cognitive Behavior Modification: An Integrative Approach. New York, Plenum, 1977
Merluzzi TV, Boltwood MD: Cognition assessment, in Comprehensive Handbook of Cognitive Therapy. Edited by Freeman A, Simon KM, Beutler LE, et al. New York, Plenum, 1989, pp 249–266
Myhr G, Payne K: Cost-effectiveness of cognitive-behavioural therapy for mental disorders: implications for pub-

lic health care funding policy in Canada. Can J Psychiatry 51:662–670, 2006

Nemeroff CB, Bremner JD, Foa EB, et al: Posttraumatic stress disorder: a state-of-the-science review. J Psychiatr Res 40:1–21, 2006

Norton PJ, Price EC: A meta-analytic review of adult cognitive-behavioral treatment outcome across the anxiety disorders. J Nerv Ment Dis 195:521–531, 2007

Persons JB: Cognitive Therapy in Practice: A Case Formulation Approach. New York, WW Norton, 1989

Plutchik R: A Psychoevolutionary Synthesis. New York, Harper and Row, 1980

Rodebaugh TL, Holaway RM, Heimberg RG: The treatment of social anxiety disorder. Clin Psychol Rev 24:883–908, 2004

Roy-Byrne PP, Craske MG, Stein MB, et al: A randomized effectiveness trial of cognitive-behavioral therapy and medication for primary care panic disorder. Arch Gen Psychiatry 62:290–298, 2005

Shafran R, Rachman S: Thought-action fusion: a review. J Behav Ther Exp Psychiatry 35:87–107, 2004

Simon KM, Fleming BM: Beck's cognitive therapy of depression: treatment and outcome, in Evaluating Behavior Therapy Outcome. Edited by Ascher LM, Turner RM. New York, Springer, 1985, pp 146–179

Stanley MA, Beck JG, Novy DM, et al: Cognitive-behavioral treatment of late-life generalized anxiety disorder. J Consult Clin Psychol 71:309–319, 2003

Taylor CB: The Nature and Treatment of Anxiety Disorders. New York, Free Press, 1988

van Boeijen CA, van Balkom AJ, van Oppen P, et al: Efficacy of self-help manuals for anxiety disorders in primary care: a systematic review. Fam Pract 22:192–196, 2005

Wells A: Cognitive Therapy of Anxiety Disorders: A Practice Manual and Conceptual Guide. New York, Wiley, 1997

Yurica C, DiTomasso RA: Cognitive distortions, in Encyclopedia of Cognitive and Behavioral Therapy. Edited by Freeman A, Felgoise SH, Nezu A, et al. New York, Kluwer, 2005, pp 117–122

Recommended Readings

Craske MG: Mastery of Your Anxiety and Panic: Therapist Guide. New York, Oxford University Press, 2006

Craske MG, Antony MM, Barlow DH: Mastering Your Fears and Phobias: Therapist Guide. New York, Oxford University Press, 2006

Foa E: Mastery of Obsessive Compulsive Disorder: Therapist Guide. New York, Oxford University Press, 2004

Foa E: Prolonged Exposure Therapy for PTSD: Therapist Guide. New York, Oxford University Press, 2007

Hope DA: Managing Social Anxiety: Therapist Guide. New York, Oxford University Press, 2006

Zinbard RE: Mastering Your Anxiety and Worry: Therapist Guide. New York, Oxford University Press, 2006

Chapter 8

Psychodynamic Concepts of Anxiety

Fredric N. Busch, M.D.
Barbara L. Milrod, M.D.
M. Katherine Shear, M.D.

Clinically, psychoanalytic concepts and psychodynamic techniques are of value in developing a well-rounded understanding of patients with anxiety disorders. In general, however, psychoanalysts have not pursued systematic testing of their treatment approaches. Although multiple case reports suggest these treatments can be effective (Busch et al. 1996; Milrod 1998; Milrod and Shear 1991; Milrod et al. 1996; Renik 1995; Stern 1995), efficacy data are limited. Only recently did one study demonstrate efficacy of a manualized psychodynamic treatment for a specific anxiety disorder (Milrod et al. 2007b). The purpose of this chapter is to give an overview of psychoanalytic theory, treatment approaches, and research in the area of anxiety disorders. Because relatively more research has been conducted on panic disorder, with and without agoraphobia, it will be a focus of this chapter, although there will be discussion of nonpanic anxiety.

Brief Historical Overview

Many psychoanalytic theoreticians and clinicians have described important aspects of the dynamics of anxiety because of its central position in psychoanalytic theory (for a summary of highlights of these theories, see Kessler 1996). Here, we outline three psychoanalysts' psychodynamic formulations of anxiety that continue to be of clinical relevance.

1. Freud (1926/1959): Two types of anxiety were delineated by Freud: The first is *traumatic anxiety*, in which the ego—which is the psychic apparatus that organizes perception, defenses, cognition, anxiety, and mood regulation—is overwhelmed by danger: an "excitation, whether of internal or external origin, which cannot be dealt with" (pp. 137, 166). The danger may carry psychological meaning. Traumatic anxiety occurs during what are described in DSM-IV-TR (American Psychiatric Association 2000) as panic episodes. The second type is *signal anxiety*, which is posited as an intrapsychic mechanism that generates smaller doses of anxiety to alert the ego to the presence of psychologically meaningful dangers. Signal anxiety acts as a stimulus to mobilize defenses and thus to prevent the breakthrough of traumatic anxiety, in which the ego is overwhelmed and unable to defend itself.

   In addition to distinguishing between traumatic and signal anxiety, Freud described a progression of central, developmentally organizing anxious fears in children. He believed that the internal dangers that are psychologically meaningful, and that can potentially lead to the eruption of normative anxiety, change with the phase of life. He outlined these traumatic or dangerous fear situations to be 1) fear of the loss of the object (e.g., mother/substitute), also described as *separation anxiety*; 2) fear of the loss of the object's love; 3) fear of castration; and 4) superego fear or, in simple terms, fear of a guilty conscience. In clinical situations with adult patients, derivatives of several or all of these developmentally organizing situational fears commonly operate simultaneously, although one or two areas may assume clinical ascendance at any given time.

2. Deutsch (1929) described the way in which unconscious angry and ambivalent aspects of intense love attachments can result in agoraphobia and the need for a phobic companion (the ambivalently held love object), partly in an unconscious attempt to prevent symbolic destruction of the love object by hostile, destructive fantasies.
3. M. Klein (1948) developed the concept of internal representations of self and others, and further described the idea that anxiety can stem from aggressive fantasies. Particular patterns of self and other, including parental, representations have been found to be present in patients with anxiety disorders (Arrindell et al. 1983; Parker 1979). Panic patients, for example, tend to view themselves as unsafe, requiring others for protection. Their perceptions add to a sense of fearful dependency on significant others; this is an intrapsychic process that is reflected in patients' interpersonal relationships.

Basic Psychodynamic Concepts That Inform an Understanding of Anxiety

To provide a clear outline of psychodynamic concepts as they pertain to the anxiety disorders, we must first define several basic psychoanalytic ideas about mental life.

The Unconscious

From a psychodynamic point of view, all of mental life exists on two levels: within the realm of consciousness and within a more inaccessible realm described as the unconscious (Freud 1893–1895/1955). Psychic or emotional symptoms arise from aspects of mental life that are, at least in part, unconscious, including unacceptable fantasies (Shapiro 1992), affects, and conflicts. For instance, clinical observations and studies indicate that patients with panic disorder often deny angry feelings and vengeful fantasies that feel as though they represent a threat to important attachment figures (Busch et al. 1991; Shear et al. 1993). Psychoanalytic treatments help patients become conscious of these affects and fantasies, articulate them, and hence render them less threatening once they have been put in verbal form and can be better understood, in order to effect symptomatic change.

The following case example illustrates anxiety symptoms that signify the symbolic representation of an unconscious fantasy.

> Ms. A, a 24-year-old woman with panic disorder, lived with the persistent unconscious fantasy/wish that she would become closer to her beloved and physically impaired brother, which she imagined would happen if she became ill, impaired, and "pathetic" herself. Many aspects of Ms. A's life, including her severe panic disorder, served to reinforce a cherished image of herself as ill. This fantasy was severely challenged when she was accepted to a prestigious graduate school, at which time she experienced profound, "unaccountable" depression and an exacerbation of her panic symptoms.
>
> While on the way to her therapist's office for the next session after her acceptance to graduate school, which also happened to be the session following her "remembering" important material that she had "forgotten" (that her brother had had a serious medical disorder throughout their childhood), she had a panic attack in the street. She needed her father to drive from another state to pick her up and bring her to her appointment. In the office, she said that she was furious with her father "because now the fact that I needed him to come and get me will make him think that he has license to treat me like I'm a pathetic, sick child."
>
> The therapist pointed out to Ms. A that she had just been discussing "another sick, pathetic child in our last session." "Oh, right," she said. "So you mean to tell me that you think this stuff about me forgetting that my brother was sick is somehow connected to my panic?"
>
> Ms. A's panic symptoms disappeared after she was able to consciously acknowledge the way in which she clung to and identified with her ill brother through her own anxiety symptoms.

Defense Mechanisms

People unconsciously avoid "unpleasure," and the ideas and feelings that produce "unpleasure" are screened from consciousness by unconscious psychological processes called *defense mechanisms* (Freud 1911/1958). Studies in which defenses have been systematically assessed indicate that the following defenses are frequently employed by panic patients: *reaction formation*, *undoing*, and *denial* (Busch et al. 1995). Reaction formation and undoing are involved in the management of attachment fears in panic patients: by unconsciously attempting to convert anger to more affiliative affects, patients reduce the threat to an attachment relationship. Somatization represents another important defense in many anxiety disorders, allowing for avoidance of fantasies and feelings through a focus on the body. In a psychoanalytic treatment, the therapist typically focuses on the meaning of defenses, in order to identify emotions and fantasies that trigger biophysiological symptoms.

The following case (Milrod et al. 1997) illustrates the use of defenses in an attempt to manage frightening angry feelings and fantasies.

> Ms. B, a 31-year-old health care provider, had the onset of panic a few days after observing a patient's sudden death. It emerged that she had found this death particularly unfair, because the patient was young and had been improving. She had the thought, "God, you can't do this to her" and then had the onset of panic, accompanied by fears of her own death and that of others close to her. Ms. B reported having struggled with feelings of unfairness throughout her life, generated by the behavior of her temperamental father toward herself, her siblings, and her mother, and jealousy of a younger sister whom she viewed as more socially adept and attractive. These frustrated feelings about her life had been strong in the months prior to panic onset, and she felt underpaid and overworked in her job and angry with her "cold and callous" boyfriend.
>
> Ms. B, however, had difficulty acknowledging her angry feelings. Demonstrating the defense of undoing, she kept taking back comments about being angry. For instance, she described holding grudges, then stated, "I'm not a vindictive person." She described fantasies of her boyfriend being injured, then stated, "But I would never hope he died." Employing reaction formation, she viewed herself as "the helping kind," always wanting to help others. Exploring with Ms. B how she had to "take back" her anger (through denial, undoing, and reaction formation), and providing the opportunity for her to express her vengeful fantasies safely, helped to relieve her anxiety.

Compromise Formation

Many aspects of mental life, including symptoms (such as anxiety), dreams, fantasies, and various aspects of character, are the result of *compromise formations* (Freud 1893–1895/1955). In brief, a compromise formation symbolically represents a compromise between a forbidden wish and the defense against the wish. Panic attacks, for example, can represent a compromise between aggressive fantasies, which are viewed as dangerous, and self-punishment for the fantasies, experienced by the patient as terror and disability. Although not recognized by the patient, aggressive wishes can be expressed by coercive efforts to control ambivalently held objects.

The following case example illustrates panic symptoms that represent a compromise formation.

> Ms. C was driving from one city to another to attend a party for her 18th birthday when she experienced her first panic attack. The attack was so severe that she had to pull off the road and call her mother in the destination city and ask her to come pick her up on the highway. It took her mother several hours to find another person to drive with her who could also drive the car back, and in the meantime Ms. C's party had to be canceled.
>
> At the moment she experienced the attack, Ms. C found herself thinking that her 18th birthday was very important to her: it symbolized her "total independence" from her family and a new ability "to get rid of them." In unraveling the onset of her illness later in psychotherapy, it became clear that in her fantasy, turning 18 and being "independent" represented the emotional equivalent of killing off her parents and siblings, all of whom enraged her. The fantasy was such a source of conflict for her, despite its appeal, that she had her first panic attack. The panic attack represented both the *wish* to be rid of her family (suddenly, Ms. C, in fantasy found herself feeling entirely alone and unable to function) and the *defense* against this wish—a sudden-onset, severe illness that made "independence" from her family (and the very existence of her birthday celebration) impossible, and effectively immobilized her in her escape/fantasy plan. Additionally, the panic represented a real way in which she punished herself for her unacceptable feelings: now she could never be free of her family. Her symptoms also effectively punished her mother, who had to spend hours canceling everything she had been planning to do in order to take care of Ms. C.

Representation of Self and Others/ Transference

In the course of development, individuals form an internalized representation of both external objects (people with whom they have significant relationships) and of themselves (M. Klein 1948). From a psychoanalytic perspective, psychic symptoms such as anxiety evolve over the course of development in relationship to developmental changes in these representations. Current relationships with other people are affected by perceptions of developmentally central relationships that continue to exert compelling unconscious influence.

Patterns of perceptions of significant others typically emerge in the relationship with the therapist; this psychological phenomenon of *transference* (Freud 1905/1953) is a cornerstone of psychodynamic theory and practice. In any clinical psychiatric or psychological practice, focus on the transference can prove helpful to patients in recognizing underlying, organizing fantasies that surround the therapeutic relationship, regardless of the type of treatment in which the patient is engaged or the therapeutic orientation of the therapist. From a psychodynamic perspective, the transference situation has far-reaching effects and necessarily influences therapeutic outcome. Patients with anxiety disorders commonly experience tremendous distress at times of separation from the significant people in their lives, including their treating therapists. Consequently, anxiety symptoms can worsen when ongoing psychiatric treatment, regardless of the modality, is temporarily or permanently discontinued. These separations and termination, in an even more extreme way, can provide important opportunities for patients to better articulate, understand, and manage their conflicts about autonomy in the context of the transference.

The next case example illustrates the centrality of the transference phenomenon in a psychiatric treatment distant from psychodynamic psychiatry. A psychopharmacologist who specializes in the treatment of panic disorder reported this case:

> Ms. D, a patient with panic disorder who had been receiving treatment from the psychopharmacologist for years, had been taking very high doses of benzodiazepines. She and her physician had been engaged in a very slow and gradual taper of the drug because her panic attacks had remitted. She was in the middle of this taper, continuing on a substantially high dose of benzodiazepines, and had been tolerating the taper well. The pharmacologist lowered her dose again in a "microscopic decrement" before *leaving for a vacation.* Ms. D had "the worst panic attack in my life," for which, years later, she still has "not forgiven" him.

Benzodiazepine taper is well known to be difficult in this patient population because withdrawal syndromes and rebound anxiety are common. Thus, benzodiazepine tapers are best accomplished over a period of months. Nonetheless, in the Cross-National Collaborative Panic Study discontinuation phase, most of the patients who received alprazolam experienced their most severe withdrawal syndromes and rebound anxiety at the very end of the drug discontinuation phase or during the first week in which they were medication free (Pecknold et al. 1988). Ms. D was in neither situation. However, this patient was experiencing another equally common panic-related phenomenon: anxiety when being separated from the important objects in her life—in this case, her psychopharmacologist. Even in the context of a pharmacological treatment, some degree of focus on the transference situation might have prevented the panic attack.

Clinical Psychodynamic Approach to the Anxious Patient

The initial focus in a psychodynamically informed treatment of any anxiety disorder is to gain the information necessary to delineate specific fantasies, conflicts, and feelings underlying the symptoms. For this reason, when confronted with an anxious patient, the psychodynamically informed clinician must obtain a very detailed psychological history of the patient, including the circumstances, meanings, and feelings associated with the anxiety. A goal of the treatment is for the patient to become consciously aware of these emotional conflicts and, with this awareness, to begin to handle them differently, in ways that are verbally rather than somatically mediated.

Much has been written about the underlying meaning of panic symptoms (Kessler 1996; Milrod 1995, 2007; Milrod and Busch 1998; Milrod et al. 1997). Clinical observations indicate that fantasies surrounding separation and independence are common areas of conflict for panic patients. Several epidemiological studies provide indirect support for this finding (Leonard and Rapoport 1989; Rosenbaum et al. 1988; Weissman et al. 1984). Clinical observations also suggest that patients with panic disorder have difficulty tolerating (and at times modulating) angry feelings and thoughts (Busch et al. 1991; Shear et al. 1993). Additionally, although panic attacks often occur in the setting of conflicted hostility, for some patients the attacks take on an exciting significance of their own, beyond the commonly manifested panic about being ill, dying, or becoming "crazy." Some patients report a frightening or arousing inherent excitement associated with the attacks, often closely tied to sadomasochistic sexual conflicts (Milrod 1995; Milrod et al. 1996). Panic attacks can serve a self-punitive function, with which patients unconsciously atone for guilty transgressions. Finally, the panic experience can represent a specific unconscious fantasy or memory (Freud 1893–1895/1955; Milrod 1995).

The following case example illustrates the underlying meaning of panic symptoms in a woman who was recently married.

> Ms. E, a 25-year-old newly married woman, presented in a constant state of severe panic and agoraphobia, which made it impossible for her to leave her apartment without a companion. She was unable to eat, had lost 15 pounds, and was sleeping only a few hours each night in intermittent spurts. She had not responded to several medication trials, including benzodiazepines, tricyclics, selective serotonin reuptake inhibitors, and, finally, chlorpromazine.
>
> Ms. E reported having been well until 3 months before her marriage, the day she first tried on her wedding dress after it had been made. Her most prominent symptoms during panic attacks were severe nausea, although she never vomited, and dizziness, symptoms she described as "being like the first trimester of pregnancy." Because of the nature of her symptoms, she had been given pregnancy tests on numerous visits to medical emergency rooms, all of which had negative results.
>
> Ms. E's panic and agoraphobia ultimately remitted after 6 months of thrice-weekly psychodynamic psychotherapy. Nonetheless, from the information presented in this case example, which was obtained during the first 10 minutes of her first contact, the following important dynamic information became clear, simply as a result of careful focus on the time and place of her initial symptoms and a brief discussion of her fantasies about the meanings of her symptoms: 1) Ms. E had some mixed feelings of which she was not aware about getting married, and 2) Ms. E thought of her panic attacks as being, somehow, oddly like the first part of a pregnancy. Given that these two ideas co-occurred with the onset of her illness, it seemed highly likely that one of the elements of her strong unconscious mixed feelings about getting married concerned her new potential to become pregnant once she was married. These dynamisms in fact proved to be of central importance later in her treatment and in her symptoms' disappearance, and formed the starting place for the therapist to approach the patient.

In working psychodynamically with patients who have severe symptoms like those described in the case of Ms. E, clinicians must refrain from joining in patients' severe anxiety and must impart the idea that symptoms are understandable psychological phenomena. The goal of psychodynamically informed psychotherapy for the treatment of anxiety disorders is to determine how the symptoms make sense as psychological phenomena and, thus, to help patients to recognize their own feelings and thoughts in a more complete way than they had been able to before.

Psychoanalytic Perspectives on Nonpanic Anxiety Disorders

Many aspects of the general psychodynamic understanding of anxiety as it has been described thus far in this chapter are applicable to a psychoanalytic view and approach to other anxiety disorders. Psychoanalytically oriented clinicians have commonly focused on underlying characterological difficulties and pervasive unconscious fantasies and conflicts rather than on specific symptomatic presentations. Psychodynamic constellations have been suggested for some specific anxiety disorders (Leahy et al. 2005), and there is a large psychoanalytic and psychodynamic literature about posttraumatic stress disorder (Freud 1920/1955; Horowitz 1999; Kanas et al. 1994; Marmar et al. 1995; Weiss and Marmar 1993). Only more recently have psychoanalysts focused on developing treatment approaches to specific anxiety disorders, but there has been little in the way of systematic assessment of treatment outcome other than for panic disorder with and without agoraphobia.

A Psychodynamic Formulation and Treatment for Panic Disorder

A psychodynamic formulation for panic disorder with and without agoraphobia was developed from the psychoanalytic precepts about anxiety and from psychological studies and clinical observations of panic patients (Busch et al. 1991; Shear et al. 1993). Personality traits, including dependence and difficulty in being assertive, appear to predispose to the onset of panic disorder, which is then triggered by particular life stressors (D.F. Klein 1964; Kleiner and Marshall 1987). Marks (1970) reported that most agoraphobic patients had been described as "soft, anxious, shy, and dependent" before the onset of panic disorder (p. 541). D.F. Klein (1964) determined that half of the patients in his early study "seem to have suffered from a chronically high separation anxiety level throughout life and to have developed panic attacks under conditions where they were peculiarly vulnerable" (pp. 405–406). Many studies suggest that acute stressors, described in the literature as "life events," frequently occur just prior to panic onset (Faravelli 1985; Last et al. 1984; Milrod et al. 2004; Roy-Byrne et al. 1986). Despite the DSM-IV-TR description of panic attacks as coming "out of the blue" (p. 431), from a psychodynamic perspective, the meaning of these events to the individual (including their unconscious significance) and the affects triggered in response to these events play a central role in the development of panic attacks.

Milrod et al. (1997) developed a manualized treatment, Panic-Focused Psychodynamic Psychotherapy (PFPP). The treatment targets the core dynamics of panic disorder, including separation anxiety, abandonment fears, and difficulty in managing ambivalence and conflicted rage. Psychodynamic techniques of clarification, confrontation, interpretation, and focus on the transference are employed, but PFPP differs from traditional psychodynamic psychotherapy in its pursuit of the unconscious significance of the symptoms of a specific psychiatric disorder.

Review of Psychodynamic Research on Anxiety Disorders

The fields of psychodynamic psychiatry and psychoanalysis lag far behind the general psychiatric community in the area of systematic outcome research. Psychoanalysis and general psychiatry have traditionally had separate literatures, training goals, and views of the role that research should have in determination of clinical care for patients. In the field of psychoanalysis, the literature has revolved around detailed individual case presentations, which have been viewed as research tools that have carried the ability to demonstrate effectiveness. Psychoanalytic treatments have been thought of as too complex to study in a systematic manner (Green 1996, 2000). Research has been considered potentially disruptive to psychoanalytic treatments, adversely affecting the transference and the psychoanalytic process. Brief treatments, the frequently necessary and expedient focus of psychotherapy studies, have generally been avoided because they are considered to be inadequate to address the underlying neurotic structure that leads to symptoms (Freud 1919/1955; Greenacre 1954). In recent years, there has been an increasing recognition of the importance of outcome research (Fonagy 2003; Fonagy et al. 2005; Gabbard et al. 2003) and a growing recognition that psychoanalytic treatments can be studied in the same fashion as other psychotherapies.

Panic Disorder

In a pilot study, Wiborg and Dahl (1996) demonstrated that 26 weekly sessions of psychodynamic psychotherapy, in addition to clomipramine, significantly reduced relapse rates at 6- and 18-month follow-up among patients with DSM-III-R (American Psychiatric Association 1987) panic disorder in comparison with patients treated with clomipramine alone (9% relapse in the combined treatment group vs. 91% in the clomipramine alone group).

Panic-Focused Psychodynamic Psychotherapy Studies

In an open trial of PFPP, 21 patients with primary DSM-IV (American Psychiatric Association 1994) panic disorder with or without agoraphobia were treated with twice-weekly, 12-week, 24-session psychoanalytic psychotherapy (Milrod et al. 2000, 2001). The findings revealed that 16 of 21 experienced remission of panic and agoraphobia. Treatment completers with comorbid major depression also experienced remission of depression (n=8). Improvements in symptoms and psychosocial function were substantial (within-group effect size=2.08 in the primary outcome measure, the Panic Disorder Severity Scale [PDSS; Shear et al. 1997]) and consistent across all measured areas. Symptomatic gains and improvements in psychosocial function were maintained over 6 months. The results of this trial indicated that PFPP was a promising nonpharmacological treatment for panic disorder.

Milrod et al. (2007b) conducted a randomized, controlled trial of 49 patients with primary DSM-IV panic disorder with or without agoraphobia, comparing PFPP with a less active psychotherapy for panic disorder, Applied Relaxation Therapy (ART) (Cerny et al. 1984). Patients entering the study who had been receiving medication (18%) agreed to keep the dose and type of medication constant. Patients were not permitted to enter the study while in another psychotherapy. Those with severe agoraphobia, major depression, and personality disorder comorbidities were included. Subjects were excluded for psychosis, bipolar disorder, and substance abuse (6 months remission necessary). Patients were diagnosed on the Anxiety Disorders Interview Schedule (Brown et al. 1995).

PFPP and ART treatments were each 24 sessions long, with twice-weekly visits. ART started with a three-session rationale and explanation about panic disorder. ART utilizes progressive muscle relaxation techniques and exposure. Progressive muscle relaxation training involves focusing attention on particular muscle groups, tensing the muscle group for 5–10 seconds, attending to sensations of tension, and then relaxing the muscles. Discrimination training, generalization, relaxation by recall, and cue-controlled relaxation (pairing the relaxed state to the word "relax") followed. One session addressed relaxation-induced panic. Home practice was required twice daily. By week 6, subjects applied relaxation skills to anxiety situations in a graduated manner. Adherence ratings were performed on three videotapes from each treatment (available from the authors). These assessments indicated that adherence to the manualized treatments was high.

The treatment groups were matched on demographic and clinical variables (severity of panic, length of illness, comorbid disorders) other than gender. A higher proportion of men were in the ART group (47% vs. 15%; two-tailed Fisher's exact text, P=0.03). PFPP had a significantly higher response rate than ART (73% vs. 39%; P=0.016), using a standard definition of "response"—a 40% decrease in the total PDSS score from baseline (Barlow et al. 2000). Subjects in the PFPP condition experienced significantly greater improvement in panic disorder symptoms as measured by the PDSS (P=0.002), and psychosocial function as measured by the Sheehan Disability Scale (Shear et al. 1997) (P=0.014). The Hamilton Depression Rating Scale (Hamilton 1960) (P=0.07) and the Hamilton Anxiety Rating Scale (Hamilton 1959) (P=0.58) did not reveal significant differences between treatments.

PFPP demonstrated efficacy in this first randomized, controlled trial of a psychoanalytic psychotherapy as a sole intervention for DSM-IV-TR panic disorder and agoraphobia. PFPP was well tolerated, with a 7% (2 of 26 subjects) dropout rate. The strong response to treatment occurred despite inclusion in the study of patients with severe agoraphobia and comorbid major depression, making for a relatively sicker and, thus, possibly more generalizable group of panic patients, compared with some other outcome studies focusing on patients with panic disorder (Barlow et al. 2000; Clark et al. 1994; Craske et al. 1991; Fava et al. 1995; Marks et al. 1993). At this writing, a study is in progress comparing PFPP directly with CBT and ART (B. Milrod and J.P. Barber, unpublished; National Institute of Mental Health grant R01 MH070918/01–5).

Preliminary moderator analyses in the PFPP randomized, controlled trial demonstrated that patients with Cluster C personality disorder comorbidity, diagnosed on the Structured Clinical Interview for DSM-II (SCID-II; First et al. 1994b), responded better to PFPP than patients who did not have Cluster C comorbidity (Milrod et al. 2007a). This finding suggests that PFPP may be particularly useful for a population of patients (those with panic disorder with Cluster C comorbidity) that may or may not be as effectively treated with CBT. A study of *reflective function* (Rudden et al. 2006), conducted in conjunction with the PFPP randomized, controlled trial, indicated that a measure of awareness of the link between emotional experience and symptoms, panic-specific reflective functioning (PSRF), increased significantly from baseline to posttreatment in patients treated with PFPP, but not in those treated with ART. The degree of change in PSRF did not correlate with degree of symptomatic change as measured by the PDSS. Further assessments of this potential mediator have been included in the design of the comparative evaluation of PFPP, cognitive-behavioral therapy, and ART.

Posttraumatic Stress Disorder

Brom et al. (1989) compared 112 patients with posttraumatic stress disorder (PTSD), diagnosed according to DSM-III criteria (American Psychiatric Association 1980), who were randomly assigned to receive one of three treatments: psychodynamic psychotherapy (n=29), hypnotherapy (n=29), or trauma desensitization (derived from systematic desensitization [n=31]), or designated to a wait-list control group (n=23). Mean treatment lengths were 18.8 sessions for psychodynamic psychotherapy, 14.4 for hypnotherapy, and 15 for trauma desensitization. Posttraumatic symptoms were assessed with the Symptom Checklist–90 (Arrindell and Ettema 1981) and the Impact of Event Scale (Horowitz et al. 1979). There were 12 dropouts spread evenly among the three treatment conditions. All three treatment groups showed significant improvement in trauma-related symptoms from baseline and in comparison with the control group.

Social Phobia

Knijnik et al. (2004) studied psychodynamic group therapy in 40 patients with primary generalized social phobia, diagnosed on SCID-IV (First et al. 1995), compared with a supportive group therapy, in a 12-week randomized, controlled trial. Patients receiving medication underwent a 4-week washout prior to the study. There were five dropouts from each group, caused by scheduling problems. The treatments consisted of 12-weekly group sessions of a manualized psychodynamic approach (available from the authors) compared with a group that received treatment based on educational and supportive approaches. Patients were rated with the Clinical Global Impression scale (Guy 1976), the Liebowitz Social Anxiety Scale (Heimberg et al. 1999), and the Hamilton Anxiety Rating Scale (Hamilton 1959). There were no significant baseline differences in demographic characteristics between the two groups. Patients in both groups demonstrated a significant improvement on all three measures with treatment. Subjects receiving psychodynamic group therapy showed significant improvement, compared with those receiving treatment based on educational and supportive approaches, on the Liebowitz scale but not on the other measures.

Generalized Anxiety Disorder

Crits-Christoph and his colleagues studied a manualized (Crits-Christoph et al. 1995), interpersonally oriented psychodynamic treatment for generalized anxiety disorder (GAD), initially in an open trial of 26 patients (Crits-Christoph et al. 1996). Patients met either 1) DSM-III-R criteria (SCID-P; Spitzer et al. 1990) for GAD (*n*=21) or 2) DSM-III-R criteria for anxiety not otherwise specified and DSM-IV criteria for GAD (*n*=5). The treatment consisted of 16 weekly sessions of supportive-expressive psychotherapy, followed by 3 monthly booster sessions. Outcome measures included the Hamilton Anxiety Rating Scale (Ham-A; Hamilton 1959), Hamilton Rating Scale for Depression (Ham-D; Hamilton 1960), Beck Anxiety Inventory (Beck et al. 1988a), Beck Depression Inventory (Beck et al. 1988b), and Penn State Worry Questionnaire (Meyer et al. 1990). Results indicated a significant reduction across outcome measures, including measures of GAD symptoms. At termination, 79% of patients no longer met criteria for GAD. In a follow-up pilot study, Crits-Christoph et al. (2005) studied 31 patients with DSM-IV (SCID-IV; First et al. 1994a) diagnoses of GAD treated in a randomized, controlled trial with either the manualized supportive-expressive GAD-specific treatment (*n*=15) or a manualized supportive psychotherapy for GAD (Borkovec and Matthews 1988) (*n*=16). There was 1 dropout from the supportive-expressive psychotherapy and 2 from supportive therapy. The researchers found the GAD-specific treatment to be superior to supportive psychotherapy in remission rates of GAD, defined as a Ham-A score of less than 7.

Psychodynamic Research on Anxiety in Children and Adolescents

Two studies in the area of child and adolescent psychiatry indirectly document some salutary effects of psychodynamic treatment for patients with anxiety disorders, although additional research is necessary. Heinicke and Ramsey-Klee (1986) evaluated the relative effects of once-weekly versus four-times-weekly psychodynamic psychotherapy or psychoanalysis on 15 boys, ages 7–10 years, with DSM-III overanxious disorder and problems at school. Patients were systematically evaluated with a series of psychological tests (e.g., the Revised Stanford-Binet Intelligence Scale, the Wide Range Achievement Test, and the Rorschach inkblot test) and a series of ratings of psychological functioning (e.g., defensive functioning, object relationships, and frustration tolerance) based on diagnostic interviews and test results, before treatment, at treatment termination, and at 2-year follow-up. Both groups showed significant improvements in levels of anxiety, but those who received four-times-weekly therapy experienced additional important characterological and coping-skills gains.

Fonagy and Target (1996) performed a retrospective review of the Anna Freud Case Center's 196 child and adolescent patients who had received diagnoses of anxiety disorders and assigned DSM-III-R diagnoses to patients from detailed clinical reports. Patients received psychoanalysis 4 or 5 times weekly or psychodynamic psychotherapy once or twice weekly. By treatment termination, including treatments of at least 6 months duration, average Children's Global Assessment Scale scores (a measure of overall functioning scored from 0 to 100) improved 13.7 points, indicating a significant overall average improvement in level of functioning. A positive correlation was found between frequency of treatment and degree of clinical improvement. A confound of this study was that children who were initially evaluated as being more impaired were assigned to the more intensive treatment condition.

Combining Psychodynamic Treatments With Medication

Although some anxious patients wish to start medication quickly to diminish the discomfort they experience, there remains a core of highly anxious patients who are too frightened of medication to consider taking it (Cross-National Collaborative Panic Study 1992; Hofmann et al. 1998). Although medication should be considered and discussed as an efficacious treatment option with patients, in many cases it may not be necessary. Evidence suggests that for many patients, psychodynamic psychotherapy for panic disorder can be an effective treatment alone (Milrod 1995; Milrod and Shear 1991; Milrod et al. 1996, 2000, 2007b; Renik 1995; Stern 1995). In the PFPP efficacy study (Milrod et al. 2007b), subjects who entered the study agreed to keep medication doses constant, and the use of medication (by 18% of patients) showed no effect on outcome in either treatment condition.

Psychodynamic treatments can be effectively combined with antianxiety medication (Milrod and Busch

1998; Wiborg and Dahl 1996). In more severe cases, in which patients feel too impaired by anxiety to be able to think clearly, medication can aid psychotherapy by relieving severe anxiety, thus permitting patients to more productively explore the underlying significance of the symptoms. In psychoanalytically based treatments, therapist and patient should discuss emotional meanings of taking medication (Milrod and Busch 1998).

Conclusion

Despite a wealth of theoretical and clinical conceptions concerning anxiety, professionals in the fields of psychoanalysis and psychoanalytic therapy have been slow to undertake efficacy studies to determine the effect of psychodynamic interventions, alone or in combination with other treatments, on anxiety disorders. We remain hopeful that the recent outcome study demonstrating the efficacy of PFPP for panic disorder will encourage more randomized, controlled trials of psychodynamic treatments to better assess the appropriate place of psychodynamic psychotherapy among the available treatments for anxiety disorders. Understanding for whom a treatment works and its mechanisms of change can lead to the development of more specific interventions for individual patients.

◀ Key Clinical Points ▶

- Psychodynamic models conceptualize anxiety disorders as developing from wishes, feelings, and fantasies, often unconscious, that are experienced as frightening or intolerable.
- In psychodynamic psychotherapy, therapist and patient work to identify and reappraise emotional conflicts, rendering them less threatening.
- Psychodynamic approaches, though widely used, have received little in the way of systematic assessment, but psychoanalytic clinicians have increasingly realized the importance of undertaking such studies.
- A manualized psychodynamic approach to panic disorder has demonstrated efficacy when compared with a less active treatment.
- Further studies will help to determine the role of psychodynamic psychotherapy among the available treatments for anxiety disorders.

References

American Psychiatric Association: Diagnostic and Statistical Manual of Mental Disorders, 3rd Edition. Washington, DC, American Psychiatric Association, 1980

American Psychiatric Association: Diagnostic and Statistical Manual of Mental Disorders, 3rd Edition, Revised. Washington, DC, American Psychiatric Association, 1987

American Psychiatric Association: Diagnostic and Statistical Manual of Mental Disorders, 4th Edition. Washington, DC, American Psychiatric Association, 1994

American Psychiatric Association: Diagnostic and Statistical Manual of Mental Disorders, 4th Edition, Text Revision. Washington, DC, American Psychiatric Association, 2000

Arrindell W, Ettema H: [Dimensional structure, reliability, and validity of the Dutch version of the Symptom Checklist (SCL-90): data based on a phobic and "normal" population] (in Dutch). Nederlands Tijdschrifi voor de Psychologie 36:77–108, 1981

Arrindell W, Emmelkamp PMG, Monsma A, et al: The role of perceived parental rearing practices in the etiology of phobic disorders: a controlled study. Br J Psychiatry 143:183–187, 1983

Barlow DH, Gorman JM, Shear MK, et al: Cognitive-behavioral therapy, imipramine, or their combination for panic disorder. JAMA 283:2529–2536, 2000

Beck AT, Epstein N, Brown G, et al: An inventory for measuring clinical anxiety: psychometric properties. J Consult Clin Psychol 56:893–897, 1988a

Beck AT, Steer RA, Garbin MG: Psychometric properties of the Beck Depression Inventory: twenty five years later. Clin Psychol Rev 8:77–100, 1988b

Borkovec TD, Matthews AM: Treatment of nonphobic anxiety disorders: a comparison of nondirective, cognitive, and coping desensitization therapy. J Consult Clin Psychol 56:877–884, 1988

Brom C, Kleber RJ, Defares PB: Brief psychotherapy for posttraumatic stress disorders. J Consult Clin Psychol 57:607–612, 1989

Brown TA, DiNardo P, Barlow DH: Anxiety Disorders Interview Schedule for DSM-IV: Lifetime Version (ADIS-IV-L). New York, Graywinds Publications, 1995

Busch F, Cooper AM, Klerman GL, et al: Neurophysiological, cognitive-behavioral, and psychoanalytic approaches to panic disorder: toward an integration. Psychoanal Inq 11:316–332, 1991

Busch F, Shear MK, Cooper AM, et al: An empirical study of defense mechanisms in panic disorder. J Nerv Ment Dis 183:299–303, 1995

Busch F, Milrod B, Cooper A, et al: Grand rounds: panic-focused psychodynamic psychotherapy. J Psychother Pract Res 5:72–83, 1996

Cerny JA, Vermilyea BB, Barlow DH, et al: Anxiety Treatment Project Relaxation Treatment Manual. Unpublished manual, 1984

Clark DM, Salkovskis PM, Hackman A, et al: A comparison of cognitive therapy, applied relaxation, and imipramine in the treatment of panic disorder. Br J Psychiatry 164:759–769, 1994

Craske MG, Brown TA, Barlow DH: Behavioral treatment of panic disorder: a two-year follow-up. Behav Ther 22:289–304, 1991

Crits-Christoph P, Crits-Christoph K, Wolf-Pacacio D, et al: Brief supportive-expressive psychotherapy for generalized anxiety disorder, in Dynamic Therapies for Psychiatric Disorders (Axis I). Edited by Barber JP, Crits-Christoph P. New York, Basic Books, 1995, pp 43–83

Crits-Christoph P, Connolly MB, Azarian K, et al: An open trial of brief supportive-expressive psychotherapy in the treatment of generalized anxiety disorder. Psychotherapy 33:418–430, 1996

Crits-Christoph P, Connolly Gibbons MB, Narducci J, et al: Interpersonal problems and the outcome of interpersonally oriented psychodynamic treatment of GAD. Psychotherapy: Theory/Research/Practice/Training 42:211–224, 2005

Cross-National Collaborative Panic Study, Second Phase Investigators: Drug treatment of panic disorder: comparative efficacy of alprazolam, imipramine, and placebo. Br J Psychiatry 160:191–202, 1992

Deutsch H: The genesis of agoraphobia. Int J Psychoanal 10:51–69, 1929

Faravelli C: Life events preceding the onset of panic disorder. J Affect Disord 9:103–105, 1985

Fava GA, Zielezny M, Savron G, et al: Long-term effects of behavioral treatment for panic disorder with agoraphobia. Br J Psychiatry 166:87–92, 1995

First MB, Spitzer RL, Gibbon M, et al: Structured Clinical Interview for DSM–IV Axis I Disorders, Patient Edition (SCID-I/P). Washington, DC, American Psychiatric Press, 1994a

First MB, Spitzer RL, Gibbon M, et al: Structured Clinical Interview for DSM-IV Axis II Personality Disorders (SCID-II), Version 2.0. New York, Biometrics Research Department, New York State Psychiatric Institute, 1994b

First MB, Spitzer RL, Williams JBW, et al: Structured Clinical Interview for DSM-IV (SCID-I) (User's Guide and Interview), Research Version. New York, Biometrics Research Department, New York State Psychiatric Institute, 1995

Fonagy P: Genetics, developmental psychopathology, and psychoanalytic theory: the case for ending our (not so splendid) isolation. Psychoanal Inq 23:218–247, 2003

Fonagy P, Target M: Predictors of outcome in child psychoanalysis: a retrospective study of 763 cases at the Anna Freud Centre. J Am Psychoanal Assoc 44:27–77, 1996

Fonagy P, Roth A, Higgitt A: Psychodynamic psychotherapies: evidence-based practice and clinical wisdom. Bull Menninger Clin 69:1–58, 2005

Freud S: Studies on hysteria (1893–1895), in Standard Edition of the Complete Psychological Works of Sigmund Freud, Vol 2. Translated and edited by Strachey J. London, Hogarth Press, 1955, pp 1–181

Freud S: Fragment of an analysis of a case of hysteria (1905), in Standard Edition of the Complete Psychological Works of Sigmund Freud, Vol 7. Translated and edited by Strachey J. London, Hogarth Press, 1953, pp 3–122

Freud S: Formulations on the two principles of mental functioning (1911), in Standard Edition of the Complete Psychological Works of Sigmund Freud, Vol 12. Translated and edited by Strachey J. London, Hogarth Press, 1958, pp 213–226

Freud S: Lines of advances in psychoanalytic therapy (1919), in Standard Edition of the Complete Psychological Works of Sigmund Freud, Vol 17. Translated and edited by Strachey J. London, Hogarth Press, 1955, pp 157–168

Freud S: Beyond the pleasure principle (1920), in Standard Edition of the Complete Psychological Works of Sigmund Freud, Vol 18. Translated and edited by Strachey J. London, Hogarth Press, 1955, pp 3–64

Freud S: Inhibitions, symptoms and anxiety (1926), in Standard Edition of the Complete Psychological Works of Sigmund Freud, Vol 20. Translated and edited by Strachey J. London, Hogarth Press, 1959, pp 77–175

Gabbard GO, Gunderson JG, Fonagy P: The place of psychoanalytic treatments within psychiatry. Arch Gen Psychiatry 59:505–510, 2003

Green A: What kind of research for psychoanalysis? International Psychoanalysis: Newsletter of the International Psychoanalytic Association 5:10–14, 1996

Green A: Science and science fiction in infant research, in Clinical and Observational Research: Roots of a Controversy. Edited by Sandler J, Sandler A-M, Davies R. London, Karnac Books, 2000, pp 41–72

Greenacre P: The role of transference: practical considerations in relation to psychoanalytic therapy. J Am Psychoanal Assoc 2:671–684, 1954

Guy W: Assessment Manual for Psychopharmacology. Washington, DC, U.S. Government Printing Office, 1976

Hamilton M: The assessment of anxiety states by rating. Br J Med Psychol 32:50–55, 1959

Hamilton M: A rating scale for depression. J Neurol Neurosurg Psychiatry 23:56–62, 1960

Heimberg RG, Horner KJ, Juster HR, et al: Psychometric properties of the Liebowitz Social Anxiety Scale. Psychol Med 29:199–212, 1999

Heinicke C, Ramsey-Klee D: Outcome of child psychotherapy as a function of frequency of session. J Am Acad Child Adolesc Psychiatry 25:247–253, 1986

Hofmann SG, Barlow DH, Papp LA, et al: Pretreatment attrition in a comparative treatment outcome study on panic disorder. Am J Psychiatry 155:43–47, 1998

Horowitz MJ: Essential Papers on Posttraumatic Stress Disorder. New York, New York University Press, 1999

Horowitz MJ, Wilner N, Alvarez W: Impact of Event Scale: a measure of subjective stress. Psychosom Med 41:209–218, 1979

Kanas N, Schoenfeld F, Marmar C, et al: Process and content in a long-term PTSD therapy group for Vietnam veterans. Group 18:78–88, 1994

Kessler RJ: Panic disorder and the retreat from meaning. J Clin Psychoanal 5:505–528, 1996

Klein DF: Delineation of two drug-responsive anxiety syndromes. Psychopharmacologia 5:397–408, 1964

Klein M: A contribution to the theory of anxiety and guilt. Int J Psychoanal 29:114–123, 1948

Kleiner L, Marshall WL: The role of interpersonal problems in the development of agoraphobia with panic attacks. J Anxiety Disord 1:313–323, 1987

Knijnik DZ, Kapczinski F, Chachamovich E, et al: Psychodynamic group treatment for generalized social phobia. Rev Bras Psiquiatr 26:77–81, 2004

Last CG, Barlow DH, O'Brien GT: Precipitants of agoraphobia: role of stressful life events. Psychol Rep 54:567–570, 1984

Leahy RL, McGinn LK, Busch FN, et al: Anxiety disorders, in Oxford Textbook of Psychotherapy. Edited by Gabbard GO, Beck JS, Holmes J. Oxford, England, Oxford University Press, 2005, pp 136–161

Leonard HL, Rapoport JL: Anxiety disorders in childhood and adolescence, in American Psychiatric Press Review of Psychiatry, Vol 8. Edited by Tasman A, Hales RE, Frances AJ. Washington, DC, American Psychiatric Press, 1989, pp 162–179

Marks IM: Agoraphobic syndrome (phobic anxiety state). Arch Gen Psychiatry 23:538–553, 1970

Marks IM, Swinson RP, Basoglu M, et al: Alprazolam and exposure alone and combined in panic disorder with agoraphobia: a controlled study in London and Toronto. Br J Psychiatry 162:776–787, 1993

Marmar CR, Weiss DS, Pynoos RS: Dynamic psychotherapy of post-traumatic stress disorder, in Neurobiological and Clinical Consequences of Stress: From Normal Adaptation to Post-Traumatic Stress Disorder. Edited by Friedman MJ, Charney DS, Deutch AY. Philadelphia, PA, Lippincott-Raven, 1995, pp 495–506

Meyer TJ, Miller ML, Metzger RL, et al: Development and validation of the Penn State Worry Questionnaire. Behav Res Ther 28:487–495, 1990

Milrod B: The continued usefulness of psychoanalysis in the treatment armamentarium for panic disorder. J Am Psychoanal Assoc 43:151–162, 1995

Milrod B: Unconscious pregnancy fantasies as an underlying dynamism in panic disorder. J Am Psychoanal Assoc 46:673–690, 1998

Milrod B: Emptiness in agoraphobia patients. J Am Psychoanal Assoc 55:1007–1026, 2007

Milrod B, Busch F: Integrating the use of medication with psychodynamic psychotherapy in the treatment of panic disorder. Psychoanal Inq 18:702–715, 1998

Milrod B, Shear MK: Dynamic treatment of panic disorder: a review. J Nerv Ment Dis 179:741–743, 1991

Milrod B, Busch F, Hollander E, et al: A twenty-three year old woman with panic disorder treated with psychodynamic psychotherapy. Am J Psychiatry 153:698–703, 1996

Milrod B, Busch F, Cooper A, et al: Manual of Panic-Focused Psychodynamic Psychotherapy. Washington, DC, American Psychiatric Press, 1997

Milrod B, Busch F, Leon AC, et al: Open trial of psychodynamic psychotherapy for panic disorder: a pilot study. Am J Psychiatry 157:1878–1880, 2000

Milrod B, Busch F, Leon AC, et al: A pilot open trial of psychodynamic psychotherapy for panic disorder. J Psychother Pract Res 10:239–245, 2001

Milrod B, Leon, AC, Shear MK: Can interpersonal loss events precipitate panic disorder? (Letter to editor). Am J Psychiatry 161:758–759, 2004

Milrod B, Leon AC, Barber JP, et al: Do comorbid personality disorders moderate panic-focused psychotherapy? An exploratory examination of the APA Practice Guideline. J Clin Psychiatry 68:885–891, 2007a

Milrod B, Leon AC, Busch F, et al: A randomized controlled clinical trial of psychoanalytic psychotherapy for panic disorder. Am J Psychiatry 164:265–272, 2007b

Parker G: Reported parental characteristics of agoraphobics and social phobics. Br J Psychiatry 135:555–560, 1979

Pecknold JC, Swinson RP, Kuck K, et al: Alprazolam in panic disorder and agoraphobia: results from a multicenter trial, III: discontinuation effects. Arch Gen Psychiatry 45:429–436, 1988

Renik O: The patient's anxiety, the therapist's anxiety, and the therapeutic process, in Anxiety as Symptom and Signal. Edited by Roose SP, Glick RA. Hillsdale, NJ, Analytic Press, 1995, pp 121–130

Rosenbaum JF, Biederman J, Gerstein M, et al: Behavioral inhibition in children of parents with panic disorder and agoraphobia. Arch Gen Psychiatry 45:463–470, 1988

Roy-Byrne PP, Geraci M, Uhde TW: Life events and the onset of panic disorder. Am J Psychiatry 143:1424–1427, 1986

Rudden M, Milrod B, Target M, et al: Reflective functioning in panic disorder patients: a pilot study. J Am Psychoanal Assoc 54:1339–1343, 2006

Shapiro T: The concept of unconscious fantasy. J Clin Psychoanal 1:517–524, 1992

Shear MK, Cooper AM, Klerman GL, et al: A psychodynamic model of panic disorder. Am J Psychiatry 150:859–866, 1993

Shear MK, Brown TA, Barlow DH, et al: Multicenter Collaborative Panic Disorder Severity Scale. Am J Psychiatry 154:1571–1575, 1997

Spitzer RL, Williams JBW, Gibbon M, et al: Structured Clinical Interview for DSM-III-R, Patient Edition (With Psychotic Screen), Version 1.0. Washington, DC, American Psychiatric Press, 1990

Stern G: Anxiety and resistance to changes in self-concept, in Anxiety as Symptom and Signal. Edited by Roose SP, Glick RA. Hillsdale, NJ, Analytic Press, 1995, pp 105–120

Weiss DS, Marmar CR: Teaching time-limited dynamic psychotherapy for post-traumatic stress disorder and pathological grief. Psychotherapy 30:587–591, 1993

Weissman MM, Leckman JF, Merikangas KR, et al: Depression and anxiety disorders in parents and children. Arch Gen Psychiatry 41:845–852, 1984

Wiborg IM, Dahl AA: Does brief dynamic psychotherapy reduce the relapse rate of panic disorder? Arch Gen Psychiatry 53:689–694, 1996

Recommended Readings

Freud S: Inhibitions, symptoms and anxiety (1926), in Standard Edition of the Complete Psychological Works of Sigmund Freud, Vol 20. Translated and edited by Strachey J. London, Hogarth Press, 1959, pp 77–175

Horowitz MJ: Essential Papers on Posttraumatic Stress Disorder. New York: New York University Press, 1999

Leahy RL, McGinn LK, Busch FN, et al: Anxiety disorders, in Oxford Textbook of Psychotherapy. Edited by Gabbard GO, Beck JS, Holmes J. Oxford, Oxford University Press, 2005, pp 136–161

Milrod B, Busch F, Cooper A, et al: Manual of Panic-Focused Psychodynamic Psychotherapy. Washington, DC, American Psychiatric Press, 1997

Milrod B, Busch F, Leon AC, et al: Open trial of psychodynamic psychotherapy for panic disorder: a pilot study. Am J Psychiatry 157:1878–1880, 2000

Chapter 9

Evolutionary Concepts of Anxiety

Myron A. Hofer, M.D.

For the past century or more, psychiatry has been divided by a shifting alignment of opposing theoretical views on the nature and origins of mental illness. However, rapid progress in our understanding of evolution over the past decade now offers an opportunity for psychiatry to find a central conceptual base in an advanced evolutionary theory that integrates the social, psychological, and biological levels of organization in a developmental framework. These advances involve discoveries in several areas: the regulation of gene expression during development; the fossil record of evolution; the application of DNA mapping to phylogeny; field studies that for the first time observe, in detail, the ongoing process of rapid evolutionary change; our understanding of the interaction between developmental and evolutionary processes; the maturation of the field of sociobiology; and the discovery of laboratory models of anxiety in a range of organisms representing our phylogenetically distant ancestors.

In addition to advances in the field of evolution, major changes have taken place in our concept of the emotions—changes that facilitate application of the new evolutionary concepts to anxiety. In traditional theory, emotions were considered discrete entities, each defined by certain characteristic behavioral and physiological response patterns (Darwin 1872/1965; Izard 1977; Lewis and Brooks-Gunn 1979). In development and in evolution, emotions were believed to emerge as units and to follow the appearance of new cognitive advances or structures. The newer view is a functional or transactional one (Campos et al. 1994; Lazarus 1991). Emotions are seen as processes existing at the interface of the organism and its transactions with the environment. They are defined in terms of particular characteristics of the functional relationships between the organism and the environment, serving to regulate (establish, maintain, or disrupt) these relationships. Different families of emotions can be defined in terms of the nature, dynamics, and adaptive role of those transactions, rather than in terms of certain invariant features of the response. In development and in evolution, each family of emotions emerges gradually, together with its cognitive components, following growth in the complexity of the organism.

Thus, in this chapter, I view anxiety as an organized group of adaptive functions by which an organism senses, evaluates, and responds to cues of danger in its external (or internal) environment. Anxiety disorders can be approached in research and treatment as failures of these adaptive processes, at any one of a number of

The author's research described in this chapter is supported by a Research Scientist Award and a project grant from the National Institute of Mental Health and by The Sackler Institute for Developmental Psychobiology at Columbia University.

possible points in their development and function. In the first section of the chapter, I review recent advances in our understanding of evolution in relation to development insofar as this knowledge can be applied to the origins of anxiety. I then use these concepts to describe the organization of prototypical anxiety states in four very different contemporary species, representing major steps in the evolution of anxiety as we know it.

New Advances in Understanding Evolution and Development

To consider the evolution of any behavior or mental state, we must first deal with the skeptic's question: how can you even talk about the evolution of something like anxiety that leaves no fossil record? Evidence in the rapidly expanding fossil record (Eldredge and Gould 1972) and in DNA evidence for the timing of divergence of vertebrate lineages (e.g., Kumar and Hedges 1998) has modified evolutionary theory in a way that allows us to use evidence from contemporary mammals to infer how anxiety manifested itself in our phylogenetic ancestors and how it evolved. This modification is a shift away from the view of evolution as having progressed with the slow, incremental effect of cumulative small changes. In the old *"phyletic gradualism,"* no contemporary species was thought to closely resemble our distant ancestors. But extensive fossil evidence now shows that once a species has evolved, it rarely undergoes major change. The evolution of new species occurs only at intervals of many millions of years, and in relatively rapid (20,000–40,000 years) spurts, occurring in a small subpopulation at the geographic border of the species range where selection pressures are likely to be the strongest. This view has been termed *punctuated equilibrium* (Eldredge 1989). It does not mean that we can simply assume that a rat, a marine invertebrate, or a microbe that we study in the laboratory today is a precise replica of a creature existing much earlier in phylogeny. But the conservative nature of evolution has resulted in a stability over hundreds of millions of years of numerous genes and their regulatory elements, cell structures, biochemical mechanisms, intercellular messengers, and major features of neural circuitry. Thus, by studying contemporary species we are likely to obtain useful insights into the probable workings of our distant ancestors' adaptive responses, even of their brain states, the precursors of anxiety. The second part of this chapter illustrates such an approach in detail.

Sociobiology

The application of evolutionary concepts to our understanding of emotions, begun by Darwin (1872/1965) with the publication of *The Expression of the Emotions in Man and Animals*, strongly influenced many later developments in psychology, such as psychoanalysis and ethology. More recently, Haldane (1932/1993), Hamilton (1964), Trivers (1974), and Wilson (1975) brought about a synthesis of ethology, evolutionary biology, and population genetics, which Wilson called *sociobiology*. Comparative psychology and ecology have been transformed as a result (Alcock 2001), but the application of this thinking to psychiatric illness has been delayed by a reluctance within the field to accept the idea of genetic influences on aspects of the human mind and personality and/or by a concept of illness limited to the medical models of infectious, nutritional, and degenerative disease; environmental toxins; and sporadic single gene mutations. However, there are signs of an awakening interest within medicine, and psychiatry in particular, to the usefulness of an evolutionary approach (McGuire and Troisi 1998; Nesse and Williams 1996). This approach is becoming more widespread with the rapid advance of genetics in psychiatry.

Evolutionary Approaches

The *existence* of evolution over millennia can be supported by the geological, genetic, and fossil record. However, the *mechanism* of evolution—natural selection—is primarily supported by evidence provided in the remarkable variation in domesticated species (Darwin 1868/1998), in the range of available laboratory animals resulting from selective breeding by scientists (DeFries et al. 1981), and in the field studies of selection under the natural pressures of yearly climatic change (Grant 1986). Examples of rapid evolution under experimental selection for anxiety traits are described later in this chapter, and in papers by Suomi (1997), Brunelli et al. (1997), Scheiner (2002), and Brunelli and Hofer (2007). Because these forms of selection have been shown to alter behavioral and biological traits of small groups of animals in a rapid and powerful manner over a few generations, this constitutes the most direct evidence we have regarding how the emotions and anxiety itself may have evolved over geological time.

In contrast to the evolution of new species (macroevolution), individual traits show rapid changes in intensity or form within species under changing environmental pressures (microevolution). Variation produced in this manner can create extremes in a trait such as anxiety, and such changes are thought to form the basis for human temperamental differences in vulnerability to anxiety disorders (Marks and Nesse 1994).

An evolutionary process that may allow us to understand how the incapacitating forms of disintegrative anxiety were not eliminated immediately by natural selection is the property of evolution to operate through trade-off and compromise. A favorite example is the evolution of incapacitating sickle cell anemia (a disease that occurs in only those who are homozygous for the trait), in an evolutionary trade-off for the resistance to malaria conferred on the far greater number who are heterozygous and are therefore unaffected with the sickle cell abnormality in their hemoglobin. In a similar way, evolution may have allowed the capacity for extreme forms of anxiety, such as those constituting clinical anxiety disorders, to evolve in some individuals as a trade-off for the advantage conferred by more moderate and adaptive levels of the same trait in most individuals. Another view, described below, emphasizes the role of development in creating the variation necessary for selection to act. Extreme forms of anxiety may be thought of as a by-product of this property of development. Individuals with extreme and maladaptive anxiety disorder may be present today because they are protected by civilized society.

Development and Evolution

New discoveries in the genetic mechanisms of early development in recent years have provided the basis for an integration of the fields of evolutionary and developmental biology (for a review, see Carroll 2005), as predicted many years earlier by Gottlieb (1987). In this view, development is seen as a major source of potentially adaptive variation for selection to act upon in the course of evolution. We have learned that genes are not only instruments of inheritance in evolution but are also targets of molecular signals originating both within the organism and in the environment outside it. These signals regulate development. Rapid progress in understanding these molecular genetic mechanisms has revealed an unexpected potential for plasticity that can enable a relatively few evolutionarily conserved cellular processes to be linked together by differential gene expression into a variety of adaptive patterns that respond to environmental changes and genetic mutations. The resulting plasticity allows a variety of developmental pathways, evident in both behavior and physiology, to be generated from the same genome. This discovery of a central role for the regulation of gene expression in development has at last provided a specific mechanism for the frustratingly vague, and much debated, concept of gene-environment interaction in the origin of adult behavior patterns and vulnerability to mental illness.

We know surprisingly little about the development of anxiety in the individual, but this may well be an area in which new evolutionary concepts can be helpful to our gaining an understanding of human anxiety. For it is becoming evident, from molecular/genetic as well as new fossil evidence, that one of the most powerful mechanisms for producing rapid, major changes in evolution is through alterations in the developmental paths of individual traits (West-Eberhard 2003). For example, each system within the organism and each behavioral trait has its own developmental schedule for expression, which is strongly shaped by genetic timing mechanisms (*heterochrony*). When one of these regulatory genes is altered by selection or mutation, the developmental schedule for that trait is shifted in relation to others. A single mutation in the timing of gene expression can have major effects on the phenotype, which is not lethal because of accommodation by the regulatory nature of other developing systems. In this way, the principle of heterochrony serves to unite the processes of evolution with those of development and helps us understand the heterogeneity of the manifestations of anxiety over the course of development and within individuals of a given age.

Such processes at work during hominid evolution, in response to a varied range of environmental demands at different ages, may help account for the variation in the forms and manifestations of anxiety throughout development in today's population. For example, Marks and Nesse (1994) related the appearance of stranger anxiety at about age 6 months in a broad range of human cultures and child-rearing practices to the appearance of the capacity for rapid crawling and exploratory behavior at that age, which can expose the infant to potentially dangerous strangers. Infanticide by unrelated males is a widespread reproductive strategy in primates as well as other species (Hrdy 1977), and is likely to have been a strong selective force in human evolution. Thus, from the appearance of particular forms of anxiety at different ages, a *developmental path* may be traced back to age-specific evolutionary forces in our distant past. An example of the formation of such a developmental path in the rat, using experimental selection over generations, is described later in this chapter (see subsection "Evolution and Development of an Anxious Temperament," under "Development of Anxiety in a Small Mammal").

Developmental Plasticity and the Evolution of Alternative Phenotypes

One of the major difficulties that psychiatrists have with evolutionary accounts of the origin of major mental illnesses is that given the obvious incapacitating consequences of these conditions on their patients, these effects should have led to their disappearance from the gene pool in the more hostile environments of our prehistoric past. It is easy to contend that although evolution may have given us adaptive patterns of response, it cannot account for clinical conditions such as panic disorder. How can evolution account for such extreme forms of behavior, without the intervention of a pathological process or a recent gene mutation? This question has several possible answers, one of which goes back to a principal line of evidence used by Darwin (1859/1976) in the first chapter of *The Origin of Species by Means of Natural Selection*. In the two volumes he published a decade later, Darwin (1868/1998) presented the most compelling evidence for his theory. Overwhelming evidence indicates that when plant seeds or young animals are brought from their natural environments in the wild into the conditions of domestication, a remarkable increase occurs in the degree of variation among individual members, with the appearance of new traits or the exaggeration of traits seen in the wild. Although he could suggest no mechanism at the time, Darwin reasoned that these new variants appeared because of the relaxation of the harsh and limiting selective pressures on the developing young in the wild and because of the developmental effects of the novel environments of domestication, such as high levels of nutrition, that facilitated the expression of novel traits. Today, we know that such facilitation is caused by the unmasking of latent developmental pathways and of novel genes that had previously remained unexpressed (Kirschner and Gerhart 2005). With the pervasive relaxation of natural selective pressures brought about by civilization, and in response to the novel environments thrust on humans by technological change, it appears likely that conditions are present for the expression of great variability in human traits. It is intriguing to speculate that patients with incapacitating anxiety may well represent extreme examples of the results of the increased variation of humans under the influence of civilization.

Developmental plasticity has resulted in the evolution of alternative phenotypes, each adapted to a different kind of environment in which the young develop. As Simpson and Belsky (2008) have theorized, different early attachment patterns are likely to have evolved because of their adaptive value in two naturally occurring extremes of environment. On the one hand, high levels of close and responsive parenting devoted to a relatively few offspring, and a secure pattern of exploratory behavior and low anxiety levels in the offspring and adults, will enhance *reproductive fitness* in the next generation, when environmental conditions are stable and resource levels are high. On the other hand, short intervals between births, a maximum number of offspring, less investment in each child in favor of a rapid return to sexual activity, short intervals between pregnancies (resulting in young with anxious, insecure attachment patterns), and high levels of anxiety in the young would result in higher levels of survival and reproductive fitness in a harsh, chaotic, and threatening environment with low levels of resources.

Mechanisms for Long-Term Maternal Effects on an Anxious Phenotype

The evolution of anxiety appears to have been embedded in the evolution of a closely coordinated pattern of associated adaptive behaviors that are transmitted across generations as *alternative phenotypes*. The plasticity of development makes it possible for a rapid switch between these very different anxiety phenotypes to occur in as little as one generation when environments suddenly change. This contrasts with the many generations required for natural selection to produce such adaptive effects in response to a major environmental shift. Recent research in animals and humans is beginning to reveal the mechanisms for these different patterns of behaviors that are closely associated with various levels of anxiety. Clinically, we refer to such patterns as different *temperaments* or *personalities*. One result of this research has been the discovery of the role of differences in parenting patterns as a crucial "switch" for the alternative developmental pathways. The parents' response to their environmental conditions plays a predictive role in the pre-adaptation of the young to the changed conditions. The evidence for this comes from both human and animal studies, but I briefly review the animal research, which is more recent and more capable of revealing the molecular/genetic mechanisms.

The discovery of specific interactions between maternal and infant behavior that regulate individual physiological and behavioral systems of the infant throughout early development (reviewed in Hofer 1994) led to the study of the long-term effects of different patterns and levels of maternal behavior on anxiety-related physiology and behavior in adult offspring. In a series of studies, Meaney (2007) and his group (Cameron et al. 2005) found two alternative phenotypes in the offspring of mothers with naturally occurring high and low levels of maternal licking, grooming, and high-arched nursing position within his laboratory colony. The long-term effects of these two patterns of mother-infant interaction were as evident in pups cross-fostered at birth to mothers of the opposite type as in the mother's own offspring, making a strong genetic interpretation seem unlikely. Low levels of maternal interaction resulted in more fearful adult offspring with heightened startle responses and intense adrenocortical responses to stress. The capacity of these adults for avoidance learning was enhanced, whereas their spatial learning and memory were relatively impaired, reflected in slower hippocampal synapse growth. Young adults in this group also showed more rapid sexual maturation (vaginal opening), greater sexual receptivity, more rapidly repeated sexual encounters, and a higher rate of pregnancy following mating than offspring of high-level-interaction mothers. These differences appear to be suited to a harsh, unpredictable, and threatening environment containing few resources—an environment in which intense defensive responses, fearful avoidance of threats, and early, increased sexual activity is likely to result in maximal survival and more offspring born in the next generation. Strikingly, the two different maternal behavior patterns were also transmitted to their daughters in the next generation, as described later in this section. High levels of mother-infant interaction, in turn, lead to the development of exploratory behavior, rather than fear of novelty, a predisposition to learn spatial maps rather than avoidance responses, lower levels of adrenocortical responses, and slower sexual development—traits that would be a liability in very harsh environments but that allow optimal adaptation to a stable, supportive environment with abundant new opportunities and resources.

In a remarkable series of cell biological studies, Meaney and his colleagues (Diorio and Meaney 2007) were able to trace the effects of maternal behaviors to the hippocampal cell membrane receptors that sense the level of adrenocortical hormone and inhibit the hormonal response to stress in the adult (a form of feedback inhibition, as in a thermostat). Next, they found that the genes responsible for the synthesis of these receptors in the infant offspring of the high- or low- licking/grooming mothers were differently regulated by their specific transcription factors. Moreover, the rates of genetic expression of these signal molecules were, in turn, modified by changes within the chromatin structure that surrounds and controls which genes will be available for activation. These findings link variation within normally occurring levels of mother-infant interactions to molecular processes regulating gene expression in the developing young. The complex molecular structure chromatin, which supports and surrounds the long, thin DNA strands, includes several mechanisms for silencing some genes and opening others to activation (gene transcription) in response to outside signals. Two genes in the brain regions known to be involved in adrenocortical responses showed evidence of this kind of epigenetic modification (methylation and deacetylation) of their chromatin proteins (Weaver et al. 2006), and the adrenocortical changes could be reversed by specifically blocking these epigenetic modifications.

Champagne, a member of Meaney's group (Champagne et al. 2006), went on to find that mothers with high and low interaction levels pass these different maternal behavior patterns on to their daughters, along with the different levels of adult adrenocortical and fear responses. This transgenerational effect on maternal behavior is beginning to be linked to the effects of maternal interaction patterns on the 1-week-old pups' developing brain systems (estrogen-induced oxytocin receptors) in the area most central to maternal behavior that is expressed much later, in adulthood. The effects of such a transgenerational mechanism link environmental stress acting on mothers—predicting a harsh environment for the next generation—to changes in anxiety levels in offspring (Champagne and Meaney 2006). Therefore, if pregnant mothers of the high-licking-and-grooming line are exposed to prenatal immobilization stress, they will show *low* levels of these maternal behaviors and their offspring will develop into the high-anxiety phenotype.

Environmental stresses play a central role in the expression of anxiety and in the precipitation of episodes of mental illness, and, in fact, stressful events and situations may best be defined as those closely resembling major selection pressures under which humankind has evolved—those events that threaten our survival and reproductive fitness (H. Weiner 1992). It has become increasingly clear in recent field studies of natural selection that behavioral responses to stress can be the "leading edge" of evolution, in the sense that the organism's behavior is often responsible for its moving into a new environment or using a new food source and that in this way, modification of behavior often precedes the evolution of new structural and physiological traits (Grant 1986; J. Weiner 1994). Thus, the behavioral and emotional anxiety responses to stress, which in extreme forms constitute mental illness, may be at the center of the evolutionary story as initiators of evolutionary change, not simply as products of it. In this way, environmental change and the highly variable behavioral responses of organisms to it have been central actors in the evolution of anxiety.

Psychiatric opinion is divided at present along a continuum, ranging from a belief that pathological genetic and environmental events of comparatively recent origin are primarily responsible for the clinical anxiety disorders to a view of these conditions as representing long-evolved adaptive responses that are triggered by inappropriate cues or in maladaptive intensity. The evidence described in this chapter is presented to show how an evolutionary perspective can illuminate both clinical and research approaches to the anxiety disorders. It is predicted that when the etiology of the anxiety disorders is finally understood, a major component will involve variation in individual vulnerability that is a legacy of our evolution.

Major Steps in the Evolution of Anxiety

Looking beyond the processes of evolution, we can see that we have shared with other species the problems in living, even more than the solutions. It is therefore illuminating to observe, in present-day species that represent our phyletic heritage, different kinds of solutions to the common problem of avoiding danger. The role of specific signal cues, the importance of memory for the context of stressful events, the occurrence of anxiety in the setting of early separation, and the adaptive value of states of enhanced attention to clues of danger are all illustrated in the examples below. I have chosen a single-celled organism, a marine invertebrate, a common vertebrate mammal, and a nonhuman primate. With these examples, I hope to illustrate some of the aspects of anxiety that are likely to have evolved first, and those that appear to be later acquisitions, in species that occupy steps in evolution similar to those taken by our ancestors over hundreds of millions of years.

Minimal Necessary Conditions in Bacteria

The essential elements within which an anxiety state might evolve would consist of the following: a means to detect signals, a means to discriminate those that denote danger, and the capacity to initiate behavior that results in avoidance of that danger. Anxiety, as we currently understand it, occurs somewhere within the matrix of those capacities. Definitions of anxiety require several attributes in addition to these basic functions, but if we are looking within the whole phylogeny for when the simplest forms of anxiety first appeared, organisms with this sort of basic equipment would be the place to start. Because of our use of words such as *detect*, *discriminate*, and *initiate* to refer to our own conscious processes, these capabilities would appear, at first glance, to require the evolution of animals with complex brains. However, in reality, much simpler processes can be used to carry out the essential functions outlined, which can be found in single-cell organisms such as motile bacteria with thin, hairlike flagella. This places the starting point for our evolutionary search at the period between 2 billion and 600 million years ago (Margulis 1993), before the great Cambrian "explosion" of life in which the major animal phyla first appeared about 580 million years ago. The discovery of complex behavior in present-day typhoid and coliform bacteria and the elucidation of the underlying biochemical mechanisms by Daniel Koshland (1980) provide a vivid demonstration that adaptive behavior in response to signals of danger does not require consciousness or even a brain.

Motile bacteria are equipped with five to seven whiplike flagella that drive them forward through the fluids that surround them. These flagella are attached to the cell membrane in a way that permits them to rotate like propellers. Koshland found that these cell membranes also contain up to 30 receptors. Flagella and receptors are both widely distributed over the surface of the cell membrane and are functionally linked through a series of intracellular biochemical pathways that are enzyme-regulated. The receptors respond to specific molecules and control the actions of the flagella, so that the bacterium can either move forward or stop. For example, in response to certain molecules in the water acting at the membrane receptors, the flagella all rotate in the same direction, forming a tight bundle that effectively drives the bacterium forward with a single corkscrew-like action. In response to other molecules, the flagella alternately rotate clockwise and counterclockwise. This causes the flagella to fly apart and then exert inconsistent and discordant forces at the various individual flagellar attachment sites on the cell membrane, so that the bacterium stops and then "tumbles" in place.

This simple system allows the bacterium to move forward in a relatively straight line, stop, and then move off again in what is likely to be a new direction determined randomly by the orientation of the bacterium at the moment that uniform flagellar rotation resumes. The bacterium can then approach sources of one kind of molecular signal (e.g., sugar), but also stop and change direction when another kind of specific signal molecule (e.g., a toxin) binds to a receptor. By trial and error, it will thus gradually move away from the source of a signal that it is predisposed to avoid. The receptor, its transmembrane protein linkage, and its intracellular signaling mechanism embody the components that are familiar to us as the basis for communication within the brain by neurotransmitter molecules. In the bacterium, they directly control the behavior of the cell in which they exist. Koshland found that some of the membrane receptors are "constitutive" and do not change with the environment, whereas others are "inducible" by exposure of the bacteria to high concentrations of certain molecules. Nine genes play a role in the formation of receptor types. Thus, responses of the cell are affected by hereditary, environmental, and probabilistic factors in the life processes of cell division, mobility, and replication of the organism. Bacteria in a given culture can be shown to have highly individual response properties despite being identical in heredity and general environment, and these differences remain for the lifetime of the cell.

The presence of multiple receptors and of time-dependent intracellular enzyme systems allows a limited degree of integration and flexibility in responses. For example, when both attractant and repellent molecules are present, bacteria respond as an algebraic function of both influences. After weak stimuli, a return to previous functioning is more rapid than after strong stimuli, and suppression of tumbling in response to positive (e.g., nutrient) gradients is long-lasting, whereas initiation of tumbling in response to negative (e.g., toxic) gradients is extremely rapid in onset. However, the only form of learning appears to be habituation, and bacterial memory is extremely short (about half a second).

A single-celled organism clearly has evolved the machinery for an organized behavioral repertoire with some fairly sophisticated capabilities. It can approach weak stimuli that are beneficial, and it can flee from very strong stimuli and those that signal danger. When it stops and tumbles in response to the loss of a positive signal or the presence of a negative signal, is it anxious? Certainly we would not want to say so, even though the mental picture of a tumbling creature with flagellar hairs standing on end may be intuitively persuasive. A change in behavioral state has taken place in the bacterium that differs from anxiety, primarily in the simplicity of the information and memory processes taking place and in the narrowness of the repertoire of responses available. We have a scaled-down, highly simplified prototype for anxiety, which is capable of producing some of the behaviors seen in anxious humans. The presence of these behaviors in so primitive an organism gives us an idea of how basic a state resembling anxiety has been for survival of life forms.

Two Types of Acquired Anxiety in an Invertebrate

Hundreds of millions of years after the first bacteria, the marine invertebrates emerged in the Cambrian period, 500 million years ago. Members of this order exist today in a physical form that has remained essentially unchanged, according to the fossil record. A modern representative of the class is *Aplysia californicus*, the sea hare studied with such success by Eric Kandel and his colleagues. Through the specialization of cellular function, the organization of groups of these cells into component organs, and the integration of organs into a self-contained system, evolution has enormously increased the variety of behaviors and the range of signals available. This complex organization now has different functional states that are specialized for responding to certain types of signals and for carrying out one or another set of behaviors. Examples of such states are hunger and sexual arousal. After some consideration, we may want to call these *motivational* or *emotional states*. The range of signals has been expanded by a crucial new addition, the capacity to detect and represent the contingencies between signals and events, to learn, and to remember. Through the organization of groups of cells specialized for signal processing, this simple nervous system can now respond to an event in terms of its past experience as well as its current environmental input.

The sea hare (*Aplysia*) normally flees from contact with its natural predator the starfish, a response also carried out (less reliably and efficiently) by the typhoid bacillus in response to a similar chemical signal. Kandel and colleagues (reviewed in Kandel 1983) showed that a chemical stimulus that *Aplysia* normally ignored, shrimp juice, could be made a signal for an escape response by associating it repeatedly with electric shock, the laboratory equivalent of a starfish attack. But they went further by showing that after such an experience, shrimp juice, when encountered a second time, induced a state change in *Aplysia* during which other defensive responses not involved in the original training, such as gill withdrawal and the release of protective clouds of ink, were enhanced. This state change also involved a reduction in appetitive behaviors such as feeding. An innocuous event had thus become a signal eliciting an anticipatory state in which responses to threat were exaggerated and what we might call pleasurable behaviors were inhibited; a simple form of anticipatory anxiety had been induced.

The sea hare in the experiments described above behaved normally after training if shrimp juice was not present. In the second procedure, a prototype of chronic anxiety was produced in which the animal showed a persistent state of altered responsiveness similar to that induced by shrimp juice but without requiring a danger signal. A series of unavoidable electrical shocks was used (sensitization), which produced a change in response repertoire over several weeks following the traumatic events. During this persistent state, defensive and escape responses were exaggerated and responses to positive events were blunted; an abnormal behavioral repertoire had been established that resembled a form of chronic diffuse anxiety.

These two simple paradigms, one for anticipatory signaled anxiety and the other for chronic generalized anxiety, became the focus of intense efforts to determine the neural and molecular mechanisms for the altered states and their novel behavioral responses. The neurotransmitter serotonin, the components of the biochemical cascade, and the enzyme protein kinase identified by those studies are conserved by evolution and are key elements underlying brain activity in higher animals, including humans. The short- and long-term presynaptic facilitation found to underlie anticipatory and chronic anxiety-like states in *Aplysia* has become a particularly promising model for understanding the molecular mechanisms for memory. This is a turn of events that Freud would enjoy, considering his emphasis on the role of remembered states in human anxiety.

Development of Anxiety in a Small Mammal

Next, we come to the age of the dinosaurs, 100–200 million years ago, when our ancestors, small terrestrial mammals, were found on dry land scurrying through the undergrowth of the forest floor, out of sight of the great reptiles. Only the most adaptive of these survived the great extinction of species that brought an end to the age of the dinosaurs 65 million years ago. Of today's small mammals, one of the most successful orders is the rodents, and a domesticated strain, the laboratory rat, is the species of animal we know the most about, next to the human. For this reason, and because it has been the subject of my own research, I have chosen this animal to represent an evolutionary innovation introduced by our early mammalian ancestors.

Paul MacLean studied the probable evolution of the brain that accompanied the splitting off of mammals from reptilian ancestors 250 million years ago. He argued that the evolution of the limbic system of the brain in mammals distinguishes them from all modern reptiles, endowing mammals with a set of novel behaviors and brain structures. According to MacLean (1985), the three crucial behavioral attributes that evolved with the mammals are play, parental behavior, and the separation cry, all of which, he pointed out, are absent in most modern-day reptiles. MacLean provided neuroanatomical and neurophysiological evidence supporting his theory that the presence of these behaviors in modern-day mammals is made possible by the specialized neural networks of the limbic system and their connections to the cerebral cortex and the midbrain. The evolution of social relationships based on mutual attachment in mammals provides a new set of behaviors, motivational systems, and dangers within which a new variant of anxiety can evolve. The infant's separation cry is a communication to the mother with adaptive value; it is also a manifestation of a state of distress that may constitute the first innate anxiety state to evolve.

Here, the cues are not learned as they are in the sea hare, because rat infants respond with loud (60–90 dB) calls, in the ultrasonic frequency range, to their first experienced separation. Evolution has endowed mammalian infants with a response to a set of cues (isolation from conspecifics) that represent the potential for several actual dangers. The uncertain nature of the dangers and the sudden loss of their familiar and responsive companions add new dimensions to this form of anxiety that were not present in the simpler forms of anxiety elicited in marine invertebrates (discussed previously). The evolution of prolonged immaturity of offspring and the related period of close parental care created the basis for a new form of anxiety in this relatively primitive mammal, a form that seems to resemble the separation anxiety we are familiar with in children and even in adult humans.

The Separation Call

In 1956, an Austrian ethologist, Wolfgang Schleidt, and his student Zippelius discovered that young mice emitted series of short pulses (each 0.1–0.3 seconds) of very-high-frequency sound (40–50 kHz), similar to the then recently discovered ultrasonic pulses of bats which had provided an animal analogue for the sonar developed by the Allies for antisubmarine patrol in World War II (Zippelius and Schleidt 1956). The emphasis of early research into this phenomenon was on the environmental events (such as cold, rough handling, altered substrate odor or texture, and novelty) to which rat or mouse infants were responding when they emitted these ultrasonic vocalizations and on the maternal search and retrieval behaviors they elicited. I became interested in this calling behavior after I found that rat pups showed other behavioral and physiological responses to separation from their mother (reviewed in Hofer 1996). In a series of studies, Harry Shair and I first found that pups emitted these calls, even in the home cage nest, if all their littermates and their mother were removed, showing that separation from social companions was a key element in eliciting these vocalizations (Hofer and Shair 1978). Next, we found that if pups were alone in an unfamiliar place, they would greatly reduce or cease calling when a littermate or their mother was placed with them, even if she was completely passive (anesthetized).

We now had a behavioral indicator for a state induced rapidly by separation—one that could be roughly quantified by using an ultrasonic detector. And we had a means of rapidly terminating the state by what appeared to be a form of contact comfort. Because the separation-induced state depended on the effect social companions had on pups, we embarked on a search for the cues to which the pup was responding in this contact comfort response and the sensory pathways by which the pup was processing this information (Hofer and Shair 1980, 1991). We found that after the neonatal period, pups appeared to be responding to texture, odor, and temperature in a cumulative fashion, with contour and size as additional factors.

But as scientific skeptics, we wondered whether rat pups really experience separation negatively and whether the state induced by separation involves a change in the way the pups respond to new information, as was found during the state induced by sensitization in *Aplysia,* and as is familiar to us from our own experiences with anxiety. Experiments by researchers interested in early learning have given affirmative answers to both of these questions. Isolated rat pups will learn difficult maze problems to get back to their mothers (Kenny and Blass 1977), and for a separated pup, merely experiencing short periods of contact with the mother acts as a powerful reinforcer (Amsel et al. 1977). Furthermore, cues associated with separation are strongly avoided when encountered subsequently (Smith et al. 1985). These findings show that rat pups dislike separation and are strongly predisposed to respond to cues associated with reunion. In addition, Norman Spear's group found a variety of associations, discriminations, and tasks that rat pups learned less well when they were separated from their home cages than when they were provided with familiar nest cues during the learning experience (summarized in Spear et al. 1985). This was not a simple generalized interference with functioning, however. As is the case in human anxiety, rat pups form some associations more readily when isolated. They learned to associate novel tastes and odors with illness and then avoid those cues (taste aversion learning) two to three times more strongly when separated than when the learning took place in the home cage.

These striking effects of social isolation and of home cage contextual cues are not seen in older juvenile and adult rats. Thus, growing evidence indicates that altered information processing is specific to young rats. Perceptual and cognitive alterations characteristic of the state of anxiety are present in a simple form in the sea hare, and involve more complex manifestations as we move on to animals such as the rodent and primate with more elaborate brains.

Brain Mechanisms

For those most interested in the neurobiological mechanisms of anxiety, studies on drugs and neuropeptide modulators have provided the most compelling evidence that the isolation distress state of young rats provides a useful animal model of anxiety. Pharmacological studies by a number of different groups have found that most major classes of drugs that are useful in human anxiety have powerful and selective inhibitory effects on isolation-induced ultrasonic calls in rat pups, usually without affecting other behaviors or inducing signs of sedation. Even more convincing evidence is that synthetic compounds known to produce severe anxiety in human volunteers (such as pentylenetetrazol and the inverse-agonist benzodiazepines) greatly increase the call rate in isolated pups and can even elicit calling in the home cage when the pup is with its familiar littermates (for reviews, see Hofer 1996; Miczek et al. 1991).

The benzodiazepines were the first anxiolytics found to be effective for isolation distress in rat pups, and Insel et al. (1989) found autoradiographic evidence that an endogenous ligand at the γ-aminobutyric acid (GABA)–benzodiazepine receptor complex in the cerebral cortex and hippocampus may play a role in rat pup isolation distress. Morphine and the more recently synthesized specific μ and δ opiate receptor ligands decrease calling, whereas a specific κ receptor ligand increases calling in isolated pups (Carden et al. 1991). κ opiate receptor activation even causes pups in the home cage nest to vocalize vigorously. Thus, endogenous opiates may play a role in both the initiation and the reduction of isolation distress. This possibility is strengthened by our finding that naltrexone, an opiate receptor blocker, prevents companion comfort response to littermates in young rats (Carden and Hofer 1990). That finding suggests that social companions exert some of their comforting effect by stimulating endogenous μ and/or δ opiate release in young that have become displaced from the nest.

Winslow and Insel (1990) showed that rat pups respond to clinically effective anxiolytic drugs that are active primarily on the serotonin system, such as the reuptake inhibitor clomipramine and the serotonin type 1A (5-HT_{1A}) receptor agonist buspirone. Neuropeptides such as cholecystokinin (implicated in human satiety), which are known to reduce anxiety in humans, reduce ultrasonic calling in young rats (Weller and Blass 1988). Insel (1992) proposed oxytocin as a neuropeptide underlying a broad range of affiliative behaviors. Oxytocin is present in maternal milk and may well be absorbed by nursing pups. When given to isolated rat pups, it reduces calling.

Evolution of Early Separation Anxiety

How did vocalization first evolve as a manifestation of the infant's separation state, so that the mother's retrieval behavior could then act selectively to enhance survival of vocal young and establish this important mother-infant communication system? To answer this question, we should recall 1) the close natural association of cold temperature with displacement from the mother and home nest in small mammals and 2) the fact that cold ambient temperature is a major cue for the elicitation of isolation calls in isolated rat pups.

We found more direct evidence for the evolution of the separation call from a physiological response to cold exposure. When rat pups were made severely hypothermic (25°C below normal) and recovered spontaneously at room temperature (a routine surgical anesthesia procedure), we found, to our great surprise, that they started to emit ultrasonic vocalizations (USVs) when they were still comatose, at surgical levels of anesthesia (Hofer and Shair 1992). These hypothermic ultrasounds are produced by the same laryngeal mechanism as isolation calls, and have similar acoustic properties. Although they are emitted at a slower tempo than isolation calls because of the slow respiratory rates of pups at such low temperatures, rat mothers will respond to hearing these calls by searching, and will use them as directional cues (Brunelli et al. 1994).

However, this behavior may not have originated in evolution as a signal to the mother, but rather in a very different physiological role. We found that when pups made hypothermic were afterwards devocalized by laryngeal nerve section and were no longer able to generate positive intrapulmonary pressure (to produce USVs) by breathing against a closed larynx, they did not rewarm nearly as fast as vocal pups and developed pulmonary edema, failing to recover at all in some cases. These findings closely parallel the pulmonary edema that regularly occurs during rewarming from accidental severe hypothermia in humans and the use of positive-pressure respiratory therapy in its treatment. They tend to support the hypothesis (Blumberg and Alberts 1990) that infant rat USV represents an "exaptation," in which a physiological regulatory response that originally evolved as an adaptation to cold later became co-opted by the evolutionary process to function in a new role as a signaling response in parent-infant communication. Our language today represents an ancient association of social separation and cold in phrases such as "left out in the cold," and the use of "warm" or "cold" to describe emotional closeness or distance. These terms may not be simply modern metaphors, but testimony to an ancient role for the separation cry during periods in our evolution when thermal stresses were unavoidable and the underlying laryngeal activity may have acted as a strong physiological selection factor promoting survival after severe hypothermia.

The nature of later evolutionary selection pressure is evident in the sensory and perceptual adaptations of rodent mothers to these ultrasonic vocalizations, physiological adaptations (such as an auditory-frequency response threshold tuned to the exact frequency of infant USV, 45 kHz) that underlie their sensitive and specific search, retrieval, and caregiving responses (Ehret 1992). But the infant's isolation call can also be used by predators to locate vulnerable infants. Not surprisingly, predator odors dramatically suppress ultrasonic vocalizations in isolated pups—a specific fear response (Takahashi 1992).

The evolution of the infant separation cry has apparently involved an evolutionary "trade-off," a ratio of risk to benefit that is thought to have shaped many behaviors. In this case, the theory predicts that in environments with many predators, and thus the likelihood of attracting a predator before their mother finds them, infants that show *less* separation-induced vocalization will gradually increase in the population. However, when nest disruption occurs frequently (e.g., through flooding) and fewer predators exist, high rates of isolation calling, and more rapid and certain maternal retrieval, will be more advantageous.

Evolution and Development of an Anxious Temperament

To explore these hypothetical evolutionary processes, we have been conducting an experiment in the laboratory that simulates them: selectively breeding adult rats that, as 10-day-old infants, had shown relatively high or relatively low rates of ultrasonic vocalization responses to separation. We found that in as few as five generations, two distinct lines emerged that differed significantly on this infantile trait from a randomly bred control line. Cross-fostering of "high-line" and "low-line" pups at birth to mothers of the opposite line revealed no evidence of postnatal maternal influences on 10-day isolation calling rates (Brunelli et al. 1997). Clearly, this manifestation of early separation anxiety has a strong hereditary basis. As there have been no other systematic studies of selective breeding for an infant behavior trait (that we have been able to discover), we did not know how repeated selection might affect the earlier and later development of this early anxiety response in descendants. Furthermore, we wondered whether other traits related to vocalization, or to an underlying anxiety state, might also be affected through their genetic, physiological, or behavioral links to the systems controlling the infants' vocal response to separation.

We found (Hofer et al. 2001) that infants' calling during isolation was strikingly elevated in high-line pups, starting as early as 3 days of age—a week before the age at which selection had been carried out. Low-line pups' calling during isolation, in contrast, was moderately decreased at this early age. The greatest difference between high and low lines was at the age of repeated selection, 10 days postnatal. Response differences were much less evident at 14 days, and the lines converged as the response ceased to occur at 18–20 days postnatal. Thus, selection had resulted in the high-line pups showing retention (and exaggeration) of the high response rates of newborn pups throughout their development, right up to and including the age of selection (10 days), and the low-line pups showing a more rapid decline than normally occurs from 3 to 10 days of age. In conclusion, selection at 10 days of age appeared to be acting on the whole developmental trajectory of the vocal response to separation, shifting it in time—either delaying or hastening the normal developmental decline in response intensity with age.

In more recent studies, we found a number of other behaviors and physiological responses at different ages in the high- and low-line rodents that have been altered by selection (Brunelli and Hofer 2007). Those differences appear to form coherent groups of traits. In the high-line juvenile group, tested in isolation at 18 days postnatal (when calling rarely occurs), both defecation/urination and sympathetically mediated heart rate acceleration were greater than among pups in the control groups. Among 30-day-old adolescents, rough-and-tumble play behavior and the short, high-frequency vocalizations that accompany it were reduced compared with the first few play bouts in randomly bred control pups. High-line adults were significantly slower to emerge into an open-test box and avoided the center area more completely than the low-line rodents. In addition, high-line adults showed a much more quiet, passive response to the Porsolt Swim Test, a pattern associated with depression-like states in rodents.

As low-line pups developed to 18 days of age, they showed the greatest heart rate acceleration to isolation testing and a much-delayed return to baseline (both due primarily to major vagal withdrawal). Low-line adolescents were deficient on all play behaviors on all days of testing and emitted the fewest play calls. As adults, the low-line rats were quicker to emerge into the open area, explored its center more than the high-line group, and were more active in the swim test. When confronted with another strong male, 70% of low-line males engaged in aggressive behavior compared with 30% of randomly bred controls.

These groups of traits suggest a characterization of the high-line rats as anxious and passive, whereas the low-line rats were exploratory, active, and aggressive. Apparently, selection for high and low rates of infant calling during isolation selects for a lifelong developmental path involving associated traits. Two alternative phenotypes, or temperaments, were created by selection at a single point early in development, almost as if organized developmental paths were available that the pup could be set upon when alleles for the different infantile anxiety traits were gradually collected by selection. These results resemble those previously described in which different maternal behavior patterns had long-term developmental effects on offspring anxiety and a specific group of associated traits in adulthood. Thus, the developmental paths or structures for two (or more) anxiety-related phenotypes, each with adaptive potential, are latent within the genetic/environmental potential of this species. One can be realized through repeated selection of genetic alleles over 15 or 20 generations, and the other in a more rapid response that is mediated through induced differences in maternal behavior acting on genomic regulation of offspring in the next two generations.

Primate Anxiety

Looking back into our recent past, 10–20 million years ago, our ancestors were likely to have resembled modern-day Old World monkeys and apes. The brains and behavior of these animals (which share 90%–99% of our genes) are uncannily similar to those of humans. Studies on rhesus macaques, for example, have allowed us to verify clinically derived hypotheses relating the powerful effects of both environmental events and genetic constitution on the etiology of severe and crippling anxiety states in individual monkeys. The studies documented, under natural conditions, the transition from evolutionarily adaptive forms of anxiety to lasting, incapacitating states resulting in substantial mortality. This work, described in other chapters on animal models of individual disorders, extends the conceptual bridge that I have tried to portray in this chapter between evolution and clinical psychiatry, and between normal and pathological anxiety.

Suomi and his colleagues (reviewed in Suomi 1997) described a subpopulation (20%) of rhesus monkeys living under natural conditions on an island in the Caribbean; this subpopulation had most of the signs of a mild generalized anxiety disorder. As infants, they showed less exploratory behavior than peers, and as juveniles, when the mother left for hours or days in the breeding season, they showed enhanced agitation, followed by lethargy, a fetal-like huddled posture, and social withdrawal. The great majority of their age-mates showed little response or actually increased their social interactions with peers in the mother's absence. Here, both anxiety and depressive behavior were enhanced in a subgroup of monkeys, as is found clinically in a subgroup of humans. As adolescents, males in the vulnerable subpopulation left their social group later than other males and were less able to establish new affiliations.

Recent research (Suomi 2006) begins to suggest possible specific genetic bases for this vulnerability in a minority of individuals. Monkeys with a variant of the serotonin transporter gene (short allele of 5-HTT) showed excessive cortisol responses to early separation if, and only if, they were subjected to rearing with peers rather than with their mothers. This gene and the monoamine oxidase A gene have specific alleles that confer vulnerability to anxiety and depression if harsh and/or depriving early rearing environments are present in those individuals, a finding that has now also been found in recent genetic epidemiologic studies in humans (Caspi et al. 2002). The anxiety-prone temperamental characteristics of this subgroup are greatly exaggerated by rearing conditions of inadequate mothering, as when they are experimentally reared with peers instead of with their mother. Their physical, motor, and social-behavioral repertoires develop adequately, but their tendency toward anxious withdrawal and avoidance is so greatly enhanced that as young adults, they drop to the bottom of dominance hierarchies within the social structure of their group. These anxiety-prone characteristics are clearly heritable, as shown by selective breeding studies. But they are also sharply modified by variations in maternal behavior during rearing: if they are fostered to unusually nurturant and experienced mothers, then the expression of the anxious traits is prevented.

What do these findings in nonhuman primates tell us about evolutionary processes in the origin of clinical anxiety disorder in humans? First, heritable traits predisposing to anxiety appear to be distributed within populations so as to leave an appreciable number of individuals at an end of the distribution that could be classified as an anxious phenotype. The variation of anxiety traits within a population allows a wide range for natural selection to act on, but anxious individuals are present in considerable numbers, even when living conditions are optimal for several generations. Second, in harsher conditions, the anxiety-prone subpopulation is likely to have a selective advantage, and these genes would then become even more common in the population. Third, inadequate mothering, which might occur under severe conditions (e.g., maternal death, and rearing primarily by age-mates), serves to increase expression of the anxious genotype. This mechanism further amplifies the capacity of the population to adapt to chronically threatening conditions. Persistent anxiety (high levels of arousal, searching for cues for danger, and high levels of avoidance of potentially damaging encounters) confers an adaptive advantage over less anxious individuals under such conditions.

Evolutionary Clues Found in Human Panic Disorder

Evolutionary approaches to obsessive-compulsive disorder, panic disorder, and other human anxiety disorders have been reviewed by Stein and Bouwer (1997). The most fully described and best documented of these—panic disorder—has been found to have properties that suggest it might have evolved from an adaptive physiological response in our ancestors, similar to the hypothesized evolution of the separation call from an adaptive response to hypothermia in infant rats described earlier in this chapter. Klein (1993) proposed that the precipitation of acute symptoms of anxiety in patients with panic disorder, and in some persons without panic disorder, by carbon dioxide (CO_2) inhalation, may represent an adaptive "suffocation alarm." Klein hypothesized that in some individuals the threshold level of this alarm system is lowered to the point that normal or even low levels of partial pressure of CO_2 (pCO_2) in the circulation can trigger acute anxiety, a "false suffocation alarm." This could be enhanced when other cues to possible suffocation, such as closed exits, crowds, or immobilization, are also present. When the person is further sensitized, through genetic or environmental mechanisms, the alarm and the panic response may occur spontaneously. He proposed that panic may be more primitive than other forms of anxiety, and that it also differs in that it is a response to an endogenous cue (pCO_2) rather than an external threat. Klein pointed out that the hyperventilation and frequent yawns and sighs in patients between panic episodes may constitute tests monitoring for signs of rising blood pCO_2. If CO_2 is not rapidly lowered and symptoms eased as a result of these respiratory maneuvers, suffocation could be imminent. Klein also suggested that another distinctive feature of panic attacks, the lack of adrenal cortical response, may derive from the maladaptive consequences of hypercortisolemia in hypoxic conditions, as would be found in suffocation.

The association of adult panic disorder with separation anxiety in childhood and the precipitating conditions of separation and loss in adulthood are also interesting from an evolutionary point of view. A calling response of infants when isolated from familiar surroundings and companions is remarkably consistent across mammalian species. It is found also among birds, a parallel evolutionary line with separate origins 60 million years ago, in which parental care is also a major feature of the evolved developmental plan. In those species in which this separation cry has been studied pharmacologically (guinea pigs, rats, mice, and monkeys), the evidence consistently supports a similarity between isolation calling and adult anxiety responses. Increased calling has been found in response to experimental anxiogenic compounds, and decreased calling has been found in response to clinically useful anxiolytic drugs (see subsection "Brain Mechanisms," under "Development of Anxiety in a Small Mammal" earlier in this chapter). The neural substrates for anxiety thus seem to appear early both in evolution and in development. One of the most effective classes of anxiolytic compounds (e.g., morphine) acts at the μ opiate receptor. At this brain site, decreased sensitivity to endogenous CO_2 and decreased responsiveness to exogenous cues such as social isolation both follow activation of the receptor by μ opioid compounds. Thus, separation and loss may involve a neural substrate that is also activated by endogenous and exogenous cues for impending suffocation, and thus for panic attacks as well.

Conclusion

By examining the examples from widely diverse life forms described in this chapter, we can gain an appreciation of the differences that have evolved in how organisms successfully use a behavioral state—anxiety—in avoiding threats to their survival. Anxiety appears to represent a stage in the process by which an individual responds to the presence of threats to its survival. This stage is omitted in the rapid responses to imminent injury that are mediated by sensorimotor reflex pathways. As soon as animals evolved more than one kind of response to danger and receptors that could detect cues before imminent injury, it became advantageous for them to enter an intervening state between stimulus and response. In this state, information processing and response thresholds could be specialized for assessing and responding to those cues for danger. Thus, anxiety allowed individuals to respond in ways that were particularly well suited to a variety of dangers and timed to be maximally effective. The very early evolution of specific information-processing capability, in the form of the membrane receptors of bacteria, emphasizes the central role of evaluative processes as forerunners of altered cognitive processing in anxiety. With the advent of the marine invertebrates, a pattern of selective enhancement of certain behavioral responses and inhibition of other behaviors evolved as part of their intervening anxiety state. The very early appearance of learning and memory in the simple neural networks of the first marine animals is now widely appreciated.

This combination of capacities, both to learn and to enter a specialized information-processing and motor response state, was likely a basic prerequisite for survival from early stages of evolution. It marks the origin of the capacity for the state we call "anxiety" as very old indeed. One could say that all that has happened in the course of our own evolution has been the addition of massive degrees of complexity to each element in the simple invertebrate system outlined earlier in this chapter. But increases in complexity have a way of creating new emergent properties. The evolution of increasingly complex social structure has added a whole new host of dangers and demands that are not present for bacteria or sea hares. The evolution of the limbic system of the brain has made possible an enormous amplification of the kinds of possible intervening emotional states, creating a variety of qualitatively different anxieties. The evolution of the cerebral cortex has vastly expanded capabilities for learning and memory so that long-past experiences, as well as recent ones, play important roles in eliciting anxiety and in shaping the processing of information during the state. The extent of parallel processing that has become possible in the primate brain has increased the extent of self-regulation within the system to the point that self-awareness and what we call "consciousness" has emerged. This creates a whole new order of response to anxiety—namely, the inner subjective experience of it. Finally, the advent of symbolic communication in language has made it possible for us to convey that experience to one another. Symbolic communication, in turn, has led to a wealth of verbal interactions that can alleviate or perpetuate anxiety and allow us to avoid or create new dangers.

Developmental research that models evolutionary processes through repeated selection in laboratory studies has shown us that evolution has created alternative developmental pathways to different adult anxiety phenotypes in mammals. As revealed by selective breeding for an infant anxiety trait (the rodent maternal separation call), different developmental paths have evolved, characterized by a cluster of different traits at different ages, that are associated with and express high or low levels of anxiety (reviewed in Brunelli and Hofer 2007). Two different groups of traits and their developmental paths each form a coherent pattern, embodying a complex adaptative repertoire, from infant to adult, resembling what we call *temperament* or *personality* in humans. The traits have evidently evolved in these animals' past history through the survival value and reproductive success of these developmental pathways under different extremes of environment and social ecology that have occurred during mammalian evolution. These alternative developmental pathways are currently available to animals (and presumably also to humans) in response to long-term changes in environment over 10 to 20 generations, as in our experiments.

Similar alternative adult phenotypes, however, can also be triggered much more rapidly by predictive environmental cues acting through rapidly induced changes in maternal behavior that affect the adult offspring in the next generation, as shown in the recent animal model studies of Michael Meaney and his group (Cameron et al. 2005; Diorio and Meaney 2007; Meaney 2007). These studies strongly support the proposed basis for human infant and parental attachment patterns described by Simpson and Belsky (2008). In the animal studies, the source of the trigger for the development of the alternative phenotypes in adult offspring can be unambiguously traced to the influence of different mother-infant interaction patterns. The mechanism for the differences in anxiety phenotypes, in turn, has been shown to be a novel epigenetic process through which lasting and widespread changes in levels of gene expression in specific areas of the offsprings' brains are produced through a long-term, or even permanent, alteration in the protein structure of the chromatin "packaging" in which the DNA is embedded. Furthermore, these changes can be transmitted to the next generation through maternal behavioral interactions affecting gene expression within the developing brain systems of her infants that will later determine their maternal behavior as adults. In this way, a single-generation developmental change can be passed on to successive generations through non-Lamarckian mechanisms that do not involve the germ cell DNA.

As our understanding of genetic mechanisms involved in the expression of behavior and in predisposition to mental illness grows exponentially in the coming years, so will our insight into the evolution of the behaviors and states of mind that are the subject of this volume. We can begin to see the outlines of what lies ahead, but there is much more to be learned than we know today. I hope that we will continue to view this state of affairs with more curiosity and anticipation than anxiety.

◀ Key Clinical Points ▶

- The transition from anxious personality to anxiety disorder will result when genetic vulnerability and life experiences combine to raise anxiety to crippling levels that are nonadaptive in the person's present environment.
- Highly complex social interactions can either intensify anxiety or preserve the life and comfort of the patient with anxiety disorder.
- Insights into the evolution of anxiety can be clinically useful. Once a patient can be led to realize that his or her symptoms are part of the history of human nature, that these responses can even be advantageous in certain situations, and that the real problem lies in their occurrence at the wrong time and place, this understanding can help alleviate the confusion, shame, and hopelessness that burden so many patients with anxiety disorders.

References

Amsel A, Radek CC, Graham M, et al: Ultrasound emission in infant rats as an indicant of arousal during appetitive learning and extinction. Science 197:786–788, 1977

Alcock J: The Triumph of Sociobiology. New York, Oxford University Press, 2001

Blumberg MS, Alberts JR: Ultrasonic vocalizations by rat pups in the cold: an acoustic by-product of laryngeal braking? Behav Neurosci 104:808–817, 1990

Brunelli SA, Hofer MA: Selective breeding for infant rat separation-induced ultrasonic vocalizations: developmental precursors of passive and active coping styles. Behav Brain Res 182:193–207, 2007

Brunelli SA, Shair HN, Hofer MA: Hypothermic vocalizations of rat pups *(Rattus norvegicus)* elicit and direct maternal search behavior. J Comp Psychol 108:298–303, 1994

Brunelli SA, Vinocur DD, Soo-Hoo D, et al: Five generations of selective breeding for ultrasonic vocalization (USV) responses in N:NIH strain rats. Dev Psychobiol 31:225–265, 1997

Cameron N, Parent C, Champagne F, et al: The programming of individual differences in defensive responses and reproductive strategies in the rat through variations in maternal care. Neurosci Biobehav Rev 29:843–865, 2005

Campos JJ, Mumme DL, Kermoian R, et al: A functionalist perspective on the nature of emotion. Monogr Soc Res Child Dev 59:284–303, 1994

Carden SE, Hofer MA: Socially mediated reduction of isolation distress in rat pups is blocked by naltrexone but not by RO 15–1788. Behav Neurosci 104:457–463, 1990

Carden SE, Barr GA, Hofer MA: Differential effects of specific opioid receptor agonists on rat pup isolation calls. Brain Res Dev Brain Res 62:17–22, 1991

Carroll S: Endless Forms Most Beautiful: The New Science of Evo-Devo. New York, WW Norton, 2005

Caspi A, McClay J, Moffitt TE, et al: Role of genotype in the cycle of violence in maltreated children. Science 297:851–854, 2002

Champagne FA, Meaney MJ: Stress during gestation alters postpartum maternal care and the development of the offspring in a rodent model. Biol Psychiatry 59:1227–1235, 2006

Champagne FA, Weaver IC, Diorio J, et al: Maternal care associated with methylation of the estrogen receptor-alpha1b promoter and estrogen receptor-alpha expression in the medial preoptic area of female offspring. Endocrinology 147:2909–2915, 2006

Darwin C: The Origin of Species by Means of Natural Selection (1859). New York, Penguin Books, 1976

Darwin C: The Variation of Animals and Plants Under Domestication (1868). Baltimore, MD, Johns Hopkins University Press, 1998

Darwin C: The Expression of the Emotions in Man and Animals (1872). Chicago, IL, University of Chicago Press, 1965

DeFries JC, Hyde JS, Lynch C, et al: The design of selection experiments, in National Institute on Alcohol Abuse and Alcoholism Research Monograph 6: Development of Animal Models as Pharmacogenetic Tools (DHHS Publ No ADM 81-1133). Edited by McClearn GE, Dietrich RA, Erwin VG. Rockville, MD, Alcohol, Drug Abuse and Mental Health Administration, 1981, pp 269–275

Diorio J, Meaney MJ: Maternal programming of defensive responses through sustained effects on gene expression. J Psychiatry Neurosci 32:275–284, 2007

Ehret G: Preadaptations in the auditory systems of mammals for phoneme perception, in The Auditory Processing of Speech: From Sounds to Words. Edited by Schouten MEH. Berlin, Germany, Gruyter, 1992, pp 99–112

Eldredge N: Time Frames: The Evolution of Punctuated Equilibria. Princeton, NJ, Princeton University Press, 1989

Eldredge N, Gould SJ: Punctuated equilibria: an alternative to phyletic gradualism, in Models in Paleobiology. Edited by Schopf TJM. San Francisco, CA, Freeman, Cooper, 1972, pp 82–115

Gottlieb G: The developmental basis of evolutionary change. J Comp Psychol 101:262–271, 1987

Grant PR: Ecology and Evolution of Darwin's Finches. Princeton, NJ, Princeton University Press, 1986

Haldane JBS: The Causes of Evolution (1932). Princeton, NJ, Princeton University Press, 1993

Hamilton WD: The genetical theory of social behavior, I, II. J Theor Biol 7:1–52, 1964

Hofer MA: Early relationships as regulators of infant physiology and behavior. Acta Paediatr Suppl 397:9–18, 1994

Hofer MA: Multiple regulators of ultrasonic vocalization in the infant rat. Psychoneuroendocrinology 21:203–217, 1996

Hofer MA, Shair HN: Ultrasonic vocalization during social interaction and isolation in 2-week-old rats. Dev Psychobiol 11:495–504, 1978

Hofer MA, Shair HN: Sensory processes in the control of isolation-induced ultrasonic vocalization by 2 week old rats. J Comp Physiol Psychol 94:271–279, 1980

Hofer MA, Shair HN: Trigeminal and olfactory pathways mediating isolation distress and companion comfort responses in rat pups. Behav Neurosci 105:699–706, 1991

Hofer MA, Shair HN: Ultrasonic vocalization by rat pups during recovery from deep hypothermia. Dev Psychobiol 25:511–528, 1992

Hofer MA, Shair HN, Masmela JR, et al: Developmental effects of selective breeding for an infantile trait: the rat pup ultrasonic isolation call. Dev Psychobiol 39:231–246, 2001

Hrdy SB: Infanticide as a primate reproductive strategy. Am Sci 65:40–49, 1977

Insel TR: Oxytocin—a neuropeptide for affiliation: evidence from behavioral, receptor autoradiographic and comparative studies. Psychoneuroendocrinology 17:3–35, 1992

Insel TR, Gelhard RE, Miller LP: Rat pup isolation distress and the brain benzodiazepine receptor. Dev Psychobiol 22:509–525, 1989

Izard C: Human Emotions. New York, Plenum, 1977

Kandel ER: From metapsychology to molecular biology: explorations into the nature of anxiety. Am J Psychiatry 140:1277–1293, 1983

Kenny JT, Blass EM: Suckling as incentive to instrumental learning in preweanling rats. Science 196:898–899, 1977

Kirschner MW, Gerhart JC: The Plausibility of Life: Resolving Darwin's Dilemma. New Haven, CT, Yale University Press, 2005

Klein DF: False suffocation alarms, spontaneous panics, and related conditions: an integrative hypothesis. Arch Gen Psychiatry 50:306–317, 1993

Koshland DE Jr: Bacterial chemotaxis in relation to neurobiology. Annu Rev Neurosci 3:43–75, 1980

Kumar S, Hedges SB: A molecular timescale for vertebrate evolution. Nature 392:917–922, 1998

Lazarus RS: Emotion and Adaptation. New York, Oxford University Press, 1991

Lewis M, Brooks-Gunn J: Social Cognition and the Acquisition of Self. New York, Plenum, 1979

MacLean PD: Brain evolution relating to family, play, and the separation call. Arch Gen Psychiatry 42:405–417, 1985

Margulis L: Symbiosis in Cell Evolution. New York, WH Freeman, 1993

Marks IM, Nesse RM: Fear and fitness: an evolutionary analysis of anxiety disorders. Ethol Sociobiol 15:247–261, 1994

McGuire M, Troisi A: Darwinian Psychiatry. New York, Oxford University Press, 1998

Meaney MJ: Environmental programming of phenotypic diversity in female reproductive strategies. Adv Genet 59:173–215, 2007

Miczek KA, Tornatsky W, Vivian JA: Ethology and neuropharmacology: rodent ultrasounds, in Animal Models in Psychopharmacology (Advances in Pharmacological Sciences). Edited by Olivier B, Mos J, Slangen JL. Basel, Switzerland, Springer Verlag, 1991, pp 409–427

Nesse RM, Williams CG: Why We Get Sick: The New Science of Darwinian Medicine. New York, Vintage Books, 1996

Scheiner SM: Selection experiments and the study of phenotypic plasticity. J Evol Biol 15:889–898, 2002

Simpson JA, Belsky J: Attachment theory within a modern evolutionary framework, in Handbook of Attachment. Edited by Shaver PR, Cassidy J. New York, Guilford, 2008, pp 131–157

Smith GJ, Kucharski D, Spear NE: Conditioning of an odor aversion in preweanlings with isolation from home nest as the unconditioned stimulus. Dev Psychobiol 18:421–434, 1985

Spear N, Kucharski D, Hoffman H: Contextual influences on conditioned taste aversions in the developing rat. Ann NY Acad Sci 443:42–53, 1985

Stein DJ, Bouwer C: A neuroevolutionary approach to the anxiety disorders. J Anxiety Disord 11:409–429, 1997

Suomi SJ: Early determinants of behaviour: evidence from primate studies. Br Med Bull 53:170–184, 1997

Suomi SJ: Risk, resilience, and gene x environment interactions in rhesus monkeys. Ann NY Acad Sci 1094:52–62, 2006

Takahashi LK: Ontogeny of behavioral inhibition induced by unfamiliar adult male conspecifics in preweanling rats. Physiol Behav 52:493–498, 1992

Trivers RL: Parent-offspring conflict. Am Zool 14:249–264, 1974

Weaver IC, Meaney MJ, Szyf M: Maternal care effects on the hippocampal transcriptome and anxiety-mediated behaviors in the offspring that are reversible in adulthood. Proc Natl Acad Sci USA 103:3480–3485, 2006

Weiner H: Perturbing the Organism: The Biology of Stressful Experience. Chicago, IL, University of Chicago Press, 1992

Weiner J: The Beak of the Finch. New York, Vintage Books, 1994

Weller A, Blass EM: Behavioral evidence for cholecystokinin-opiate interactions in neonatal rats. Am J Physiol 255:R901–R907, 1988

West-Eberhard MJ: Developmental Plasticity and Evolution. New York, Oxford University Press, 2003

Wilson EO: Sociobiology: The New Synthesis. Cambridge, MA, Harvard University Press, 1975

Winslow JT, Insel TR: Serotonergic and catecholaminergic reuptake inhibitors have opposite effects on the ultrasonic isolation calls of rat pups. Neuropsychopharmacology 3:51–59, 1990

Zippelius HM, Schleidt WM: Ultraschall-laute bei jungen Mausen [Ultrasonic vocalization in infant mice]. Naturwissenschaften 43:502, 1956

Recommended Readings

Alcock J: The Triumph of Sociobiology. New York, Oxford University Press, 2001

Brunelli SA, Hofer MA: Selective breeding for infant rat separation-induced ultrasonic vocalizations: developmental precursors of passive and active coping styles. Behav Brain Res 182:193–207, 2007

Cameron N, Parent C, Champagne F, et al: The programming of individual differences in defensive responses and reproductive strategies in the rat through variations in maternal care. Neurosci Biobehav Rev 29:843–865, 2005

Carroll S: Endless Forms Most Beautiful: The New Science of Evo-Devo. New York, WW Norton, 2005

Kirschner MW, Gerhart JC: The Plausibility of Life: Resolving Darwin's Dilemma. New Haven, CT, Yale University Press, 2005

McGuire M, Troisi A: Darwinian Psychiatry. New York, Oxford University Press, 1998

Weaver IC, Meaney MJ, Szyf M: Maternal care effects on the hippocampal transcriptome and anxiety-mediated behaviors in the offspring that are reversible in adulthood. Proc Natl Acad Sci USA 103:3480–3485, 2006

Weiner H: Perturbing the Organism: The Biology of Stressful Experience. Chicago, IL, University of Chicago Press, 1992

Chapter 10

Combined Treatment of Anxiety Disorders

Maryrose Gerardi, Ph.D.
Kerry Ressler, M.D., Ph.D.
Barbara Olasov Rothbaum, Ph.D.

In this chapter, we examine the empirical research on combined treatment for each of the major anxiety disorders. By *combined treatment* we refer to some form of psychotherapy, most commonly short-term cognitive-behavioral therapy (CBT), combined with pharmacological treatment. We also review some of the newer forms of combination therapy, in which treatment is approached from a nontraditional model. Combined pharmacological treatments will not be addressed in this context.

The success of psychotherapy and medication in the treatment of anxiety disorders would reasonably indicate that the combination of both would be an even more effective treatment intervention. However, this has not been the case, particularly with the more traditional medications such as the newer antidepressants and anxiolytics. In a systematic review of the literature on combined pharmacotherapy and CBT approaches for the anxiety disorders (Foa et al. 2002), there was not much supporting evidence for any advantage of combined approaches. Similarly, a literature review of relevant studies by Black (2006) showed that although combined treatment for anxiety disorders is commonly recommended, empirical support for this approach is limited. We explore the empirical evidence regarding combined treatment for individual anxiety disorder diagnostic categories and include combined strategies with more novel medication approaches.

Cognitive-Behavioral Therapy Overview

CBT has shown impressive efficacy in treating individuals with anxiety disorders and has often been considered a first-line treatment for anxiety (see Chapter 7, "Cognitive-Behavioral Concepts of Anxiety," in this volume). Most of the CBT approaches for treatment of anxiety can be divided into 1) exposure and 2) anxiety management. Many CBT treatments include some form of exposure therapy, which is recommended for most, if not all, the anxiety disorders. Exposure therapy has its basis in the animal studies literature on extinction training. During extinction training, the feared stimuli are presented repeatedly with no aversive consequences; the fear decreases until, ideally, the stimuli no longer engender fear. In general, exposure therapy involves confrontation with feared stimuli in a therapeutic manner (Rothbaum et al. 2007). For the exposure to be therapeutic, the anxiety must be activated and changed. Desired changes include decreased symptoms of anxiety and arousal (i.e., responses), and decreased estimates of danger (i.e., meaning). Ways in which stimuli can be presented include imaginally (in imagination), in vivo (in real life), and in virtual reality.

The other major CBT approach to treating anxiety is anxiety management training (AMT). Exposure helps address excessive avoidance, whereas AMT helps address excessive arousal. The two most popular components of AMT are *cognitive restructuring* and *relaxation*. In cognitive restructuring, the patient's cognitive errors are made explicit, and means of correcting these errors are taught. Relaxation techniques often include breathing retraining and/or deep muscle relaxation.

Review of the Literature

The criteria selected for studies to be included in our review were that patients in the study had received an established diagnosis and the study included at least two treatment groups, one of which had received pharmacotherapy or CBT (with or without pill placebo) and the other of which had been treated with a combination of CBT plus medication (as in Foa et al. 2002). Included studies permitted tests of combined versus monotherapy and employed adequate methodology (including random assignment; sample sizes large enough for statistical power; use of manualized therapy with adequate treatment quality, dose, and duration to allow for symptom reduction; blind independent evaluation by a trained assessor; and essential statistics for calculating within-group effect sizes). We will now turn to reviewing the literature on combined pharmacotherapy and psychotherapy studies, the majority of which met these criteria, first reviewing the more traditional anxiety disorders and their associated medical treatments, then turning our attention to novel approaches.

Panic Disorder

Panic disorder is characterized by repeated, unexpected, discrete episodes of intense fear and discomfort, accompanied by physical and cognitive changes (Allen and Barlow 2006) (see Chapter 21, "Phenomenology of Panic Disorder," in this volume). The benefits of CBT in the treatment of panic disorder are well documented (e.g., Barlow 2002). According to Foa et al. (2002), CBT challenges the patient's threat interpretations of events and replaces these with more realistic ones. Within the emotional processing theory proposed by Foa and Kozak (1986), fear is a cognitive structure in memory that supports adaptive behavior when faced with a realistically threatening situation, but which becomes pathologic when associations among stimulus, response, and meaning do not reflect reality (i.e., harmless stimuli or responses assume threat meaning). For example, in panic disorder, individuals erroneously interpret physiological responses associated with panic as dangerous. This misinterpretation leads to anxiety and, usually, to avoidance behavior. CBT is thought to modify the fear structure by correcting these misinterpretations.

Medications, including selective serotonin reuptake inhibitors (SSRIs), tricyclic antidepressants, monoamine oxidase inhibitors (MAOIs), and benzodiazepines have also been successful in treating this disorder (e.g., Van Etten and Taylor 1998) (see Chapter 23, "Pharmacotherapy for Panic Disorder," in this volume). However, in a combined treatment model, the reduction of anxiety by certain medications may block the fear activation necessary for cognitive changes aimed at disconfirming catastrophic beliefs about anxiety-related bodily responses (Foa et al. 2002).

Three of the studies evaluated combined approaches for panic disorder. The first compared alprazolam, exposure therapy, and alprazolam plus exposure therapy in the treatment of panic disorder with agoraphobia (Marks et al. 1993). In this study, 154 patients were randomly assigned to one of four conditions: exposure (six 2-hour sessions of therapist-aided exposure and self-directed homework exposure) plus alprazolam, exposure plus placebo, relaxation (psychological placebo in this study) plus alprazolam, and relaxation plus placebo. Treatment lasted for 8 weeks, with alprazolam and placebo tapered over the following 8 weeks. Both exposure conditions produced greater improvement at posttreatment on measures of phobic avoidance than did alprazolam or placebo conditions. However, at 5-month follow-up, exposure treatment plus placebo outcome was reported as superior to all other conditions.

The second study included 77 patients with a diagnosis of panic disorder with agoraphobia, randomly assigned to 16 weeks of either CBT (cognitive restructuring, imaginal, and in vivo exposure; exposure to anxiety-related physical sensations; and self-exposure homework) plus buspirone, or CBT plus placebo (Cottraux et al. 1995). Results indicated no treatment differences between groups at posttreatment and at follow-up, again suggesting that the main effect in this study was the CBT and not the medication augmentation.

The third study examined CBT, imipramine, and the combination of the two in the treatment of panic disorder. In the study, 312 patients were randomly assigned to CBT plus imipramine, CBT plus placebo, CBT alone, imipramine alone, and placebo alone (Barlow et al. 2000). CBT consisted of eleven 50-minute panic-control treatment sessions (cognitive restructuring, exposure to interoceptive cues, and breathing retraining) over the course of 3 months; medication management consisted of 30-minute sessions over the same time frame. Monthly maintenance treatment was offered to treatment responders over the following 6 months, for a total of 9 months participation. CBT plus imipramine was found to be superior to CBT alone at both the 3- and 9-month assessments. However, at 6 months following treatment discontinuation, CBT groups without imipramine evidenced a superior outcome compared with the group receiving the combined treatment.

Research on combined treatment for panic disorder suggests that the combination of medication and CBT may interfere with long-term gains. However, the results with imipramine may not generalize to other medications, and further research is needed. Necessary cognitive changes may be impeded by medication if gains are attributed to medication or if medication hampers CBT disconfirmation of erroneous beliefs associated with anxiety-related physical responses (Foa et al. 2002).

Obsessive-Compulsive Disorder

The fear structure of individuals with obsessive-compulsive disorder (OCD) often involves erroneous interpretation of safe external stimuli as dangerous (Foa et al. 2002). OCD is characterized by recurrent, intrusive, and distressing thoughts, images, and urges, along with ritualized behaviors or thoughts used to reduce related distress. We include four randomized, controlled trials of combined pharmacological and psychotherapeutic treatment for this disorder.

In the first trial, the investigators compared exposure and ritual prevention (8 sessions of imaginal exposure plus in vivo exposure homework, followed by 16 sessions of therapist-guided, in vivo exposure plus ritual prevention) plus fluvoxamine, exposure and ritual prevention plus placebo, and fluvoxamine alone, in a 24-week treatment of 60 patients diagnosed with OCD (Cottraux et al. 1990). A 4-week medication taper followed. No group differences were detected, as measured by reduction of daily rituals greater than or equal to 30%, at either posttreatment or follow-up.

The second study compared exposure and ritual prevention (3-week assessment and 4-week treatment, which involved six 3-hour therapist-assisted sessions that included cognitive restructuring and homework) plus fluvoxamine to exposure and ritual prevention plus placebo in the treatment of 58 patients diagnosed with OCD (Hohagen et al. 1998). As measured by total score on the Yale-Brown Obsessive Compulsive Scale (Y-BOCS; Goodman et al. 1989), both groups improved significantly from pretreatment to posttreatment, with no significant differences between groups. Percentage of responders, defined by 35% improvement in total Y-BOCS score, indicated an advantage for the combined treatment.

Cognitive therapy, exposure and ritual prevention, fluvoxamine plus cognitive therapy, fluvoxamine plus exposure and ritual prevention, and wait-list were compared in 117 patients in the third study on OCD (Van Balkom et al. 1998). In the combined treatments, fluvoxamine was administered for 8 weeks, followed by 10 sessions of CBT (both cognitive therapy and exposure and ritual prevention conditions) over 8 weeks; wait-list condition was 8 weeks in length. Using the Y-BOCS as the outcome measure, all four active treatment conditions were found to be superior to wait-list at both midtreatment and posttreatment, with no significant differences revealed among active treatments.

In a double-blind, randomized trial, Foa et al. (2005) included a pill placebo condition when comparing clomipramine, exposure and ritual prevention, and clomipramine plus ritual prevention in the treatment of 122 adult outpatients with OCD. This study was conducted at three treatment centers that had expertise in one of the treatment conditions. Exposure and ritual prevention was conducted across 4 weeks (imaginal and in vivo exposure, including therapist home visits and daily homework), with 8-week maintenance sessions. Clomipramine was administered for 12 weeks, up to a maximum dose of 250 mg/day. Results, as measured by Y-BOCS total score and improvement on the Clinical Global Impression Scale (CGI; Guy 1976) at week 12, indicated that all active treatments were superior to placebo. Exposure and ritual prevention results did not differ from exposure and ritual prevention plus clomipramine results, and both were superior to clomipramine alone.

An additional study compared cognitive-behavioral group therapy (2-hour sessions over 12 weeks), including psychoeducation, exposure and response prevention, correction of cognitive distortions, relapse prevention techniques, and homework assignments (e.g., Cordioli et al. 2003) in a randomized clinical trial with sertraline (100 mg) in 56 outpatients diagnosed with OCD (Sousa et al. 2006). Cognitive-behavioral *group* therapy was found to be significantly more effective in global reduction of symptoms and in reducing the intensity of compulsions, as measured by the Y-BOCS. The study authors also reported that the percentage of patients who obtained full remission was significantly higher among those treated with cognitive-behavioral group therapy (32%) versus those treated with sertraline (4%). Limitations of this study include the small sample size, the lack of a placebo control group, and the lack of a group receiving combined treatment with sertraline and cognitive-behavioral group therapy. Additional well-controlled studies in this area are warranted.

Overall, the reviewed studies indicate no clear advantage for combined treatment with traditional antidepressant or anxiolytic medication over CBT alone in the treatment of OCD.

Social Phobia

Social phobia, also referred to as *social anxiety disorder*, is characterized by persistent fear in social and/or performance situations (see Chapter 25, "Phenomenology of Social Anxiety Disorder," in this volume). CBT treatment of social phobia has been largely based on the cognitive model (Clark and Wells 1995; Rapee and Heimberg 1997), in which the following four maintenance processes are highlighted: 1) an increase in self-focus attention and monitoring, and a reduction in observation of other people and their responses; 2) the use of misleading internal information to make negative inferences about how one appears to others; 3) the use of safety behaviors that are intended to prevent feared catastrophes but instead have negative consequences; and 4) the use of negatively biased anticipatory and post-event processing. It is interesting to note that one study indicated individual CBT may be superior to group CBT for this disorder (Stangier et al. 2003).

Validated pharmacotherapy for social phobia includes benzodiazepines, MAOIs, and SSRIs (Hood and Nutt 2001), with SSRIs being the most extensively studied (Hidalgo et al. 2001) (see Chapter 27, "Pharmacotherapy for Social Anxiety Disorder," in this volume). Serotonin-norepinephrine reuptake inhibitors (SNRIs) have also been found to be efficacious (Liebowitz et al. 2003).

There are only three randomized, controlled trials that involve combined treatments for social phobia. In a primary-care-based study, sertraline, exposure therapy plus sertraline, exposure therapy plus placebo, and placebo were compared in the treatment of 387 patients diagnosed with social phobia (Blomhoff et al. 2001). Exposure therapy consisted of nine 20-minute sessions of assignments for self-exposure homework and feedback regarding progress, including identification of goals and coping strategies. Treatment length was 16 weeks. Medication treatment (sertraline 50–150 mg) also occurred over 16 weeks and consisted of 10 visits. Both groups had a final posttreatment visit at week 24. Response to treatment, based on CGI scale self and investigator ratings, indicated that patients in all active treatment groups improved significantly more than placebo-treated patients at week 12; but at weeks 16 and 24, only improvement in the groups treated with sertraline remained significantly superior to placebo. However, no significant response differences were discovered between the active treatment groups. It should also be noted that exposure was in the form of instructions for self-exposure, and did not occur in sessions.

A randomized, placebo-controlled trial treating 60 patients diagnosed with generalized social phobia was conducted using cognitive therapy (weekly self-exposure assignments), fluoxetine (up to 60 mg) plus self-exposure, or placebo plus self-exposure (Clark et al. 2003). At 16 weeks posttreatment, the medication blind was broken and both the cognitive therapy and fluoxetine plus self-exposure patients entered a 3-month "booster" phase. Outcome was assessed with the employment of a social-phobia composite score based on seven individual social phobia measures. Significant improvements were evidenced in all three treatment conditions, with cognitive therapy revealing superiority to fluoxetine plus self-exposure and placebo plus self-exposure at midtreatment and posttreatment. Results for fluoxetine plus self-exposure and placebo plus self-exposure did not differ significantly. Notably, results revealing that cognitive therapy was the superior treatment were reascertained at the end of the booster period and at 12-month follow-up.

In a randomized, double-blind, placebo-controlled trial conducted at two academic sites, Davidson et al. (2004) compared fluoxetine (10–60 mg), comprehensive cognitive-behavioral group therapy (14 weekly group sessions with 5–6 participants, which included social skills training, exposure to simulated situations, cognitive restructuring, and in vivo homework assignments), placebo, and combined fluoxetine and cognitive-behavioral group therapy in the treatment of 295 outpatients diagnosed with generalized social phobia. Primary outcome measures were the Brief Social Phobia Scale (Davidson et al. 1997b) and the CGI Scale. Results indicated that by the final visit, all active treatments were found to show significantly better results than placebo but did not differ from each other. The authors conclude that there was no evidence of greater benefit of combined treatment over monotherapy, which seems to be the case for social anxiety disorder in general.

Generalized Anxiety Disorder

The hallmark of generalized anxiety disorder (GAD) is excessive worry, along with chronic anxiety and multiple somatic symptoms (see Chapter 11, "Phenomenology of Generalized Anxiety Disorder," in this volume). Studies exploring treatments for GAD have focused on the cognitive components of worry, such as intolerance of uncertainty, erroneous beliefs about worry, poor problem orientation, and cognitive avoidance (Behar and Borkovec 2006; Ladouceur et al. 2000). Medication interventions that have been efficacious in the treatment of this disorder include benzodiazepines, SSRIs, and SNRIs (Baldwin et al. 2006) (see Chapter 13, "Pharmacotherapy for Generalized Anxiety Disorder," in this volume).

There is only one study of combined treatment for GAD. In a controlled study, 101 outpatients diagnosed with GAD were randomly assigned to one of five conditions: diazepam (5 mg) alone, placebo alone, cognitive-behavioral therapy, diazepam plus CBT, and placebo plus CBT (Power et al. 1990). Pill groups received 6 weeks of medication 3 times per day, and then had a graded withdrawal period. CBT consisted of 7 treatment sessions over a 9-week period, a time period equivalent to the pill conditions. Treatment focused on modification of automatic thoughts and irrational assumptions, and included training in progressive muscle relaxation, along with homework that involved graded exposure exercises. Outcome measures were self, psychologist, and general practitioner ratings on a 7-point scale measuring severity of illness and change in symptoms. The study authors noted that there was a high level of agreement among these ratings. All active treatments were evaluated as superior to placebo. Combined diazepam plus CBT produced the best results on almost all measures at posttreatment, but active treatment results did not significantly differ from one another. Initial treatment gains for all patients receiving CBT were maintained at follow-up, with these patients less likely to receive subsequent psychiatric or psychological treatment 6 months after completion of the study. However, initial moderate treatment gains among patients in the group receiving diazepam were not well maintained at follow-up. Based on the small amount of evidence available, it is difficult to make any conclusion about the efficacy of a combined approach to treatment of GAD; there does not appear to be an advantage to a combined approach.

Posttraumatic Stress Disorder

There is evidence for the effectiveness of both pharmacological and psychotherapeutic treatment interventions for posttraumatic stress disorder (PTSD). PTSD is characterized by exposure to a traumatic event, followed by symptoms of physiological arousal, avoidance, and reexperience of the trauma (see Chapter 30, "Phenomenology of Posttraumatic Stress Disorder," in this volume). Cognitive-behavioral therapy, and specifically *prolonged exposure* (PE), has the largest amount of empirical support in the literature (Rothbaum et al. 2000) for the treatment of PTSD. Well-controlled studies examining the efficacy of PE have revealed that 60%–95% of participants who received PE no longer met criteria for PTSD following treatment (Foa et al. 2003). Other effective psychological interventions include *eye movement desensitization and reprocessing* (Shapiro 1995) and *cognitive processing therapy* (Resick et al. 2002).

Studies have widely confirmed the efficacy of SSRIs as pharmacological treatment for PTSD (e.g., Davidson et al. 2001), and more recently, SNRIs have also been found to be effective and well tolerated (Davidson et al. 2006) (see Chapter 32, "Pharmacotherapy for Posttraumatic Stress Disorder," in this volume).

Rothbaum et al. (2006) conducted a multicenter investigation of augmentation of sertraline with PE in the treatment of PTSD. In the study, 88 male and female outpatients diagnosed with PTSD were treated with open-label sertraline (up to 200 mg or the maximum tolerated by week 6) for 10 weeks in phase I, then were randomly assigned to receive continuation with sertraline alone or to receive augmentation with PE (10 twice-weekly sessions of 90–120 minutes) in phase II. PE included psychoeducation about trauma reactions, breathing exercises, in vivo exposure, prolonged imaginal exposure, and homework that involved listening to a tape of the imaginal exposure recorded in session. Results indicated that 5 additional weeks of treatment with sertraline alone did not result in further improvement on measures of PTSD severity, depression, and general anxiety. Augmentation with PE did result in further reduction of PTSD severity as measured by the Structured Interview for PTSD (Davidson et al. 1997a), but not in depression as measured by the Beck Depression Inventory (Beck et al. 1961), or general anxiety as measured by the state portion of the State-Trait Anxiety Inventory (Speilberger et al. 1970). The beneficial effect of PE augmentation was observed among medication partial (weaker) responders. There were no significant differences at the end of treatment between groups on PTSD severity.

This sole study of combined treatment for PTSD indicates some advantage for medication partial responders in adding CBT, but did not compare CBT alone to the combined approach.

Novel Treatments for Anxiety Disorders

In this section we briefly assess nontraditional approaches to the treatment of anxiety disorders.

Advances in animal research elucidating neurotransmitters involved in fear extinction (Davis and Myers 2002) have led to the exploration of combination treatment strategies for anxiety disorders, with a focus on the enhancement of *extinction learning* that occurs in CBT. Extinction learning refers to the reduction of fear to a cue previously paired with an aversive event when that cue is presented repeatedly in the absence of the aversive event. In this model, pharmacotherapy is aimed at improving the learning that takes place during CBT (specifically exposure-based therapy), and not at treating the symptoms of anxiety (Davis et al. 2006).The glutamatergic *N*-methyl-D-aspartate (NMDA) receptor has been found to be critically involved in learning and memory (e.g., Bear 1996; Newcomer and Krystal 2001), and this learning may be augmented by the NMDA partial agonist D-cycloserine (DCS). DCS has been shown in animal studies to facilitate the extinction of learned fear and to produce generalized extinction (Davis et al. 2006). DCS has been approved by the U.S. Food and Drug Administration for the treatment of tuberculosis for more than 20 years. The side-effect profile of DCS has been examined across three studies. Results indicate there are no adverse effects of single-pill administrations of DCS in dosages ranging from 15–500 mg per administration, with 3–7 days between administrations.

Specific Phobia

The first clinical test of a treatment for a specific phobia in humans that combined DCS with exposure therapy was performed by Ressler et al. (2004). The 28 participants diagnosed with acrophobia were randomly assigned to three treatment groups (double blind): placebo plus virtual reality exposure (VRE) therapy, DCS (50 mg) plus VRE therapy, or DCS (500 mg) plus VRE therapy. The lower dose was chosen on the basis of doses used in past research on DCS as a cognitive enhancer in Alzheimer's disease and schizophrenia (e.g., Randolph et al. 1994; Tuominen et al. 2005), and the higher dose was chosen based on evidence of tolerability when used in the treatment of tuberculosis. There were no significant differences in primary outcome measures between the group receiving 50 mg and the group receiving 500 mg, so those groups were combined for subsequent analyses. Participants underwent two therapy sessions (suboptimal exposure) and were instructed to take a single pill 2–4 hours before the therapy session, for a total of two pills during the course of the study. Posttreatment assessments occurred at 1 week and at 3 months after the second therapy session. At both assessments, participants who received DCS in conjunction with VRE therapy had significantly enhanced decreases in fear within the virtual environment. This group also reported significantly more improvement than the placebo group in their overall acrophobic symptoms at 3-month follow-up, and skin conductance fluctuations (a psychophysiological measure of anxiety) were significantly decreased in this group (Ressler et al. 2004).

Social Phobia

In a randomized, double-blind, placebo-controlled evaluation, 27 outpatients diagnosed with social anxiety disorder participated in a five-session treatment (Hofmann et al. 2006). The first session was psychoeducational, and the following five sessions consisted of stepwise social exposures, with 50 mg DCS or placebo received 1 hour prior to each exposure session. Treatment was delivered across clinicians in individual and group formats. Participants who received DCS augmentation demonstrated significantly greater improvement at posttreatment and at follow-up evaluation.

Notably, a replication study has been performed (*N*=56) following a very similar design to the Hofmann study. Guastella and colleagues (2008) found that patients administered DCS (50 mg) as an adjunct to exposure therapy reported greater improvement on measures of symptom severity, dysfunctional cognitions, and life impairment from social anxiety in comparison with placebo-treated patients. Effect sizes were mostly in the medium range.

Obsessive-Compulsive Disorder

Kushner et al. (2007) examined the use of DCS 125 mg to accelerate reduction of obsession-related distress in patients diagnosed with OCD undergoing extinction-based exposure therapy. In a randomized, double-blind trial, subjects were given either DCS or placebo 2 hours before 10 exposure/ritual prevention therapy sessions. There were 25 subjects who completed treatment. Results indicated that DCS helped to decrease the number of exposure sessions required to achieve clinical milestones. After four sessions (versus the 10–15 sessions typical in OCD therapy), patients in the DCS group (*n*=14) reported a significantly greater decrease in obsession-related distress compared with the placebo group (*n*=11). Results indicated that those given placebo were about six times more likely to drop out of the exposure/ritual prevention therapy as those given DCS.

In another randomized, double-blind, placebo-controlled trial of DCS 100 mg compared with placebo augmentation of behavior therapy (10 sessions, twice per week) for 23 patients with OCD, the investigators found that, relative to the placebo group, OCD symptoms in the DCS group were significantly improved at midtreatment, and depressive symptoms were significantly further improved at posttreatment (Wilhelm et al. 2006).

Notably, these results were not replicated in another study of 24 patients by Storch et al. (2007). The investigators found that there were no significant group differences found across outcome variables, and the rate of improvement did not differ between groups. But there were several important differences between the two studies showing positive results and the study showing no improvement. In the study conducted by Storch and colleagues 1) the DCS was given 4 hours before the therapy began, 2) the dose used was higher than in the other studies (250 mg), and 3) all subjects received twelve sessions of 90-minute therapy. Together, these differences may be important in terms of 1) timing of dosing (too-early dosing may lead to the peak drug effect not being coincident with the emotional learning processes that take place during psychotherapy), 2) dose of drug (too high a dose may activate the antagonist properties of this NMDA partial agonist), and 3) a floor effect, in which all subjects show improvement and thus no "drug-by-therapy" effect can be observed. Therefore, this study, which did not reveal improvement in patients receiving DCS, may highlight some significant variables that must be accounted for in designing combined treatment studies.

Panic Disorder

Tolin et al. (2006) conducted a randomized, double-blind, placebo-controlled trial of DCS compared to placebo in combination with brief CBT for panic disorder. Following two sessions of psychoeducation and cognitive restructuring, a single dose of DCS (50 mg) or placebo was administered prior to each of three sessions of exposure-based treatment (interoceptive exposure in and out of the therapist's office). Outcome measures including the Panic Disorder Severity Scale and CGI scale indicated clinically and statistically significant differences between groups at posttreatment, with the DCS group evidencing greater reduction of panic symptoms and CGI scores and having more patients in remission. These differences were less clear at 1-month follow-up.

Posttraumatic Stress Disorder

Although no studies have been published to date on the effect of combining D-cycloserine with CBT for PTSD, at this writing several are in progress in the United States, including studies by Difede (Weill Cornell Medical Center, New York), Litz (Boston University), Marmar (University of California, San Francisco), and Rothbaum (Emory University, Atlanta).

Summary

In contrast to the more traditional medications (e.g., antidepressants and anxiolytics) combined with CBT for anxiety, the novel medication approaches outlined in this section do seem to afford some advantages when combined with CBT. More importantly, the theoretical rationale of these new approaches is fundamentally different from that of the earlier combined treatment studies. In previous studies, both with antidepressant and anxiolytic medication, the goal was primarily to achieve an additive effect with therapy and medication. The new approaches aim to combine psychotherapy with a cognitive enhancer medication that will specifically improve the efficacy of the emotional learning process that takes place in psychotherapy and possibly make these new emotional memories more robust, stable, and long-lasting.

Conclusion

Given the lackluster performance of combination approaches, with outcomes of significant relapse upon discontinuation of traditional medications, CBT has often been recommended as a first-line approach in the treatment of patients with anxiety disorders. However, if CBT is not readily available, SSRIs or SNRIs are a good first treatment. If these medications do not produce an adequate response, and if CBT is available, it is reasonable to augment treatment of partial medication responders with CBT. In addition, for patients presenting with anxiety and significant comorbid depression, the combining of medication treatment for depression with CBT for anxiety would be a logical approach.

Key Clinical Points

- Several different strategies may be considered for combining pharmacotherapy and psychotherapy, and each presents challenges and advantages.
- If antidepressant medication and psychotherapy are combined and are both begun at the same time, this presents the problem of time-to-response, generally about 4 weeks, for the medication. It may make more sense to combine these approaches sequentially, starting first with the antidepressant, so that the patient is receiving medication for at least 4 weeks before commencing psychotherapy.
- Anxiolytic medications other than the antidepressants usually have a much quicker onset of action; therefore, these drugs can be combined with psychotherapy from the outset. However, there is some evidence that these medications may impede CBT, especially exposure therapy.
- In the case of the more novel medication approaches, the drug is not expected to afford any benefits in and of itself; medication is only effective in combination with exposure therapy, so both should be administered at the same time.

References

Allen LB, Barlow DH: Treatment of panic disorder, in Pathological Anxiety, Emotional Processing in Etiology and Treatment. Edited by Rothbaum BO. New York, Guilford, 2006, pp 166–180

Baldwin DS, Huusom AKT, Maehlum E: Escitalopram and paroxetine in the treatment of generalized anxiety disorder. Br J Psychiatry 189:264–272, 2006

Barlow DH: Anxiety and Its Disorders: The Nature and Treatment of Anxiety and Panic, 2nd Edition. New York, Guilford, 2002

Barlow DH, Gorman JM, Shear MK, et al: Cognitive-behavioral therapy, imipramine, or their combination for panic disorder: a randomized controlled trial. JAMA 283:2529–2536, 2000

Bear MF: A synaptic basis for memory storage in the cerebral cortex. Proc Natl Acad Sci USA 93:13453–13459, 1996

Beck AT, Ward CH, Mendelson M, et al: An inventory for measuring depression. Arch Gen Psychiatry 4:561–571, 1961

Behar E, Borkovec TD: The nature and treatment of generalized anxiety disorder, in Pathological Anxiety: Emotional Processing in Etiology and Treatment. Edited by Rothbaum BO. New York, Guilford, 2006, pp 181–196

Black DW: Efficacy of combined pharmacotherapy and psychotherapy versus monotherapy in the treatment of anxiety disorders. CNS Spectr 11(suppl):29–33, 2006

Blomhoff S, Haug TT, Hellstrom K, et al: Randomised controlled general practice trial of sertraline, exposure therapy, and combined treatment in generalized social phobia. Br J Psychiatry 179:23–30, 2001

Clark DM, Wells A: A cognitive model of social phobia, in Social Phobia: Diagnosis, Assessment and Treatment. Edited by Heimberg R, Liebowitz M, Hope DA, et al. New York, Guilford, 1995, pp 69–93

Clark DM, Ehlers A, McManus F, et al: Cognitive therapy versus fluoxetine in generalized social phobia: a randomized placebo-controlled trial. J Consult Clin Psychol 71:1058–1067, 2003

Cordioli AV, Heldt E, Bochi DB, et al: Cognitive behavioral group therapy in obsessive compulsive disorder: a randomized clinical trial. Psychother Psychosom 72:211–216, 2003

Cottraux J, Mollard E, Bouvard M, et al: A controlled study of fluvoxamine and exposure in obsessive-compulsive disorder. Int Clin Psychopharmacol 5:635–641, 1990

Cottraux J, Note ID, Cungi C, et al: A controlled study of cognitive-behavior therapy with buspirone or placebo in panic disorder with agoraphobia. Br J Psychiatry 167:635–641, 1995

Davidson JR, Malik MA, Travers J: Structured interview for PTSD (SIP): psychometric validation for DSM-IV criteria. Depress Anxiety 5:127–129, 1997a

Davidson JR, Miner CM, de Veaugh Geiss J, et al: The Brief Social Phobia Scale: a psychometric evaluation. Psychol Med 27:161–166, 1997b

Davidson JR, Rothbaum BO, van der Kolk BA, et al: Multicenter, double-blind comparison of sertraline and placebo in the treatment of posttraumatic stress disorder. Arch Gen Psychiatry 58:485–492, 2001

Davidson JR, Foa EB, Huppert D, et al: Fluoxetine, comprehensive cognitive behavioral therapy, and placebo in generalized social phobia. Arch Gen Psychiatry 61:1005–1013, 2004

Davidson JR, Baldwin D, Stein DJ, et al: Treatment of posttraumatic stress disorder with venlafaxine extended release: a 6 month randomized controlled trial. Arch Gen Psychiatry 63:1158–1165, 2006

Davis M, Myers KM: The role of glutamate and gamma-aminobutyric acid in fear extinction: clinical implications for exposure therapy. Biol Psychiatry 52:998–1007, 2002

Davis M, Ressler K, Rothbaum BO, et al: Effects of D-cycloserine on extinction: translation from preclinical to clinical work. Biol Psychiatry 60:369–375, 2006

Foa EB, Kozac MJ: Emotional processing of fear: Exposure to corrective information. Psychol Bull 99:20–35, 1986

Foa EB, Franklin ME, Moser J: Context in the clinic: how well do cognitive-behavioral therapies and medications work in combination? Biol Psychiatry 52:987–997, 2002

Foa EB, Rothbaum BO, Furr JM: Is the efficacy of exposure therapy for posttraumatic stress disorder augmented with the addition of other cognitive behavior therapy procedures? Psychiatr Ann 33:47–53, 2003

Foa EB, Liebowitz MR, Kozak MJ, et al: Randomized, placebo-controlled trial of exposure and ritual prevention, clomipramine, and their combination in the treatment of obsessive-compulsive disorder. Am J Psychiatry 162:151–161, 2005

Goodman WK, Price LH, Rasmussen SA, et al: The Yale-Brown Obsessive-Compulsive Scale, I: development, use, and reliability. Arch Gen Psychiatry 46:1006–1011, 1989

Guastella AJ, Richardson R, Lovibond PF, et al: A randomized controlled trial of D-cycloserine enhancement of exposure therapy for social anxiety disorder. Biol Psychiatry 63:544–549, 2008

Guy W: ECDEU Assessment Manual for Psychopharmacology (Publ No ADM 76-338). Washington, DC, Department of Health, Education, and Welfare, 1976

Hidalgo RB, Barnett SD, Davidson JRT: Social anxiety disorder in review: two decades of progress. Int J Neuropsychopharmacol 4:279–298, 2001

Hofmann SG, Meuret AE, Smits JA, et al: Augmentation of exposure therapy with D-cycloserine for social anxiety disorder. Arch Gen Psychiatry 63:298–304, 2006

Hohagen F, Winkelmann G, Rashce-Rauchle H, et al: Combination of behavior therapy with fluvoxamine in comparison with behavior therapy and placebo: results of a multicentre study. Br J Psychiatry 173:71–78, 1998

Hood SD, Nutt DJ: Psychopharmacological treatments: an overview, in International Handbook of Social Anxiety. Edited by Crozier WR, Alden LE. London, Wiley, 2001, pp 471–504

Kushner MG, Kim SW, Donohue C, et al: D-cycloserine-augmented exposure therapy for obsessive compulsive disorder. Biol Psychiatry 62:835–838, 2007

Ladouceur R, Dugas MJ, Freeston MH, et al: Efficacy of a cognitive behavioral treatment for generalized anxiety disorder: evaluation in a controlled clinical trial. J Consult Clin Psychol 68:957–964, 2000

Liebowitz MR, Allgulander C, Mangano R, et al: Comparison of venlafaxine-XR and paroxetine in the short-term treatment of SAD. Poster presented at the U.S. Psychiatric and Mental Health Congress, Orlando, FL, November 2003

Marks IM, Swinson RP, Basaglu M, et al: Alprazolam and exposure alone and combined in panic disorder with agoraphobia: a controlled study in London and Toronto. Br J Psychiatry 152:522–534, 1993

Newcomer JW, Krystal JH: NMDA receptor regulation of memory and behavior in humans. Hippocampus 11:529–542, 2001

Power KG, Simpson RJ, Swanson V, et al: Controlled comparison of pharmacological and psychological treatment of generalized anxiety disorder in primary care. Br J Gen Pract 40:289–294, 1990

Randolph C, Roberts JW, Tierney MC, et al: D-cycloserine treatment of Alzheimer disease. Alzheimer Dis Assoc Disord 603:207–214, 1994

Rapee RM, Heimberg RG: A cognitive behavioral model of anxiety in social phobia. Behav Res Ther 35:741–756, 1997

Resick PA, Nishith P, Weaver T, et al: A comparison of cognitive processing therapy, prolonged exposure, and a waiting condition for the treatment of posttraumatic stress disorder in female rape victims. J Consult Clin Psychol 70:867–879, 2002

Ressler KJ, Rothbaum BO, Tannenbaum L, et al: Cognitive enhancers as adjuncts to psychotherapy: use of D-cycloserine in phobics to facilitate extinction of fear. Arch Gen Psychiatry 61:1136–1144, 2004

Rothbaum BO, Meadows EA, Resick P, et al: Cognitive-behavioral treatment: position paper summary for the ISTSS Treatment Guidelines Committee. J Trauma Stress 13:558–563, 2000

Rothbaum BO, Cahill SP, Foa EB, et al: Augmentation of sertraline with prolonged exposure in the treatment of posttraumatic stress disorder. J Trauma Stress 19:625–638, 2006

Rothbaum BO, Foa EB, Hembree E: Reclaiming Your Life From a Traumatic Experience: Client Workbook. New York, Oxford University Press, 2007

Shapiro F: Eye Movement Desensitization and Reprocessing: Basic Principles, Protocols and Procedures. New York, Guilford, 1995

Sousa MB, Isolan LR, Oliveira RR, et al: A randomized clinical trial of cognitive behavioral group therapy and sertraline in the treatment of obsessive compulsive disorder. J Clin Psychiatry 67:1133–1139, 2006

Spielberger CD, Gorsuch RL, Lechene RE, et al: State-Trait Anxiety Inventory (Self-Evaluation Questionnaire). Palo Alto, CA, Consulting Psychologists Press, 1970

Stangier U, Heidenreich T, Peitz M, et al: Cognitive therapy for social phobia: individual versus group treatment. Behav Res Ther 41:991–1007, 2003

Storch EA, Merlo LJ, Bengtson M, et al: D-cycloserine does not enhance exposure-response prevention therapy in obsessive-compulsive disorder. Int Clin Psychopharmacol 22:230–237, 2007

Tolin DF, Pearlson GD, Krystal JH, et al: A controlled trial of D-cycloserine with brief CBT for panic disorder. Paper presented at the 40th annual convention of the Association for Behavioral and Cognitive Therapies, Chicago, IL, November, 2006

Tuominen HJ, Tiihonen J, Wahlbeck K: Glutamatergic drugs for schizophrenia: a systematic review and meta-analysis. Schizophr Res 72:225–234, 2005

Van Balkom AJ, de Haan E, van Oppen P, et al: Cognitive and behavioral therapies alone and in combination with fluvoxamine in the treatment of obsessive-compulsive disorder. J Nerv Ment Dis 186:492–499, 1998

Van Etten ML, Taylor S: Comparative efficacy of treatments for post-traumatic stress disorder: a meta-analysis. Clin Psychol Psychother 5:126–144, 1998

Wilhelm S, Buhlmann U, Tolin D, et al: Augmentation of behavior therapy with D-cycloserine for obsessive-compulsive disorder. Paper presented at the 40th annual convention for the Association for Behavioral and Cognitive Therapies, Chicago, IL, 2006

Recommended Readings

Anxiety Disorders Association of America: http://www.adaa.org/GettingHelp/treatment.asp

Davis M, Barad M, Otto M, et al: Combining pharmacotherapy with cognitive behavioral therapy: traditional and new approaches. J Trauma Stress 19:571–581, 2006

Foa EB, Hembree E, Rothbaum BO: Prolonged Exposure Therapy for PTSD: Emotional Processing of Traumatic Experiences, Therapist Guide. New York, Oxford University Press, 2007

Pull CB: Combined pharmacotherapy and cognitive-behavioural therapy for anxiety disorders. Curr Opin Psychiatry 20:30–35, 2007

Rothbaum BO (ed): Pathological Anxiety: Emotional Processing in Etiology and Treatment of Anxiety. New York, Guilford, 2006

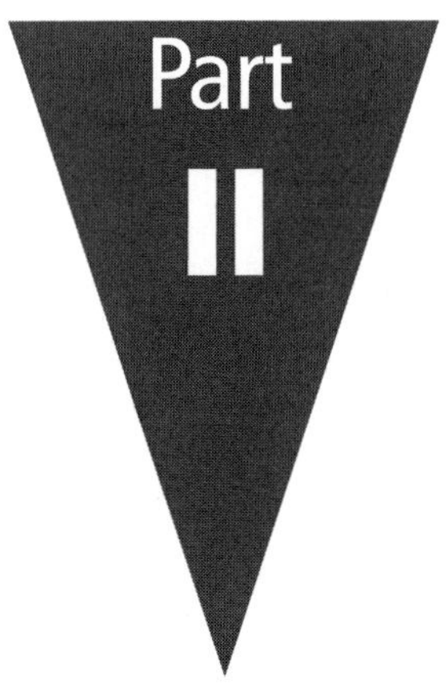

Generalized Anxiety Disorder

Chapter 11

Phenomenology of Generalized Anxiety Disorder

Laszlo A. Papp, M.D.

Generalized anxiety disorder (GAD) is a disabling, chronic condition that is common in many medical settings. However, it remains one of the least researched anxiety disorders, for numerous reasons. First, because the diagnostic category of GAD was first introduced in DSM-III in 1980, studies conducted before that date have limited relevance and questionable validity; substantive revisions of the diagnostic criteria in later editions of DSM (see "Diagnosis" subsection of this chapter) made longitudinal data collection challenging. Second, because treatment resistance in GAD is not uncommon, patients and therapists are reluctant to engage in the prolonged and frequently unsuccessful therapeutic process that could yield much-needed information. Third, because the diverse symptoms of GAD can mimic a variety of medical conditions, GAD patients are usually seen by non–mental health specialists. Psychiatric referral, if made, is frequently delayed. Finally, because "pure" GAD without comorbid conditions is uncommon, the interpretation of studies with heterogeneous comorbid samples is difficult.

Collecting information on GAD in populations with special needs, such as children, women, and older patients, is especially challenging. A possible explanation is the reluctance of both investigators and relatives to "expose" the elderly, children, and women of childbearing potential to research. However, regulatory agencies, yielding to public demands, have begun to emphasize the need to include these patient groups in research studies. The recognition that GAD accounts for a very sizable proportion of all mental illness, that comorbid GAD complicates more than half of all psychiatric and medical conditions, and that GAD is associated with substantially increased disability and medical cost (Judd et al. 1998; Maser 1998; Olfson and Gameroff 2007; Olfson et al. 1997) should mobilize the field.

Epidemiology

The diagnostic criteria for GAD in DSM-IV (retained in DSM-IV-TR; American Psychiatric Association 1994, 2000) are more inclusive than those in previous editions of DSM. As a result, prevalence rates of GAD have been revised upward. Although rates remain highly dependent on the method of interviewing used to obtain them (e.g., family history, first- or second-degree relatives or index-pair informants, direct interviewing, training and experience of the interviewers

Supported in part by National Institute of Mental Health grants MH53582, MH30906, and MH077156 and by Independent Scientist Award MH01397 (L.A. Papp).

[Rougemont-Buecking et al. 2008]), the more recently reported rates seem to reflect clinical reality.

The largest survey of DSM-III GAD was conducted in 1983–1984 as part of the Epidemiologic Catchment Area (ECA) study (Blazer et al. 1991b). The 1-year prevalence rate for GAD, excluding other disorders, was 3.8%. Given the high rate of comorbidity in GAD, the rate dropped to 2.7% when comorbid depression and panic were excluded, and to 1.7% when all other comorbid conditions were excluded. The ECA data also showed that GAD was about twice as prevalent in women as in men. Without comorbid panic and depression, GAD was found to be more prevalent among African Americans. When no exclusions were made, prevalence was highest in people younger than age 30 years.

Five other community-based studies examined the prevalence of DSM-III GAD. In the United States, the point, 1-year, and lifetime prevalence rates were 2.5%, 4%, and 6.4%, respectively (Uhlenhuth et al. 1983; Weissman et al. 1978). Current prevalence of 1.5% and 1-year prevalence of 5.2% were reported from Europe (Angst and Dobler-Mikola 1985), whereas two studies conducted in Asia (Hwu et al. 1989; Lee et al. 1990a, 1990b) found that the 1-year prevalence of GAD ranged from 3.4% to 8.6%, and the lifetime prevalence ranged from 2.9% to 10.5%; rates were lowest among city dwellers. As in the ECA study, Asian women with GAD outnumbered men 2 to 1. In contrast to the U.S. study, however, age comparisons in the Asian samples showed increasing rates of prevalence over time (2.9% for ages 18–24 years vs. 4.3% for ages 45–65 years).

In Florence, Italy, Faravelli et al. (1989) assessed a community sample of 1,110 adults for both DSM-III and DSM-III-R (American Psychiatric Association 1987) anxiety disorders. GAD was the most frequently reported disorder, but prevalence rates declined significantly when the more stringent DSM-III-R criteria were used. The lifetime prevalence rates for DSM-III and DSM-III-R GAD were 5.4% and 3.9%, and the point prevalence rates were 2.8% and 2.0%, respectively. Overall, rates were lower than those reported in other surveys. Possible explanations include the use of psychiatrists, rather than lay interviewers, as diagnosticians and the use of a hierarchical diagnostic model, which allowed only one possible diagnosis per case. Wacker et al. (1992) used both DSM-III-R and ICD-10 criteria to compare the prevalence of GAD in a survey of residents in Basel, Switzerland. They found that the lifetime prevalence of DSM-III-R GAD was 1.9%; the ICD-10 prevalence rate was 9.2%, more than four times greater.

The largest study of DSM-III-R GAD was conducted by Wittchen et al. (1994). They used data collected from the U.S. National Comorbidity Survey, which included 8,098 community-based respondents between ages 15 and 54 years. The current prevalence of GAD was 1.6%, the 1-year prevalence was 3.1%, and the lifetime prevalence was 5.1%. Consistent with previous surveys, GAD was twice as common in women as in men. In addition, GAD was more common in those who were unemployed, separated, divorced, widowed, and older than 24 years. Of those with lifetime GAD, 90% reported at least one other lifetime DSM disorder (most often, depression and panic), and of those with current GAD, 65% reported current comorbid disorders (most commonly, depression, panic, and agoraphobia). Similar to the percentage reported by Wacker et al. (1992), lifetime prevalence of GAD according to ICD-10 criteria was significantly higher (8.9%). The discrepancy may be attributed, in part, to the higher symptom thresholds required by DSM-III-R for diagnosis. The ICD-10 system requires only four symptoms (as opposed to six in DSM-III-R) and does not stipulate that worries must be excessive or unrealistic.

Rates of DSM-IV-defined GAD, although varying significantly among the few surveys, are more comparable with those based on ICD-10 criteria. Some argue that the two diagnostic systems identify different groups of patients with GAD (Slade and Andrews 2001). This may explain the similar prevalence in spite of significantly discrepant diagnostic criteria. For instance, unlike DSM-IV, the ICD-10 diagnosis of GAD requires symptoms of autonomic arousal and does not allow comorbid panic/agoraphobia, social phobia, or obsessive-compulsive disorder. DSM-IV sets a higher threshold of severity than ICD-10 by requiring excessive worry, significant distress or impairment, and 6 months of duration.

An Australian household survey of 10,641 adults, using the Composite International Diagnostic Interview to identify GAD as defined by DSM-IV, revealed a 1-month prevalence of 2.8% and a 12-month prevalence of a whopping 36% (Hunt et al. 2002). The differences in rating instrument used and the training of the interviewers might explain this highly discrepant percentage. In the group with 1-month DSM-IV GAD, comorbidity was 68%. In a sample of 2,847 households in Singapore, the General Health Questionnaire and Schedules for Clinical Assessment in Neuropsychiatry were used to generate DSM-IV GAD diagnoses (Lim et al. 2005). Lifetime prevalence of GAD was 3.3%, and current prevalence was 3.0%. Female-to-male ratio was 3.6:1. As expected, high comorbidity was reported for major depression, dysthymia, panic disorder, and social phobia.

The U.S. National Comorbidity Survey Replication study (NCS-R; Kessler et al. 2005) reported a DSM-IV GAD lifetime prevalence rate of 5.6% and a 12-month prevalence rate of 3.0%. With a required minimum symptom duration of at least 1 month (compared with the 6 months required by DSM-IV), the respective rates increased to 9.1% and 4.5%. When subjects with a 1-month minimum symptom duration were included and the "excessiveness" criterion was not included, the rates in this study were even higher (12.8% and 6.2%, respectively). Claiming improved validity, the authors advocated lowering the duration and eliminating the controversial term "excessive" for the next editions of DSM. Confirming evidence of improved validity, specificity, and predictive validity may justify these revisions.

Epidemiology in Youths

As in adult populations, changing diagnostic criteria of GAD in youths (see "Diagnosis" subsection later in this chapter) have resulted in reports of highly variable prevalence rates. Anderson et al. (1987) examined DSM-III disorders in 792 eleven-year-old New Zealand children. They found a 1-year prevalence of overanxious disorder of 2.9%, with a male-to-female ratio of 1.7:1. In this sample, overanxious disorder was more common than simple phobia (2.4%), depression (1.8%), and social phobia (0.9%), but less prevalent than separation anxiety disorder (3.5%). Four years later, overanxious disorder became the most prevalent disorder (5.9%) in the same cohort (McGee et al. 1990), and the sex ratio was reversed (female-to-male, 1.9:1).

Studies in which DSM-III-R criteria were used found similar incidence rates. In a large sample of Canadian adolescents, the lifetime prevalence of overanxious disorder was 3.6% (Bowen et al. 1990), nearly identical to the rate (3.7%) found by Whitaker et al. (1990). In a clinic sample of 188 children ages 5–18 years with anxiety disorders, 13% had DSM-III-R overanxious disorder (9.6% had panic disorder, 27% had separation anxiety disorder, 19.7% had simple phobia, and 15% had social phobia). The mean age at onset for overanxious disorder was 8.8 years in this group. Rates in males and females did not differ significantly (Last et al. 1992). In contrast, among adolescents in the Whitaker study ranging between ages 14 and 17 years (disregarding the DSM-III minimum age requirement of 18 years), the male-to-female ratio was 1.8:4.6, which is consistent with the literature on rates of GAD among adults.

One of the largest surveys of DSM-III-R overanxious disorder in adolescents came from the Virginia Twin Study of 2,762 white twins ages 8–16 years (Simonoff et al. 1997). This survey found a 3-month prevalence of overanxious disorder of 4.4%, the most common disorder along with simple phobia (also 4.4%). Overanxious disorder in this sample was almost twice as common in girls as in boys (5.6:3.1). The study also found that prevalence rates increased with age; the rate was 2.6% among 8- to 10-year-olds, 4.4% among 11- to 13-year-olds, and 10.7% among 14- to 16-year-olds. Overanxious disorder was found to be comorbid with one other disorder in 68% of cases, and 14% were comorbid with two or more. Phobias were the most common co-occurring disorders (57%), followed by separation anxiety disorder with depression (14%) and depression (13%).

A longitudinal community study of 1,420 children followed three cohorts of children (ages 9, 11, and 13 years) with yearly interviews to age 16 (Costello et al. 2003). Using the Child and Adolescent Psychiatric Assessment, investigators reported a 3-month prevalence of 2.4% for any DSM-IV anxiety disorder. The highest prevalence, 4.6%, was found in the 9-year-old children; the lowest prevalence was 0.9%, among the 12-year-olds. The predicted cumulative prevalence of any DSM-IV anxiety disorder by age 16 was 9.9%. Comorbidity was high: 25.1% of those with any anxiety disorder had a comorbid depressive disorder.

Epidemiology in the Elderly

Anxiety disorders are common in the elderly. Epidemiological surveys identified generalized anxiety disorder (GAD) as one of the most prevalent anxiety disorders in late life (Beekman et al. 1998; Kessler et al. 2005). Kessler and colleagues (1999) confirmed that the severe disability associated with late-life GAD is comparable with, but independent of, depression, which is often a comorbid condition. In a large majority of elderly patients with another anxiety disorder diagnosis, GAD is also a frequent comorbid condition (Brawman-Mintzer et al. 1993; Brown and Barlow 1992; Hassan and Pollard 1994). Taken together, these findings suggest that the rate of clinically significant anxiety problems may be as high as 20% among elderly individuals (Sheikh 1992).

Uhlenhuth et al. (1983) found a 1-year prevalence of DSM-III GAD of 7.1% in 442 subjects ages 65–79 years. This rate was lower than that for those ages 50–64 (8.6%) but higher than that for those ages 18–34 (5.8%) and 35–49 (4.7%). The same study found that GAD was the most common disorder in elderly patients—more than triple the rate for panic and phobias and 20% more common than major depression.

Another survey (Copeland et al. 1987) examined a sample of 841 subjects (about half in the United Kingdom and half in the United States) ages 65 years and older and found much lower incidence rates (0.7% in New York City and 1.1% in London). However, they used a non-DSM-III, computer-based diagnostic system that employed a strict diagnostic hierarchy and included the older "anxiety neurosis" category, as opposed to GAD. Using a generalized anxiety scale constructed for their study, Lindesay et al. (1989) surveyed 890 low-income elderly people (65 years or older) living at home in London. They found a 1-month prevalence rate of 3.7% for generalized anxiety (2.5% in men and 4.5% in women).

Blazer et al. (1991a) examined data from the Durham, North Carolina, site of the ECA study, which included 2,993 community-dwelling subjects 18 years of age and older. They found 6-month and lifetime prevalence rates for DSM-III GAD of 1.9% and 4.6%, respectively, for those age 65 and older (vs. 3.1% and 6.7% for those between ages 45 and 64 years). These rates were greater than those for subjects with panic disorder (0.04% and 0.30%), social phobia (1.3% and 2.6%), and obsessive-compulsive disorder (1.84% and 1.98%) but lower than rates for subjects with simple phobia (9.6% and 16.1%) and agoraphobia (5.2% and 8.4%).

The high rate of variability in reported prevalence rates for GAD in elderly patients, as in most populations, may be the result of methodological factors such as differences in survey methods, case definition, and hierarchical versus nonhierarchical approaches to diagnosis (Flint 1994). In addition, underreporting of anxiety disorders by the elderly may be caused by diminished recall ability, higher rates of anxiolytic medication use, and institutionalization.

Clinical Features

Diagnosis

First described in DSM-III (American Psychiatric Association 1980), GAD, along with atypical anxiety disorder, was considered a residual category reserved for disorders not meeting criteria for any other anxiety disorder. According to DSM-III, patients with generalized anxiety had a persistent, increased level of diffuse anxiety of at least 1 month duration and manifested symptoms from three of four categories: motor tension, autonomic hyperactivity, apprehensive expectation, and vigilance and scanning.

DSM-III-R (American Psychiatric Association 1987) extended the duration of symptoms necessary to meet criteria for GAD from 1 to 6 months, emphasized the importance of excessive or unrealistic worry, and required the presence of at least 6 of 18 anxiety symptoms. DSM-III-R also eliminated some of the hierarchical rules and allowed the diagnosis of GAD in the presence of other Axis I disorders.

The DSM-IV diagnostic criteria for GAD (1994; reprinted in DSM-IV-TR [American Psychiatric Association 2000]) are listed in Table 11–1. DSM-IV-TR defines GAD as including at least 6 months of excessive and uncontrollable anxiety associated with somatic symptoms such as restlessness, fatigue, irritability, muscle tension, sleep disturbance, or difficulty concentrating. The criteria for somatic symptoms have been simplified, and the emphasis has shifted to the pervasive and uncontrollable nature of the worry. The anxiety impairs functioning and is not limited to another Axis I disorder or due to substance use or a medical condition. In evaluating the excessive nature of the worry, the sociocultural context, including the age and sex of the person, is emphasized. The current diagnostic hierarchy considers major depression the primary diagnosis when it is comorbid with GAD. This rule may need to be modified. Recent epidemiological data suggest that when comorbid with major depression, GAD meets the definition of "primary" diagnosis just as frequently as depression does (Moffitt et al. 2007b).

Parallel with the changes in the consecutive DSMs, the anxiety categories in the *International Classification of Diseases* (ICD) have been revised as well. Although ICD-9 (World Health Organization 1977) acknowledged only generic "anxiety states" under the category "Neurotic Disorders," ICD-10 (World Health Organization 1992) is more compatible with DSM-IV (American Psychiatric Association 1994) terminology. One of the most important differences between the two diagnostic systems is DSM-IV's requirement that the worry be "excessive." Eliminating the excessive worry and 6-month duration requirements in the next edition of DSM is under consideration. New data suggest that relaxing these criteria could further improve validity of the GAD diagnosis (see previous section, "Epidemiology," in this chapter).

The strict phenomenological approach first implemented in DSM-III represented a conscious effort to steer clear of theoretical debates concerning the etiology of anxiety. But neuroscience is making significant progress in understanding its biological basis. For exam-

TABLE 11–1. DSM-IV-TR diagnostic criteria for generalized anxiety disorder

A. Excessive anxiety and worry (apprehensive expectation), occurring more days than not for at least 6 months, about a number of events or activities (such as work or school performance).

B. The person finds it difficult to control the worry.

C. The anxiety and worry are associated with three (or more) of the following six symptoms (with at least some symptoms present for more days than not for the past 6 months). **Note:** Only one item is required in children.

(1) restlessness or feeling keyed up or on edge

(2) being easily fatigued

(3) difficulty concentrating or mind going blank

(4) irritability

(5) muscle tension

(6) sleep disturbance (difficulty falling or staying asleep, or restless unsatisfying sleep)

D. The focus of the anxiety and worry is not confined to features of an Axis I disorder, e.g., the anxiety or worry is not about having a panic attack (as in panic disorder), being embarrassed in public (as in social phobia), being contaminated (as in obsessive-compulsive disorder), being away from home or close relatives (as in separation anxiety disorder), gaining weight (as in anorexia nervosa), having multiple physical complaints (as in somatization disorder), or having a serious illness (as in hypochondriasis), and the anxiety and worry do not occur exclusively during posttraumatic stress disorder.

E. The anxiety, worry, or physical symptoms cause clinically significant distress or impairment in social, occupational, or other important areas of functioning.

F. The disturbance is not due to the direct physiological effects of a substance (e.g., a drug of abuse, a medication) or a general medical condition (e.g., hyperthyroidism) and does not occur exclusively during a mood disorder, a psychotic disorder, or a pervasive developmental disorder.

ple, it is now feasible to select a symptom of an anxiety disorder such as fear or worry and examine its neuroanatomy and neurochemistry (LeDoux 1996). Because these symptoms frequently cut across diagnostic categories, future DSMs may have to accommodate a dimensional diagnostic system as well.

Diagnosis in Youths

The diagnosis of GAD in children and adolescents has been controversial. The DSM-III term for GAD in patients younger than 18 years was *overanxious disorder*. Defined as excessive or unrealistic worry (DSM-III-R) or generalized and persistent anxiety (DSM-III) lasting 6 months or longer, overanxious disorder was diagnosed in the presence of any four of seven possible symptoms:

1. Excessive or unrealistic worry about future events
2. Excessive or unrealistic worry about the appropriateness of past behavior
3. Excessive or unrealistic worry about competence in one or more areas (e.g., athletic, academic, social)
4. Frequent somatic complaints, such as headaches or stomachaches, for which no physical basis can be established
5. Marked self-consciousness
6. Excessive need for reassurance about a variety of concerns
7. Marked feelings of tension or inability to relax

In contrast to DSM-III, according to DSM-III-R, patients younger than age 18 years could receive diagnoses of either overanxious disorder or GAD, but GAD took precedence as a diagnosis when patients were older than age 18 years and met criteria for both disorders. DSM-III-R allowed overanxious disorder to be diagnosed after age 18 years as well, providing that the patient's symptoms did not meet criteria for GAD.

In DSM-IV, overanxious disorder was subsumed under the diagnosis of GAD. Thus, the criteria for GAD in children are now the same as for adults, with one exception: children can present with only one of six symptoms (vs. three of six for adults) in addition to excessive worry. The accumulating evidence that children and adolescents may respond to medications in ways that are different from adults (e.g., increased suicidal ideation) should warrant a more refined characterization of anxiety disorders in youths; symptomatic differences might predict outcome and guide treatment choice.

Current recommendations for the next edition of DSM range from making the criteria identical to those for adults to arguing for a single nonspecific anxiety diagnosis that differentiates subtypes only by the number of symptoms and possibly severity. This latter argument is partially supported by high comorbidity. Verduin and Kendall (2003) reported that among 199 children ages 8–13 years assessed at an anxiety disorders clinic, those diagnosed with DSM-III-R or DSM-IV GAD, separation anxiety disorder, or social phobia, 74% of those with primary separation anxiety disorder and 57% of those with primary social phobia also met criteria for GAD. It has been suggested that in younger patients, DSM-IV anxiety disorders may simply represent different dimensions with highly overlapping symptoms (Muris et al. 2002).

Diagnosis in the Elderly

It is becoming clear that the current criteria are frequently inadequate for characterizing GAD in older patients. Diagnosing anxiety in this population can be difficult. Comorbid psychiatric conditions that can mask and/or produce anxiety in the elderly include mood disorders and dementia (Alexopoulos 1991; Reisberg et al. 1987). An additional complication is that a primary medical condition (e.g., endocrine abnormality, nutritional deficiency, or secreting tumor) may be causal (McCullough 1992).

Evidence indicates that clinically significant anxiety problems in the elderly often elude identification by conventional methods, and are actually more prevalent than in the young (Kessler et al. 2005). Surveys that focus on anxiety symptoms rather than anxiety disorders indicate steadily increasing rates of anxiety as individuals age (Sallis and Lichstein 1982). Use of anxiolytic drugs increases with age (Rifkin et al. 1989; Salzman 1985), with some studies showing that as many as 20% of the noninstitutionalized elderly and 30% of the medically hospitalized elderly use benzodiazepines (Parry et al. 1973; Salzman 1991; Shaw and Opit 1976). Also, 20%–25% of the elderly experience insomnia "often" or "always." Research indicates that anxiety is the factor most often associated with insomnia in the elderly (Morgan et al. 1988); therefore, a significant proportion of nighttime benzodiazepine use in elderly patients may reflect anxiety in addition to a sleep problem. Finally, the elderly are subjected to an increasing number of real-life stressors (e.g., illness, disability, widowhood, financial decline, and social isolation) that are known to foster anxiety (Hassan and Pollard 1994). These stressors have been shown to predict ill health among the elderly, particularly stress-related disorders such as headache, gastrointestinal distress, hypertension, and cardiovascular disease (Deberry 1982). Often, ill health brings the elderly patient to the attention of the medical practitioner, and the concomitant or underlying anxiety disorder is frequently overlooked (Turnbull 1989). In sum, the unique manifestations of GAD in older patients will require modified diagnostic criteria.

Symptoms

The symptoms of GAD are numerous and highly variable. Signs of motor tension, autonomic hyperactivity, and hyperarousal are frequently the presenting problems. Patients complain of restlessness, inability to relax, and fatigue. The motor tension results in frequent headaches and chronic muscle pain in the shoulder, neck, and lower back. A DSM-IV-TR companion book provides a case vignette describing a typical patient with GAD (Papp 2004).

Pathological worry has been identified as the pathognomonic feature of GAD. The nature of pathological worry, however, has been subjected to research only recently. Therefore, only limited data are available on the characteristics of worry in actual clinical samples. GAD patients consistently report a greater number of worry areas compared with patients with other anxiety disorders and nonanxious control subjects, but the particular patterns of worry content are highly variable and do not consistently identify patients with GAD (Roemer et al. 1997). Studies show that patients with GAD share the same concerns as nonanxious control subjects, such as concerns about family and interpersonal relationships, work, school, finances, and health (Craske et al. 1989; Roemer et al. 1997; Sanderson and Barlow 1990).

Some investigators suggest that the manifest content of the worry is unimportant. They argue that the worry is simply a distraction and serves to protect patients from their "real" problems. Indeed, GAD subjects do believe that worry serves to distract them from more emotional topics (Borkovec and Roemer 1995). The role of emotional trauma in the pathogenesis of GAD may also be supported by the finding that these patients have more exposure to potentially traumatizing events in their pasts than nonanxious control subjects (Roemer et al. 1996). This hypothesis, akin to the "unconscious conflict" paradigm of psychodynamic thinking, needs further support.

GAD worry has been distinguished from "normal" worry by being perceived as significantly more uncontrollable and unrealistic. Patients with GAD spend more of the day worrying than nonanxious control subjects (60% vs. 18%). Reliance on the perception of control alone, however, may be misleading. An objective measure of thought suppression has shown that although patients with GAD have significantly less mental control over intrusive thoughts concerning their "main worry" than they do over their own neutral cognitions, contrary to expectation, they have no more actual "main worry" intrusions than do nonanxious control subjects (Becker et al. 1998).

The one content area that has consistently distinguished GAD patients from others is excessive worry over minor matters (e.g., daily hassles and time management) (Craske et al. 1989; Roemer et al. 1997; Sanderson and Barlow 1990). This criterion has proven to be a necessary, if not sufficient, feature for a diagnosis of GAD. A negative answer to the question "Do you worry excessively about minor matters?" effectively ruled out the diagnosis of (DSM-IV) GAD in subjects (0.94 negative predictive power vs. 0.36 positive predictive power) (R. DiNardo, unpublished analysis, cited in Brown 1993). On the other hand, patients who do not consider their worry excessive or uncontrollable, frequently suffer from GAD that is otherwise indistinguishable from and just as disabling as a full-symptom GAD. The excessive nature of the worry may not be a necessary criterion of GAD; it is not required by ICD-10. Similarly, the duration criterion of 6 months may exclude patients with an otherwise identical condition. Many consider GAD a chronic but fluctuating illness with several active episodes occurring for as briefly as 1 month (Rickels and Rynn 2001a, 2001b).

GAD patients do not lack problem-solving *skills* but do have poorer problem *orientation* (i.e., response-set involving sense of control, problem-solving confidence, and approach vs. avoidance), and have significantly more difficulty tolerating ambiguity, compared with control subjects (Davey 1994; Ladouceur et al. 1998). Low tolerance of uncertainty might also predict more severity and could differentiate GAD from other anxiety and mood disorders (Dugas et al. 2005, 2007). Individuals with GAD also show a cognitive bias for threat-related information. Studies employing the modified Stroop task, in which a subject's speed at naming the colors that different words are printed in is measured, consistently revealed that patients with GAD were slower than nonanxious control subjects in color-naming negative or threat-related words (Martin et al. 1991; Mathews and MacLeod 1985; Mogg et al. 1989, 1995).

Comorbidity

The symptoms of generalized anxiety are present in most anxiety and mood disorders, but only about 20% of the patients with depression and 10% of those with another anxiety disorder meet the criteria for the full syndrome of GAD. More than two-thirds of patients with the principal diagnosis of GAD have an additional Axis I disorder, with social phobia, depression, or panic leading the list (Borkovec et al. 1995; Wittchen et al. 1994). A recent survey among primary care patients showed that 89% of those with GAD met criteria for a comorbid psychiatric disorder as well (Olfson et al. 1997).

A New Zealand birth cohort study of 1,037 males and females followed to age 32 years showed that both pure GAD and GAD comorbid with major depression, but not pure major depression, were preceded by most of the 13 risk factors chosen to assess domains of family history, early trauma, childhood behavior, and personality (Moffitt et al. 2007a). Comorbidity was also associated with early onset, more recurrence, and more treatment, suggesting that the diagnosis of GAD, with or without depression, was associated with more severity. In the comorbid group, each condition, depression or GAD alone or comorbid GAD and depression, occurred first in about one-third of the cases (Moffitt et al. 2007b). These findings are at variance with the theory that a more disabling and more severe depression usually follows a relatively less severe GAD. If these results were confirmed, major depression should not warrant the primary designation when comorbid with GAD. Comorbidity is also discussed in this chapter in the sections "Epidemiology" and "Differential Diagnosis."

Course

The course of GAD is chronic, with fluctuating severity and symptom patterns (see Chapter 14, "Psychotherapy for Generalized Anxiety Disorder," in this volume). It usually begins in a person's early 20s, but, because of the overwhelmingly retrospective data, there is much controversy about age at onset. Although most agree that onset after age 60 years is rare, some investigators believe onset could occur much earlier than in the 20s. Patients with onset of GAD before age 10 years may represent a separate category that characterizes a more malignant type of the disorder. Although questions remain about whether these various types are sufficiently distinct, late-onset GAD is usually characterized by rapid onset following a clearly identifiable major stress. Early-onset GAD is more likely to develop gradually, presents with comorbid depression and other Axis I and Axis II disorders (Shores et al. 1992), and follows a more chronic course. These patients have a frequent history of childhood fears, school problems, and behavioral inhibition. Middle-aged patients report, on average, a 20-year history of significant baseline anxiety with frequent exacerbations. When GAD remains untreated, prolonged remission is unusual. Treated or untreated, the long-term outcome of GAD is variable. Severity is dependent on several factors, including the existence of GAD with comorbid Axis I and Axis II disorders, environmental support, the biology of the disorder, and the duration of the illness.

Evaluation

Rating Scales

Historically, the interrater reliability of the GAD diagnosis had been low compared with most anxiety disorders. The standard assessment tools were not diagnostic instruments and did not discriminate among the various anxiety disorders, or between anxious depression and an anxiety disorder. For the most part, efforts to provide a distinct measure of anxiety independent of other psychopathology, such as depression, had been largely unsuccessful. Most ratings of anxiety show substantial correlation with measures of depression.

The sources of poor reliability for current GAD were inconsistent ratings of the anxiety symptoms, poor and inconsistent recall by patients, and disagreements on the nature of GAD worry. With statistics ranging from 0.27 to 0.57 (DiNardo et al. 1993; Mannuzza et al. 1989), estimates of the stability of the GAD diagnosis were clearly compromised. The most common reason given for interrater disagreement was related to severity, as opposed to the presence or absence of GAD.

Because of controversy surrounding the diagnostic agreement, several investigators have questioned the validity of the GAD category. However, emerging consensus based on distinct course, specific treatment response, and family studies showing a higher risk of developing GAD in first-degree relatives of patients with GAD confirmed the legitimacy of the diagnosis. Data from two large national surveys also suggested that the magnitude of role impairment from GAD was comparable with that of depression, and that GAD-related disability occurred independently from comorbid depression or other comorbid conditions (Kessler et al. 1999). Although not yet supported by biological data, reports from field trials and clinical experience also suggested that GAD is a distinct anxiety disorder (see Chapter 2, "Classification of Anxiety Disorders," in this volume).

More recent statistics (0.83) have indicated much better reliability of GAD diagnoses with no significant effect of coexistent depressive disorders (cited in Barlow and Wincze 1998). Indicating renewed interest, a 7-item anxiety scale (GAD-7) was developed and tested as a screening instrument in primary care (Spitzer et al. 2006). As reflected by both self-rated questionnaire responses and phone interviews with mental health professionals, the scale demonstrated good reliability as well as criterion, construct, factorial, and procedural validity. In spite of significant overlap, factor analyses successfully differentiated symptoms of depression and anxiety. It was also confirmed that GAD and depression symptoms had differing but independent effects on functional impairment and disability.

For now, considering the continued controversy over DSM criteria for GAD, the inclusion of an assessment package containing several rating instruments is well justified (e.g., Penn State Worry Questionnaire; State-Trait Anxiety Inventory; Hamilton Rating Scale for Anxiety, Clinical Global Impression and Improvement scales). This approach allows the collection of data on subjects who are defined as anxious according to psychometric criteria but ruled out for a GAD diagnosis by DSM criteria, or vice versa (Gorenstein et al. 1999). Identifying symptom patterns within the GAD category could lead to both more valid and more specific diagnoses. Because understanding the course and phenomenology of GAD depends on interrater and test-retest reliability, further improvement in this area is a priority.

Differential Diagnosis

Nonpathological Anxiety

Among the anxiety disorders, GAD is probably the one most similar to "normal" anxiety. As described in DSM-IV-TR, the anxiety of patients with GAD is more pervasive and affects routine daily activities, resulting in functional impairment. Nonpathological anxiety, on the contrary, usually is facilitating and does not manifest as disabling physical symptoms and catastrophic cognitive processes. As described earlier in this chapter, research on the nature of GAD worry has begun to delineate the phenomenology of pathological worry.

Depression

Unquestionably, the most difficult and controversial differential diagnosis is between depression and anxiety. Depression, particularly dysthymia, and GAD share many features: insidious onset, protracted course with periodic exacerbations, and chronic dysphoric affect. The symptoms frequently represent the prodromal phase to major depression or panic disorder. Severe depressive symptoms, suicidality, and hopelessness are more characteristic of depression, whereas high ratings on vigilance, scanning, and somatization, specifically respiratory symptoms, indicate anxiety disorder. The analysis of cognitive content (anxious anticipation vs.

anticipated happiness) also differentiates patients with GAD and those with major depression. Although similar personality factors have been described in the two disorders, the suggestion that these similar features may explain the overlap has not been substantiated. For the many cases when differentiation seems impossible, the category of mixed anxiety-depression has been suggested.

Hypochondriasis

Another challenging diagnostic task is to distinguish between the health concerns of a patient with GAD and the disease conviction of a patient with hypochondriasis. In the absence of clear hierarchical rules, when disease conviction is present and the patient meets criteria for GAD, both conditions should be diagnosed.

Panic Disorder

The most obvious distinguishing symptom of panic disorder is the presence of panic attacks. The age at onset is similar to that of GAD, but there is a sharp contrast between the sudden, unexpected panic attack marking the beginning of panic disorder and the insidious, vague complaints at the onset of GAD. Panic attacks may also occur in GAD, but they are rare, usually less severe, and not the leading symptoms. Patients with panic disorder are more disabled by their symptoms than patients with GAD, and they seek treatment earlier. Patients with panic disorder complain more of fearful, catastrophic thoughts, focusing on acute cardiopulmonary symptoms, whereas GAD manifests as less specific, chronic discomfort involving multiple organ systems. Low tolerance of uncertainty by patients with GAD might also differentiate them from patients with panic disorder (Dugas et al. 2005).

Personality Disorders

Compared with the average rate of personality disorders of 10% in the general population, the rate of personality disorders in patients with GAD is close to 50%. Treatment resistance in GAD may be associated with an even higher rate of comorbid personality disorder. Although no specific personality disorder has been identified as typically comorbid with GAD, avoidant, dependent, and obsessive-compulsive personality disorders and traits are common in patients with GAD. Some theories suggest that these personality disorders are complications of the anxiety disorder or represent a vulnerability to develop an anxiety disorder. However, a prospective study revealed no difference in the rate of baseline personality disorder between patients who later developed depression and those who developed an anxiety disorder. This finding would suggest that premorbid personality disorders do not predispose to anxiety disorders. However, personality traits frequently improve with anxiety disorder–specific treatments, suggesting that some personality disorders may be secondary to an anxiety disorder. These treatment results also challenge the validity of strictly differentiating Axis I and Axis II diagnoses.

Substance-Related Disorders

Self-medication is the most frequently suggested paradigm to explain the high rate of comorbidity between anxiety and substance use. Although anxiety disorders, including GAD, are common in alcoholic patients, patients with GAD are less likely to self-medicate with alcohol and other substances than are patients with panic disorder and social phobia. However, up to two-thirds of patients receiving treatment for alcohol problems report clinically significant anxiety, including GAD (Grant et al. 2005). In most cases GAD develops after the alcohol problem. Alcohol and other substance withdrawal states are indistinguishable from the autonomic symptoms of GAD. Prolonged exposure to alcohol and other substances can lead to the same gastrointestinal, acid-base, and sleep disturbances described by patients with GAD.

Conclusion

GAD is a challenging diagnostic and treatment dilemma. Notwithstanding changing diagnostic criteria, epidemiological surveys suggest that the disorder is one of the most prevalent psychiatric conditions. While clinicians attempt to identify response patterns, course, and predictors of response in rigorous double-blind studies, neuroscientists focus on the neurochemistry and neuroanatomy of select features of DSM categories, such as the excessive worry seen among individuals with GAD. The synthesis of the results of basic and clinical neuroscience and DSM-based treatment and epidemiological studies will likely improve our understanding of the nature of GAD and lead to better treatment.

Key Clinical Points

- Generalized anxiety disorder is distinct and common, but the severe disability associated with it is still underappreciated.
- The diagnosis of GAD can be made reliably, even in the presence of many comorbid conditions.
- The epidemiology and symptoms of GAD are likely to differ significantly by age and gender.

References

Alexopoulos GS: Anxiety and depression in the elderly, in Anxiety in the Elderly. Edited by Salzman C, Lebowitz BD. New York, Springer, 1991, pp 63–77

American Psychiatric Association: Diagnostic and Statistical Manual of Mental Disorders, 3rd Edition. Washington, DC, American Psychiatric Association, 1980

American Psychiatric Association: Diagnostic and Statistical Manual of Mental Disorders, 3rd Edition, Revised. Washington, DC, American Psychiatric Association, 1987

American Psychiatric Association: Diagnostic and Statistical Manual of Mental Disorders, 4th Edition. Washington, DC, American Psychiatric Association, 1994

American Psychiatric Association: Diagnostic and Statistical Manual of Mental Disorders, 4th Edition, Text Revision. Washington, DC, American Psychiatric Association, 2000

Anderson JC, Williams S, McGee R, et al: DSM-III disorders in preadolescent children: prevalence in a large sample from the general population. Arch Gen Psychiatry 44:69–76, 1987

Angst J, Dobler-Mikola A: The Zurich study: anxiety and phobia in young adults. Eur Arch Psychiatry Neurol Sci 235:171–178, 1985

Barlow DH, Wincze J: DSM-IV and beyond: what is generalized anxiety disorder? Acta Psychiatr Scand Suppl 383:23–29, 1998

Becker ES, Rinck M, Roth WT, et al: Don't worry and beware of white bears: thought suppression in anxiety patients. J Anxiety Disord 12:39–55, 1998

Beekman AT, Bremmer HA, Deeg DJ, et al: Anxiety disorders in later life: a report from the Longitudinal Aging Study Amsterdam. Int J Geriatr Psychiatry 13:717–726, 1998

Blazer D, George LK, Hughes D: The epidemiology of anxiety disorders: an age comparison, in Anxiety in the Elderly: Treatment and Research. Edited by Salzman C, Lebowitz BD. New York, Springer, 1991a, pp 17–30

Blazer DG, Hughes D, George LK, et al: Generalized anxiety disorder, in Psychiatric Disorders in America: The Epidemiologic Catchment Area Study. Edited by Robins LN, Regier DA. New York, Free Press, 1991b, pp 180–203

Borkovec TD, Roemer L: Perceived functions of worry among generalized anxiety disorder subjects: distraction from more emotionally distressing topics? J Behav Ther Exp Psychiatry 26:25–30, 1995

Borkovec TD, Abel JL, Newman H: Effects of psychotherapy on comorbid conditions in generalized anxiety disorder. J Consult Clin Psychol 63:479–483, 1995

Bowen RC, Offord DR, Boyle MH: The prevalence of overanxious disorder and separation anxiety disorder: results from the Ontario Child Health Study. J Am Acad Child Adolesc Psychiatry 29:753–758, 1990

Brawman-Mintzer O, Lydiard RB, Emmanuel N, et al: Psychiatric comorbidity in patients with generalized anxiety disorder. Am J Psychiatry 150:1216–1218, 1993

Brown TA, Barlow DH: Comorbidity among anxiety disorders: implications for treatment and DSM-IV. J Consult Clin Psychol 60:835–844, 1992

Copeland JRM, Gurland BJ, Dewey ME, et al: Is there more dementia, depression and neurosis in New York? A comparative study of the elderly in New York and London using the computer diagnosis AGECAT. Br J Psychiatry 151:466–473, 1987

Costello EJ, Mustillo S, Erkanli A, et al: Prevalence and development of psychiatric disorders in childhood and adolescence. Arch Gen Psychiatry 60:837–844, 2003

Craske MG, Rapee RM, Jackel L, et al: Qualitative dimensions of worry in DSM-III-R generalized anxiety disorder subjects and nonanxious controls. Behav Res Ther 27:397–402, 1989

Davey GCL: Worrying, social problem solving abilities, and problem-solving confidence. Behav Res Ther 32:327–330, 1994

Deberry S: An evaluation of progressive muscle relaxation on stress related symptoms in a geriatric population. Int J Aging Hum Dev 14:255–269, 1982

DiNardo PA: MacArthur reanalysis of generalized anxiety disorder (unpublished manuscript), 1991. Cited in Brown TA, O'Leary TA, Barlow DH: Generalized anxiety disorder, in Clinical Handbook of Psychological Disorders,

2nd Edition. Edited by Barlow DH. New York, Guilford, 1993, pp 137–188

DiNardo P, Moras K, Barlow DH, et al: Reliability of DSM-III-R anxiety disorder categories using the Anxiety Disorders Interview Schedule–Revised (ADIS-R). Arch Gen Psychiatry 50:251–256, 1993

Dugas MJ, Marchand A, Ladouceur R: Further validation of a cognitive-behavioral model of generalized anxiety disorder: diagnostic and symptom specificity. J Anxiety Disord 19:329–343, 2005

Dugas MJ, Savard P, Gaudet A, et al: Can the components of a cognitive model predict the severity of generalized anxiety disorder? Behav Ther 38:169–178, 2007

Faravelli C, Guerrini Degl'Innocenti B, Giardinelli L: Epidemiology of anxiety disorders in Florence. Acta Psychiatr Scand 79:308–312, 1989

Flint AJ: Epidemiology and comorbidity of anxiety disorders in the elderly. Am J Psychiatry 151:640–649, 1994

Gorenstein EE, Papp LA, Kleber MS: Cognitive-behavioral treatment of anxiety in later life. Cogn Behav Practice 6:305–320, 1999

Grant BF, Hasin DS, Stinson FS, et al: Prevalence, correlates, comorbidity, and comparative disability of DSM-IV generalized anxiety disorder in the USA: results from the National Epidemiologic Survey on Alcohol and Related Conditions. Psychol Med 35:1747–1759, 2005

Hassan R, Pollard CA: Late-life-onset panic disorder: clinical and demographic characteristics of a patient sample. J Geriatr Psychiatry Neurol 7:86–90, 1994

Hunt C, Issakidis C, Andrews G: DSM-IV generalized anxiety disorder in the Australian National Survey of Mental Health and Well-Being. Psychol Med 32:649–659, 2002

Hwu HG, Yeh EK, Chang LY: Prevalence of psychiatric disorders in Taiwan defined by the Chinese Diagnostic Interview Schedule. Acta Psychiatr Scand 79:136–147, 1989

Judd LL, Kessler RC, Paulus HP, et al: Comorbidity as a fundamental feature of generalized anxiety disorders: results from the National Comorbidity Study (NCS). Acta Psychiatr Scand Suppl 393:6–11, 1998

Kessler RC, DuPont RL, Berglund P, et al: Impairment in pure and comorbid generalized anxiety disorder and major depression at 12 months in two national surveys. Am J Psychiatry 156:1915–1923, 1999

Kessler RC, Berglund P, Demler O, et al: Lifetime prevalence and age-of-onset distributions of DSM-IV disorders in the National Comorbidity Survey Replication. Arch Gen Psychiatry 62:593–602, 2005

Ladouceur R, Blais F, Freeston MH, et al: Problem solving and problem orientation in generalized anxiety disorder. J Anxiety Disord 12:139–152, 1998

Last CG, Perrin S, Hersen M, et al: DSM-III-R anxiety disorders in children: sociodemographic and clinical characteristics. J Am Acad Child Adolesc Psychiatry 31:1070–1076, 1992

LeDoux JE: The Emotional Brain: The Mysterious Underpinnings of Emotional Life. New York, Simon and Schuster, 1996

Lee CK, Kwak YS, Yamamoto J, et al: Psychiatric epidemiology in Korea, part I: gender and age differences in Seoul. J Nerv Ment Dis 178:242–246, 1990a

Lee CK, Kwak YS, Yamamoto J, et al: Psychiatric epidemiology in Korea, part II: urban and rural differences. J Nerv Ment Dis 178:247–252, 1990b

Lim L, Ng TP, Chua HC, et al: Generalised anxiety disorder in Singapore: prevalence, comorbidity and risk factors in a multi-ethnic population. Soc Psychiatry Psychiatr Epidemiol 40:972–979, 2005

Lindesay J, Briggs K, Murphy E: The Guy's/Age Concern Survey: prevalence rates of cognitive impairment, depression and anxiety in an urban elderly community. Br J Psychiatry 155:317–329, 1989

Mannuzza S, Fyer AJ, Martin MS, et al: Reliability of anxiety assessment, I: diagnostic agreement. Arch Gen Psychiatry 46:1093–1101, 1989

Martin M, Williams RM, Clark DM: Does anxiety lead to selective processing of threat-related information? Behav Res Ther 29:147–160, 1991

Maser JD: Generalized anxiety disorder and its comorbidities: disputes at the boundaries. Acta Psychiatr Scand Suppl 393:12–22, 1998

Mathews A, MacLeod C: Discrimination of threat cues without awareness in anxiety states. J Abnorm Psychol 95:131–138, 1985

McCullough PK: Evaluation and management of anxiety in the older adult. Geriatrics 47:35–39, 1992

McGee R, Feehan M, Williams S, et al: DSM-III disorders in a large sample of adolescents. J Am Acad Child Adolesc Psychiatry 29:611–619, 1990

Moffitt TE, Caspi A, Harrington H, et al: Generalized anxiety disorder and depression: childhood risk factors in a birth cohort followed to age 32. Psychol Med 37:441–452, 2007a

Moffitt TE, Harrington H, Caspi A, et al: Depression and generalized anxiety disorder: cumulative and sequential comorbidity in a birth cohort followed prospectively to age 32 years. Arch Gen Psychiatry 64:651–660, 2007b

Mogg K, Mathews A, Weinman J: Selective processing of threat cues in anxiety states: a replication. Behav Res Ther 27:317–324, 1989

Mogg K, Bradley BP, Millar N, et al: A follow-up study of cognitive bias in generalized anxiety disorder. Behav Res Ther 33:927–935, 1995

Morgan K, Dallosso H, Ebrahim S, et al: Characteristics of subjective insomnia in the elderly living at home. Age Ageing 17:1–7, 1988

Muris P, Schmidt H, Engelbrecht P, et al: DSM-IV-defined anxiety disorder symptoms in South African children. J Am Acad Child Adolesc Psychiatry 41:1360–1368, 2002

Olfson M, Gameroff MJ: Generalized anxiety disorder, somatic pain and health care costs. Gen Hosp Psychiatry 29:310–316, 2007

Olfson M, Fireman B, Weissman MM, et al: Mental disorders and disability among patients in primary care group practice. Am J Psychiatry 154:1734–1740, 1997

Papp LA: Discussion of "Edgy Electrician" [Generalized anxiety disorder: evaluation and treatment], in Treatment Companion to the DSM-IV-TR Case Book. Edited by Spitzer RL, First MB, Gibbon M, et al. Washington, DC, American Psychiatric Publishing, 2004, pp 137–142

Parry HJ, Balter MB, Mellinger GD, et al: National patterns of psychotherapeutic drug use. Arch Gen Psychiatry 28:769–783, 1973

Reisberg B, Borenstein J, Salob SP, et al: Behavioral symptoms in Alzheimer's disease: phenomenology and treatment. J Clin Psychiatry 48(suppl):9–15, 1987

Rickels K, Rynn M: Overview and clinical presentation of generalized anxiety disorder. Psychiatr Clin North Am 24:1–17, 2001a

Rickels K, Rynn M: What is generalized anxiety disorder? J Clin Psychiatry 62(suppl):4–14, 2001b

Rifkin A, Seshagiri DM, Basawaraj K, et al: Benzodiazepine use and abuse by patients at outpatient clinics. Am J Psychiatry 146:1331–1332, 1989

Roemer L, Molina S, Litz BT, et al: Preliminary investigation of the role of previous exposure to potentially traumatizing events in generalized anxiety disorder. Depress Anxiety 4:134–138, 1996

Roemer L, Molina S, Borkovec TD: An investigation of worry content among generally anxious individuals. J Nerv Ment Dis 185:314–319, 1997

Rougemont-Buecking A, Rothen S, Jeanprêtre N, et al: Inter-informant agreement on diagnoses and prevalence estimates of anxiety disorders: direct interview versus family history method. Psychiatry Res 157:211–223, 2008

Sallis JF, Lichstein KL: Analysis and management of geriatric anxiety. Int J Aging Hum Dev 15:197–211, 1982

Salzman C: Geriatric psychopharmacology. Annu Rev Med 36:217–228, 1985

Salzman C: Pharmacologic treatment of the anxious elderly patient, in Anxiety in the Elderly: Treatment and Research. Edited by Salzman C, Lebowitz BD. New York, Springer, 1991, pp 149–173

Sanderson WC, Barlow DH: A description of patients diagnosed with DSM-III-R generalized anxiety disorder. J Nerv Ment Dis 178:588–591, 1990

Shaw SM, Opit LJ: Need for supervision in the elderly receiving long-term prescribed medication. BMJ 1:505–507, 1976

Sheikh JI: Anxiety disorders and their treatment. Clin Geriatr Med 8:411–426, 1992

Shores MM, Glubin T, Cowley DS, et al: The relationship between anxiety and depression: a clinical comparison of generalized anxiety disorder, dysthymic disorder, panic disorder, and major depression. Compr Psychiatry 33:237–244, 1992

Simonoff E, Pickles A, Meyer JM, et al: The Virginia Twin Study of Adolescent Behavioral Development: influences of age, sex, and impairment on rates of disorder. Arch Gen Psychiatry 54:801–808, 1997

Slade T, Andrews G: DSM-IV and ICD-10 generalized anxiety disorder: discrepant diagnoses and associated disability. Soc Psychiatry Psychiatr Epidemiol 36:45–51, 2001

Spitzer RL, Kroenke K, Williams JB, et al: A brief measure for assessing generalized anxiety disorder: the GAD-7. Arch Intern Med 166:1092–1097, 2006

Turnbull JM: Anxiety and physical illness in the elderly. J Clin Psychiatry 50(suppl):40–45, 1989

Uhlenhuth EH, Balter MB, Mellinger GD, et al: Symptom checklist syndromes in the general population: correlations with psychotherapeutic drug use. Arch Gen Psychiatry 40:1167–1173, 1983

Verduin TL, Kendall PC: Differential occurrence of comorbidity within childhood anxiety disorders. J Clin Child Adolesc Psychol 32:290–295, 2003

Wacker HR, Mullejans R, Klein KH, et al: Identification of cases of anxiety disorders and affective disorders in the community according to ICD-10 and DSM-III-R by using the Composite International Diagnostic Interview (CIDI). Int J Methods Psychiatr Res 2:91–100, 1992

Weissman MM, Myers JK, Harding PS: Psychiatric disorders in a US urban community: 1975–1976. Am J Psychiatry 135:459–462, 1978

Whitaker A, Johnson J, Shaffer D, et al: Uncommon troubles in young people: prevalence estimates of selected psychiatric disorders in a nonreferred adolescent population. Arch Gen Psychiatry 47:487–496, 1990

Wittchen H-U, Zhao S, Kessler RC, et al: DSM-III-R generalized anxiety disorder in the National Comorbidity Survey. Arch Gen Psychiatry 51:355–364, 1994

World Health Organization: International Classification of Diseases, 9th Revision. Geneva, Switzerland, World Health Organization, 1977

World Health Organization: International Statistical Classification of Diseases and Related Health Problems, 10th Revision, Vol 1. Geneva, Switzerland, World Health Organization, 1992

Recommended Readings

Kessler RC, Berglund P, Demler O, et al: Lifetime prevalence and age-of-onset distributions of DSM-IV disorders in the National Comorbidity Survey Replication. Arch Gen Psychiatry 62:593–602, 2005

Moffitt TE, Harrington H, Caspi A, et al: Depression and generalized anxiety disorder: cumulative and sequential comorbidity in a birth cohort followed prospectively to age 32 years. Arch Gen Psychiatry 64:651–660, 2007

Papp LA: Generalized anxiety disorder: evaluation and treatment, in Treatment Companion to the DSM-IV-TR Case Book. Edited by Spitzer RL, First MB, Gibbon M, et al. Washington, DC, American Psychiatric Publishing, 2004, pp 137–142

Rickels K, Rynn M: Overview and clinical presentation of generalized anxiety disorder. Psychiatr Clin North Am 24:1–17, 2001

Spitzer RL, Kroenke K, Williams JB, et al: A brief measure for assessing generalized anxiety disorder: the GAD-7. Arch Intern Med 166:1092–1097, 2006

Chapter 12

Pathogenesis of Generalized Anxiety Disorder

Jeffrey D. Lightfoot, Ph.D.
Steven Seay Jr., M.S.
Andrew W. Goddard, M.D.

Generalized anxiety disorder (GAD) is a relatively new diagnosis that was first defined in the *Diagnostic and Statistical Manual of Mental Disorders*, Third Edition (American Psychiatric Association 1980). GAD is characterized by excessive and uncontrollable anxiety and worry and is often considered the most "basic" anxiety disorder because its core features manifest in other anxiety disorders (Brown et al. 2001). Although individuals with GAD do not differ from healthy individuals with regard to the content of their worries, they tend to grossly overpredict the occurrence of negative outcomes (Barlow 1988; G. Butler and Mathews 1987). Physical symptoms associated with GAD include motor tension and vigilance (Brawman-Mintzer et al. 1994; Marten et al. 1993), and individuals with GAD commonly report irritability, feelings of restlessness, muscle tension, fatigability, and sleep and concentration difficulties (Marten et al. 1993). In this chapter, we review biological and psychosocial factors that are thought to play a role in the development and maintenance of the disorder. The biological section includes contributions from genetics, neurochemistry, and neurophysiology, and the psychosocial section explores intrapsychic, social, and learning accounts of the disorder. We then attempt to integrate these main areas to provide an etiological model of GAD.

Biological Factors

Genetics

Early studies investigating the genetics of GAD found that 19.5% of the first-degree relatives of patients with GAD also met diagnostic criteria for the disorder, compared with 3.5% of control subjects' relatives (Noyes et al. 1987). However, data from twin studies have been equivocal. Although Kendler et al. (1992b) found that the heritability of GAD was 30% in pairs of female twins, Andrews et al. (1990) found no significant differences in concordance rates between monozygotic twins and dizygotic twins. In a review of the genetics of anxiety disorders, Hettema et al. (2001a) looked at the magnitude of familial aggregation and the relative etiological contributions of genetics versus environment and found strong support for familial aggregation. The majority of familial risk was associated with genetics (30%–40%), but the largest proportion of variance in liability was related to individual environmental factors (see also Kendler 1996; Mackintosh et al. 2006). One longitudinal study conducted over 8 years suggested an even higher heritability rate of 50%–60% (Kendler et al. 1992a). Notably, this genetic link appears to be consistent across genders (Hettema et al. 2001b).

Alterations in serotonin metabolism and the regulation of serotonin transporters have been implicated in these overall findings. Findings from one study suggest that the serotonin transporter (5-HTT) gene-linked polymorphic region SS genotype (short/short) is higher in patients with GAD than in controls (68% vs. 49%), and the frequency of the short allele is also observed at a higher rate in patients with GAD (You et al. 2005). Interestingly, this polymorphism may be specific to anxiety (Tadic et al. 2003). Although genetic factors may contribute significantly to the pathogenesis of GAD, a genetic diathesis is unlikely to be sufficient for phenotypic expression in all cases. Moreover, genetic differences can arise due to environmental factors and do not necessarily reflect an inherent vulnerability to disease. Adoption studies and chromosomal analysis will help clarify these issues.

Neurochemistry

Norepinephrine

Norepinephrine is a catecholamine that acts both as a hormone and as a neurotransmitter. The main norepinephrine nucleus in the brain, the locus coeruleus, has been shown to be activated by stress and has been implicated in fear behavior, vigilance, and attentional processes (Aston-Jones et al. 1997; Chrousos and Gold 1992). Perhaps not surprisingly, norepinephrine has been the focus of neurochemical studies of GAD.

A study by R.J. Mathew et al. (1980) found that patients with GAD had higher plasma catecholamine levels than did controls; however, a subsequent study failed to replicate these findings (R.J. Mathew et al. 1982a). Methodological confounds (e.g., venipuncture-induced stress) might account for this discrepancy. In a study using an indwelling catheter, Munjack et al. (1990) found no significant differences in catecholamine levels between controls and patients with GAD. Likewise, no difference was found between controls and patients with GAD in plasma levels of the catecholamine degradation enzymes catechol-*O*-methyltransferase, dopamine β-hydroxylase, and monoamine oxidase (Khan et al. 1986). A comparison study by Kelly and Cooper (1998) showed a gradient of plasma norepinephrine levels in which controls had the lowest levels, followed by increasing levels measured in patients with GAD, patients with depression, and patients with melancholia. Although only the plasma levels observed in patients with melancholia significantly exceeded those observed in controls, the results suggest at least some evidence for sympathetic hyperactivity in patients with GAD.

Interestingly, several studies have reported increased noradrenergic activity in patients with GAD. Sevy et al. (1989) found that patients with GAD had increased levels of plasma norepinephrine and its metabolite 3-methoxy-4-hydroxyphenylglycol (MHPG) relative to control subjects and patients with major depression. This study also found that in GAD, the number of α_2 adrenoreceptors was decreased, which implies possible chronic activation of this system. Levels of another norepinephrine metabolite, vanillylmandelic acid, also were increased in patients with GAD, and increases in urine excretion of this metabolite correlated with increased anxiety levels (Garvey et al. 1995). To better understand the role of norepinephrine in GAD, assessment of norepinephrine function in the central nervous system (CNS) has been necessary.

Most studies involving norepinephrine activity in the CNS have focused on the inhibitory α_2-adrenergic receptor. Inhibition of this presynaptic inhibitory receptor has the net result of increasing noradrenergic activity and anxiety behaviors in animals (Redmond 1987). Although human studies with the α_2-adrenergic antagonist yohimbine found that patients with panic disorder and posttraumatic stress disorder were abnormally sensitive to the drug, this finding did not generalize to GAD (Charney et al. 1989). Another set of studies used clonidine, an α_2-adrenergic receptor agonist that decreases locus coeruleus firing and has anxiolytic properties, and yohimbine to quantify the relative number of α_2-adrenergic receptors in patients with GAD and control subjects. Both of these studies were interested in the α_2 binding sites on platelets, which have many of the same receptors found in the CNS. These studies suggested that patients with GAD had fewer α_2-adrenergic receptors than did control subjects (Cameron et al. 1990; Sevy et al. 1989). Another study noted a blunted growth hormone response to clonidine in patients with GAD, suggesting that these patients have decreased postsynaptic α_2-adrenergic receptor sensitivity and that this may be attributable to a downregulation of α_2 receptors (Abelson et al. 1991; Schittecatte et al. 1995). This decrease in inhibitory receptors and receptor sensitivity suggests that GAD might be characterized by hyperactivity in the locus coeruleus and chronically elevated levels of the catecholamines (Sevy et al. 1989).

Serotonin

Another neurotransmitter implicated in the etiology of GAD is serotonin, which is widely distributed in the brain. Deakin and Graeff (1991) proposed that two distinct serotonergic routes arise from the dorsal raphe nucleus: 1) an "ascending" route that travels to the amygdala and frontal cortex is associated with conditioned fears, and serves as a model for GAD, and 2) a "descending" route that travels to the periaqueductal gray matter and is involved in unconditioned fears (e.g., panic). Following the GAD route, potentially threatening situations might increase synaptic serotonin, which would allow cortical and limbic regions to use this input to assess the situation and formulate a response (Handley 1995). However, studies with serotonin synthesis inhibitors, such as *p*-chlorophenylalanine (PCPA), have inconsistently indicated that these agents are anxiolytic and that decreased serotonergic activity also is associated with anxiety (Brody 1970; Geller and Blum 1970). Hence, serotonin levels in themselves may not explain the onset of anxiety.

Garvey et al. (1995) found that elevated urinary levels of the serotonin metabolite 5-hydroxyindoleacetic acid (5-HIAA) predicted higher anxiety levels in GAD, implying increased serotonin metabolism in anxious patients with GAD. Conversely, the serotonin synthesis inhibitor PCPA has been shown to be anxiogenic in humans, implying an association between decreased serotonin levels and anxiety. Because the relationship between serotonin levels and anxiety has been inconsistent, empirical attention has also focused on serotonin receptor subtypes. Preclinical trials have supported the role of 5-hydroxytryptamine (serotonin) receptor subtypes 5-HT_{2C} and 5-HT_{2A} in GAD (Khan et al. 1986). Furthermore, patients with GAD have shown hypersensitivity to the mixed postsynaptic 5-HT_2/5-HT_{2A} agonist/antagonist *m*-chlorophenylpiperazine (*m*-CPP; Germine et al. 1992).

Several serotonergic agents are efficacious in the treatment of GAD. Imipramine, trazodone, and venlafaxine inhibit the reuptake of serotonin and appear to be effective in treating GAD (Davidson 1998; Rickels et al. 1993). 5-HT_{1A} agonists, such as the partial agonist buspirone, also have been shown to be anxiolytic, and this anxiolysis appears to be associated with the serotonergic properties of the drugs (Eison et al. 1986; Taylor 1990). Moreover, despite having similar efficacy to benzodiazepines, buspirone does not impair cognition or psychomotor function, induce sedation or muscle relaxation, or cause physiological withdrawal (A.F. Jacobson et al. 1985; Laakmann et al. 1998; Pecknold et al. 1989). However, the 5-HT_3 antagonist ondansetron has demonstrated only limited efficacy in the treatment of GAD (Freeman et al. 1997). Preliminary data also show that atypical neuroleptics block 5-$HT_{2A/C}$ receptors (e.g., risperidone; Brawman-Mintzer et al. 2006). Hence, clinical studies in humans support the role of serotonin in GAD, although the exact etiological role of the neurotransmitter remains unclear. The finding of increased serotonin metabolites in patients with GAD supports a serotonin overactivation model of GAD, whereas similar findings with the serotonin synthesis inhibitor PCPA support a serotonin underactivation model of GAD.

Gamma-Aminobutyric Acid

Gamma-aminobutyric acid (GABA) is the primary inhibitory neurotransmitter in the CNS and is found in most parts of the brain. The benzodiazepines and anxiolytics that are agonists at the receptor-associated benzodiazepine site increase the affinity of GABA for its binding site and cause the $GABA_A$ receptor complex to be more responsive to available GABA. Farabollini et al. (1996) found that the number of benzodiazepine receptors in the hippocampus and cortex decreased in animals following stress. In humans, most work examining the relationship between GAD and GABA has focused on the effects of administering benzodiazepines. Because of the link between antianxiety treatments and GABA, the GABA-benzodiazepine system has been a logical focus of research into the pathophysiology of anxiety (Nutt 2001).

Patients with GAD appear to have a decreased density of platelet benzodiazepine binding sites, but the receptor density was found to have increased after chronic administration of diazepam (Weizman et al. 1987). Similar results have been found in studies of lymphocytes, in which benzodiazepine binding site density normalized in patients with GAD following diazepam treatment (Ferrarese et al. 1990; Rocca et al. 1991). However, peripheral and central benzodiazepine receptors are distinct, so it is difficult to conclude what significance to assign to findings in these studies (Brawman-Mintzer and Lydiard 1997). Central benzodiazepine receptor function can be studied by measuring the velocity of saccadic eye movements, which are under the control of central benzodiazepine receptors in the superior colliculus and pons. Patients with GAD have been shown to have a reduced sensitivity of saccadic eye movements, implying downregulation of these receptors (Cowley et al. 1991). However, this abnormality is nonspecific and is also found in patients with obsessive-compulsive disorder and panic disorder (Roy-Byrne et al. 1996). Another study of the central benzodiazepine receptors found that benzodiazepine binding is significantly decreased in the left temporal pole of patients with GAD, and the density distribution of these cerebral benzodiazepine receptors is more homogeneous than in control subjects (Tiihonen et al. 1997).

Thus, both preclinical and clinical data implicate decreased benzodiazepine function in GAD. This decrease is consistent with impairment in the capacity of patients with GAD to respond to endogenous anxiolytic ligands that activate the benzodiazepine receptor. Whether this is a state or trait abnormality is unknown. Therefore, atypical antipsychotics and some of the newer anticonvulsants have been suggested for the treatment of GAD, but the support for these approaches currently relies on anecdotal evidence and case reports (Gorman 2003). One agent, pregabalin, has been examined in controlled trials. Pande (2003), Rickels et al. (2005), and Montgomery et al. (2006) found that the anxiolytic effect of pregabalin was comparable to that of lorazepam in terms of both symptom reduction and speed of effect. Several other GABA-potentiating agents, including vigabatrin, topiramate, tiagabine, and gabapeptin, hold promise as anxiolytics. However, all are currently supported only by pilot data. Further assessment of the GABA neuronal system, molecular genetics, and neuroimaging techniques is warranted to determine the precise nature of GABA-related dysfunction in GAD.

Glutamate

Preclinical studies have shown that the amygdala plays a key role in fear circuitry and that its pathways can affect the acquisition and expression of fear conditioning (Garakani et al. 2006). The lateral amygdala seems to be responsible for key elements of fear conditioning (Blair et al. 2001; Shumyatsky et al. 2002), and disruptions of this area can interfere with the acquisition of conditioned fear and conditioned fear memories (Blair et al. 2005; Goosens and Maren 2001; Wallace and Rosen 2001). It has been proposed that this memory consolidation occurs when calcium enters the cell through *N*-methyl-D-aspartate (NMDA) receptors and through voltage-gated calcium channels (Bauer et al. 2002). Current application of these findings to humans is limited. Memantine, a noncompetitive NMDA receptor antagonist, is used to enhance memory in patients with Alzheimer's disease and has also been found to have anxiolytic properties in some animal studies (Bertoglio and Carobrez 2003, 2004) but not in others (B.H. Harvey et al. 2005; Karcz-Kubicha et al. 1997). However, studies of lamotrigine, a glutamate antagonist, found positive results (Hertzberg et al. 1999; Mizra et al. 2005; Rickels et al. 2005), leading to potential approval as an anxiolytic agent by the U.S. Food and Drug Administration. Glutamate may also play a key role in the extinction of fears through the activation of NMDA receptors in the amygdala. Partial NMDA agonists such as D-cycloserine have been shown to facilitate extinction (Ledgerwood et al. 2005; Walker et al. 2002). Because of these findings, glutamate has been further examined as a specific pathway in the treatment of GAD. For example, in an open-label trial of riluzole, glutamatergic agents were found to provide rapid anxiolytic effects (S.J. Mathew et al. 2005).

Cholecystokinin

Cholecystokinin (CCK) is one of the most abundant peptide neurotransmitters in the brain. A high density of cholecystokinin receptors is found in the hippocampus, the brain stem, and regions implicated in fear behavior in animals (i.e., limbic system, basal ganglia, and cortex). Of the several cholecystokinin peptides, the neurotransmitters CCK_4 and CCK_8 have been of most interest (Lydiard 1994). Two types of cholecystokinin receptors have been described: CCK_A, which is found in the viscera and some brain regions, and CCK_B, which is widely distributed in the brain and appears more directly involved in animal models of anxiety (Harro et al. 1993). CCK_B antagonists block the anxiogenic properties of cholecystokinin agonists in animal fear paradigms (Woodruff and Hughes 1991).

Studies of the CCK_B receptor have implicated it in the pathogenesis of anxiety. A CCK_B agonist, pentagastrin, induced a panic attack in 71% of patients with GAD versus 14% of controls (Brawman-Mintzer et al. 1995, 1997). This finding, however, is not specific because similar findings have been obtained in patients with panic disorder and social phobia, suggesting that cholecystokinin dysfunction may contribute to general anxiety proneness. Moreover, human studies of CCK_B antagonists in GAD have been disappointing. Receptor binding alone, however, does not convey the entire story. The administration of CCK_8 in animals stimulates the release of adrenocorticotropic hormone (ACTH) and cortisol (Kamilaris et al. 1992), and a study in humans found that these two stress reactants became elevated after administration of the mixed $CCK_{B/A}$ agonist pentagastrin (Abelson et al. 1994). However, increased CCK_8 binding is also associated with chronic treatment with diazepam, and CCK_8 may be involved in anxiety regulation but perhaps in an antagonistic manner to the role of CCK_4 (Harro et al. 1993). Thus, the cholecystokinin system appears to be involved early in the processes of anxiety induction.

The cholecystokinin system also may indirectly modulate anxiety in GAD through its interactions with other systems. For instance, cholecystokinin may contribute to anxiety through its influence on the noradrenergic system. Cholecystokinin activates neurons in the locus coeruleus via peripheral cholecystokinin receptors in vagal afferent pathways (Monnikes et al. 1997). Selective destruction of noradrenergic nerve terminals in the locus coeruleus results in an increased cholecystokinin receptor density in the frontal cortex and hippocampus, two regions that receive input from the locus coeruleus (Harro et al. 1993). In addition, the cholecystokinin system may influence anxiety through its interaction with the GABA system. Cholecystokinin is localized in GABA-synthesizing neurons in the cortex, hippocampus, and basolateral amygdala (Harro et al. 1993). Benzodiazepines selectively antagonize CCK_8-induced activation of rat hippocampal pyramidal cells, but the benzodiazepine antagonist flumazenil does not appear to antagonize the effect of CCK_4 in healthy subjects (Bradwejn et al. 1994). Bradwejn et al. (1994) theorized that both benzodiazepines and the cholecystokinin system act on GABA in opposing but separate mechanisms.

Hypocretins are recently discovered neuropeptides that originate in the hypothalamus with excitatory afferents to noradrenergic, serotonergic, and GABAergic neurons that increase corticotropin-releasing hormone secretion and that appear to have anxiolytic properties (Singareddy and Uhde 2006). Allopregnanolone is a neurosteroid that acts as a positive modulator of GABA receptors and is a powerful anxiolytic, anticonvulsant, and anesthetic agent. Griffin and Mellon (1999) reported that selective serotonin reuptake inhibitors (SSRIs), particularly fluoxetine, sertraline, and paroxetine, could alter concentrations of allopregnanolone in humans.

Neuropeptide Y is produced in the hypothalamus and plays a role in central regulation of the anterior pituitary and appetitive functions. Horvath et al. (1997) found that about one-third of the neuropeptide Y–producing arcuate nucleus perikarya co-expressed GABA, and proposed that this heterogeneity in the neuropeptide Y–producing perikarya of the hypothalamus may help explain some of the adverse effects seen in GAD. An examination of the possible import of this relationship was found when Guidi et al. (1999) examined neuropeptide Y plasma levels and immunological changes during stress. They found a significant negative correlation between measures of acute stress and lymphocyte proliferation, interleukin-2 production, and an increase in plasma cortisol levels. However, levels of neuropeptide Y did not differ from baseline.

Substance P is another target of investigation. Substance P facilitates the evoked release of glutamate and likely contributes to anxiety through ion channels (Maneuf et al. 2001). Studies of pregabalin found that substance P was significantly reduced, possibly through potent binding to the voltage-gated calcium channels (Pande et al. 2003), likely resulting in anxiolytic effects. Although several studies have suggested a role for substance P, its value as a therapeutic target remains unclear.

Endocrine Function

The multiple components of the endocrine system modulate the body's metabolism. One of the many roles of the endocrine system is to respond to stress and reestablish homeostasis; hence, the endocrine system, especially the hypothalamic-pituitary-adrenal (HPA) axis, has been a major interest with respect to human anxiety disorders such as GAD.

Corticotropin-releasing factor (CRF), which is released from the paraventricular nucleus of the hypothalamus, modulates ACTH release and has been implicated in stress and fear behaviors and cognitive responses to stress (Nemeroff 2004). Both acute and chronic stress increase CRF levels in the locus coeruleus and periventricular hypothalamic areas (P.D. Butler et al. 1990). CRF-secreting neurons are modulated by neurotransmitters such as norepinephrine and serotonin, which potentiate release of CRF. Rodents administered CRF decrease exploration and increase activities such as sniffing, indicating an increase in arousal (Chrousos and Gold 1992). In humans, however, cerebrospinal fluid levels of CRF are not significantly different among persons with GAD, panic disorder, obsessive-compulsive disorder, and no psychiatric diagnosis, suggesting that the three disorders have no tonic abnormality related to CRF secretion (Fossey et al. 1996). However, CRF may be episodically hypersecreted and may initiate fear responses in some contexts. Moreover, cerebrospinal fluid levels do not reflect localized CRF function in the brain, and these regional differences may be significant in anxiety disorders. The findings in animal studies support the role of CRF in the induction of anxiety, but human data have been negative thus far. Further studies in humans must be done before this agent is ruled out as a contributor to anxiety. The development of specific CRF-1 antagonists by industry may offer new tools to probe CRF in GAD and other disorders.

The stress reactant cortisol also has been a focus of research in GAD. Rosenbaum et al. (1983) found no significant difference in 24-hour urinary-free cortisol levels between patients with GAD and psychiatrically healthy control subjects. However, results from several other studies implied that patients with GAD have elevated cortisol levels. Between 27% and 38% of patients with GAD are nonsuppressors on the dexamethasone suppression test (Avery et al. 1985; Tiller et al. 1988). These findings must be viewed in light of the high comorbidity of GAD and depression because of the possibility that the combination provides a unique stress response in terms of ACTH and cortisol release (Young et al. 2004). Tiller et al.'s (1988) finding that patients with GAD reverted to suppressors after successful nondrug treatment (i.e., behavior therapy) of their GAD supports the view that patients with GAD have chronic hypercortisolemia. This finding is supported by the observation that rats exposed to chronic stress or exogenous steroids showed a decrease in hippocampal corticosteroid receptor density. Corticosteroid receptors in the hippocampus inhibit the secretion of stress-induced glucocorticoids by the HPA axis (L. Jacobson and Sapolsky 1991). Therefore, chronic stress leads to a heightened stress response to future dangers. In conclusion, the HPA axis appears overactivated in GAD and possibly plays a role in perpetuating the disorder.

Another endocrine system examined in relation to the pathogenesis of GAD is the thyroid axis. Patients with thyroid dyscrasias often present with anxiety that may be mistaken for GAD. However, thyroid function does not appear to differ between patients with and patients without GAD (Munjack and Palmer 1988), and the levels of thyrotropin-releasing factor do not appear to be significantly different between these groups (Fossey et al. 1993).

Carbon Dioxide and Lactate

When the body is faced with danger, one of the responses is hyperventilation. Adaptive reasons behind this reflex may be to exhale carbon dioxide (CO_2), induce a respiratory alkalosis, and compensate for the metabolic acidosis being created by rising levels of lactate. Clinical studies have shown that inducing these conditions by infusing lactate (Pitts and McClure 1967) or hyperventilating is panicogenic in anxiety patients (Bass et al. 1987). Patients who inhale CO_2 have similar results (Gorman et al. 1988). These anxiogenic techniques, therefore, can be useful tools in the study of anxiety disorders.

Both CO_2 and lactate are used to provoke anxiety symptoms and have played an important role in differentiating GAD from panic disorder. Results from studies by R.J. Mathew and Wilson (1987), Gorman et al. (1988), and Holt and Andrews (1989) indicate that many patients with panic disorder had panic attacks while inhaling 5% CO_2 but that patients with GAD did not. However, Verburg et al. (1995) found that when inhaling 35% CO_2, patients with GAD had less anxiety and fewer panic attacks than patients with panic disorder. Both groups had a similar increase in somatic symptoms. A study involving sodium lactate infusion found that patients with GAD were more likely than patients with panic disorder to report increased anxiety, although individuals with panic disorder continued to have a higher rate of panic attacks (Cowley et al. 1988). The results of these challenges show that GAD and panic disorder not only are discrete disorders but also share a common sensitivity to certain physiological stressors. These findings also imply that both of these disorders might derive from the dysregulation of a self-preservation response.

Neurophysiology

Physiological Parameters

GAD has been associated with alterations of respiratory and cardiovascular function. In a study by Hoehn-Saric et al. (1989), the resting respiratory rate, pulse rate, and blood pressure of women with GAD did not differ significantly from those of control subjects. This finding was supported by other data that showed that after the administration of yohimbine, patients and psychiatrically healthy controls had no differences in blood pressure or heart rate (Charney et al. 1989). However, another study reported that patients with GAD had lower systolic blood pressure than control subjects after standing (Cameron et al. 1990), suggesting that subtle autonomic dysfunction occurs in patients with GAD. In addition, Aström (1996) reported that worry shortens interbeat intervals recorded on electrocardiogram (ECG) and decreases the mean differences of cardiac interbeat differences. In this study, patients with GAD had shorter interbeat intervals on an ECG than did control subjects. Aström theorized that patients with

GAD have lowered cardiac vagal control. Whether this alteration is a cause or an effect of GAD is unclear, because, as in all biological studies of GAD, the study patient often enters the protocol already in an anxious state. In another paper, Brawman-Mintzer and Lydiard (1997) suggested that patients with GAD had autonomic inflexibility. The authors theorized that these patients have a weakened response to stress and require longer recovery from a stressor. Overall, the data support the idea that the chronic worry of GAD is accompanied by specific chronic alterations in the autonomic system.

Patients with GAD also have abnormal electroencephalographic (EEG) findings, which may imply a relationship to other syndromes. The EEG sleep profile of GAD indicates a decrease in slow-wave sleep (primarily stage 4) but none of the rapid eye movement (REM) sleep disturbances characteristic of major depression. This same sleep profile is seen in patients with dysthymia and may indicate a relationship between these two chronic disorders (Arriaga and Paiva 1990–1991). Notably, the low-voltage alpha-wave changes seen in many of the anxiety disorders, including GAD, occur in a variety of medical, neurological, and psychiatric disorders (Spiegel et al. 1986). The abnormal EEG profile observed in GAD therefore lacks the specificity to help define the disturbance.

Studies measuring other parameters have found other possible physiological differences in patients with GAD compared with healthy control subjects. Several studies have found an increased startle reflex in patients with posttraumatic stress disorder, and anecdotal evidence indicates that patients with GAD also exhibit this increased sensitivity (Grillon et al. 1997). The skin conductance of patients with GAD is similar to that of control subjects but takes longer to return to baseline following psychological stress (Hoehn-Saric et al. 1989), a finding that supports the autonomic inflexibility theory discussed in this section.

Neuroimaging Studies

Results from a number of studies have indicated no difference in baseline cerebral blood flow between patients with GAD and healthy controls (Drevets et al. 1997; Tiller et al. 1988). However, studies examining changes in blood flow tell a different story. Patients with left hemisphere lesions were likely to develop a combination of anxious and depressed symptoms, whereas patients with right hemisphere lesions developed only anxiety (Aström 1996). Positron emission tomography (PET) showed that anxiety scores correlated with changes in glucose metabolism in the limbic system and basal ganglia, although no significant difference was found between the right and left parahippocampal gyrus. PET scans of patients with GAD showed a relative increase in glucose metabolism in parts of the occipital, right posterior temporal lobe, left inferior gyrus, cerebellum, and right frontal gyrus, and a relative decrease in the basal ganglia, temporal lobe, and cingulate gyrus (Wu et al. 1991). In this same study, Wu et al. (1991) found that during vigilance tasks, patients with GAD had a relative increase in basal ganglia and right parietal metabolism, with decreased metabolism in the right temporal and occipital lobes. Benzodiazepine administration did not normalize this pattern; thus, stimulus processing may be dysfunctional in patients with GAD, contributing to the cognitive bias toward chronic worrying. In addition, studies of EEG patterns have supported the role of the centroparietal and occipital regions in anxiety (Grillon and Buchsbaum 1987). Thus, imaging studies imply that multiple regions of the brain contribute to GAD and that the basal ganglia and the occipital and temporal lobes have been implicated most consistently.

In a normal brain, function and blood flow are closely coupled, and increased arousal is associated with an increase in cerebral blood flow (R.J. Mathew et al. 1982b). Hence, patients with GAD might be expected to have abnormal increased cerebral blood flow. However, only one study found that people with low baseline anxiety had an increase in cerebral blood flow as their level of anxiety increased, whereas those with high baseline anxiety had a decrease in cerebral blood flow as they became more anxious, perhaps consistent with loss of the capacity to mount an adaptive stress response (Gur et al. 1987). Decreased cerebral blood flow with benzodiazepines has also been observed (R.J. Mathew and Wilson 1991), but this effect was more likely the result of decreased metabolic rates in the cortex, limbic system, and basal ganglia with these drugs (Wu et al. 1991).

Findings of a decrease in cerebral blood flow in anxiety patients under stress have been inconsistent, however. In an earlier study, R.J. Mathew et al. (1982b) found no differences in cerebral blood flow patterns between patients with GAD and controls. Later, R.J. Mathew and Wilson (1991) found that the decreases in cerebral blood flow in patients with GAD did not correlate with the patients' level of anxiety. Still later, they found that the response to CO_2 and epinephrine in patients with GAD distinguished their degree of cerebral blood flow from others. Those patients with the most severe anxious response to 5% CO_2 and epinephrine had less of an increase in cerebral blood flow than did those with less of an anxious response (R.J. Mathew et al. 1997). Similar to Brawman-Mintzer and Lydiard (1997), who introduced the autonomic inflexibility theory, R.J. Mathew et al. (1997) attributed this difference to the more severely anxious patients having a pronounced sympathetic response, which limits hypercapnic cerebral vasodilation. These findings support the view that cerebral blood flow may be altered in patients with GAD and that paradoxically these hyperaroused individuals have a decrease in blood flow during stress.

Imaging studies of GAD are still in their infancy but already show that a complex pattern of interactions occurs between brain regions in patients with GAD. The inconsistent findings of measures such as metabolic activity and blood flow across studies indicate that variables such as anxiety level at the time of the scan may have a profound effect. Another possibility is that the inconsistent participation of regions such as the occipital and left inferior frontal lobes reflects different manifestations of worry, such as visual versus verbal cues for anxiety. Also, differences of methods could be important in this newly developing field. Although a great deal remains to be learned, imaging studies have been fruitful in illustrating aberrant brain metabolism in patients with GAD. Possible future directions in neuroimaging include studying the sequence of metabolic changes in GAD, better delineating the quality of the anxiety state with the regions involved, and comparing pre- and posttreatment scans of patients receiving medications that work at different receptors.

Psychosocial Factors

Whatever role biology may hold in the hierarchy of contributors to GAD, the patient's own internal process, experience, and means of coping with a chronic state of anxiety certainly play a major role in maintaining, if not precipitating, this disorder. In this section, we highlight several findings about the life experiences, personality traits, cognitive processing, and coping skills of patients with GAD (note that psychodynamic theories are not discussed because Chapter 8 in this volume, "Psychodynamic Concepts of Anxiety," is dedicated to this subject). A unifying belief among many of the psychological theories of GAD is that dysfunctional worries can stem from early experience.

Childhood/Developmental Issues

Early life events have been linked to GAD when such experiences are traumatic or involve the need for vigilance against possible threats to the child and/or caregiver (Safren et al. 2002). *Behavioral inhibition* is defined as a tendency to be shy and timid in novel situations (Hirshfeld et al. 1992). Children with behavioral inhibition have higher rates of childhood anxiety disorders, and behavioral inhibition may also predict later anxiety disorders in adulthood (Rosenbaum et al. 1993). Although several authors have proposed theories of how childhood behavioral inhibition may manifest as an anxiety disorder in adulthood, additional longitudinal studies are needed to test these theories.

Some investigators have examined parenting factors in relation to GAD. Retrospective studies of adults with GAD have consistently found that they viewed their parents as rejecting and controlling, where *controlling* is defined as overinvolvement of a parent (Rapee 1997). The obvious limitation to these studies is that they were done retrospectively and may reflect more of the patients' perceptions of their childhoods than their actual experiences. However, psychiatric symptoms may be more significantly influenced by the perception than the realities of child rearing (Parker 1983). Studies in which anxious children are questioned about their parenting have had less consistent results, but other work indicates that anxious children's families are less cohesive and more enmeshed compared with control subjects' families (Rapee 1997). Rapee (1997) proposed that excessive protection from a parent conveys to the child that the world is a dangerous place and reduces the child's opportunity to explore and learn.

The effect of trauma and its possible contribution to GAD has been a subject of great interest. The idea that a child who experiences some catastrophic event will grow up more fearful and apprehensive than his or her peers seems intuitively plausible. However, not all studies support this. Raskin et al. (1982) found that patients with GAD and panic disorder did not differ from each other in the amount of childhood abuse or separation. This finding implies that traumatic events do not necessarily contribute to the development of chronic worry. However, Windle et al. (1995) found a significant association between physical and sexual abuse and the development of adult psychiatric disorders, particularly

GAD. The findings of these two studies are not necessarily contradictory in that other factors aside from the trauma may determine who will develop chronic anxiety and who will develop severe, episodic anxiety.

Personality

One perspective on GAD is to not view it as a disorder as much as a constellation of maladaptive personality traits. Trait anxiety could be defined as a relatively stable disposition to respond to a wide range of situations with state anxiety (Spielberger 1972). Some investigators argue that GAD can be considered to be a manifestation of a high-anxiety trait. The tendency to worry is highly correlated with trait anxiety (Borkovec et al. 1983) but not necessarily state anxiety (Saklofske and Eysenck 1983). Trait anxiety also is associated with an elevated estimate of threat (G. Butler and Mathews 1987)—a phenomenon with implications that are discussed below, in the section "Information Processing in Generalized Anxiety Disorder." Although Rapee (1985) stated that GAD arises from a trait disposition, he acknowledged that GAD in some cases does not occur until after childhood. He theorized that adult-onset anxiety arises from a life stressor causing anxiety characteristics to become more severe or from a change in life that might lead to attitude changes. He proposed that following an attitude change, what was once seen as a way of life could become viewed as a problem.

Thus, GAD could be envisioned as the result of a coping style that enlists high arousal and worry at the least amount of stress. These suggestions are bolstered by a study by Hettema et al. (2004) that found substantial overlap between genetic factors that influence neuroticism and GAD. Additionally, Massion et al. (2002) found that the presence of personality disorders predicted a 30% lower likelihood of remission in GAD. Patients with GAD appear to differ from others both in coping styles and in approach to potentially threatening situations.

In contrast to the disease model of GAD, the model described in this section suggests that GAD can be best explained by shared personality traits that reflect longstanding characteristics of individuals with GAD. A weakness of this theory is that these studies have observed a limited number of characteristics and assumed that the unique features seen in patients with GAD explain the etiology of the disorder when, in fact, these same characteristics could have been a consequence of the disorder.

Cognitive-Behavioral Theory

Cognitive-behavioral theory proposes that patients with GAD have developed a set of catastrophic automatic thoughts that are self-reinforcing and prevent the person from approaching novel situations without great trepidation. The patient's focus of worries cascades, and the person finds it progressively harder to cope with his or her concerns about the future. Worry is an understandable reaction to the possibility of future danger and may be reinforced as a coping behavior. However, the anxious patient overestimates the probability and severity of feared events, and this overestimation is responsible for maintaining the anxiety disorder and creating unnecessary avoidance. The anxious patient overattends to potentially threatening stimuli, and this biased attention propagates his or her feeling of being in danger. Patients engage in avoidance or escape behaviors, which prevent them from encountering evidence that would contradict their pessimistic predictions; thus, patients continue to hold these beliefs (D.M. Clark 1988). Although selective attention to emotionally laden material may be characteristic of a normal state of heightened arousal, in anxiety disorders, the attention appears to be more intensely focused and often centers on some idiosyncratic belief (Martin et al. 1991). Thus, selectively focusing on threatening stimuli propagates the symptoms of GAD.

Other theorists have emphasized the role of automatic cognitions in anxiety and mood disorders (Beck et al. 1985). These automatic cognitions are recurrent thoughts that the patient either has throughout the day or reverts to in stressful situations. Beck proposed that these automatic cognitions involve anticipated harm or danger to personal domain. In depressed patients, these thoughts tend to focus on loss or failures (Beck et al. 1987), whereas in anxious patients, these automatic thoughts tend to be more situational, future oriented, and probabilistic (Beck and Clark 1988). These cognitions about harm and danger are particularly predictive of developing anxiety (D.A. Clark et al. 1989).

The cognitive-behavioral perspective proposes that patients with GAD selectively focus and ruminate on potentially threatening situations and, therefore, these patients should improve if these ruminations are challenged and if the patient is educated about the inaccuracy of the level of danger perceived in a situation. Cognitive-behavioral treatment for GAD has been shown to improve symptoms of the disorder and is based on the idea that automatic pessimistic thoughts are a mechanism by which the chronic worry of GAD persists

(A.G. Harvey and Rapee 1995). Although this theory does not explain what leads to the development of these ruminations, it does provide an effective, theory-driven model for treating the symptoms of GAD.

Information Processing

One role of the brain is to filter out unnecessary information and to develop a memory based on the remaining data. In the previous section, on cognitive-behavioral theory, we focused on how anxious patients appear to overfocus on anxious memories. However, another approach would be to determine how anxious patients process information. Information-processing theories of anxiety disorders are concerned with which data are not filtered out and how that leads to the development of anxious memories.

Patients with GAD appear to process threatening information differently from other people in that they have an apparent memory bias for mood-congruent threat information (Coles et al. 2007). Studies found that patients with GAD allocate extensive attentional resources to threatening stimuli and detect such information rapidly and effectively (MacLeod et al. 1986). One study found that patients with GAD consistently write down the threatening version of a homophone (e.g., "die" instead of "dye"), and this tendency to use the threatening spelling correlated with trait but not state anxiety (Mathews et al. 1989). In a study by Mogg et al. (1987), control subjects and patients with GAD were asked to memorize a word list and later recall it. Patients with GAD tended not to remember the threatening words, suggesting that some inhibitory process interfered with proper storage of memory of threat. Mathews et al. (1989) argued that this inhibitory processing may be somewhat voluntary and helps to prevent extensive elaboration. In this same paper, the authors reported that trait anxiety is not correlated with threat bias on word stem completion tasks but is correlated with threat bias on cued recall. Finally, Coles et al. (2007) found significant differences in self-selected word lists generated by patients with GAD and by control subjects, as well as evidence of an explicit memory bias for threat words. These findings suggest that patients with GAD allocate extensive attentional resources to potential threats, so even ambiguous conditions are more likely to be interpreted as threatening.

Barlow (1988) proposed another model of attentional narrowing in anxiety disorders. He suggested that negative life events trigger stress-related neurobiological reactions. This process leads the person to focus on life events, even minor ones, and to react to these events with negative affect. This negative affect derives from stress-related neurobiological reactions and a belief that events are proceeding in an unpredictable fashion. This, in turn, leads the person to shift his or her focus from the task at hand to self-evaluation, which only leads to further arousal. The person begins a spiral of further vigilance and narrowing of attention to the focus of concern and his or her inability to cope with it. This theory is supported by a finding that erroneous interpretation of information correlates with the pathogenic effect of cholecystokinin in anxious patients (Alouja et al. 1997). However, other studies do not support this theory. Lack of control alone appears to be insufficient to develop distress (England and Dickerson 1988). Rapee (1991) theorized that the coupling of this lack of control with a focus on potential threats leads to distress in patients with GAD. What both of these theories support, however, is that the symptoms of GAD are potentiated by a persistent focus on worries.

In summary, patients with GAD appear to both attend to and process information in a manner that potentiates, and possibly initiates, the disorder. This relatively new area of research may be a fertile link between the previously discussed biological findings and the clinical presentation of GAD.

Affect Theory

As discussed earlier in this chapter, patients with GAD often have mood disorders as well. The distinction between mood and anxiety symptoms can often be blurred, and these two categories of disorders may share a similar etiological basis. Therefore, another hypothesis to explain the etiology of GAD proposes that this syndrome is a disorder of affect.

Watson and Tellegen (1985) proposed a two-dimensional model of affect composed of positive and negative affect. They defined *positive affect* as the extent to which a person feels a zest for life and *negative affect* as the extent to which a person feels upset or unpleasantly aroused. Their theory holds that people with high negative affect experience more negative emotion and have negative views of the world, causing them to focus on negative aspects of self, others, and the world. Those with negative affect also ruminate about their mistakes and failures. Watson et al. (1988) argued that anxious patients have a high degree of negative affect, and their degree of positive affect fails to play the sort of role that it plays in depression, in which the low positive and high negative affects result in this disorder. Tellegen (1985), however, proposed that both disorders result from an aberration of negative affect. If the negative affect has a strong fear component, the person will become anxious, and if sadness and fatigue are more evident, then depression will develop. This fear component also can be conceptualized as an "orienting or questioning mode," which leads the anxious person to focus on the uncertainties of future events and circumstances. These theories share a good deal in common with cognitive-behavioral models and likely have similar clinical implications.

Avoidance Theory

The hallmark feature of GAD is worry, which has been hypothesized to be the key functional feature that underpins biases in information processing, memory, problem solving, and interpretation of ambiguity. Although worry is not unique to GAD, the use of worry as a mechanism of avoidance may be what sets GAD apart, because worry is the primary strategy to avoid negative affect and feeds the broad domains in which biases are exhibited (Aikins and Craske 2001). Indeed, Borkovec et al. (2004) proposed that when a human anticipates a significant problem, he or she will be highly motivated to solve it, and that worry is a highly evolved ability to adapt to future dangers.

According to learning theory, individuals develop anxiety to nonthreatening situations because of punishment associated with past experiences involving those situations. Indeed, Mowrer's (1947) two-stage theory of fear states that fear is gained through classical conditioning and then maintained through operantly conditioned avoidance. This simple proposition actually forms the basis for modern cognitive-behavioral therapeutic approaches, which attempt to alter existing reactions to feared stimuli and to exhaust the fear value of those stimuli through repeated exposures. However, this approach has been less successful in treating GAD, where the cues are diffuse rather than discrete. Bandura (1969) argued that the reason for this lack of success is that the fear cues are internal and the avoidance of internal fear cues might well play a role in the maintenance of anxiety. This suggestion was supported by a study that found that attention deployed toward or away from anxiety-provoking stimuli during exposure treatment significantly influenced the rate of between-session extinction (Grayson 1982).

Worry as a mechanism of avoidance was further supported by a study that found a significant difference in cognition between patients with GAD and control subjects during relaxation (Freeston et al. 1994). Subjects with GAD reported much higher levels of thought and much lower levels of imagery than control subjects. However, when fear-inducing topics were used in relaxation sessions, control subjects also used more thought and less imagery. Avoidance theory argues that when aversive images occur or when threatening stimuli are detected, the shifting of attention to worrisome thinking results in escape or avoidance of the fear response (Borkovec et al. 2004). In other words, worry is an attempt to avoid the feared images or stimuli themselves, as well as to avoid unpleasant somatic responses that would otherwise be elicited. Such a response would make classic extinction of fears impossible and would explain both the propagation and maintenance of anxiety in persons with GAD.

Self-Efficacy

Implicit in the act of worrying is the belief that the focus of concern is so overwhelming that it is beyond one's ability to cope. Earlier in this chapter, in "Cognitive-Behavioral Theory," we discussed how patients with GAD selectively attend to and process stressful stimuli. However, the degree to which someone worries about a particular stressor is subjective. The level of threat may be determined not only by the stimuli and how they are processed but also by how well the person believes he or she can cope with the situation. Self-efficacy is concerned with the patient's beliefs about his or her ability to exercise control over events. In a disorder in which worry is the cardinal symptom, GAD may result from low self-efficacy.

Self-doubt may underlie many of the symptoms of GAD. Individuals who doubt their capability to complete a task have reduced effort and often settle prematurely on mediocre solutions, thereby reinforcing their belief that they could not adequately handle the situation (Bandura 1989). Bandura (1989) also noted that those who believe that they are incapable of managing threatening situations tend to perceive the situation as more perilous than it is and to dwell on their own inadequacies to deal with it. This reaction leads to higher levels of stress and anxiety. In anxious patients, the perception of self-efficacy is closely related to the degree of distress in a given situation (Kent and Gibbons 1987). These findings suggest that GAD may be a disorder of self-efficacy.

The phenomenon of relaxation-induced anxiety also might be explained by the GAD patient's low self-efficacy. Heide and Borkovec (1984) used the term *relaxation-induced anxiety* to describe the finding that techniques such as progressive relaxation, biofeedback, and meditation can initiate or exacerbate anxiety in some individuals. These authors theorized that because generalized anxiety states result from a fear of loss of control, relaxation techniques that entail relinquishing this control leave the anxious person without whatever active coping skills he or she had developed. The same coping skills, however, may be the source of the constant tension and anxiety experienced by those with GAD. Interestingly, Heide and Borkovec found that the specific techniques that provoked relaxation-induced anxiety differed among individuals. Therefore, GAD not only might be a disorder of poor self-efficacy but also might stem from maladaptive coping strategies.

Etiological Models

Both biological and psychosocial factors appear to contribute to the development and maintenance of GAD. Although much of the prior discussion seems to argue against a single explanatory model for GAD, the nature of GAD as the "basic" anxiety disorder has led to attempts to develop conceptual models to facilitate further research and treatment. Indeed, Barlow (1988) termed this fundamental process "anxious apprehension," which refers to a mood state in which one prepares to cope with upcoming negative events and that is associated with high negative affect, chronic hyperarousal, a lack of control, and an attentional bias toward threat-related stimuli. The primary features of GAD are considered dimensions of vulnerability in etiological models (L.A. Clark et al. 1994). Kendler (1996) suggested that events involving danger are distinctly associated with developing anxiety; in contrast, facing great loss is associated with developing depression.

An alternative theory integrating this information hypothesizes a behavioral inhibition system (Gray 1988). This theory proposes that the septohippocampal area is responsible for processing threat-relevant stimuli. The presence of danger activates the behavioral inhibition system, resulting in increased arousal and inhibition of all regular behaviors. Noradrenergic and serotonergic stimulation of the septohippocampal region further activates this system. Gray proposed that this increased state of vigilance is analogous to GAD. Therefore, drugs that reduce noradrenergic or serotonergic input into the septohippocampal area will treat anxiety. A weakness of this theory is that some drugs that have been helpful in the treatment of GAD, such as buspirone and the SSRIs, increase serotonin function with chronic administration.

A model of anxiety proposed by Goddard and Charney (1997) focuses on the central role of the amygdala in the regulation of anxiety. Electrical stimulation of the amygdala elicits fearlike behaviors in animals and is associated with severe physiological changes consistent with anxiety (Kaada 1972). Anatomically, the amygdala's extensive network of afferent and efferent pathways provides access to the other areas of the brain involved with anxiety. This theory proposes that sensory input is processed in the cortices, entorhinal cortex, limbic area (amygdala and hippocampus), and brain stem structures (nucleus paragigantocellularis and locus coeruleus). Threatening stimuli are processed in the context of past and present experiences, and the processing areas of the orbitofrontal cortex and the amygdala choose an anxiety response. Next, this response is implemented by the locus coeruleus, hippocampus, dorsal motor nucleus of the vagus, parabrachial nucleus, trigeminal nucleus, facial motor nucleus, striatum, and periaqueductal gray. The strength of this theory is its ability to integrate the numerous areas implicated in the development of anxiety. A limitation is that it fails to address which factors predispose someone to a specific disorder. However, additional research into the role of specific neural structures is required before this question can be answered. The amygdala model of anxiety, however, offers a model by which the neural structures initiate and propagate anxiety disorders.

Cloninger (1986) proposed a model in which inherited abnormalities in neurotransmitter systems cause personality traits that could manifest as GAD. Cloninger focused on three aspects of personality—novelty seeking, harm avoidance, and reward dependence—that he argued are determined by monoamine activity. Several studies support the idea that novelty seeking is associated with low basal dopaminergic activity, harm avoidance is seen in individuals with high serotonergic activity, and reward dependence results from low basal noradrenergic activity (Cloninger 1986). Cloninger used the Tridimensional Personality Questionnaire to draw several conclusions about the relationship of these traits and the development of chronic anxiety. In particular, he hypothesized that extremely high or low levels of harm avoidance predispose individuals to chronic anxiety because low harm avoidance increases the risk of aversive events (such as trauma), and the person learns that the world is not a safe place; whereas high harm avoidance predisposes individuals to overestimate risk and leads them to constantly perceive danger. Cloninger further suggested that specific combinations of these traits led to "somatic anxiety" or "cognitive anxiety." Those with somatic anxiety have high novelty seeking but not harm avoidance, whereas those with cognitive anxiety have low novelty seeking and low reward dependence. Cloninger proposed that GAD is the result of chronic cognitive anxiety. In one study, harm avoidance was slightly elevated and reward dependence slightly lowered in patients with GAD, but their novelty seeking was not different from that of control subjects (Starcevic et al. 1996). This assertion is also supported by a study that found an association between a polymorphism in a region that regulates the expression of the serotonin transporter and anxiety-related personality traits, particularly harm avoidance (Lesch et al. 1996). Assuming that Cloninger's ideas about specific monoamines being associated with traits are correct, this study supports the idea that norepinephrine and serotonin play some role in GAD, whereas dopamine does not.

Both Barlow (1988) and Borkovec (1994) suggested that early experiences of uncontrollability represent a psychological vulnerability in that childhood histories of trauma and insecure attachment may be very important. Borkovec (1991, 1994) proposed the most widely recognized psychosocial model of GAD in which he regarded worry as a mostly conceptual but also verbal/behavioral attempt to avoid future aversive events and imagery. This process is experienced by the person with GAD as both negative and uncontrollable, and is associated with perceptions that the world is dangerous and that the individual may not be able to cope. Several studies have confirmed that worry is associated with high levels of thought and low levels of imagery, but Borkovec further asserted that worry itself is negatively reinforcing because it is associated with the avoidance of even more threatening images or somatic responses (Brown et al. 2001). According to Borkovec et al.'s (2004) model, worry provides short-term relief from more distressing levels of anxiety but has long-term consequences in the form of emotional and behavioral inhibition and the persistence of anxiety-producing cognitions. Therefore, the avoidant nature of worry hinders effective problem solving of real concerns, but because the worry is perceived as uncontrollable, the person with GAD is caught in increasing negative affect and cognitive intrusions. This leads to the pathological nature of the worry and the functional consequences associated with the disorder.

Clearly, several lines of thought have generated a variety of models that to a greater or lesser extent include the biological and psychosocial underpinnings of GAD. However, none of the current models provides an overarching description of the process that leads from genetics through early life experiences and into later patterns of physiological and cognitive response that results in generalized anxiety. Much work continues as the relationships between and transitions from various etiological components of generalized anxiety disorder are explored.

Conclusion

GAD is characterized by chronic worry and somatic tension. In this chapter, we explored the range of biological and psychosocial theories and integrated these ideas into potential etiological models to explain the development and maintenance of this disorder. Biological factors seem to play a significant role in GAD. Genetic factors appear to predispose individuals to the development of GAD but do not yet account for all cases. Several studies have found aberrations in the norepinephrine system, suggestive of norepinephrine overactivity in GAD. The serotonin system also has been an area of interest. GABA plays a significant regulatory role throughout the brain, and its role in the release of several neurotransmitters (including cholecystokinin) may be important in the initiation and propagation of GAD. The cholecystokinin system also may be involved early in the induction of anxiety and potentially acts on the GABA system in a way that opposes benzodiazepines. Patients with GAD appear to have other pathophysiological lesions as well. The HPA axis tends to be overactivated in GAD, whereas the thyroid axis appears unaffected. These patients also have shorter interbeat variability on ECG, which may be the result of an inflexible response to stress and a requirement for a prolonged time to recover from a stressor. Neuroimaging studies also demonstrate differences between patients with GAD and control subjects.

Psychosocial factors such as child rearing, trauma, temperament, and information processing may play roles in the initiation and propagation of this disorder. Inasmuch as GAD is influenced by both biological and psychosocial factors, several authors have proposed models that combine these facets. Barlow (2000) proposed that negative life events lead to neurobiological reactions, which lead to anxious patients who limit their focus to only potentially threatening stimuli. Kendler (1996) theorized that major depression and anxiety have identical genetic causes and that significant life events determine which disorder will develop. Gray (1988) proposed a behavioral inhibition system, which theorizes that anxiety results when norepinephrine and serotonin overstimulate the septohippocampal region. Charney et al. (1989) proposed that the amygdala is the central structure in anxiety and that stimuli are processed and cognitively responded to via pathways that all communicate with the amygdala. Cloninger (1986) proposed a set of neurochemically driven personality traits that, in concert, lead to the development of GAD. Finally, Borkovec (1983) proposed a model of worry as a means of avoidance that allows a person to cope with short-term discomforts at the cost of ongoing anxiety and the inability to generate meaningful responses to many more difficult situations. At this point, none of these models can sufficiently explain the development of GAD. More research is required in the genetics, biochemistry, anatomy, stimulus processing, and premorbid history of GAD before a more definitive model can be generated.

◀ Key Clinical Points ▶

- Generalized anxiety disorder is a relatively new diagnostic category, having been formalized in DSM-III. Although some controversy remains about the validity of this category versus trait conceptions of anxiety, the development of the diagnostic construct GAD has facilitated studies into its epidemiology and etiopathogenesis. GAD has since been determined to be a high-prevalence, chronic anxiety syndrome with morbidity and illness burden that approximate levels seen in major depressive disorder.
- Biological factors have been implicated in the pathogenesis of GAD. Family and twin studies indicate that genetic factors account for 30%–40% of the variance of causative factors contributing to the genesis of GAD. Neurochemical and imaging studies have implicated dysregulation in the serotonin, norepinephrine, GABA, glutamatergic, and peptide (corticotropin-releasing factor, cholecystokinin, neuropeptide Y) transmitter systems in the pathophysiology of GAD. Components of the human fear circuit that may be of particular relevance to GAD include the medial prefrontal cortex (subserving fear extinction processes), the amygdala (risk assessment processing), the bed nucleus of the stria terminalis (implicated in contextual fear), and the insula cortex (an area integrating interoceptive stimuli).
- Antecedent psychosocial risk factors for adult GAD include behavioral inhibition in childhood, high trait neuroticism, and high levels of obsessive-compulsive personality traits. More recent psychological theories of GAD have underscored the role of worry as a defensive coping strategy (affect avoidance), the contribution of cognitive bias to threat stimuli, and the role of deficits in self-efficacy resulting in exaggerated self-doubt.

References

Abelson JL, Glitz D, Cameron OG, et al: Blunted growth hormone response to clonidine in patients with generalized anxiety disorder. Arch Gen Psychiatry 25:141–152, 1991

Abelson JL, Nesse RM, Vinik AL: Pentagastrin infusions in patients with panic disorder, II: neuroendocrinology. Biol Psychiatry 36:84–96, 1994

Aikins DE, Craske MG: Cognitive theories of generalized anxiety disorder. Psychiatr Clin North Am 24:57–74, 2001

Alouja A, Shlik J, Vasar V, et al: Emotional and cognitive factors connected with response to cholecystokinin tetrapeptide in healthy volunteers. Psychiatry Res 66:59–67, 1997

American Psychiatric Association: Diagnostic and Statistical Manual of Mental Disorders, 3rd Edition. Washington, DC, American Psychiatric Association, 1980

Andrews G, Stewart S, Allen R, et al: The genetics of six neurotic disorders: a twin study. J Affect Disord 19:23–29, 1990

Arriaga F, Paiva T: Clinical and EEG sleep changes in primary dysthymia and generalized anxiety: a comparison with normal subjects. Neuropsychobiology 24:109–114, 1990–1991

Aston-Jones G, Rajkowski J, Kubiak P: Conditioned responses of monkey locus coeruleus neurons anticipate acquisition of discriminative behavior in a vigilance task. Neuroscience 80:697–715, 1997

Aström M: Generalized anxiety disorder in stroke patients: a 3-year longitudinal study. Stroke 27:270–275, 1996

Avery DH, Osgodd TB, Ishiki DM, et al: The DST in psychiatric outpatients with generalized anxiety disorder, panic disorder, or primary affective disorder. Am J Psychiatry 142:844–848, 1985

Bandura A: Principles of Behavior Modification. New York, Holt, Rinehart & Winston, 1969

Bandura A: Human agency in social cognitive theory. Am Psychol 44:1175–1184, 1989

Barlow DH: Anxiety and Its Disorders: The Nature and Treatment of Anxiety and Panic. New York, Guilford Press, 1988

Barlow DH: Unraveling the mysteries of anxiety and its disorders from the perspective of emotion theory. Am Psychol 55:1247–1263, 2000

Bass C, Kartsounis L, Lelliott P: Hyperventilation and its relation to anxiety and panic. Integr Psychiatry 5:274–282, 1987

Bauer EP, Schafe GE, LeDoux JE: NMDA receptors and L-type voltage-gated calcium channels contribute to long-term potentiation and different components of fear memory formation in the lateral amygdala. J Neurosci 22:5239–5249, 2002

Beck AT, Clark CA: Anxiety and depression: an information processing perspective. Anxiety Research 1:23–36, 1988

Beck AT, Emery G, Greenberg RL: Anxiety Disorders and Phobias: A Cognitive Perspective. New York, Basic Books, 1985

Bertoglio LJ, Carobrez AP: Anxiolytic-like effects of NMDA/glycine-B receptor ligands are abolished during the elevated plus-maze trial 2 in rats. Psychopharmacology 170:335–342, 2003

Bertoglio LJ, Carobrez AP: Scopolamine given pre-Trial 1 prevents the one-trial tolerance phenomenon in the elevated plus-maze Trial 2. Behav Pharmacol 15:45–54, 2004

Blair HT, Schafe GE, Bauer EP, et al: Synaptic plasticity in the lateral amygdala: a cellular hypothesis of fear conditioning. Learn Mem 8:229–242, 2001

Blair HT, Sotres-Bayon F, Moita MA, et al: The lateral amygdala processes the value of conditioned and unconditioned aversive stimuli. Neuroscience 133:561–569, 2005

Borkovec TD: The nature, functions, and origins of worry, in Worrying: Perspectives in Theory, Assessment, and Treatment. Edited by Davey GCL, Tallis F. New York, Wiley, 1994, pp 5–34

Borkovec TD, Robinson E, Pruzinsky T, et al: Preliminary exploration of worry: some characteristics and processes. Behav Res Ther 21:9–16, 1983

Borkovec TD, Shadick RN, Hopkins M: The nature of normal versus pathological worry, in Chronic Anxiety and Generalized Anxiety Disorder. Edited by Rapee R, Barlow DH. New York, Guilford, 1991, pp 29–51

Borkovec TD, Alcaine O, Behar E: Avoidance theory of worry and generalized anxiety disorder, in Generalized Anxiety Disorder: Advances in Research and Practice. Edited by Heimberg RG, Turk CL, Mennin DS. New York, Guilford, 2004, pp 77–108

Bradwejn J, Koszycki D, Couetoux du Tertre A, et al: Effects of flumazenil on cholecystokinin-tetrapeptide-induced panic symptoms in healthy volunteers. Psychopharmacology 114:257–261, 1994

Brawman-Mintzer O, Lydiard RB: Biological basis of generalized anxiety disorder. J Clin Psychiatry 58 (suppl 3):16–25; discussion 26, 1997

Brawman-Mintzer O, Lydiard RB, Crawford MM, et al: Somatic symptoms in generalized anxiety disorder with and without comorbid psychiatric disorders. Am J Psychiatry 151:930–932, 1994

Brawman-Mintzer O, Lydiard RB, Villarreal G, et al: Biological findings in GAD: CCK B agonist challenge. Paper presented at the 15th national conference of the Anxiety Disorders Association of America, Pittsburgh, PA, April 1995

Brawman-Mintzer O, Lydiard RB, Bradwejn J, et al: Effects of the cholecystokinin agonist pentagastrin in patients with generalized anxiety disorder. Am J Psychiatry 154:700–702, 1997

Brawman-Mintzer O, Knapp RG, Nietert PJ: Adjunctive risperidone in generalized anxiety disorder: a double-blind, placebo-controlled study. J Clin Psychiatry 66:1321–1325, 2005

Brody JF Jr: Behavioral effects of serotonin depletion and of p-chlorophenylalanine (a serotonin depletory) in rats. Psychopharmacologia 17:14–33, 1970

Brown TA, O'Leary TA, Barlow DH: Clinical Handbook of Psychological Disorders: A Step-by-Step Treatment Manual, 3rd Edition. New York, Guilford, 2001

Butler G, Mathews A: Anticipatory anxiety and risk perception. Cognit Ther Res 11:551–565, 1987

Butler PD, Nemeroff CB, Chappel PB: Corticotropin-releasing factor as a possible cause of comorbidity in anxiety and depressive disorders, in Comorbidity of Mood and Anxiety Disorders. Edited by Mader JD, Cloninger CR.

Washington, DC, American Psychiatric Press, 1990, pp 413–435

Cameron OG, Smith CB, Lee MA, et al: Adrenergic status in anxiety disorders: platelet alpha 2-adrenergic receptor binding, blood pressure, pulse, and plasma catecholamines in panic and generalized anxiety disorder patients and in normal subjects. Biol Psychiatry 28:3–20, 1990

Charney DS, Woods SW, Heninger GR: Noradrenergic function in generalized anxiety disorder: effects of yohimbine in healthy subjects and patients with generalized anxiety disorder. Psychiatry Res 27:173–182, 1989

Chrousos GP, Gold PW: The concepts of stress and stress system disorders: overview of physical and behavioral homeostasis. JAMA 267:1244–1252, 1992

Clark DA, Beck AT, Brown G: Cognitive mediation in general psychiatric outpatients: a test of the content-specificity hypothesis. J Pers Soc Psychol 56:958–964, 1989

Clark DM: A cognitive model of panic, in Panic: Psychological Perspectives. Edited by Rachman S, Majer J. Hillsdale, NJ, Erlbaum, 1988, pp 71–89

Clark LA, Watson D, Mineka S: Temperament, personality, and the mood and anxiety disorders. J Abnorm Psychol 103:103–116, 1994

Cloninger CR: A unified biosocial theory of personality and its role in the development of anxiety states. Psychiatr Dev 3:167–226, 1986

Coles ME, Turk CL, Heimberg RG: Memory bias for threat in generalized anxiety disorder: the potential importance of stimulus relevance. Cogn Behav Ther 36:65–72, 2007

Cowley DS, Dager SR, McClellan J, et al: Response to lactate infusion in generalized anxiety disorder. Biol Psychiatry 24:409–414, 1988

Cowley DS, Roy-Byrne PP, Hommer D, et al: Benzodiazepine sensitivity in anxiety disorders. Biol Psychiatry 29:57A, 1991

Davidson JRT: Alternative treatments for anxiety: an introduction and overview. Paper presented at the annual meeting of the Anxiety Disorders Association of America, Boston, MA, April 1998

Deakin JF, Graeff FG: 5-HT and mechanisms of defence. J Psychopharmacol 5:305–315, 1991

Drevets WC, Price JL, Simpson JR Jr, et al: Subgenual prefrontal cortex abnormalities in mood disorders. Nature 386:824–827, 1997

Eison AS, Eison MS, Stanley M, et al: Serotonergic mechanisms in the behavioral effects of buspirone and gepirone. Pharmacol Biochem Behav 24:701–707, 1986

England S, Dickerson M: Intrusive thoughts: unpleasantness not the major cause of uncontrollability. Behav Res Ther 26:279–282, 1988

Farabollini F, Fluck E, Albonetti ME, et al: Sex differences in benzodiazepine binding in the frontal cortex and amygdala of the rat 24 hours after restraint stress. Neurosci Lett 218:177–180, 1996

Ferrarese C, Appollonio I, Frigo M, et al: Decreased density of benzodiazepine receptors in lymphocytes of anxious patients: reversal after chronic diazepam treatment. Acta Psychiatr Scand 82:169–173, 1990

Fossey MD, Lydiard RB, Ballenger JC, et al: Cerebrospinal fluid thyrotropin-releasing hormone concentrations in patients with anxiety disorders. J Neuropsychiatry Clin Neurosci 5:335–337, 1993

Fossey MD, Lydiard RB, Ballenger JC, et al: Cerebrospinal fluid corticotrophin-releasing factor concentrations in patients with anxiety disorders and normal comparison subjects. Biol Psychiatry 39:703–707, 1996

Freeman AM 3rd, Westphal JR, Norris GT, et al: Efficacy of ondansetron in the treatment of generalized anxiety disorder. Depress Anxiety 5:140–141, 1997

Freeston MH, Rheaume J, Letarte H, et al: Why do people worry? Pers Individ Dif 17:791–802, 1994

Garakani A, Mathew SJ, Charney DS: Neurobiology of anxiety disorders and implications for treatment. Mt Sinai J Med 73:941–949, 2006

Garvey MJ, Noyes R Jr, Woodman C, et al: The association of urinary 5-hydroxyindoleacetic acid and vanillylmandelic acid in patients with generalized anxiety. Neuropsychobiology 31:6–9, 1995

Geller I, Blum K: The effects of t-HTP on para-chlorophenylalanine (p-CPA) attenuation of conflict behavior. Eur J Pharmacol 9:319–324, 1970

Germine M, Goddard AW, Woods SW, et al: Anger and anxiety responses to m-chlorophenylpiperazine in generalized anxiety disorder. Biol Psychiatry 32:457–461, 1992

Goddard AW, Charney DS: Toward an integrated neurobiology of panic disorder. J Clin Psychiatry 58 (suppl 2):4–11, 1997

Goosens KA, Maren S: Contextual and auditory fear conditioning are mediated by the lateral, basal, and central amygdaloid nuclei in rats. Learn Mem 8:148–155, 2001

Gorman JM: New molecular targets for antianxiety interventions. J Clin Psychiatry 64 (suppl 3):28–35, 2003

Gorman JM, Fyer MR, Goetz R, et al: Ventilatory physiology of patients with panic disorder. Arch Gen Psychiatry 45:31–39, 1988

Gray JA: The neurobiological basis of anxiety, in Handbook of Anxiety Disorder. Edited by Last CG, Hersen M. New York, Pergamon, 1988, pp 10–37

Grayson JB, Foa EB, Steketee G: Habituation during exposure treatment: distraction vs. attention-focusing. Behav Res Ther 20:323–328, 1982

Griffin LD, Mellon SH: Selective serotonin reuptake inhibitors directly alter activity of neurosteroidogenic enzymes. Proc Natl Acad Sci USA 96:13512–13517, 1999

Grillon C, Buchsbaum MS: EEG topography of response to visual stimuli in generalized anxiety disorder. Electroencephalogr Clin Neurophysiol 66:337–348, 1987

Grillon C, Dierkier L, Merikangas KR: Startle and risk for anxiety and depression. J Am Acad Child Adolesc Psychiatry 36:925–932, 1997

Guidi L, Tricerri A, Vangeli M, et al: Neuropeptide Y plasma levels and immunological changes during academic stress. Biol Psychiatry 40:188–195, 1999

Gur RC, Gur RE, Resnick SM, et al: The effect of anxiety on cortical cerebral blood flow and metabolism. J Cereb Blood Flow Metab 7:173–177, 1987

Handley SL: 5-Hydroxytryptamine pathways in anxiety and its treatment. Pharmacol Ther 66:103–148, 1995

Harro J, Vasar E, Bradwejn J: CCK in animal and human research on anxiety. Trends Pharmacol Sci 14:244–249, 1993

Harvey AG, Rapee RM: Cognitive-behavioral therapy for generalized anxiety disorder. Psychiatr Clin North Am 18:859–870, 1995

Harvey BH, Bothma T, Nel A, et al: Involvement of the NMDA receptor, NO-cyclic GMP and nuclear factor K-beta in an animal model of repeated trauma. Hum Psychopharmacol 20:367–373, 2005

Heide F, Borkovec TD: Relaxation induced anxiety: mechanism and theoretical implications. Behav Res Ther 22:1–12, 1984

Hertzberg MA, Butterfield MI, Feldman ME, et al: A preliminary study of lamotrigine for the treatment of posttraumatic stress disorder. Biol Psychiatry 45:1226–1229, 1999

Hettema JM, Neale MC, Kendler KS: A review and meta-analysis of the genetic epidemiology of anxiety disorders. Am J Psychiatry 158:1568–1578, 2001a

Hettema JM, Prescott CA, Kendler KS: A population-based twin study of generalized anxiety disorder in men and women. J Nerv Ment Dis 189:413–420, 2001b

Hettema JM, Prescott CA, Kendler KS: Genetic and environmental sources of covariation between generalized anxiety disorder and neuroticism. Am J Psychiatry 161:1581–1587, 2004

Hirshfeld DR, Rosenbaum JF, Biederman J, et al: Stable behavioral inhibition and its association with anxiety disorder. J Am Acad Child Adolesc Psychiatry 31:103–111, 1992

Hoehn-Saric R, McLeod DR, Zimmerli WD: Somatic manifestations in women with generalized anxiety disorder: psychophysiological responses to psychological stress. Arch Gen Psychiatry 46:1113–1119, 1989

Holt PE, Andrews G: Provocation of panic: three elements of the panic reaction in four anxiety disorders. Behav Res Ther 27:253–261, 1989

Horvath TL, Bechmann I, Naftolin F, et al: Heterogeneity in the neuropeptide Y–containing neurons of the rat arcuate nucleus: GABAergic and non-GABAergic subpopulations. Brain Res 756:283–286, 1997

Jacobson AF, Dominguez RA, Goldstein BJ, et al: Comparison of buspirone and diazepam in generalized anxiety disorder. Pharmacotherapy 5:290–296, 1985

Jacobson L, Sapolsky R: The role of the hippocampus in feedback regulation of the hypothalamic-pituitary-adrenocortical axis. Endocr Rev 12:118–134, 1991

Kaada BR: Stimulation and regional ablation of the amygdaloid complex with reference to functional representations, in The Neurobiology of the Amygdala. Edited by Eleftheriou BE. New York, Plenum, 1972, pp 205–281

Kamilaris TC, Johnson EO, Calogero AK, et al: Cholecystokinin-octapeptide stimulates hypothalamic-corticotropin-releasing hormone. Endocrinology 139:1764–1774, 1992

Karcz-Kubicha M, Jessa M, Nazar M, et al: Anxiolytic activity of glycine-B antagonists and partial agonists—no relation to intrinsic activity in the patch clamp. Neuropharmacology 36:1355–1367, 1997

Kelly CB, Cooper SJ: Differences in variability in plasma noradrenaline between depressive and anxiety disorders. J Psychopharmacol 12:161–167, 1998

Kendler KS: Major depression and generalized anxiety disorder: same genes, (partly) different environments—revisited. Br J Psychiatry Suppl 30:68–75, 1996

Kendler KS, Karkowski LM, Prescott CA: Fears and phobias: reliability and heritability. Psychol Med 29:539–553, 1992a

Kendler KS, Neale MC, Kessler RC, et al: Generalized anxiety disorder in women: a population-based twin study. Arch Gen Psychiatry 49:267–272, 1992b

Kent G, Gibbons R: Self-efficacy and the control of anxious cognitions. J Behav Ther Exp Psychiatry 18:33–40, 1987

Khan A, Lee E, Dager S, et al: Platelet MAO-B activity in anxiety and depression. Biol Psychiatry 21:847–849, 1986

Laakmann G, Schule C, Lorkowski G, et al: Buspirone and lorazepam in the treatment of generalized anxiety disorder in outpatients. Psychopharmacology 136:357–366, 1998

Ledgerwood L, Richardson R, Cranney J: D-Cycloserine facilitates extinction of learned fear: effects on reacquisition and generalized extinction. Biol Psychiatry 57:841–847, 2005

Lesch KP, Bengel D, Heils A, et al: Association of anxiety-related traits with a polymorphism in the serotonin transporter gene regulatory region. Science 274:1527–1531, 1996

Lydiard RB: Neuropeptides and anxiety: focus on cholecystokinin. Clin Chem 40:315–318, 1994

Mackintosh MA, Gatz M, Wetherell JL, et al: A twin study of lifetime generalized anxiety disorder (GAD) in older adults: genetic and environmental influences shared by neuroticism and GAD. Twin Res Hum Genet 9:30–37, 2006

MacLeod C, Mathews A, Tata P: Attentional bias in emotional disorders. J Abnorm Psychol 95:15–20, 1986

Maneuf YP, Hughes J, McKnight AT: Gabapentin inhibits the substance P-facilitated K(+)-evoked release of [(3)H] glutamate from rat caudal trigeminal nucleus slices. Pain 93:191–196, 2001

Marten PA, Brawn TA, Barlow DH, et al: Evaluation of the ratings comprising the associated symptom criterion of DSM-III-R generalized anxiety disorder. J Nerv Ment Dis 181:676–682, 1993

Martin M, Williams RM, Clark DM: Does anxiety lead to selective processing of threat-related information? Behav Res Ther 29:147–160, 1991

Massion AO, Dyck IR, Shea MT, et al: Personality disorders and time to remission in generalized anxiety disorder, social phobia, and panic disorder. Arch Gen Psychiatry 59:434–440, 2002

Mathew RJ, Wilson WH: Cerebral blood flow changes induced by CO_2 in anxiety. Psychiatry Res 23:285–294, 1987

Mathew RJ, Wilson WH: Evaluation of the effects of diazepam and an experimental anti-anxiety drug on regional cerebral blood flow. Psychiatry Res 40:125–134, 1991

Mathew RJ, Ho BT, Kralik P, et al: Catechol-*O*-methyltransferase and catecholamines in anxiety and relaxation. Psychiatry Res 3:856–891, 1980

Mathew RJ, Ho BT, Francis DJ, et al: Catecholamines and anxiety. Acta Psychiatr Scand 65:142–147, 1982a

Mathew RJ, Weinman ML, Caghorn JL: Anxiety and cerebral blood flow, in The Biology of Anxiety. Edited by Mathew RJ. New York, Brunner/Mazel, 1982b, pp 23–33

Mathew RJ, Wilson WH, Humphreys D, et al: Cerebral vasodilation and vasoconstriction associated with acute anxiety. Biol Psychiatry 41:782–795, 1997

Mathew SJ, Amiel JM, Coplan DJ, et al: Open-label trial of riluzole in generalized anxiety disorder. Am J Psychiatry 162:2379–2381, 2005

Mathews A, Richards A, Eysenck M: Interpretation of homophones related to threat in anxiety states. J Abnorm Psychol 98:31–34, 1989

Mizra NR, Bright JL, Stanhope KJ, et al: Lamotrigine has an anxiolytic-like profile in the rat conditioned emotional response test of anxiety: a potential role for sodium channels? Psychopharmacology 180:159–168, 2005

Mogg K, Mathews A, Weinman J: Memory bias in clinical anxiety. J Abnorm Psychol 96:94–98, 1987

Monnikes H, Lauer G, Arnold R: Peripheral administration of cholecystokinin activates c-fos expression in the locus coeruleus/subcoeruleus nucleus, dorsal vagal complex and paraventricular nucleus via capsaicin-sensitive vagal afferents and CCK-A receptors in the rat. Brain Res 770:277–288, 1997

Montgomery SA, Tobias K, Zornberg GL, et al: Efficacy and safety of pregabalin in the treatment of generalized anxiety disorder: a 6-week, multicenter, randomized, double-blind, placebo-controlled comparison of pregabalin and venlafaxine. J Clin Psychiatry 67:771–782, 2006

Mowrer OH: On the dual nature of learning: a re-interpretation of "conditioning" and "problem-solving." Harv Educ Rev 17:102–148, 1947

Munjack DJ, Palmer R: Thyroid hormones in panic disorder, panic disorder with agoraphobia, and generalized anxiety disorder. J Clin Psychiatry 49:229–231, 1988

Munjack DJ, Baltazar PL, DeQuattro V, et al: Generalized anxiety disorder: some biochemical aspects. Psychiatry Res 32:35–43, 1990

Nemeroff CB: Early life adversity, CRF dysregulation, and vulnerability to mood and anxiety disorders. Psychopharmacol Bull 38 (suppl 1):14–20, 2004

Noyes R, Clarkson C, Crowe RR, et al: A family study of generalized anxiety disorder. Am J Psychiatry 144:1019–1024, 1987

Nutt DJ: Neurobiological mechanisms in generalized anxiety disorder. J Clin Psychiatry 62 (suppl 11):22–27, 2001

Pande AC, Crockatt JG, Feltner DE, et al: Pregabalin in generalized anxiety disorder: a placebo-controlled trial. Am J Psychiatry 160:533–540, 2003

Parker G: Parental Overprotection: A Risk Factor in Psychosocial Development. Sydney, Australia, Grune & Stratton, 1983

Pecknold JC, Matas M, Howarth BG, et al: Evaluation of buspirone as an antianxiety agent: buspirone and diazepam versus placebo. Can J Psychiatry 34:766–771, 1989

Pitts FN, McClure JN: Lactate metabolism in anxiety neurosis. N Engl J Med 277:1329–1336, 1967

Rapee R: Distinctions between panic disorder and generalized anxiety disorder: clinical presentation. Aust N Z J Psychiatry 19:227–232, 1985

Rapee R: Generalized anxiety disorder: a review of clinical features and theoretical concepts. Clin Psychol Rev 11:419–440, 1991

Rapee R: Potential role of childrearing practices in the development of anxiety and depression. Clin Psychol Rev 17:47–67, 1997

Raskin M, Peeke HVS, Dickman W, et al: Panic and generalized anxiety disorders. Arch Gen Psychiatry 39:687–689, 1982

Redmond DE: Studies of the nucleus locus coeruleus in monkeys and hypotheses for neuropsychopharmacology, in Psychopharmacology: The Third Generation of Progress. Edited by Meltzer HY. New York, Raven, 1987, pp 967–975

Rickels K, Downing R, Schweitzer E, et al: Antidepressants for the treatment of generalized anxiety disorder: a placebo-controlled comparison of imipramine, trazadone, and diazepam. Arch Gen Psychiatry 50:884–895, 1993

Rickels K, Pollack MH, Feltner DE, et al: Pregabalin for treatment of generalized anxiety disorder: a 4-week, multicenter, double-blind, placebo-controlled trial of pregabalin and alprazolam. Arch Gen Psychiatry 62:1022–1030, 2005

Rocca P, Ferrero P, Gualerzi A, et al: Peripheral-type benzodiazepine receptors in anxiety disorders. Acta Psychiatr Scand 84:537–544, 1991

Rosenbaum AH, Achatzberg AF, Jost FA 3rd, et al: Urinary free cortisol levels in anxiety. Psychosomatics 24:835–837, 1983

Rosenbaum JF, Biederman J, Bolduc-Murphy EA, et al: Behavioral inhibition in childhood: a risk factor for anxiety disorders. Harv Rev Psychiatry 1:2–16, 1993

Roy-Byrne P, Wingerson DK, Rant A, et al: Reduced benzodiazepine sensitivity in patients with panic disorder: comparison with patients with obsessive-compulsive disorder and normal subjects. Am J Psychiatry 153:1444–1449, 1996

Safren SA, Gershuny BS, Marzol P, et al: History of childhood abuse in panic disorder, social phobia, and generalized anxiety disorder. J Nerv Ment Dis 190:453–456, 2002

Saklofske DH, Eysenck SB: Impulsiveness and venturesomeness in Canadian children. Psychol Rep 52:147–152, 1983

Schittecatte M, Garcia-Valentin J, Charles G, et al: Efficacy of the "clonidine REM suppression test (CREST)" to separate patients with major depression from controls: a comparison with currently proposed biological markers of depression. J Affect Disord 33:151–157, 1995

Sevy S, Papadimitriou GN, Surmont DW, et al: Noradrenergic function in generalized anxiety disorder, major depressive disorder, and healthy subjects. Biol Psychiatry 25:141–152, 1989

Shumyatsky G, Tsvetkov E, Malleret G, et al: Identification of a signaling network in lateral nucleus of amygdala important for inhibiting memory specifically related to learned fear. Cell 111:905–918, 2002

Singareddy R, Uhde T: Differential effects of hypocretins on noise-alone versus potentiated startle responses. Physiol Behav 89:650–655, 2006

Spiegel R, Koberle S, Allen SR: Significance of slow wave sleep: considerations from a clinical viewpoint. Sleep 9:66–79, 1986

Spielberger CD: Anxiety as an emotional state, in Anxiety: Current Trends in Theory and Research, Vol 1. Edited by Spielberger CD. New York, Academic Press, 1972, pp 24–49

Starcevic V, Uhlenhuth E, Fallon S, et al: Personality dimensions in panic disorder and generalized anxiety disorder. J Affect Disord 37:75–79, 1996

Tadic A, Rujescu D, Szegedi A, et al: Association of a MAOA gene variant with generalized anxiety disorder, but not with panic disorder or major depression. Am J Med Genet B Neuropsychiatr Genet 117B:1–6, 2003

Taylor DP: Serotonin agents in anxiety. Ann N Y Acad Sci 600:545–557, 1990

Tellegen A: Structures of mood and personality and their relevance to assessing anxiety, with an emphasis on self-report, in Anxiety and the Anxiety Disorders. Edited by Tuma AH, Maser J. Hillsdale, NJ, Erlbaum, 1985, pp 681–706

Tiihonen J, Kuikka J, Rasanen P, et al: Cerebral benzodiazepine receptor binding and distribution in generalized anxiety disorder: a fractal analysis. Mol Psychiatry 2:463–471, 1997

Tiller JW, Biddle N, Maguire KP, et al: The dexamethasone suppression test and plasma dexamethasone in generalized anxiety disorder. Biol Psychiatry 23:261–270, 1988

Verburg K, Griez E, Meijer J, et al: Discrimination between panic disorder and generalized anxiety disorder by 35% carbon dioxide challenge. Am J Psychiatry 152:1081–1083, 1995

Walker DL, Ressler KJ, Lu KT, et al: Facilitation of conditioned fear extinction by systematic administration of intra-amygdala infusions of D-cycloserine as assessed with fear-potentiated startle in rats. J Neurosci 22:2343–2351, 2002

Wallace KJ, Rosen JB: Neurotoxic lesions of the lateral nucleus of the amygdala decrease conditioned fear but not unconditioned fear of a predator odor: comparison with electrolytic lesions. J Neurosci 21:3619–3627, 2001

Watson D, Tellegen A: Toward a consensual structure of mood. Psychol Bull 98:219–235, 1985

Watson D, Clark LA, Carey G: Positive and negative affectivity and their relation to anxiety and depressive disorders. J Abnorm Psychol 97:346–353, 1988

Weizman R, Tanne Z, Granek M, et al: Peripheral benzodiazepine binding sites on platelet membranes are increased during diazepam treatment of anxious patients. Eur J Pharmacol 138:289–292, 1987

Windle M, Windle RC, Scheidt DM, et al: Physical and sexual abuse and associated mental disorders among alcoholic inpatients. Am J Psychiatry 152:1322–3128, 1995

Woodruff GN, Hughes J: Cholecystokinin antagonists. Annu Rev Pharmacol Toxicol 31:469–501, 1991

Wu JC, Buchsbaum MS, Hershey TG, et al: PET in generalized anxiety disorder. Biol Psychiatry 29:1181–1199, 1991

You JS, Hu SY, Chen B, et al: Serotonin transporter and tryptophan hydroxylase gene polymorphisms in Chinese patients with generalized anxiety disorder. Psychiatr Genet 15:7–11, 2005

Young EA, Abelson JL, Cameron OG: Effect of comorbid anxiety disorders on the hypothalamic-pituitary-adrenal axis response to a social stressor in major depression. Biol Psychiatry 56:113–120, 2004

Recommended Readings

Ballenger JC, Davidson JR, Lecrubier Y, et al: Consensus statement on generalized anxiety disorder from the International Consensus Group on Depression and Anxiety. J Clin Psychiatry 62 (suppl 11):53–58, 2001

Hettema JM, An SS, Neale MC, et al: Association between glutamic acid decarboxylase genes and anxiety disorders, major depression, and neuroticism. Mol Psychiatry 11:752–762, 2006 [erratum published in: Mol Psychiatry 11(8)794, 2006]

Poulton R, Andrews G, Millichamp J: Gene-environment interactions and the anxiety disorders. Eur Arch Psychiatry Clin Neurosci 258(2):65–68, 2008

Stein MB: Neurobiology of generalized anxiety disorder. J Clin Psychiatry 70 (suppl 2):15–19, 2009

Chapter 13

Pharmacotherapy for Generalized Anxiety Disorder

Michael Van Ameringen, M.D., FRCPC
Catherine Mancini, M.D., FRCPC
Beth Patterson, B.Sc.N., B.Ed.
William Simpson, B.Sc.
Christine Truong, B.Sc.

Initially considered to be a residual category to be used when no other diagnosis could be made, generalized anxiety disorder (GAD) now represents a distinct clinical entity that is recognized as such in the widely used *Diagnostic and Statistical Manual of Mental Disorders*, 4th Edition, Text Revision (DSM-IV-TR) (American Psychiatric Association 2000) and *International Statistical Classification of Diseases and Related Health Problems*, 10th Revision (ICD-10) (World Health Organization 1992). The diagnostic nomenclature of GAD has evolved considerably since its inclusion in DSM-III (American Psychiatric Association 1980), marked by a shift from psychoanalytic theories of neurosis to a more research-based concept that anxiety is a product of the interaction of neurobiology, psychological factors, and environmental stressors (Rickels and Rynn 2001). This issue is of great importance when examining the GAD treatment literature, because the description of GAD in DSM-III and that in DSM-IV-TR are of quite different disorders.

The evaluation of pharmacological treatments for GAD has spanned a broad range of drug classes. Industry has turned to GAD as proof of concept of the anxiolytic properties of a drug; virtually every class of psychotropic agent has been tested for efficacy in patients with this disorder. Benzodiazepines have long been the mainstay of the treatment of anxiety and anxiety disorders (Cowley et al. 1995; van Steveninck et al. 1997). Selective serotonin reuptake inhibitors (SSRIs) and serotonin-norepinephrine reuptake inhibitors (SNRIs) have emerged as the gold standard treatment for anxiety disorders. Anticonvulsants have been widely used in the treatment of mood disorders; in anxiety disorders such as GAD, these medications have shown promise as an alternative first-line treatment. Other agents such as antipsychotics, azapirones, beta-blockers, and antihistamines have also been evaluated as GAD treatments. In this chapter, we review the current evidence for the efficacy of pharmacotherapy across a variety of drug classes in treating GAD, relying primarily on reports from randomized, controlled trials. We examine short-term studies, long-term studies, relapse prevention studies, studies in elderly and treatment-resistant patients, and novel pharmacological approaches to treating GAD.

Medication Treatments

Short-Term Studies (1–12 Weeks)

Benzodiazepines

Benzodiazepines are the most prescribed anxiolytic medications and have a long history of use in the treatment of GAD. Benzodiazepines work mainly by modulating the effects of the neurotransmitter γ-aminobutyric acid (GABA). Ultimately, these medications bind to specific benzodiazepine receptors, increasing GABA's inhibitory effects and causing an overall decrease in psychological and physiological arousal (Costa 1979). When first introduced, benzodiazepines were hailed by many as a safer and equally efficacious alternative to the barbiturate class of medications (Lader 1991), offering advantages such as rapid therapeutic onset as well as sedative and anticonvulsant properties. In comparison to their predecessors, the barbiturates, benzodiazepines are also less toxic in high concentrations and have lower potential for overdose and use in suicide attempts (Lader 1991).

For the treatment of nonspecific anxiety symptoms, chlordiazepoxide, diazepam, clorazepate, lorazepam, and oxazepam have all been shown to be more efficacious than placebo (Greenblatt and Shader 1974). In randomized, controlled trials focused specifically on the treatment of GAD, clorazepate (Rickels et al. 1988a, 1988b), lorazepam (Rickels et al. 1988a), and diazepam (Rickels et al. 1983) were superior to placebo. These results, however, are based on DSM-III GAD criteria, a factor that limits their generalizability. As mentioned earlier, in the introduction to this chapter, DSM-III diagnostic criteria for GAD differ significantly from those in more recent DSM versions. Although the benzodiazepines showed efficacy in these early studies, their results are not directly transferable to current definitions of GAD; therefore, no distinct conclusions can be drawn. Comparator trials, particularly those using the anticonvulsant agent pregabalin, were the first controlled trials of benzodiazepines using DSM-IV criteria for GAD (Feltner et al. 2003; Pande et al. 2003; Rickels et al. 2005). Results of these randomized, controlled trials indicated that alprazolam and lorazepam were superior to placebo; these studies are discussed in detail in later sections of this chapter.

Despite their demonstrated efficacy in GAD and rapid therapeutic onset, benzodiazepines have many disadvantages. Because many benzodiazepines have a rather short half-life, patients require more frequent dosing than with other anxiolytic medications. Also, some data suggest that compared to antidepressants, benzodiazepines may be associated with high rates of relapse following treatment discontinuation (Schweizer et al. 1995). Other drawbacks to these agents include possible rebound anxiety; the ineffectiveness of benzodiazepines in the treatment of comorbid conditions commonly found with GAD, such as depression; and the potential for dependence in patients with comorbid substance abuse. Significant side effects, such as persistent attentional, psychomotor, cognitive, and memory effects, have been associated with benzodiazepine treatment (Thomas 1998). The use of benzodiazepines as a first-line treatment for GAD is no longer recommended (Baldwin et al. 2005; Canadian Psychiatric Association 2006). For the short term, the benzodiazepine class of medications has two primary advantages: rapid onset of treatment effect on GAD symptoms (in particular somatic complaints) and low cost.

Azapirones

Buspirone. Buspirone, an azapirone derivative, is a partial 5-hydroxytryptamine (serotonin) type 1A (5-HT_{1A}) receptor agonist approved for use in GAD in 1986 by the U.S. Food and Drug Administration (Gammans et al. 1992). It has anxiolytic efficacy similar to that of the benzodiazepines (Rickels et al. 1982) but appears to have a better safety profile (Rakel 1990). Unlike the benzodiazepines, azapirones do not have sedative, muscle relaxant, or anticonvulsant properties. In addition, the potential for abuse or withdrawal effects from these agents is limited, and cognitive, memory, or psychomotor impairments have not been associated with azapirones. Other advantages of azapirones include negligible overdose toxicity, absence of respiratory depressant properties, no serious drug interaction effects, and no anticholinergic or cardiotoxic effects. Azapirones have the additional benefit of being well tolerated by elderly patients (Jann 1988; Lader 1987; Napoliello and Domantay 1991).

Sramek et al. (1996) found buspirone (15–45 mg/day) superior to placebo in a 6-week randomized, double-blind, parallel-group study of 162 patients with GAD and coexisting mild depressive symptoms. Compared with patients treated with placebo, patients treated with buspirone had a significantly greater reduction in Hamilton Anxiety Scale (Ham-A) total scores from baseline (P<0.03), as well as a greater reduction on their Hamilton Rating Scale for Depression (Ham-D) scores from baseline (P<0.05). In general, the incidence of adverse events was similar for both treatment groups.

In another randomized, double-blind comparative study, Sramek et al. (1997) evaluated the efficacy and safety of buspirone (30 mg/day) administered twice daily (bid) versus three times daily (tid) in patients with GAD. No appreciable difference in efficacy or safety was found for 15 mg bid (n=57) or 10 mg tid (n=62). In fact, both treatment groups achieved significant improvement on the Ham-A and Clinical Global Impression Improvement Scale (CGI-I) (P<0.0001). Consistent results were found in a later study that compared similar buspirone regimens (30 mg/day bid vs. tid) with a placebo (Sramek et al. 1999).

In a 6-week randomized, double-blind, parallel-group study conducted by Majercsik et al. (2003), 52 male patients with a DSM-IV (American Psychiatric Association 1994) diagnosis of GAD and a Ham-A score >15 were treated with either buspirone (30 mg/day) (n=33) or placebo (n=19). Compared with patients treated with placebo, patients treated with buspirone demonstrated a highly significant reduction in Ham-A scores (P<0.0001). Full recovery (defined as Ham-A scores<15) was evident in two (10%) of the placebo-treated patients by the end of the study, compared with 16 (48%) of the buspirone-treated group.

Tollefson et al. (1992) investigated 51 patients dually diagnosed with generalized anxiety and alcohol abuse/dependence in a randomized, double-blind, placebo-controlled trial of buspirone versus placebo. Buspirone was superior to placebo as an anxiolytic, was well tolerated, and was associated with both a reduction in the number of days desiring alcohol and an overall clinical global improvement. This study suggests that buspirone may be an effective treatment strategy for "anxious" or "mixed anxious-depressive" patients with comorbid alcoholism.

Using a retrospective analysis of pooled efficacy data, Gammans et al. (1992) compared buspirone (10–60 mg/day) with placebo in 520 patients with GAD. Buspirone demonstrated significant improvement over baseline in total Ham-A scores compared with placebo (P≤0.001) in patients with GAD and in patients with GAD and comorbid depressive symptoms. Furthermore, patients with GAD and coexisting depressive symptoms of at least moderate intensity responded at least as well or better to buspirone therapy as did those with GAD who had less severe depressive symptoms.

Finally, several studies have compared the anxiolytic effects of buspirone and other pharmacological agents. A large amount of this research directly compares buspirone with several different benzodiazepines. Buspirone has been found to be equal in efficacy to both lorazepam (Laakmann et al. 1998) and clorazepate (Goldberg and Finnerty 1982) but to be more effective at preventing relapse after treatment discontinuation (Laakmann et al. 1998) and to produce fewer sedative side effects (Goldberg and Finnerty 1982). Direct comparison of buspirone with alprazolam, however, has shown alprazolam to be more effective in both onset of treatment effects and frequency of adverse events (Enkelmann 1991). Further comparison of buspirone with the benzodiazepine class was conducted by Ansseau et al. (1990), examining buspirone and oxazepam. Results indicated that although both were superior to placebo, oxazepam was more effective after 2 weeks, and both medications displayed similar relapse characteristics following discontinuation. Several studies have directly compared buspirone with diazepam, with mixed results. Some studies found diazepam to be superior to buspirone (Fontaine et al. 1987), whereas others indicated equal efficacy (Cohn et al. 1989; Goldberg and Finnerty 1982; Wheatley 1982). In general, buspirone was shown to be superior to diazepam in controlling sedation and preventing symptom relapse after treatment discontinuation (Fontaine et al. 1987; Goldberg and Finnerty 1982; Wheatley 1982).

Davidson et al. (1999) examined the effects of buspirone and of the SNRI venlafaxine and found venlafaxine to be superior to both buspirone and placebo (see "Venlafaxine," later in this chapter, for a detailed review). In another study, Pollack et al. (1997) found that buspirone was equal in efficacy to abecarnil but provided a lower frequency of relapse upon study completion (see "Abecarnil," later in the chapter, for a more detailed review).

Taken together, these controlled trials of buspirone seem to indicate that buspirone is equal in efficacy to more traditional benzodiazepines. Buspirone may provide lower relapse rates upon treatment termination, as well as lower levels of sedation during the treatment period.

Gepirone. Gepirone is a partial 5-HT_{1A} agonist, with the potential to display anxiolytic effects (Eison et al. 1986). The therapeutic value of gepirone for GAD was examined in a placebo-controlled trial with diazepam conducted by Rickels et al. (1997). In this study, 198 patients with GAD, as defined by DSM-III (at least 1 month duration, Ham-A≥20), were randomly assigned to receive gepirone (10–45 mg/day) or diazepam (10–45 mg/day) for a period of 8 weeks. Analysis using the Ham-A, CGI-I, and CGI Severity Scale (CGI-S) as the primary efficacy measures indicated that significant reductions in anxiety were seen with diazepam versus placebo beginning at week 1 ($P<0.05$), but reductions in anxiety were not seen for gepirone versus placebo until weeks 6–8 ($P<0.05$), indicating a significant delay in therapeutic onset. Based on attrition rates, diazepam was significantly superior to gepirone and placebo. Upon study completion, patient retention was 66% for diazepam, 42% for gepirone, and 58% for placebo ($P<0.05$). The authors concluded that gepirone was largely ineffective when compared with diazepam and placebo.

Beta-Blockers

Propranolol. Propranolol is a nonselective beta-blocker that blocks the action of epinephrine on both β_1 and β_2 adrenoreceptors, potentially producing anxiolytic effects (Noyes 1985). Meibach et al. (1987) compared the efficacy and safety of propranolol (80, 160, or 320 mg/day) with chlordiazepoxide (30, 45, or 75 mg/day) and placebo in a 3-week double-blind study of 212 patients with anxiety (unspecified) whose symptoms warranted daily treatment with an anxiolytic. Patients in all groups demonstrated significant improvement in their level of anxiety at all time points compared with their baseline level, as measured by the Ham-A and Covi Anxiety Scale. At week 1, patients taking propranolol or chlordiazepoxide were significantly better than those taking placebo ($P\leq0.05$); at week 2, only propranolol was superior to placebo ($P\leq0.05$); and by week 3, neither drug was significantly more effective than placebo. The incidence of side effects was similar for the two active drugs. Discontinuation of treatment was not associated with adverse side effects in any treatment group. The results from this study do not support the use of propranolol in the treatment of GAD.

Antihistamines

Hydroxyzine. Hydroxyzine is a H_1 receptor antagonist, as well as a mild 5-HT_2 receptor antagonist, and has been shown to possess some anxiolytic properties (Kubo et al. 1987). To date, only a handful of randomized, controlled trials have examined the effectiveness of hydroxyzine in treating GAD. The first study was conducted by Darcis et al. (1995), who examined over 100 patients with GAD as defined by DSM-III-R (American Psychiatric Association 1987). Patients were randomly assigned to 4 weeks of hydroxyzine (50 mg/day) or placebo. The mean change in Ham-A score from baseline (primary outcome measure) was significant ($P\leq0.001$) in favor of hydroxyzine at week 4 (end of treatment) and at week 5 (after 1 week of no treatment). The only side effect showing significant differences between the two groups was drowsiness, experienced significantly more often by the hydroxyzine group.

In a second study, Lader and Scotto (1998) compared hydroxyzine (50 mg/day) with buspirone (20 mg/day) and placebo in a 4-week randomized, controlled, double-blind study of 241 patients with GAD diagnosed using DSM-IV. Pairwise comparisons on Ham-A scores were conducted between all groups (hydroxyzine-placebo, buspirone-placebo, hydroxyzine-buspirone); significant differences in improvement were observed only within the hydroxyzine-placebo group ($P=0.015$). Upon medication termination, both buspirone and hydroxyzine patients continued to improve, and no rebound effects of withdrawal symptoms were observed.

Hydroxyzine has also been examined in a randomized, double-blind, parallel-group study comparing hydroxyzine (50 mg/day), bromazepam (6 mg/day), and placebo (Llorca et al. 2002) in 334 patients with GAD diagnosed using DSM-IV. Compared with placebo, hydroxyzine demonstrated significant improvement in Ham-A total score from baseline (primary efficacy measure) ($P=0.019$). The study was not sufficiently powered to compare the two medication groups; however, bromazepam also demonstrated a significant difference from placebo in change of Ham-A score, baseline adjusted means ($P\leq0.03$). Hydroxyzine and bromazepam had higher rates of response ($\geq$50% reduction in Ham-A score) than placebo ($P\leq0.01$ for both groups vs. placebo), as well as higher rates of remission (Ham-A total score $\leq$10) (hydroxyzine, $P\leq0.03$; bromazepam, $P\leq0.01$). Both medications exhibited similar side-effect profiles, with drowsiness as the most common side effect, but side effects appeared at a higher frequency in the bromazepam group. The authors concluded that long-term treatment with hydroxyzine was a comparable alternative treatment to benzodiazepines for reducing anxiety, due in part to a lower incidence of drowsiness.

Although the results of randomized, controlled trials indicate potential efficacy of hydroxyzine in GAD, the medication is not typically used as a first-line agent due to its significant sedative properties and the lack of demonstrated efficacy in common comorbid conditions found with GAD. It may, however, have a place in treatment-resistant cases.

Tricyclic Antidepressants

Generally, the tricyclic antidepressants are believed to work by inhibiting the reuptake of excitatory neurotransmitters (norepinephrine, serotonin, and dopamine). In addition to increasing excitatory impulses, the tricyclic antidepressants are also believed to affect H_1 and muscarinic receptors (Feighner 1999).

Of the tricyclic agents examined in treating patients with GAD, imipramine appears to be the only agent that has consistently shown greater response rates than placebo (Rickels and Rynn 2002). Three randomized, controlled studies involving imipramine have shown its effectiveness in the treatment of GAD. In two of these studies (Rickels et al. 1993; Rocca et al. 1997), imipramine was used as a comparator drug. In the study by Rickels et al. (1993), imipramine (25–200 mg/day), trazodone (50–400 mg/day), and diazepam (5–40 mg/day) were compared in an 8-week double-blind, placebo-controlled study of 230 patients with GAD diagnosed using DSM-III. Diazepam was found to be superior in the short term, showing the most improvement over the first 2 weeks according to the Ham-A total score (primary efficacy measure) ($P<0.01$); however, by week 8, only imipramine demonstrated a statistically significant improvement compared with placebo ($P<0.01$). Upon study completion, moderate to marked clinical improvement (CGI-I≤2) was reported by 73% of patients treated with imipramine, 69% of patients treated with trazodone, and 66% of patients treated with diazepam ($P<0.026$). The results seem to suggest that all GAD treatments were equally effective, with imipramine showing potentially greater efficacy according to the primary outcome measure.

The final randomized trial of imipramine was conducted by Hoehn-Saric et al. (1988). In this study, patients with DSM-III–diagnosed GAD of 6-month duration were randomly assigned to receive imipramine (25–300 mg/day) or alprazolam (1.5–6 mg/day) for a period of 6 weeks. Fifty-two patients completed the study. Results from a repeated-measures analysis of covariance (ANCOVA) indicated that over the first 2 weeks, alprazolam was superior to imipramine in reducing somatic complaints ($P<0.05$), whereas imipramine was superior in reducing psychic symptoms ($P<0.05$). After 6 weeks, no significant differences in efficacy between the two medications were observed. However, imipramine patients reported higher incidences of undesirable side effects.

Despite the potential efficacy of tricyclic antidepressants in long-term use, their blockage of H_1 histamine receptors, α_1 adrenoceptors, and muscarinic receptors decreases their tolerability as well as their potential for lethality in overdose, which limits their use as a first-line treatment in patients with GAD (Baldwin and Polkinghorn 2005).

Research has shown potential benefits of using tricyclic antidepressants in the treatment of GAD. These agents have demonstrated equal efficacy to newer antidepressants (SSRIs and SNRIs) and have not been associated with the dependence and withdrawal symptomatology observed with benzodiazepines. However, due to the less desirable tolerability profile of tricyclic antidepressants, they have been largely replaced by other classes of medications and are reserved for use as second-line treatment or for treatment-refractory GAD.

Opipramol. Opipramol, a drug widely prescribed in Germany, is a tricyclic compound with no reuptake-inhibiting properties. However, it is an effective dopamine (D_2), 5-HT_2, and H_1 receptor blocker and thus shows potential for use as an antidepressant in the treatment of GAD (Bischoff et al. 1986). In a 4-week randomized, controlled trial, Moller et al. (2001) randomly assigned 307 patients diagnosed with GAD using the ICD-10 to receive opipramol (200 mg/day), alprazolam (2 mg/day), or placebo. Primary efficacy was measured via changes in Ham-A total score. Upon study completion, average Ham-A scores were 13.1 for patients taking opipramol, 12.6 for those taking alprazolam, and 16.2 for those taking placebo. Both active treatments exhibited significant superiority over placebo ($P<0.02$). No significant differences between groups were observed, with the exception of sleep disturbances in the placebo group (significance value not reported). Overall, the authors concluded that opipramol appears to have anxiolytic properties nearly equal to those of alprazolam; however, the mechanism by which the medication achieves this effect is still unknown and warrants more research.

Selective Serotonin Reuptake Inhibitors

The primary mechanism of action of the SSRIs is through blockade of the reuptake of serotonin. What sets these medications apart from other serotonin modulators is their ability to selectively block certain serotonin receptor subtypes (Feighner 1999).

Escitalopram. The SSRI escitalopram has been shown to be effective in short-term trials (Baldwin et al. 2006; Davidson et al. 2004; Goodman et al. 2005), long-term trials (Bielski et al. 2005), and relapse prevention studies (Allgulander et al. 2006; Bakish et al. 2006; Davidson et al. 2005). We review the short-term studies in this section, but the long-term and relapse prevention studies are reviewed in later sections of this chapter.

Davidson et al. (2004) conducted an 8-week study of escitalopram in 307 outpatients with GAD diagnosed using DSM-IV. Patients with baseline Ham-A scores ≥18 were randomly assigned to double-blind treatment with escitalopram (10 mg/day for 4 weeks, then flexibly dosed at 10–20 mg/day) or placebo. Escitalopram was significantly superior to placebo, based on all outcome measures, including total Ham-A scores. Mean change in Ham-A scores from baseline (primary efficacy measure) was −11.3 for patients taking escitalopram but only −7.4 for those taking placebo ($P<0.001$). Escitalopram was generally well tolerated, and a low incidence of adverse events was observed.

In another randomized, controlled trial, Goodman et al. (2005) examined the efficacy of escitalopram in treating GAD using nearly identical methodology as Davidson et al. (2004) used. Data were pooled across three separate trials. In total, 856 patients (ages 18–80 years) with a noncomorbid primary diagnosis of GAD were randomly assigned to receive escitalopram (10 mg/day for 4 weeks, then flexibly dosed to 20 mg/day) or placebo for a period of 8 weeks. Primary treatment efficacy was measured via the change in total Ham-A scores from baseline over the 8-week period. Full treatment response was defined as at least a 50% reduction in Ham-A scores or a CGI-I score of 1 or 2. Escitalopram patients were found to have had a significantly greater reduction of all primary outcome measures at endpoint ($P<0.05$). Pooled analysis of secondary outcome measures indicated that escitalopram was superior to placebo beginning in week 1 or 2 and continuing until week 8 ($P<0.05$). Additionally, escitalopram patients were significantly more likely to be identified as responders (47.5%, $P<0.001$) and remitters (26.4%, $P<0.001$) than were patients taking placebo (28.6% responders; 14.1% remitters).

In a study comparing escitalopram and paroxetine in treating patients with a DSM-IV diagnosis of GAD, 681 patients were randomly assigned to one of five groups—placebo, escitalopram (5, 10, 20 mg/day), and paroxetine (20 mg/day)—for a period of 12 weeks (Baldwin et al. 2006). The primary outcome measures were Ham-A, CGI-S, and CGI-I. Treatment with escitalopram at 10-mg and 20-mg dosages was superior to placebo ($P=0.006$, $P=0.022$) and to paroxetine ($P\leq 0.05$) at week 12 on the primary efficacy measure (change in total Ham-A score), whereas treatment with escitalopram at 5 mg was not consistently superior to placebo, nor was treatment with paroxetine. Response (≥50% reduction in Ham-A) was significantly greater for escitalopram 20 mg versus placebo at week 12 ($P<0.05$). Escitalopram 20 mg also had a significantly greater proportion of responders (80%) at week 12 than did paroxetine (60%) ($P<0.05$). All three dosages of escitalopram resulted in significantly greater rates of remission (Ham-A total score ≤7) than placebo at week 12 ($P<0.05$); remission rates in the group taking escitalopram 10 mg (48%) were significantly greater than in the paroxetine group (33%) ($P<0.05$). Treatment was generally well tolerated, but patient withdrawal due to adverse events was significantly higher for the groups taking paroxetine and escitalopram 20 mg ($P<0.01$). Based on these results, the authors concluded that escitalopram was the superior pharmacological intervention for GAD in this study, citing its higher tolerability and efficacy compared to paroxetine.

Paroxetine. The efficacy of paroxetine in the treatment of GAD was initially demonstrated by Rocca et al. (1997) in a comparator trial with imipramine and diazepam. Results from short-term trials (Hewett et al. 2001; Pollack et al. 2001; Rickels et al. 2003), comparator trials (Baldwin et al. 2006; Ball et al. 2005; Bielski et al. 2005; Kim et al. 2006; Rosenthal 2003), and relapse prevention studies (Stocchi et al. 2003) confirm these initial findings. In this section, we review the short-term trials of paroxetine. Relapse prevention studies are examined in later sections.

In an 8-week study, Rocca et al. (1997) compared treatment with paroxetine and treatment with either imipramine or diazepam in 81 patients with GAD. Results showed a significant improvement on primary efficacy measures (Ham-A, Ham-D, and CGI) for all three drugs, with no significant differences between the groups at endpoint. The authors noted, however, that the onset of therapeutic action varied substantially. Diazepam showed fast initial relief during the first 2 weeks of therapy, but diazepam was surpassed by imipramine and paroxetine at week 4.

Pollack et al. (2001) examined 324 patients with GAD in an 8-week randomized, controlled trial of paroxetine and placebo. Patients taking paroxetine (20–50 mg/day) showed significantly larger reductions in anxiety as evidenced by mean change in Ham-A total scores ($P<0.01$) (primary outcome measure). Remission rates for paroxetine patients (36%) were also significantly higher ($P=0.009$) than for placebo patients (22.7%). The study medication was well tolerated, with a low incidence of adverse events.

In an 8-week study by Hewett et al. (2001), 364 subjects with GAD were randomly assigned to receive to flexibly dosed paroxetine (20–50 mg/day) or placebo. No significant difference was demonstrated between the paroxetine and placebo groups on the primary efficacy measure of change in total Ham-A score; however, the paroxetine group had significantly lower CGI-S scores (*P*=0.05).

Further research involving paroxetine was conducted by Rickels et al. (2003), who randomly assigned 566 patients with a DSM-IV diagnosis of GAD to treatment with paroxetine (20 or 40 mg/day) or placebo for 8 weeks. Comparison of mean change in Ham-A scores from baseline (primary outcome measure) indicated a significant advantage of paroxetine 20 mg (–12.5) and 40 mg (–12.2) over placebo (–9.3) (*P*<0.001). In addition, patients treated with paroxetine, compared with placebo, showed significantly greater levels of response (CGI-I≤2) (20 mg: 62%, 40 mg: 68%, placebo: 46%; *P*<0.001) as well as remission (Ham-A score≤7) (20 mg: 30%, 40 mg: 36%, placebo: 20%; *P*=0.004).

Sertraline. To date, three multicenter studies have been conducted to explore the efficacy and safety of sertraline in the treatment of patients with GAD (Allgulander et al. 2004; Brawman-Mintzer et al. 2006a; Morris et al. 2003). Morris et al. (2003) examined the efficacy of sertraline versus placebo in a 12-week study of 188 adult outpatients with a DSM-IV diagnosis of GAD. Sertraline (flexible dosages of 50–150 mg/day) resulted in significantly greater improvement than placebo on all efficacy measures, including the primary efficacy measure, Ham-A total score (*P*<0.0001). At the end of the study treatment, patients treated with sertraline achieved significantly greater rates of response (CGI-I≤2) over placebo in both the completers (73% vs. 46%; *P*<0.0001) and the last-observation-carried-forward (LOCF) sample (63% vs. 37%; *P*<0.0001). A significantly greater rate of remission (Ham-A=7) occurred in the group treated with sertraline (37%) than in the group taking placebo (23%) (*P*<0.01), and the attrition rate due to adverse events was lower for patients taking sertraline (8.2%) than for those taking placebo (10.0%).

The efficacy of sertraline was examined by Allgulander et al. (2004) in a 12-week study of 330 patients diagnosed with GAD based on DSM-IV criteria. Upon enrollment, patients were randomly assigned to receive flexible dosages of sertraline (50–150 mg/day) or placebo. Sertraline (mean dosage 95.1 mg/day) was superior to placebo beginning at week 4 (*P*<0.0001) and at endpoint, according to the primary efficacy measure of mean change in Ham-A scores (sertraline: –11.7, placebo: –8.0; *P*<0.0001) as well as secondary measures of the CGI-S (sertraline: –1.56, placebo: –0.90; *P*<0.0001) and CGI-I scores (sertraline: 2.30, placebo: 3.00; *P*<0.0001). Response rates (CGI-I≤2) for sertraline were significantly higher (*P*<0.001) than for placebo beginning at week 4 and remained so until study completion. Similarly, remission rates (Ham-A≤7) were significantly higher for sertraline (31%, *P*=0.002) than for placebo (18%) at endpoint.

In a randomized, double-blind, placebo-controlled study of GAD, sertraline (50–200 mg/day) produced a statistically significant reduction in anxiety symptoms, as measured by change in the primary outcome measure of the Ham-A total score (–12.71 sertraline vs.–11.15 placebo, *P*=0.032) (Brawman-Mintzer et al. 2006a). Response rates were also significantly higher for the sertraline group than the placebo group when response was defined as Ham-A ≥50% score decrease (59.2% vs. 48.2%, *P*=0.050) and approached significance when response was defined as CGI-I ≤2 (64.6% vs. 54.3%, *P*=0.057). The mean dosage at study endpoint was 149.1 mg/day (SD=59.0). Sexual side effects (including decrease or loss of libido and male sexual dysfunction) were the only side effects reported significantly more often by subjects receiving sertraline than by subjects receiving placebo (*P*<0.001).

Steiner et al. (2005) examined gender differences of clinical presentation and response to sertraline treatment of GAD. Adult outpatients who met DSM-IV criteria for GAD were randomly assigned to 12 weeks of double-blind treatment with flexible dosages of sertraline (50–150 mg/day) (*n*=182; female 59%) or placebo (*n*=188; female 51%). Women and men with GAD showed similar clinical presentations, except that women had an earlier age at onset and reported more somatic anxiety symptoms. For both men and women, treatment with sertraline resulted in greater change from baseline to endpoint on the Ham-A compared with placebo (adjusted change± standard error: men,–12.1 ± 0.9 vs. –8.8±0.9; women, –11.4±0.8 vs. –7.1±0.9; *P*<0.001); the interaction between gender and treatment group was not significant, and the average change from baseline to endpoint was not significantly different for men compared with women. The response rates (defined as CGI-I ≤2 at endpoint) for patients taking sertraline versus placebo were significantly different (*P*<0.0001) in both men (64% vs. 40%) and women (62% vs. 34%). Response rates showed no significant interaction between gender and treatment, and there was no significant difference in the response rates by gender.

In a 12-week double-blind study, sertraline treatment (flexible dosages of 50–150 mg/day) resulted in significant and rapid improvement in quality of living and work productivity for adult outpatients with a DSM-IV diagnosis of GAD (Sjodin et al. 2003). Outcome measures included the Quality of Life Enjoyment and Satisfaction Questionnaire (Q-LES-Q), with normal quality of life defined as a Q-LES-Q score within 10% of community norms. Compared with patients taking placebo, sertraline-treated patients had significantly greater improvements on the Q-LES-Q (P<0.0001), and improvements were consistent across all scale items. Significant improvements were also found on functional impairment scales: the Endicott Work Productivity Impairment Scale and a visual analogue scale (perceived state of health). At baseline, 11.8% reported normal Q-LES-Q scores. At the end of the study, normal Q-LES-Q scores were higher in completers (51%); responders (66%); and remitters, defined as those with Ham-A=7 (71%). Improvement of depressive symptoms, as defined by a change in score on the Montgomery-Åsberg Depression Rating Scale (MADRS), was found to be the only predictor of improved quality of life (P<0.001).

Ball et al. (2005) compared the efficacy of sertraline (25–100 mg/day) and paroxetine (10–40 mg/day) in an 8-week double-blind, parallel-group study of 55 patients with a DSM-IV diagnosis of GAD. Primary outcome measures consisted of the Ham-A and CGI scales. Both treatment groups responded positively and displayed significant reductions in total Ham-A scores (P<0.001), with an overall reduction averaging 56%±28% for the sertraline group and 57%±28% for the paroxetine group, with no significant differences between the two groups. Remission (CGI-S=1) was achieved by 40% of patients taking paroxetine and 46% of patients taking sertraline (NS), with no significant differences between the groups. In addition, no comorbidity-by-medication interaction occurred, and the presence of a comorbid disorder did not affect the Ham-A scores in the intention-to-treat (ITT) group. No significant differences in tolerability were observed between groups, and the authors concluded that both paroxetine and sertraline were efficacious treatments for GAD.

Serotonin-Norepinephrine Reuptake Inhibitors

Venlafaxine. The SNRI venlafaxine extended release (ER) has shown promising results in the treatment of GAD, as evidenced by results from several randomized, controlled trials. In short-term trials, all but two (Nimatoudis et al. 2004; Rickels et al. 2000b) have compared venlafaxine with other agents as well as placebo (Davidson et al. 1999; Hartford et al. 2007; Kim et al. 2006; Montgomery et al. 2006). The efficacy of venlafaxine has also been evaluated in long-term trials (Allgulander et al. 2001; Gelenberg et al. 2000; Hackett et al. 1999), childhood treatment (Rynn et al. 2007), and treatment of elderly patients (Katz et al. 2002). Venlafaxine was one of the first agents to obtain an indication for the treatment of GAD in North America. Rickels et al. (2000b) evaluated the effectiveness of venlafaxine ER (75, 150, 225 mg/day) versus placebo in 377 patients with a DSM-IV diagnosis of GAD for a period of 8 weeks in a randomized, double-blind, controlled trial. Based on four primary outcome measures—Ham-A total and psychic anxiety scores, CGI-S, and CGI-I—venlafaxine ER was shown to be effective in relieving anxious symptomology; however, only the 225-mg/day dosage demonstrated significant difference from placebo on all measures. The mean CGI-I score at endpoint was 2.22 for the group taking venlafaxine ER 225 mg/day versus 2.61 for the group taking placebo.

In an examination of venlafaxine ER, Nimatoudis et al. (2004) evaluated remission rates (Ham-A ≤7) and Ham-A total score reductions in 46 patients with a DSM-IV diagnosis of GAD. Patients were randomly assigned to 8 weeks of treatment with venlafaxine ER (75 or 150 mg/day) or placebo. Upon study completion, remission was achieved by 62.5% of venlafaxine ER patients compared with only 9.1% of placebo patients (P=0.0006). Reduction in total Ham-A scores was also significantly greater for venlafaxine ER patients (–19.2) than for placebo patients (–10.8) (P<0.001).

Davidson et al. (1999) compared venlafaxine ER, buspirone, and placebo for the treatment of GAD. In this 8-week study, 365 patients with GAD diagnosed using DSM-IV were assigned to venlafaxine ER (75 or 150 mg/day), buspirone (30 mg/day), or placebo. Primary outcome measures consisted of Ham-A total and psychic anxiety and anxious mood scores and CGI scores. Adjusted mean Ham-A total scores were greater for all treatment groups than for the placebo group for all time points; however, these differences failed to reach significance. At week 8, Ham-A psychic anxiety scores and anxious mood scores were significantly lower (P<0.05) for both venlafaxine ER groups compared with the placebo group; however, the scores of the buspirone and placebo groups showed no difference. Based on CGI scores, venlafaxine ER 75 mg/day was found to be significantly superior to placebo at all time points after week 2 ($P<0.01$). The proportion of treatment responders, based on a 50% reduction in Ham-A scores, was not significant between groups at any time point; however, venlafaxine ER 75 mg/day and buspirone indicated significant rates of response, defined as CGI-I ≤2, compared with placebo ($P\leq 0.03$, $P\leq 0.04$, respectively).

In a direct comparison of paroxetine (10–40 mg/day) and venlafaxine ER (37.5–225 mg/day) conducted by Kim et al. (2006), 60 patients with a DSM-IV diagnosis of GAD were entered into an 8-week double-blind, randomized, controlled study. Primary outcome measures consisted of the total Ham-A score and CGI Scale scores. Repeated-measures analyses of variance of both Ham-A and CGI-I scores indicated a significant decrease in anxiety symptoms over time ($P<0.0001$), but no differences were found between the groups. Response (≥50% Ham-A score reduction) rates were high, with no significant difference between the groups: 90.5% for venlafaxine ER and 92% for paroxetine. Remission (Ham-A ≤7) rates were 33.3% for venlafaxine ER and 36% for paroxetine, also with no group difference.

Duloxetine. Duloxetine is another dual reuptake inhibitor of both serotonin and norepinephrine. Based on a pooled sample of over 1,100 patients diagnosed with GAD using DSM-IV criteria, duloxetine was found to be an efficacious treatment for reducing the severity of anxiety symptoms associated with GAD (Allgulander et al. 2007). One of three studies in the pooled sample compared a 9-week fixed-dosage treatment with duloxetine (60 or 120 mg/day) with placebo (Koponen et al. 2007). The second study compared a 10-week flexible-dosage treatment with duloxetine (60–120 mg/day) with placebo (Rynn et al. 2008). The third study compared flexibly dosed duloxetine with an active comparator, venlafaxine (75–225 mg/day), and with placebo (Hartford et al. 2007). Results from each of these studies indicated that patients taking duloxetine compared with placebo showed significant improvement on the primary efficacy measure, although in the third study the rates of remission (Ham-A≤7) were significantly greater for venlafaxine ER over placebo (30% vs.19%, $P\leq 0.05$) but not for duloxetine over placebo. Compared with placebo-treated patients, duloxetine-treated patients had a significantly greater mean reduction on the Ham-A total score ($P\leq 0.001$). Ham-A response and remission rates were significantly greater with duloxetine treatment (51% response, 30% remission) than with placebo treatment (33% response, 20% remission) ($P\leq 0.001$ both comparisons). Duloxetine-treated patients also showed greater functional improvement than placebo-treated patients on the Sheehan Disability Scale (SDS) global function and domain scores ($P\leq 0.001$). Treatment-emergent adverse events of nausea, dizziness, dry mouth, fatigue, constipation, insomnia, somnolence, hyperhydrosis, and decreased libido occurred in ≥5% of the duloxetine group, which was twice the rate in the placebo group (Allgulander et al. 2007).

In a later review of the same pooled analysis, Endicott et al. (2007) looked specifically at the efficacy of duloxetine treatment for improving functional outcomes for patients with GAD. The main functional outcome measure for each study was the SDS. Duloxetine-treated patients improved significantly compared with placebo-treated patients on SDS global functioning (study 1 [fixed dosage], $P\leq 0.001$; studies 2 and 3 [flexible dosage], $P\leq 0.01$) and on SDS work, social life, and family/home responsibility scores (P values ranged from ≤0.05 to ≤0.001). At treatment endpoint, a greater percentage of duloxetine-treated patients than placebo-treated patients had obtained SDS global functioning scores in the normative range (P values ranged from ≤0.05 to ≤0.001). Duloxetine-treated patients also reported greater increases in quality of life, well-being, and health compared with the placebo group on the other functional measures (P values ranged from ≤0.05 to ≤0.001).

Other Antidepressants

Agomelatine. Agomelatine has a novel mechanism of action, affecting primarily the hormone melatonin, which is involved in the maintenance of circadian rhythms. Agomelatine acts as an MT_1 and MT_2 agonist while also being a 5-HT_{2C} antagonist (Zupancic and Guilleminault 2006). In a randomized, double-blind, placebo-controlled study, D.J. Stein et al. (2007) examined the efficacy of agomelatine in the treatment of GAD, using the Ham-A and CGI scales as primary outcome measures. For a treatment period of 12 weeks, 121 nondepressed patients with GAD were treated with flexible dosages (20–50 mg/day). At study endpoint, Ham-A scores for agomelatine patients were significantly lower than for placebo controls ($P=0.04$). In addition, rates of response (50% Ham-A reduction) and remission (Ham-A≤7) were significantly higher in agomelatine patients than in placebo ($P=0.026$ and

P=0.027, respectively). Agomelatine patients did not differ significantly from placebo controls in the incidence of treatment-related adverse events or discontinuation symptoms. Agomelatine displayed a highly desirable tolerability profile when compared with traditional SSRIs. Although more research is required, agomelatine may prove to be a valuable treatment option for GAD because it displays comparable levels of efficacy to SSRIs with the apparent absence of significant adverse events, such as sleep disturbances and sexual dysfunction.

Bupropion. Bupropion is an antidepressant that acts as a norepinephrine and dopamine reuptake inhibitor as well as a nicotinic agonist. This agent belongs to the chemical class of aminoketones and is similar in structure to phenethylamines (Ascher et al. 1995). In a double-blind, placebo-controlled comparison by Bystritsky et al. (2005), 32 outpatients with GAD were given either bupropion ER (300 mg/day) or escitalopram (20 mg/day). Primary outcome measures consisted of total Ham-A scores, Ham-D scores, and socioeconomic status measures. Upon study completion, a marked reduction in Ham-A scores was seen in both treatment groups. The average Ham-A scores were 11.06 and 4.54 for escitalopram and bupropion, respectively. These values suggest a significant advantage for bupropion ($P<0.005$) over escitalopram in the treatment of GAD. The authors concluded that these promising results suggest a potential benefit for the use of bupropion in the treatment of GAD. However, these results need to be interpreted with caution because the efficacy of bupropion still needs to be demonstrated in placebo-controlled trials and in studies with larger sample sizes.

Antipsychotics

Traditional or typical antipsychotic medications act primarily on the dopamine system and have been used for many years in the treatment of psychosis and schizophrenia. These agents have been associated with significant side effects, most notably extrapyramidal symptoms as well as tardive dyskinesia, which can occur with prolonged use (Seeman 2002). In contrast, the atypical antipsychotics represent a new generation of antipsychotic agents that possess more desirable tolerability profiles. These newer medications bind less strongly to D_2 dopamine receptors, allowing for more transient effects and reducing the incidence of extrapyramidal side effects (Seeman 2002). Recently, interest has been shown in the potential anxiolytic properties of these atypical agents and in particular their use in treating GAD that is resistant to more traditional forms of treatment. Although, to date, few randomized, controlled trials have been conducted examining this drug class, most investigations involve refractory cases of GAD and are discussed in detail in the "Treatment-Refractory GAD" section later in this chapter.

Trifluoperazine. Trifluoperazine is a typical antipsychotic known to have an early onset of action and a relatively long duration of activity (Ayd 1959; Moyer and Conner 1958). Moreover, it produces a minimum of autonomic and endocrine side effects (Ayd 1959; Moyer and Conner 1958). In a double-blind, placebo-controlled multicenter trial, Mendels et al. (1986) examined the effectiveness of trifluoperazine in the short-term treatment of 415 outpatients with a diagnosis of moderate to severe GAD, as defined by DSM-III. Patients were randomly assigned to receive either trifluoperazine (n=207) or placebo (n=208) for 4 weeks. Each week, patients were evaluated with the Ham-A, Hopkins Symptom Checklist (HSCL), and CGI Scale. At all points of comparison for all rating scales used in the study, the average scores were significantly lower for the trifluoperazine treatment group than for the placebo group (Ham-A, $P<0.05$; HSCL, $P<0.001$; and CGI scores, $P<0.001$).

Quetiapine. Quetiapine is an atypical antipsychotic medication that has been shown to be effective in treating schizophrenia and bipolar disorder (Calabrese et al. 2005; Small et al. 1997). Use of antipsychotics to treat GAD is often reserved for patients with treatment-resistant or treatment-refractory GAD. Three acute randomized, controlled trials of monotherapy quetiapine in GAD treatment have been completed, as well as one relapse prevention study. In a 6-week study of 38 patients with a primary diagnosis of GAD (Ham-A≥20), Brawman-Mintzer et al. (2006b) examined the efficacy of quetiapine monotherapy in the treatment of GAD. Patients were randomly assigned to receive quetiapine (25–300 mg/day) or placebo. Primary efficacy was assessed through baseline to endpoint changes in total Ham-A scores. Results indicated that patients taking quetiapine had significantly reduced Ham-A total and psychic anxiety scores compared with placebo at weeks 2 and 4 ($P<0.05$), but not at endpoint. Both response (>50% Ham-A reduction) and remission (Ham-A ≤7) rates were higher for quetiapine (57.9% and 42.1%) than for placebo (36.8% and 21.1%) but were not statistically significant.

In the second study, patients were randomly assigned to receive 10 weeks of quetiapine (50 or 150 mg/day), paroxetine, or placebo. All active treatments were found to be significantly better than placebo based on the primary outcome measure (change from baseline to week 8 on Ham-A, $P<0.05$) and response rates (≥50% reduction on Ham-A, $P<0.05$). Remission rates (Ham-A ≤7) were significantly better for the quetiapine 150 mg/day group ($P<0.01$) and the paroxetine group ($P<0.05$) than the placebo group (Chouinard et al. 2007).

In the third study, patients were randomly assigned to receive 10 weeks of quetiapine (50, 150, or 300 mg/day) or placebo. Only the quetiapine 50 and 150 mg/day dosages were significantly better than placebo based on the primary outcome measure (change from baseline to week 8 on Ham-A, $P<0.001$) and response rates (≥50% reduction on Ham-A, $P<0.05$). Remission rates (Ham-A ≤7) were significantly higher for the group receiving quetiapine 150 mg/day than for the placebo group ($P<0.05$) (Joyce et al. 2008).

Based on the small amount of evidence regarding the efficacy of adjunctive antipsychotics in the treatment of GAD, these agents appear promising, especially for those patients who are resistant to traditional treatment. However, we caution readers to keep in mind that the evidence supporting the use of antipsychotics in GAD is limited primarily to one agent (quetiapine). Additionally, the safety and tolerability profiles for atypical antipsychotic medications (particularly for the development of weight gain, changes in glucose and lipid levels, and diabetes) make them less desirable as current first-line treatments.

Anticonvulsants

Abnormalities in both GABA systems and glutamatergic systems have been associated with various anxiety disorders. A dysfunction in $GABA_A$ receptor binding is also thought to play a role in anxiety disorders, stemming from the observation of diminished response to exogenous benzodiazepines in individuals with anxiety (T.A. Smith 2001). Various anticonvulsant agents are thought to modulate GABA and glutamate, and therefore treating anxious patients with such agents may restore the homeostasis between these two neurotransmitters and decrease neuronal overexcitability, particularly in the amygdala.

Pregabalin. Pregabalin is a structural analog to GABA, although it is not active at GABA receptors and it does not acutely alter GABA uptake or degradation (Frampton and Foster 2006). It has a novel mechanism of action, in that it binds to the delta subunit of voltage-dependent calcium channels in central nervous system tissues (Fink-Jensen et al. 1992), and acts as a presynaptic modulator of several excitatory neurotransmitters.

Pande et al. (2003) compared the effectiveness and tolerability of pregabalin to those of lorazepam and placebo in patients with GAD. In this study, 276 patients were randomly assigned to four treatment groups for double-blind drug therapy of pregabalin (150 mg/day and 600 mg/day), lorazepam (6 mg/day), and placebo. The high-dosage pregabalin and lorazepam groups demonstrated similar anxiolytic effects (based on Ham-A scores). Significant improvements from baseline to endpoint were found on the Ham-A for all active treatment groups. There were also significantly more responders (≥50% decrease in Ham-A) among the patients receiving 600 mg/day of pregabalin (46%) and lorazepam (61%) than among those given placebo (27%). Although the side effects of pregabalin and lorazepam were similar, patients in the pregabalin treatment group found the side effects to be more tolerable.

In a double-blind, fixed-dosage, parallel-group, placebo- and active-controlled study, Feltner et al. (2003) compared 271 patients randomly assigned to receive pregabalin 50 mg tid, pregabalin 200 mg tid, lorazepam 2 mg tid, or placebo for 4 weeks. Adjusted mean change scores on the Ham-A (primary outcome measure) were significantly improved for patients taking pregabalin 200 mg tid (difference of 3.90 between drug and placebo; $P\leq0.0013$ [ANCOVA]) or lorazepam (difference of 2.35; $P\leq0.0483$ [ANCOVA]), with a significant difference between the pregabalin 200 mg tid and placebo groups at week 1 of treatment ($P\leq0.0001$ [ANCOVA]). The results of this study suggest that pregabalin is effective and safe in short-term treatment for GAD.

Similar results were found in a double-blind, placebo-controlled, active-comparator trial in which 454 patients were randomly assigned to 4 weeks of treatment with pregabalin (300, 450, or 600 mg/day), alprazolam (1.5 mg/day), or placebo, each dosed on a thrice-daily schedule (Rickels et al. 2005). Response at endpoint was defined as ≥50% reduction in the Ham-A total score. Pregabalin and alprazolam produced a significantly greater reduction in mean ± SE Ham-A total score at LOCF endpoint compared with placebo: pregabalin 300 mg (12.2 ± 0.8, $P<0.001$), 450 mg (11.0 ± 0.8, $P=0.02$), and 600 mg (11.8 ± 0.8, $P=0.002$); alprazolam (10.9 ± 0.8, $P=0.02$); and placebo (8.4 ± 0.8).

By week 1 and at LOCF endpoint, the three pregabalin groups and the alprazolam group had significantly ($P<0.01$) improved Ham-A psychic anxiety symptoms compared with the placebo group. Ham-A somatic anxiety symptoms were also significantly ($P<0.02$) improved in the 300- and 600-mg pregabalin groups compared with the placebo group, but not in the 450-mg pregabalin group (week 1, $P=0.06$; week 4, $P=0.32$) or alprazolam group (week 1, $P=0.21$; week 4, $P=0.15$). Of the five treatment groups, the 300-mg/day pregabalin group was the only medication group that differed statistically in global improvement at treatment endpoint not only from the placebo group but also from the alprazolam group.

Likewise, Pohl et al. (2005) evaluated the anxiolytic efficacy of twice-daily versus three-times-daily dosing of pregabalin in 341 patients with GAD. Outpatients with GAD were randomly assigned to 6 weeks of double-blind treatment with pregabalin (200 mg/day bid, 400 mg/day bid, 450 mg/day tid) or placebo. Mean improvement in endpoint Ham-A total score was significantly greater for pregabalin 200 mg/day ($P=0.006$), 400 mg/day ($P=0.001$), and 450 mg/day ($P=0.005$) compared with placebo (LOCF). Pairwise comparisons of twice-daily versus three-times-daily dosing found no difference in Ham-A change score at endpoint. Improvement on both psychic and somatic factors of the Ham-A was rapid: significant improvement for patients taking pregabalin versus placebo was achieved as early as the first assessment at week 1, with ≥30% reduction in Ham-A score and equal or greater improvement for every subsequent visit in ≥38% of patients in all three pregabalin dosage groups ($P\leq0.001$). The results from this study indicate that pregabalin is an effective treatment for GAD, with similar efficacy and comparable tolerability from twice-daily and thrice-daily dosing.

Montgomery et al. (2006) showed that pregabalin was safe, well tolerated, and rapidly efficacious across both the physical-somatic and the emotional symptoms of GAD in a 6-week randomized, double-blind, placebo-controlled multicenter comparison of pregabalin and venlafaxine. Outpatients ($N=421$) were randomly assigned to receive pregabalin (400 or 600 mg/day), venlafaxine (75 mg/day), or placebo. Pregabalin at both dosages (400 mg/day, $P=0.008$; 600 mg/day, $P=0.03$) and venlafaxine ($P=0.03$) produced significantly greater improvement in Ham-A total scores at LOCF endpoint than did placebo. Only the pregabalin 400 mg/day treatment group experienced significant improvement in all a priori primary and secondary efficacy measures. Pregabalin in both dosage treatment groups (400 mg/day, $P<0.01$; 600 mg/day, $P<0.001$) significantly improved Ham-A total scores at week 1, with significant improvement continuing through LOCF endpoint. Statistically significant improvement began at week 2 for venlafaxine.

In an 8-week trial, Kasper et al. (2009) examined the anxiolytic efficacy and speed of onset of efficacy of pregabalin (300–600 mg/day) and venlafaxine ER (75–225 mg/day) versus placebo in patients with a DSM-IV diagnosis of GAD. In the intent-to-treat analysis ($N=374$), treatment with pregabalin was associated with a significantly greater mean change in the Ham-A total score at LOCF endpoint than placebo (–14.5±0.9 vs. –11.7±0.9; $P=0.028$); however, treatment with venlafaxine ER did not significantly differ from placebo. In addition, the pregabalin group showed an early onset of improvement, with significantly greater mean change in the Ham-A by day 4 (5.3±0.5) when compared with both placebo (–3.4±0.5; $P=0.008$) and venlafaxine ER (–2.9± 0.5; $P=0.0012$).

The results from these positive large-scale placebo-controlled trials indicate that pregabalin is a very reasonable first-line alternative treatment to the SSRIs and SNRIs for treating patients with GAD. Further study of pregabalin's ability to treat commonly comorbid conditions, such as depressive symptoms and other anxiety disorders, and further comparator trials would allow for a better understanding of its role and place in treating GAD.

Tiagabine. Tiagabine is the only selective GABA reuptake inhibitor (SGRI) currently available. It increases the synaptic GABA availability by selective inhibition of the GAT-1 GABA transporter, the most abundant GABA transporter (Borden et al. 1994; Fink-Jensen et al. 1992). It has been indicated for add-on treatment of partial seizures.

In a double-blind, placebo-controlled trial examining tiagabine monotherapy (mean dosage 10.5 mg/day) for GAD, 272 patients were randomly assigned to receive tiagabine or placebo for 8 weeks of treatment (Pollack et al. 2005). In the completers analysis ($n=198$), a significant reduction on the primary outcome measure (Ham-A score) was demonstrated; however, in ITT analysis, the difference did not reach statistical significance. Fifty-seven percent of patients in the tiagabine group were considered responders (CGI-I≤2), compared with 44% of those in the placebo group ($P=0.08$). Tiagabine reduced symptoms of GAD according to the observed case and mixed models repeated-measures (MMRM) analyses, but not on the primary outcome measure (the mean reduction in Ham-A total score from baseline to endpoint) with the LOCF analysis. In post hoc MMRM analysis, a significant difference in the mean reduction in Ham-A total score over the efficacy evaluation period was found, favoring tiagabine over placebo (P<0.01). Tiagabine had an early onset of effect, as shown by significant reduction from baseline in mean Ham-A total score compared with placebo at week 1 (observed cases, P<0.05). Although tiagabine did not separate from placebo in the ITT analysis, the improvements seen in the observed cases indicate that tiagabine may reduce symptoms in GAD.

In a combined analysis of three additional randomized, controlled trials of tiagabine (one fixed-dosage trial at 4, 8, or 12 mg/day and two flexible-dosage trials at 4–16 mg/day), no significant difference from placebo was found in the change in Ham-A score (primary efficacy measure) with any tiagabine dosage (LOCF). In a small subsample of patients in the flexible-dosage studies, the change in Ham-A score reached significance only at week 10. The authors concluded that tiagabine was not an effective treatment for GAD (Pollack et al. 2008). The anxiolytic effects of tiagabine in GAD, therefore, are not supported by evidence from randomized, controlled trials.

Other Agents

Abecarnil. Abecarnil is a novel β-carboline with no universally accepted mechanism of action. It is believed to partially or selectively bind to the benzodiazepine receptors, thereby potentially modulating GABA activity (Stephens et al. 1993). In a double-blind, placebo-controlled multicenter evaluation, Lydiard et al. (1997) examined the effects, safety, and tolerability of abecarnil and alprazolam in the treatment of GAD. In this study, 180 patients with GAD, diagnosed using DSM-III-R criteria, were randomly assigned to receive abecarnil (3–9 mg/day), alprazolam (1.5–4.5 mg/day), or placebo for a 4-week treatment period, followed by a 1- to 2-week taper period. Primary outcome measures consisted of the Ham-A, the Covi Anxiety Scale, the Raskin Scale for Depression, the HSCL, and the Physicians Withdrawal Checklist. Statistically significant reductions in Ham-A scores compared to placebo were observed in week 1 for alprazolam (P=0.001) and in week 2 for abecarnil (P=0.001). LOCF analysis indicated statistically significant reductions in Ham-A scores for both alprazolam and abecarnil versus placebo (P=0.038 and P=0.026, respectively). Adverse events between medications were similar, with significantly more alprazolam patients experiencing sedation than abecarnil and placebo patients (P<0.05). Treatment retention based on CGI-I scores was comparable for abecarnil and placebo, but significantly lower for alprazolam patients (P<0.03). The researchers thus concluded that both abecarnil and alprazolam are adequate short-term treatments for GAD, but recognized the potential advantage of abecarnil due to fewer adverse events and a better tolerability profile.

Abecarnil has been investigated as an alternative to benzodiazepines as a short-term treatment for patients with GAD. Rickels et al. (2000a) conducted a double-blind, placebo-controlled comparison of abecarnil and diazepam in 302 patients with GAD diagnosed using DSM-III-R criteria. Upon entering the 6-week study, patients were randomly assigned to receive abecarnil (7.5–17.5 mg/day), diazepam (15–35 mg/day), or placebo. Primary efficacy was measured through changes in Ham-A and CGI Scale scores. LOCF analysis upon study completion indicated a significant reduction in Ham-A scores compared to placebo for diazepam (P<0.001) but not for abecarnil. Week-by-week analysis indicated that both abecarnil and diazepam were significantly superior to placebo beginning at week 1 (P<0.05), with diazepam showing a slight advantage to abecarnil, although this difference failed to reach statistical significance. CGI scores (when compared with placebo) also indicated significant clinical improvement with diazepam (P<0.01) but not abecarnil at study endpoint. Adverse events consisted mainly of drowsiness, headache, and dizziness for all treatment groups. Diazepam caused significantly greater levels of discontinuation symptoms than did placebo (P<0.02) and abecarnil (P<0.01). Given these mixed results, abecarnil warrants further evaluation to support its use for the treatment of GAD.

Lesopitron. Farre and Frigola (1994) suggested that lesopitron acts as a ligand for central serotonin 5-HT_{1A} receptors, thereby potentially inducing anxiolytic effects. Fresquet et al. (2000) examined the efficacy of lesopitron in the treatment of 161 patients with GAD, who were randomly assigned to receive lesopitron (40–80 mg/day), lorazepam (2–4 mg/day), or placebo for a period of 6 weeks. Primary efficacy was measured via changes in total Ham-A scores and ratings on the CGI scales. Lorazepam demonstrated statistically significant reductions (compared with placebo) on all Ham-A subscales and CGI scales upon study completion ($P<0.05$); insignificance was observed with Ham-A total scores and Ham-A anxious mood scores in the lorazepam group. Statistical significance against placebo was observed only for the lesopitron group on the Ham-A somatic score, Ham-A anxious mood score, and CGI-I score. Adverse events were mild to moderate and consisted mainly of somnolence, headache, and dyspepsia. The authors noted that the results from this randomized, controlled trial were inconclusive because no treatment was unanimously efficacious on the primary outcome measures.

Meta-Analyses

Schmitt et al. (2005) conducted a meta-analysis of antidepressants in the treatment of GAD for randomized, controlled trials up to May 2002. Of the eight studies included, the antidepressants imipramine, venlafaxine, and paroxetine were found to be superior to placebo in treating GAD. The calculated number needed to treat (NNT) for the overall group was 5.15. By individual drug class, the NNT for imipramine was 4.07; for venlafaxine, 5.06; and for paroxetine, 6.7. The NNT for sertraline was 1.62; however, the sample size was small (N=22) and included children and adolescents. The pooled relative risk (RR) for nontreatment response was 0.70 (95% confidence interval [CI] 0.62–0.79), favoring antidepressant treatment. The calculated RR for nontreatment response for each antidepressant was as follows: imipramine, 0.67 (95% CI 0.50–0.91); venlafaxine, 0.68 (95% CI 0.46–0.99); paroxetine, 0.72 (95% CI 0.56–0.92); and paroxetine versus imipramine, 1.73 (95% CI 0.31–9.57). The RR for sertraline versus placebo was not included. The RR for dropouts for any antidepressant was 0.95 (95% CI 0.84–1.09). Similarly, when individual antidepressants were considered, no differences were found between individual treatments and the placebo group. Likewise, no significant differences occurred in dropout rates between patients taking the older antidepressant (imipramine) and those taking newer agents (venlafaxine and paroxetine). Overall, side effects were more common in the drug-treated than in the placebo-treated groups. Data for more than one trial were available only for venlafaxine.

Mitte et al. (2005) also conducted a meta-analysis of pharmacotherapy for GAD in the available literature up to May 2002 and included the results of 48 studies (and 26 drugs) in the analysis. The analysis revealed that pharmacotherapy was superior to placebo in the short-term treatment of patients with GAD. The mean effect sizes were 0.32 for benzodiazepines, 0.30 for buspirone, 0.33 for venlafaxine, and 0.20 for paroxetine, with no significant differences between drug classes. The mean unweighted dropout rate across all drugs was 24.4% (standard deviation [SD]=15.57). The dropout rate was significantly lower for benzodiazepines (20.5%; SD=14.30) compared with azapirones (30.7%, SD=17.96) but not compared with pill placebo (30.2%, SD=22.32). No significant differences were found between completer and ITT analysis, between fixed and flexible dosages, between studies using a placebo run-in or not, or between studies using different diagnostic criteria sets. Overall, results suggest that benzodiazepines and azapirones were more favorable in the short-term treatment of GAD.

Mitte (2005) examined the efficacy of cognitive-behavioral therapy (CBT) for GAD in a meta-analysis comparing CBT to pharmacological treatment (namely benzodiazepines). A total of 65 studies were included, six of which compared the two interventions directly. No significant differences in efficacy were found between CBT and pharmacotherapy across all six studies. The effect size for CBT with no treatment control was 0.82 (95% CI 0.62–1.01); for CBT with a placebo control, 0.57 (95% CI 0.30–0.85); and for CBT with pharmacotherapy, 0.33 (95% CI 0.02–0.67). Comparison of CBT and pharmacotherapy revealed a significantly lower dropout rate for CBT ($P<0.01$), indicating that CBT is better tolerated by patients. The results of this meta-analysis indicate that CBT is at least as effective as pharmacotherapy in the treatment of GAD.

In a more recent meta-analysis, Hidalgo et al. (2007) compared 21 double-blind, placebo-controlled trials of medications treating GAD (diagnosed with DMS-III-R, DSM-IV, or ICD-10) and using Ham-A score change from baseline as the main efficacy measure. The authors found that when comparing all drugs versus placebo, the mean effect size was 0.39. On an individual basis, pregabalin emerged with the highest effect size of 0.5, followed by hydroxyzine, 0.45; venlafaxine, 0.42; benzodiazepine (alprazolam, diazepam, lorazepam), 0.38; SSRI (paroxetine, sertraline, fluvoxamine, and escitalopram), 0.36; buspirone, 0.17; and kava kava and homeopathic preparations, –0.31.

Based on the results of these meta-analyses, pregabalin seems to have the greatest effect size and should be considered a first-line treatment. However, the SSRIs and SNRIs should also be considered first-line treatments due to their reasonable effect size, broad spectrum of efficacy across common comorbid conditions, and good tolerability.

Predictors of Treatment

Few studies have examined predictors of treatment outcome for patients with GAD. Early studies of GAD, using DSM-III and DSM-III-R criteria, indicated potential predictors of poor treatment outcome, including the presence of a personality disorder, recurrent episodes, older age, and poor relationships (Seivewright et al. 1998; Yonkers et al. 2000). In addition, DeMartinis et al. (2000) suggested that previous use of benzodiazepines may increase patient attrition from treatment with buspirone. Pollack et al. (2003) examined predictors of outcome of GAD in a pooled analysis of short- and long-term studies using venlafaxine ER (*N*=1,839). A history of substance abuse was found to be a strong predictor of response such that it predicted a positive response in placebo-treated patients. Comorbid sleep disturbance (based on DSM-IV criteria) also predicted significant positive response in placebo-treated patients and was a significant but less robust predictor in patients taking venlafaxine ER as well. Restlessness was found to be a predictor of poor response and lack of remission in either treatment condition. Finally, poor concentration was found to be a positive predictor of short-term remission in the placebo group only. Other factors such as sex, age, history of depression or panic disorder, prior use of benzodiazepines (or no prior use), easy fatigability, muscular tension, and irritability were found to be only modest predictors of outcome.

Long-Term Treatment

Examination of the long-term efficacy of pharmacological treatment of GAD is particularly important due to GAD's chronic course and association with significant functional impairment. Long-term randomized, controlled trials have evaluated the efficacy and safety of venlafaxine, escitalopram, and pregabalin in the treatment of GAD.

Hackett et al. (1999) examined fixed dosages of venlafaxine ER (37.5, 75, and 150 mg) in 544 patients for up to 168 days. Primary efficacy measures consisted of mean change in baseline total Ham-A score and CGI scores. Results indicated that all three dosage levels provided statistically significant reductions in anxiety measures (*P* values were not reported in the publication). Significant advantages of venlafaxine ER (75 and 150 mg/day) compared with placebo were observed beginning at week 2 and continued for 6 months. In addition, treatment with the highest dosage of venlafaxine (150 mg/day) was significantly superior to the lowest dosage (37.5 mg/day) beginning at week 8 and continuing up to 6 months.

Further examination of the long-term usage of venlafaxine ER was conducted by Gelenberg et al. (2000). In this 28-week randomized, controlled trial, 251 patients with a primary diagnosis of GAD, based on DSM-IV criteria, were randomly assigned to receive either venlafaxine ER (75, 150, 225 mg/day) or placebo. Primary efficacy was assessed through Ham-A total and psychic anxiety scores, as well as CGI scores. Upon study completion, venlafaxine ER was found to be significantly superior to placebo on all primary outcome measures (total Ham-A: –13.4 vs. –8.7; psychic anxiety: –7.4 vs. –4.2; CGI-I score: 2.2 vs. 3.0; all $Ps<0.001$) and was evident as early as week 1 ($P<0.01$). Response rates (Ham-A decrease≥40% from baseline or CGI-I=1 or 2) were also significantly higher for venlafaxine ER than placebo, beginning at week 2 (42% vs. 21%, $P<0.001$) and continuing through week 28 (69% or higher vs. 42%–46%, $P<0.001$). The authors concluded that venlafaxine was likely safe and efficacious for both short- and long-term treatment of GAD.

The long-term treatment of GAD with venlafaxine ER was also assessed by Allgulander et al. (2001). In this 24-week randomized, placebo-controlled study, 529 patients with a DSM-IV diagnosis of GAD were treated with venlafaxine ER (37.5, 75, 150 mg/day) or placebo. Primary efficacy measures consisted of Ham-A total, psychic anxiety factor, and anxiety subscale scores. CGI scales were also used as primary outcome measures. At the 8-week mark, compared with placebo, venlafaxine ER 75 mg/day and 150 mg/day caused significantly greater reductions in Ham-A scores ($P<0.017$). Upon study completion at 24 weeks, all treatment groups produced significantly greater reductions compared with placebo on all primary efficacy measures ($P<0.017$), except venlafaxine ER 37.5 mg/day had an insignificant reduction on CGI-I scales compared with placebo. In addition, the group taking 150 mg/day was significantly better than the group taking 37.5 mg/day on the Ham-A anxiety subscale and psychic anxiety factor scores ($P<0.017$). No significant differences were found between groups in overall frequency of adverse events. All side effects were similar to those previously reported in the literature, and their incidence was dosage dependent. Overall, the authors concluded that treatment with venlafaxine ER was effective in managing GAD, in both short- and long-term settings. These long-term results are important because GAD is highly chronic and can persist for many years.

The long-term use of escitalopram in treating GAD was first demonstrated in a study by Davidson et al. (2005). In this study, patients from three 8-week randomized, controlled trials of nearly identical methodology were pooled. Patients completing 8 weeks of double-blind treatment were then given the option of continuing for 24 weeks of open-label treatment with flexibly dosed escitalopram (10–20 mg/day). Treatment with escitalopram led to overall improvement across all efficacy measures. Based on LOCF analysis, 76% of patients completing open-label treatment were responders (compared with 49% entering the open-label phase) and 49% were considered remitters. The conclusions from this study suggest that escitalopram has long-term efficacy in treating GAD, although the lack of a placebo arm in the long-term phase limits the conclusions that can be made.

In a study by Bielski et al. (2005), 121 patients were randomly assigned to receive either escitalopram (10–20 mg/day) or paroxetine (20–50 mg/day) in a 24-week long-term study of GAD. Total Ham-A scores were used as the primary outcome measure. Upon study completion, a reduction in Ham-A scores was seen for both groups (−15.3 and −13.3 for escitalopram and paroxetine, respectively). No significant differences in Ham-A reduction were seen between treatment groups (P=0.13). A significant difference was observed between groups in terms of withdrawal due to adverse events. Overall, only 6.2% of escitalopram patients withdrew due to adverse events, compared with 22.6% of paroxetine patients (P=0.02). The mean dosage of escitalopram was 14.4 mg/day compared with 29.9 mg/day of paroxetine. The authors concluded based on the results of this study that escitalopram had a more favorable tolerability profile and was a superior first-line treatment for GAD.

Relapse Prevention Studies

Within the current literature, paroxetine, escitalopram, duloxetine, quetiapine XR, and pregabalin have been examined in relapse prevention of GAD. Stocchi and colleagues (2003) examined paroxetine (20–50 mg/day) in a 24-week relapse prevention study. Adults (N=652) with a DSM-IV diagnosis of GAD entered single-blind treatment with paroxetine (20–50 mg/day) for a period of 8 weeks. Those classified as responders (CGI-S≤3 or a drop in baseline score≥2) were then randomly assigned to 24 weeks of treatment with either their current dosage of paroxetine or placebo. Primary efficacy was assessed by examining the proportion of patients relapsing (CGI-S increase≥2 from baseline to a score of 4 or more or withdrawal due to lack of efficacy) during the double-blind treatment phase. Scores on the Ham-A were used as a secondary outcome measure. Results indicated that paroxetine patients were significantly less likely to relapse (10.9%) than placebo patients (39.9%, P<0.001). Furthermore, patients who switched from paroxetine to placebo at week 8 were 4.7 times more likely to relapse than those remaining on paroxetine. Upon study completion, 73.0% of paroxetine patients had achieved full remission (Ham-A≤7) compared with only 34.4% of placebo patients (P<0.001). The authors concluded that the results obtained from this study demonstrate the maintained efficacy of paroxetine in the long-term treatment of GAD.

Two studies have examined the effectiveness of escitalopram in relapse prevention. In a study of 491 patients with GAD diagnosed using DSM-IV, Allgulander et al. (2006) examined relapse rates with escitalopram treatment. Upon admission into the study, patients received 12 weeks of open-label treatment with escitalopram 20 mg/day. Responders (Ham-A total score ≤10) were then randomly assigned either to continue taking 20 mg/day escitalopram or to receive placebo for a minimum of 24 but up to 76 weeks. The primary efficacy measure was time to relapse (Ham-A≥15 or as judged by investigator) during the double-blind period. Results for the open-label period indicated substantial reductions in total Ham-A score (mean change 27.3±6.6). During the double-blind phase, escitalopram showed significant effects relative to placebo in time required to relapse (P<0.001). Relapse occurred in 56% of placebo patients but only 19% of escitalopram patients, representing a significant difference (P<0.001). Further analysis indicated that placebo patients were 4.04 times more likely to relapse than escitalopram patients. This led the authors to conclude that escitalopram 20 mg/day showed significant benefits over placebo in the prevention of relapse in GAD.

Bakish et al. (2006) also examined the efficacy of escitalopram in 107 patients with a primary diagnosis of GAD. Patients were treated in an open-label fashion with escitalopram (20 mg/day) for a period of 12 weeks. Of these, 72 patients were considered responders (Ham-A≤10) and were randomly assigned to double-blind treatment with either escitalopram (20 mg/day) or placebo for a minimum of 24 weeks. Relapse was defined as an increase in Ham-A scores such that the total score was ≥15. Results indicated that escitalopram significantly improved time to relapse (P<0.014). Within the escitalopram group, 33% of patients relapsed, compared with 64% of the placebo group ($P<0.01$). Risk of relapse was also found to be 2.33 times greater for placebo patients than escitalopram patients ($P<0.018$). These results led the authors to conclude that escitalopram was effective in the long-term treatment of GAD. However, caution must be taken in interpreting these results, because the sample size for this study was relatively small.

W. Smith et al. (2002) investigated the long-term efficacy of pregabalin in 624 adult patients with a DSM-IV diagnosis of GAD and a mean Ham-A score of 25.2. The patients received open-label pregabalin 150 mg tid for 8 weeks. Responders who had a Ham-A score≤11 for the week 7 and 8 visits were then randomly assigned to double-blind treatment with either pregabalin ($n=168$) or placebo ($n=170$) for an additional 26 weeks. The primary efficacy parameter was time to relapse, defined as one of the following: 1) Ham-A≥20 and diagnosis of GAD at two successive visits 1 week apart; 2) CGI-I rated *much worse* or *very much worse* and a diagnosis of GAD at two successive visits 1 week apart; or 3) symptomatic worsening of anxiety that required clinical intervention. A significant difference was seen between pregabalin and placebo groups in time to relapse ($P=0.0001$). Significantly more pregabalin-treated patients maintained efficacy through the double-blind period (endpoint CGI-I≤5) compared with double-blind baseline (pregabalin 57.1%, placebo 36.5%; $P=0.001$). Statistical significance in favor of pregabalin was also demonstrated on the Ham-A and on the SDS (total score and subscales). Pregabalin was well tolerated, with no unexpected adverse events occurring during the 8 months of the study. The results of this study clearly demonstrate the efficacy of pregabalin for the prevention of relapse of GAD during long-term treatment.

Davidson et al. (2007) examined duloxetine (flexible dosage) in the prevention of relapse in adults with GAD. In this study, 887 patients were treated with open-label duloxetine (60–120 mg/day) for 26 weeks, and nonresponders were randomly assigned to double-blind duloxetine or placebo for an additional 26 weeks. Duloxetine was found to be significantly superior to placebo in terms of rates of relapse (13.7% vs. 41.8%, $P\leq0.001$). Placebo-treated patients had significant worsening of their GAD symptoms on all primary and secondary efficacy measures ($P\leq0.001$ on all comparisons). In patients who did relapse, duloxetine-treated patients had a longer time to relapse than placebo-treated patients ($P\leq0.001$). The authors concluded that duloxetine was very effective for long-term treatment and prevention of relapse in patients with GAD.

The efficacy of quetiapine ER monotherapy has also been examined in relapse prevention in a study of GAD (Katzman et al. 2008). Following 12–18 weeks of open-label treatment with quetiapine ER (50, 150, or 300 mg/day), 433 patients (Ham-A ≤12, MADRS ≤16, CGI-S ≤3) were randomly assigned to continue on quetiapine or switch to placebo. Primary outcome measure was "time to event," which was defined as time to recurrence of anxiety symptoms (maximum 52 weeks). Quetiapine ER–treated patients had significantly reduced risk of an anxiety event ($P<0.0001$) compared with placebo-treated patients, implying increased time to event. Twenty-two (10.8%) patients in the quetiapine ER group versus 84 (38.9%) in the placebo group experienced a symptom recurrence ($P<0.001$). Ham-A total score was also significantly reduced at study endpoint for quetiapine ER versus placebo ($P<0.001$), and depressive symptoms (MADRS) and overall symptom severity (CGI-S) were significantly lower in the quetiapine group than in the placebo group. Quetiapine was well tolerated and did not demonstrate an increased risk of serious adverse events.

Special Populations

Pharmacotherapy of GAD in Elderly Patients

Because treatment of GAD in elderly patient populations poses unique challenges, treatment options must be carefully evaluated to ensure their maximum effectiveness. In determining treatments, physicians also should consider age-related difficulties (declining physical health, bereavement, etc.) experienced by elderly patients. Although benzodiazepines have been used in the treatment of older GAD patient cohorts, their long-term use and their sedative, cognitive, and muscle relaxant properties are not always beneficial. A handful of studies have investigated the effectiveness of other pharmacological agents in elderly patients with GAD.

More specifically, studies of the SNRIs venlafaxine and duloxetine (Davidson et al. 2008; Katz et al. 2002), the SSRI citalopram (Lenze et al. 2005), and the anticonvulsant pregabalin (Bobes Garcia et al. 2007) have been conducted using older patient populations (the data on venlafaxine and duloxetine are derived from subanalyses of samples that included elderly patients). The current literature on elderly patients with GAD supports the use of pregabalin, citalopram, and venlafaxine, all of which have demonstrated superior efficacy to placebo. These studies are detailed elsewhere in this volume (Chapter 35, "Anxiety Disorders in the Elderly").

Patients With Treatment-Refractory GAD

The empirical evidence is meager concerning next-step treatments and strategies for patients with treatment-refractory GAD. Open-label evidence has suggested the efficacy of ziprasidone (Snyderman et al. 2005), adjunctive risperidone (Simon et al. 2006), and tiagabine monotherapy (with paroxetine as positive control) (Rosenthal 2003), and several positive case reports have suggested the use of tiagabine, levetiracetam, and gabapentin.

Risperidone

In a study conducted by Brawman-Mintzer et al. (2005), the effect of adjunctive risperidone (0.5–1.5 mg/day) was examined in a 5-week double-blind, placebo-controlled trial in 40 patients with GAD who were considered nonresponders (Ham-A≥18) to their current anxiolytic treatment. The most common medications being taken by patients were benzodiazepines, sertraline, and buspirone; however, many patients were taking multiple medications at the time of risperidone augmentation. Adjunctive treatment with risperidone was significantly more effective at reducing total Ham-A scores (primary efficacy measure) from baseline than was placebo (−9.8±5.5 vs. −6.2±4.9; *P*=0.34, LOCF). Response (CGI-I≤2) rates were higher in the risperidone group, but the rates did not differ significantly from placebo. Some of the limitations of this study include the small sample size and short treatment duration, as well as the heterogeneity of the anxiolytic medications being taken by patients. A wide variety of medications were examined as baseline treatment, leaving the generalizability of these results in question.

Olanzapine

In a randomized, controlled study conducted by Pollack et al. (2006), patients remaining symptomatic after 6 weeks of treatment with fluoxetine (20 mg/day) were randomly assigned to receive 6 weeks of olanzapine (mean dosage 8.7±7.1 mg/day) or placebo augmentation. Olanzapine resulted in a greater proportion of treatment responders based on a CGI-S endpoint score of 1 or 2 (*P*<0.05) or a 50% reduction in Ham-A score (*P*<0.05). No other outcome measures showed statistically significant differences for olanzapine compared to placebo. Patients receiving olanzapine augmentation experienced significant weight gain compared with patients receiving placebo augmentation (11.0±5.1 vs. −0.7±2.4 pounds; *t*=6.32, *P*<0.001). Although the results from this study appeared promising, limitations included the small sample size, as well as the high incidence of weight gain associated with olanzapine.

Quetiapine

In another augmentation study, patients with GAD were prospectively treated with open-label controlled-release paroxetine (up to 62.5 mg/day) for 10 weeks. Those remaining symptomatic (Ham-A≥7) were randomly assigned to receive quetiapine (25–400 mg/day) or placebo for an additional 8 weeks. Quetiapine augmentation demonstrated no significant benefit over placebo on the primary outcome measure (change from baseline to endpoint on Ham-A) (Simon et al. 2008).

Cognitive-Behavioral Therapy

In studies comparing CBT and control conditions, CBT has been shown to be an effective treatment for patients with GAD. CBT yielded moderate to large effect sizes in the meta-analysis by Mitte (2005). In studies included in this meta-analysis, which compared pharmacotherapy and CBT, no significant differences were found between these two treatment modalities. Given that CBT is a highly efficacious treatment, it should be considered as an alternate treatment for GAD, especially in nonresponders to pharmacotherapy. In addition, CBT may be a useful augmenting strategy to pharmacotherapy, although the efficacy of combining pharmacotherapy and CBT for GAD has not been well evaluated, with the exception of one preliminary study (Black 2006).

Novel and Experimental Approaches

Increasing numbers of people are turning to alternative therapies to either complement or replace conventional medicine (Eisenberg et al. 1993, 1998). Such alternative approaches include homeopathic treatment with kava kava, valerian, passionflower, and ginkgo biloba.

Kava Kava

Kava kava (*Piper methysticum*) is a popular herbal medicine sometimes used in the naturopathic treatment of anxiety (Singh and Singh 2002). Although some randomized, controlled trials have been conducted, they are predominantly in the German literature, and many examine anxiety in general rather than GAD. To date, two randomized, controlled trials have been conducted examining the use of kava kava specifically in GAD.

Analysis of the use of kava kava for treating patients with GAD was conducted by Boerner et al. (2003) in an 8-week double-blind comparison with buspirone and opipramol. A total of 129 outpatients with GAD diagnosed using ICD-10 criteria (Ham-A≥19) were randomly assigned to receive kava kava (400 mg/day), buspirone (10 mg/day), or opipramol (100 mg/day). Primary efficacy was measured via baseline to endpoint change in Ham-A scores and proportion of responders (>50% reduction from baseline Ham-A score). Results indicated that mean reductions in primary efficacy measures did not differ significantly between groups upon study completion. Analysis of response and remission (Ham-A<9) rates revealed no significant differences between treatment groups at endpoint, although the authors reported that two-thirds of all patients were fully remitted after week 8. Thus, the authors concluded that acute treatment with kava kava appeared to be equally effective to treatment with either buspirone or opipramol in patients with GAD.

The second randomized, controlled trial examining kava kava was conducted by Connor et al. (2006). In this study, the authors pooled results of three randomized, controlled trials (one published and two unpublished) of kava kava in patients with a DSM-IV diagnosis of GAD. Two of the pooled studies examined kava kava against placebo, whereas the third examined kava kava against both venlafaxine ER and placebo. In the total pooled sample of 64 patients, 28 were randomly assigned to receive kava kava (140–280 mg/day), 6 to receive venlafaxine ER (37.5–225 mg/day), and 30 to receive placebo. Primary efficacy was measured via baseline to endpoint changes in Ham-A total scores, Hospital Anxiety and Depression Scale (HADS) scores, and Sheehan Disability Inventory (SDI) scores. Results from the pooled analysis revealed a significant effect of placebo on Ham-A total scores ($P<0.04$), a significant treatment-by-study interaction on SDI scores ($P<0.04$) for placebo, and a trend toward significance on the HADS scores ($P<0.07$) for placebo. Kava kava was observed to have a trend toward significance on Ham-A scores in only one study ($P=0.05$). Additionally, the authors noted several limitations, namely small sample size and differing baseline Ham-A criteria across the three studies (Ham-A≥12–20 at baseline). Therefore, the authors concluded that kava kava did not show any significant clinical benefit in the treatment of GAD. This, coupled with reports of severe hepatotoxicity (Russmann et al. 2001) while taking kava kava, places the drug's usefulness in the treatment of GAD into question.

Valerian

Valerian (*Valeriana officinalis*) is an herbal medicine commonly used for insomnia (Donath et al. 2000) and also used for anxiety. Miyasaka et al. (2006) reviewed studies of the efficacy of valerian in the treatment of anxiety disorders. Of these studies, only one randomized, controlled trial focused specifically on GAD (Andreatini et al. 2002). In this 4-week double-blind, randomized, controlled trial, 36 patients with GAD diagnosed using DSM-III-R criteria were randomly assigned to valerian (50–150 mg/day), diazepam (2.5–7.5 mg/day), and placebo groups. Primary efficacy was measured via changes in Ham-A scores and the State Trait Anxiety Inventory (STAI) ratings. Upon study completion, a significant reduction was observed in total Ham-A scores from baseline ($P<0.05$) for all treatment groups. However, no significant differences were achieved between groups, although final Ham-A scores for valerian and diazepam were comparable and lower than placebo (14.6 and 14.2 vs. 16.0). Based on patient-rated STAI scores, diazepam was the only treatment to achieve significant reductions in anxious symptoms from baseline ($P<0.05$).

Passionflower

Passionflower (*Passiflora incarnata*) is a large flowering plant that has traditionally been used for its sedative, sleep-inducing properties (Bergner 1995). Akhondzadeh et al. (2001) examined passionflower extract in a double-blind, randomized trial. In this study, 36 patients diagnosed with GAD using DSM-IV criteria (Ham-A≥14) were randomly assigned to receive oxazepam (30 mg/day) or passionflower extract (45 drops/day) for a period of 4 weeks. Primary efficacy was assessed through changes in total Ham-A scores. Results indicated that treatment with either medication resulted in significant reductions in Ham-A scores from baseline ($P<0.001$), with no significant differences observed between groups at study endpoint. Treatment with passionflower was significantly superior to oxazepam at day 4 ($P=0.008$); however, this difference was only transient. No significant differences were observed in the incidence of adverse events, except that oxazepam patients reported higher levels of job performance impairment

(P=0.049). Based on these preliminary results, no evidence is available to support the use of passionflower extract in the treatment of GAD.

Ginkgo Biloba

Ginkgo biloba special extract EGb 761 is registered in Germany as an antidementia medication for use in elderly patients. It reportedly enhances cognitive and social functioning in elderly patients (Kanowski et al. 1996). Its potential anxiolytic properties were assessed in a recent randomized, controlled trial. Woelk et al. (2007) examined 82 patients with GAD, diagnosed using DSM-III-R criteria, who were randomly assigned to receive EGb 761 (240 or 480 mg/day) or placebo for a period of 4 weeks. Primary efficacy was measured via changes in Ham-A total scores. Upon study completion, results indicated that EGb 761 was superior to placebo (based on Ham-A total scores) at both dosage levels (240 mg/day, P=0.04; 480 mg/day, P=0.004). Response rates (>50% reduction in Ham-A total score) with both EGb 761 dosages were higher than with placebo (44% high dosage and 39% low dosage vs. 22% placebo). This trend was also observed in regard to remission (Ham-A≤7) rates (9% high dosage and 8% low dosage vs. 5% placebo) (significance levels not reported). The authors concluded that EGb 761 demonstrated specific dose-dependent anxiolytic activity that was superior to the placebo effect traditionally observed in psychoactive drug trials. These results suggest the potential usefulness of this specific herbal extract, although large-scale randomized, controlled trials are still required.

Summary

There has been a lack of efficacy shown in placebo-controlled studies of herbal remedies in GAD. As a result, herbal remedies are not recommended as treatments for GAD.

Conclusion

Our review of the pharmacotherapy of GAD gives support to a broad range of treatments. For an effective synthesis of this literature, summarizing the data based on levels of evidence is helpful. As detailed in the Canadian Clinical Practice Guidelines (Canadian Psychiatric Association 2006), levels of evidence are ranked from 1 to 4 as follows: 1) meta-analysis or replicated randomized, controlled trial that includes a placebo condition (the highest level of evidence); 2) at least one randomized, controlled trial with placebo or active comparison condition; 3) uncontrolled trial with at least 10 or more subjects; and 4) anecdotal reports or expert opinions. Level 1 evidence has been demonstrated with the following compounds: the antidepressants paroxetine, sertraline, escitalopram, venlafaxine, duloxetine, and imipramine; the benzodiazepines diazepam, alprazolam, bromazepam, and lorazepam; the azapirone buspirone; the anticonvulsant pregabalin; and the antihistamine hydroxyzine. The current published treatment guidelines suggest starting with one of the efficacious SSRIs (paroxetine, sertraline, or escitalopram) or the SNRI venlafaxine as a first-line treatment (Baldwin et al. 2005; Canadian Psychiatric Association 2006). However, with the most recent data from the meta-analysis of pharmacological treatments for GAD (Hidalgo et al. 2007), pregabalin should also be considered a first-line agent. At this time, no empirical data are available to suggest the next-step treatment should an individual have a partial response or nonresponse to the first treatment trial. Therefore, switching to a different class of drug is a reasonable next step. The GAD treatment literature also lacks any real direction as to treatment resistance.

Unlike other anxiety disorders, GAD is a relatively infrequent disorder in the first two decades of life, with the lifetime prevalence of GAD increasing steadily, particularly in women after their mid-20s. Although few prevalence studies have involved individuals over the age of 65 years, elderly individuals in the general population appear to have high rates of GAD (Beekman et al. 2000). Only a small number of studies have examined the treatment of GAD in this age group, although some good preliminary evidence supports the use of venlafaxine, citalopram, and pregabalin. Treatment of GAD in elderly patients is an area that clearly needs more investigation.

Patients with GAD experience a high degree of comorbidity, with up to 91% presenting with at least one additional diagnosis (Sanderson and Barlow 1990). High rates of comorbidity have been found in patients with GAD attending both psychiatric facilities and primary care practices (D.J. Stein 2001). In general, GAD with comorbidity results in a less favorable treatment outcome, with higher rates of health care service use, illness burden, and treatment nonresponse (D.J. Stein 2001; D.J. Stein and Hollander 2002). The current body of literature has unfortunately excluded GAD with comorbidity, likely limiting the applicability of the data to regular clinical populations. The response rates in the current literature may not have been as positive had GAD with comorbidity been studied. Future investigations need to evaluate or include GAD with comorbidity.

Given the broad range of agents found to be efficacious in treating GAD, developing predictors of response would be helpful in guiding clinicians. The burgeoning field of genetics and the identification of genetic polymorphisms may contribute to more effective clinical treatment of GAD, such as has already occurred in the areas of depression and social phobia (M.B. Stein et al. 2006).

Nevertheless, the future of GAD as it is currently known is in question. The definition and classification of GAD in the next revision of DSM may create further challenges in the treatment of this intricate disorder.

◀ Key Clinical Points ▶

- A wide variety of pharmacological agents have demonstrated efficacy in generalized anxiety disorder.
- Balancing efficacy, broad spectrum of action, safety, and tolerability as important concerns, clinicians should consider SSRIs, SNRIs, and pregabalin as first-line treatments for GAD.
- Given the lack of information on treatment resistance or partial response, the use of an alternative first-line treatment is a reasonable approach before moving to second-line treatments, such as benzodiazepines, imipramine, quetiapine, hydroxyzine, or buspirone.
- Cognitive-behavioral therapy is also an effective alternative treatment; however, it may not be readily available in all communities. Combining CBT with pharmacotherapy may be a promising strategy for treatment resistance but is as yet unproven.

References

Akhondzadeh S, Naghavi HR, Vazirian M, et al: Passionflower in the treatment of generalized anxiety: a pilot double-blind randomized controlled trial with oxazepam. J Clin Pharm Ther 26:363–367, 2001

Allgulander C, Hackett D, Salinas E: Venlafaxine extended release (ER) in the treatment of generalised anxiety disorder: twenty-four-week placebo-controlled dose-ranging study. Br J Psychiatry 179:15–22, 2001

Allgulander C, Dahl AA, Austin C, et al: Efficacy of sertraline in a 12-week trial for generalized anxiety disorder. Am J Psychiatry 161:1642–1649, 2004

Allgulander C, Florea I, Trap Huusom AK: Prevention of relapse in generalized anxiety disorder by escitalopram treatment. Int J Neuropsychopharmacol 9:495–505, 2006

Allgulander C, Hartford J, Russell J, et al: Pharmacotherapy of generalized anxiety disorder: results of duloxetine treatment from a pooled analysis of three clinical trials. Curr Med Res Opin 23:1245–1252, 2007

American Psychiatric Association: Diagnostic and Statistical Manual of Mental Disorders, 3rd Edition. Washington, DC, American Psychiatric Association, 1980

American Psychiatric Association: Diagnostic and Statistical Manual of Mental Disorders, 3rd Edition, Revised. Washington, DC, American Psychiatric Association, 1987

American Psychiatric Association: Diagnostic and Statistical Manual of Mental Disorders, 4th Edition. Washington, DC, American Psychiatric Association, 1994

American Psychiatric Association: Diagnostic and Statistical Manual of Mental Disorders, 4th Edition, Text Revision. Washington, DC, American Psychiatric Association, 2000

Andreatini R, Sartori VA, Seabra ML, et al: Effect of valepotriates (valerian extract) in generalized anxiety disorder: a randomized placebo-controlled pilot study. Phytother Res 16:650–654, 2002

Ansseau M, Papart P, Gerard MA, et al: Controlled comparison of buspirone and oxazepam in generalized anxiety. Neuropsychobiology 24:74–78, 1990

Ascher JA, Cole JO, Colin JN, et al: Bupropion: a review of its mechanism of antidepressant activity. J Clin Psychiatry 56:395–401, 1995

Ayd FJ: Trifluoperazine therapy for everyday psychiatric problems. Curr Ther Res Clin Exp 18:17–28, 1959

Bakish D, Huusom AKT, Legault M: Escitalopram prevents relapse in generalized anxiety disorder: an analysis of data from Canadian patients participating in a multinational clinical study. Int J Neuropsychopharmacol 9:S185–S186, 2006

Baldwin DS, Polkinghorn C: Evidence-based pharmacotherapy of generalized anxiety disorder. Int J Neuropsychopharmacol 8:293–302, 2005

Baldwin DS, Anderson IM, Nutt DJ, et al: Evidence-based guidelines for the pharmacological treatment of anxiety disorders: recommendations from the British Association for Psychopharmacology. J Psychopharmacol 19:567–596, 2005

Baldwin DS, Huusom AK, Maehlum E: Escitalopram and paroxetine in the treatment of generalised anxiety disorder: randomised, placebo-controlled, double-blind study. Br J Psychiatry 189:264–272, 2006

Ball SG, Kuhn A, Wall D, et al: Selective serotonin reuptake inhibitor treatment for generalized anxiety disorder: a double-blind, prospective comparison between paroxetine and sertraline. J Clin Psychiatry 66:94–99, 2005

Beekman AT, de Beurs E, van Balkom AJ, et al: Anxiety and depression in later life: co-occurrence and communality of risk factors. Am J Psychiatry 157:89–95, 2000

Bergner P: Passionflower. Medical Herbalism 7:13–14, 1995

Bielski RJ, Bose A, Chang C: A double-blind comparison of escitalopram and paroxetine in the long-term treatment of generalized anxiety disorder. Ann Clin Psychiatry 17:65–69, 2005

Bischoff S, Heinrich M, Sonntag JM, et al: The D-1 dopamine receptor antagonist SCH 23390 also interacts potently with brain serotonin (5-HT2) receptors. Eur J Pharmacol 129:367–370, 1986

Black D: Efficacy of combined pharmacotherapy and psychotherapy versus monotherapy in the treatment of anxiety disorders. CNS Spectr 11:29–33, 2006

Bobes Garcia J, Montgomery S, Baldinetti F, et al: Pregabalin for the treatment of generalized anxiety disorder (GAD): efficacy and safety in elderly patients. Eur Psychiatry 22:S280, 2007

Boerner RJ, Sommer H, Berger W, et al: Kava-kava extract LI 150 is as effective as opipramol and buspirone in generalised anxiety disorder—an 8-week randomized, double-blind multi-centre clinical trial in 129 out-patients. Phytomedicine 10 (suppl 4):38–49, 2003

Borden LA, Murali Dhar TG, Smith KE, et al: Tiagabine, SK&F 89976-A, CI-966, and NNC-711 are selective for the cloned GABA transporter GAT-1. Eur J Pharmacol 269:219–224, 1994

Brawman-Mintzer O, Knapp RG, Nietert PJ: Adjunctive risperidone in generalized anxiety disorder: a double-blind, placebo-controlled study. J Clin Psychiatry 66:1321–1325, 2005

Brawman-Mintzer O, Knapp RG, Rynn M, et al: Sertraline treatment for generalized anxiety disorder: a randomized, double-blind, placebo-controlled study. J Clin Psychiatry 67:874–881, 2006a

Brawman-Mintzer O, Nietert PJ, Rynn MA, et al: Quetiapine monotherapy in patients with GAD. Paper presented at the annual meeting of the American Psychiatric Association, Toronto, Canada, May 2006b

Bystritsky A, Kerwin L, Eiduson S, et al: A pilot controlled trial of bupropion vs. escitalopram in generalized anxiety disorder (GAD). Neuropsychopharmacology 30:S101, 2005

Calabrese JR, Keck PE Jr, Macfadden W, et al: A randomized, double-blind, placebo-controlled trial of quetiapine in the treatment of bipolar I or II depression. Am J Psychiatry 162:1351–1360, 2005

Canadian Psychiatric Association: Clinical practice guidelines: management of anxiety disorders. Can J Psychiatry 51 (8, suppl 2):9S–91S, 2006

Chouinard G, Bandelow B, Ahokas A, et al: Once-daily extended release quetiapine fumarate (quetiapine XR) monotherapy in generalized anxiety disorder: a phase III, double-blind, placebo-controlled study. Poster presented at the annual meeting of the American College of Neuropsychopharmacology, Boca Raton, FL, December 2007

Cohn JB, Rickels K, Steege JF: A pooled, double-blind comparison of the effects of buspirone, diazepam and placebo in women with chronic anxiety. Curr Med Res Opin 11:304–320, 1989

Connor KM, Payne V, Davidson JR: Kava in generalized anxiety disorder: three placebo-controlled trials. Int Clin Psychopharmacol 21:249–253, 2006

Costa E: Molecular mechanisms in the receptor action of benzodiazepines. Annu Rev Pharmacol 19:531–545, 1979

Cowley DS, Roy-Byrne PP, Radant A, et al: Benzodiazepine sensitivity in panic disorder: effects of chronic alprazolam treatment. Neuropsychopharmacology 12:147–157, 1995

Darcis T, Ferreri M, Natens J, et al: A multicenter double-blind placebo-controlled study investigating the anxiolytic efficacy of hydroxyzine in patients with generalized anxiety. Hum Psychopharmacol 10:181–187, 1995

Davidson JR, DuPont RL, Hedges D, et al: Efficacy, safety, and tolerability of venlafaxine extended release and buspirone in outpatients with generalized anxiety disorder. J Clin Psychiatry 60:528–535, 1999

Davidson JR, Bose A, Korotzer A, et al: Escitalopram in the treatment of generalized anxiety disorder: double-blind, placebo controlled, flexible-dose study. Depress Anxiety 19:234–240, 2004

Davidson JR, Bose A, Wang Q: Safety and efficacy of escitalopram in the long-term treatment of generalized anxiety disorder. J Clin Psychiatry 66:1441–1446, 2005

Davidson J, Wittchen H, Llorca P, et al: Duloxetine 60 to 120 mg once daily for the prevention of relapse in adults with generalized anxiety disorder: a double-blind placebo-controlled trial. Poster presented at the annual meeting of the American College of Neuropsychopharmacology, Boca Raton, FL, December 2007

Davidson JR, Allugalnder C, Pollack MH, et al: Efficacy and tolerability of duloxetine in elderly patients with generalized anxiety disorder: a pooled analysis of four randomized, double-blind, placebo-controlled studies. Hum Psychopharmacol 23:519–526, 2008

DeMartinis N, Rynn M, Rickels K, et al: Prior benzodiazepine use and buspirone response in the treatment of generalized anxiety disorder. J Clin Psychiatry 61:91–94, 2000

Donath F, Quispe S, Diefenbach K, et al: Critical evaluation of the effect of valerian extract on sleep structure and sleep quality. Pharmacopsychiatry 33:47–53, 2000

Eisenberg DM, Kessler RC, Foster C, et al: Unconventional medicine in the United States: prevalence, costs, and patterns of use. N Engl J Med 328:246–252, 1993

Eisenberg DM, Davis RB, Ettner SL, et al: Trends in alternative medicine use in the United States, 1990–1997: results of a follow-up national survey. JAMA 280:1569–1575, 1998

Eison AS, Eison MS, Stanley M, et al: Serotonergic mechanisms in the behavioral effects of buspirone and gepirone. Pharmacol Biochem Behav 24:701–707, 1986

Endicott J, Russell JM, Raskin J, et al: Duloxetine treatment for role functioning improvement in generalized anxiety disorder: three independent studies. J Clin Psychiatry 68:518–524, 2007

Enkelmann R: Alprazolam versus buspirone in the treatment of outpatients with generalized anxiety disorder. Psychopharmacology 105:428–432, 1991

Farre AJ, Frigola J: Lesopitron dihydrochloride. Future Drugs 19:51–55, 1994

Feighner JP: Mechanism of action of antidepressant medications. J Clin Psychiatry 60 (suppl 4):4–11, 1999

Feltner DE, Crockatt JG, Dubovsky SJ, et al: A randomized, double-blind, placebo-controlled, fixed-dose, multicenter study of pregabalin in patients with generalized anxiety disorder. J Clin Psychopharmacol 23:240–249, 2003

Fink-Jensen A, Suzdak PD, Swedberg MD, et al: The gamma-aminobutyric acid (GABA) uptake inhibitor, tiagabine, increases extracellular brain levels of GABA in awake rats. Eur J Pharmacol 220:197–201, 1992

Fontaine R, Beaudry P, Beauclair L, et al: Comparison of withdrawal of buspirone and diazepam: a placebo controlled study. Prog Neuropsychopharmacol 11:189–197, 1987

Frampton JE, Foster RH: Pregabalin: in the treatment of generalised anxiety disorder. CNS Drugs 20:685–693, 2006

Fresquet A, Sust M, Lloret A, et al: Efficacy and safety of lesopitron in outpatients with generalized anxiety disorder. Ann Pharmacother 34:147–153, 2000

Gammans RE, Stringfellow JC, Hvizdos AJ, et al: Use of buspirone in patients with generalized anxiety disorder and coexisting depressive symptoms: a meta-analysis of 8 randomized, controlled studies. Neuropsychobiology 25:193–201, 1992

Gelenberg AJ, Lydiard B, Rudolph RL, et al: Efficacy of venlafaxine extended-release capsules in nondepressed outpatients with generalized anxiety disorder. JAMA 283:3082–3088, 2000

Goldberg HL, Finnerty R: Comparison of buspirone in two separate studies. J Clin Psychiatry 43:87–91, 1982

Goodman WK, Bose A, Wang Q: Treatment of generalized anxiety disorder with escitalopram: pooled results from double-blind, placebo-controlled trials. J Affect Disord 87:161–167, 2005

Greenblatt DJ, Shader RI: Benzodiazepines in Clinical Practice. New York, Raven Press, 1974

Hackett D, Desmet A, Salinas EO: Dose-response efficacy of venlafaxine XR in GAD. Poster presented at 11th World Congress of Psychiatry, Hamburg, Germany, August 1999

Hartford J, Kornstein S, Liebowitz M, et al: Duloxetine as an SNRI treatment for generalized anxiety disorder: results from a placebo and active-controlled trial. Int Clin Psychopharmacol 22:167–174, 2007

Hewett K, Adams A, Bryson H, et al: Generalized anxiety disorder: efficacy of paroxetine. Paper presented at the 7th World Congress of Biological Psychiatry, Berlin, Germany, July 2001

Hidalgo RB, Tupler LA, Davidson JR: An effect-size analysis of pharmacologic treatments for generalized anxiety disorder. J Psychopharmacol 21:864–872, 2007

Hoehn-Saric R, McLeod DR, Zimmerli WD: Differential effects of alprazolam and imipramine in generalized anxiety disorder: somatic versus psychic symptoms. J Clin Psychiatry 49:293–301, 1988

Jann MW: Buspirone: an update on a unique anxiolytic agent. Pharmacotherapy 8:100–116, 1988

Joyce M, Khan A, Atkinson S, et al: Efficacy and safety of extended release quetiapine fumarate (quetiapine XR) monotherapy in patients with generalized anxiety disorder (GAD). Poster presented at the annual meeting of the American Psychiatric Association, Washington, DC, May 2008

Kanowski S, Herrmann WM, Stephan K, et al: Proof of efficacy of the ginkgo biloba special extract EGb 761 in outpatients suffering from mild to moderate primary degenerative dementia of the Alzheimer type or multi-infarct dementia. Pharmacopsychiatry 29:47–56, 1996

Kasper S, Herman B, Nivoli G, et al: Efficacy of pregabalin and venlafaxine XR in generalized anxiety disorder: results of a double-blind, placebo-controlled 8-week trial. Int Clin Psychopharmacol 24:87–96, 2009

Katz IR, Reynolds CF 3rd, Alexopoulos GS, et al: Venlafaxine ER as a treatment for generalized anxiety disorder in older adults: pooled analysis of five randomized placebo-controlled clinical trials. J Am Geriatr Soc 50:18–25, 2002

Katzman M, Brawman-Mintzer O, Reyes E, et al: Extended release quetiapine fumerate (quetiapine XR) monotherapy in long-term treatment of generalized anxiety disorder (GAD): efficacy and tolerability results from a randomized, placebo-controlled trial. Biol Psychiatry 63:141S, 2008

Kim TS, Pae CU, Yoon SJ, et al: Comparison of venlafaxine extended release versus paroxetine for treatment of patients with generalized anxiety disorder. Psychiatry Clin Neurosci 60:347–351, 2006

Koponen H, Allgulander C, Erickson J, et al: Efficacy of duloxetine for the treatment of generalized anxiety disorder: implications for primary care physicians. Prim Care Companion J Clin Psychiatry 9:100–107, 2007

Kubo N, Shirakawa O, Kuno T, et al: Antimuscarinic effects of antihistamines: quantitative evaluation by receptor-binding assay. Jpn J Pharmacol 43:277–282, 1987

Laakmann G, Schule C, Lorkowski G, et al: Buspirone and lorazepam in the treatment of generalized anxiety disorder in outpatients. Psychopharmacology 136:357–366, 1998

Lader M: Assessing the potential for buspirone dependence or abuse and effects of its withdrawal. Am J Med 82:20–26, 1987

Lader M: History of benzodiazepine dependence. J Subst Abuse Treat 8:53–59, 1991

Lader M, Scotto JC: A multicentre double-blind comparison of hydroxyzine, buspirone and placebo in patients with generalized anxiety disorder. Psychopharmacology 139:402–406, 1998

Lenze EJ, Mulsant BH, Shear MK, et al: Efficacy and tolerability of citalopram in the treatment of late-life anxiety disorders: results from an 8-week randomized placebo-controlled trial. Am J Psychiatry 162:146–150, 2005

Llorca PM, Spadone C, Sol O, et al: Efficacy and safety of hydroxyzine in the treatment of generalized anxiety disorder: a 3-month double-blind study. J Clin Psychiatry 63:1020–1027, 2002

Lydiard RB, Ballenger JC, Rickels K: A double-blind evaluation of the safety and efficacy of abecarnil, alprazolam, and placebo in outpatients with generalized anxiety disorder. Abecarnil Work Group. J Clin Psychiatry 58 (suppl 11):11–18, 1997

Majercsik E, Haller J, Leveleki C, et al: The effect of social factors on the anxiolytic efficacy of buspirone in male rats, mice and men. Prog Neuropsychopharmacol 27:1187–1199, 2003

Meibach RC, Dunner D, Wilson LG, et al: Comparative efficacy of propranolol, chlordiazepoxide, and placebo in the treatment of anxiety—a double-blind trial. J Clin Psychiatry 48:355–358, 1987

Mendels J, Krajewski TF, Huffer V, et al: Effective short-term treatment of generalized anxiety disorder with trifluoperazine. J Clin Psychiatry 47:170–174, 1986

Mitte K: Meta-analysis of cognitive-behavioral treatments for generalized anxiety disorder: a comparison with pharmacotherapy. Psychol Bull 131:785–795, 2005

Mitte K, Noack P, Steil R, et al: A meta-analytic review of the efficacy of drug treatment in generalized anxiety disorder. J Clin Psychopharmacol 25:141–150, 2005

Miyasaka LS, Atallah AN, Soares BG: Valerian for anxiety disorders. Cochrane Database Syst Rev, Issue 4, Art. No.: CD004515. DOI: 10.1002/14651858.CD004515.pub2, 2006

Moller HJ, Volz HP, Reimann IW, et al: Opipramol for the treatment of generalized anxiety disorder: a placebo-controlled trial including an alprazolam-treated group. J Clin Psychopharmacol 21:59–65, 2001

Montgomery SA, Tobias K, Zornberg GL, et al: Efficacy and safety of pregabalin in the treatment of generalized anxiety disorder: a 6-week, multicenter, randomized, double-blind, placebo-controlled comparison of pregabalin and venlafaxine. J Clin Psychiatry 67:771–782, 2006

Morris PLP, Dahl AA, Kutcher SP, et al: Efficacy of sertraline for the acute treatment of generalized anxiety disorder (GAD). Eur Neuropsychopharmacol 13:S375, 2003

Moyer JH, Conner PK: Clinical and laboratory observations on two trifluoromethyl phenothiazine derivatives. J Lab Clin Med 51:185–197, 1958

Napoliello MJ, Domantay AG: Buspirone: a worldwide update. Br J Psychiatry Suppl 12:40–44, 1991

Nimatoudis I, Zissis NP, Kogeorgos J, et al: Remission rates with venlafaxine extended release in Greek outpatients with generalized anxiety disorder: a double-blind, randomized, placebo controlled study. Int Clin Psychopharmacol 19:331–336, 2004

Noyes R Jr: Beta-adrenergic blocking drugs in anxiety and stress. Psychiatr Clin North Am 8:119–132, 1985

Pande AC, Crockatt JG, Feltner DE, et al: Pregabalin in generalized anxiety disorder: a placebo-controlled trial. Am J Psychiatry 160:533–540, 2003

Pohl RB, Feltner DE, Fieve RR, et al: Efficacy of pregabalin in the treatment of generalized anxiety disorder: double-blind, placebo-controlled comparison of bid versus tid dosing. J Clin Psychopharmacol 25:151–158, 2005

Pollack MH, Worthington JJ, Manfro GG, et al: Abecarnil for the treatment of generalized anxiety disorder: a placebo-controlled comparison of two dosage ranges of abecarnil and buspirone. J Clin Psychiatry 58 (suppl 11):19–23, 1997

Pollack MH, Zaninelli R, Goddard A, et al: Paroxetine in the treatment of generalized anxiety disorder: results of a placebo-controlled, flexible-dosage trial. J Clin Psychiatry 62:350–357, 2001

Pollack MH, Meoni P, Otto MW, et al: Predictors of outcome following venlafaxine extended-release treatment of DSM-IV generalized anxiety disorder: a pooled analysis of short- and long-term studies. J Clin Psychopharmacol 23:250–259, 2003

Pollack MH, Roy-Byrne PP, Van Ameringen M, et al: The selective GABA reuptake inhibitor tiagabine for the treatment of generalized anxiety disorder: results of a placebo-controlled study. J Clin Psychiatry 66:1401–1408, 2005

Pollack MH, Simon NM, Zalta AK, et al: Olanzapine augmentation of fluoxetine for refractory generalized anxiety disorder: a placebo controlled study. Biol Psychiatry 59:211–215, 2006

Pollack MH, Tiller J, Xie F, et al: Tiagabine in adult patients with generalized anxiety disorder: results from three randomized, double-blind, placebo-controlled, parallel-group studies. J Clin Psychopharmacol 28:308–316, 2008

Rakel RE: Long-term buspirone therapy for chronic anxiety: a multicenter international study to determine safety. South Med J 83:194–198, 1990

Rickels K, Rynn M: Overview and clinical presentation of generalized anxiety disorder. Psychiatr Clin North Am 24:1–17, 2001

Rickels K, Rynn M: Pharmacotherapy of generalized anxiety disorder. J Clin Psychiatry 63:9–16, 2002

Rickels K, Weisman K, Norstad N, et al: Buspirone and diazepam in anxiety: a controlled study. J Clin Psychiatry 43:81–86, 1982

Rickels K, Case WG, Downing RW, et al: Long-term diazepam therapy and clinical outcome. JAMA 250:767–771, 1983

Rickels K, Fox IL, Greenblatt DJ, et al: Clorazepate and lorazepam: clinical improvement and rebound anxiety. Am J Psychiatry 145:312–317, 1988a

Rickels K, Schweizer E, Csanalosi I, et al: Long-term treatment of anxiety and risk of withdrawal: prospective comparison of clorazepate and buspirone. Arch Gen Psychiatry 45:444–450, 1988b

Rickels K, Downing R, Schweizer E, et al: Antidepressants for the treatment of generalized anxiety disorder: a placebo-controlled comparison of imipramine, trazodone, and diazepam. Arch Gen Psychiatry 50:884–895, 1993

Rickels K, Schweizer E, DeMartinis N, et al: Gepirone and diazepam in generalized anxiety disorder: a placebo-controlled trial. J Clin Psychopharmacol 17:272–277, 1997

Rickels K, DeMartinis N, Aufdembrinke B: A double-blind, placebo-controlled trial of abecarnil and diazepam in the treatment of patients with generalized anxiety disorder. J Clin Psychopharmacol 20:12–18, 2000a

Rickels K, Pollack MH, Sheehan DV, et al: Efficacy of extended-release venlafaxine in nondepressed outpatients with generalized anxiety disorder. Am J Psychiatry 157:968–974, 2000b

Rickels K, Zaninelli R, McCafferty J, et al: Paroxetine treatment of generalized anxiety disorder: a double-blind, placebo-controlled study. Am J Psychiatry 160:749–756, 2003

Rickels K, Pollack MH, Feltner DE, et al: Pregabalin for treatment of generalized anxiety disorder: a 4-week, multicenter, double-blind, placebo-controlled trial of pregabalin and alprazolam. Arch Gen Psychiatry 62:1022–1030, 2005

Rocca P, Fonzo V, Scotta M, et al: Paroxetine efficacy in the treatment of generalized anxiety disorder. Acta Psychiatr Scand 95:444–450, 1997

Rosenthal M: Tiagabine for the treatment of generalized anxiety disorder: a randomized, open-label, clinical trial with paroxetine as a positive control. J Clin Psychiatry 64:1245–1249, 2003

Russmann S, Lauterburg BH, Helbling A: Kava hepatotoxicity. Ann Intern Med 135:68–69, 2001

Rynn MA, Riddle MA, Yeung PP, et al: Efficacy and safety of extended-release venlafaxine in the treatment of generalized anxiety disorder in children and adolescents: two placebo-controlled trials. Am J Psychiatry 164:290–300, 2007

Rynn M, Russell J, Erickson J, et al: Efficacy and safety of duloxetine in the treatment of generalized anxiety disorder: a flexible dose, progressive titration, placebo-controlled trial. Depress Anxiety 25:182–189, 2008

Sanderson WC, Barlow DH: A description of patients diagnosed with DSM-III-R generalized anxiety disorder. J Nerv Ment Dis 178:588–591, 1990

Schmitt R, Gazalle KF, de Lima MS, et al: The efficacy of antidepressants for generalized anxiety disorder: a systematic review and meta-analysis. Rev Bras Psiquiatr 27:18–24, 2005

Schweizer E, Rickels K, Uhlenhuth EH: Issues in the long-term treatment of anxiety disorders, in Psychopharmacology: The Fourth Generation of Progress. Edited by Bloom FE, Kupfer DJ. New York, Raven Press, 1995, pp 1349–1359

Seeman P: Atypical antipsychotics: mechanism of action. Can J Psychiatry 47:27–38, 2002

Seivewright H, Tyrer P, Johnson T: Prediction of outcome in neurotic disorder: a 5-year prospective study. Psychol Med 28:1149–1157, 1998

Simon NM, Hoge EA, Fischmann D, et al: An open-label trial of risperidone augmentation for refractory anxiety disorders. J Clin Psychiatry 67:381–385, 2006

Simon NM, Connor KM, LeBeau RT, et al: Quetiapine augmentation of paroxetine CR for the treatment of refractory generalized anxiety disorder: preliminary findings. Psychopharmacology 197:675–681, 2008

Singh YN, Singh NN: Therapeutic potential of kava in the treatment of anxiety disorders. CNS Drugs 16:731–743, 2002

Sjodin I, Kutcher SP, Ravindran A, et al: Efficacy of sertraline in improving quality of life and functioning in generalized anxiety disorder (GAD). Eur Neuropsychopharmacol 13:S365–S366, 2003

Small JG, Hirsch SR, Arvanitis LA, et al: Quetiapine in patients with schizophrenia: a high- and low-dose double-

blind comparison with placebo. Seroquel Study Group. Arch Gen Psychiatry 54:549–557, 1997
Smith TA: Type A gamma-aminobutyric acid (GABAA) receptors subunits and benzodiazepines binding site sensitivity. Br J Biomed Sci 58:111–121, 2001
Smith W, Feltner D, Kavoussi R: Pregabalin in generalized anxiety disorder: long term efficacy and relapse prevention. Eur Neuropsychopharmacol 12:S350, 2002
Snyderman SH, Rynn MA, Rickels K: Open-label pilot study of ziprasidone for refractory generalized anxiety disorder. J Clin Psychopharmacol 25:497–499, 2005
Sramek JJ, Fresquet A, Marion-Landais G, et al: Establishing the maximum tolerated dose of lesopitron in patients with generalized anxiety disorder: a bridging study. J Clin Psychopharmacol 16:454–458, 1996
Sramek JJ, Frackiewicz EJ, Cutler NR: Efficacy and safety of two dosing regimens of buspirone in the treatment of outpatients with persistent anxiety. Clin Ther 19:498–506, 1997
Sramek JJ, Hong WW, Hamid S, et al: Meta-analysis of the safety and tolerability of two dose regimens of buspirone in patients with persistent anxiety. Depress Anxiety 9:131–134, 1999
Stein DJ: Comorbidity in generalized anxiety disorder: impact and implications. J Clin Psychiatry 62 (suppl 11):29–34, 2001
Stein DJ, Hollander E: Anxiety Disorders Comorbid With Depression: Social Anxiety Disorder, Post-Traumatic Stress Disorder, Generalized Anxiety Disorder and Obsessive-Compulsive Disorder. London, Martin Dunitz, 2002
Stein DJ, Ahokas A, Fabiano A, et al: Agomelatine in generalized anxiety disorder: a randomized, placebo-controlled study with a possibility for blinded-dose adjustment. Fundam Clin Pharmacol 21:80, 2007
Stein MB, Seedat S, Gelernter J: Serotonin transporter gene promoter polymorphism predicts SSRI response in generalized social anxiety disorder. Psychopharmacology 187:68–72, 2006
Steiner M, Allgulander C, Ravindran A, et al: Gender differences in clinical presentation and response to sertraline treatment of generalized anxiety disorder. Hum Psychopharmacol 20:3–13, 2005
Stephens DN, Terski L, Jones GH, et al: Abecarnil: a novel anxiolytic with mixed full agonist/partial agonist properties in animal models of anxiety and sedation, in Anxiolytic β-Carbolines: From Molecular Biology to the Clinic. Edited by Stephens DN. New York, Springer-Verlag, 1993, pp 79–95
Stocchi F, Nordera G, Jokinen RH, et al: Efficacy and tolerability of paroxetine for the long-term treatment of generalized anxiety disorder. J Clin Psychiatry 64:250–257, 2003
Thomas RE: Benzodiazepine use and motor vehicle accidents: systematic review of reported association. Can Fam Physician 44:799–808, 1998
Tollefson GD, Montagueclouse J, Tollefson SL: Treatment of comorbid generalized anxiety in a recently detoxified alcoholic population with a selective serotonergic drug (buspirone). J Clin Psychopharmacol 12:19–26, 1992
van Steveninck AL, Wallnofer AE, Schoemaker RC, et al: A study of the effects of long-term use on individual sensitivity to temazepam and lorazepam in a clinical population. Br J Clin Pharmacol 44:267–275, 1997
Wheatley D: Buspirone: multicenter efficacy study. J Clin Psychiatry 43:92–94, 1982
Woelk H, Arnoldt KH, Kieser M, et al: Ginkgo biloba special extract EGb 761 in generalized anxiety disorder and adjustment disorder with anxious mood: a randomized, double-blind, placebo-controlled trial. J Psychiatr Res 41:472–480, 2007
World Health Organization: International Statistical Classification of Diseases and Related Health Problems, 10th Revision. Geneva, World Health Organization, 1992
Yonkers KA, Dyck IR, Warsaw M, et al: Factors predicting the clinical course of generalized anxiety disorder. Br J Psychiatry 176:544–549, 2000
Zupancic M, Guilleminault C: Agomelatine: a preliminary review of a new antidepressant. CNS Drugs 20:981–992, 2006

Recommended Readings

Bandelow B, Zohar J, Hollander E, et al.: World Federation of Societies of Biological Psychiatry (WFSBP) Guidelines for Pharmacological Treatment of Anxiety, Obsessive-Compulsive and Post-Traumatic Stress Disorders—First Revision. World J Biol Psychiatry 9:248–312, 2008
Mathew SJ, Hoffman EJ: Pharmacotherapy for generalized anxiety disorder, in Oxford Handbook of Anxiety and Related Disorders. Edited by Antony MM, Stein MB. New York, Oxford University Press, 2008, pp 350–363
Van Ameringen M, Pollack M: Generalized Anxiety Disorder. New York, Oxford University Press, 2009

Chapter 14

Psychotherapy for Generalized Anxiety Disorder

Jonathan D. Huppert, Ph.D.
William C. Sanderson, Ph.D.

As discussed in other chapters in this volume, generalized anxiety disorder (GAD) is a relatively common disorder that is associated with significant distress and functional impairment. Recent advances in both pharmacotherapy and psychotherapy have resulted in a greater likelihood of providing effective treatment. However, reports suggest that people with GAD respond less robustly compared with those who have other anxiety disorders, which highlights the need for continued work in understanding the nature and treatment of GAD. In this chapter, we provide an overview of empirically based psychotherapeutic treatment of GAD. First, we briefly describe the history of psychosocial approaches to GAD, which have been predominantly cognitive-behavioral. Next, we elucidate the psychological mechanisms associated with GAD that appear to be involved in the maintenance of the disorder and, thus, must be addressed in treatment. We then provide a review of the treatment outcome literature relevant to GAD, and briefly review how treatment has been applied to special populations such as children and older adults. Finally, an overview of empirically supported psychological treatment strategies is provided. This chapter ends with a treatment algorithm to suggest what techniques to use and when to use them.

The Nature of Generalized Anxiety Disorder

GAD is a relatively new diagnosis, transformed from a "wastebasket" diagnosis pertaining to anyone with anxiety whose symptoms did not meet criteria for any other anxiety disorder listed in DSM-III (American Psychiatric Association 1980) to an independent diagnosis, more "carved at its joints" in DSM-III-R and DSM-IV (American Psychiatric Association 1987, 1994) (see also Chapter 11, "Phenomenology of Generalized Anxiety Disorder," in this volume). Until the advent of DSM-III-R in 1987, the development of treatment for GAD was aimed at treating "anxious neurotics." Two primary techniques were utilized: relaxation or biofeedback to address physiological tension and arousal (Rice and Blanchard 1982), and cognitive therapy to address the anxious thoughts associated with GAD (Beck 1976). Most CBT treatment protocols developed since then continue to integrate these two major strategies. However, as a result of greater precision in the definition of GAD and an increased understanding of the nature of worry and anxiety (Heimberg et al. 2004), newer treatment protocols also include strategies to address these recently identified components (e.g., techniques to minimize experiential avoidance, techniques to enhance problem solving).

Worry

The diagnosis of GAD depends on the existence of two core symptoms: worry (i.e., preoccupation with negative events occurring in the future) and physiological hyperarousal (e.g., muscle tension, sleep disturbance, feeling keyed up). Clearly, worry is frequently the most prominent symptom of GAD and is considered the cardinal feature of the disorder. Worry is a cognitive activity often referred to as anxious apprehension. It is elicited by the perception of *potential* future danger (Craske 2003) such as "What if I fail the licensing exam I am taking next week and as a result I am not able to get a job?" Worry is often accompanied by behavior directed at gaining control to avoid the occurrence of the negative event (Rapee 1991; e.g., "What can I do to prevent failing the exam?"). Indeed, the appropriate "function" of worry will lead one to take action to decrease the likelihood of potential negative outcomes (e.g., increase studying to avoid failing the exam), thereby decreasing the anxiety.

Although worry in itself is not pathological, and is in fact very common in the population at large, individuals diagnosed with GAD suffer from excessive worry; that is, reporting worry most of the day, nearly every day (Brown et al. 1993; Dupuy et al. 2001). Even though worry often activates attempts at problem solving in nearly everyone, individuals with GAD lack confidence in their solutions, thereby leading to continued worry (Davey 1994). This raises an important issue to consider: if worry is a ubiquitous experience, how does it differ in individuals with GAD versus those without the disorder? There are two main aspects of pathological worry that differentiate it from "normal" worry (descriptive studies such as Ruscio and Borkovec 2004 and information-processing studies such as Mathews 1990 provide supportive evidence). First, pathological worry appears to be uncontrollable. In a study by Abel and Borkovec (1995), all (100%) of the patients with GAD described their worry as uncontrollable, in comparison with none of the control subjects. Second, pathological worry is excessive for a given situation, in that patients overestimate the threat in their environment, especially when interpreting ambiguous cues (Mathews 1990). In fact, these two features may be the result of GAD patients' intolerance of uncertainty, leading to more excessive and uncontrollable worry (Dugas et al. 1998). In addition, anxious subjects tend to selectively attend to threatening, personally relevant stimuli (Mathews 1990). The overprediction of danger may lead patients with GAD to worry more often than others because they perceive their environment as more threatening. Frequently, the implied belief is that worry will make the world more controllable and predictable. For example, one patient stated, "When I fly in an airplane, I worry that the plane will crash. If I stopped worrying about it, it probably would crash." Consistent with this feature, worriers report five major functions of worry: 1) superstitious avoidance of catastrophes, 2) actual avoidance of catastrophes, 3) avoidance of deeper emotional topics, 4) coping preparation, and 5) motivating devices (Borkovec 1994).

Research has demonstrated that pathological worry has a functional role for patients with GAD. Ironically, worry inhibits autonomic arousal in patients with GAD when they are shown aversive imagery (Borkovec and Hu 1990). Worrying may allow for the avoidance of aversive imagery, the latter being associated with a greater emotional state (Borkovec et al. 1991). Thus, worry may be maintained by both the avoidance of certain affective states and the reduction of anxious states through the decrease in arousal that occurs along with worry (see Borkovec et al. 2004 for a review). Counterintuitively, relaxation has been shown to increase the amount of worry in some patients with GAD (Borkovec et al. 1991). In these patients, relaxation may signal a lack of control, triggering an increase in anxiety, or these patients may sit quietly with their thoughts, causing greater exposure to their worries.

In addition, individuals with GAD often have a heightened sense of the likelihood of negative events (i.e., increased risk perception) and often exaggerate the negative consequences that would occur (Brown et al. 1993). Patients with GAD and control subjects appear to worry about similar topics (Sanderson and Barlow 1990), although patients with GAD tend to worry more frequently about minor matters (Brown et al. 1994). Spheres of worry endorsed by patients with GAD include concerns about family, health, social matters, finances, work, and world events. The topics of worry may change with age and life situation.

Physiological Hyperarousal

In addition to worry, patients with GAD experience unpleasant somatic sensations associated with physiological hyperarousal. The presence of physiological arousal is seen as a component of the *"fight-or-flight"* response that is activated by GAD patients' perceptions of danger. Although both the cognitive and the somatic sensations usually increase during the course of a "worry episode," for the most part these symptoms are relatively chronic, and not limited to episodes of worry. The most common somatic symptom reported by patients with GAD is muscle tension. Other common symptoms include irritability, restlessness, feeling keyed up or on edge, difficulty sleeping, fatigue, and difficulty concentrating.

Characteristics of Patients With Generalized Anxiety Disorder

GAD is a relatively chronic disorder that begins in childhood (Brown et al. 1994). In view of these and other similar data, some argue that in contrast to other anxiety disorders, a subtype of GAD (chronic, pervasive symptoms since childhood) may be better conceptualized as an underlying personality trait that increases one's vulnerability to developing anxiety disorders (Sanderson and Wetzler 1991). Along this line, Barlow (2002) considers GAD the "basic anxiety disorder." GAD-like symptoms typically start in childhood, but often, a major stressor at some point in the individual's life will exacerbate symptoms and raise the condition to a clinical disorder. For example, one common example of a trigger we see clinically is becoming a parent. It appears that the increased responsibility and desire for perfection in child rearing may exacerbate these traits to the point of interference and distress.

New conceptualizations of GAD have focused on interpersonal deficits that may have developed in childhood (Crits-Christoph et al. 2005; Newman et al. 2004). In fact, interpersonal difficulties and concerns appear to be common triggers for worry episodes. Along this line, Sanderson and Barlow (1990) found that the majority of patients with GAD suffer from clinically significant social evaluative concerns. Other recent conceptualizations have focused on emotion regulation problems in individuals with GAD (e.g., Mennin et al. 2005). It is likely that the interpersonal and emotion regulation deficits interact to create difficulties (e.g., Erickson and Newman 2007). Other common characteristics of GAD patients include perfectionism, extraordinary need for control in their environment, difficulty tolerating ambiguity, and feelings of increased personal responsibility for negative events that occur or are predicted to occur in their environment (Wells 1994).

Differentiating Generalized Anxiety Disorder From Other Disorders

Accurate diagnosis is an essential first step in providing the appropriate treatment for a particular disorder. In fact, differentiating GAD from other anxiety disorders can be extremely complicated. First, worry (or anticipatory anxiety) is a relatively generic feature of anxiety disorders (e.g., patients with panic disorder often worry about future panic attacks, patients with social anxiety disorder worry about embarrassing themselves in forthcoming social situations). In addition, a high level of comorbidity exists among the anxiety disorders, and GAD in particular, which requires one to consider diagnosing multiple disorders to account for the full range of psychopathology displayed by the individual (Sanderson and Wetzler 1991). To do this, the clinician must distinguish between symptoms that can be subsumed within GAD versus those that are signs of an additional, independent disorder. The primary distinction to be made in differential diagnosis is not the presence of worry per se, but the *focus* of the worry. Patients with GAD experience uncontrollable worry about multiple areas of their life. Common worries include minor matters, work and family responsibilities, money, health, safety, and the well-being of significant others. Moreover, patients with GAD often end up worrying about their worry (known as *metaworry*; Wells 1994). We will review differential diagnostic considerations below, with an emphasis on the distinctions that are relevant to CBT treatment (see Chapter 11, "Phenomenology of Generalized Anxiety Disorder," for other considerations of differential diagnosis).

Panic Disorder

Patients with panic disorder are worried about having a panic attack or about the consequences of experiencing certain bodily sensations. Their focus is on internal states. What makes the differential diagnosis particularly confusing is that the worry experienced by patients with GAD can lead to a panic attack. However, unlike patients with panic disorder, patients with GAD are concerned primarily about some future event, not about the negative consequences of having a panic attack or the symptoms of anxiety per se. Some patients with GAD focus on the physical symptoms of their anxiety, and this can lead one to think that the preoccupation with bodily sensations is a sign of panic disorder. However, there is a distinction between distress about the presence of bodily sensations (e.g., muscle tension) and catastrophic misinterpretations of such sensations (e.g., my heart racing means I am having a heart attack). Another distinction is the course of onset of worry compared with that of panic symptoms. The onset of a panic attack is sudden, and its peak typically lasts for several minutes, whereas the onset and course of GAD-related anxiety are usually longer and more stable.

Social Anxiety Disorder

Social concerns are a common area of worry for patients with GAD, and these patients are often assigned a comorbid diagnosis of social anxiety disorder (social phobia) (Sanderson et al. 1990). For diagnosis of GAD, additional concerns beyond the social evaluative fears must be present. As opposed to the concerns of individuals with social anxiety disorder, interpersonal concerns in individuals with GAD frequently include interactions with close friends and relatives (e.g., "Did I say something wrong to my wife?") and are not as focused on rejection by others specifically because of inadequate content or behaviors (i.e., saying or doing things that are perceived as strange or unintelligent). In contrast to patients with social anxiety disorder, the evaluative concerns of patients with GAD extend beyond fears of embarrassment. In addition, patients with GAD are less likely than patients with social anxiety disorder to engage in significant overt avoidance (e.g., not going to parties, not meeting new people, not talking to people) or social anxiety–specific safety behaviors (e.g., censoring one's thoughts, staying on the edge of groups, rehearsing sentences in one's mind before speaking) that are focused on the prevention of negative evaluations and embarrassment.

Obsessive-Compulsive Disorder

Although differentiation between cases of obsessive-compulsive disorder (OCD) and GAD seems obvious because of the behavioral rituals that are unique to OCD (Brown et al. 1994), some cases still can be extremely difficult to differentiate. This is especially true of patients with OCD who do not have overt compulsions (i.e., have only mental rituals). In these cases, a distinction must be made between the obsessions and the worries. To do so, it is necessary to assess the focus of concern. The nature of obsessions tends to be unrealistic and often takes an "if-then" form (e.g., "If I don't cancel the thought that my child will be hurt in a car accident by imagining him safe at home, then he will be in a car accident"). In contrast, worry associated with GAD is usually focused on future negative events that are potentially more realistic; and it is more likely to be specified in a "what if" fashion, without a consequence being stated (e.g., "What if I am in a car accident on the highway and my children are injured?" or "What if I become ill?"). In research examining the distinction, nonanxious subjects reported that worry lasts longer and is more distracting (Wells and Morrison 1994). Worry also usually takes the form of predominantly verbal thoughts as opposed to images (Wells and Morrison 1994). Although compulsive behaviors are associated with OCD, patients with GAD often engage in reassurance-seeking and checking that can be somewhat ritualistic and superstitious (i.e., similar to compulsive behavior; Schut et al. 2001). In addition, patients with GAD may report feeling compelled to act to neutralize their worries (Wells and Morrison 1994; e.g., to call one's wife at work to lessen a worry about something happening to her). However, these behaviors are not as consistent, methodical, or ritualized as compulsive behaviors in patients with obsessive-compulsive disorder.

Mood Disorders

A differentiation must also be made between GAD and mood disorders, especially major depression and dysthymia. According to DSM-IV-TR, if GAD symptoms are present only during the course of a depressive episode, then GAD is not diagnosed as a comorbid disorder. More often than not, anxiety symptoms occur within the context of depression; thus, GAD is diagnosed as a separate disorder only when the symptoms have occurred at least at some point independent of depression. However, regardless of DSM exclusionary criteria, the nature of cognitions associated with each disorder can be distinguished: ruminations (common in depressive disorders) tend to be negative thought patterns about past events, whereas worries (associated with GAD) tend to be negative thought patterns about future events. This is consistent with theoretical conceptualizations of anxiety and depression, which posit that depression is a reaction to uncontrollable, inescapable negative events, leading to feelings of hopelessness and helplessness and deactivation, whereas anxiety is a reaction to uncontrollable negative events that the person attempts or plans to escape from (for a more detailed explanation, see Barlow 2002). The high comorbidity rates, symptom overlap, and genetic similarities between GAD and depressive disorders (see Huppert, in press, for a review) support the notion that GAD and depression may have a common underlying predisposition. In fact, it has been suggested that GAD be moved into a category of dysphoric disorders in DSM-V and not be included among the anxiety disorders (Watson 2005).

Review of Treatment Outcome Studies

In our previous review of GAD (Huppert and Sanderson 2002), we reviewed meta-analyses and studies conducted between 1987 and 2000. Since 2000, several reviews have been written about the treatment of GAD (Borkovec and Ruscio 2001; Covin et al. 2008; Gould et al. 2004; Hunot et al. 2007; Mitte 2005; Roemer et al. 2002; Rygh and Sanderson 2004; Siev and Chambless 2007; Westen and Morrison 2001). As in earlier reviews, the efficacy of cognitive-behavioral therapy (CBT) and related strategies (e.g., cognitive restructuring, relaxation training) has received the most supportive evidence when used to alleviate worry and anxiety. In fact, the Task Force of the Division of Clinical Psychology of the American Psychological Association, which is involved with identifying empirically supported treatments, found that the only psychosocial treatment with sufficient research support to be labeled "empirically supported treatment" is CBT (Chambless et al. 1998; Woody and Sanderson 1998). Independent reviews of treatments for GAD by the National Institute for Clinical Excellence in the United Kingdom (McIntosh et al. 2004) and by the International Consensus Group on Anxiety and Depression (Ballenger et al. 2001) concluded that CBT is equivalent to medication as a first-line treatment. Furthermore, Dutch guidelines for treatment of anxiety by primary care physicians also recommend CBT (van Boeijen et al. 2005). These treatment recommendations are based on the accumulated literature demonstrating the efficacy of CBT for GAD as well as support for the cost-effectiveness of such treatments (Heuzenroeder et al. 2004). Although there is some preliminary evidence suggesting short-term psychodynamic treatments for anxiety disorders may be effective (Crits-Christoph et al. 2005; Ferrero et al. 2007), adequate controlled studies have yet to be conducted. Therefore, consistent with the empirical literature, our review emphasizes CBT.

Previous Reviews

Borkovec and Ruscio (2001) conducted a meta-analysis of treatment outcome studies for GAD. Their primary conclusion was that CBT for patients with GAD is more efficacious in treating both anxious and depressive symptoms than no treatment or nonspecific control conditions, and that the combination of cognitive and behavioral strategies tends to be better than either alone. Specifically, they reported large between-group effect sizes for acute CBT when compared with no treatment, medium effect sizes when compared with placebo or alternative therapies, and small effect sizes when compared with cognitive or behavioral therapy alone. Nonspecific treatments (e.g., supportive psychotherapy) were reported to have large within-group effect sizes, but smaller than CBT. The authors also found that long-term follow-up suggested smaller, but sustained, advantages of CBT over other treatments. Similar conclusions about the efficacy of CBT for GAD were reported by Gould et al. (2004). However, in their review, Hunot et al. (2007) concluded that it is difficult to determine whether CBT is substantially more effective than supportive therapy. A meta-analysis by Mitte (2005) in which CBT was compared to medications revealed that, overall, CBT was superior to no treatment or placebo control conditions and was similar in effectiveness to medications. However, further analyses suggested that medications for GAD may be somewhat more effective than CBT, even though CBT may be more tolerable than medications (based on lower dropout rates). In her conclusions, Mitte stated that it is clear CBT for GAD has specific treatment effects beyond common factors. Most reviews conclude that approximately 50% of patients receiving CBT are categorized as responders.

Newer Studies

As shown in Table 14–1, during the period 2000–2007, 17 outcome studies on GAD were published. A few of these studies presented follow-up data to previously conducted trials; most included CBT and at least one other treatment group, a minimum of a 6-month follow-up assessment, and a variety of outcome measures, usually a combination of self-report and clinician-rated measures. For Table 14–1, we calculated percentage improvement in anxiety and worry by subtracting posttreatment averages from pretreatment averages and then dividing by the pretreatment averages. Data were gathered from information provided in the published reports. Self-report and clinician-rated measures were separated, because each type of information can be substantially different (i.e., a clinician may see improvement when a patient does not, or vice versa). Whether authors noted improvement, no change, or relapse during follow-up periods is noted next in the table. Finally, the rate of dropout is presented in the last column. Note that many percentages of improvement were calculated by using treatment-completer analyses; these results could have been substantially different if intent-to-treat analyses had been used. We do not review each study

TABLE 14–1. Results of recent psychosocial treatment outcome studies of generalized anxiety disorder

Study and follow-up period	Conditions (treatment length in sessions)	*N*	% Improvement in anxiety (IE; SRs)	% Drops	Follow-up
Durham et al. (1994,[a] 1999, 2003)	CBT (8 or 20)	38	IE: 55%; SR: 30%	10%	+
1-year and 8–10-year follow-ups	PSA (8 or 20)	39	IE: 40%; SR: 4%	24%	0/–
	BT (8)	22	IE:44%; SR: 15%	27%	0
Bowman et al. (1997); Floyd et al. (2002)	SET (CBT self-help)	19	IE: 33%; SR: 20%	11%	0
2-year follow-up	Wait-list	19	IE: –3%; SR: 4%	5%	
Crits-Christoph et al. (1996, 2004, 2005)	SEP (16)	61[b]	IE: 44%; SR: 57%	1	0
6-month follow-up	NDT (16)	16	N/R	2	N/A
Ladouceur et al. (2000)	CBT (16)	14	IE: 47%; SR: 42%	0	0
1-year follow-up	Wait-list	12	IE: 9%; SR: 4%	0	
Ost and Breitzholz (2000)	CT (12)	18	IE: 47%; SR: 21%	5%	0
1-year follow-up	AR (12)	15	IE: 47%; SR: 20%	12%	0
Bond et al. (2002)	CBT (7)+ PBO	12	IE: 48%	N/R	N/A
No follow-up	NDT (7)+ PBO	14	IE: 44%	N/R	N/A
	CBT (7)+ buspirone	11	IE: 56%	N/R	N/A
	NDT (7)+ buspirone	7	IE: 51%	N/R	N/A
Arntz (2003)	CT (12)	25	SR: 18%	20%	0
6-month follow-up	AR (12)	20	SR: 20%	15%	0
Borkovec et al. (2002)	CT (14)	25	IE: 66%; SR: 26%	8%	0
2-year follow-up	AR (14)	26	IE: 57%; SR: 27%	15%	0
	CBT (14)	25	IE: 64%; SR: 28%	4%	0
Dugas et al. (2003)	CBT (14 group 2 hours)	25	IE: 47%; SR: 40%	8%	0
2-year follow-up	Wait-list	27	IE: 9%; SR: 8%	7%	
Durham et al. (2004)	CBT good prognosis (5)	29	IE: 41%; SR: 11%	34%	0
6-month follow-up	CBT poor prognosis (10)	27	IE: 35%; SR: 21%	33%	0
	CBT poor prognosis (20)	30	IE: 33%; SR: 13%	40%	0

TABLE 14–1. Results of recent psychosocial treatment outcome studies of generalized anxiety disorder *(continued)*

Study and follow-up period	Conditions (treatment length in sessions)	*N*	% Improvement in anxiety (IE; SRs)	% Drops	Follow-up
Linden et al. (2005)	CBT (24 sessions)	36	IE: 35%; SR: 15%	14%	0
4 months treatment, 8-month follow-up	Contact control (CCG)	36	IE: 6%; SR: 3%	11%	N/A
Fava et al. (2005)	CBT (8)	10	IE: 32%; SR: 48%	20%	0
1-year follow-up	CBT+ well-being (4+4)	10	IE: 54%; SR: 90%	20%	0
Wells and King (2006)	CT (2–12)	10	SR: 61%	0%	0
12-month follow-up					
Ferrero et al. (2007)	PSD (12 sessions)	34	IE: 29%	3%	0
3 months treatment, 9-month follow-up	Medication	33	IE: 43%	15%	0
	PSD+ medication	20	IE: 27%	10%	0
Zinbarg et al. (2007)	CBT (12)	8	IE: 55%; SR: 39%	12%	N/A
No follow-up	Wait-list	10	IE: 0%; SR: 4%	0%	
Roemer and Orsillo (2007)	ABT (16 sessions)	19	IE: 54%; SR: 49%	16%	0/–
3-month follow-up					
Evans et al. (2008)	MBCT (8, group)	12	SR: 41%	8%	N/A
No follow-up					

Note. 0=no change from end of treatment; –=some loss of gains after treatment; +=continued improvement after treatment; 0/–=nonsignificant loss of gains after treatment; ABT=acceptance-based behavior therapy; AR=applied relaxation; BT=behavior therapy; CBT=cognitive-behavioral therapy; CT=cognitive therapy; IE=independent evaluator ratings; MBCT=mindfulness-based cognitive therapy; N/A=not applicable; NDT=nondirective supportive therapy; N/R=not reported; PBO=placebo; PSA=psychoanalytic therapy; PSD=Adlerian psychodynamic therapy; SEP=supportive-expressive psychodynamic therapy; SR=self-report ratings.

[a]In the Durham et al. (1994) study there were five conditions, but because of the similarities in outcomes between long (20 sessions) and short (8 sessions) treatments, these were combined in the table.
*This is a combined sample from an open trial and a randomized, controlled trial.

here because many of them are included in the previous discussion of meta-analytic reviews.

The 17 studies can be divided into numerous categories: studies examining the efficacy of CBT versus wait-list conditions, dismantling designs that examined relaxation versus cognitive therapy (and/or their combination), studies attempting to improve CBT outcomes by adding other techniques, and studies examining psychodynamic therapies. Some of these studies also provided analyses to determine predictors of treatment outcome, which will be discussed later. Studies varied in terms of the length of treatment sessions employed and in the number of treatment sessions included. As in our review of studies that were published during the 1990s (Huppert and Sanderson 2002), percentage of improvement was rated consistently greater by "blind" clinicians than by patients' self-reports. According to independent evaluators, CBT yielded from 30% to 66% improvement in anxiety, and self-report measures yielded between 11% and 61% improvement. With regard to follow-up, all but one study revealed no significant changes (either deterioration or improvement) from posttreatment to follow-up. However, one study did show statistically significant continued improvement after acute treatment (i.e., improvement from posttreatment to follow-up). With regard to comparisons with other treatments, overall, CBT was seen as significantly more effective than the wait-list control condition, and results for those who received CBT after being in the wait-list group showed they improved similarly to those who initially received CBT (Bowman et al. 1997; Ladouceur et al. 2000). Dismantling studies that examine the separate components of CBT found that cognitive therapy, relaxation, and their combination yielded similar effect sizes (see also Siev and Chambless 2007).

To date, attempts to improve outcome by adding or modifying techniques have yielded variable results, with some findings showing more promise than others. Durham and colleagues (1994, 2004) have examined longer- versus shorter-duration CBT, with mixed findings. Durham et al. (1994) suggested that 16 sessions of CBT may be more effective than 8 sessions. However, in a second study in which patients were a priori categorized into those likely to have good versus poor outcome, Durham et al. (2004) found that providing more CBT (20 vs. 10 sessions) to individuals predicted to have poor outcome did not improve outcomes. In contrast, providing short-duration CBT (6 sessions) to individuals predicted to have good outcomes worked quite well (equivalent to those receiving more sessions, in the group predicted to have poor outcomes), and improvement continued at follow-up (see Table 14–1). Borkovec et al. (2002) modified typical CBT by including 2-hour sessions for all conditions. Although they found somewhat larger effect-sizes compared with other studies using this treatment in the short run (at posttreatment), the results were not substantially better than previous findings at follow-up. As a result of this study and their clinical experiences, Borkovec et al. (2002) suggested the need to examine alternative strategies to CBT, such as addition of interpersonal and emotion-focused techniques, rather than just an increase in the amount of CBT. Indeed, Newman et al. (2008) have completed a trial of CBT alone compared with an integrated CBT plus interpersonal and emotion-focused therapy. Preliminary results suggest that CBT alone was as effective as the integrated treatment at posttreatment and at 1-year follow-up. However, for a subgroup of patients, advantages of the integrated treatment in anxiety symptom reduction at 2-year follow-up emerged (Newman et al. 2008).

At present, perhaps the area receiving the greatest amount of attention within the CBT field is the incorporation of *mindfulness meditation* and *acceptance-based techniques* into, or instead of, standard CBT approaches. These techniques have been examined in the treatment of GAD as well. Unfortunately, preliminary results from initial trials in which the outcomes are compared with other CBT trials have not supported the notion that these strategies provide an additional benefit. The inclusion of mindfulness and acceptance-based techniques (Evans et al. 2008; Roemer and Orsillo 2007) does not appear to enhance the efficacy of CBT for GAD (see Table 14–1).

Two therapeutic strategies that appear to be promising additions to CBT are the addition of well-being exercises (i.e., focusing on improving quality of life and positive aspects of one's life; cf. Fava et al. 2005) and meta-cognitive therapy (i.e., focusing specifically on positive and negative beliefs about worry, thought control strategies, and other techniques; Wells and King 2006). Table 14–1 provides more details of these and other studies modifying CBT.

Three studies have examined the efficacy of psychodynamic treatments for GAD. Although two of these studies are predominantly nonrandomized trials, the fact that they include psychodynamic treatment, which is a commonly utilized approach in clinical practice, merits their extensive consideration. Therefore, more details about these studies are described, although this should not be seen as an endorsement of these techniques over CBT approaches that have been studied more extensively. Each study used a different school of psychodynamic thought (psychoanalytic/classical Freudian, neo-Freudian interpersonal, Adlerian). Durham et al. (1994, 1999, 2003) were the only investigators to examine both cognitive and psychodynamic therapies for GAD. Crits-Christoph et al. (1996) conducted an open trial examining the effects of short-term psychodynamic therapy for GAD, for which 1-year follow-up data are available (Crits-Christoph et al. 2004). The group also published a randomized trial suggesting that nondirective, supportive therapy was as effective as their psychodynamic approach (Crits-Christoph et al. 2005). They presented their data in a combined sample. In addition, Ferrero et al. (2007) reported on a trial of short-term Adlerian psychodynamic therapy. Each of the treatments yielded improvements in symptoms, although the degree of improvement differed.

Durham et al. (1994) compared cognitive therapy (Beck et al. 1985) to anxiety management (a behavioral technique) and to psychoanalytic therapy. A total of 110 patients with GAD were divided into five groups: 1) brief CBT (average of 9 sessions), 2) extended CBT (average of 14 sessions), 3) brief analytic therapy (average of 8 sessions), 4) extended analytic therapy (average of 16 sessions), and 5) anxiety management training (average of 8 sessions). Results of this study indicated that patients who received any form of CBT improved most and those who received psychoanalytic psychotherapy improved least, with the group receiving anxiety management showing levels of improvement somewhere in between. Patients who received psychoanalytic treatment deteriorated on three measures (although not significantly), whereas patients in the CBT groups improved on all measures at posttreatment and 6-month follow-up, and the anxiety management group maintained gains. Follow-up data revealed that patients continued to improve after CBT or anxiety management was terminated. Follow-up data at 1 year and 8–10 years have been published (Durham et al. 1999, 2003). At 1 year, CBT continued to show superiority to psychoanalytic therapy in terms of symptom reduction, response rates, and overall functioning, and there were some advantages found for more intensive CBT over fewer sessions. Anxiety management continued to be a bit less effective than CBT and more effective than psychoanalytic therapy. At the 8–10-year follow-up, many differences between CBT and psychoanalytic treatment on anxiety and response measures had disappeared, though functioning and global symptom measures continued to indicate CBT was superior. It is interesting to note that a greater number of patients who received psychoanalytic therapy sought further treatment between the posttreatment and follow-up assessments.

This study had several strengths. First, the authors measured patients' expectancies of recovery through therapy, which showed that patients in both CBT and relaxation training had greater expectations of improvement than did those in the psychoanalytic groups after the third treatment session. In addition, they used well-trained therapists who were strong believers in their respective theoretical perspectives, thus eliminating experimental bias (allegiance effects) for any one treatment. However, the study had several weaknesses as well. The researchers did not conduct adherence or competency ratings to ensure that the therapists in fact provided the said treatment components. In addition, few therapists were used in the study and, as a result, it was possible that some of the treatment differences could have been due to therapist differences.

Crits-Christoph et al. (1996, 2004, 2005) conducted an open clinical trial and a small randomized trial of a short-term psychodynamically oriented treatment for GAD called supportive-expressive psychodynamic therapy (SEP). The authors used treatment manuals, adherence ratings, and therapists carefully trained in a psychodynamic treatment to target problems specifically thought to arise in GAD. SEP is grounded in psychodynamic theory, positing that anxiety is related to conflictual interpersonal attachment patterns and incomplete processing of past traumatic events. The treatment focused on conflicts in relationships through examining the interpersonal desires of the patient (wishes), reactions of others to these desires, and consequences of these reactions. Relationships explored included current and past relationships, as well as the therapeutic relationship. In SEP, the proposed mechanism of change is through working with the patient on exploring alternative methods of coping with feelings and interpersonal conflicts. SEP orients the therapist to deal with specific GAD-oriented wishes, mechanisms of defense, and resistances. In addition, the influence of termination on the patient is explored in depth.

A total of 61 patients with GAD (diagnosed by structured interview) were treated by therapists trained in SEP (Crits-Christoph et al. 2005). Posttreatment measures indicated significant improvement in all areas. There was less change in specific areas of interpersonal functioning (dominant and overly nurturing styles) than expected. Overall, effect sizes were similar to those calculated for CBT and nondirective psychotherapy. A subset of these patients was part of an unpublished randomized trial comparing SEP with nondirective supportive therapy (see Borkovec and Costello 1993, in which CBT was superior to the same treatment). No differences in outcome were found on continuous measures. However, the quality of the response among patients receiving SEP was better than among those receiving the nondirective therapy (i.e., more were considered to be remitters), and the variability of response was less. Thus, preliminary data suggest that this new, innovative psychodynamic therapy may be effective for patients with GAD, and is certainly worthy of further investigation.

Another psychodynamic approach, Adlerian psychodynamic therapy (APT), was examined in a clinical trial by Ferrero et al. (2007). Patients with GAD were assigned to either APT, medication management, or the combination, based on clinical judgment of what was best for the patient by the treating psychiatrist. Results suggested that all three conditions were effective, although the percentage of improvement was somewhat lower than in CBT treatment trials. Given the lack of random assignment, it is difficult to make firm conclusions from this study. However, it appeared that APT was quite effective in reducing anxiety and depression and improving quality of life. In addition, there was no difference in outcome in the APT condition for those with Axis II disorders and those without, whereas for medication treatment, there appeared to be poorer response among patients with Axis II disorders. Overall, the results complement the findings of Crits-Christoph et al. (2005), demonstrating that short-term dynamic therapy focused on interpersonal issues can be therapeutic for individuals with GAD. Clearly, more research is needed on these psychodynamic treatments, especially controlled trials, as well as investigation into the mechanism of action of psychodynamic treatment and whether or not it differs from that of CBT (Ablon and Jones 2002).

Effect of Comorbidity on Outcome of Generalized Anxiety Disorder

Given the high rate of comorbidity in GAD (Sanderson and Barlow 1990), it is important to determine the impact of additional diagnoses on treatment outcome. Although many of the treatment studies described above have included patients with a variety of comorbid diagnoses, only four published studies have specifically examined the effect of comorbid disorders on the treatment of GAD. Borkovec et al. (1995) found that comorbid anxiety disorders tended to remit when treatment focused on GAD. Of 55 patients with a principal diagnosis of GAD, 23 (41.8%) were rated as having at least one clinically significant comorbid Axis I diagnosis (patients with major depression had been ruled out of the study, thus decreasing the overall rate of comorbidity). At a 12-month follow-up, only two patients retained a clinically significant comorbid diagnosis, suggesting that in most cases, comorbid anxiety disorders may not need to be addressed directly. This may be largely a result of the fact that the treatment for GAD may be useful in reducing other anxiety symptoms as well. For example, learning cognitive restructuring as applied to worry in GAD may ultimately be generalized by the patient and used for coping with other anxiety symptoms. Ladouceur et al. (2000) reported that their sample of 26 patients included individuals with multiple comorbid diagnoses—most commonly, specific phobia and social phobia. At pretreatment, patients had an average of 1.6 additional diagnoses, whereas at posttreatment and follow-up, they had significantly fewer (an average of 0.4) additional diagnoses.

Sanderson et al. (1994) examined the influence of personality disorders on outcome in an open trial and found that CBT treatment effects were equivalent for GAD patients with and without personality disorders. However, patients with personality disorders were more likely to drop out of treatment. A total of 32 patients with diagnoses of GAD were separated into two groups, based on whether or not they had a concurrent personality disorder. Of the 32 patients, 16 were diagnosed with a personality disorder and 16 without. Of the 10 dropouts (those not receiving what was defined as a minimal dose of treatment), 7 were given a diagnosis of a personality disorder at the pretreatment evaluation. Effect sizes of treatment completers in both groups were similar to those mentioned by Borkovec and Ruscio (2001). In light of these data, it appears that attention should be paid to issues related to dropout in patients with personality disorders (e.g., difficulties forming therapeutic relationships, which is a consistent theme in a subgroup of GAD patients, as noted above).

Analogous to the finding in the Borkovec et al. (1995) study, a number of studies have focused on changes in comorbidity rates in treated patients with principal diagnoses of panic disorder. Brown et al. (1995) reported that GAD remitted when the focus of treatment was on the principal diagnosis of panic disorder in patients with a comorbid diagnosis of GAD. Of 126 patients with panic disorder, 32.5% received an additional diagnosis of GAD. Comorbidity did not appear to influence completer status, but did appear to influence initial severity of panic (i.e., those with a comorbid disorder had more severe panic disorder). Of the 57 patients available for follow-up analyses, 26.3% were given diagnoses of GAD at pretreatment, whereas only 7.0% were given such diagnoses at posttreatment, 8.8% at 3-month follow-up, and 8.8% at 24-month follow-up. Thus, 11 of 15 (73.3%) patients did not meet criteria for a clinical diagnosis of GAD at posttreatment, and gains were maintained throughout follow-up assessments. Similar findings have been found by Tsao and colleagues in three studies (2005). Once again, considering that the strategies used in CBT for panic disorder are similar to those used for GAD, it is not surprising that the treatment would generalize to other anxiety symptoms as well (Sanderson and McGinn 1997).

Predictors of Outcome

Durham and colleagues (2004) have been highly systematic in examining predictors of treatment outcome. In two studies, they found that predictors of poor outcome include greater initial severity, low socioeconomic status, comorbidity, history of previous treatment, and relationship difficulties. The last is consistent with studies by Borkovec et al. (2002) and Zinbarg et al. (2007), both of which found pretreatment interpersonal style or hostile communication patterns with partners to be predictive of treatment outcome. In addition, Durham et al. (2004) found that the therapeutic alliance was a good predictor of acute outcome but a much less significant predictor of long-term outcome.

Special Populations

Older Adults

Although controversy exists as to whether or not the typical onset of GAD tends to be earlier versus later in life (Barlow 2002), it is safe to say that a significant percentage of older adults (i.e., >age 60 years), perhaps as high as 7% of the population, suffer from GAD (Flint 1994). Given that the vast majority of treatment trials on GAD examine considerably younger subjects (in fact, some exclude individuals over age 65), it cannot be assumed that the effectiveness of treatment found in those trials applies to older adults. Thus, a body of research has emerged examining the efficacy of CBT, as described above, for GAD in older adults (e.g., Stanley et al. 1996, 2003a; Wetherell et al. 2003). Clearly, the treatment with the most consistent support for late-life GAD is CBT (Ayers et al. 2007), with approximately half of patients achieving a significant improvement (Wetherell et al. 2005). Although these results are promising, it is important to note that, overall, responder rates in studies of GAD in older adults have been somewhat lower than those reported in the literature on younger adults (Stanley et al. 2003b). In light of this finding, a study by Mohlman et al. (2003) is particularly interesting. In a preliminary uncontrolled study, they tested an "enhanced version" of CBT that included learning and memory aids designed to make the therapy more effective for elderly patients (e.g., homework reminder and troubleshooting calls) and found it to be superior to standard CBT. Investigating this modification in controlled trials is certainly warranted, and may eliminate the gap between response rates in younger and older adults suffering from GAD.

Children

Although there are no studies examining the efficacy of CBT in an exclusive sample of children diagnosed with GAD, several trials have evaluated CBT on mixed samples, often including children with GAD, overanxious disorders, and social anxiety disorder. For example, a large study by Kendall et al. (2004) included 94 children who had an anxiety disorder—55 of whom were diagnosed with GAD. Data revealed significant improvement in anxiety symptoms from pretreatment to posttreatment. In a thorough review of the literature on CBT for childhood anxiety disorders, Chorpita and Southam-Gerow (2006) concluded that CBT has "very strong empirical support" for childhood GAD. It is worth noting that although the treatment closely resembles the intervention package utilized for adults (i.e., it includes cognitive and behavioral components), the child intervention by Kendall (1990), labeled the Coping Cat Program, has been modified to be more child-friendly.

CBT Techniques for Generalized Anxiety Disorder

As should be clear by now, CBT is the only psychotherapeutic approach with strong empirical support from controlled research studies. Although there may be some subtle differences in treatment packages employed within these studies, for the most part, there are several common "essential" elements contained in almost every CBT manual for GAD. (For detailed descriptions of these techniques, see: Rygh and Sanderson 2004;

Zinbarg et al. 2006.) These methods include psychoeducation, self-monitoring, cognitive restructuring, relaxation, worry exposure, worry behavior control, and problem solving. Of course, these techniques should be delivered in the context of a good psychotherapeutic atmosphere that includes all of the nonspecific effects of therapy (e.g., a good therapeutic relationship, positive expectancy, warmth). Each technique is briefly described below.

Psychoeducation

As in most cognitive-behavioral treatments, psychoeducation about GAD is an important aspect of therapy. Several rationales exist for starting treatment with education about anxiety and worry. First, we believe that knowledge is an important factor in change. Many patients who have come in for treatment have never been told their diagnosis and frequently have misconceptions about their disorder (e.g., that anxiety will lead to psychosis) and misunderstandings about common responses (e.g., physiological, emotional) to worry and stress (e.g., that all worry is bad or that increased heart rate means that you are more likely to have a heart attack). In addition, some patients want a greater understanding of why they are anxious and what they can do about it. So the first step in CBT treatment is educating patients about the biopsychosocial model of anxiety (Rygh and Sanderson 2004; Borkovec et al. 2004). Many patients experience great relief in knowing that their experiences are not uncommon, that a considerable amount of scientific knowledge exists about the etiology and phenomenology of GAD, and that effective treatments designed specifically for their difficulties are available. Finally, providing education about GAD is a way to review the treatment rationale (i.e., what the purpose of each treatment strategy is) and thus may facilitate treatment compliance.

We recommend that psychoeducation be provided first in a written form (e.g., via a Web site on GAD such as the one available through the National Institute of Mental Health (http://www.nimh.nih.gov/health/topics/generalized-anxiety-disorder-gad/index.shtml) and then followed up in session. During the session, questions are answered and the information is reviewed in a manner that makes the information personally relevant to the patient.

Self-Monitoring

Self-monitoring is one of the most basic yet essential parts of CBT. Monitoring is used as both an assessment procedure (to identify the context and content of worry) and a treatment strategy. (Becoming aware of patterns and focusing on worry and anxiety may lead to reduction in worry and anxiety.) The basic concept of monitoring is that each time the patient feels worried or anxious, he or she should record when and where the anxiety began and the intensity of the experience, including symptoms that were present. The patient can monitor his or her experience on a full sheet of paper that describes the entire week or record one situation or day at a time. The amount of information gathered may vary with each patient, according to each individual's abilities and needs. It should be noted that avoidance of monitoring is seen as detrimental to treatment, because of the likelihood that the patient is avoiding anxiety. Thus, we prefer to simplify and problem-solve to attain compliance rather than eliminate the monitoring altogether.

To enhance compliance, the therapist should inform the patient of the reasoning behind the monitoring: to help elicit specific patterns that occur and lead to worry episodes, to obtain a good estimate of current symptoms, to be able to notice effects of treatment on symptoms, and to further examine worry (e.g., cognitions, behaviors). The basic aspects of worry monitoring are date, time began, time ended, place, event (trigger), average anxiety (from 1 [minimal] to 8 [extremely distressing]), peak anxiety (1–8), average depression (1–8), and topics of worry. Once cognitive restructuring is introduced, monitoring the specific thought process involving worries is added.

Cognitive Therapy: Restructuring the Worry

As stated earlier, worry is a predominantly cognitive process, thereby making cognition an important aspect to address. Cognitive therapy is an effective strategy for this purpose. Patients with anxiety disorders, and with GAD in particular, overestimate the likelihood of negative events and underestimate their ability to cope with difficult situations (A.T. Beck et al. 1985). These "cognitive distortions" can play a major role in the vicious cycle of anxiety, and they accentuate the patient's feelings of danger and threat. Thus, cognitive therapy targets the faulty appraisal system and attempts to guide the patient toward more realistic, logical thinking.

The idea of cognition and its influence on anxiety are reviewed with the patient in the introduction to therapy and in the psychoeducation discussion. Threaded throughout the biopsychosocial model is the theme that cognition plays a major role in eliciting and perpetuating the cycle of anxiety. Cognitive restructuring is introduced in detail by discussing the concepts of automatic thoughts, anxious predictions, and the maintenance of anxiety through unchallenged/unchecked negative predictions about the future.

Automatic thoughts are described as learned responses to cues that can occur so quickly that they may be outside of one's awareness. However, these cognitions can create, maintain, and escalate anxiety if their content contains information with a danger-related theme. Thus, the patient is taught to observe his or her own thoughts at the moment of anxiety (or immediately after), to assess what cues may have brought on the feeling, and to elaborate on what thoughts were going through his or her mind. The goal is to bring the thoughts into awareness. Initially, the thoughts are not immediately challenged but collected as data to determine common thoughts that occur during worry. In addition to self-monitoring during anxiety episodes, anxious cognitions are accessed within the therapy session through Socratic questioning (asking questions to lead the patient to uncover his or her thoughts during anxiety-provoking situations), role-playing (if worry occurred during a social interaction, playing the role of the friend and replaying the event in the session), and imagery (trying to visualize a worry-provoking event to access thoughts and fears). Increases in levels of anxiety either in or outside of the session are opportune times to monitor "hot" cognitions. This often needs to be modeled by filling out a thought record and helping the patient elicit thoughts (e.g., "I won't be able to do the homework right") in session before patients can accurately monitor their thoughts for homework. It is often helpful to warn patients that monitoring thoughts can provoke anxiety because one is focusing on anxious cognitions. It should be explained that exposure to such thoughts, while uncomfortable, is necessary for change.

Once thoughts have been monitored sufficiently to determine frequency and themes, categories of distorted thinking are introduced. Several cognitive distortions have been identified as common in patients with GAD, the three most common being probability overestimation, catastrophizing, and all-or-none (black-and-white) thinking (A.T. Beck et al. 1985; Brown et al. 1993).

Frequently, many distortions exist within one statement. In our clinical experience, it can be very helpful to address all of the distortions in each statement. This will help the patient have a fully loaded armamentarium against anxious thoughts. A patient may remain anxious after challenging a thought-focus on a single type of distortion because he or she is still apprehensive about another distortion. Thus, we believe that the most effective strategy is to thoroughly process all cognitive distortions. For example, a patient presents with a worry statement that he is not going to be able to pay the rent on time because he thinks that his paycheck will come in the mail late. We would have the patient evaluate the probability that he will not pay the rent, based on past experiences of receiving his paycheck, evaluate the consequences of his paying the rent late, and evaluate his belief that if he is one day late with the rent, it is as if he will never pay it. Thus, the one worry may contain all three categories of distortions. Challenging in this fashion focuses on automatic thoughts. This may be sufficient for some patients, but for others it may be necessary to examine core beliefs (i.e., consistent thought patterns about oneself, the environment, or the future; J.S. Beck 1995).

Relaxation

Relaxation exercises are an important component of most CBT-oriented treatments for GAD. The function of these exercises is to reduce the physiological correlates of worry and anxiety by lowering the patient's overall arousal level. Relaxation reduces arousal, but it may play other roles as well. First, it may help broaden the focus of one's attention; anxiety tends to narrow attentional focus (Barlow et al. 1996). As a result of its anxiety-reducing property, relaxation may widen the scope of attention and thereby increase the patient's ability to consider alternatives in an anxiety-provoking situation. In addition, relaxation may serve as a distraction. Distraction is not effective as a sole method, because by constantly avoiding anxious cognitions, the patient is subtly supporting the belief that his or her thoughts are threatening and/or harmful. However, distraction can be an effective tool when the GAD patient is "stuck" in a worry pattern and needs to break the perseverating thoughts. Finally, contrary to the concepts described above and to conventional wisdom, which assumes that relaxation is solely a coping strategy, relaxation may at times facilitate the activation of anxious thoughts that are otherwise not being processed (Borkovec and Whisman 1996), thereby assisting in exposure to the anxious thoughts. This may explain why some patients describe becoming more anxious when initially engaging in relaxation exercises. Specifically, worrying prevents the processing of other, more fearful information (see Borkovec and Hu 1990), and relaxation helps reduce this "protective" worry and thus may ultimately aid in exposure to fearful thoughts, ideas, or images that were not fully processed through or evoked by worrying.

Whether for any of the reasons cited above or for other reasons not discussed here, relaxation clearly helps patients with GAD. Most recent methods of teaching relaxation have adapted a flexible concept rather than insisting on any particular approach. Thus, although progressive muscle relaxation techniques are emphasized for most patients and have the most empirical support, if a patient prefers another method and is able to use it effectively, then we recommend continued use of that strategy. At times, a combination of relaxation techniques can also be encouraged, depending on the needs of the patient. Accordingly, yoga, transcendental or other types of meditation, and tai chi are all acceptable, especially if the patient is already engaged in such activities and/or if progressive muscle relaxation does not appear effective.

There are several caveats to be noted about conducting progressive muscle relaxation. First, the goal is to have the patient feel relaxed. Although similar procedures are used to help patients with insomnia, the goal here is not to have the person fall asleep. Second, this procedure is similar to those used in initiating a hypnotic trance; because of this, patients may react to the procedure with anxiety, fearing a "loss of control." It is important to explain to the patient that the difference between hypnosis and relaxation, as used in CBT for GAD, is that in progressive muscle relaxation, the focus is on awareness of bodily sensations. Hypnosis has the goal of distraction to the point of reaching a trance state. This would be counterproductive in treating GAD because, as discussed in this section, these patients are already distracted from aversive states through worry. Our goal is facilitated exposure to worry-provoking stimuli, not avoidance.

Worry Exposure

As noted above, the perpetuation of worry in GAD patients may be caused by incomplete processing of the worry, which may be a result of avoiding focusing on the worry itself. Instead of focusing on a worry that will increase anxiety in the short run, patients attempt to avoid fully processing the worry through various behaviors (discussed in the next section), as well as through constant shifting of worries. For this reason, Brown et al. (1993) described a technique in which patients purposely expose themselves to both worry and images associated with the worry for an extended period. The concept is to have the patient activate the worst possible outcome in order to process it and habituate to the anxiety associated with it. Habituation of the anxiety is facilitated through cognitive challenging after the patient focuses on the image for 20–30 minutes. Similar procedures (called *cognitive exposure*) are used to facilitate intolerance of uncertainty in the treatment developed by Dugas et al. (2003). Borkovec et al. (1983) developed a similar technique referred to as *stimulus control.* In this approach, patients are asked to postpone worrying when it begins to happen, make a list of the worries that occur, and then set aside an hour in the evening to focus exclusively on the worries. This exercise allows for a concentrated effort to process the worry, and theoretically it will result in habituation to the content of worry, thereby decreasing anxiety and the worry process itself. Even though there are subtle differences between worry exposure and stimulus control, the basic mechanism of action may be the same, namely, cognitive processing and habituation. If the function of worry is similar to that of agoraphobia or compulsions, in that it reduces the overall anxiety experience in the short run, then repeated exposure will cause extinction of the specific worry or the underlying fears.

Worry Behavior Control

Many patients who worry may behave in certain ways to try to avoid it. Although it is an aversive experience, uncontrollable worry may serve the function of avoiding an even more intolerable experience (i.e., by focusing on the worry instead of the other experience). Behaviors that facilitate the avoidance of the worry itself may then result in avoidance of both the anxiety created by worry and the experience avoided through worrying. According to this explanation, the patient's preoccupation with worry distracts him or her from the original source of the negative state (e.g., fear, depression). Therefore, eliminating worry behaviors allows the patient to fully experience and process the worry.

To prevent worry behaviors, the patient carefully monitors what he or she does when he or she notices the onset of worry. Both subtle and explicit variants of these avoidance behaviors are detected through careful monitoring, assessment, and questioning. Then, in a technique similar to that of response prevention used in the treatment of obsessive-compulsive disorder, the patient is asked to refrain from these behaviors and instead to use the techniques described earlier to cope with the worry. If many behaviors are involved, or if the patient is too anxious to just give up the worry behaviors, hierarchies are created to assist the patient in systematically giving up the behaviors, starting with easier ones and moving on to more difficult behaviors, making the task considerably less overwhelming (e.g., checking the child's forehead once daily to see if he has a fever, then every other day, and so on).

Problem Solving

Teaching problem solving is a classic CBT approach for many disorders. Dugas and colleagues (1998, 2003) outline two main problems for individuals with GAD. They suggest that the core problem of GAD is the intolerance of uncertainty, and that this has an impact on two types of problems that GAD patients face. The first type are "unrealistic problems." These problems cannot be solved rationally and must be dealt with via *worry exposure* (for example, for a person who continually worries about his or her health, there is no way to rationally guarantee that the person will never become ill, so exposure to the fear is recommended). The second type of problem is "catastrophic thinking" about real issues. For example, consider a person who worries about losing his job because he received some negative feedback on an evaluation. In this case, there are steps that can be taken—a problem-solving approach—to reduce the likelihood of this negative outcome. Often, GAD patients become so focused on the catastrophic outcome and on attempting to avoid the anxiety associated with it that they lose their natural ability to problem-solve. Therefore, problem solving must be deliberately instituted. Problem solving includes identification of the problem, goal setting, generation of alternative solutions, selection of a solution, and implementation and evaluation. The goal in introducing these steps is not just to solve the problem being focused on, but to help the patient learn better problem-solving skills and learn that there are often multiple solutions to problems.

Future Directions

As noted in this chapter, the techniques of challenging worries through cognitive restructuring, worry exposure, and problem solving are not sufficient for all patients with GAD. If we conceptualize worry as a reaction generated in order to avoid a more intense underlying affective state, then elimination of worry will be helpful to only those patients who have sufficient coping skills and strategies to deal with whatever affect they experience. For example, just as exposure is helpful in agoraphobia, most cognitive-behavioral treatments of panic work by providing coping skills that will be used instead of avoidance strategies. If some patients with GAD are avoiding affect (Mennin et al. 2005), then simply eliminating the worry through relaxation and cognitive techniques will not work unless they are taught other strategies for dealing with the triggers for the affect. Borkovec et al. (2004) proposed that interpersonal strategies (i.e., Safran and Segal 1990) be tested, in addition to cognitive techniques, to determine whether processing of interpersonal difficulties facilitates activation and modification of affective structures (Foa and Kozak 1986). In addition, others have suggested working more directly on emotion regulation strategies through CBT techniques (Huppert and Alley 2004), emotion-focused therapy techniques (Mennin 2004), or acceptance and mindfulness techniques (Roemer and Orsillo 2007). Promising research has been conducted in the area of adding concepts of well-being and/or approaching valued, positive experiences (Fava et al. 2005).

Along these lines, some have suggested applying schema-focused therapy to those patients who have not responded to traditional CBT (McGinn et al. 1994). This approach focuses on addressing underlying "early maladaptive schemas," which theoretically influence current symptomatology. Schemas are defined as persistent beliefs one develops about the self, based on formative experiences (which are often recurrent). Negative or faulty interpretations of positive and negative life experiences may lead to lifelong cognitive, behavioral, and emotional patterns of interacting with others and the environment. Based on our observations of patients with GAD, we hypothesize that they may have schemas that include unrelenting standards (the belief that one needs to be the best or perfect at everything one does), vulnerability to harm (the belief that the world is a dangerous place and one can easily be hurt in it), and emotional inhibition (the belief that expressing one's emotions is dangerous to the self or others and must be prevented). We have previously hypothesized that patients who are CBT nonresponders may fit into the characterological model of GAD; thus, an approach that focuses on the aforementioned schemas may be warranted (McGinn et al. 1994). However, at this point, the idea is based on our clinical experience and not on research data. Our recommendation for treating GAD is to begin with the standard CBT approach, and then apply the schema-focused approach to those patients who have not responded.

Finally, as an overall approach to treatment, a stepped-care approach should be further examined. The basic idea of a stepped-care approach is to provide treatment in "steps," depending on need. Given the promising outcomes of self-help programs for some patients with GAD (White 1998a), as well as the benefit of CBT provided in group format (White 1998b), these are both reasonable first-line approaches and can be followed by more intensive CBT methods for those patients who do not respond to the initial intervention. The stepped-care approach highlights the need for more research on modifying standard CBT treatment to address treatment-refractory illness (Durham et al. 2004). Modification of standard treatment raises not only the prospect of providing more intensive CBT, but also the question of whether alternative approaches, such as mindfulness/acceptance-based or psychodynamic approaches, can improve outcome in patients with CBT-refractory GAD.

Conclusion

Considerable progress has been made in understanding the nature and treatment of GAD, especially given that GAD only became an independent Axis I disorder in 1987. In fact, this progress is largely a result of the continued refinement of the diagnosis from DSM-III to DSM-III-R and, more recently, DSM-IV, in which GAD went from a residual disorder to an independent disorder with worry advanced as its cardinal feature. With a focus on the nature and function of worry, clinical researchers have been able to develop treatments that specifically target the putative underlying psychopathological mechanisms. Demonstrating the process of developing empirically derived treatments, investigators have not been satisfied with treatment results from standard CBT packages (which appear to help approximately 50% of patients), and though unsuccessful to date in finding strategies to significantly improve CBT treatment, they continue to develop and test new strategies. These continuing research efforts suggest a promising future in the treatment of GAD.

◀ Key Clinical Points ▶

- Substantial evidence suggests that cognitive-behavioral therapy for generalized anxiety disorder is effective, helping approximately 50% of GAD patients achieve significant symptom reduction and high end-state functioning.
- CBT typically consists of psychoeducation, self-monitoring, relaxation, and cognitive restructuring.
- Additional techniques such as worry exposure, problem solving, and focusing on improving positive aspects of one's life are also potentially helpful.

References

Abel JL, Borkovec TD: Generalizability of DSM-III-R generalized anxiety disorders to proposed DSM-IV criteria and cross validation of proposed changes. J Anxiety Disord 9:303–315, 1995

Ablon JS, Jones EE: Validity of controlled clinical trials of psychotherapy: findings from the NIMH treatment of depression collaborative research program. Am J Psychiatry 159:775–783, 2002

American Psychiatric Association: Diagnostic and Statistical Manual of Mental Disorders, 3rd Edition. Washington, DC, American Psychiatric Association, 1980

American Psychiatric Association: Diagnostic and Statistical Manual of Mental Disorders, 3rd Edition, Revised. Washington, DC, American Psychiatric Association, 1987

American Psychiatric Association: Diagnostic and Statistical Manual of Mental Disorders, 4th Edition. Washington, DC, American Psychiatric Association, 1994

Arntz A: Cognitive therapy versus applied relaxation as treatment of generalized anxiety disorder. Behav Res Ther 41:633–646, 2003

Ayers CR, Sorrell JT, Thorp SR, et al: Evidence-based psychological treatment for late-life anxiety. Psychol Aging 22:8–17, 2007

Ballenger J, Davidson JRT, Lecrubier Y, et al: Consensus statement on generalised anxiety disorder from the international consensus group on depression and anxiety. J Clin Psychiatry 62:53–58, 2001

Barlow DH: Anxiety and Its Disorders, 2nd Edition. New York, Guilford, 2002

Barlow DH, Chorpita BF, Turovsky J: Fear, panic, anxiety, and disorders of emotion, in Nebraska Symposium on Motivation: Perspectives on Anxiety, Panic, and Fear, Vol 43. Edited by Hope DA. Lincoln, University of Nebraska Press, 1996, pp 251–328

Beck AT: Cognitive Therapy and the Emotional Disorders. New York, New American Library, 1976

Beck AT, Emery G, Greenberg RL: Anxiety Disorders and Phobias: A Cognitive Perspective. New York, Basic Books, 1985

Beck JS: Cognitive Therapy: Basics and Beyond. New York, Guilford, 1995

Bond AJ, Wingrove J, Curran HV, et al: Treatment of generalised anxiety disorder with a short course of psychological therapy, combined with buspirone or placebo. J Affect Disord 72:267–271, 2002

Borkovec TD: The nature, functions, and origins of worry, in Worrying: Perspectives on Theory, Assessment and Treatment. Edited by Davey GCL, Tallis F. New York, Wiley, 1994, pp 5–33

Borkovec TD, Costello E: Efficacy of applied relaxation and cognitive-behavioral therapy in the treatment of generalized anxiety disorder. J Consult Clin Psychol 61:611–619, 1993

Borkovec TD, Hu S: The effect of worry on cardiovascular response to phobic imagery. Behav Res Ther 28:69–73, 1990

Borkovec TD, Ruscio AM: Psychotherapy for generalized anxiety disorder. J Clin Psychiatry 62:37–42, 2001

Borkovec TD, Whisman MA: Psychosocial treatment for generalized anxiety disorder, in Long-Term Treatments of Anxiety Disorders. Edited by Mavissakalian MR, Prien RF. Washington, DC, American Psychiatric Press, 1996, pp 171–199

Borkovec TD, Wilkinson L, Folensbee R, et al: Stimulus control applications to the treatment of worry. Behav Res Ther 21:153–158, 1983

Borkovec TD, Shadick RN, Hopkins M: The nature of normal and pathological worry, in Chronic Anxiety: Generalized Anxiety Disorder and Mixed Anxiety-Depression. Edited by Rapee RM, Barlow DH. New York, Guilford, 1991, pp 29–51

Borkovec TD, Abel JL, Newman H: Effects of psychotherapy on comorbid conditions in generalized anxiety disorder. J Consult Clin Psychol 63:479–483, 1995

Borkovec TD, Newman MG, Pincus AL, et al: A component analysis of cognitive behavioral therapy for generalized anxiety disorder and the role of interpersonal problems. J Consult Clin Psychol 70:288–298, 2002

Borkovec TD, Alcaine O, Behar E: Avoidance theory of worry and generalized anxiety disorder, in Generalized Anxiety Disorder: Advances in Research and Practice. Edited by Heimberg RG, Turk CL, Mennin DS. New York, Guilford, 2004, pp 77–108

Bowman D, Scogin F, Floyd M, et al: Efficacy of self-examination therapy in the treatment of generalized anxiety disorder. J Consult Clin Psychol 44:267–273, 1997

Brown TA, O'Leary TA, Barlow DH: Generalized anxiety disorder, in Clinical Handbook of Psychological Disorders, 2nd Edition. Edited by Barlow DH. New York, Guilford, 1993, pp 137–188

Brown TA, Barlow DH, Liebowitz MR: The empirical basis of generalized anxiety disorder. Am J Psychiatry 151:1272–1280, 1994

Brown TA, Antony MM, Barlow DH: Diagnostic comorbidity in panic disorder: effect on treatment outcome and course of comorbid diagnoses following treatment. J Consult Clin Psychol 63:408–418, 1995

Chambless DL, Baker MJ, Baucom DH, et al: Update on empirically validated therapies, II. Clin Psychol 51:3–16, 1998

Chorpita BF, Southam-Gerow M: Fears and anxieties, in Treatment of Child Disorders, 3rd Edition. Edited by Mash EJ, Barkley RA . New York, Guilford, 2006, pp 271–335

Covin R, Ouimet AJ, Seeds PM, et al: A meta-analysis of CBT for pathological worry among clients with GAD. J Anxiety Disord 22:108–116, 2008

Craske MG: Origins of Phobias and Anxiety Disorders: Why More Women Than Men. Amsterdam, The Netherlands, Elsevier, 2003

Crits-Christoph PC, Connolly MB, Azarian K, et al: An open trial of brief supportive-expressive psychotherapy in the treatment of generalized anxiety disorder. Psychotherapy 33:418–430, 1996

Crits-Christoph PC, Gibbons, MBC, Crits-Christoph K: Supportive-expressive psychodynamic therapy, in Generalized Anxiety Disorder: Advances in Research and Practice. Edited by Heimberg RG, Turk CL, Mennin DS. New York, Guilford, 2004, pp 293–319

Crits-Christoph PC, Gibbons MBC, Narducci J, et al: Interpersonal problems and the outcome of interpersonally oriented psychodynamic Treatment of GAD. Psychotherapy: Theory, Research, Practice, Training 42:211–224, 2005

Davey GCL: Pathological worrying as exacerbated problem-solving, in Worrying: Perspectives on Theory, Assessment and Treatment. Edited by Davey GCL, Tallis F. New York, Wiley, 1994, pp 35–59

Dugas MJ, Gagnon F, Ladouceur R, et al: Generalized anxiety disorder: a preliminary test of a conceptual model. Behav Res Ther 36:215–226, 1998

Dugas MI, Ladouceur RLE, Ereeston M, et al: Group cognitive-behavioral therapy for generalized anxiety disorder: treatment outcome and long-term follow-up. J Consult Clin Psychol 71:821–825, 2003

Dupuy JB, Beaudoin S, Rhéaume J, et al: Worry: daily self-report in clinical and non-clinical populations. Behav Res Ther 39:1249–1255, 2001

Durham RC, Murphy T, Allan T, et al: Cognitive therapy, analytic psychotherapy and anxiety management training for generalized anxiety disorder. Br J Psychiatry 165:315–323, 1994

Durham RC, Fisher PL, Treliving LR, et al: One year follow-up of cognitive therapy, analytic psychotherapy and anxiety management training for generalized anxiety disorder: symptom change, medication usage and attitudes to treatment. Behav Cogn Psychother 27:19–35, 1999

Durham RC, Chambers JA, MacDonald RR, et al: Does cognitive-behavioural therapy influence the long-term outcome of generalized anxiety disorder? An 8–14 year follow-up of two clinical trials. Psychol Med 33:499–509, 2003

Durham RC, Fisher PL, Dow MGT, et al: Cognitive behaviour therapy for good and poor prognosis generalized anxiety disorder: a clinical effectiveness study. Clin Psychol Psychother 11:145–157, 2004

Erickson TM, Newman MG: Interpersonal and emotional processes in generalized anxiety disorder analogues during social interaction tasks. Behav Ther 38:364–377, 2007

Evans S, Ferrando S, Finder M, et al: Mindfulness-based cognitive therapy for generalized anxiety disorder. J Anxiety Disord 22:716–721, 2008

Fava GA, Ruini C, Rafanelli C, et al: Well-being therapy of generalized anxiety disorder. Psychother Psychosom 74:26–30, 2005

Ferrero A, Pierò A, Fassina S, et al: A 12-month comparison of brief psychodynamic psychotherapy and pharmacotherapy treatment in subjects with generalised anxiety disorders in a community setting. Eur Psychiatry 22:530–539, 2007

Flint AJ: Epidemiology and comorbidity of anxiety disorders in the elderly. Am J Psychiatry 151:640–649, 1994

Floyd M, McKendree-Smith N, Bailey E, et al: Two-year follow-up of self-examination therapy for generalized anxiety disorder. J Anxiety Disord 16:369–375, 2002

Foa EB, Kozak MJ: Emotional processing of fear: exposure to corrective information. Psychol Bull 99:20–35, 1986

Gould RA, Safren SA, Washington DO, et al: A meta-analytic review of cognitive-behavioral treatments, in Generalized Anxiety Disorder: Advances in Research and Practice. Edited by Heimberg RG, Turk CL, Mennin DS. New York, Guilford, 2004, pp 248–264

Heimberg RG, Turk CL, Mennin DS: Generalized Anxiety Disorder: Advances in Research and Practice. New York, Guilford, 2004

Heuzenroeder L, Donnelly M, Haby MM, et al: Cost-effectiveness of psychological and pharmacological interventions for generalized anxiety disorder and panic disorder. Aust N Z J Psychiatry 38:602–612, 2004

Hunot V, Churchill R, Teixeira V, et al: Psychological therapies for generalised anxiety disorder. Cochrane Database Syst Rev 24:CD001848, 2007

Huppert JD: Anxiety disorders and depression, in Oxford Handbook of Anxiety and Related Disorders. Edited by Antony MM, Stein MB. New York, Oxford University Press, 2009, pp 576–586

Huppert JD, Alley AC: The clinical application of emotion research in generalized anxiety disorder: some proposed procedures. Cogn Behav Pract 11:387–392, 2004

Huppert JD, Sanderson WC: Psychotherapy for generalized anxiety disorder, in Textbook of Anxiety Disorders. Edited by Stein DJ, Hollander E. Washington DC, American Psychiatric Press, 2002, pp 163–178

Kendall PC: Coping Cat Workbook. Ardmore, PA, Workbook Publishing, 1990

Kendall PC, Safford S, Flannery-Schroeder E, et al: Child anxiety treatment: outcomes in adolescence and impact on substance use and depression at 7.4-year follow-up. J Consult Clin Psychol 72:276–287, 2004

Ladouceur R, Dugas MJ, Freeston MH, et al: Efficacy of a cognitive-behavioral treatment for generalized anxiety disorder: evaluation in a controlled clinical trial. J Consult Clin Psychol 68:957–964, 2000

Linden M, Zubraegel D, Baer T, et al: Efficacy of cognitive behaviour therapy in generalized anxiety disorders: results of a controlled clinical trial (Berlin CBT-GAD Study). Psychother Psychosom 74:36–42, 2005

Mathews A: Why worry? The cognitive function of anxiety. Behav Res Ther 28:455–468, 1990

McGinn LK, Young JE, Sanderson WC: When and how to do long-term therapy without feeling guilty. Cogn Behav Pract 2:187–212, 1994

McIntosh A, Cohen A, Turnbull N, et al: Clinical Guidelines and Evidence Review for Panic Disorder and Generalised Anxiety Disorder. Sheffield, London, University of Sheffield/London: National Collaborating Centre for Primary Care, 2004

Mennin DS: Emotion regulation therapy for generalized anxiety disorder. Clin Psychol Psychother 11:17–29, 2004

Mennin DS, Heimberg RG, Turk CL, et al: Preliminary evidence for an emotion dysregulation model of generalized anxiety disorder. Behav Res Ther 43:1281–1310, 2005

Mitte K: Meta-analysis of cognitive-behavioral treatments for generalized anxiety disorder: a comparison with pharmacotherapy. Psychol Bull 131:785–795, 2005

Mohlman J, Gorenstein EE, Kleber M, et al: Standard and enhanced cognitive-behavior therapy for late-life generalized anxiety disorder: two pilot investigations. Am J Geriatr Psychiatry 11:24–32, 2003

Newman MG, Castonguay LG, Borkovec TD, et al: Integrative psychotherapy, in Generalized Anxiety Disorder: Advances in Research and Practice. Edited by Heimberg RG, Turk CL, Mennin DS. New York, Guilford, 2004, pp 320–350

Newman MG, Castonguay LG, Fisher AJ, et al: Interpersonal and emotion processing focused treatment in generalized anxiety disorder. Paper presented at the annual meeting of the Society for Psychotherapy Research, Barcelona, Spain, June 2008

Ost LG, Breitholtz E: Applied relaxation vs. cognitive therapy in the treatment of generalized anxiety disorder. Behav Res Ther 38:777–790, 2000

Rapee RM: Psychological factors involved in generalized anxiety, in Chronic Anxiety: Generalized Anxiety Disorder and Mixed Anxiety-Depression. Edited by Rapee RM, Barlow DH. New York, Guilford, 1991, pp 76–94

Rice KM, Blanchard EB: Biofeedback in the treatment of anxiety disorders. Clin Psychol Review 2:557–577, 1982

Roemer L, Orsillo SM: An open-trial investigation of an acceptance-based behavior therapy for generalized anxiety disorder. Behav Ther 38:72–85, 2007

Roemer L, Orsillo SM, Barlow DH: Generalized anxiety disorder, in Anxiety and Its Disorders: The Nature and Treatment of Anxiety and Panic, 2nd Edition. Edited by Barlow DH. New York, Guilford, 2002, pp 477–515

Ruscio AM, Borkovec TD: Experience and appraisal of worry among high worriers with and without generalized anxiety disorder. Behav Res Ther 42:1469–1482, 2004

Rygh JL, Sanderson WC: Treating Generalized Anxiety Disorder: Evidence-Based Strategies, Tools, and Techniques. New York, Guilford, 2004

Safran JD, Segal ZV: Interpersonal Process in Cognitive Therapy. New York, Basic Books, 1990

Sanderson WC, Barlow DH: A description of patients diagnosed with DSM-III-R generalized anxiety disorder. J Nerv Ment Dis 178:588–591, 1990

Sanderson WC, McGinn LK: Psychological treatment of anxiety disorder patients with comorbidity, in Treatment Strategies for Patients With Psychiatric Comorbidity. Edited by Wetzler S, Sanderson WC. New York, Wiley, 1997, pp 105–134

Sanderson WC, Wetzler S: Chronic anxiety and generalized anxiety disorder: issues in comorbidity, in Chronic Anxiety: Generalized Anxiety Disorder and Mixed Anxiety-Depression. Edited by Rapee RP, Barlow DH. New York, Guilford, 1991, pp 119–135

Sanderson WC, DiNardo PA, Rapee RM, et al: Syndrome comorbidity in patients diagnosed with a DSM-III-R anxiety disorder. J Abnorm Psychol 99:308–312, 1990

Sanderson WC, Beck AT, McGinn LK: Cognitive therapy for generalized anxiety disorder: significance of comorbid personality disorders. Journal of Cognitive Psychotherapy: An International Quarterly 8:13–18, 1994

Schut AJ, Castonguay LG, Borkovec TD: Compulsive checking behaviors in generalized anxiety disorder. J Clin Psychol 57:705–715, 2001

Siev J, Chambless DL: Specificity of treatment effects: cognitive therapy and relaxation for generalized anxiety and panic disorders. J Consult Clin Psychol 75:513–522, 2007

Stanley MA, Beck JG, Glassco JD: Treatment of generalized anxiety in older adults: a preliminary comparison of cognitive-behavioral and supportive approaches. Behav Ther 27:565–581, 1996

Stanley MA, Beck JG, Novy DM, et al: Cognitive-behavioral treatment of late-life generalized anxiety disorder. J Consul Clin Psychol 71:309–312, 2003a

Stanley MA, Hopko DR, Diefenbach GJ, et al: Cognitive-behavior therapy for late-life generalized anxiety disorder in primary care: preliminary findings. Am J Geriatr Psychiatry 11:92–96, 2003b

Tsao JCI, Mystkowski JL, Zucker BG, et al: Impact of cognitive-behavioral therapy for panic disorder on comorbidity: a controlled investigation. Behav Res Ther 43:959–970, 2005

van Boeijen CA, van Oppen P, Van Balkom AJ, et al: Treatment of anxiety disorders in primary care practice: a randomised controlled trial. Br J Gen Pract 55:763–769, 2005

Watson D: Rethinking the mood and anxiety disorders: a quantitative hierarchical model for DSM-V. J Abnorm Psychol 114:522–536, 2005

Wells A: Attention and the control of worry, in Worrying: Perspectives on Theory, Assessment and Treatment. Edited by Davey GCL, Tallis F. New York, Wiley, 1994, pp 91–114

Wells A, King P: Metacognitive therapy for generalized anxiety disorder: an open trial. J Behav Ther Exp Psychiatry 37:206–212, 2006

Wells A, Morrison AP: Qualitative dimensions of normal worry and normal obsessions: a comparative study. Behav Res Ther 32:867–870, 1994

Westen D, Morrison K: A multidimensional meta-analysis of treatments for depression, panic, and generalized anxiety disorder: an empirical examination of the status of empirically supported therapies. J Consult Clin Psychol 69:875–899, 2001

Wetherell JL, Gatz M, Craske MG: Treatment of generalized anxiety disorder in older adults. J Consult Clin Psychol 71:31–40, 2003

Wetherell JL, Lenze EJ, Stanley MA: Evidence-based treatment of geriatric anxiety disorders. Psychiatr Clin North Am 28:871–896, 2005

White J: "Stress control" large group therapy for generalized anxiety disorder: two year follow-up. Behav Cogn Psychother 26:237–246, 1998a

White J: Stresspac: three year follow-up of a controlled trial of a self-help package for the anxiety disorders. Behavioural and Cognitive Psychotherapy 26:133–141, 1998b

Woody SR, Sanderson WC: Manuals for empirically supported treatments: 1998 update from the Task Force on Psychological Interventions. Clin Psychol 51:17–21, 1998

Zinbarg RE, Craske MG, Barlow DH: Mastery of Your Anxiety and Worry (Therapist Guide), 2nd Edition. New York, Oxford University Press, 2006

Zinbarg RE, Lee JE, Yoon KL: Dyadic predictors of outcome in a cognitive-behavioral program for patients with generalized anxiety disorder in committed relationships: a "spoonful of sugar" and a dose of nonhostile criticism may help. Behav Res Ther 45:699–713, 2007

Recommended Readings

Heimberg RG, Turk CL, Mennin DS: Generalized Anxiety Disorder: Advances in Research and Practice. New York, Guilford, 2004

Hunot V, Churchill R, Teixeira V, et al: Psychological therapies for generalised anxiety disorder. Cochrane Database Syst Rev 24:CD001848, 2007

Leahy RL: The Worry Cure: Seven Steps to Stop Worry Stopping You. New York, Random House, 2005

Rygh JL, Sanderson WC: Treating Generalized Anxiety Disorder: Evidence-Based Strategies, Tools, and Techniques. New York, Guilford, 2004

Zinbarg RE, Craske MG, Barlow DH: Mastery of Your Anxiety and Worry (Therapist Guide), 2nd Edition. New York, Oxford University Press, 2006

Web Sites of Interest

Anxiety Disorders Association of America: Generalized anxiety disorder (GAD). Available at http://www.adaa.org/GettingHelp/AnxietyDisorders/GAD.asp. Accessed March 26, 2009.

Association for Advancement of Behavior Therapy: Anxiety. Available at http://www.abct.org/docs/dMembers/FactSheets/ANXIETY%200907.pdf. Accessed March 26, 2009.

National Institute of Mental Health: Generalized anxiety disorder (GAD). Available at http://www.nimh.nih.gov/health/topics/generalized-anxiety-disorder-gad/index.shtml. Accessed March 26, 2009.

Anxiety Disorders Treatment Center: General anxiety: summary. Available at http://anxieties.com/gad.php. Accessed March 26, 2009.

Mixed Anxiety-Depression

Chapter 15

Mixed Anxiety-Depressive Disorder

An Undiagnosed and Undertreated Severity Spectrum?

Jan Fawcett, M.D.
Rebecca P. Cameron, Ph.D.
Alan F. Schatzberg, M.D.

Mixed anxiety-depressive disorder, a diagnostic category proposed in DSM-IV (American Psychiatric Association 1994) for further study, is characterized by dysphoria combined with other depressive and anxiety symptoms that are subthreshold for a diagnosis of a primary affective or anxiety disorder (Table 15–1). This diagnosis follows the lead of the World Health Organization, which included a similar subsyndromal diagnosis with anxious and depressed features, mixed anxiety-depressive disorder, in ICD-10 (World Health Organization 1992c). The category "mixed anxiety-depressive disorder" reflects a fresh attempt to address several clinical phenomena that have been underrecognized in recent DSMs: anxiety and depression frequently co-occur; patients' disorders do not always fit neatly into the primary diagnostic categories, such as major depression and generalized anxiety disorder (GAD); and subsyndromal symptoms may be clinically significant.

Another form of anxiety-depression has also been recognized in the literature (Clayton et al. 1991; Fava et al. 2008). This has taken the form of full-criteria major depression with a high level of anxiety—usually accompanied by diagnoses of one or more comorbid anxiety disorders—that predicted a poorer treatment outcome and a higher risk of suicidality and suicide. This form of anxiety-depression will also be reviewed, as well as recent studies of the common co-occurrence of GAD with major depressive disorder which have led to suggestions that GAD be classified in the mood disorders section in DSM-V. There is growing recognition that full-syndrome forms of major depressive disorder with comorbid anxiety disorders or comorbid severe anxiety may distinguish a different outcome (including an increased risk of suicide) and may present another, more severe form of anxiety. This recognition may call for a redefinition, delineating a more severe form of mixed anxiety-depressive disorder, or a severity spectrum of mixed anxiety-depression, rather than the subsyndromal syndrome initially studied in preparation for DSM-IV.

Prior to DSM-III (American Psychiatric Association 1980), the concept of mixed anxiety-depressive disorders had been widely accepted, as evidenced in diagnostic labels such as anxiety-depressive neurosis (Shammas 1977), psychoneurotic depressive illness

TABLE 15–1. DSM-IV-TR research criteria for mixed anxiety-depressive disorder

A. Persistent or recurrent dysphoric mood lasting at least 1 month.

B. The dysphoric mood is accompanied by at least 1 month of four (or more) of the following symptoms:

(1) difficulty concentrating or mind going blank

(2) sleep disturbance (difficulty falling or staying asleep, or restless, unsatisfying sleep)

(3) fatigue or low energy

(4) irritability

(5) worry

(6) being easily moved to tears

(7) hypervigilance

(8) anticipating the worst

(9) hopelessness (pervasive pessimism about the future)

(10) low self-esteem or feelings of worthlessness

C. The symptoms cause clinically significant distress or impairment in social, occupational, or other important areas of functioning.

D. The symptoms are not due to the direct physiological effects of a substance (e.g., a drug of abuse, a medication) or a general medical condition.

E. All of the following:

(1) criteria have never been met for major depressive disorder, dysthymic disorder, panic disorder, or generalized anxiety disorder

(2) criteria are not currently met for any other anxiety or mood disorder (including an anxiety or mood disorder, in partial remission)

(3) the symptoms are not better accounted for by any other mental disorder

with associated anxiety or anxiety-depressive syndromes (Houck 1970), anxiety masquerading as depression, or depression with prominent features of anxiety (Verner 1969). The use of earlier psychopharmacological agents (benzodiazepines and tricyclic antidepressants [TCAs]) with seemingly more specific effects for anxious or depressive symptoms, and the emphasis in DSM-III on differential categorical classification, encouraged an exaggerated dichotomy between the two broad diagnostic categories that has persisted.

Despite somewhat successful attempts to separate a variety of anxiety and depressive syndromes, the distinction between GAD and major depression has never been clear-cut, and genetic evidence suggests that these two disorders are outcomes of the same underlying diathesis (Kendler 1996; Kendler et al. 1992). In 1983, Fawcett and Kravitz found that among patients diagnosed with major depression, 29% were found to have co-occurring panic attacks, and more than 60% scored at least moderate psychic anxiety, as measured by the Schedule for Affective Disorders and Schizophrenia–Change Version (SADS-C) ratings. Although, as characterized in DSM-IV, mixed anxiety-depressive disorder reflects symptomatology below diagnostic thresholds for existing anxiety and mood diagnoses (except the residual categories of anxiety disorder not otherwise specified and depressive disorder not otherwise specified), the syndrome appears to have clinically important implications for patients' distress and disability and, potentially, for their treatability. However, the inclusion of mixed anxiety-depressive disorder does not resolve the issue of overlap between anxiety and depression (in particular, GAD and major depression). Rather, it describes a syndrome with milder symptoms of this overlapping construct. We review the development of this new category (about which many research questions remain unresolved, including course, prognosis, and appropriate treatment) in the context of the long-standing debate about the distinction between anxiety and depressive disorders, particularly GAD and major depression.

History of Combined Anxiety-Depressive Syndromes

1960s–1970s: Development of Specific Psychopharmacological Agents

Anxiety and Depression as Overlapping Constructs

Anxiety and depression were not as stringently differentiated in the era prior to DSM-III, when it was widely accepted that many patients presented for treatment with symptoms of both disorders. For example, Roth et al. (1972) noted that "a wide range of workers drawn from many schools of thought have (explicitly or implicitly) upheld the view that anxiety states and depressive disorders merge insensibly with one another or belong to different parts of a single continuum of affective disturbance" (pp. 147–148).

Dichotomization of Anxiety and Depression

The concept of two separate classes of disorders was increasingly accepted by clinicians during the 1960s and 1970s. Roth et al. (1972), in a seminal study, investigated the difficulty of differentiating between depressed and anxious patients and found that they could be distinguished despite areas of overlap. Factor analysis of symptoms suggested that two factors appeared to depict patients with either panic disorder or major depression with melancholia, and a third, residual factor corresponded to GAD and depression. Historical data and social functioning indicated that the anxious group was more disturbed and disabled by their symptoms. This study's findings led to incorporation of the distinction between panic disorder and major depression in DSM-III. However, the study results did not help to resolve the debate regarding the existence of a mixed anxiety-depressive disorder.

The development of pharmacological agents with relatively specific antidepressant or anxiolytic effects, particularly TCAs and benzodiazepines, supported the dichotomization of depression and anxiety. Initial confusion over whether benzodiazepines should be considered an antidepressant class of drugs gave way over time to evidence that they were primarily and specifically useful for anxiety symptoms. In contrast, TCAs were found to be primarily useful for depressive symptoms and for endogenous or severe depression, although data did emerge as to their effectiveness in panic disorder as well.

Rickels and Downing (1972) and Rickels et al. (1970) found that depressed outpatients classified on relative degree of depression and anxiety differed in their treatment responses to a TCA, a minor tranquilizer, a combination, or placebo. Patients with high levels of depression and high levels of anxiety responded best to a combined regimen of amitriptyline and chlordiazepoxide, whereas amitriptyline alone was indicated for patients with high depression and low anxiety, and chlordiazepoxide was most effective for patients with low depression and high anxiety. Patients with low depression and low anxiety showed no difference in response among the three active treatments and placebo (Rickels et al. 1970). Results for outpatients diagnosed with neurosis and identified as having low-level depression and low-level anxiety support the newly proposed category of mixed anxiety-depressive disorder.

In the late 1970s, we reviewed the efficacy of benzodiazepines and TCAs in the treatment of depressive disorders (Schatzberg 1978; Schatzberg and Cole 1978). We suggested then the need to differentiate endogenous from nonendogenous depression, noting that nonendogenous depressive syndromes resemble neurotic anxiety disorders. *Endogenous depression* was defined as depression with symptoms including diurnal variation; terminal insomnia; decreased interest, pleasure, and energy; psychomotor retardation; and lack of reactivity to the environment. Nonendogenous depression was considered more heterogeneous, but it could include histrionic behavior, anxiety, anger, obsessionality, reversed diurnal variation, early insomnia, and variable responses to external stimuli. This latter syndrome is less easily distinguishable from anxiety states, which also are frequently accompanied by mild depressive symptoms. We suggested a continuum ranging from anxiety states to endogenous depression, with nonendogenous depression being intermediate between the two. We also concluded that TCAs should be the drug of first choice for either type of depression or a mixed type. Benzodiazepines could be considered as an initial adjunctive treatment for specific symptoms, such as difficulty falling asleep, or for side effects of TCAs, such as agitation.

The Advent of DSM-III and Changes in DSM-III-R: Categorical Classification

Multiple Models of the Possible Relationship Between Generalized Anxiety and Depression

Today, several models of the relationship between anxiety and depression exist (Stahl 1993; Stavrakaki and Vargo 1986). The unitary position suggests that anxiety and depression are aspects of the same disorder but differ quantitatively or temporally. In the pluralistic model, anxiety and depression are viewed as distinct disorders. A third position maintains that mixed anxiety and depression is distinct from both primary anxiety and primary depression.

A fourth position, put forward by Clayton et al. (1991) and Fava et al. (2006), suggests a type of full-criteria major depression accompanied by significant levels of anxiety that could meet criteria for the full range of anxiety disorders. This combination results in a poorer treatment outcome. In fact, N.M. Simon et al. (2007) reported that five epidemiological studies, two clinical studies of unipolar major depression, and two clinical studies of bipolar disorders have shown a higher risk of suicidal behaviors and, in one study, a higher rate of suicide in patients with comorbid anxiety or anxiety disorders (Table 15–2).

A major issue in developing such models is the frequent comorbidity among anxiety disorders and between anxiety and depression. Anxiety and depression can be comorbid in a variety of ways: comorbidity of full-syndrome disorders; one full-syndrome condition

TABLE 15–2. Studies linking suicidal behavior and severe psychic anxiety/anxiety disorders in depressed patients/probands

Study	Finding
Fawcett et al. 1990	Severe psychic anxiety (>5) on SADS-C psychic anxiety scale was significantly associated with suicide over 1 year in MDD.
Clayton et al. 1991	Depressed subjects with higher ratings for anxiety took longer to recover.
Hall et al. 1999	90% of suicide-attempt patients interviewed after admission of severe suicide attempt expressed severe anxiety over the month before the attempt.
Busch et al. 2003	76% of inpatients had at least 3 days of severe anxiety/agitation within 7 days prior to suicide.
Wunderlich et al. 1998	Comorbidity, especially anxiety disorders, increases the risk of suicide attempts more than any DSM-IV diagnosis.
Sareen et al. 2005	The data clearly indicate that comorbid anxiety disorders amplify the risk of suicide in mood disorders.
Foley et al. 2006	Suicidal risk was greatest in association with current depression plus generalized anxiety disorder (OR 468.5).
Boden et al. 2007	Any anxiety disorder increased the risk of suicide attempts by 5.65 times. Rates of suicidal behavior increased with the number of anxiety disorders present.
Bolton et al. 2008	Presence of one or more anxiety disorders at baseline was significantly associated with subsequent onset suicide attempts (OR 2.2).
Fava et al. 2004	46% met criteria for anxious depression of Ham-D subscale of 7 or greater. These patients had more severe depression and increased rates of suicidal ideation.
Fava et al. 2006	Individuals with anxious depression were more likely to endorse IDS-C30 items concerning melancholic endogenous features, both before and after adjusting for baseline severity of depression.
N.M. Simon et al. 2007	In bipolar patients, a lifetime anxiety disorder doubled the odds of a past suicide attempt and current anxiety. Comorbidity more than doubled the odds of current suicide ideation.
G.E. Simon et al. 2007	Comorbid anxiety disorder was associated with significantly higher risk of suicide attempt (HR 1.4) and suicide death (HR 1.81).

Note. Ham-D=Hamilton Rating Scale for Depression; HR=hazard ratio; IDS-C30=Inventory of Depressive Symptomatology–Clinician-Rated; MDD=major depressive disorder; OR=odds ratio; SADS-C=Schedule for Affective Disorders and Schizophrenia–Change.

with significant subsyndromal overlay from the other; or a residual category of mixed, subsyndromal symptoms.

In a study of comorbidity, Wetzler and Katz (1989) discussed the problems of differentiating anxiety and depression. They distinguished two conceptual stances: a dimensional approach and a categorical approach. In the dimensional approach, anxiety and depression are considered separate, continuous constructs, whereas in the categorical approach, anxiety and depression are viewed as syndromes that characterize different groups of patients. They noted that different questions are raised and different statistical techniques would be used to analyze questions flowing from these contrasting approaches. In addition, they ascertained that attempting to separate depression and anxiety is a somewhat artificial undertaking, given the frequent co-occurrence of the two syndromes. They studied a multivantaged approach combining self-report data with nurses' and doctors' ratings of anxiety and depressed mood, and found that different vantage points yielded different results for the distinction between these syndromes. Doctors' ratings were best able to distinguish anxiety and depression among severely depressed patients, whereas patients' self-reports reflected temporal distinctions in improvement within symptom clusters in response to treatment. Given the complexity of the relation between anxiety and depression, multiple vantage points have the potential to increase validity in psychological measurement of these two constructs.

DSM-III, DSM-III-R, and Comorbidity

Changes in classifications from DSM-II (American Psychiatric Association 1968) through DSM-IV have reflected then-current views and further influenced our conceptualizations of anxiety, depression, and their overlap. DSM-III contained a more elaborate system for classifying anxiety and depressive disorders than did DSM-II, with more subtypes under each broad syndrome and more specific criteria for each diagnostic category. DSM-III also implemented exclusion criteria that prioritized diagnoses of depression over diagnoses of anxiety. DSM-III-R (American Psychiatric Association 1987) eliminated this hierarchy for anxiety disorders, thereby making it easier for comorbid anxiety and mood disorders to be diagnosed as such. Despite such efforts, a debate remains about the differentiation of GAD and major depression, and this debate is only heightened by the somewhat arbitrary criteria. For example, the difference in duration of symptoms required for diagnosis of the two disorders (6 months for GAD vs. 2 weeks for major depression) still makes it difficult to assess the true extent of overlap in symptom presentation. In fact, except for the distinction in duration of symptoms, GAD and major depression, as defined in DSM-IV, could easily be applied to the same clinical presentation if both dysphoria and worry were present.

Despite efforts to include dimensional constructs, as reflected in Axis V, the DSMs have primarily used a categorical approach to psychopathology. Residual categories, such as depressive disorder not otherwise specified and the recently proposed mixed anxiety-depressive disorder and minor depressive disorder, offer a method for recognizing clinically significant distress or impairment occurring at lower levels of symptom severity within a diagnostic group. However, it remains to be seen whether a more truly dimensional approach would more accurately and usefully reflect psychiatric phenomena.

Generalized Anxiety Disorder Differentiation

In his review of the literature on GAD and comorbidity, Maser (1998) noted the shifting diagnostic criteria for GAD over time, with respect to both the duration of symptoms (1 month in DSM-III, yielding a 45% prevalence of GAD in a probability sample; 6 months in DSM-III-R and DSM-IV, yielding a 9% prevalence) and the hierarchical rules disallowing GAD from being diagnosed as a comorbid disorder with other anxiety and depressive disorders (present in DSM-III but gradually eliminated in subsequent DSMs). Epidemiologic Catchment Area data indicated a 1-year prevalence of GAD alone of 1.30%–2.23%; GAD in the presence of other disorders was diagnosed in 3.42%–4.94% of the sample. In addition, the number of symptoms used to define GAD changed from DSM-III-R to DSM-IV, again with the likelihood that prevalence rates and comorbidity findings would be affected. However, Carter et al. (2001) studied German adults and found only minor differences in prevalence and comorbidity rates for DSM-IV GAD versus DSM-III-R GAD.

Maser (1998) further noted that obtaining comorbidity data from clinical samples confounds questions about the nature and frequency of comorbidity with the fact that treatment-seeking populations are more likely to be experiencing comorbidity and are more likely to be relatively severe cases. With these limitations in mind, he reviewed studies that found that 91% of the clinic patients with GAD had at least one comorbid condition. In this sample, 41% of the clinic patients with GAD had a mood disorder (usually dysthymia). In other clinical samples, rates of comorbid mood disorders ranged from 9% to 45% for major depression and from 29% to 69% for mood disorders defined more broadly (e.g., including dysthymia).

Alternative Conceptualizations

Evidence From Psychometric Studies of Self-Report Instruments: Affect Dimensions

Increasing evidence indicates that depression and anxiety do have common dimensional features or risk factors (e.g., genetics), although discriminating characteristics may also exist. Clark and Watson (1991) and Watson et al. (1988) investigated a tripartite model, in which measures of negative affect, positive affect, and hyperarousal were used to differentiate depression and anxiety (see Chapter 5, "Anxious Traits and Temperaments," in this volume). Studies have shown that low-state positive affect is a specific feature of depression, whereas positive affect is largely unrelated to anxiety. Hyperarousal or autonomic arousal corresponds to the physiological symptoms of anxiety, such as pounding heart, feelings of constriction, and light-headedness. This feature is highly relevant to panic disorder and is less clearly temperamental. Negative affect is a common risk factor for both depression and anxiety, and it may reflect, in part, the overlap in phenomenological distress between these two disorders.

Findings From Genetic Studies

Kendler (1996; Kendler et al. 1992) examined genetic and environmental contributions to the frequent comorbidity of GAD and major depression. Lifetime diagnosis was used for the first study, and 1-year follow-up prevalence was used for the second. In a sample of approximately 1,000 female twin pairs, Kendler et al.

(1992) found that GAD (diagnosed according to modified DSM-III-R criteria) and major depression (as defined by DSM-III-R criteria) share a common genetic diathesis. Furthermore, shared environmental experiences, such as shared aspects of family environment, played no role in the etiology of major depression or GAD. Instead, individual-specific experiences were responsible for whether the genetic diathesis was expressed as major depression or GAD. Kendler (1996) replicated these findings and suggested that different stressful life events might be responsible for the occurrence of major depression and GAD.

Generalized Anxiety Disorder as Anxious Temperament Type

Akiskal (1998) suggested that GAD could be reconceptualized as the extreme manifestation of an anxious temperament type, called generalized anxious temperament. This constellation of traits represents a vigilant stance focused on harm avoidance and is considered narrower in scope than either neuroticism or negative affectivity. It may be associated with increased risk for depression and other disorders (e.g., phobias, substance use). Evidence in support of this view includes the finding that GAD symptoms (e.g., worry, nausea) are lifelong and traitlike, rather than acute, for many individuals. Acute life events may thus provoke a more severe episode (GAD) in the context of long-standing symptoms (generalized anxious temperament).

In 1990, Fawcett et al. found that severe psychic anxiety, panic attacks, and severe (global) insomnia, measured prospectively by SADS-C ratings, were associated with the occurrence of suicide over a follow-up period of 12 months, whereas standard predictors of suicide such as recent or prior suicide attempts, suicidal ideation, and severe hopelessness did not show a correlation with suicide over the 1-year period but did demonstrate a correlation with suicide as an outcome during a 2- to 10-year follow-up period. This work suggested a change in focus from the presence of comorbid anxiety disorders to severity of the anxiety symptoms, estimated on the basis of patients' inability to distract themselves from anxious ruminations, perceived intensity of the anxiety, and proportion of waking consciousness taken up by the anxiety experience, using the SADS-C measure. A subsequent study of 76 inpatient suicide cases by Busch et al. (2003) found an association of suicide with periods of severe anxiety or agitation recorded in hospital chart notes, and a study of 100 consecutive suicide attempts requiring admission from a city hospital emergency room by Hall et al. (1999) found that 90% of these patients suffering from depression had experienced severe anxiety in the month prior to their severe suicide attempt (see Table 15–2).

Advent of Selective Serotonin Reuptake Inhibitors

The development of selective serotonin reuptake inhibitors and other new compounds has provided clinicians with access to treatments that are safer and better tolerated than older categories of antidepressants. Over time, evidence has accumulated that these drugs are effective in treating depression, anxious depression, panic, and, more recently, GAD. The ability of these drugs to address a range of symptoms facilitates their use in primary care settings, where clinicians may not have the time to clarify complex differential diagnoses. However, this versatility may have negative repercussions for accumulating clinical data on questions such as differential course and prognosis of different presentations of anxiety and depression and may reduce the apparent need for referrals to psychiatrists and other mental health specialists. The broad applicability of newer pharmacological agents may raise questions about distinctions in the underlying biochemical dysregulation of anxiety and depression.

Are Generalized Anxiety Disorder and Major Depression Distinct Presentations of the Same Disorder?

In conclusion, patients often experience symptoms of both anxiety and depression, although our diagnostic system is still evolving toward characterizing these syndromes in a conceptually meaningful and clinically useful way. The use of categorical diagnoses and somewhat arbitrary criteria for diagnoses may hinder our ability to capture the nuances of the relations between these two broad symptom areas. However, research on comorbidity, affect dimensions, genetics, course of illness, and psychopharmacology is contributing to our understanding of the relation between depression and anxiety.

The Development of DSM-IV and the Introduction of Mixed Anxiety-Depressive Disorder

Changes in DSM-IV

Two changes to DSM are reshaping our conceptualization of the relation between generalized anxiety and depression (Stahl 1993). First, GAD was redefined from its former status as a residual anxiety diagnosis (i.e., diagnosed only in the absence of any other anxiety disorder) to a generalized anxiety syndrome with symptoms of mild depression that are less severe than the symptoms of anxiety. Thus, GAD has become more explicitly a mixed disorder. In addition, from DSM-III-R onward, GAD has been defined as a chronic disorder, with a minimum of 6 months' duration to warrant the diagnosis. Second, mixed anxiety-depressive disorder has been introduced and defined as a stable core of subsyndromal symptoms that do not reach the threshold for diagnosis of GAD, major depression, or any other full-syndrome disorder. It is unclear whether this syndrome is in fact a stable disorder or whether, under stress, it can be exacerbated, leading to an overt anxiety or depressive disorder.

The DSM-IV-TR (American Psychiatric Association 2000) criteria for mixed anxiety-depressive disorder are somewhat different from the ICD-10 criteria. ICD-10 defines mixed anxiety-depressive disorder as comprising symptoms of both anxiety and depression, with neither more salient than the other and neither at a level that would warrant a separate diagnosis (World Health Organization 1992c). The ICD-10 clinical descriptions (World Health Organization 1992a) offer further specificity by requiring that autonomic symptoms be present and that a significant life change not be associated with the onset of symptoms (in which case, the diagnosis should be adjustment disorder). Finally, the ICD-10 research criteria suggest that researchers may wish to develop their own criteria within the guidelines described above (World Health Organization 1992b).

Effect of Subsyndromal States on Functioning

Many researchers have documented the effect of subsyndromal states on disability. Johnson et al. (1992) carried out an epidemiological survey and found that threshold diagnoses of major depression or dysthymia resulted in increased service use and social morbidity (medication use, impaired physical and emotional health, time lost from work, and attempted suicide). However, the presence of subthreshold depressive symptoms resulted in higher levels of service use and social morbidity as well, and on a population basis, subthreshold symptomatology resulted in greater social impairment and service cost than did diagnosable disorders. Other researchers (Gotlib et al. 1995; Wells et al. 1989) have obtained similar findings, and Roy-Byrne (1996) concluded that despite a tendency to view GAD as mild, GAD and mixed anxiety-depressive disorder are associated with significant social impairment and role-functioning limitations.

Effect of Comorbid Anxiety Disorders/Severe Anxiety With Full-Syndrome Major Depression on Outcome and Suicidal Behavior

Studies cited in Table 15–2 have documented the significance of comorbid severe anxiety and anxiety disorders with major depression in both unipolar and bipolar disorders. These studies show that the risks of poor outcome and suicidal behavior are significantly higher with mixed anxiety depression in its full syndromal state. Taking this with the evidence of documented effects of subsyndromal depression and anxiety presents a very significant severity spectrum—at the mild end, worth recognizing and treating to prevent chronic suffering and disability; at the more severe end, a mixed anxiety syndrome capable of leading to poor treatment response and even death through suicide.

Preparations for DSM-IV

The recognition of high levels of comorbidity of full-syndrome anxiety and depressive disorders, as well as the ICD-10 inclusion of a subsyndromal mixed disorder, prompted the planners of DSM-IV to consider several questions related to revising existing diagnoses or adding new ones. The work group charged with considering the possibility of including a mixed anxiety-depression diagnosis in DSM-IV delineated two relevant issues (Moras 1989, as cited in Moras et al. 1996). The first issue was whether to include a diagnosis that would correspond to the ICD-10 diagnosis of mixed anxiety-depressive disorder. The second issue was whether DSM-IV diagnoses should be altered to better reflect the overlap between anxiety and depression or whether a new diagnosis should be included to reflect empirical knowledge about comorbid anxiety and depressive disorders. Literature reviews were undertaken to answer these questions.

Evidence for a Subsyndromal Category

Katon and Roy-Byrne (1991) examined literature based on community samples, primary care samples, and psychiatric samples to determine whether a patient population with clinically important symptoms of anxiety and depression that fell below the thresholds for specific DSM-III-R diagnoses (consistent with the ICD-10 description of mixed anxiety-depressive disorder) existed. With respect to community samples, their review found that diagnosable mood disorders occurred in 3%–8% of the population (based on Epidemiologic Catchment Area data), that subsyndromal depression occurred in

13%–20% of the population, and that community members who experienced depressive symptoms were more likely to have mixed anxious-depressive profiles than more purely depressive profiles.

In their review of studies that used primary care samples, Katon and Roy-Burne found higher rates of distress (40%) than diagnosable disorder (25%), suggesting a 15% prevalence of subsyndromal, distressed patients in these settings. Furthermore, the patients with mixed-symptom profiles in this setting did have deficits in functioning.

Finally, a review of studies of psychiatric populations found a subgroup of patients with chronic anxiety and depression (general neurotic syndrome) that was stable, except that increased stress could result in acute exacerbations leading to diagnosable levels of symptoms.

Taken together, these findings suggested that a subsyndromal, mixed-symptom disorder does exist, that it results in meaningful functional impairment, and that it represents a higher risk of developing more severe disorders. Unresolved questions included determination of appropriate criteria, the possibility of lowering the threshold on existing diagnoses to capture this group, and resolution of issues of course and prognosis.

Diagnosis Based on the Tripartite Model

As described earlier in this chapter, Clark and Watson (1991, cited in Moras et al. 1996) presented a new dimensional model for characterizing depressive and anxious syndromes, based on patients' symptomatology with respect to the dimensions of negative affect, positive affect, and hyperarousal. The mixed anxiety-depression category proposed by Clark and Watson represents a more severe symptom profile than the mixed anxiety-depression category currently proposed in DSM-IV-TR. Other authors have called this type of symptom mixture *panic-depressive disorder* or *mixed mood disorder* (Akiskal 1990; Moras et al. 1996). Findings by Kring et al. (2007) supported the tripartite model in a study of 41 patients treated for depression with cognitive therapy. They found that nearly two-thirds of the variance in anxiety change was accounted for by changes in depression and negative affect, and just over three-fourths of the variance in depression was accounted for by changes in anxiety and negative affect, indicating that much of the change in anxiety and depression across the course of treatment is shared in common.

A Possible Comorbid Diagnostic Category

In his review of the literature on comorbidity, Moras (1989, as cited in Moras et al. 1996) focused on concurrent comorbidity rather than lifetime comorbidity. He selected major depression and dysthymia from the mood disorders, and included a range of anxiety disorders, such as agoraphobia, panic disorder, GAD, obsessive-compulsive disorder, social phobia, simple phobia, and posttraumatic stress disorder. He found that comorbidity rates varied, but that, generally, patients with anxiety disorders were more likely to have a concomitant depressive diagnosis than were depressed patients to have an anxiety disorder. He concluded that the data did not support the creation of mixed diagnoses that would reflect current understandings of comorbidity.

The work group concluded that field trials should be conducted for the proposed mixed-symptom, subsyndromal disorder; that existing diagnoses should not be changed to reflect comorbidity; and that research should be conducted on the Clark and Watson tripartite model of depression and anxiety to prepare for DSM-V revisions.

Field Trial for Mixed Anxiety-Depressive Disorder

The DSM-IV field trial (Zinbarg et al. 1994) for mixed anxiety-depression was designed to answer four questions: 1) Do patients with subsyndromal symptoms and functional impairment exist? 2) Does medical pathology, rather than psychopathology, account for their functional deficits? 3) What is the breakdown of this population with respect to anxiety symptoms, depressive symptoms, or mixed symptoms? and 4) What is the best way to operationalize the criteria for any subsyndromal diagnosis?

Patients (*N*=666) were studied at five primary care medical sites and two mental health sites, chosen to yield a range of demographic characteristics of the patient population. Patients presenting to primary care clinics were screened for subjective distress with the General Health Questionnaire and the Medical Outcomes Study/Rand Short-Form General Health Survey. Those whose scores were at or above the cutoff and half as many patients whose scores were below the cutoff were interviewed in depth. Every patient presenting to the psychiatry clinics was interviewed. In-depth evaluations used included the Anxiety Disorders Interview Schedule—Revised, the mixed anxiety-depression field trial revision of the Hamilton Anxiety Scale and the Hamilton Rating Scale for Depression, and the chronic disease score.

In addition to DSM-III-R diagnoses with previously established criteria sets, diagnoses of anxiety disorder not otherwise specified and depressive disorder not otherwise specified (i.e., sufficiently distressed or impaired to be considered a probable or definite "case" but not better fitting another diagnostic category) were identified. Patients with not-otherwise-specified diagnoses constituted 11.7% of the patients surveyed, making that group the third-largest diagnostic group after those with panic disorder (29.1%) and GAD (20.2%), just ahead of the group with major depression (11.6%). They were characterized by high levels of impairment or distress (80% met criteria for definite caseness).

A principal-components analysis of the Hamilton symptom ratings (anxiety and depression) on all patients yielded three factors, which the investigators labeled *anxiety* (e.g., tension, apprehension), *physiological arousal* (e.g., tachycardia, choking), and *depression* (e.g., helplessness, diminished libido). These components were used to define symptom scales. A fourth symptom scale was constructed of items loading on both the anxiety and the depression components. This scale was labeled *negative affect* and included items such as irritability and fatigue. It is important to note that this symptom scale does not equate to the trait construct *negative affect*, but the investigators considered their findings to be consistent with Clark and Watson's (1991) work identifying three factors (negative affect, positive affect, and hyperarousal) that underlie the constructs of anxiety and depression as measured by self-report instruments.

Patients in the largest diagnostic groups (anxiety or depression not otherwise specified, panic disorder with agoraphobia, GAD, major depression, and no diagnosis) were analyzed according to the symptom scales described earlier. These analyses indicated that the patients with anxiety or depression not otherwise specified could be identified with the negative affect scale. Profile analyses suggested that this negative affect scale characterized the subsyndromal group and differentiated it from the other groups of more established disorders. Although altering the criteria for GAD or major depression would be an alternative that would include many of these patients in existing categories, mixed anxiety-depressive disorder was seen as a more accurate and useful category for these patients. First, mixed anxiety-depressive disorder makes explicit the mixed-symptom profile with which these patients present, and second, it increases the likelihood that a diagnosis will be made for these patients. Thus, a proposed criteria-set for DSM-IV included symptoms reflective of the overlap between depression and anxiety.

Investigators concluded that at least as many patients had subsyndromal affective symptoms (defined as meeting criteria for anxiety disorder not otherwise specified or for depressive disorder not otherwise specified) as had symptoms meeting criteria for certain well-delineated diagnostic categories; that these patients had meaningful levels of functional impairment; that nonspecific mixed-symptom profiles were the most common pattern of subsyndromal disorder; and that these patients could be distinguished from patients with GAD, major depression, and panic disorder with agoraphobia.

What Do We Know About Subsyndromal Mixed Anxiety-Depressive Disorder?

Given the decision to include mixed anxiety-depressive disorder as a proposed category in DSM-IV, and given the ongoing debate over how to account for comorbidity and overlap between anxiety and depression, epidemiological data and data on clinical course are needed. Although defining a subsyndromal diagnosis of mixed anxiety-depressive disorder does not resolve the big questions about continuity between risk factors, symptoms, and syndromes, or about the appropriateness of considering anxiety and depression to be separate or overlapping constructs, it does potentially afford an opportunity to characterize a distressed and impaired group that is not currently a focus of attention. Moreover, at this point, little has been established about mixed anxiety-depressive disorder patients. Information on sex, age at onset, chronicity, course, and treatment is scarce or nonexistent. On the other hand, we do have some information on the prevalence of mixed anxiety-depressive disorder (based on different criteria sets) in various settings (Table 15–3).

Wittchen and Essau (1993) reported results of the Munich Follow-Up Study, including data from a general population sample. They assessed depression and dysthymia, as well as panic disorder, agoraphobia, and simple and social phobias, but not GAD. They found that the prevalence of mixed anxiety-depressive disorder, based on the ICD-10 definition (i.e., the presence of subsyndromal anxiety and subsyndromal depression), was 0.8% in their epidemiological sample, less than that of pure subsyndromal categories (21.9% subsyndromal anxiety and 2.4% subsyndromal depression). In addition, Wittchen and Essau found that comorbid depression and anxiety, whether above or below diagnostic thresholds, were associated with higher levels of subjective suffering, functional impairment, and health service use than were pure disorders.

Roy-Byrne et al. (1994) used data from the field trial to describe the sample of 267 patients drawn from five

TABLE 15–3. Prevalence of mixed anxiety-depressive disorder in specific settings

Reference	Sample type	*N*	Prevalence (%)
Wittchen and Essau (1993)	Epidemiological	1,366	0.8
Roy-Byrne et al. (1994)	Primary care	267	5.1
Sartorius and Üstün (1995)	Primary care	25,916	1.3
Stein et al. (1995)	Primary care	501	2.0

Note. Definitions of mixed anxiety-depressive disorder vary; see text.

primary care settings in the United States, France, and Australia. A brief screen, followed by a structured interview, revealed that 5.1% of the patients had subsyndromal symptoms of anxiety and depression (defined as depression not otherwise specified or anxiety not otherwise specified, based on DSM-III-R criteria), accompanied by functional impairment. This prevalence rate was comparable with the prevalence of mood disorders in this sample and was about one-fourth the prevalence of anxiety disorders. In addition, the subsyndromal patients demonstrated functional impairments comparable with those of the anxiety and mood disorder groups.

Stein et al. (1995) studied 501 primary care patients who denied having a current psychiatric diagnosis or receiving current psychiatric treatment. Of these, 78 (15.6%) were systematically interviewed after screening positive for distress on the Beck Depression Inventory and/or the Beck Anxiety Inventory. Of the patients interviewed, 12.8% met the authors' criteria for mixed anxiety-depressive disorder (2.0% of the larger sample). In contrast to DSM-IV requirements, patients with previous diagnoses of anxiety or mood disorders were not excluded from the mixed anxiety-depressive disorder category. In contrast to the ICD-10 definition, autonomic symptoms were not required for a diagnosis of mixed anxiety-depressive disorder. For comparison, 44.9% of the interviewed sample met criteria for any depressive or anxiety diagnosis (7.0% of the larger sample). Mixed anxiety-depressive disorder patients reported levels of disability comparable with those of full-syndrome anxiety or mood disorder patients.

Another investigation of the prevalence of mixed anxiety-depressive disorder, as defined in ICD-10, was conducted by Sartorius and Üstün (1995); they used a large data set of 25,916 patients in general health care facilities in 14 countries. A sample of 5,379 patients, including those who scored high and low on the General Health Questionnaire, received in-depth evaluations. In this sample, the rate of depressive disorders was 11.8%, and the rate of anxiety disorders was 10.2%. The prevalence rates of subthreshold depression and subthreshold anxiety were 6.5% and 5.0%, respectively. Although there was some variability from country to country, the overall rate of mixed anxiety-depressive disorder was 1.3%.

In their review of the literature, Boulenger et al. (1997) estimated that the prevalence of mixed anxiety-depressive disorder ranged from 0.8% to 2.5% in epidemiological studies and from 5% to 15% in primary care settings. Furthermore, they concluded that longitudinal evidence supported the conceptualization of mixed anxiety-depressive disorder as a risk factor for full-syndrome depressive and anxiety disorders.

Controversy About Adding Mixed Anxiety-Depressive Disorder Category

Several authors have addressed the need for and potential problems with adding a new category of mixed anxiety-depressive disorder (Boulenger et al. 1997; Katon and Roy-Byrne 1991; Roy-Byrne 1996; Wittchen and Essau 1993). Beyond providing for compatibility with ICD-10, several arguments for adding mixed anxiety-depressive disorder to the DSM classification have been offered:

- Mixed anxiety-depressive disorder is seen in primary care settings, particularly because anxious and depressed patients tend to present somatic symptoms to their physicians. Identifying this group of patients may help physicians identify patients in need of intervention and may reduce excessive or inappropriate medical use. Providing appropriate treatment is particularly important, because subthreshold symptomatology can have a marked effect on distress and disability.
- Mixed anxiety-depressive disorder may represent a prodromal or residual phase of a more severe disorder, so identifying this at-risk group may facilitate the development of secondary preventive interventions.

- Mixed anxiety-depressive disorder may be a more appropriate diagnosis than adjustment disorder for some patients who do not identify a precipitating stressor or who may be particularly reactive to stress (Liebowitz 1993).
- Mixed anxiety-depressive disorder may comprise a spectrum ranging from subsyndromal anxiety-depression to full-syndrome major depression with severe anxiety or comorbid anxiety disorders, representing a disorder that is very important to recognize and that requires special treatment in order to avoid poor response or even suicide.

Potential problems with the diagnosis of mixed anxiety-depressive disorder have also been raised. The diagnostic category of mixed anxiety-depressive disorder may increase the risk of trivializing distress that is severe enough to affect functioning (Stahl 1993), may overlap too much with adjustment disorder or other DSM diagnoses (Liebowitz 1993), or may become a "wastebasket" category and thus discourage more careful diagnosis. These problems could ultimately impede research and reduce the identification of major depression and other diagnoses requiring prompt, serious, and specific intervention (Liebowitz 1993; Preskorn and Fast 1993). In addition, mixed anxiety-depressive disorder may be an unstable diagnosis leading to episodes of traditional affective or anxiety disorders. Minor depression may provide a subsyndromal diagnostic category adequate to meet clinical needs (Liebowitz 1993). Other authors argue that more effort should be put into distinguishing anxious from depressed patients (rather than combining them into one category) and offer strategies for making the appropriate primary diagnosis (Clayton 1990; Preskorn and Fast 1993).

Implications of an Anxiety-Depression Spectrum Diagnosis for DSM-V

A concept of mixed anxiety-depressive disorder may well recognize a syndrome associated with significant suffering and disability. But given the evidence that full-syndrome major depression with comorbid anxiety is associated with poor treatment outcome and increased risk of suicidal behavior, it should be asked whether the introduction into DSM-V of a new diagnosis implying a less severe, though treatment-worthy, anxiety-depressive syndrome would inappropriately reduce the perceived risk associated with full-syndrome major depression associated with severe comorbid anxiety. One solution would be to establish a category for mixed anxiety-depression with agreed-upon dimensions of severity, which would imply different treatment approaches. Such an approach would present the advantage of introducing the concept of symptom severity (as opposed to only identifying the number of symptoms) back into the DSM diagnostic system as a meaningful dimension to guide treatment decisions, while still recognizing the presence of a mixed anxiety-depression category. This would require agreement on and utilization of an accepted dimensional measure of the severity of anxiety and depression for patients classified in this category.

Primary Care

It has long been recognized that anxiety and depression are associated with somatic symptoms influencing medical use (Roth et al. 1972). Primary care providers currently prescribe the majority of anxiolytic and antidepressant medications. Negative publicity about benzodiazepine dependence may have reduced the willingness of primary care providers to treat anxiety. Somatic symptoms may be seen as an acceptable route for seeking treatment for anxiety. In contrast, depression may be considered more legitimate and more treatable. It will be important to continue to gather evidence about somatization and medical use among patients with mixed anxiety-depressive disorder.

Clinical Course and Treatment

As alluded to earlier in this chapter, an important and unresolved question about patients meeting criteria for mixed anxiety-depressive disorder has to do with the stability of the diagnosis versus its status as a risk factor for more severe psychiatric illness.

In addition, appropriate and efficacious treatments for mixed anxiety-depressive disorder need to be established. Drawing on the treatment literature for major depression and anxiety disorders, selective serotonin reuptake inhibitors are effective for symptoms of both anxiety and depression. Beginning in the 1980s, the treatment of unipolar conditions has shifted from short-term to continuation therapy to maintenance therapy. If mixed anxiety-depressive disorder proves to be a chronic disorder that responds to selective serotonin reuptake inhibitors, then maintenance therapy is likely to be indicated.

Boulenger et al. (1997) suggested that patients who have residual symptoms following a previously diagnosable disorder should conform to existing approaches to chronic conditions. In any event, according to DSM-IV criteria, these patients would not receive a diagnosis of mixed anxiety-depressive disorder. Nevertheless, the researchers pointed out that it is less clear how to treat mixed anxiety-depressive disorder in patients who have never had a psychiatric diagnosis in the past. Given the lack of research, particularly with DSM-IV criteria, they suggest that treatments used for mild anxiety and depression be considered.

Despite the lack of conclusive findings on treatment of mixed anxiety-depressive disorder, Zajecka and Ross (1995) and Boulenger et al. (1997) offered tentative recommendations. First, all of the major groups of antidepressants can be considered, because they all have some degree of anxiolytic and antidepressant effects. Second, buspirone may be useful, because it may have antidepressant effects at higher doses than are typically given for GAD. Buspirone is more effective for treating the psychological symptoms than the somatic symptoms of anxiety—and psychological symptoms are more typical in mixed anxiety-depressive disorder. Third, there may be a role for benzodiazepines in treating mixed anxiety-depressive disorder, but they may be insufficient if depressive symptoms are severe and if rebound and withdrawal effects are a concern. These authors further reviewed evidence that benzodiazepines are less effective for mild anxiety than for severe anxiety. Finally, combination treatments may be warranted, and cognitive-behavioral psychotherapeutic approaches, including anxiety management, applied relaxation, and cognitive restructuring, that have been established as beneficial in treating GAD may be applicable to mixed anxiety-depressive disorder.

A pilot study by Lang (2003) found that brief cognitive-behavioral intervention was effective in 35 patients presenting with anxiety-depression. In a study by Ninan et al. (2002), a combination of the Cognitive-Behavioral Analysis System of Psychotherapy and nefazodone was found to be superior to either treatment alone in 801 patients with major depression. In patients assessed with high levels of comorbid anxiety by the Hamilton Anxiety Scale and the Inventory of Depressive Symptomatology Self-Report (IDS-SR-30), nefazodone, either alone or in combination with the Cognitive-Behavioral Analysis System of Psychotherapy, was most effective. In studying primary care patients with major depression and lifetime anxiety disorders, Brown et al. (1996) found that patients presenting with this combination of disorders tended to terminate treatment more frequently and, although they showed recovery, took much longer to attain it than patients with depression without comorbid anxiety disorders. Silverstone and Salinas (2001) found that venlafaxine was effective in treating patients with major depressive disorder and comorbid GAD, but showed a prolonged onset of effect in this group. Last, Andrescu et al. (2007) reported higher rates of recurrence of late-life depression with anxiety, measured on the Brief Symptom Inventory: 29% recurrence in the group with low-level anxiety with pharmacotherapy, and 58% recurrence in the high-level anxiety group treated with pharmacotherapy.

For the more severe forms of mixed anxiety-depression, there is evidence that augmentation of antidepressants or mood stabilizers with clonazepam (Smith et al. 1998, 2002; Londborg et al. 2000), and, in more recent findings, with atypical antipsychotic agents such as quetiapine and olanzapine (Hirschfeld et al 2006; Houston et al. 2006; McIntyre et al. 2007), may significantly reduce severe anxiety symptoms with ruminations as well as agitation. Suicide may be associated with high levels of psychic anxiety and agitation in patients with severe mixed anxiety-depression, and in some cases may be averted by reductions in these symptoms. Literature supporting the anxiolytic effect of pregabalin as similar to that of benzodiazepines (Feitner et al. 2003; Montgomery et al. 2006; Pande et al. 2003; Rickels et al. 2005) suggests that this agent may be useful as an adjunct to antidepressant medications in treating more severe forms of mixed anxiety-depression. Treatment should continue after symptoms have abated, and patients should be monitored for the development of full-syndrome disorders.

Other authors have investigated the use of psychotherapy in patients with mixed-symptom profiles. For example, Moras et al. (1993) described two case studies of treatment for comorbid GAD or anxiety disorder not otherwise specified and major depression. They adapted and integrated existing treatments for panic disorder (cognitive-behavioral therapy; Barlow 1992, as cited in Moras et al. 1993) and major depression (interpersonal therapy; Klerman et al. 1983, as cited in Moras et al. 1993) and found that the approach was promising in one case and less so in the other. Other researchers are investigating the effectiveness of an integration of cognitive-behavioral approaches for depression and anxiety among distressed primary care patients.

Conclusion

Mixed anxiety-depression is a subsyndromal combination of depression and anxiety, which, untreated, has been shown to result in significant disability. In addition, numerous studies have demonstrated the clinical significance of a full-syndrome major depressive disorder with comorbid severe anxiety symptoms or anxiety disorders, resulting in more difficult course, higher relapse rates, and increased risk of suicide attempts and suicide.

We have traced the historical progression of conceptualizations of the diagnostic distinctions between anxiety and depression over the past 30 years, focusing on GAD and depression. Early on, anxiety neurosis was redefined as either panic disorder or GAD, and both anxiety and depression have given rise to more differentiated and more specifically defined disorders. As hierarchical diagnostic rules were relaxed, researchers began to investigate and document the high rates of comorbidity between anxiety and depression. However, shifting criteria for GAD, in particular, have contributed to difficulties in combining findings from studies conducted under the different versions of DSMs.

Following the lead of ICD-10, a mixed-symptom, subsyndromal diagnostic category of mixed anxiety-depressive disorder was included in DSM-IV for further study. This reflects our increasing recognition of the common occurrence and disabling effect of subsyndromal states, as well as the consistent observations of co-occurring symptoms. However, many questions remain unanswered about mixed anxiety-depressive disorder, including the demographic breakdown of patients with mixed anxiety-depressive disorder; the range of severity, the course, stability, and prognosis associated with the mixed anxiety-depressive disorder diagnosis along a range of severity of symptoms; and the optimal treatment for mixed anxiety-depressive disorder. Researchers need to address these questions. In addition, fundamental questions of continuity between GAD and major depression must be resolved. These questions have implications for the issue of whether categorical or dimensional approaches best describe the clinical syndromes of anxiety and depression. The diagnosis of mixed anxiety-depressive disorder associated with a dimension of severity may facilitate research on these questions of continuity and discontinuity. A diagnostic system that focuses on the co-occurrence of anxiety with depression could lead to more focused treatment of anxiety symptoms or disorders associated with depression, which may have important effects on improved outcomes, decreased disability, and reduced suicidal behavior and suicidal death in patients manifesting mixed anxiety-depression symptoms. A possible approach being considered for DSM-V is the addition of behavioral severity dimensional ratings to indicate severity of anxiety and depression across diagnostic categories, in addition to categorical diagnoses.

◀ Key Clinical Points ▶

- In its subsyndromal form, mixed anxiety-depression is a significant cause of impairment. In the case of severe anxiety accompanying a full-syndromal depression, it has been associated with poorer treatment response and outcome, as well as a heightened risk for suicidal behavior and suicide.
- Anxious full-syndromal depression may predict familial occurrence in first-degree relatives.
- The presence of mixed anxiety-depression predicts impairment, course, treatment outcome, and familiality. Therefore, a plausible argument can be made that mixed anxiety-depression should be recognized as a separate diagnosis.
- The existence of a separate diagnosis for mixed anxiety-depression would help focus the clinician's attention on treating comorbid anxiety as well as depression, which could result in a reduction in impairment, improved quality of recovery, and reduced suicide risk.
- Because there is a mild form of mixed anxiety-depression as well as a full syndromal form of major depression, and because of the higher risks associated with the more severe form, these disorders should be distinguished by a meaningful severity descriptor to avoid the assumption that patients with mixed anxiety and depressive symptoms should be diagnosed with the milder form.
- Distinguishing between the mild and full-syndromal forms is especially important because the frequency of the full-syndrome form is about 50%, as indicated in reports from the Sequenced Treatment Alternatives to Relieve Depression (STAR*D) (Fava et al. 2008).
- This diagnostic designation utilizing dimensional severity ratings may also focus attention on more effective treatments for comorbid anxiety associated with depression.

References

Akiskal HS: Toward a clinical understanding of the relationship of anxiety and depressive disorders, in Comorbidity of Mood and Anxiety Disorders. Edited by Maser JD, Cloninger CR. Washington, DC, American Psychiatric Press, 1990, pp 597–607

Akiskal HS: Toward a definition of generalized anxiety disorder as an anxious temperament type. Acta Psychiatr Scand 98(suppl):66–73, 1998

American Psychiatric Association: Diagnostic and Statistical Manual of Mental Disorders, 2nd Edition. Washington, DC, American Psychiatric Association, 1968

American Psychiatric Association: Diagnostic and Statistical Manual of Mental Disorders, 3rd Edition. Washington, DC, American Psychiatric Association, 1980

American Psychiatric Association: Diagnostic and Statistical Manual of Mental Disorders, 3rd Edition, Revised. Washington, DC, American Psychiatric Association, 1987

American Psychiatric Association: Diagnostic and Statistical Manual of Mental Disorders, 4th Edition. Washington, DC, American Psychiatric Association, 1994

American Psychiatric Association: Diagnostic and Statistical Manual of Mental Disorders, 4th Edition, Text Revision. Washington, DC, American Psychiatric Association, 2000

Andrescu C, Lenze EJ, Dew MA, et al: Effects of comorbid anxiety on treatment response and relapse risk in late-life depression: controlled study. Br J Psychiatry 190:344–349, 2007

Barlow DH: Cognitive behavioral approaches to panic disorder and social phobia. Bull Menninger Clin 56 (2, suppl):A14–A24, 1992

Boden JM, Fergusson DM, Horwood LJ, et al: Anxiety disorders and suicidal behaviors in adolescence and young adulthood: findings from a longitudinal study. Psychol Med 37:431–440, 2007

Bolton JM, Cox BJ, Afifi TO, et al: Anxiety disorders and risk of suicide attempts: findings from the Baltimore Epidemiologic Catchment area follow-up study. Depress Anxiety 25:477–481, 2008

Boulenger J-P, Fournier M, Rosales D, et al: Mixed anxiety and depression: from theory to practice. J Clin Psychiatry 58(suppl):27–34, 1997

Brown C, Shulberg HC, Madonia MJ, et al: Treatment outcomes for primary care patients with major depression and lifetime anxiety disorders. Am J Psychiatry 153:1293–1300, 1996

Busch KA, Fawcett J, Jacobs DC: Clinical correlates of inpatient suicide. J Clin Psychiatry 64:14–19, 2003

Carter RM, Wittchen HU, Pfister H, et al: One-year prevalence of subthreshold and threshold DSM-IV generalized anxiety disorder in a nationally representative sample. Depress Anxiety 13:78–88, 2001

Clark LA, Watson D: Tripartite model of anxiety and depression: psychometric evidence and taxonomic implications. J Abnorm Psychol 100:316–336, 1991

Clayton PJ: The comorbidity factor: establishing the primary diagnosis in patients with mixed symptoms of anxiety and depression. J Clin Psychiatry 51(suppl):35–39, 1990

Clayton PJ, Grove WH, Coryell W, et al: Follow-up and family study of anxious depression. Am J Psychiatry 148:1512–1517, 1991

Fava M, Alpert JE, Carmin CN, et al: Clinical correlates and symptom patterns of anxious depression among patients with major depressive disorder in STAR*D. Psychol Med 34:1299–1308, 2004

Fava M, Rush AJ, Alpert JE, et al: What clinical and symptom patterns of comorbid disorders characterize outpatients with anxious major depressive disorder? A replication and extension. Can J Psychiatry 51:823–835, 2006

Fava M, Rush AJ, Alpert JE, et al: Difference in treatment outcome in outpatients with anxious vs. nonanxious depression: a STAR*D report. Am J Psychiatry 165:342–351, 2008

Fawcett J, Kravitz HM: Anxiety syndromes and their relationship to depressive illness. J Clin Psychiatry 44:8–11, 1983

Fawcett J, Scheftner WA, Fogg L, et al: Time-related predictors of suicide in major affective disorder. Am J Psychiatry 147:1189–1194, 1990

Feitner DE, Crockett JG, Dubovosky SJ, et al: A randomized, double-blind, placebo-controlled, fixed dose multicenter study of pregabalin in patients with generalized anxiety disorder. J Clin Psychopharmacol 23:240–249, 2003

Foley DL, Goldston DB, Costello EJ, et al: Proximal risk factors for suicidality in youth: the Great Smoky Mountains study. Arch Gen Psychiatry 63:1017–1024, 2006

Gotlib IH, Lewinsohn PM, Seeley JR: Symptoms versus a diagnosis of depression: differences in psychosocial functioning. J Consult Clin Psychol 63:90–100, 1995

Hall RC, Platt DE, Hall RC: Suicide risk assessment: a review of risk factors for suicide in 100 patients who made severe suicide attempts: evaluation of suicide risk in a time of managed care. Psychosomatics 40:18–27, 1999

Hirschfeld RM, Weister RM, Raines SR, et al: Quetiapine in the treatment of anxiety in patients with bipolar I or II depression: a secondary analysis from a randomized, double-blind, placebo-controlled study. J Clin Psychiatry 67:355–362, 2006

Houck J: Combined therapy in anxiety-depressive syndromes, II: comparative effects of amitriptyline and Limbitrol (chlordiazepoxide-amitriptyline). Dis Nerv Syst 31:421–426, 1970

Houston JP, Ahi J, Moyers AL, et al: Reduced suicidal ideation in bipolar I disorder mixed-episode patients in a placebo-controlled trial of olanzapine combined with lithium or divalproex. J Clin Psychiatry 67:1246–1252, 2006

Johnson J, Weissman MM, Klerman GL: Service utilization and social morbidity associated with depressive symptoms in the community. JAMA 267:1478–1483, 1992

Katon W, Roy-Byrne PP: Mixed anxiety and depression. J Abnorm Psychol 100:337–345, 1991

Kendler KS: Major depression and generalized anxiety disorder: same genes, (partly) different environments—revisited. Br J Psychiatry 168(suppl):68–75, 1996

Kendler KS, Neale MC, Kessler RC, et al: Major depression and generalized anxiety disorder: same genes, (partly) different environments? Arch Gen Psychiatry 49:716–722, 1992

Klerman GL: The efficacy of psychotherapy as the basis for public policy. Am Psychol 38:929–934, 1983

Klerman GL, Vaillant GE, Spitzer RL, et al: A debate on DSM-III. Am J Psychiatry 141:539–553, 1984

Kring AM, Persons JB, Thomas C: Changes in affect during treatment for depression and anxiety. Behav Res Ther 45:1753–1764, 2007

Lang AJ: Brief intervention for co-occurring anxiety and depression in primary care: a pilot study. Int J Psychiatry Med 33:141–154, 2003

Liebowitz MR: Mixed anxiety and depression: should it be included in DSM-IV? J Clin Psychiatry 54(suppl):4–7, 1993

Londborg PD, Smith WT, Glaudin V, et al: Short term cotherapy with clonazepam and fluoxetine: anxiety, sleep disturbance and core symptoms of depression. J Affect Disord 61:73–79, 2000

Maser JD: Generalized anxiety disorder and its comorbidities: disputes at the boundaries. Acta Psychiatr Scand Suppl 393:12–22, 1998

McIntyre A, Gendron A, McIntyre A: Quetiapine adjunct to selective serotonin reuptake inhibitors of venlafaxine in patients with major depression, comorbid anxiety, and residual depressive symptoms: a randomized, placebo controlled pilot study. Depress Anxiety 24:487–494, 2007

Montgomery SA, Tobias K, Zornberg GL, et al: Efficacy and safety of pregabalin in the treatment of generalized anxiety disorder: a 6 week, multicenter, randomized, double-blind, placebo-controlled comparison of pregabalin and venlafaxine. J Clin Psychiatry 67:771–782, 2006

Moras K: Diagnostic comorbidity in the DSM-III and DSM-III-R anxiety and mood disorder: implications for the DSM-IV. Review paper for the DSM-IV Generalized Anxiety Disorder and Mixed Anxiety Depression

Work Group. Center for Stress and Anxiety Disorders, University at Albany, State University of New York, 1989
Moras K, Telfer LA, Barlow DH: Efficacy and specific effects data on new treatments: a case study strategy with mixed anxiety-depression. J Consult Clin Psychol 61:412–420, 1993
Moras K, Clark LA, Katon W, et al: Mixed anxiety-depression, in DSM-IV Sourcebook, Vol 2. Edited by Widiger TA, Frances AJ, Pincus HA, et al. Washington, DC, American Psychiatric Association, 1996, pp 623–643
Ninan PT, Rush AJ, Crits-Christoph P, et al: Symptomatic and subsyndromal anxiety in chronic forms of major depression: effect of nefazodone, cognitive behavioral analysis system of psychotherapy, and their combination. J Clin Psychiatry 63:434–444, 2002
Pande AC, Crockett JG, Feitner DE, et al: Pregabalin in generalized anxiety disorder: a placebo-controlled trial. Am J Psychiatry 160:533–540, 2003
Preskorn SH, Fast GA: Beyond signs and symptoms: the case against a mixed anxiety and depression category. J Clin Psychiatry 54(suppl):24–32, 1993
Rickels K, Downing RW: Methodological aspects in the testing of antidepressant drugs, in Depressive Illness: Diagnosis, Assessment, Treatment, International Symposium, St. Moritz. Edited by Kielholz P. Stuttgart, Germany, Huber Berne, 1972, pp 84–99
Rickels K, Hesbacher P, Downing RW: Differential drug effects in neurotic depression. Dis Nerv Syst 31:468–475, 1970
Rickels K, Pollack MH, Feitner DE, et al: Pregabalin for the treatment of generalized anxiety disorder: a 4-week, multicenter, double-blind, placebo-controlled trial of pregabalin and alprazolam. Arch Gen Psychiatry 62:1022–1030, 2005
Roth M, Gurney C, Garside RF, et al: Studies in the classification of affective disorders: the relationship between anxiety states and depressive illnesses, I. Br J Psychiatry 121:147–161, 1972
Roy-Byrne P: Generalized anxiety and mixed anxiety-depression: association with disability and health care utilization. J Clin Psychiatry 57(suppl):86–91, 1996
Roy-Byrne P, Katon W, Broadhead WE, et al: Subsyndromal ("mixed") anxiety-depression in primary care. J Gen Intern Med 9:507–512, 1994
Sareen J, Cox BJ, Afifi TO, et al: Anxiety disorders and risk for suicidal ideation and attempts. Arch Gen Psychiatry 62:1249–1257, 2005
Sartorius N, Üstün TB: Mixed anxiety and depressive disorder. Psychopathology 28(suppl):21–25, 1995
Schatzberg AF: Benzodiazepines in depressive disorders: a clinical guide. South Med J 71(suppl):18–23, 1978
Schatzberg AF, Cole JO: Benzodiazepines in depressive disorders. Arch Gen Psychiatry 35:1359–1365, 1978
Shammas E: Controlled comparison of bromazepam, amitriptyline, and placebo in anxiety-depressive neurosis. Dis Nerv Syst 38:201–207, 1977
Silverstone PH, Salinas E: Efficacy of venlafaxine extended release in patients with major depressive disorder and generalized anxiety disorder. J Clin Psychiatry 62:523–529, 2001
Simon GE, Hunkeler E, Fireman B, et al: Risk of suicide attempts and suicide death in patients treated for bipolar disorder. Bipolar Disord 9:526–530, 2007
Simon NM, Zalta AK, Otto NW, et al: The association of comorbid anxiety disorders with suicide attempts and suicidal ideation in outpatients with bipolar disorder. J Psychiatr Res 41:255–264, 2007
Smith WT, Londborg PD, Glaudin V, et al: Short term augmentation of fluoxetine with clonazepam in the treatment of depression: a double-blind study. Am J Psychiatry 155:1339–1345, 1998
Smith WT, Londborg PD, Glaudin V, et al: Is extended clonazepam cotherapy of fluoxetine effective for outpatients with major depression? J Affect Disord 70:251–259, 2002
Stahl SM: Mixed anxiety and depression: clinical implications. J Clin Psychiatry 54(suppl):33–38, 1993
Stavrakaki C, Vargo B: The relationship of anxiety and depression: a review of the literature. Br J Psychiatry 149:7–16, 1986
Stein MB, Kirk P, Prabhu V, et al: Mixed anxiety-depression in a primary-care clinic. J Affect Disord 34:79–84, 1995
Verner JV: Comparison of imipramine and chlordiazepoxide in treatment of the depressed and anxious patient. J Fla Med Assoc 56:15–21, 1969
Watson D, Clark LA, Carey G: Positive and negative affectivity and their relation to anxiety and depressive disorders. J Abnorm Psychol 97:346–353, 1988
Wells KB, Stewart A, Hays RD, et al: The functioning and well-being of depressed patients: results from the Medical Outcomes Study. JAMA 262:914–919, 1989
Wetzler S, Katz MM: Problems with the differentiation of anxiety and depression. J Psychiatr Res 23:1–12, 1989
Wittchen H-U, Essau CA: Comorbidity and mixed anxiety-depressive disorders: is there epidemiologic evidence? J Clin Psychiatry 54(suppl):9–15, 1993
World Health Organization: The ICD-10 Classification of Mental and Behavioural Disorders: Clinical Descriptions and Diagnostic Guidelines. Geneva, Switzerland, World Health Organization, 1992a
World Health Organization: The ICD-10 Classification of Mental and Behavioural Disorders: Diagnostic Criteria for Research. Geneva, Switzerland, World Health Organization, 1992b
World Health Organization: International Statistical Classification of Diseases and Related Health Problems, 10th Revision, Vol 1. Geneva, Switzerland, World Health Organization, 1992c
Wunderlich U, Bronisch T, Wittchen HU, et al: Comorbidity patterns in adolescents and young adults with suicide attempts. Eur Arch Psychiatry Clin Neurosci 248:87–95, 1998

Zajecka JM, Ross JS: Management of comorbid anxiety and depression. J Clin Psychiatry 56(suppl):10–13, 1995

Zinbarg RE, Barlow DH, Liebowitz M, et al: The DSM-IV field trial for mixed anxiety-depression. Am J Psychiatry 151:1153–1162, 1994

Recommended Readings

*The references listed in Table 15–2 should be useful in further understanding the effect of comorbid anxiety on the outcome of depression. Clayton et al. (1991) skillfully discuss the background and significance of severe anxiety in depression. Publications from the Sequenced Treatment Alternatives to Relieve Depression (STAR*D) (e.g., Fava et al. 2004, 2008) clearly show the effect of comorbid anxiety on outcome. And a study by Stordal et al. (2008) further emphasizes the role of anxious depression in increasing the risk for suicide. The original findings of a correlation between acute suicides and severity of anxiety, as opposed to other standard risk factors—prior attempt, hopelessness, suicidal ideation—that show more long-term risk (Fawcett et al. 1990) is further supported by a study of 76 inpatient suicides (Busch et al. 2003). Together, these studies emphasize the crucial role played by severe anxiety in the outcome of depression and help emphasize the importance of detection and treatment of comorbid anxiety in the management of depressive illness.*

Busch KA, Fawcett J, Jacobs DC: Clinical correlates of inpatient suicide. J Clin Psychiatry 64:14–19, 2003

Clayton PJ, Grove WH, Coryell W, et al: Follow-up and family study of anxious depression. Am J Psychiatry 148:1512–1517, 1991

Fava M, Alpert JE, Carmin CN, et al: Clinical correlates and symptom patterns of anxious depression among patients with major depressive disorder in STAR*D. Psychol Med 34:1299–1308, 2004

Fava M, Rush AJ, Alpert JE, et al: Difference in treatment outcome in outpatients with anxious vs. nonanxious depression: a STAR*D report. Am J Psychiatry 165:342–351, 2008

Fawcett J, Scheftner WA, Fogg L, et al: Time-related predictors of suicide in major affective disorder. Am J Psychiatry 147:1189–1194, 1990

Stordal E, Morken G, Mykleton A, et al: Monthly variation in the prevalence of comorbid depression and anxiety in the general population at 63–65 degrees North: The HUNT study. J Affect Disord 106:273–278, 2008

Obsessive-Compulsive Disorder/ Related Disorders

Chapter 16

Phenomenology of Obsessive-Compulsive Disorder

Jane L. Eisen, M.D.
Agustin G. Yip, M.D., Ph.D.
Maria C. Mancebo, Ph.D.
Anthony Pinto, Ph.D.
Steven A. Rasmussen, M.D.

Historical Considerations

Obsessive-compulsive disorder (OCD), an intriguing and often debilitating syndrome characterized by the presence of obsessions and compulsions (Table 16–1), is not a newly observed disorder. Numerous descriptions of obsessions and compulsions can be found in a variety of sources dating back hundreds of years; this literature has been reviewed by Berrios (1995), as summarized here. One account, written in 1621 by Robert Burton in *The Anatomy of Melancholy,* depicts an individual who "dared not go over a bridge, come near a pool, rock, steep hill, lie in a chamber where cross beams were, for fear he be tempted to hang, drawn or precipitate himself. In a silent auditorium as at a sermon, he [was] afraid he shall speak aloud at unawares, something indecent, unfit to be said" (Burton 1883, quoted in Berrios 1995).

Another example, written in 1791, is Boswell's description of Dr. Johnson's "peculiarity...it appeared to me some superstitious habit, which [he] had contracted early... that was his anxious care to go out or in at a door or passage, by a certain number of steps from a certain point, or at least so that either his right or his left foot (I am not certain which) should constantly make the first actual movement when he came close to the door or passage" (Boswell 1791, quoted in Berrios 1995).

From the beginning, obsessive-compulsive behaviors were often explained in social and religious terms (Berrios1995; Mora1969). The evolution from *behavior* to *disorder* originated in France and Germany during the second half of the nineteenth century. OCD was first classified as insanity, as a "reasoning or instinctive monomania...an involuntary, irresistible, and instinctive activity" in which the subject was "chained to actions that neither reason nor emotion have originated, that conscience rejects, and will cannot suppress" (Esquirol 1838). Several decades later, Morel (1866) classified OCD as a *délire emotif* (disease of the emotions), which he considered to be a neurosis, an illness which originated in the autonomic nervous system (Berrios 1995).

At the beginning of the twentieth century, Pierre Janet (1903), having observed more than 300 individuals with this disorder, described OCD symptoms in terms that are clearly recognizable to clinicians over 100 years

TABLE 16–1. DSM-IV-TR diagnostic criteria for obsessive-compulsive disorder

A. Either obsessions or compulsions:

Obsessions as defined by (1), (2), (3), and (4):

(1) recurrent and persistent thoughts, impulses, or images that are experienced, at some time during the disturbance, as intrusive and inappropriate and that cause marked anxiety or distress

(2) the thoughts, impulses, or images are not simply excessive worries about real-life problems

(3) the person attempts to ignore or suppress such thoughts, impulses, or images, or to neutralize them with some other thought or action

(4) the person recognizes that the obsessional thoughts, impulses, or images are a product of his or her own mind (not imposed from without as in thought insertion)

Compulsions as defined by (1) and (2):

(1) repetitive behaviors (e.g., hand washing, ordering, checking) or mental acts (e.g., praying, counting, repeating words silently) that the person feels driven to perform in response to an obsession, or according to rules that must be applied rigidly

(2) the behaviors or mental acts are aimed at preventing or reducing distress or preventing some dreaded event or situation; however, these behaviors or mental acts either are not connected in a realistic way with what they are designed to neutralize or prevent or are clearly excessive

B. At some point during the course of the disorder, the person has recognized that the obsessions or compulsions are excessive or unreasonable. **Note:** This does not apply to children.

C. The obsessions or compulsions cause marked distress, are time consuming (take more than 1 hour a day), or significantly interfere with the person's normal routine, occupational (or academic) functioning, or usual social activities or relationships.

D. If another Axis I disorder is present, the content of the obsessions or compulsions is not restricted to it (e.g., preoccupation with food in the presence of an eating disorder; hair pulling in the presence of trichotillomania; concern with appearance in the presence of body dysmorphic disorder; preoccupation with drugs in the presence of a substance use disorder; preoccupation with having a serious illness in the presence of hypochondriasis; preoccupation with sexual urges or fantasies in the presence of a paraphilia; or guilty ruminations in the presence of major depressive disorder).

E. The disturbance is not due to the direct physiological effects of a substance (e.g., a drug of abuse, a medication) or a general medical condition.

Specify if:

With Poor Insight: if, for most of the time during the current episode, the person does not recognize that the obsessions and compulsions are excessive or unreasonable

later (translated by Pitman 1987). He characterized the development of frank obsessions and compulsions as being preceded by a period he termed *psychasthenic state,* characterized by a sense that actions are performed incompletely (and the associated need to do them perfectly), a strong focus on order and uniformity, indecisiveness, and restricted emotional expression. According to his observations, people with this disorder proceeded through two more stages of symptomatology. The second stage, *forced agitations,* included an increased need for perfection, accompanied by the development of behaviors we would now describe as symmetry, repeating, and checking compulsions. Tics also emerged during this second phase of the illness, as well as specific fears/phobias. In the third stage, *frank obsessions and additional compulsions* were described by Janet, with mention of aggressive, religious, and sexual thoughts that were extremely distressing to the patient.

At the same time that Janet was contributing to our conceptualization of OCD, Freud was offering groundbreaking observations of individuals struggling with obsessions and compulsions (Freud 1895/1962, 1909/1955). However, OCD was considered a rare disorder until relatively recently. Fueled by the findings from several epidemiological surveys conducted in the 1980s, which documented surprisingly high prevalence rates of OCD, in recent years there has been tremendous interest and a rapid growth in the understanding of the clinical features and treatment of this disorder.

In this chapter, we review the current state of knowledge of the epidemiology, clinical features, and evaluation of OCD.

Epidemiology

Although psychiatric literature has long contained striking descriptions of patients with debilitating obsessions and compulsions, until the mid-1980s OCD was considered extremely rare. This perception was based on an epidemiological study by Rudin (1953), who estimated OCD prevalence to be 5 in 10,000 in the general population. Several studies conducted in the 1950s and 1960s to examine the frequency of psychiatric diagnoses in inpatient and outpatient settings reinforced the notion that OCD occurred rarely; OCD made up a small minority (1%–4%) of disorders in the total patient pool (Ingram 1961; Kringlin 1965; Pollitt 1957). Some investigators believed that Rudin's figures were probably an underestimate, given that patients often did not seek treatment because of fear or shame. In a more recent study, Hantouche et al. (1995) found that 9.2% of 4,364 psychiatric outpatients received a diagnosis of OCD, and 17% were reported to have obsessive-compulsive symptoms. These higher figures most likely represent a combination of improved recognition by clinicians and increasing numbers of patients seeking treatment.

The results of a large psychiatric epidemiological study, the national Epidemiologic Catchment Area (ECA) survey, conducted in the United States in 1984, painted a very different picture of the prevalence of OCD. In this study, OCD was the fourth most common psychiatric disorder, following the phobias, substance use disorders, and major depression, with a 6-month point prevalence of 1.6% and a lifetime prevalence of 2.5% (Myers et al. 1984; Robins et al. 1984).

Most recently, the National Comorbidity Survey Replication (NCS-R) (Kessler et al. 2005a, 2005b) published point estimates broadly comparable with those of the ECA survey: 12-month prevalence was reported to be 1.2% and lifetime prevalence 2.3%.

The same instrument that was used in the ECA survey was used in studies in diverse cultures, including those of Puerto Rico, Canada, Germany, Taiwan, New Zealand, and Korea, as part of the Cross-National Collaborative Group (Weissman et al. 1994). OCD lifetime prevalence rates (ranging between 1.9% in Korea and 2.5% in Puerto Rico) and annual prevalence rates (ranging between 1.1% in Korea and 1.8% in Puerto Rico) were remarkably consistent across these cultures, with the exception of Taiwan's. The prevalence rates in Taiwan were substantially lower (0.7% lifetime prevalence) than those in the other sites, paralleling Taiwan's low rates for other psychiatric disorders (Weissman et al. 1994). Although it is possible that this population does in fact have low rates of mental illness across the board, methodological differences (e.g., a systematic bias in the diagnostic instrument) seem a more plausible explanation for these findings. Tadai et al. (1995) measured the prevalence of OCD in 424 Japanese students by using the Maudsley Obsessional-Compulsive Inventory and found that 1.7% had symptoms that met DSM-III-R (American Psychiatric Association 1987) criteria for OCD.

Some studies have failed to support the ECA findings. Degonda et al. (1993) investigated the longitudinal course of OCD and obsessive-compulsive symptoms over an 11-year period in a Swiss cohort. The prevalence of DSM-III (American Psychiatric Association 1980) OCD in the study was considerably lower than 1%. When a lower diagnostic threshold based on obsessive-compulsive symptoms and social impairment was used, the weighted lifetime prevalence rate for OCD at age 30 years was 5.5%. Distinguishing between subthreshold OCD and full-criteria OCD is critical in determining prevalence in both epidemiological and clinical studies. Rachman and DeSilva (1978) reported that a high percentage of the non-OCD population has some obsessions and compulsions. Most children also go through developmental stages characterized by obsessive-compulsive or superstitious behavior. Determining the relation between subthreshold OCD (minor obsessions and compulsions) and full-criteria OCD (i.e., symptoms cause significant distress or impairment in functioning) is key to identifying homogeneous groups for assessment of course, prognosis, treatment response, familial transmission, and prevalence.

Some studies in adolescent populations have supported the ECA findings. Using a modified Leyton Obsessional Inventory, Flament and colleagues (1988) screened 5,000 high school students. Those who scored above a predetermined cutoff on the scale were interviewed by a psychiatrist who was an expert in childhood OCD. Of the total 5,000 students, 15 (0.3%) were given DSM-III-R diagnoses of OCD. The average age of the subjects was 15.4 years, whereas the average age at onset of the disorder is around 20 years. When an age correction was applied, the point prevalence estimate for the general population was 1%. In a similar two-stage study, Valleni-Basile et al. (1994) screened 3,283 adolescents with a self-report screening questionnaire, followed by the Schedule for Affective Disorders and Schizophrenia for School-Aged Children. The 1-year incidence rates of OCD and subclinical OCD were 0.7% and 8.4%, respectively. Douglass et al. (1995) found that the 1-year prevalence rate of OCD in 930 18-year-olds, as measured by the Diagnostic Interview Schedule (DIS), was 4%. In a similar epidemiological study, Apter et al. (1996) studied 861 Israelis who were16 years old during pre-induction military screening. In the sample, 8% reported spending more than an hour daily on obsessions and/or compulsions.

Fontenelle et al. (2006) conducted a systematic overview of the descriptive epidemiology of OCD along methodological lines. They posited that the heterogeneity of findings across studies is at least partially explained by several a priori methodologically informed decisions (such as choice of diagnostic instrument for case finding), apart from the intrinsic characteristics of study populations. Studies using the DIS, such as the ECA study (Robins et al. 1984) and the Cross-National Group study by Weissman et al. (1994) described above, reported broadly comparable rates. The NCS-R rates (Kessler et al. 2005a, 2005b), using the Composite International Diagnostic Interview (CIDI), which is modeled closely after the DIS (see section "Evaluation: Rating Scales" in this chapter), also showed similar results. The DIS and CIDI, being rigidly structured interview schedules conducted by lay interviewers, have been criticized as overly lenient and open to interpretation by lay personnel and, therefore, likely to systematically inflate case finding. For example, Stein et al. (1997) found a 1-month prevalence for OCD of 3.1% when the CIDI was used in telephone assessments conducted by lay personnel. A much lower figure, 0.6%, was found when a reappraisal by mental health professionals employing the Structured Clinical Interview for DSM Disorders (SCID) was conducted (Fontenelle et al. 2006).

Demographic Features

Sex Distribution

Women appear to develop OCD slightly more frequently than do men. In two large clinical studies, 55% of the sample were women (Pinto et al. 2006; Rasmussen and Eisen 1988) In the DSM-IV (American Psychiatric Association 1994) field trial, 51% of the 431 subjects with OCD were women (Foa and Kozak 1995). Similarly, epidemiological samples have found a slightly higher prevalence of OCD in women. In the ECA study, the lifetime prevalence of OCD in women was 2.9%, compared with 2% found in men (Karno et al. 1988). In the Cross-National Collaborative Group study, the lifetime ratio of females to males ranged from 1.8 to 1.2, with the exception of Germany (with a finding of more men than women) and New Zealand (with an unusual ratio of 3.8:1) (Weissman et al. 1994). A study that assessed the presence of comorbid disorders characterized by psychosis (schizophrenia, delusional disorder) or psychotic-like features (schizotypal personality disorder) in 475 patients with OCD found a different sex ratio. Of the OCD patients without one of these comorbid disorders, 56% were women, whereas 85% of those with one of these comorbid psychotic disorders were men (Eisen and Rasmussen 1993).

A predominance of males has also been observed in child and adolescent OCD clinical populations (Geller et al. 1998). In a National Institute of Mental Health study of 70 subjects with OCD between ages 6 and 18 years, 47 (67%) were males (Leonard et al. 1989). This finding may be a result of the fact that males develop OCD at a younger age than females. Genetic data have shown a significantly higher frequency of OCD in relatives of patients who develop OCD before age 14 years, suggesting that in addition to sex distribution, there are differences between pediatric OCD and adult OCD (Bellodi et al. 1992; Nestadt et al. 2000). Among participants in our Brown Longitudinal Obsessive Compulsive Study (BLOCS, a National Institute of Mental Health–funded observational study of the course of OCD in a large clinical sample of individuals with primary OCD), significantly more juveniles than adults were male (67% vs. 45%; χ^2=10.77, P=0.001). When the gender distributions of each group were examined separately, there was a significant male preponderance among juveniles, but not among adults with a juvenile onset of OCD (Mancebo et al. 2008).

Marital Status

Patients being treated for OCD are less likely to be married when compared to the general population. In the ECA study, for example, Karno et al. (1988) found that OCD was more prevalent among divorced or separated subjects than among those who were married or single (this finding was not specific to OCD, however). This is true of clinical populations across several countries (Çilli et al. 2004; Fontenelle and Hasler 2008; Fontenelle et al. 2004).

In the BLOCS, our ongoing observational follow-up study of the course of OCD, less than half (44%) of the first 293 adult participants were married, and 36% had never been married (Pinto et al. 2006). These rates are similar to those reported in two previous studies of OCD outpatients in which 43%–48% of adults with

OCD had never married (Attiullah et al. 2000; Rasmussen and Eisen 1991). A study comparing marital status in OCD patients with that in a matched group of patients with major depression found no significant differences between the two groups (Coryell 1981). Although marital status was not found to be a predictor of course in several follow-up studies, a prospective study of 107 subjects with OCD found that being married significantly increased the probability of partial remission, with married patients more than twice as likely to remit as unmarried ones (Steketee et al. 1999).

Treatment Seeking

Few people with OCD are in contact with a mental health professional, and those receiving appropriate treatments are fewer still. Torres et al. (2007) analyzed service use by adults with OCD living in private households in Great Britain from the British Survey of Psychiatric Morbidity of 2000 (N=8,580). They found that persons with OCD (n=114) were more likely than persons with other neuroses (n=1,395) to be receiving treatment (40% compared with 23%, P<0.001). However, those with OCD alone (n=38) were much less likely than those with OCD and a comorbid disorder to be in treatment (14% compared with 56%, P<0.001). In the previous year, 9.4% of persons with OCD had seen a psychiatrist and 4.6% had seen a psychologist. Of these persons, 5% were receiving cognitive-behavioral therapy, 2% were taking selective serotonin reuptake inhibitors, and 10% were taking tricyclics.

Intake data from the BLOCS cohort of treatment-seeking adults with a primary diagnosis of OCD indicated that the majority of individuals reported receiving serotonin reuptake inhibitors. At study entry, 79% of the 293 adults were receiving serotonin reuptake inhibitors and 62% had achieved at least the minimum recommended dose (Mancebo et al. 2006); 14% were also receiving a neuroleptic. Of this sample, 55% reported attending at least one session of cognitive-behavioral therapy at some point, but only 38% reported receiving the minimum recommended number of 13 sessions of lifetime cognitive-behavioral therapy (Mancebo et al. 2006).

Clinical Features

Clinical Vignette

A 40-year-old woman presents with a recent increase in the frequency and duration of cleaning and checking rituals that she has been performing since she was 16 years old. She now spends between 2 and 3 hours a day washing her hands, washing herself in the shower, and checking doors and stoves before leaving her home. In addition, she has difficulty discarding magazines and newspapers, utility and credit card bills, and junk mail.

She fears that if she were to deviate from her routine, something "bad" might happen to her father, who has advanced Alzheimer's disease and is in a nursing home.

In the past month, she has not been able to get to work on time because it takes her half an hour to complete rituals in her car (checking dashboard parts) in the office parking lot. Once at her desk, she spends 15 minutes ordering and rearranging her handbag, making sure everything is "accounted for." Her work productivity has suffered, her colleagues have made snide comments about her "habits," and she is at risk of losing her job. Her life is restricted, and her family members are upset about her behavior. She is severely "depressed and frustrated," and feels she "cannot go on living like this."

Diagnosis

The diagnosis of OCD requires a psychiatric examination and history. DSM-IV-TR defines OCD as the presence of either obsessions or compulsions (Criterion A) that cause marked distress, are time-consuming, or interfere with social or occupational functioning (Criterion C). Although other Axis I diagnoses may be present, the obsessive-compulsive symptoms must not be secondary to another disorder (Criterion D). Most patients recognize these symptoms to be unreasonable or excessive at some point during the course of illness (Criterion B), although this criterion does not apply to children or adults with poor insight (American Psychiatric Association 2000; see Table 16–1).

Symptoms

Obsessions (intrusive, inappropriate, and disturbing ideas, thoughts, or images) and compulsions (repetitive or ritualized behaviors to reduce anxiety) constitute the core clinical symptoms of OCD. Historical descriptions of obsessions and compulsions, beginning with scrupulosity in the fifteenth century and continuing into the twentieth century in the writings of Janet (1903) and Freud (1895/1962, 1909/1955), are strikingly consistent with current clinical presentations of OCD. Several investigators have systematically characterized obsessions and compulsions based on the content of the obsession or the specific compulsive behavior. Hodgson and Rachman (1977) developed the Maudsley Obsessional-Compulsive Inventory, a 30-item true-false questionnaire about obsessive-compulsive symptoms. This inventory focused predominantly on checking and cleaning compulsions. Goodman and colleagues (1989a, 1989b) developed the Yale-Brown Obsessive Compulsive Scale Symptom Checklist (Y-BOCS-SC) of specific obsessions and compulsions. This checklist includes 60 specific obsessions and compulsions and organizes them into 15 categories. The original obsession categories are aggressive, sexual, religious, somatic, symmetry, contamination, hoarding, and miscellaneous. The compulsion categories are checking, ordering and arranging, counting, repeating rituals, cleaning, hoarding and collecting, and miscellaneous.

Recent data from the BLOCS are presented in Table 16–2 (Pinto et al. 2006). In adults, the most common obsession is fear of contamination, followed by over-responsibility for harm (e.g., fire or accidents), aggressive obsessions, and need for symmetry. The most common compulsion is checking, followed by washing, repeating routine activities, and ordering/arranging (see Table 16–2). Children and adolescents with OCD present with similar OCD symptoms but may show some developmental differences (Geller et al. 2001). For example, sexual, religious, and aggressive obsessions appear to emerge in adolescence. Miscellaneous types of compulsions such as rituals involving other people (usually family members) and tic-like compulsions (touching, tapping, or rubbing) are common among children and adolescents and adults with a juvenile onset of OCD (Geller et al. 2001; Rosario-Campos et al. 2001).

OCD Symptom Subtypes

The following descriptions of contamination, over-responsibility for harm, symmetry, somatic obsessions, sexual and aggressive obsessions, mental compulsions, and hoarding illustrate the clinical presentation of these symptoms.

Contamination. Contamination obsessions are the most frequently encountered obsessions in OCD. Such obsessions are usually characterized by a fear of dirt or germs. Contamination fears may also involve toxins or environmental hazards (e.g., asbestos or lead) or bodily waste or secretions. Patients usually describe a feared consequence from contacting a contaminated object (e.g., spreading disease or contracting an illness themselves). However, the fear is occasionally based not on a fear of disease but on a fear of the sensory experience of not being clean. The content of the contamination obsession and the feared consequence commonly changes over time—for example, a fear of cancer may be replaced by a fear of a sexually transmitted disease.

Many patients with contamination fears use avoidance, in addition to excessive washing, to prevent contact with contaminants. The fear structure for contamination is similar to that seen in specific phobias: precipitation by a specific external trigger, high level of anxiety, and a well-developed and coherent cognitive framework. In some cases, a specific feared object and the associated avoidance become more generalized, a pattern also described in specific phobias. Unlike individuals with specific phobias, those with contamination obsessions usually worry that they will inadvertently cause others to be harmed or to become ill.

Washing is the compulsion most commonly associated with contamination obsessions. This behavior usually occurs after contact with the feared object; however, proximity to the feared stimulus is often sufficient to engender severe anxiety and washing compulsions, even though the contaminated object has not been touched. Most patients with washing compulsions perform these rituals in response to a fear of contamination, but these behaviors occasionally occur in response to a drive for perfection or a need for symmetry. Some patients, for example, repeatedly wash themselves in the shower until they "feel right" or must wash their right arm and then their left arm the same number of times.

Over-responsibility for harm. Patients who have the symptom over-responsibility for harm are plagued by the concern that they will be responsible for a dire event as a result of their carelessness. They may, for example, worry that they will start a fire because they neglected to turn off the stove before leaving the house. Such patients often describe doubting their own perceptions. Excessive doubt and associated feelings of excessive responsibility frequently lead to checking rituals. Patients may spend several hours checking their home before they leave. As is the case for contamination obsessions, over-responsibility for harm also can lead to marked avoidance behavior. Some patients become housebound to avoid the responsibility of leaving the house potentially unlocked.

Over-responsibility for harm is also embedded in the cognitive framework of several other obsessions. Patients with aggressive obsessions may be plagued by the doubt that they inadvertently harmed someone without knowing that they did so.

Patients may adopt several strategies to limit the time they spend checking; these may include counting the

TABLE 16–2. Frequency of current obsessions and compulsions among BLOCS participants

	Children (*n*=20) (%)	Adolescents (*n*=44) (%)	Adults (*n*=293) (%)
Obsessions			
Contamination	11 (55.0)	30 (68.2)	169 (57.5)
Over-responsibility for harm	9 (45.0)	25 (59.1)	164 (56.0)
Need for symmetry	13 (65.0)	26 (59.1)	140 (47.8)
Aggressive	3 (15.0)	21 (47.7)	133 (45.5)
Hoarding	8 (40.0)	12 (27.3)	86 (29.4)
Somatic	5 (25.0)	8 (18.2)	77 (26.3)
Religious	4 (20.0)	12 (27.3)	77 (26.3)
Sexual	1 (5.0)	11 (25.0)	39 (13.3)
Miscellaneous	5 (25.0)	13 (29.5)	167 (57.0)
Compulsions			
Checking	14 (70.0)	26 (59.1)	202 (68.9)
Washing/cleaning	7 (35.0)	24 (54.5)	176 (60.1)
Repeating	13 (65.0)	26 (59.1)	165 (56.3)
Ordering	12 (60.0)	26 (59.1)	127 (43.3)
Hoarding	8 (40.0)	9 (20.5)	83 (28.3)
Counting	2 (10.0)	5 (11.4)	76 (25.9)
Miscellaneous	18 (90.0)	40 (90.9)	176 (60.1)

Note. BLOCS=Brown Longitudinal Obsessive Compulsive Study.
Most adults and children with OCD have multiple obsessions and compulsions over time, with a particular fear or concern dominating the clinical picture at any one time. The presence of pure obsessions without compulsions is unusual. Patients who appear to have obsessions alone frequently have reassurance rituals or unrecognized mental compulsions (such as repetitive, ritualized praying) in addition to their obsessions. Pure compulsions are extremely rare. In the DSM-IV field trial, 91% of the 411 patients with DSM-III-R OCD were classified as having "mixed obsessions and compulsions," 8.5% were classified as having "predominantly obsessions," and 0.5% were classified as having "pure compulsions" (Foa and Kozak 1995). With the Yale-Brown Obsessive Compulsive Symptom Checklist, the findings were more striking: only 2.1% had obsessions without compulsions, and 1.7% had compulsions without obsessions. Pure compulsions, although unusual in adult patients, do occur in children with OCD, especially in the very young (e.g., ages 6–8 years) (Swedo et al. 1989).

number of times they check or involving a family member to observe the checking ritual so they can be reassured later that they actually completed the checking task.

Need for symmetry. Need for symmetry is a drive to order or arrange things "perfectly," to do and undo certain motor actions in an exact sequence, or to perform certain behaviors symmetrically or in a balanced way. Patients describe an urge to repeat motor acts until they achieve a "just right" feeling that the act has been completed perfectly. These patients can be divided into two groups: 1) those with primary magical thinking and 2) those with primary obsessive slowness. Individuals with primary magical thinking report obsessional worries about feared consequences to their loved ones. They perform certain ordering and arranging compulsions to prevent harm to loved ones from occurring. Patients who have primary obsessive slowness take an inordinate amount of time to complete even the simplest of tasks (Rachman and Hodgson 1980). Unlike most patients with OCD, those with obsessive slowness may not experience their symptoms as ego-dystonic. Instead, they seem to have lost their goal directedness in favor of completing a given subroutine perfectly. The basal ganglia control motor planning and, therefore, coordinate motor subroutines, as well as what MacLean (1985) termed the "master routine." It is therefore tempting to speculate that these patients have some frontal-limbic basal ganglia dysfunction that interferes with their goal directedness, rendering them incapable of distinguishing the importance of subroutines and overall goal-directed behavior.

Patients with symmetry obsessions and compulsions often describe feeling uneasy or unsettled, rather than fearful or anxious, when things are not lined up "just so" or "perfectly." In that sense, these patients can be seen as at the extreme end of the spectrum of compulsive personality, in which the need for every detail to be "perfect" or "just so" is greatest. Their description of rising tension followed by relief after the act is more similar to the subjective sensory experience of patients with tics than to the anxiety experienced by other patients with OCD without comorbid tic disorders. Investigators have used numerous terms, such as *sensory phenomena* (Miguel et al. 1995, 1997, 2000), *just right* perceptions (Leckman et al. 1994), and *not just right* experiences (Coles et al. 2003, 2005), to describe these sensations (see later subsection "Approaches to OCD Subtyping"). Patients with obsessional slowness and/or extreme perfectionism may not respond to behavior therapy interventions, which may be related to this lack of subjective anxiety.

The desire to "even up" or balance movements may be present in patients with tapping or touching rituals. Patients may, for example, feel that the right side of the chair must be tapped after the left side has been tapped. Such urges and behaviors are also frequently seen in patients with comorbid tic disorders (Holzer et al. 1994; Leckman et al. 1994; Miguel et al. 1995, 1997, 2000), who may, for example, describe an urge to have a tic on the right side of their body after experiencing a tic on the left side.

Somatic obsessions. Somatic obsessions (i.e., the irrational and persistent fears of developing a serious life-threatening illness) may be seen in a variety of disorders, including OCD, hypochondriasis, major depression, and panic disorder. Several features may be useful in distinguishing OCD with somatic obsessions from hypochondriasis. Patients with OCD usually have other past or current classic OCD obsessions, are more likely to engage in classic OCD compulsions, such as checking and reassurance seeking, and generally do not experience somatic and visceral symptoms of illness. Somatic obsessions are more easily distinguished from somatization disorder, in that patients with somatic obsessions usually focus on one illness at a time and are not preoccupied with a diverse, apparently unrelated array of somatic symptoms.

In contrast to many patients with contamination obsessions, patients with somatic obsessions are usually worried about their own health rather than the well-being of others. Common somatic obsessions include a fear of cancer or venereal disease and a fear of developing acquired immunodeficiency syndrome (AIDS). Checking compulsions that consist of checking and rechecking the body part of concern or of reassurance-seeking are commonly associated with this fear.

Sexual and aggressive obsessions. Patients with sexual or aggressive obsessions are plagued by fears that they might commit a sexually unacceptable act, such as molestation, or harm others. They often fear not only that they will commit a dreadful act in the future but also that they have already committed such an act. Patients are typically horrified by the content of their obsessions and are reluctant to divulge them. It is quite striking that the content of these obsessions tends to consist of ideas that patients find particularly abhorrent.

Individuals with these highly distressing obsessions frequently carry out checking and confession or reassurance rituals. They may report themselves to the police or repeatedly seek out priests to confess their imagined crimes. An unsolved murder case in the media may cause tremendous anxiety and lead to extensive reassurance rituals. Patients may repeatedly tell their therapist, spouse, or close friend some terrible thought or deed that they feel they have committed as a way of seeking reassurance that they are really not capable of doing what they are worried about. Sometimes they leave the therapist's office after having sought reassurance for the whole hour, only to call back later to add an insignificant detail they earlier omitted confessing. Guilt and anxiety are the dominant affective symptoms. Patients may think that they should be jailed for their thoughts (both to protect them from what they think they might do and because they feel they deserve to be punished).

Patients may also use extensive avoidance to prevent obsessions (e.g., removing all sharp implements, such as scissors and knives, from the house or avoiding all television programs with references to violence, such as the news).

Mental compulsions. Traditionally, obsessions have been considered mental events (e.g., thoughts, images), whereas compulsions have been thought of as observable behaviors (e.g., washing or checking). More recently, on the basis of systematic investigation by researchers and cognitive-behavioral therapists, this view has shifted to the prevailing concept that obsessions are mental events that cause distress and compulsions are either behavioral or mental acts that are performed to neutralize or reduce obsessional distress. Mental compulsions, therefore, are neutralizing thoughts, such as mental counting or praying, which decrease anxiety caused by obsessions. Mental rituals were the third most common type of compulsion, after hand-washing and checking, in the DSM-IV field trial (Foa and Kozak 1995). In that study of 431 subjects with OCD, almost 80% reported having both behavioral and mental compulsions. However, less than 1% reported having only mental compulsions.

Taking a careful inventory of mental rituals and distinguishing them from obsessions is particularly important when the patient is engaged in exposure treatment. Behavior therapy comprises differing techniques for these symptoms: exposure is used for obsessions, and response prevention is used for compulsions. In addition, because mental rituals and avoidance often take the place of overt motor behavior, the patient may extinguish his or her overt rituals with no significant improvement in outcome.

Hoarding. Compulsive hoarding is characterized by the acquisition of and inability to discard items, even though they appear (to others) to have no value. This behavior is usually driven by obsessional fears of losing important items that the individual believes will be needed later, distorted beliefs about the importance of possessions, excessive acquisition, and exaggerated emotional attachments to possessions (Frost and Gross 1993; Saxena 2007). Patients frequently report that their living and work spaces are taken over by clutter and that their hoarding behavior causes significant impairment in social and occupational functioning.

One of the major developments in OCD nosology in recent years is the proposition that compulsive hoarding is a discrete entity, with a characteristic profile of core symptoms (classically, urges to save, difficulty discarding, and excessive acquisition; but also indecisiveness, perfectionism, procrastination, difficulty organizing tasks, and avoidance) that are not strongly correlated with other OCD symptoms (Frost and Hartl 1996); distinct susceptibility genes (Samuels et al. 2007); and unique neurobiological abnormalities that differ from those in nonhoarding OCD (Saxena 2007). The unique profile of hoarding suggests that both pharmacological and behavioral treatment approaches should be adapted to address this specific symptom.

Poor insight. Interest in the role of insight in OCD has increased in recent years. Traditionally, awareness of the senselessness or unreasonableness of obsessions (often referred to as *insight*) and the accompanying or resultant struggle against the obsessions (referred to as *resistance*) have been generally accepted as fundamental to the diagnosis of OCD. However, numerous descriptions of OCD patients who are completely convinced of the reasonableness of their obsessions and of the need to perform compulsions have appeared in the psychiatric literature during the past century (Kozak and Foa 1994). Insel and Akiskal (1986) described several such patients and presented the hypothesis that patients with OCD have varying degrees of insight and resistance, with obsessive-compulsive psychosis at one extreme of a hypothesized continuum. They also noted a fluidity between neurotic (i.e., associated with insight) and psychotic states in these patients.

The range of insight in OCD has been investigated systematically in several studies. Eisen and Rasmussen (1993) found that 14% of 475 patients with DSM-III-R OCD also had psychotic symptoms. Moreover, 6% showed lack of insight and high conviction about the reasonableness of the obsessions as their *only* psychotic symptom. Lelliott et al. (1988) used an interview that evaluated several insight-related parameters, including fixity of beliefs underlying the obsession, bizarreness, resistance, and degree of control. The fixity dimension included several constructs: strength of the belief in the feared situation, how the patient thought others viewed the belief, and the patient's response to evidence that contradicted the belief. A full range of responses was found in the 43 patients assessed, which led the authors to conclude that good insight in OCD is not necessarily present and that insight spans a spectrum from good to absent (i.e., delusional thinking).

In the DSM-IV field trial, insight was assessed by asking patients whether they feared consequences other than anxiety if they did not perform their compulsions (Foa and Kozak 1995). Results revealed that 58% believed that harmful consequences would occur. The degree of certainty that their obsessions were reasonable ranged across the entire spectrum of insight: most were uncertain whether they actually needed to perform their compulsions to avoid harm; however, 4% were certain, and 25% were mostly certain.

To reflect the results of these various studies, DSM-IV established a new OCD specifier: *with poor insight*. This specifier applies "when, for most of the time during the current episode, the individual does not recognize that the obsessions or compulsions are excessive or unreasonable" (DSM-IV-TR, American Psychiatric Association 2000, p. 458). In addition, DSM-IV acknowledges that the beliefs that underlie OCD obsessions can be delusional and notes that in such cases, an additional diagnosis of delusional disorder or psychotic disorder not otherwise specified may be appropriate.

Although these changes were made in DSM-IV, no generally accepted, reliable, and valid method was available to differentiate degrees of insight. To address the need for a scale that measures insight in OCD and other psychiatric disorders, Eisen et al. (1998) developed the Brown Assessment of Beliefs Scale (BABS), a seven-item, semistructured interview with specific probes and anchors that measure various dimensions of delusionality. Items include conviction, perception of others' views of the belief, explanation of differing views, fixity, rejection of views, and insight. This scale, which has established reliability and validity, may prove useful in phenomenological, prognostic, and treatment studies of OCD. Comparing the clinical characteristics of OCD and body dysmorphic disorder, Phillips et al. (2007) found that 2% of patients with OCD were categorized as delusional, versus 27.3% of patients with body dysmorphic disorder.

Whether insight is an important predictor of prognosis and treatment response in OCD is an intriguing question that has received very little investigation. The available literature on insight as a predictor of response to behavior therapy is conflicting. Two studies found that patients with overvalued ideas did not respond to behavior therapy as well as did patients with good insight (Foa 1979; Neziroglu et al. 1999a, 1999b). Other studies found that patients with high levels of conviction about their obsessions and the need to perform compulsions responded just as robustly as patients with good insight to behavioral intervention (Foa et al. 1983; Hoogduin and Duivenvoorden 1988; Lelliott et al. 1988).

The literature regarding the role of insight in pharmacological treatment is inconsistent as well. A study examining insight before and after open treatment with sertraline in 71 patients with OCD reported 1 patient (1.4%) with delusional OCD and 14 patients (19.7%) with poor insight, as defined by the BABS at baseline (Eisen et al. 2001). No correlation was found between the degree of insight in OCD at baseline and response to sertraline. Patients with poor insight at baseline were just as likely to respond to sertraline as patients with better insight. However, more recently, poor insight was identified as a predictor of poor treatment response (Ravi Kishore 2004). Further investigation regarding the role of insight in both pharmacological and behavioral treatment is warranted.

Approaches to OCD subtyping. To advance our understanding of the clinical, neurobiological, and genetic features of OCD, there has been an effort to identify meaningful subtypes of this heterogeneous disorder. Proposed strategies for subtyping include identification of comorbidity, specifically with the tic disorders, and identification of subtypes by clinical presentation. Research groups have analyzed data collected with the Y-BOCS-SC to identify subtypes of obsessions and compulsions that cluster together on factor analysis (Hasler et al. 2007; Leckman et al. 1997). Baer (1994) applied principal-components analysis to 107 patients with OCD who completed the Y-BOCS-SC and examined the correlations between the factor scores and the presence of comorbid tic or personality disorders. They found three independent symptom subtypes or factors: 1) symmetry/hoarding, which had high factor loading from symmetry and saving obsessions and ordering, hoarding, repeating, and counting compulsions; 2) contamination/checking, which had high factor loading from contamination and somatic obsessions, and cleaning and checking compulsions; and 3) pure obsessions, which had high factor loading from aggressive, sexual, and religious obsessions. The symmetry/hoarding factor was the only factor found to be related to comorbid Tourette syndrome or chronic tic disorder. Patients who scored high on symmetry/hoarding had a relative risk that was 8.5 times higher for having a chronic tic disorder than did those who scored low on this factor.

Another early study that used factor analysis of the Y-BOCS-SC in two independent groups of patients identified four factors: 1) obsessions and checking, 2) symmetry and ordering, 3) cleanliness and washing, and 4) hoarding (Leckman et al. 1997). As in the previous study, patients with chronic tic disorders scored significantly higher on symmetry and ordering factors in the total study group.

More recently, Mataix-Cols et al. (2005) conducted a systematic overview that identified 12 factor-analytic studies involving more than 2,000 patients. At least four "symptom dimensions" were consistently identified across these studies: 1) symmetry/ordering, 2) hoarding, 3) contamination/cleaning, and 4) obsessions/checking. They posited that the dimensions were associated with distinct patterns of comorbidity, genetic transmission, neural substrates, and treatment response. The evidence supporting the hoarding dimension appeared particularly robust (see discussion of Pinto 2008, below).

Pinto et al. (2007a) proposed a dimensional structure of OCD symptoms based on an exploratory factor analysis using intake data of 293 adults with primary OCD enrolled in the BLOCS. Applying principal-components analysis to the proportion of current symptoms endorsed in each of the Y-BOCS-SC categories produced a five-factor solution: 1) symmetry/ordering, 2) hoarding, 3) doubt/checking, 4) contamination/cleaning, and 5) taboo thoughts (aggressive, sexual, and religious obsessions). The resulting five factors correspond to widely accepted and long-held OCD symptom themes dating back to Janet's descriptions in 1903 of incompleteness (*les sentiments d'incomplétude*), forbidden thoughts, and doubt (*folie du doute*) (Pitman 1987).

To further validate this model, Pinto et al. (2008) independently replicated these five factors in a separate data set, using data on individual symptoms (rather than symptom categories) from 485 adults with lifetime OCD enrolled in the OCD Collaborative Genetics Study. These analyses indicated that the same underlying structure of OCD symptoms holds in both a sample of individuals with OCD and a sample of affected family members. When testing the familiality of the derived factors in affected sibling pairs, significant sib-sib associations were found for four of the five factors, with the hoarding and taboo thoughts factors being the most robustly familial ($r_{ICC} \geq 0.2$).

A different approach used to identify meaningful subtypes in OCD based on symptoms has been developed by Rasmussen and Eisen (1998). They hypothesized that this disorder has three core features: 1) abnormal risk assessment, 2) pathological doubt, and 3) incompleteness. These features cut across phenomenological subtypes such as checking, washing, and the need for symmetry, although some symptom subtypes are more closely associated with one core feature than another.

The core features appear to relate to both the clinical features of OCD and their connection with comorbid disorders. Patients with abnormalities in risk assessment have high levels of anxiety associated with their symptoms. In addition, they are more likely to have comorbid Axis I panic disorder, generalized anxiety disorder, or social phobia; avoidant and dependent personality features; and a family history of an anxiety disorder. In contrast, patients with incompleteness are more likely to manifest low levels of anxiety, comorbid multiple tics or habit disorders such as skin picking, and obsessive-compulsive personality features, specifically perfectionism and indecisiveness. Further empirical validation of this proposed subtyping according to core features is necessary and may have important implications for diagnosis and treatment. Summerfeldt (2004) has continued to investigate incompleteness and has suggested modifications of traditional exposure and response prevention techniques that may be particularly helpful in treating individuals whose OCD symptoms are driven by a sense of incompleteness. Other researchers have also actively investigated this putative core feature/subtype, using other related terms (mentioned previously) such as "just right experiences" (Coles et al. 2003; Leckman et al. 1993, 1994) and "sensory phenomena" (Miguel et al. 1995, 1997, 2000; Rosario-Campos 2001). Further research on this proposed subtype is critically important to advance our knowledge regarding the most effective treatment approaches for those individuals whose OCD symptoms are primarily driven by a sense of incompleteness.

Comorbidity

The coexistence of mood disorders, other anxiety disorders, and psychotic symptoms with obsessive-compulsive symptoms was reported in earlier psychiatric literature (Kringlin 1965; Pollitt 1957; Stengel 1945). In the ongoing BLOCS, 70% of children, 80% of adolescents, and 91% of adults met criteria for at least one other lifetime Axis I disorder at entry into the study (Mancebo et al. 2008; Pinto et al. 2006). Lifetime rates for major depressive disorder were 74%, and 52% of adults had at least one other anxiety disorder. More than one-third of the adult sample also met criteria for a comorbid personality disorder, the most common being obsessive-compulsive and avoidant personality disorders (Pinto et al. 2006).

Depressive symptoms have been the most common comorbid syndrome, both in clinical studies that were completed before 1985 without the benefit of standardized diagnostic criteria or reliable structured instruments and in more recent studies that assessed comorbidity more systematically. In our initial study of 100 patients with primary OCD being seen in an OCD clinic, 67% had a lifetime history of major depression, and 31% met criteria for current major depression (Rasmussen and Eisen 1988). Over the course of their illness, most patients reported that depression developed *after* their OCD symptoms occurred—thus, they were classified as having secondary depression. A minority (8%) of the patients had concurrent onset of their obsessive-compulsive symptoms with their depressive episodes. Although it may be difficult to distinguish a primary from a secondary diagnosis, some patients with

OCD view their depressive symptoms as occurring secondary to the demoralization and hopelessness accompanying their OCD symptoms, and they report that they would not be depressed if they did not have OCD. However, other patients view their major depressive symptoms as occurring independently of their OCD symptoms. OCD symptoms may be less severe when these patients cycle into an episode of major depression because they feel too apathetic to be as concerned with their obsessions and too fatigued to perform compulsions. However, OCD symptoms intensify in some patients during depressive episodes.

In the ECA study, respondents who had both lifetime OCD and major depressive disorder frequently reported the onset of OCD before the onset of major depressive disorder (Karno et al. 1988). In the NCS-R study, major depressive disorder was found to be frequently comorbid with OCD. Although specific temporal associations were not analyzed, the average age at onset for major depressive disorder was later than that for OCD (Kessler et al. 2005a, 2005b; reviewed in Fontenelle and Hasler 2008).

Until relatively recently, obsessive-compulsive features were rarely, if ever, described in mania. Over the past decade, however, numerous studies have documented comorbidity between OCD and bipolar disorders by assessing the frequency of obsessions and compulsions in individuals with bipolar disorders as well as ascertaining the frequency of these mood disorders in patients with OCD. In the ECA sample, Chen and Dilsaver (1995) found that 21% of the patients with bipolar disorder, 12.2% of the patients with unipolar depression, and 5.9% of the patients with other disorders had OCD. Krüger et al. (1995) found that 35% of both bipolar and unipolar depressed patients had an obsessive-compulsive syndrome. Angst et al. (2004) reported an increased prevalence of OCD or obsessive-compulsive syndromes among subjects ascertained as having bipolar spectrum disorders, bipolar type II disorder, or "minor bipolar disorder" in a large Swiss cohort. Of 204 subjects with OCD referred to an academic anxiety disorders clinic, Maina and colleagues (2007) indicated that 10.3% met criteria for bipolar disorders, particularly bipolar II. Another study comparing clinical characteristics of those OCD patients with and without bipolar disorder noted the worsening of OCD symptoms during depressive episodes and improvement during the hypomanic/mania episodes (Zutshi et al. 2007).

Other anxiety disorders also frequently coexist with OCD. In several studies, researchers have assessed the frequency of OCD among patients in treatment for other anxiety disorders. In a study of 60 patients with panic disorder diagnosed with the Schedule for Affective Disorders and Schizophrenia, Lifetime Version, modified for anxiety disorders and personal interviews, Breier et al. (1986) found that 17% had DSM-III OCD. Subsequent studies by Mellman and Uhde (1986) and Barlow (1988) confirmed these initial findings of the overlap between panic disorder and OCD. In the Harvard/Brown Anxiety Research Project (HARP), a prospective study of course in 711 patients with panic disorder, social phobia, and/or generalized anxiety disorder, 11% had comorbid OCD at baseline (Steketee et al. 1999).

This comorbidity has also been assessed by reports on the frequency of other anxiety disorders in clinical OCD samples. Relatively high lifetime rates of social phobia (18%), panic disorder (12%), and specific phobia (22%) were reported in a sample of 100 subjects with primary OCD (i.e., those who sought treatment for OCD) (Rasmussen and Eisen 1988). In the ongoing BLOCS, social phobia (28%) and specific phobia (22%) were the most common comorbid anxiety disorders. This high frequency of current and lifetime anxiety disorders suggests that OCD patients are vulnerable to many types of anxiety. The high prevalence of anxiety states in these patients may be caused by common developmental and temperamental traits whose phenotypic expression is secondary to shared genotypic and psychosocial factors. Of particular interest in this regard is the high lifetime prevalence of separation anxiety in this group of patients. In the BLOCS cohort, 12% of adults with a juvenile onset of OCD and 23% of juveniles met lifetime criteria for separation anxiety disorder (Mancebo et al. 2008). Research has supported the idea that separation anxiety disorder in childhood is linked with increased risk for anxiety disorders, including OCD, in adulthood (Bruckl et al. 2007; Lipsitz et al. 1994).

Attention has been focused on the relation between tics and OCD. Leckman et al. (1993) found that patients with Tourette syndrome had high rates of comorbid OCD and obsessive-compulsive symptoms (30%–40% reporting obsessive-compulsive symptoms). Conversely, approximately 20% of patients with OCD had a lifetime history of multiple tics and 5%–10% had a lifetime history of Tourette syndrome (Leckman et al. 1994). This subgroup had an earlier age at onset and family pedigrees that are loaded for both Tourette syndrome and OCD (Pauls et al. 1995). An Israeli cross-sectional study reported that the rates of Tourette syndrome and transient and chronic motor tics in adolescents with OCD were significantly higher than those of age-matched control subjects without OCD (Zohar et al. 1992). A subsequent prospective study of 976 children in upstate New York revealed that the presence of tics in childhood and early adolescence predicted an increase in OCD symptoms in late adolescence and early adulthood (Peterson et al. 2001). In addition to genetic comorbidity data linking OCD and tic disorders, some evidence suggests that these disorders are linked phenomenologically, as noted earlier in this chapter; certain OCD symptoms such as symmetry and ordering are more common in patients with OCD and tic disorders than in patients with OCD alone (Labad et al. 2007).

Several studies have found significant comorbidity between anorexia nervosa and OCD. In one study, 17% of 100 OCD subjects were found to have a lifetime history of an eating disorder (Rasmussen and Eisen 1988). Conversely, in a series of 93 subjects with an eating disorder, 37% met criteria for comorbid OCD, with Y-BOCS scores of 16 or higher (Thiel et al. 1995). A number of additional studies have shown substantial rates of OCD in individuals with anorexia (Godart et al. 2006; Rastam et al. 1995; Salbach-Andrae et al. 2008).

The relationship between schizophrenia and OCD has been assessed by a number of investigators over the past two decades. Frequencies of comorbidity between the two disorders have ranged from 7.8% to 40.5% (Berman et al. 1995; Eisen et al. 1997; Fenton and McGlashan 1986; Porto et al. 1997). Differences in the findings may be based on criteria used to define OCD and obsessive-compulsive symptoms. Regardless of this range, it seems clear that a subgroup of patients with schizophrenia has co-occurring obsessions and compulsions. Assessment of prognosis and neuropsychological testing are two approaches that have been used to characterize this subgroup. Fenton and McGlashan (1986) found that 10% of the schizophrenic patients in a Chestnut Lodge (Rockville, Maryland) follow-up study had prominent obsessive-compulsive symptoms. These "obsessive-compulsive schizophrenics" tended to have a more chronic course and a greater frequency of social or occupational impairment, compared with a matched sample of schizophrenic patients without obsessive-compulsive features. A study in which neuropsychological testing was conducted in two groups of patients with schizophrenia—those with and those without OCD—found that the group with comorbid OCD performed worse in visuospatial skills, delayed nonverbal memory, and cognitive shifting abilities—cognitive areas thought to be impaired in OCD (Berman et al. 1998). De Haan et al. (2005) studied 113 consecutively hospitalized patients with recent-onset schizophrenia or related disorders. They found that patients with acute recent-onset schizophrenia and OCD had more severe depressive and less severe negative symptoms at baseline, compared with patients without comorbid OCD. These differences were no longer significant after 6 weeks of treatment, although obsessive-compulsive symptom severity remained constant among a subset of schizophrenic subjects with either OCD or subthreshold obsessive-compulsive symptoms. A recent study in which the role of insight was investigated in individuals with both schizophrenia and obsessive-compulsive symptoms revealed that a majority of patients (48 patients, 84.2%) exhibited good or fair insight into their obsessive-compulsive symptoms. Interestingly, in the schizo-obsessive group, insight into obsessive-compulsive symptoms was positively correlated with awareness of schizophrenia, but not with awareness of delusions (Poyurovsky et al. 2007).

Comorbidity between these two disorders has also been assessed cross-sectionally and in follow-up in an examination of the frequency of psychotic symptoms in a group of patients with primary OCD. Retrospective follow-up studies in which the subsequent development of schizophrenia in patients with OCD were examined have produced varying results, with rates ranging from 0.7% to as high as 12.3% (Ingram 1961; Kringlin 1965; Lo 1967; Muller 1953; Pollitt 1957; Rosenberg 1968). These studies, however, were methodologically limited, in that none of them were prospective, diagnoses were made by chart review, and standardized diagnostic criteria were not used, which probably resulted in the inclusion of affective psychoses. In reviewing this literature, Goodwin et al. (1969) concluded that subjects with OCD were at no greater risk for developing schizophrenia than individuals in the general population. In a study with a cross-sectional design, Eisen and Rasmussen (1993) identified 67 of 475 (14%) OCD subjects as having psychotic symptoms. These 67 subjects were quite heterogeneous: 18 (4% of the larger cohort) had comorbid schizophrenia, 8 (2%) had comorbid delusional disorder unrelated to OCD, and 14 (3%) had comorbid schizotypal personality disorder. In the remaining 27 patients (6% of the larger cohort), the only psychotic symptom present was a delusional conviction about the reasonableness of the obsessions (i.e., delusional OCD, or OCD without insight). Notably, the 27 subjects without insight were similar to the OCD patients without any psychotic symptoms (i.e., OCD with insight) in terms of epidemiological and clinical features such as course of illness. Similarly, treatment studies of patients with OCD and comorbid schizotypal personality disorder have shown a poorer prognosis and poorer response to psychotropic medications for the comorbid group (Jenike et al. 1986). Thus, it appears important to differentiate OCD plus a comorbid psychotic disorder, which may have a relatively poor outcome, from delusional OCD, which may be more similar to OCD with insight and without comorbid psychosis.

Finally, comorbidity between Axis II disorders and OCD has been reported. The most commonly reported comorbid personality disorder diagnoses in OCD have been dependent, avoidant, passive-aggressive, and obsessive-compulsive personality disorders. Most recently, obsessive-compulsive (24.6%) and avoidant (15.3%) were found to be the most common personality disorders in the latest BLOCS (Pinto et al. 2006). Comorbid schizotypal, paranoid, and borderline personality disorders are found less commonly in OCD, but appear to be associated with poor outcome (Baer et al. 1992).

The comorbidity between obsessive-compulsive personality disorder (OCPD) and OCD is particularly interesting. Janet (1903) viewed all obsessional patients as having a premorbid personality causally related to pathogenesis of the disorder. However, as described above, several studies revealed that a significant percentage of OCD patients do not have premorbid compulsive personalities. In seven studies reviewed by Black (1974), marked obsessional traits were found in 31% of 254 obsessional patients, moderate traits were found in 40%, and no obsessional traits were found in 29%. All of these studies were completed before the introduction of DSM-III, so comparisons among studies are difficult because of variations in methodology and sample selection.

Studies completed after the introduction of DSM-III have also reported varied rates of comorbidity of OCPD and OCD. A study in which researchers applied DSM-III-R criteria showed that OCPD was found in 25% of the subjects with OCD; the higher rate of OCPD found with DSM-III-R criteria may reflect changes in the criteria set between DSM-III and DSM-III-R (Baer et al. 1990). Even the DSM-III-R rate shows that the comorbidity of OCD and OCPD is relatively low, a finding that is at odds with earlier studies in which it was postulated that OCD and OCPD are closely related disorders on a continuum of severity. A possible explanation for this disparity lies in the varied criteria used to make the diagnosis of OCPD. A study using the Structured Interview for the DSM-III Personality Disorders (SID-P) in 114 patients with DSM-III OCD revealed that most patients had difficulty with perfectionism and indecisiveness (82% and 70%, respectively) (Eisen and Rasmussen 1991). In contrast, the other traits constituting OCPD (i.e., restricted ability to express warmth, rigidity, and excessive devotion to work) were not seen as frequently (32%, 32%, and 18%, respectively). In fact, these traits were no more common in OCD patients than in non-OCD control subjects, suggesting that these traits are not developmental antecedents for OCD.

More recently, Coles et al. (2008) examined the validity of using comorbid OCPD to identify a subtype of individuals with OCD by drawing on a cohort of treatment-seeking patients with primary and current DSM-IV OCD (N=238). Slightly more than one-quarter of subjects (n=65; 27%) met criteria for comorbid OCPD. As compared with OCD without OCPD subjects, the OCD plus OCPD subjects had a significantly younger age at onset of first obsessive-compulsive symptoms and had higher rates of symmetry and hoarding obsessions and of cleaning, ordering, repeating, and hoarding compulsions. Subjects with OCD plus OCPD had higher rates of comorbid anxiety disorders and avoidant personality disorder. The OCD plus OCPD subjects also had significantly lower global, and specifically social, functioning, despite a lack of significant differences on overall severity of OCD symptoms. The authors concluded that individuals with both OCD and OCPD have distinct clinical characteristics (e.g., age at onset of initial obsessive-compulsive symptoms, the types of obsessions and compulsions they experience, and psychiatric comorbidity) and may represent a specific subset of the OCD population.

Differential Diagnosis

The DSM-IV-TR (American Psychiatric Association 2000) criteria for OCD are listed in Table 16–1. Even if the diagnosis of OCD is frequently straightforward, it may, at times, be difficult to distinguish OCD from depression, psychosis, anxiety disorders, and severe OCPD.

Patients with OCD frequently have comorbid depression, and these patients may be difficult to distinguish from depressed patients who have concurrent obsessive symptoms. The distinction between primary and secondary obsessions rests on the order of occurrence. In addition, depressive ruminations may present similarly to pure obsessions. Ruminations, in contrast to obsessions, are usually focused on a past incident rather than a current or future event and are rarely resisted (Hollander and Simeon 2003).

OCD and anxiety disorders may present very similarly. All these disorders are characterized by avoidant behavior, excessive fear, and intense subjective and autonomic responses to focal stimuli, and they appear to respond to similar behavioral interventions. Patients with OCD who experience high levels of anxiety may describe panic-like episodes, but these are secondary to obsessions and do not arise spontaneously, unlike in panic disorder. Individuals with OCD can never entirely avoid the obsession, whereas phobic patients have more focal external stimuli that they can successfully avoid (Hollander and Simeon 2003). The content of worry in generalized anxiety disorder usually focuses on everyday concerns, such as finances, whereas obsessions tend to involve less commonly held fears.

OCD must be distinguished from schizophrenia and other psychotic disorders. The natural history of both OCD and schizophrenia may involve chronic debilitation and functional (e.g., social and occupational) decline. There may be subtle distinctions between an obsession and a delusion that are difficult to discern. In general, an obsession is ego-dystonic, resisted, and recognized as having an internal origin; a delusion is not resisted and is believed to be external, although there are rare exceptions when individuals with obsessions lack insight into the irrationality of their concerns (see subsection "Insight" in this chapter). Both disorders may exist independently, and DSM-IV allows the diagnosis of both disorders (Hollander and Simeon 2003).

The literature supports that a distinction can be made between OCPD and OCD (Baer 1998; Baer et al. 1990, 1992; Eisen and Rasmussen 1991). The classic distinction of compulsions being ego-syntonic in OCPD as opposed to ego-dystonic in OCD is useful but not absolute. Some patients with cleaning or hoarding compulsions and those with the need for symmetry and precision or obsessive slowness who strive for perfection or completeness find their rituals ego-syntonic until the rituals begin to impair social and occupational functioning. Whether these patients should be classified as having OCPD or subthreshold OCD is a subject for further empirical study.

Course and Natural History

Age at Onset

In the BLOCS cohort of adults with OCD, the mean age at onset was 18.5 years. Men had a significantly earlier onset of illness: 19.5±9.2, compared with 22.0±9.8 for women (Pinto et al. 2006). Of the patients studied, 82% experienced the onset of significant symptoms before age 25 years, whereas fewer than 10% had onset of the disorder after age 30 years (Grant et al. 2007). Most patients described minor symptoms (i.e., obsessions and/or compulsions that do not cause significant distress or impairment) prior to the development of full criteria for OCD. Although OCD usually begins in late adolescence, prepubertal onset is not rare: 34% had onset of OCD before age 14 years, and 23% had onset before age 12 years.

Some evidence suggests that age at onset may be significant in terms of familial transmission. In a study that revealed the frequency of OCD in the first-degree relatives of 100 probands with OCD, 82% of the probands reported onset of OCD before age 18 years (Pauls et al. 1995). In this study, the rate of OCD and subthreshold OCD among relatives of the probands with onset of OCD before age 18 years was approximately twice as high as the rate of OCD in relatives of OCD probands with late onset.

Age at onset of OCD may also be a predictor of course. The vast majority of patients endorse having a chronic course once OCD occurs (see next subsection, "Course of Illness"). However, Swedo et al. (1998) described a subtype of OCD that begins before puberty and is characterized by an episodic course with intense exacerbations. Exacerbations of OCD symptoms in this subtype have been linked with group A β-hemolytic streptococcal infections, leading to the subtype designation of pediatric autoimmune neuropsychiatric disorders associated with streptococcal infections (PANDAS). Whether the course of illness in patients with PANDAS continues to be episodic into adulthood or chronic, as is the case with postpubertal onset, is not known definitively.

Course of Illness

DSM-IV and DSM-IV-TR describe the course of OCD as typically chronic with some fluctuation in the severity of symptoms over time (American Psychiatric Association 1994, 2000). Although terminology and definitions vary from study to study, overall this appears to be supported, both by studies conducted retrospectively and by more recent follow-up and prospective studies.

In follow-up studies with a retrospective design, investigators generally identified patterns of course of illness in OCD as falling into the following categories:

complete absence of obsessions and compulsions (remission), symptoms unchanged or worsening, symptoms much improved, and symptoms minimally improved with poor functioning. In these studies, it is often unclear whether patients described as "much improved" would nevertheless still meet criteria for the disorder. Another approach has been to determine the episodicity of OCD (i.e., whether this illness is characterized by distinct periods of illness and remission similar to major depressive disorder). These follow-up studies are compared in Table 16–3, with the caveat that different measures were used to assign patients to categories of course of illness. For the sake of comparison in Table 16–3, subjects considered mildly improved, but with poor functioning, were combined with subjects classified as having obsessive-compulsive symptoms that were minimally improved, were unchanged, or had worsened.

These early phenomenological and follow-up studies of OCD had several methodological limitations, including retrospective study design, small sample size, lack of standardized criteria to determine diagnosis, hospital-based samples not representative of the spectrum of the disorder found in the population as a whole, biases in inclusion and exclusion criteria, chart review rather than personal interview, absence of structured interviews, and lack of consensus on the definitions of relapse, remission, and recovery. In reviewing these studies, Goodwin et al. (1969) concluded that the course of OCD is usually chronic but variable, with fluctuations in severity of symptoms. They described depression as the most common psychiatric disorder to develop after the onset of OCD and observed that the subsequent development of schizophrenia occurs rarely, if it is adequately excluded at baseline.

In follow-up studies conducted since 1980, course of illness has been evaluated with different criteria from those used in the earlier studies described above. Patients were retrospectively assigned to the following categories: continuous, waxing and waning, deteriorative, and episodic with full remissions between episodes. Rasmussen and Tsuang (1986) conducted a study in which patients were selected based on current enrollment in an outpatient OCD clinic. Most of the 44 patients (84%) described the course of OCD as chronic or "continuous"; 6 subjects (14%) had a deteriorating course, and only 1 (2%) had an episodic course. The average duration of illness at time of assessment was more than 15 years, again suggesting the chronicity of the disorder. Because these subjects were acquired through the process of clinic referral and course was assessed retrospectively, no former OCD patients who had already recovered and remained well were included. Patients who developed other major psychiatric disorders (e.g., schizophrenia) were also unlikely to be represented in this cohort of patients in an OCD clinic.

Two studies used control groups to compare course of illness with an OCD cohort. Coryell (1981) compared the course of illness following hospitalization in 44 inpatients with OCD and 44 inpatients with major depression. He observed that although 55.6% of the patients with OCD had some improvement at follow-up, this cohort was significantly less likely to experience remission after discharge (22%) than the comparison cohort of depressed patients (64%). However, suicide occurred significantly less frequently in the cohort of patients with OCD, compared with patients with depression.

In a follow-up study, Thomsen (1995) interviewed 47 patients with OCD 6–22 years after they had been treated for OCD as children and compared their characteristics with those of a group of non-OCD psychiatric control subjects. All subjects were at least 18 years old at the time of the follow-up interview. The majority of the subjects had either no OCD symptoms (27.7%) or only subclinical obsessive-compulsive symptoms (25.5%) at follow-up; 10 subjects (21.3%) had a chronic course of OCD. In this study, researchers also assessed outcome by measuring Global Assessment Scale (Endicott et al. 1976) scores. Although the difference was not statistically significant, males with childhood-onset OCD appeared to have a poorer outcome than females: 9 of the 10 patients with Global Assessment Scale scores below 50 at follow-up were males.

More recently, investigators have used the Y-BOCS , which is designed to measure severity of obsessive-compulsive symptoms, and assessed course by assigning patients to groups by percent improvement on the Y-BOCS (Goodman et al. 1989a, 1989b). In a study conducted by Orloff et al. (1994), most of the 85 subjects assessed 1–3 years after baseline evaluation were considered much improved at follow-up, based on chart review; 33% had a greater than 75% decrease in Y-BOCS score. The mean follow-up Y-BOCS score was in the range of mild to minimal obsessions and compulsions that did not cause interference with functioning (Y-BOCS score=10.1±7.0). This improvement in obsessive-compulsive symptoms compared with baseline symptomatology may reflect the availability of effective behavioral and pharmacological treatments for OCD,

TABLE 16–3. Retrospective follow-up studies of obsessive-compulsive disorder (OCD)

Reference	*N*	Mean follow-up (years)	Well (%)	Much improved (%)	Minimally improved, unchanged, or worse (%)	Comments
Lewis 1936	50	>5	32	14	44	10% episodic course
Pollitt 1957	67[a]	3.4	24	36	37	Mostly outpatients
Ingram 1961	29	5.9	7	21[b]	72	Inpatients
Kringlin 1965	80	13–20	0	24	76	Inpatients
Grimshaw 1965	100	5	40	24	35	Inpatients
Lo 1967	88	3.9	23	50	27	Inpatients and outpatients, diagnostic heterogeneity
Coryell 1981	44	≥0.5	22	55	22	Inpatients
Thomsen 1995	47	6–22	28	47	25	Childhood OCD

[a]Leukotomized.
[b]One patient nonleukotomized; five patients leukotomized.

such as exposure and response prevention techniques and selective serotonin reuptake inhibitors (SSRIs). In fact, 99% of the subjects had received at least a 10-week trial of an SSRI, and 45% had received some behavior therapy (although only 16% received at least 20 hours of behavior therapy). Notably, most patients were still receiving medication at the time of follow-up, with clear relapses in those patients who discontinued medication, suggesting that maintenance of improvement in obsessive-compulsive symptoms over time may require continued treatment.

In another follow-up study conducted in Austria, researchers assessed 62 inpatients who met ICD-8/9 (World Health Organization 1977) criteria for OCD after structured interviews (Demal et al. 1993). This study's findings were consistent with those of earlier studies: episodic course with complete remission (11.3%), episodic with partial remission (24.4%), deteriorative (9.7%), continuous and unchanging (27.4%), and continuous with improvement (24.4%). Demal and colleagues used the Y-BOCS to rate current obsessive-compulsive symptom severity and found that 29.1% had Y-BOCS scores in the normal range, 20.9% had scores in the subclinical range (8–15), and 50.0% had scores in the clinical range (16–40).

A prospective naturalistic study of course of OCD in adults was conducted, in which data were collected on 66 subjects over the course of 2 years (Eisen et al. 1995). Of the subjects meeting full criteria for OCD at the start of the study, 57% still met full criteria for OCD after 2 years. Although some of these subjects showed considerable improvement in the severity of their obsessive-compulsive symptoms, many nonetheless had continued significant impairment because of obsessions and/or compulsions. Only 12% had minimal or no symptoms (Y-BOCS scores≤8). The remainder of the subjects (31%) had obsessions and compulsions that persisted but did not meet full criteria, and might be classified as being in partial remission or much improved. Survival analysis estimated a 47% probability of achieving at least partial remission during the 2-year study period. However, if more stringent criteria were used to define remission (i.e., patients had only occasional or no obsessions and compulsions for 8 consecutive weeks), the probability of achieving remission was only 12%. Almost half the patients (48%) who achieved partial or full remission subsequently relapsed. These findings are consistent with those of most previous studies of OCD, which found that most people who meet full criteria for this disorder continue to have obsessions and compulsions, even though they may show considerable improvement in both the intensity of their symptoms and the corresponding degree of impairment.

Skoog and Skoog (1999) studied the course of illness among 251 patients with OCD (diagnosed according to Schneiderian criteria) in Göteborg, Sweden, for more than 40 years. Improvement was observed in 83%, including recovery in 48% (complete recovery, 20%; recovery with subclinical symptoms, 28%). Among those who recovered, 38% had done so during the first decade of follow-up; 48% had OCD for more than 30 years. Subjects whose symptoms included early age at onset, both obsessive and compulsive symptoms, low social functioning, and a chronic course at baseline were associated with a worse outcome, as were magical obsessions and compulsive rituals. Qualitative symptom changes within the OCD occurred in 58% of the patients. The authors concluded that after several decades, most individuals with OCD improve, although most patients continue to have clinical or subclinical symptoms.

More recently, the first 214 adult BLOCS subjects with OCD were followed prospectively for 2 years. One-quarter of the sample experienced periods of subclinical OCD symptoms during the prospective period. However, full remission was rare, which is consistent with the view of OCD as a chronic and persistent illness. Earlier onset of OCD, greater severity of symptoms at intake, older age at intake, and being male were each associated with a decreased likelihood of remission over the course of 2 years (Pinto et al. 2007b).

Over the past two decades, several studies on course of illness in childhood-onset OCD have been conducted in which a prospective design was used. In one of these studies, all students in a high school were screened for the presence of obsessions and/or compulsions. Of the 5,596 high school students screened, 59 were identified as having OCD, subclinical OCD, other psychiatric disorders with obsessive-compulsive symptoms, or OCPD (Flament et al. 1988). These teenagers were reinterviewed 2 years after the initial interview by raters blind to the baseline diagnosis (Berg et al. 1989). Of the 12 subjects with initial diagnoses of OCD, 5 (42%) still met full criteria for OCD. Those subjects with initial diagnoses of OCD at baseline and subclinical OCD at the 2-year interview (8%) might be analogous to the subjects described in other studies as being much improved or in partial remission. Only 1 subject with an initial diagnosis of OCD had no diagnosis after 2 years. Of interest is the development of psychiatric symptoms in the 15 students with subclinical OCD at baseline: at follow-up, 27% met full criteria for OCD, 27% continued to have subclinical OCD, 27% developed other psychiatric disorders with obsessive-compulsive features, and only 1 subject received no diagnosis.

In another study of OCD in children conducted prospectively, 25 children with OCD 2–7 years after initial evaluation were assessed (Flament et al. 1990). The majority of subjects (68%) still met criteria for OCD at follow-up, and 28% were considered completely well (with no obsessions or compulsions). More than half the subjects had a lifetime history of major depression, and 44% had been diagnosed as having another anxiety disorder, in addition to OCD (e.g., social phobia or separation anxiety); 5 patients had OCPD, and 22 patients developed psychotic symptoms (diagnosed as atypical psychosis or schizophreniform disorder).

A third study on the course of illness in children with OCD assessed the effect of treatment on course. Following participation in a controlled trial of clomipramine and a variety of interim interventions, 54 children and adolescents were reinterviewed after 2–7 years (Leonard et al. 1993). At follow-up, most patients were only mildly symptomatic, and obsessive-compulsive symptoms were more severe in only 10 subjects at reassessment—so that, as a whole, the cohort had improved. However, only 3 subjects (6%) were considered to be in true remission (defined as no obsessions or compulsions and no medication), and 23 subjects (43%) still met full criteria for OCD. In addition, most patients were taking medication at follow-up, which again suggests that maintenance of improvement in OCD may require ongoing pharmacological intervention.

To synthesize findings from varied studies on course of illness in adults and children, it may be important to separate the best possible outcome (full remission, symptom-free) from what is described as "much improved" or "improved." The episodic pattern of full remission (and sometimes later recurrence), when it is clearly identified as such, appears to occur in about 10%–15% of OCD patients, although this proportion may increase somewhat as follow-up is extended for several years. In most studies, a smaller proportion (6%–14%) seems to follow a deteriorating course. Most patients presumably follow a course marked by chronicity, with some symptom fluctuation over time but without clear-cut remissions or deterioration. Those fortunate patients who experience complete remission of their obsessive-compulsive symptoms are very much in the minority.

Evaluation: Rating Scales

As with most psychiatric disorders, the diagnosis of OCD rests on purely clinical grounds (i.e., psychiatric examination and history). Yet formal assessments, in the form of structured interviews, self-report and significant-other-report questionnaires, and clinical rating scales, play an important adjunctive role in research, administrative (e.g., health care delivery documentation/coding), and clinical settings (e.g., screening, formal testing to diagnose according to DSM or similar criteria, symptom severity monitoring). The most frequently used instruments relevant to OCD are reviewed here.

A number of general psychiatric interview schedules include OCD modules. Among the most extensively used are the SCID-I and DIS/CIDI. OCD-specific measures include the Y-BOCS and the OVIS. These measures are described below.

The Structured Clinical Interview for for DSM-IV Axis I Disorders (SCID-I; First et al. 1996) is a semistructured, clinician-administered interview designed to diagnose 33 psychiatric disorders by DSM-IV criteria. The list comprises mood disorders, psychotic disorders, substance use disorders, anxiety disorders (including OCD), somatoform disorders, and eating disorders. Diagnoses are made on a lifetime (ever present) and current (meets diagnostic criteria in the past month) basis, and subthreshold diagnoses are noted. The SCID's modular nature allows selective use for confirming a diagnosis suspected after a clinical evaluation (First et al. 1996; Rush et al. 2000). To our knowledge, no psychometric data have been published on the SCID-I for OCD as operationalized in DSM-IV.

The Diagnostic Interview Schedule (DIS; Robins et al. 1996) was developed for lay interviewers to assess current and lifetime psychiatric disorders according to DSM-III criteria in the landmark National Institute of Mental Health ECA study, which produced an estimate of OCD prevalence that was much higher than had previously been reported (see "Epidemiology" section in this chapter). It has been revised (the DIS-IV) to yield diagnoses on the basis of DSM-IV diagnostic criteria (Robins et al. 1996). The DIS is the forerunner of the Composite International Diagnostic Interview (CIDI; Kessler and Ustan 2004), which was designed to address the need for an epidemiological interview schedule applicable to cross-cultural comparisons of psychiatric disorders. The CIDI produces diagnoses that meet both *International Classification of Diseases* (ICD—standard nomenclature and nosology in most of the rest of the world) and DSM-IV criteria (Rush et al. 2000). The most recent version was used in the NCS-R (Kessler and Merikangas 2004) (see "Epidemiology" section for OCD lifetime and 12-month prevalence estimates). Both instruments are highly structured interviews administered by verbatim reading of questions with forced-response choices concerning psychopathological symptoms (Rush et al. 2000).

The Yale-Brown Obsessive Compulsive Scale (Y-BOCS; Goodman et al. 1989a, 1989b), a 10-item, clinician-administered scale with specific probes and anchors, assesses severity of five domains for obsessions and compulsions. These domains include *time, distress, interference, resistance,* and *control.* Each domain is rated from 0 (no symptoms) to 4 (extreme symptoms). The Y-BOCS has established reliability (Cronbach's alpha, 0.69–0.91 total scale and 0.51–0.85 subscales for internal consistency; intraclass correlation coefficient [ICC], 0.80–0.99 and 0.81–0.97 for interrater and test-retest reliability, respectively) and validity (e.g., moderate convergence between total scale and subscale Y-BOCS and questionnaire measures of OC symptoms; *r*, 0.33–0.62). It is widely accepted as the major outcome measure for OCD, having been shown to be sensitive to change with pharmacological and psychosocial treatments for OCD. The symptom checklist included with Y-BOCS captures 53 of the most common obsessive and compulsive symptoms. The patient is asked to endorse which specific obsessions and compulsions apply to him or her. The Y-BOCS is not a diagnostic instrument, because it does not specifically assess whether diagnostic criteria for OCD have been met. Notably, individuals who present with either obsessions or compulsions exclusively may score spuriously low on the Y-BOCS total scale, despite severe symptoms. Specifying subscale scores circumvents this problem (Goodman et al. 1989a, 1989b).

The Brown Assessment of Beliefs Scale (BABS), a 7-item semistructured interview, assesses the degree and presence of delusional thinking. This scale was developed for use across psychiatric disorders and has been used to measure insight/degree of delusionality in OCD, as well as other disorders (Eisen et al. 1998, 2001, 2004; Phillips et al. 2001, 2007; Steinglass et al. 2007). BABS items are scored on a 5-point scale and assess the following dimensions of delusional thinking during the past week: *conviction, perception of others' views, explanation of differing views, fixity, attempt to disprove beliefs, insight,* and *ideas/delusions of reference.* The BABS has acceptable interrater and test-retest reliability (ICC for total score, 0.96 and 0.95, respectively), as well as internal consistency (Cronbach's alpha=0.87), and is sensitive to medication-induced changes in insight. Total BABS scores are significantly positively correlated with items and total scores of other scales measuring delusionality, but not with symptom severity scores, as measured by the Y-BOCS (Eisen et al. 1998).

The Over-valued Ideas Scale (OVIS; Neziroglu et al. 1999a) is a 9-item clinician-administered scale designed to quantitatively assess levels of overvalued ideas (OVI) in OCD. The scale is scored between 0 and 10 along the following domains related to obsessions/beliefs: one item each for *bizarreness, belief accuracy, fixity, reason-*

ableness, effectiveness of compulsions, pervasiveness of belief, reasons others do not share the belief, and two items assessing *stability of belief.* OVIS was found to have adequate internal consistency reliability (coefficient alpha=0.88 at baseline), test-retest reliability (r=0.86), and interrater reliability (r=0.88). Moderate to high levels of convergent validity were found with measures of obsessive-compulsive symptoms, a single-item assessment of overvalued ideas and psychotic symptoms (item 11) on the Y-BOCS. Medium levels of discriminant validity using measures of anxiety and depression were obtained in this study. Individuals determined to have high OVI showed greater stability of this pathology than those with lower OVI, suggesting that overvalued ideas are stable for extreme scorers (Neziroglu et al. 1999a).

Conclusion

Recent years have seen tremendous strides in knowledge about the etiology, epidemiology, and treatment of OCD. We now know that OCD is a common psychiatric disorder, not only in the United States but also globally. Research regarding phenomenological aspects of OCD has focused on various areas, including identification of subtypes, investigation of the relationship between OCD and OCPD, and patterns of comorbidity. Several studies that examined the course of illness in OCD found that the course is usually chronic in adults. However, increasing evidence indicates that there may be a subtype of OCD that is characterized by an episodic course, and current research is focusing on delineating that subtype more specifically. Another hypothesized subtype involves patients with both OCD and chronic tic disorders. Certain obsessions and compulsions are more common in patients with these two disorders, adding evidence to the familial transmission and treatment data suggesting that this pattern of comorbidity may identify a meaningful subtype.

Another area of focus has been the role of insight. Evidence that patients with OCD have a range of insight has been increasing. It remains to be seen whether patients with poor insight have a different treatment response and/or different course than patients with better insight.

Finally, comorbidity between OCD and schizophrenia has been of interest, particularly over the past decade. Evidence is emerging that obsessions and compulsions are more common in patients with schizophrenia than was previously thought. The effect of obsessions and compulsions on schizophrenia in terms of both treatment response and course is currently being investigated.

Despite tremendous advances in treatment of this potentially debilitating disorder, a significant percentage of OCD patients have symptoms that do not respond to standard treatment. Continued research to identify meaningful subtypes in OCD is necessary to unravel important questions about etiology and to develop specific treatment strategies for patients with treatment-refractory OCD.

◀ Key Clinical Points ▶

- Obsessive-compulsive disorder is an intriguing and often debilitating syndrome characterized by the presence of recurrent distressing thoughts, impulses, or images (obsessions) or repetitive behaviors or mental acts (compulsions).
- Previously considered extremely rare, OCD was the fourth most common psychiatric disorder (following the phobias, substance use disorders, and major depression) in the National Epidemiologic Catchment Area study, with a 6-month point prevalence of 1.6% and a lifetime prevalence of 2.5%. Its prevalence across national and ethnic populations is fairly consistent, allowing for methodological differences among studies.
- In adults, the most common obsession is fear of contamination, followed by over-responsibility for harm (e.g., fire or accidents), aggressive obsessions, and need for symmetry. The most common compulsion is checking, followed by washing, repeating routine activities, and ordering/arranging. Pure obsessions or pure compulsions are extremely rare.
- Children and adolescents with OCD present with similar OCD symptoms but may show some developmental differences.
- OCD follows a chronic waxing and waning course: most individuals with OCD improve, although many continue to have clinical or subclinical symptoms up to decades after the onset of illness.
- Factor-analytic and other approaches to OCD subtyping have potential genetic/neurobiological/etiological, treatment, and prognostic implications. For example, hoarding compulsions may be less responsive to treatment than other OCD subtypes.

References

American Psychiatric Association: Diagnostic and Statistical Manual of Mental Disorders, 3rd Edition. Washington, DC, American Psychiatric Association, 1980

American Psychiatric Association: Diagnostic and Statistical Manual of Mental Disorders, 3rd Edition, Revised. Washington, DC, American Psychiatric Association, 1987

American Psychiatric Association: Diagnostic and Statistical Manual of Mental Disorders, 4th Edition. Washington, DC, American Psychiatric Association, 1994

American Psychiatric Association: Diagnostic and Statistical Manual of Mental Disorders, 4th Edition, Text Revision. Washington, DC, American Psychiatric Association, 2000

Angst J, Gamma A, Endrass J, et al: Obsessive-compulsive severity spectrum in the community: prevalence, comorbidity, and course. Eur Arch Psychiatry Clin Neurosci 254:156–164, 2004

Apter A, Fallon TJ, King RA, et al: Obsessive compulsive characteristics: from symptoms to syndrome. J Am Acad Child Adolesc Psychiatry 35:907–912, 1996

Attiullah N, Eisen JL, Rasmussen SA: Clinical features of obsessive-compulsive disorder. Psychiatr Clin North Am 23:469–492, 2000

Baer L: Factor analysis of symptom subtypes of obsessive compulsive disorder and their relation to personality and tic disorders. J Clin Psychiatry 55(suppl):18–23, 1994

Baer L: Personality disorders in obsessive-compulsive disorder, in Obsessive-Compulsive Disorders: Practical Management, 3rd Edition. Edited by Jenike MA, Baer L, Minichiello WE. St Louis, MO, Mosby, 1998, pp 65–83

Baer L, Jenike MA, Ricciardi JN, et al: Standardized assessment of personality disorders in obsessive-compulsive disorder. Arch Gen Psychiatry 47:826–830, 1990

Baer L, Jenike MA, Black DW, et al: Effect of Axis II diagnoses on treatment outcome with clomipramine in 54 patients with obsessive compulsive disorder. Arch Gen Psychiatry 49:862–866, 1992

Barlow DH: Anxiety and Its Disorders: The Nature and Treatment of Anxiety and Panic. New York, Guilford, 1988

Bellodi L, Sciuto G, Diaferia G, et al: Psychiatric disorders in the families of patients with obsessive-compulsive disorder. Psychiatry Res 42:111–120, 1992

Berg CZ, Rapoport JL, Whitaker A, et al: Childhood obsessive compulsive disorder: a two-year prospective follow-up of a community sample. J Am Acad Child Adolesc Psychiatry 28:528–533, 1989

Berman I, Kalinowski A, Berman S, et al: Obsessive compulsive symptoms in chronic schizophrenia. Compr Psychiatry 36:6–10, 1995

Berman I, Merson A, Viegner B, et al: Obsessions and compulsions as a distinct cluster of symptoms in schizophrenia: a neuropsychological study. J Nerv Ment Dis 186:150–156, 1998

Berrios GE: Obsessive-compulsive disorder, in History of Clinical Psychiatry: The Origin and History of Psychiatric Disorders. Edited by Berrios GE, Porter RA. London, Athlone Press, 1995, pp 573–592

Black A: The natural history of obsessional neurosis, in Obsessional States. Edited by Beech HR. London, Methuen, 1974, pp 1–23

Boswell J: The Life of Dr. Johnson. London, Dent, 1791

Breier A, Charney DS, Heninger GR: Agoraphobia and panic disorder: development, diagnostic stability and course of illness. Arch Gen Psychiatry 43:1029–1036, 1986

Bruckl TM, Wittchen H, Hofler M, et al: Childhood separation anxiety and the risk of subsequent psychopathology: results from a community study. Psychother Psychosom 76:47–56, 2007

Burton R: The Anatomy of Melancholy (1621). London, Chatto and Windus, 1883

Chen YW, Dilsaver C: Comorbidity for obsessive compulsive disorder in bipolar and unipolar disorders. Psychiatry Res 59:57–64, 1995

Çilli AS, Telcioglu M, Aslin R, et al: Twelve-month prevalence of obsessive-compulsive disorder in Konya, Turkey. Compr Psychiatry 45:367–374, 2004

Coles ME, Frost RO, Heimberg RG, et al: "Not just right experiences": perfectionism, obsessive-compulsive features and general psychopathology. Behav Res Ther 41:681–700, 2003

Coles ME, Heimberg RG, Frost RO, et al: Not just right experiences and obsessive-compulsive features: experimental and self-monitoring perspectives. Behav Res Ther 43:153–167, 2005

Coles ME, Pinto A, Mancebo MC, et al: OCD with comorbid OCPD: a subtype of OCD? J Psychiatr Res 42:289–296, 2008

Coryell W: Obsessive compulsive disorder and primary unipolar depression: comparisons of background, family history, course and mortality. J Nerv Ment Dis 169:220–224, 1981

De Haan L, Hoogenboom B, Beuk N, et al: Obsessive-compulsive symptoms and positive, negative, and depressive symptoms in patients with recent-onset schizophrenic disorders. Can J Psychiatry 50:519–524, 2005

Degonda M, Wyss M, Angst J: The Zurich Study, XVIII: obsessive compulsive disorders and syndromes in the general population. Eur Arch Psychiatry Clin Neurosci 243:16–22, 1993

Demal U, Gerhard L, Mayrhofer A, et al: Obsessive-compulsive disorder and depression. Psychopathology 26:145–150, 1993

Douglass HM, Moffitt TE, Dar R, et al: Obsessive compulsive disorder in a birth cohort of 18 year olds: prevalence and predictors. J Am Acad Child Adolesc Psychiatry 34:1424–1431, 1995

Eisen JL, Rasmussen SA: OCD and compulsive traits: OCD with comorbid OCPD—a subtype of OCD?, in New Research Program and Abstracts, American Psychiatric Association 144th Annual Meeting, New Orleans, LA, May 11–16, 1991. Washington, DC, American Psychiatric Association, 1991

Eisen JL, Rasmussen SA: Obsessive compulsive disorder with psychotic features. J Clin Psychiatry 54:373–379, 1993

Eisen JL, Rasmussen SA, Goodman WK, et al: Remission and relapse in OCD: a two-year prospective study, in New Research Program and Abstracts, American Psychiatric Association 148th Annual Meeting, Miami, FL, 1995. Washington, DC, American Psychiatric Association, 1995

Eisen JL, Beer D, Pato MT, et al: Obsessive compulsive disorder in patients with schizophrenia or schizoaffective disorder. Am J Psychiatry 154:271–273, 1997

Eisen JL, Phillips K, Rasmussen SA, et al: The Brown Assessment of Beliefs Scale (BABS): reliability and validity. Am J Psychiatry 155:102–108, 1998

Eisen JL, Rasmussen SA, Phillips KA, et al: Insight and treatment outcome in obsessive-compulsive disorder. Compr Psychiatry 42:494–497, 2001

Eisen JL, Phillips KA, Coles ME, et al: Insight in obsessive compulsive disorder and body dysmorphic disorder. Compr Psychiatry 45:10–15, 2004

Endicott J, Spitzer RI, Fleiss JL, et al: The Global Assessment Scale: a procedure for measuring overall severity of psychiatric disturbance. Arch Gen Psychiatry 33:766–771, 1976

Esquirol JED: Des maladies mentales considérées sous les rapports médical, hygienique et médico-legal. Paris, Baillière, 1838

Fenton WS, McGlashan TH: The prognostic significance of obsessive-compulsive symptoms in schizophrenia. Am J Psychiatry 143:437–441, 1986

First MB, Spitzer RL, Gibbon M, et al: Structured Clinical Interview for DSM-IV Axis I Disorders, Patient Edition (SCID-I/P, version 2.0). New York, Biometrics Research, New York State Psychiatric Institute, 1996

Flament MF, Whitaker A, Rapoport JL, et al: Obsessive compulsive disorder in adolescence: an epidemiologic study. J Am Acad Child Adolesc Psychiatry 27:764–771, 1988

Flament MF, Koby E, Rapoport JL, et al: Childhood obsessive-compulsive disorder: a prospective follow-up study. J Child Psychol Psychiatry 31:363–380, 1990

Foa EB: Failure in treating obsessive-compulsives. Behav Res Ther 17:169–176, 1979

Foa EB, Kozak MJ: DSM-IV field trial: obsessive compulsive disorder. Am J Psychiatry 152:90–96, 1995

Foa EB, Grayson JB, Steketee GS, et al: Success and failure in the behavioral treatment of obsessive-compulsives. J Consult Clin Psychol 51:287–297, 1983

Fontenelle LF, Hasler G: The analytical epidemiology of obsessive-compulsive disorder: risk factors and correlates. Prog Neuropsychopharmacol Biol Psychiatry 32:1–15, 2008

Fontenelle LF, Medlowicz MV, Marques C, et al: Transcultural aspects of obsessive-compulsive disorder: a description of a Brazilian sample and a systematic review of international clinical studies. J Psychiatr Res 38:403–411, 2004

Fontenelle LF, Medlowicz MV, Versiani M: The descriptive epidemiology of obsessive-compulsive disorder. Prog Neuropsychopharmacol Biol Psychiatry 30:327–337, 2006

Freud S: On the grounds for detaching a particular syndrome from neurasthenia under the description "anxiety neurosis" (1895), in The Standard Edition of the Complete Psychological Works of Sigmund Freud, Vol 3. Translated and edited by Strachey J. London, Hogarth Press, 1962, pp 90–117

Freud S: Notes upon a case of obsessional neurosis (1909), in The Standard Edition of the Complete Psychological Works of Sigmund Freud, Vol 10. Translated and edited by Strachey J. London, Hogarth Press, 1955, pp 151–318

Frost RO, Gross RC: The hoarding of possessions. Behav Res Ther 31:367–381, 1993

Frost R, Hartl T: A cognitive-behavioral model of compulsive hoarding. Behav Res Ther 34:341–350, 1996

Geller D, Biederman J, Jones J, et al: Is juvenile obsessive-compulsive disorder a developmental subtype of the disorder? A review of the pediatric literature. J Am Acad Child Adolesc Psychiatry 37:420–427, 1998

Geller DA, Biederman J, Faraone S, et al: Developmental aspects of obsessive compulsive disorder: findings in children, adolescents, and adults. J Nerv Ment Dis 189:471–477, 2001

Godart N, Berthoz S, Rein Z, et al: Does the frequency of anxiety and depressive disorders differ between diagnostic subtypes of anorexia nervosa and bulimia? Int J Eat Disord 39:772–778, 2006

Goodman WK, Price LH, Rasmussen SA, et al: The Yale-Brown Obsessive Compulsive Scale (Y-BOCS), part I: reliability. Arch Gen Psychiatry 46:1006–1011, 1989a

Goodman WK, Price LH, Rasmussen SA, et al: The Yale-Brown Obsessive Compulsive Scale (Y-BOCS), part II: validity. Arch Gen Psychiatry 46:1012–1016, 1989b

Goodwin DW, Guze SB, Robbins E: Follow-up studies in obsessional neurosis. Arch Gen Psychiatry 20:182–187, 1969

Grant JE, Mancebo MC, Pinto A, et al: Late-onset obsessive compulsive disorder: clinical characteristics and psychiatric comorbidity. Psychiatry Res 152:21–27, 2007

Grimshaw L: The outcome of obsessional disorder: a follow-up study of 100 cases. Br J Psychiatry 111:1051–1056, 1965

Hantouche EG, Bouhassira M, Lancrenon S, et al: Prevalence of obsessive compulsive disorders in a large French patient population in psychiatric consultation. Encéphale 21:571–580, 1995

Hasler G, Pinto A, Greenberg BD, et al: Familiality of factor analysis-derived YBOCS dimensions in OCD-affected sibling pairs from the OCD Collaborative Genetics Study. Biol Psychiatry 61:617–625, 2007

Hodgson RJ, Rachman S: Obsessional-compulsive complaints. Behav Res Ther 15:389–395, 1977

Hollander E, Simeon D: Obsessive-compulsive disorder, in American Psychiatric Publishing Textbook of Clinical Psychiatry, 4th Edition. Washington, DC, American Psychiatric Publishing, 2003, pp 543–630

Holzer JC, Goodman WK, McDougle CJ, et al: Obsessive compulsive disorder with and without a chronic tic disorder. Br J Psychiatry 164:469–473, 1994

Hoogduin CA, Duivenvoorden HJ: A decision model in the treatment of obsessive-compulsive neuroses. Br J Psychiatry 152:516–521, 1988

Ingram E: Obsessional illness in mental hospital patients. J Ment Sci 107:382–402, 1961

Insel TR, Akiskal HS: Obsessive-compulsive disorder with psychotic features: a phenomenological analysis. Am J Psychiatry 143:1527–1533, 1986

Janet P: Les obsessions et la psychasthénie. Paris, Alcan, 1903

Jenike MA, Baer L, Minichiello WE, et al: Concomitant obsessive-compulsive disorder and schizotypal personality disorder. Am J Psychiatry 143:530–532, 1986

Karno M, Golding JM, Sorensen SB, et al: The epidemiology of obsessive-compulsive disorder in five US communities. Arch Gen Psychiatry 45:1094–1098, 1988

Kessler RC, Merikangas KR: The National Comorbidity Survey Replication (NCS-R): background and aims. Int J Methods Psychiatr Res 3:60–68, 2004

Kessler RC, Ustun TB: The World Mental Health (WMH) Survey Initiative Version of the World Health Organization (WHO) Composite International Diagnostic Interview (CIDI). Int J Methods Psychiatr Res 13:93–121, 2004

Kessler RC, Berglund P, Demler O, et al: Lifetime prevalence and age-of-onset distributions of DSM-IV disorders in the National Comorbidity Survey Replication (NCS-R). Arch Gen Psychiatry 62:593–602, 2005a

Kessler RC, Chiu WT, Demler O, et al: Prevalence, severity, and comorbidity of twelve-month DSM-IV disorders in the National Comorbidity Survey (NCS-R). Arch Gen Psychiatry 62:617–627, 2005b

Kozak MJ, Foa EB: Obsessions, overvalued ideas, and delusions in obsessive-compulsive disorder. Behav Res Ther 32:343–353, 1994

Kringlin E: Obsessional neurotics: a long-term follow-up. Br J Psychiatry 111:709–722, 1965

Krüger S, Cooke RG, Hasey GM, et al: Comorbidity of obsessive compulsive disorder in bipolar disorder. J Affect Disord 34:117–120, 1995

Labad J, Menchon JM, Alonso P, et al: Gender differences in obsessive-compulsive symptom dimensions. Depress Anxiety 25:832–835, 2007

Leckman JF, Walker DE, Cohen DJ: Premonitory urges in Tourette syndrome. Am J Psychiatry 150:98–102, 1993

Leckman JF, Walker DE, Goodman WK, et al: "Just right" perceptions associated with compulsive behavior in Tourette's syndrome. Am J Psychiatry 151:675–680, 1994

Leckman JF, Grice DE, Boardman J, et al: Symptoms of obsessive-compulsive disorder. Am J Psychiatry 154:911–917, 1997

Lelliott PT, Noshirvani HF, Basoglu M, et al: Obsessive-compulsive beliefs and treatment outcome. Psychol Med 18:697–702, 1988

Leonard HL, Swedo SE, Rapoport JL, et al: Treatment of childhood obsessive-compulsive disorder with clomipramine and desipramine: a double blind crossover comparison. Arch Gen Psychiatry 46:1088–1092, 1989

Leonard HL, Swedo SE, Lenane MC, et al: A 2- to 7-year follow-up study of 54 obsessive compulsive children and adolescents. Arch Gen Psychiatry 50:429–439, 1993

Lewis AJ: Problems of obsessional illness. Proc R Soc Med 29:325–336, 1936

Lipsitz JD, Martin LY, Mannuzza S, et al: Childhood separation anxiety disorder in patients with adult anxiety disorders. Am J Psychiatry 151:927–929, 1994

Lo WH: A follow-up study of obsessional neurotics in Hong Kong Chinese. Br J Psychiatry 113:823–832, 1967

MacLean PD: Brain evolution relating to family, play, and the separation call. Arch Gen Psychiatry 42:405–417, 1985

Maina G, Albert U, Pessina E, et al: Bipolar obsessive-compulsive disorder and personality disorders. Bipolar Disord 9:722–729, 2007

Mancebo MC, Eisen JL, Pinto A, et al: The Brown Longitudinal Obsessive Compulsive Study: treatments received and patient impressions of improvement. J Clin Psychiatry 67:1713–1720, 2006

Mancebo MC, Garcia AM, Pinto A, et al: Juvenile-onset OCD: clinical features in children, adolescents and adults. Poster presented at the 12th annual Brown Research Symposium on Mental Health Sciences, Providence, RI, March 27, 2008

Mataix-Cols D, do Rosario-Campos MC, Leckman JF: A multidimensional model of obsessive-compulsive disorder. Am J Psychiatry 162:228–238, 2005

Mellman TA, Uhde TW: Obsessive compulsive symptoms in panic disorder. Am J Psychiatry 144:1573–1576, 1986

Miguel EC, Coffey BJ, Baer L, et al: Phenomenology of intentional repetitive behaviors in obsessive compulsive disorder and Tourette's disorder. J Clin Psychiatry 56:246–255, 1995

Miguel EC, Baer L, Coffey BJ, et al: Phenomenological differences appearing with repetitive behaviours in obsessive-compulsive disorder and Gilles de la Tourette's syndrome. Br J Psychiatry 170:140–145, 1997

Miguel EC, do Rosário-Campos MC, Prado SH, et al: Sensory phenomena in patients with obsessive-compulsive disorder and Tourette's syndrome. J Clin Psychiatry 61:150–156, 2000

Mora G: The scrupulosity syndrome. Int J Clin Psychology 5:163–174, 1969

Morel BA: Du délire emotif. Nevrose du systeme nerveus ganglionaire viscerale. Archives Générales de Médecine 7:385–402, 1866

Muller C: Der Ubergong zwangsnevrose in Schizphrenic im Licht der Katamnese. Schweiz Arch Neurol Psychiatr 72:218–225, 1953

Myers JK, Weissman MM, Tischler GL, et al: Six month prevalence of psychiatric disorders in three communities, 1980 to 1982. Arch Gen Psychiatry 41:949–958, 1984

Nestadt G, Samuels J, Riddle M, et al: A family study of obsessive-compulsive disorder. Arch Gen Psychiatry 57:358–363, 2000

Neziroglu F, McKay KP, Yaryura-Tobias JA, et al: The Overvalued Ideas Scale: development, reliability and validity in obsessive-compulsive disorder. Behav Res Ther 37:881–902, 1999a

Neziroglu F, Stevens K, Yaryura-Tobias JA: Overvalued ideas and their impact on treatment outcome. Rev Brasileira Psiquiatr 21:209–214, 1999b

Orloff LM, Battle MA, Baer L, et al: Long term follow-up of 85 patients with obsessive compulsive disorder. Am J Psychiatry 51:441–442, 1994

Pauls DL, Alsobrook MP, Goodman W, et al: A family study of obsessive compulsive disorder. Am J Psychiatry 152:76–84, 1995

Peterson BS, Pine DS, Cohen P, et al: Prospective, longitudinal study of tic, obsessive-compulsive, and attention-deficit/hyperactivity disorders in an epidemiological sample. J Am Acad Child Adolesc Psychiatry 40:685–695, 2001

Phillips KA, McElroy SL, Dwight MM, et al: Delusionality and response to open-label fluvoxamine in body dysmorphic disorder. J Clin Psychiatry 62:87–91, 2001

Phillips KA, Pinto A, Menard W, et al: Obsessive-compulsive disorder versus body dysmorphic disorder: a comparison study of two possibly related disorders. Depress Anxiety 24:399–409, 2007

Pinto A, Mancebo, MC, Eisen JL, et al: The Brown Longitudinal Obsessive Compulsive Study: clinical features and symptoms of the sample at intake. J Clin Psychiatry 67:703–711, 2006

Pinto A, Eisen JL, Mancebo MC, et al: Taboo thoughts and doubt/checking: a refinement of the factor structure for obsessive compulsive disorder symptoms. Psychiatry Res 151:255–258, 2007a

Pinto A, Eisen JL, Mancebo MC, et al: A 2-year follow-up study of the course of obsessive compulsive disorder. Poster presented at the annual meeting of the Association for Behavioral and Cognitive Therapies, Philadelphia, PA, 2007b

Pinto A, Greenberg BD, Grados MA, et al: Further development of YBOCS dimensions in the OCD Collaborative Genetics Study: symptoms vs. categories. Psychiatry Res 160:83–93, 2008

Pitman RK: Pierre Janet on obsessive-compulsive disorder (1903). Review and commentary. Arch Gen Psychiatry 44:226–232, 1987

Pollitt JD: Natural history of obsessional states: a study of 150 cases. Br Med J 1:194–198, 1957

Porto L, Bermanzohn PC, Pollack S, et al: A profile of obsessive-compulsive symptoms in schizophrenia. CNS Spectr 2:21–25, 1997

Poyurovsky M, Faragian S, Kleinman-Balush V, et al: Awareness of illness and insight into obsessive-compulsive symptoms in schizophrenia patients with obsessive-compulsive disorder. J Nerv Ment Dis 195:765–768, 2007

Rachman S, DeSilva P: Abnormal and normal obsessions. Behav Res Ther 16:233–248, 1978

Rachman S, Hodgson RL: Obsessions and Compulsions. Englewood Cliffs, NJ, Prentice Hall, 1980

Rasmussen SA, Eisen JL: Clinical and epidemiologic findings of significance to neuropharmacologic trials in OCD. Psychopharmacol Bull 24:466–470, 1988

Rasmussen SA, Eisen JL: Phenomenology of obsessive compulsive disorder, in Psychobiology of Obsessive Compulsive Disorder. Edited by Insel J, Rasmussen SA. New York, Springer-Verlag, 1991, pp 743–758

Rasmussen SA, Eisen JL: The epidemiology and clinical features of obsessive-compulsive disorder, in Obsessive-Compulsive Disorder: Practical Management, 3rd Edition. Edited by Jenike MA, Baer L, Minichiello WE. St Louis, MO, Mosby, 1998, pp 12–43

Rasmussen SA, Tsuang MT: DSM-III obsessive compulsive disorder: clinical characteristics and family history. Am J Psychiatry 143:317–322, 1986

Rastam M, Gillberg IC, Gillberg C: Anorexia nervosa 6 years after onset, part II: comorbid psychiatric problems. Compr Psychiatry 36:70–76, 1995

Ravi Kishore V, Samar R, Janardhan Reddy YC, et al: Clinical characteristics and treatment response in poor and good insight obsessive-compulsive disorder. Eur Psychiatry 19:202–208, 2004

Robins LN, Helzer JE, Weissman MM, et al: Lifetime prevalence of specific psychiatric disorders in three sites. Arch Gen Psychiatry 41:958–967, 1984

Robins LN, Marcus L, Reich W, et al: National Institute of Mental Health Diagnostic Interview Schedule, Version IV. St Louis, MO, Department of Psychiatry, Washington University School of Medicine, 1996

Rosario-Campos MC, Leckman JF, Mercadante MT, et al: Adults with early-onset obsessive-compulsive disorder. Am J Psychiatry 158:1899–1903, 2001

Rosenberg CM: Complications of obsessional neurosis. Br J Psychiatry 114:447–478, 1968

Rudin E: Ein Beitrag zur Frage der Zwangskrankheit insebesondere ihrere hereditarenBeziehungen. Arch Psychiatr Nervenkr 191:14–54, 1953

Rush AJ, Pincus HA, First MB, et al: Handbook of Psychiatric Measures. Washington, DC, American Psychiatric Press, 2000

Salbach-Andrae H, Lenz K, Simmendinger N, et al: Psychiatric comorbidities among female adolescents with anorexia nervosa. Child Psychiatry Hum Dev 39:261–272, 2008

Samuels JF, Bienvenu OJ III, Pinto A, et al: Hoarding in obsessive-compulsive disorder: results from the OCD Collaborative Genetics Study. Behav Res Ther 45:673–686, 2007

Saxena S: Is compulsive hoarding a genetically and neurobiologically discrete syndrome? Implications for diagnostic classification. Am J Psychiatry 164:380–384, 2007

Skoog G, Skoog I: A 40-year follow-up of patients with obsessive-compulsive disorder. Arch Gen Psychiatry 56:121–127, 1999

Stein MB, Forde DR, Anderson G, et al: Obsessive-compulsive disorder in the community: an epidemiologic survey with clinical reappraisal. Am J Psychiatry 154:1120–1126, 1997

Steinglass JE, Eisen JL, Attia E, et al: Is anorexia nervosa a delusional disorder? An assessment of eating beliefs in anorexia nervosa. J Psychiatr Pract 13:65–71, 2007

Steketee G, Eisen J, Dyck I, et al: Predictors of course in obsessive-compulsive disorder. Psychiatry Res 89:229–238, 1999

Stengel E: A study of some clinical aspects of the relationship between obsessional neurosis and psychotic reaction types. J Ment Sci 91:166–187, 1945

Summerfeldt L: Understanding and treating incompleteness in obsessive-compulsive disorder. J Clin Psychol 60:1155–1168, 2004

Swedo SE, Rapoport JL, Leonard H, et al: Obsessive-compulsive disorder in children and adolescents: clinical phenomenology of 70 consecutive cases. Arch Gen Psychiatry 46:335–341, 1989

Swedo SE, Leonard HL, Garvey M, et al: Pediatric autoimmune neuropsychiatric disorders associated with streptococcal infections: clinical description of the first 50 cases. Am J Psychiatry 155:264–271, 1998

Tadai T, Nakamura M, Okazaki S, et al: The prevalence of obsessive compulsive disorder in Japan: a study of students using the Maudsley Obsessional-Compulsive Inventory and DSM-III-R. Psychiatry Clin Neurosci 49:39–41, 1995

Thiel A, Broocks A, Ohlmeier M, et al: Obsessive compulsive disorder among patients with anorexia nervosa and bulimia nervosa. Am J Psychiatry 152:72–75, 1995

Thomsen PH: Obsessive-compulsive disorder in children and adolescents: predictors in childhood for long-term phenomenological course. Acta Psychiatr Scand 92:255–259, 1995

Torres AR, Prince MJ, Bebbinggton PE, et al: Treatment seeking by individuals with obsessive-compulsive disorder from the British Psychiatric Morbidity Survey of 2000. Psychiatr Serv 58:977–982, 2007

Valleni-Basile LA, Garrison CZ, Jackson KL, et al: Frequency of obsessive compulsive disorder in a community sample of young adolescents. J Am Acad Child Adolesc Psychiatry 34:782–791, 1994

Weissman MM, Bland RC, Canino GJ, et al: The cross national epidemiology of obsessive compulsive disorder. J Clin Psychiatry 55(suppl): 5–10, 1994

World Health Organization: International Classification of Diseases, 9th Revision. Geneva, Switzerland, World Health Organization, 1977

Zohar AH, Ratzoni G, Pauls DL, et al: An epidemiological study of obsessive-compulsive disorder and related disorders in Israeli adolescents. J Am Acad Child Adolesc Psychiatry 31:1057–1061, 1992

Zutshi A, Kamath P, Reddy YC: Bipolar and nonbipolar obsessive-compulsive disorder: a clinical exploration. Compr Psychiatry 48:245–251, 2007

Recommended Readings

Berrios GE: Obsessive-compulsive disorder, in History of Clinical Psychiatry: The Origin and History of Psychiatric Disorders. Edited by Berrios GE, Porter RA. London, Athlone Press, 1995, pp 573–592 [*History*]

Eisen JL, Phillips K, Rasmussen SA, et al: The Brown Assessment of Beliefs Scale (BABS): reliability and validity. Am J Psychiatry 155:102–108, 1998 [*Evaluation, insight*]

Fontenelle LF, Medlowicz MV, Versiani M: The descriptive epidemiology of obsessive-compulsive disorder. Prog Neuropsychopharmacol Biol Psychiatry 30:327–337, 2006 [*Epidemiology, descriptive*]

Fontenelle LF, Hasler G: The analytical epidemiology of obsessive-compulsive disorder: risk factors and correlates. Prog Neuropsychopharmacol Biol Psychiatry 32:1–15, 2008 [*Epidemiology, risk factors, and comorbidity*]

Goodman WK, Price LH, Rasmussen SA, et al.: The Yale-Brown Obsessive Compulsive Scale (Y-BOCS), part I: reliability. Arch Gen Psychiatry 46:1006–1011, 1989a [*Evaluation, symptom checklist and severity*]

Goodman WK, Price LH, Rasmussen SA, et al: The Yale-Brown Obsessive Compulsive Scale (Y-BOCS), part II: validity. Arch Gen Psychiatry 46:1012–1016, 1989b [*Evaluation, symptom checklist, and severity*]

Mataix-Cols D, do Rosario-Campos MC, Leckman JF: A multidimensional model of obsessive-compulsive disorder. Am J Psychiatry 162:228–238, 2005 [*Subtypes*]

Pinto A, Mancebo MC, Eisen JL, et al: The Brown Longitudinal Obsessive Compulsive Study: clinical features and symptoms of the sample at intake. J Clin Psychiatry 67:703–711, 2006 [*Clinical features*]

Skoog G, Skoog I: A 40-year follow-up of patients with obsessive-compulsive disorder. Arch Gen Psychiatry 56:121–127, 1999 [*Natural history/course of illness*]

Chapter 17

Pathophysiology of Obsessive-Compulsive Disorders

Darin D. Dougherty, M.D.
Scott L. Rauch, M.D.
Benjamin D. Greenberg, M.D., Ph.D.

Obsessive-compulsive disorder (OCD) is a heterogeneous entity. One of the more important concepts to emerge in the past two decades of OCD research is the realization that the obvious clinical variability associated with the diagnosis likely reflects neurobiologically meaningful subtypes or dimensions of disease, in terms of both etiology and pathophysiology. In this chapter, we will review several etiological and pathophysiological models, emphasizing the ways in which disparate data may well reflect real differences among OCD subtypes. Likewise, the discussion will be extended to other diagnostic entities that may share common pathophysiological features with OCD and thus implicate a neurobiologically based obsessive-compulsive (OC) spectrum of disease. In this context, it is interesting that OCD remains categorized among the anxiety disorders, despite accruing evidence that it appears to be closely related to an array of other disorders that are scattered across DSM-IV (American Psychiatric Association 1994).

In broad terms, the shared phenomenology of OC spectrum disorders is fundamentally characterized by intrusive events leading to repetitive behaviors (Miguel et al. 1995; Rauch and Jenike 1997; Rauch et al. 1998c). In the case of OCD, the intrusive events are of a cognitive nature (obsessions) and prompt intentional repetitive behaviors (compulsions) that serve to neutralize the cognitive intrusions themselves, as well as accompanying anxiety. In an analogous fashion, the tics of Tourette syndrome (TS) are typically performed in response to sensory intrusions (Leckman et al. 1993; Miguel et al. 1995); in the minority of cases in which the tics occur spontaneously, they can be conceptualized as motor intrusions. By extension, the phenomenology of trichotillomania (TTM) may be more reminiscent of a tic, whereas body dysmorphic disorder (BDD), with its prominent cognitive intrusive phenomena, may be more akin to OCD.

On the one hand, according to this heuristic, the shared pathophysiology of OC spectrum disorders should entail some basis for intrusive events. On the other hand, the distinctions among the various disorders should reflect the differential involvement of sensorimotor versus cognitive representations. Moreover, there must be some explanation for why the repetitive behavior ultimately leads to temporary waning of the intrusive symptoms and, consequently, a temporary decrement in the drive to perform the repetitive behavior.

In this chapter, we begin by reviewing family genetic data that support a genetic vulnerability to development of OCD and that suggest a relationship between one subtype of OCD and TS. We review neurochemical models of OCD, emphasizing the role of serotonergic systems. We assess neuroendocrine factors in the pathophysiology of OCD and the issue of an immunologic etiology for some individuals with OCD or related disorders, as a putative mechanism leading to striatal pathology. We present a brief heuristic model of OCD and related disorders that is based on phenomenological characteristics and is informed by neuroanatomical considerations. We outline the relevant functional anatomy of corticostriatothalamocortical (CSTC) circuitry and review data that implicate various elements of this system in different subtypes of OCD and in other candidate OC spectrum disorders. We discuss psychological factors such as childhood and developmental factors, personality factors, cognitive-behavioral factors, information processing, cultural factors, and others, and their possible relationship to the pathophysiology of OCD. In closing, we attempt to provide an integrated view of pathogenetic models as they pertain to OCD and related disorders, and we conclude by foreshadowing future research directions in this field.

Biological Factors

Genetics of OCD and Related Disorders

The genetics of OCD and related disorders have been the subject of considerable and continuing interest. Numerous approaches have been used. These approaches and some representative results are summarized briefly below. More detailed descriptions of the status of this field and current approaches are available elsewhere Bienvenu et al. 2000; Grados and Mathews 2008; Grados and Wilcox 2007; Pauls 2008; Samuels and Nestadt 1997).

Twin Studies

Few twin studies of OCD and related disorders have been performed. Inouye (1965) reported OC symptom concordance rates of 80% (8/10) in monozygotic twin pairs compared with 50% (2/4) in dizygotic twin pairs; Carey and Gottesman (1981) reported rates of 87% (13/15) and 47% (7/15), respectively, in another series. A review of OCD twin studies (van Grootheest et al. 2005) concluded that OC symptoms are heritable, with genetic influences ranging from 45% to 65% in children and from 27% to 47% in adults. Age-at-onset data suggest that there may be OCD subgroups. One study revealed statistically validated age-at-onset cutoff points, based on two Gaussian distributions, at ages 11.1±4.1 and 23.5±11 years (Delorme et al. 2005). Prevalence of OCD in relatives of probands with pediatric OCD is about 22%, whereas only 11% of relatives of adult OCD probands have the disorder (Nestadt et al. 2000; Pauls et al. 1995). Together, these studies suggest that genetic etiologies might contribute more frequently to pathogenesis in pediatric OCD than in adult-onset cases, a finding relevant to future genetics research.

Twin studies demonstrate that concordance rates for chronic tic disorders are analogous to those in OCD. The rates across several studies varied in range, from approximately 75%–90% for monozygotic twins to 10%–20% for dizygotic twins (see Alsobrook and Pauls 1997). If OCD or TS were solely dependent on genetic factors, one would predict about 100% concordance among monozygotic twins and about 50% among dizygotic twins. Conversely, if these disorders were wholly attributable to epigenetic or nongenetic factors, one would expect little disparity between the rates for monozygotic and dizygotic twin pairs. Therefore, despite the limited data from these twin-pair case series, they are consistent with a substantial genetic component in the etiology of OCD and chronic tic disorders.

Family Studies

Family studies have established that OCD is indeed a familial disorder, and researchers have investigated the recurrence risk for OCD among relatives of affected individuals. The results of these studies have also helped to establish possible familial relationships between OCD and comorbid conditions. Most such studies use a case-control design. Affected probands and controls are first identified, and the relatives of each group are then assessed by interviewers masked to the probands' status. Such studies found as early as the 1930s that obsessional neurosis was familial. More than one-third of parents and one-fifth of siblings shared the condition (Lewis 1935). Studies in the modern era have confirmed these early findings, with broadly defined OCD present in approximately 16%–18% of relatives of affected probands, compared with 2%–3% in parents of control subjects (Black et al. 1992; Pauls et al. 1995). Nestadt et al. (2000) found the prevalence of narrowly defined OCD was 12% in relatives of OCD probands and 3% in relatives of control subjects. A meta-analysis of five studies that included 1,209 first-degree relatives indicated an increased risk of OCD among relatives of probands (8.2%) versus control subjects (2.0%; odds ratio=4.0) (Hettema et al. 2001).

With regard to the relationship between OCD and tic disorders, Pauls et al. (1995) performed several influential family genetic studies focusing on OCD and TS. In 1995, they compared prevalence rates in first-degree relatives of OCD probands with first-degree relatives of psychiatrically normal control subjects; significant differences were found with respect to OCD (10.3% vs. 1.9%), subthreshold OCD (7.9% vs. 2.0%), OCD plus subthreshold OCD (18.2% vs. 4.0%), and tics (4.6% vs. 1.0%). Moreover, the risks to relatives were higher among probands who had early-onset OCD (i.e., <19 years old). Similarly, Leonard et al. (1992) studied children and adolescents with OCD and found an earlier age of OCD onset in probands who developed comorbid TS as well as an elevated lifetime prevalence of tics in their first-degree relatives (14%). Conversely, family genetic studies have found a significantly greater prevalence of OCD in first-degree relatives of probands with TS, regardless of OCD comorbidity in the probands (Pauls et al. 1986, 1995). In two studies of TS probands for which segregation analysis was employed, Pauls and colleagues found familial patterns of TS, chronic tics, and OCD that were consistent with an autosomal dominant mode of transmission with incomplete penetrance (Pauls and Leckman 1986; Pauls et al. 1990). Two subsequent studies have ostensibly replicated these findings (Eapen et al. 1993; van de Wetering 1993). Across studies, the penetrance rates have ranged from 0.5 to 0.9 for males and 0.2 to 0.8 for females (see Alsobrook and Pauls 1997).

Interestingly, there are hints that pediatric and adult-onset OCD may display different patterns of comorbidity. In adult-onset OCD, Black et al. (1992) found that in first-degree relatives of affected individuals, the rate of OCD was low but the rate of anxiety disorders was high. This finding suggests a familial vulnerability to anxiety pathology that might not be specific to OCD when probands had adult OCD onset. Hanna et al. (2005) demonstrated that early-onset OCD is highly familial and that within OCD symptom subtypes, ordering compulsions are familial. Tics also aggregated in these families, in accordance with other studies focused on children and adolescents, which found greater familial risk of tics (9.5%–17%) compared with later-onset OCD (Bellodi et al. 1992; Chabane et al. 2005; Lenane et al. 1990; Leonard et al. 1992; Reddy et al. 2001; Riddle et al. 1990; Rosario-Campos et al. 2005). Given that only approximately half of OCD cases might be familial (Cavallini et al. 1999; Eapen et al. 1993; Nicolini et al. 1996), the family genetic contribution is likely to be weighted less in adult-onset cases. This finding suggests that other etiological factors might be involved in such sporadic (nonfamilial) cases of OCD, in addition to a possible anxiety-affective diathesis suggested by Black et al. (1992).

Linkage Studies

Linkage studies aim to identify genetic loci that are transmitted with a diagnosis in affected families. One challenge for this technique is that transmitted genetic variants need to be above a threshold level of etiological significance to be detected. Another is that mutations may be associated with a diagnosis (such as OCD) in only some families and not in others. Despite these limitations, linkage studies have suggested at least one positional candidate for OCD, on chromosome 9p24, where a glutamate transporter gene, *SLC1A1*, is located (Hanna et al. 2002). Chromosome 9p24 was also associated with OCD in other studies (see Grados and Wilcox 2007 for review). Two additional linkage studies of OCD have been published (Samuels et al. 2007; Shugart et al. 2006). These, together with other genetic approaches and refinements in OCD phenotypes, are expected to provide additional promising leads.

Candidate Gene Approaches

To the extent that OCD has a genetic origin, it is foreseeable that discrete genes responsible for conferring increased risk will ultimately be identified and fully characterized. To date, multiple studies have used association strategies focusing on genes where differences in gene product function would plausibly be involved in risk for OCD and/or course of illness or responses to treatment. These include genes coding for the serotonin transporter and its upstream promotor region (Hanna et al. 1998; Hu et al. 2006; Mundo et al. 2002) and serotonergic receptors (5-HT_{1A} [Brett et al. 1995], 5-HT_{2A} [Enoch et al. 2001], 5-HT_{2B} [Kim et al. 2000], 5-HT_{2C} [Cavallini et al. 1998], 5-HT_{1B} [Mundo et al. 2002]), as well as tryptophan hydroxylase (Walitza et al. 2005). Genes related to dopamine function studied in OCD include those related to the dopamine transporter (Billett et al. 1998; Rowe et al. 1998), postsynaptic receptors (D_2, D_3, and D_4 [Cruz et al. 1997]), and enzymes including catechol-*O*-methyltranferase (COMT) (Alsobrook et al. 2002) and monoamine oxidase A (MAO-A) (Camerena et al. 2001; Karayiorgou et al. 1999). Glutamate-related genes, including *GRIK* (glutamate receptor, ionotropic, kainate) (Delmore et al. 2004; Stewart et al., "Family-Based Association Between Obsessive-Compulsive Disorder and Glutamate Receptor

Genes GRIN2B and GRIK," unpublished manuscript), *GRIN* (Arnold et al. 2004; Stewart et al., unpublished manuscript), and *SLC-1A1* (Arnold et al. 2006; Dickel et al. 2006; Stewart et al. 2007a), have also been studied. Finally, white matter genes such as *OLIG2* (Stewart et al. 2007b) and *MOG* (Zai et al. 2004), have been studied as well. Although investigators have searched for a role for all of these genes in the pathophysiology of OCD, it is unlikely that any single gene plays a large role in the pathophysiology of OCD. Instead, OCD is likely to be related to small, cumulative effects from some of these genes. Thus far, few of the findings regarding candidate genes and OCD have been replicated in large samples.

Taken together, currently available data suggest that the risk for developing OCD is often inherited. Specifically, there appear to be at least two familial forms of OCD: one that is characterized by an early age of onset and an association with chronic tic disorders (including TS), and a second familial form that is not tic related (Alsobrook and Pauls 1997; Pauls et al. 1995). Thus, pathogenetic models of OCD and related disorders must account for an inherited component, together with epigenetic influences on expression. Moreover, in the case of tic-related OCD, pathogenetic models should explain the spectrum of clinical presentation, in terms of both phenomenology and treatment response. Finally, there is a third group of patients with OCD for whom no familial relationship is evident. These sporadic cases may well represent phenocopies of the disorder attributable to a variety etiologies, including unrecognized general medical causes (e.g., infarction, tumor); consequently, this third group is likely to reflect a high degree of pathophysiological heterogeneity as well.

Neurochemistry and Neuropharmacology of OCD and Related Disorders

Neurotransmitters mediate communication among the cells that comprise the neuroanatomical constructs discussed previously in this chapter. Furthermore, the neurochemistry and molecular biology of neuronal events form the basis of neuropsychiatric health and disease. In this section, we review the role of serotonergic and dopaminergic systems in OCD and related disorders.

Serotonin and the Pathogenesis of OCD and Related Disorders

Serotonin is a neurotransmitter that is released from neurons whose cell bodies are located within the raphe nuclei of the midbrain. Serotonergic projections from the raphe are widespread. Moreover, there are numerous different serotonergic receptor subtypes, each with its own profile in terms of distribution in brain, location on neurons, effector mechanisms (e.g., second messengers), and influences on neuronal firing (Hoyer et al. 1994). Consequently, dissection of the serotonergic system is a complex and challenging enterprise.

A serotonergic hypothesis of OCD was originally prompted by the observed differential efficacy of serotonergic reuptake inhibitors (SRIs) in alleviating OCD symptoms (Fernandez and Lopez-Ibor 1967; Greist et al. 1995; Insel et al. 1983; Leonard et al. 1989; Murphy et al. 1996; Thoren et al. 1980; Zohar and Insel 1987). There was instant appeal to the concept that SRIs might be producing their antiobsessional effects by correcting some fundamental abnormality in the serotonergic system. However, the fact that medications with serotonergic action serve as effective antiobsessionals does not necessarily mean that the serotonergic system is fundamentally dysfunctional in OCD. Rather, SRIs may act via modulation of an intact system to compensate for underlying pathophysiology in OCD that is otherwise unrelated to serotonin function. Thus, it is critical to distinguish between these different concepts; while some research efforts may speak to the hypothesis of the existence of a primary serotonergic abnormality in patients with OCD, others more directly address how and where SRIs confer their beneficial antiobsessional effects.

A considerable literature has accrued that is based on indirect measurements of serotonergic function in OCD. Numerous studies of peripheral receptor binding in the blood or concentrations of 5-HT metabolites in cerebrospinal fluid have been performed, but these studies have yielded disappointingly inconsistent results (see Barr et al. 1992 and Marazziti et al. 1994 for reviews). Furthermore, these measures do not necessarily represent accurate indicators of serotonergic function within the brain. Pharmacological challenge studies provide another indirect approach. By administering serotonergic agents and measuring endocrine or behavioral variables, investigators have attempted to assess central serotonergic sensitivities. For example, *m*-chlorophenylpiperazine (m-CPP) was found to exacerbate OCD symptoms in four studies (Hollander et al. 1992; Khanna et al. 2001; Pigott et al. 1991; Zohar et al. 1987), but not in two others (Goodman et al. 1995; Ho Pian et al. 1998). However, pharmacological challenge studies utilizing lactate (Gorman et al. 1985), carbon dioxide (Perna et al. 1995), yohimbine (Rasmussen et al. 1987), and cholecystokinin (CCK) receptor agonists (de Leeuw et al. 1996) for anxiogenic purposes have not exacerbated OCD symptoms. This suggests specific serotonergic dysfunction associated with OCD.

Methods for probing the serotonergic system in brain are necessary for directly testing a serotonergic hypothesis of OCD pathophysiology. With the advent of functional imaging receptor characterization techniques, such studies are now feasible. Thus far, most such studies have focused on the role of the serotonin transporter in the pathophysiology of OCD. Using single-photon emission computed tomography (SPECT) and [^{123}I]β-CIT, two studies (Hesse et al. 2005; Zitterl et al. 2007) have found a reduction in serotonin transporter binding in the thalamus/hypothalamus that correlated with symptom severity in OCD cohorts. One of these studies also found decreased serotonin transporter binding in the midbrain and brain stem (Hesse et al. 2005). However, another study using SPECT and [^{123}I]β-CIT found increased serotonin transporter binding in the midbrain (Pogarell et al. 2003). Lastly, one SPECT study using [^{123}I]β-CIT failed to find any difference between OCD subjects and psychiatrically healthy control subjects (van der Wee et al. 2004). One study (Simpson et al. 2003) using positron emission tomography and the serotonin transporter ligand [^{11}C]McN 5652 failed to show a difference between OCD subjects and psychiatrically healthy control subjects, whereas another (Reimold et al. 2007), utilizing the serotonin transporter ligand [^{11}C]DASB, showed reduced binding in the thalamus and midbrain of subjects with OCD when compared to psychiatrically healthy control subjects.

Finally, considerable pharmacological research has begun to clarify the therapeutic mechanisms of SRIs. Animal studies indicate that antidepressants can potentiate serotonergic transmission (Blier and de Montigny 1994). In the case of SRIs, potentiation of serotonergic transmission appears to be mediated by autoreceptor desensitization (Blier and Bouchard 1994; Blier et al. 1988). The time course of these receptor changes parallels the observed delay between initiation of SRIs and onset of therapeutic response. In an important study, Mansari et al. (1995) showed that SRI-induced changes in serotonergic transmission occur more quickly in lateral frontal cortex than in medial frontal cortex of rodents. This corresponds beautifully with the observation that the antidepressant effects of SRIs tend to occur sooner than antiobsessional effects (Fineberg et al. 1992). Furthermore, current models of mediating anatomy suggest that lateral prefrontal areas are involved in the pathophysiology of major depression, whereas medial frontal (i.e., orbitofrontal) cortex has been implicated in the pathophysiology of OCD. The ultimate neuropharmacological effects of SRIs on frontal cortex and other relevant territories remain to be fully delineated. Likewise, the relative role of different receptor subtypes (see Pineyro et al. 1994), as well as downstream effects on second messengers and genetic transcription factors (see Lesch et al. 1993), requires further study.

In summary, although there is some evidence to support a serotonergic hypothesis of OCD pathophysiology, modulation of serotonergic systems clearly plays a role in the effective pharmacotherapy of OCD with serotonergic agents. Emerging data suggest that SRIs might produce their beneficial effects, following a delay of several weeks after treatment initiation, by downregulating terminal autoreceptors (5-HT_{1D}) in orbitofrontal cortex, thereby facilitating serotonergic transmission in that region (Mansari et al. 1995). Advances in radiochemistry and pharmacology, together with contemporary in vivo neuroimaging methods, should soon provide an opportunity to directly test the serotonergic hypothesis of OCD pathophysiology. Additional studies will be necessary to clarify the precise mechanisms that underlie the antiobsessional effects of SRIs as well as those of other effective treatments, including nonpharmacological modalities.

Finally, it is not clear how this information generalizes to other OC spectrum disorders. SRIs appear to be of modest therapeutic benefit for BDD and TTM but are not typically effective for reducing the tics of TS (although they can be helpful in addressing other associated affective or behavioral manifestations). Thus, a model of SRI action in OCD must explain the observed differential efficacy across this spectrum of disorders. Given the data at hand, it may be that SRIs exert their effects by modulating corticostriatal systems at the level of cortex and with prominent effects within medial and lateral prefrontal zones. Therefore, OC spectrum disorders that entail dysfunction within the cognitive and affective corticostriatal circuits might be preferentially responsive to SRIs; chronic tics involving sensorimotor cortex may be unresponsive to such interventions.

Dopaminergic Systems and the Pathogenesis of OCD and Related Disorders

Transgenic mice expressing a neuropotentiating cholera toxin transgene in dopamine D_1 receptor–expressing neurons have been found to engage in biting and in perseverative locomotor and behavioral abnormalities consistent with animal models of OCD (Campbell et al. 1999a, 1999b). The authors suggested that the chronic potentiation of cortical and limbic D_1 neurons might be responsible for these OC behaviors (Campbell et al. 2000; McGrath et al. 2000). In addition, rats chronically treated with quinpirole (a D_2/D_3 receptor agonist) exhibit ritualistic behavior resembling checking behavior (Ben-Pazi et al. 2001; Einat and Szechtman 1995; Szechtman et al. 1998, 2001). Other studies have failed to demonstrate a link between D_2 receptors and OCD (Novelli et al. 1994).

In humans, few peripheral measures of dopamine in OCD cohorts have been performed, and none has yielded positive results. Likewise, few pharmacological probes to assess the role of dopaminergic function in the pathophysiology of OCD have been conducted. However, agents that affect dopaminergic function, such as cocaine (Koizumi 1985; McDougle et al. 1989; Rosse et al. 1993, 1994; Satel and McDougle 1991) and methylphenidate/amphetamine (Frye and Arnold 1981; Iyo et al. 1999; Koizumi 1985; Kotsopoulos and Spivak 2001; Kouris 1998; Lemus et al. 1991), have been reported to exacerbate or induce OCD symptoms. In addition, augmentation of SRIs with dopamine antagonists constitutes an effective strategy for treating OCD patients who do not respond to SRIs alone (for review, see Dougherty et al. 2007). Finally, multiple in vivo neuroimaging studies focusing on dopaminergic function in OCD have been conducted. Two such studies found increased dopamine transporter binding in the basal ganglia of OCD cohorts (Kim et al. 2003; van der Wee et al. 2004), whereas another failed to detect a difference (Pogarell et al. 2003). Another study demonstrated decreased D_2 receptor binding in the basal ganglia of an OCD cohort (Denys et al. 2004). Taken together, these findings suggest higher synaptic concentrations of dopamine in the basal ganglia in OCD patients.

Complementing the previous discussion of serotonin and its role in OCD, dopamine antagonists are effective for reducing the tics of TS as well as the manifestations of other hyperkinetic movement disorders. Conversely, dopamine agonists are known to exacerbate tics and other adventitial movements. There are considerable data implicating primary dopaminergic abnormalities in TS.

The cell bodies of dopamine-containing neurons are principally concentrated in midbrain and tegmentum and project rostrally, forming the nigrostriatal pathway as well as the mesolimbic and mesocortical systems. It has long been presumed that the therapeutic effects of dopamine antagonists in hyperkinetic movement disorders follow logically from the well-established role of dopamine in mediating motor control via the nigrostriatal system. A series of studies in the 1990s demonstrated striatal dopamine receptor abnormalities in TS. A comparison of postmortem tissue from people with TS compared with control subjects revealed higher binding rates for a dopamine transporter site ligand in the striatum (Singer et al. 1991) in TS subjects. An analogous in vivo neuroimaging study (Malison et al. 1995) demonstrated increased binding capacity for dopaminergic reuptake sites in the striatum of TS patients compared with matched controls, indicating an elevated density of available transporter sites in patients with TS. In a study of twins concordant for TS but discordant for tic severity, Wolf et al. (1996) found decreased binding capacity for dopaminergic postsynaptic receptors in the striatum of the more severely affected twins. These results imply that more severe TS is associated with either higher levels of ambient dopamine or a reduced density of postsynaptic dopamine receptor sites. Taken together, the findings from these three studies suggest that patients with TS do exhibit abnormalities of the dopaminergic system within the striatum. These preliminary findings should be interpreted cautiously, however, given that the sample sizes were small and the subjects in these studies were not neuroleptic naive. Therefore, some of the observed abnormalities may be a consequence of past exposure to antidopaminergic medications or other differences between the groups that are unrelated to TS diagnosis. Nonetheless, these data provide initial evidence supporting a dopaminergic hypothesis of TS. Specifically, TS appears to be associated with fundamental dopaminergic abnormalities within the striatum, and tic symptoms can be exacerbated by exposure to dopamimetic agents as well as attenuated by treatment with dopamine antagonist medications.

Neurochemistry Across the Obsessive-Compulsive Spectrum

Pathophysiological heterogeneity may explain why some subtypes of OCD are responsive to SRIs alone and some to SRIs plus dopamine antagonists while others are wholly unresponsive to either of these interventions. For instance, tic-related OCD appears to be relatively SRI-refractory and preferentially responsive to the combination of SRIs plus dopamine antagonists (McDougle et al. 1994a, 1994b). One possibility is that BDD and non-tic-related OCD involve primary orbitofrontal dysfunction or pathophysiology, whereas tic-related OCD and TS involve primary striatal pathology. Therefore, serotonergic modulation at the level of orbitofrontal cortex might be sufficient for antiobsessional effects in BDD or non-tic-related OCD, whereas dopaminergic modulation within the striatum synergizes with orbitofrontal serotonergic modulation to relieve tic-related OCD, and pure TS responds to dopamine modulation at the level of the striatum, but not to serotonergic modulation at orbitofrontal cortex.

Endocrine/HPA Axis Function

Because abnormalities of the hypothalamic-pituitary-adrenal (HPA) axis have been demonstrated in other anxiety disorders, some researchers have focused on HPA axis function in OCD as well. In multiple studies, investigators have examined peripheral measures of HPA axis function in patients with OCD. Other studies have been focused on corticotropin-releasing hormone (CRH) in cerebrospinal fluid of OCD cohorts with mixed results. One study found increased levels in OCD patients (Altemus et al. 1992), whereas another failed to find a difference versus healthy control subjects (Chappell et al. 1996). Another study (Gehris et al. 1990) found increased 24-hour urinary cortisol levels in OCD subjects. Finally, three studies have found increased serum concentrations of cortisol in OCD cohorts (Catapano et al. 1992; Kluge et al. 2007; Monteleone et al. 1994), with one of these (Kluge et al. 2007) also finding increased adrenocorticotropic hormone (ACTH) secretion in OCD subjects.

HPA axis challenge studies have been performed with OCD subjects as well. Dexamethasone suppression test (DST) studies in OCD cohorts have been inconsistent, with some studies demonstrating nonsuppression (Catapano et al. 1990; Cottraux et al. 1984) and others failing to find DST abnormalities (Coryell et al. 1989; Jenike et al. 1987; Liberman et al. 1985; Lucey et al. 1992; Vallejo et al. 1988). In one study, CRH challenge was associated with blunted ACTH secretion in OCD subjects (Bailly et al. 1994). Two studies (Khanna et al. 2001; Zohar et al. 1987) found hyporesponsivity of the HPA axis following m-CPP challenge, whereas two others failed to detect abnormalities (Charney et al. 1988; Hollander et al. 1992).

In summary, although HPA axis dysfunction is clearly present in other anxiety disorders, the results of studies examining HPA axis function in OCD have been inconsistent, at best. These outcomes are likely to reflect the noncentrality of HPA axis function to the pathophysiology of OCD. Nevertheless, some abnormalities have been detected as epiphenomena due to the nonspecific anxiety symptoms associated with OCD. However, further studies of the role of the HPA axis in OCD need to be conducted.

Possible Autoimmune Etiology

Over the past two decades, a fascinating scientific story has emerged regarding the potential role of autoimmune mechanisms in the pathogenesis of OCD and related disorders. It had long been appreciated that Sydenham's chorea, one manifestation of acute rheumatic fever, is accompanied by neuropsychiatric symptoms reminiscent of OCD and TS. Unlike OCD or TS, however, much about the pathogenesis of Sydenham's chorea has been known since the mid-1970s. In particular, a study by Husby et al. (1976) suggested that the damage to the basal ganglia characteristic of Sydenham's chorea is mediated by antineuronal antibodies as part of an autoimmune response to group A beta-hemolytic streptococcal (GABHS) infection. Hence, it was proposed that a similar process might cause OCD and/or TS in a subset of cases (Swedo et al. 1994). Critical clinical research initiated in the late 1980s demonstrated that OCD symptoms were common among children with Sydenham's chorea and that these symptoms often preceded motor manifestations of the disease (Swedo et al. 1989a, 1993). A series of studies involving children with OCD and TS showed that antineuronal antibodies were present in a subset of cases (Leonard et al. 1992; Rettew et al. 1992: Swedo et al. 1989b). Longitudinal study of a number of such cases indicated characteristic features of abrupt onset and discrete episodes of symptom exacerbation, which are often associated with demonstrable GABHS infection (Allen et al. 1995; Ayoube and Wannemaker 1966; Berrios et al. 1985; Swedo et al. 1998). Interestingly, a few longitudinal cases have been reported in which serial neuroimaging data demonstrate acute changes in striatal volume that parallel the clinical course (Giedd et al. 1995). Taken together, these findings led to the designation of *pediatric autoimmune neuropsychiatric disorders associated with streptococcal infections* (PANDAS). Specific criteria have been developed, based on research to date, and include 1) presence of OCD and/or a tic disorder, 2) prepubertal onset, 3) episodic course of symptom severity, 4) association with GABHS infection, and 5) association with neurological abnormalities (Allen et al. 1995; Swedo et al. 1998). The autoimmune mechanisms of pathogenesis in this subtype of OCD and related disorders suggest new possibilities in terms of early diagnosis and treatment, including prophylaxis with antibiotics or plasmapheresis (Swedo et al. 1998).

It is believed that a vulnerability to rheumatic fever, and hence PANDAS, may be inherited as an autosomal recessive trait (Gibofsky et al. 1991). A monoclonal antibody against the B lymphocyte antigen D8/17 appears to serve as a genetic marker for susceptibility to rheumatic fever; preliminary studies have indicated significantly greater D8/17 binding in cases of OCD and TS (Murphy et al. 1997; Swedo et al. 1997). Given that PANDAS cases bear striking similarity to cases of early-onset and tic-related OCD as well as TS, it is tempting to consider that PANDAS may account for a substantial proportion of childhood-onset cases of OCD and related disorders. The relative frequency of OCD and TS attributable to PANDAS, in fact, remains unknown. However, it is interesting to note that family genetic data suggest a different inheritance pattern for PANDAS than has been observed in the large pedigrees of OCD and TS studied to date.

Other Biological Factors

Although most biological factors related to the pathophysiology of OCD are discussed in other sections of this chapter, it is worth noting that OCD may also develop following birth injury (Capstick and Seldrup 1977), temporal lobe epilepsy (Kettl and Marks 1986), or head injury (McKeon et al. 1984). Specifically, damage to the basal ganglia is particularly associated with the development of OCD symptoms (Tonkonogy and Barriera 1989), as are diseases associated with degeneration of the basal ganglia (e.g., Huntington's disease and Parkinson's disease) (Cummings and Cunningham 1992; Muller et al. 1997).

Neuroanatomy and Pathophysiology of OCD and Related Disorders

Relevant Normal Neuroanatomy

Contemporary neuroanatomical models of OCD and related disorders have emphasized the role of CSTC circuitry. In a series of classic articles, Alexander and colleagues (1986) introduced and reviewed the organization of multiple, parallel, segregated CSTC circuits. Briefly, each CSTC circuit involves projections from a variety of cortical zones to specific corresponding subterritories of striatum, which, in turn, send projections via other intermediate basal ganglia targets to ramify within the thalamus. These circuits are ultimately closed via reciprocal projections from thalamus back to the very same prefrontal cortical regions from which the corticostriatal projections originated. There are several levels of complexity to consider with regard to the anatomy and function of these circuits in order to appreciate their role in the pathophysiology of OCD and related disorders. Therefore, we will begin by describing the key elements of these circuits, as well as their functional significance (Rauch et al. 1998c).

Prefrontal cortex mediates a variety of cognitive functions, including response inhibition, planning, organizing, controlling, and verifying operations. Consequently, prefrontal dysfunction is associated with disinhibition, disorganization, inflexibility, perseveration, and stereotypy (Otto 1990). Prefrontal cortex comprises several functional subterritories. Dorsolateral prefrontal cortex plays a role in learning and memory, as well as planning and other complex cognitive (i.e., executive) functions. Ventral prefrontal cortex can be further subdivided into two functional domains. Posteromedial orbitofrontal cortex is a component of the paralimbic system and plays a role in affective and motivational functions (Mesulam 1985), as discussed in later sections. Anterior and lateral orbitofrontal cortex represent the structural and functional intermediaries between the lateral prefrontal and paralimbic prefrontal zones. For instance, anterior and lateral orbitofrontal cortex seem to play a role in response inhibition and regulation of behavior based on social context, as well as other affectively tinged cognitive operations (Mesulam 1985; Zald and Kim 1996).

The *paralimbic system* is the name given to a contiguous belt of cortex that forms the functional conduit between other cortical areas and the limbic system proper. The constituents of the paralimbic belt include posteromedial orbitofrontal cortex, as well as cingulate, anterior temporal, parahippocampal, and insular cortex (Mesulam 1985). This system is believed to integrate abstracted representations of the outside world with inner emotional states, so that appropriate meaning and priority can be assigned to information as it is processed. Convergent data from human neuroimaging studies, together with previous animal and human research, suggest that the paralimbic system plays a critical role in mediating intense emotional states or arousal; in particular, this system has been implicated in anxiety (Rauch and Shin 1997; Rauch et al. 1994, 1995a, 1996, 1997a). Furthermore, it has long been appreciated that paralimbic elements serve to modulate the autonomic responses, including heart rate and blood pressure, that represent the somatic manifestations of intense affects or heightened arousal (Mesulam 1985).

The *striatum* comprises the caudate nucleus, putamen, and nucleus accumbens (also called the ventral striatum). Historically, the basal ganglia, including the striatum, were thought to play a circumscribed role, limited to the modulation of motor functions. More recently, however, a much more complicated scheme has been adopted, which recognizes the role of striatum in cognitive and affective functions as well (Houk et al. 1995).

Parallel, segregated CSTC circuits differ from one another on the basis of their distinct projection zones within cortex, striatum, and thalamus, and thus the particular type of functions each subserves. For the purposes of this review, four of these CSTC circuits are emphasized: 1) The circuit involving projections from sensorimotor cortex via the putamen subserves sensorimotor functions; 2) the corticostriatal circuit involving projections from paralimbic cortex via the nucleus accumbens subserves affective or motivational functions; 3) projections from anterior and lateral orbitofrontal cortex via ventromedial caudate nucleus constitute the ventral cognitive circuit, which is thought to mediate context-related operations and response inhibition; and 4) projections from dorsolateral prefrontal cortex via dorsolateral caudate nucleus constitute the dorsal cognitive circuit, which is thought to mediate working memory and other executive functions.

Two major branches of the CSTC circuits exist: 1) The corticothalamic branch provides a reciprocal excitatory monosynaptic communication between cortex and thalamus that purportedly mediates consciously initiated output (corticothalamic) and consciously accessible input (thalamocortical) streams; and 2) the corticostriatothalamic branch represents a collateral pathway that serves to modulate transmission at the level of the thalamus. Purportedly, the function of the striatum in this context is to process information automatically and without conscious representation. Thus, the healthy striatum, by exerting a balance of suppression and/or enhancement at the level of thalamus, serves to 1) filter out extraneous input, 2) ensure refined output, and 3) mediate stereotyped, rule-based processes without necessitating the allocation of conscious resources (Graybiel 1995; Houk et al. 1995; Rauch and Savage 1997; Rauch et al. 1995b, 1997b; Wise et al. 1996). In this way the striatum regulates the content, and facilitates the quality, of information processing within the explicit (i.e., conscious) domain by fine-tuning input and output. In addition, the striatum enhances the efficiency of the brain by carrying out some nonconscious functions, thereby reducing the computational load on conscious processing systems.

The *direct and indirect corticostriatothalamic pathways* represent a third level of complexity. Each corticostriatothalamic collateral consists of both a "direct" and an "indirect" pathway (Albin et al. 1989; Alexander et al. 1990). These two systems operate in parallel, with opposing ultimate influences at the level of the thalamus. The direct system is so named because it involves direct projections from striatum to globus pallidus interna, with a net excitatory influence on the thalamus. Conversely, the indirect system involves indirect projections from striatum via the globus pallidus externa to the globus pallidus interna and has a net inhibitory effect at the level of the thalamus. Although these two systems share many features in common, they are characterized by important neurochemical differences. Specifically, while the direct system utilizes the neuropeptide substance P as a transmitter, the indirect system utilizes enkephalin instead.

There are additional levels of complexity regarding the heterogeneity of cellular characteristics within striatal subterritories (i.e., the patch-matrix level of organization [Gerfen 1992; Graybiel 1990]). However, those concepts are tangential to the focus of this review.

The Corticostriatal Hypothesis of OCD

For the past two decades, neurobiological models of OCD have emphasized the role of frontal cortex and the striatum (Baxter et al. 1990; Cummings 1993; Insel 1992; Modell et al. 1989; Rapoport and Wise 1988; Rauch and Jenike 1993, 1997; Rauch et al. 1998c; Salloway and Cummings 1996). The scheme of corticostriatal circuitry fit well with emerging data implicating the elements of those circuits. Convergent results from neuroimaging studies indicated hyperactivity of orbitofrontal cortex, anterior cingulate cortex and (less consistently) caudate nucleus at rest, and attenuation of these abnormalities with effective treatment (see Rauch and Baxter 1998 for review). Neuropsychological studies were consistent with subtle deficits involving frontostriatal functions (see Rauch and Savage 1997 for review). Neurosurgical procedures that interrupted this circuit appeared to reduce OCD symptoms (see Cosgrove and Rauch 1995; Mindus et al. 1994). Furthermore, cases of other diseases characterized by documented striatal pathology were noted to exhibit OCD symptoms or similar clinical manifestations

(Cummings 1993; Salloway and Cummings 1996; Weilburg et al. 1989; Williams et al. 1988). There was also heuristic appeal to the hypothesis that positive feedback loops between cortex and thalamus might mediate circular, repetitive thoughts, whereas the striatum might mediate fixed action patterns in the form of repetitive behaviors or compulsions (Baxter et al. 1990, 1992; Insel 1992; Modell et al. 1989; Rauch and Jenike 1993; Rauch et al. 1998c).

Although there were several early versions of this model, each posited an overdriven corticothalamic reverberating circuit. Modell et al. (1989) proposed that a hyperactive caudate nucleus might be the cause of net excitation of the thalamus; Baxter et al. (1990) hypothesized that the apparent hyperactivity in caudate represented insufficient compensation for intrinsic striatal dysfunction, such that inhibition of the thalamus via the corticostriatothalamic collateral was inadequate. As researchers came to appreciate the ramifications of the direct and indirect systems within the corticostriatothalamic collateral branch, the models evolved. A revised version suggested that in psychiatrically healthy individuals, an appropriate balance between the direct and indirect systems enabled the collateral to optimally modulate activity at the thalamus, whereas in individuals with OCD, a shift toward dominance of the direct system could result in excitation or disinhibition at the thalamus, thereby overdriving the corticothalamic branch. Insel (1992) provided a complementary model of OCD, which focused on the role of orbitofrontal cortex as the primary component of a "worry circuit." Thus, the corticostriatal models of OCD accommodated much of the available data, as of 1993 (Cummings 1993; Rauch and Jenike 1993).

The Striatal Topography Model of OCD and Related Disorders

Baxter and colleagues (1990) were the first to clearly articulate what has come to be known as the striatal topography model of OCD and related disorders (Leckman et al. 1992; Rauch and Baxter 1998; Rauch and Jenike 1997; Rauch et al. 1998c) . As the phenomenological, familial, and neurobiological relationships between OCD and TS became appreciated, Baxter and colleagues hypothesized that the two disorders might share a fundamental pathophysiology, whereby the clinical manifestations of each disease are governed by the precise topography of dysfunction within the striatum. The researchers suggested that different corticostriatal circuits might mediate different symptoms and might therefore define a spectrum of different disease entities. Originally, they proposed that ventromedial caudate/accumbens involvement might mediate obsessions, dorsolateral caudate dysfunction might mediate compulsions, and putamen involvement might mediate the tics of TS. Subsequently, based on results of symptom provocation studies, we have proposed that the paralimbic system (including posteromedial orbitofrontal cortex) mediates affective manifestations, including the anxiety of OCD or BDD and the "urges" of TS or TTM, whereas the ventral cognitive circuit, comprising anterior and lateral orbitofrontal cortex and ventromedial caudate, mediates obsessional symptoms (Rauch and Baxter 1998; Rauch et al. 1998c). Further support for the striatal topography model comes from imaging studies that indicate structural abnormalities involving the caudate in OCD (see Jenike et al. 1996; Rauch and Baxter 1998; Robinson et al. 1995; Scarone et al. 1992; but also see Aylward et al. 1996) and the putamen in TS (Peterson et al. 1993; Singer et al. 1993) and TTM (O'Sullivan et al. 1997).

CSTC Dysfunction and the Implicit-Processing Deficit Hypothesis

The striatal topography model has further implications when elaborated from a cognitive neuroscience perspective. One scheme for understanding information processing, in the context of learning and memory, distinguishes between explicit (i.e., conscious) and implicit (i.e., nonconscious) operations (Rauch et al. 1995b, 1997b; Reber 1989, 1992; Reber and Squire 1994; Schacter and Tulving 1994). Apparently, these various information processing functions are performed by distinct and dissociable brain systems. Explicit learning and memory are primarily mediated via dorsolateral prefrontal cortex and medial temporal structures, such as the hippocampus (Schacter et al. 1996; Squire 1992; Ungerleider 1995). There are several types of implicit learning and memory. Classical conditioning (especially with regard to aversive stimuli) is mediated in part by the amygdala. Implicit learning of procedures, skills, or stereotyped serial operations is purportedly mediated via corticostriatal systems (see Mishkin and Petri 1984; Mishkin et al. 1984; Rauch and Savage 1997, 2000). Therefore, if OC spectrum disorders are fundamentally referable to striatal dysfunction, their phenomenology might best be understood as a consequence of implicit processing deficits (Rauch and Savage 2000; Rauch et al. 1998c).

From the cognitive neuroscience perspective, it is plausible that the intrusive events that are the hallmark of OCD and related disorders represent failures in filtering at the level of the thalamus, attributable to deficient modulation via the corticostriatothalamic collateral. To frame this in another way, information that is normally processed efficiently via corticostriatal systems, outside of the conscious domain (i.e., implicitly), instead finds access to explicit processing systems due to striatal dysfunction. This theory could explain the cognitive intrusions of OCD or BDD, as well as the sensorimotor intrusions of TS or TTM. Furthermore, it makes sense that these symptoms would persist or recur until they are effectively put to rest. The manner and inefficiency with which this end is achieved may depend on both the degree of dysfunction and the nature of compensatory processes.

Imaging studies have shown that striatum is reliably recruited during learning of sequential behaviors (Rauch et al. 1995b). Patients with OCD fail to show this normal pattern of striatal activation when confronted with an implicit sequence learning task and, instead, exhibit recruitment of medial temporal structures typically associated with conscious information processing (Rauch et al. 1997b).

Repetitive Behaviors and the Modulation of Thalamic Overdrive

For an individual with a pattern of striatal dysfunction, the most adaptive means for producing striatothalamic modulation might be through performance of highly ritualized thoughts or behaviors that activate adjacent striatothalamic networks that are intact. In this way, compulsions or tics may represent a compensatory, though relatively inefficient, method for recruiting the viable remnants of the corticostriatothalamic collateral. Thus, these repetitive behaviors actually serve to facilitate gating at the level of the thalamus. This would explain why the behaviors sometimes require numerous repetitions before the precipitating intrusive symptoms are put to rest.

This model also provides an explanation for the correspondence between intrusive symptoms and the repetitive behaviors performed in response to them. In this scheme, the pairing should be related principally to the topography or interconnections of the neural systems involved. Within the putamen, it makes sense that these relationships would be somatotopic, such that sensory intrusions that involve a given somatic distribution (e.g., the right shoulder) should prompt repetitive behavior in the same or a nearby somatic distribution (e.g., a shoulder or arm tic). In the case of cognitions, this mapping is less obvious and certainly is not yet empirically established. It is plausible, however, that networks that mediate cognitive representations of contamination, for instance, might be topographically near to or linked with neural networks that mediate cleaning procedures. Further, this model would provide an explanation why some patients develop rituals and also why some patients experience intrusions but never develop ritualistic behaviors; presumably, in those cases, no ritual evolves that effectively ameliorates the intrusive symptoms.

Again, in the context of an implicit sequence learning paradigm, functional imaging studies have demonstrated a characteristic pattern of thalamic deactivation in association with striatal recruitment (Rauch et al. 1998b). These findings have been interpreted as one illustration of thalamic gating. Moreover, such paradigms represent potential tools for characterizing dysfunction within this system in patients with OCD and related disorders.

Cortical Excitability in OCD and Tourette Syndrome

Although the striatal topography model of OCD and related disorders focuses on subcortical dysfunction, it is possible that primary cortical pathology is the cause in some subtypes of these disorders. Transcranial magnetic stimulation (TMS) is a noninvasive means of inducing regional neuronal activity in humans. TMS can be employed to assess the degree of neuronal inhibition in the cerebral cortex. The technique involves activating cortical motor output cells with magnetic pulses produced by a scalp electromagnetic coil. The resulting motor evoked potentials are reduced when subthreshold TMS pulses precede suprathreshold stimuli by several milliseconds. This phenomenon of intracortical inhibition is thought to be due to activation of inhibitory interneurons by the subthreshold pulse. One study revealed that intracortical inhibition was defective in patients with TS (Ziemann et al. 1997); preliminary findings from an analogous study of OCD likewise showed an intracortical inhibition deficit (Greenberg et al. 2000). These results implicate insufficient local cortical inhibition as one possible mechanism underlying the intrusive phenomena characterizing OC spectrum disorders.

The cortical excitability model of OCD and related disorders is consistent with the observed efficacy of agents that facilitate intracortical inhibition. For instance, clinical trials have suggested that benzodiazepines are therapeutic for both OCD and TS (Hewlett

1993). Furthermore, preliminary clinical data suggested that gabapentin, a neutral γ-aminobutyric acid (GABA) analog, may also be effective in OCD (Beauclair et al. 1996). Interestingly, preclinical data (Gellman and Aghajanian 1993) indicated that serotonin may act within frontal cortex by augmenting GABA transmission. This finding implies that modulation of cortical 5-HT transmission, via SRI administration, may ultimately ameliorate symptoms of OCD by enhancing intracortical inhibition.

Neuroanatomical Correlates of Factor-Analyzed Symptom Dimensions

Although PANDAS provides the potential for identifying one subtype of OC spectrum conditions with a homogeneous etiology, optimal strategies for characterizing OC spectrum subtypes based on pathophysiology and phenomenology are yet to be established. Several strategies have been employed for subtyping OCD and related disorders based on symptomatology. The approach of factor analysis has been used to determine clusters of intercorrelated OCD symptoms that can be treated as orthogonal factors for describing clinical presentation (Baer 1994; Leckman et al. 1997). Because these factors are independent of one another, it is reasonable to hypothesize that each one reflects a separate underlying aspect of pathophysiology. This modular approach to the characterization of OCD was recently tested by seeking neuroanatomical correlates of symptom severity for each factor, using positron emission tomography (Rauch et al. 1998a). In this preliminary study, the symptom factors employed included 1) checking and religious, aggressive, and sexual obsessions; 2) symmetry and ordering; and 3) washing and cleaning (Baer 1994; Leckman et al. 1997). Notably, factors 1 and 2 had previously been associated with tic-related OCD. Interestingly, Rauch et al. (1998a) found that during a nominally neutral state, factor 1 was positively correlated with bilateral striatal activity, factor 2 was negatively correlated with right caudate activity, and factor 3 was positively correlated with orbitofrontal and anterior cingulate cortical activity. Though preliminary, these results suggest that different symptom dimensions are associated with activity within different modules of the CSTC circuits of interest. In fact, the three key findings may correspond to the following: 1) increased activity within striatal neurons that participate in the direct system, 2) decreased activity within striatal neurons that participate in the indirect system, and 3) increased activity within the relevant prefrontal cortical zones. This constellation of findings resonates with the range of substrates hypothesized in the previous sections on the neuroanatomy of OCD and related disorders, and it underscores the potential pathophysiological heterogeneity of these conditions.

Psychological Factors

Childhood/Developmental Factors

OCD is associated with a bimodal onset. Anywhere from one-third to one-half of adults with OCD develop the disorder in childhood (Burke et al. 1990; Weissman et al. 1994). The mean age at onset for OCD in adulthood is between 22 and 35 years (Maj et al. 2002). Interestingly, early-onset OCD differs in many important ways from adult-onset OCD. Early-onset OCD is associated with greater severity (Fontanelle et al. 2003; Rosario-Campos et al. 2001), higher persistence rates in long-term outcome studies (Stewart et al. 2004), a higher prevalence of compulsions without obsessions (Geller et al. 1998; Rosario-Campos et al. 2001), and higher comorbidity rates with tic disorders (Eichstedt and Arnold 2001), as well as attention-deficit/hyperactivity disorder and anxiety disorders (Geller et al. 2001). Finally, early-onset OCD appears to be more common in males (Fontanelle et al. 2003; Geller et al. 1998; Tukel et al. 2005), whereas adult-onset OCD may be slightly more common in females (Burke et al. 1990; Douglass et al. 1995; Nestadt et al. 1998; Weissman et al. 1994).

Personality Factors

One way to look for a relationship between personality and OCD is to look at the prevalence of personality disorders in OCD patients. Studies that have examined this issue have reported diverse findings regarding the prevalence of comorbid Axis II diagnoses (see Baer 1998 for review). However, most studies indicate that roughly half of OCD patients have comorbid Axis II diagnoses.

A better approach is to look at personality as a dimensional factor. One widely used model categorizes personality along four temperament dimensions (novelty seeking, harm avoidance, reward dependence, and persistence) and three character dimensions (self-directedness, cooperativeness, and self-transcendence) (Cloninger 1987; Cloninger et al. 1993). All studies in which this model was used to investigate OCD subjects found higher harm-avoidance scores among OCD subjects (Alonso et al. 2008; Bejerot et al. 1998; Kusunoki et al. 2000; Lyoo et al. 2001; Pfohl et al. 1990; Richter et al. 1996); three of these studies found lower novelty-seeking (Alonso et al. 2008; Kusunoki et al. 2000; Lyoo et al. 2001) and one found high scores on reward dependence (Pfohl et al. 1990). On the character dimension, low scores on self-directedness (Alonso et al. 2008; Bejerot et al. 1998; Kusunoki et al. 2000; Lyoo et al. 2001) and cooperativeness (Alonso et al. 2008; Bejerot et al. 1998; Kusunoki et al. 2000) have been reported in OCD cohorts.

Another tool used for studying personality is the Minnesota Multiphasic Personality Inventory (MMPI; Graham 1977). There is only one published study in which the MMPI was used in an OCD cohort (Carey et al. 1986). In that study, elevations were reported in the depression, psychasthenia, schizophrenia, and psychopathic tendencies scales of OCD subjects.

Cognitive-Behavioral Factors

Although a complete review of cognitive-behavioral factors in the pathogenesis of OCD is beyond the scope of this chapter, a brief overview is useful (for a more detailed review, see Steketee et al. 1998). In short, cognitive theories of OCD have grown out of an appraisal model of the development and maintenance of stress and anxiety. In OCD, primary appraisal occurs in conjunction with the intrusive thoughts associated with obsessions, and secondary appraisal leads to faulty coping (compulsions and avoidance). Patients with OCD typically overestimate the likelihood of an unfavorable outcome in the context of primary appraisal (during obsessions) (Carr 1971, 1974), and they perform compulsive behaviors in order to reduce the perceived threat. In terms of cognitive domains, studies of patients with OCD have found an exaggerated sense of responsibility (Rachman 1993; Salkovskis 1985), overestimation of threat (Carr 1971; McFall and Wollersheim 1979), perfectionism (Guidano and Liotti 1983; McFall and Wollershiem 1979), overimportance of thoughts, need for control (Clark and Purdon 1993), and intolerance of ambiguity (Guidano and Liotti 1983).

Information Processing

Studies of information processing in OCD have revealed deficits in multiple cognitive domains, including memory and executive functioning. OCD subjects perform at the same level as psychiatrically healthy control subjects during verbal memory tasks such as the Wechsler Memory Scale's Logical Memory and Paired Associate Learning subtests, the Rey Auditory Verbal Learning Test, and the California Verbal Learning Test (Boone et al. 1991; Christensen et al. 1992; Zielinski et al. 1991). However, studies have found that OCD subjects underutilize organizational strategies during these tasks when compared with psychiatrically healthy control subjects (Deckersbach et al. 2000a, 2005; Savage et al. 2000). In terms of nonverbal memory, OCD subjects perform as well as psychiatrically healthy control subjects in copying the Rey Complex Figure Test (Martinot et al. 1990; Penades et al. 2005). However, OCD subjects demonstrate lower recall (Deckersbach et al. 2000a, 2000b) and, again, tend to underutilize organizational strategies (Deckersbach et al. 2000a; Penades et al. 2005; Savage et al. 1999) during nonverbal memory tasks. Studies of executive functioning in OCD show increased response latencies, perseveration of responses, and difficulties utilizing feedback to adapt to change (for review, see Olley et al. 2007).

Cultural Factors

Cultural factors probably are not central to the pathogenesis of OCD, given that the prevalence of OCD is fairly consistent in epidemiological studies in countries throughout the world. However, cultural factors may play an important role in the clinical presentation of OCD.

Integrating Perspectives on the Pathogenesis of OCD and Related Disorders

We have reviewed etiological and pathophysiological models that reflect current concepts regarding the pathogenesis of OCD and related disorders. It is clear that no single model will explain the full spectrum of clinical and neurobiological phenomena associated with OC spectrum disorders. On the contrary, accruing evidence implicates multiple etiologies and a true pathophysiological spectrum of disease. Consequently, a sophisticated understanding of OCD and related disorders will require an integration of the various pieces of this puzzle. We propose that neurobiologically and clinically relevant schemes for subtyping OCD, as well as for defining and subdividing populations with OC spectrum disorders, will be critical to advancements in our understanding of these diseases.

CSTC loops represent an anatomical framework within which to describe the pathogenesis of OCD and related disorders. One perspective emphasizes the circuits that are involved: dysfunction within the orbitofrontal-caudate circuit may represent a final common pathway for OCD symptoms; analogous dysfunction within the sensorimotor-putamen pathway may underlie chronic tics. Another perspective emphasizes the locus of primary pathology within these circuits. We have reviewed data that implicate striatal subterritories as primary sites of pathology (as supported by observed volumetric abnormalities and a feasible etiological scenario involving autoimmune mechanisms). TMS data suggest that defective inhibition within cortex could be primary in some cases. A third perspective acknowledges the neurochemistry superimposed on the anatomy: serotonergic medications appear to act at the level of cortex to ameliorate OCD symptoms, but not those of TS. Dopaminergic medications are purported to have their principal action within striatum; they are effective as primary treatments in TS, but only as augmentors of SRIs in a subgroup of patients with tic-related OCD. A fourth perspective focuses on the issue of etiology. Genetic factors appear to play a role in most cases of OCD and TS. However, exactly what is inherited that confers increased risk remains unclear, as do the critical epigenetic factors that influence expression, including penetrance.

PANDAS represent a prime example in which these various perspectives can be integrated to describe a phenomenological spectrum, whose genesis can likely be found in an inherited vulnerability for autoimmune destruction of striatum in the face of GABHS infection. Presumably, the topography and extent of striatal damage largely govern the clinical presentation, as well as the efficacy of conventional treatments. PANDAS are such a valuable example not only because they bridge the above perspectives but also because they underscore the potential benefits derived from delineating pathogenesis. Once the etiology and pathophysiology of a disease are better understood, the scientific community is better equipped to rationally pursue superior interventions and even prophylaxis or cure.

Conclusion

Advances in the genetics of OC spectrum disorders could be most important. Once genes that confer risk are identified, there will be enhanced potential to study subjects at risk longitudinally, thereby enabling the investigation of pathogenesis. Furthermore, with identification of at-risk individuals, early diagnosis and thus early intervention or prophylactic strategies become feasible. Although systematic efforts to map the human genome move forward at an accelerated pace, genetic studies are ultimately reliant on valid determinations of phenotype. Therefore, establishing phenotypic designations based on convergent data, including phenomenological, physiological, and etiological factors, will be crucial.

Evolving brain imaging techniques represent the most powerful tools for characterizing in vivo human neuroanatomy, neurophysiology, and neurochemistry at modest temporal and spatial resolution. Categorical approaches will aim to identify discrete subtypes of patients, based on the measures reviewed in this chapter, as well as on symptomatology and treatment response. Dimensional approaches will aim to consider these as continuous variables. Only time will tell which of these approaches is superior for describing the OC spectrum. Concretely, prospective imaging studies can generate and test hypotheses regarding the elements of neuroimaging profiles that predict treatment response for medications, behavior therapy, or other therapies. Simultaneously, phenomenological characteristics can be correlated with both brain imaging indices and treatment outcomes. Thus, by triangulating across such multifaceted data sets, it should be possible to achieve a robust and valid clinical-neurobiological basis for diagnosis and subtyping across the OC spectrum.

As various pathophysiological entities are dissected, the hope is that each one will give way to specific treatments. Basic pharmacological research will continue to explore the receptor changes and, perhaps more importantly, the downstream molecular effects of currently available therapies. Such research will progressively illuminate the salient changes that are necessary to ameliorate symptoms in each of the subtypes of the OC spectrum. Once these targets are established, it will be possible to rationally design new and, hopefully, better treatments. Although this paragraph implies a focus on pharmacotherapy, in fact an analogous process will be necessary to advance nonpharmacological treatments, including behavior therapy as well as others.

These are exciting times in psychiatric neuroscience, as the field moves closer to the promise of a diagnostic scheme that reflects pathophysiology. In this context, OCD is a model disorder: despite its historical placement among the anxiety disorders, with which OCD does share many phenomenological similarities, contemporary research is clarifying that at least one subtype of OCD is closely related to a movement disorder, and perhaps another is associated with an autoimmune etiology. Even though technical advances in neuroimaging, genetics, and pharmacology have provided new tools with which to elucidate the pathogenesis of OCD, there should be renewed enthusiasm for the essential contribution of careful phenomenological characterization. It should already be clear that OCD, as defined in DSM-IV, is not one disease, but several. Conversely, in some cases, OCD and TS may not be different diseases pathogenetically, but rather, different faces of the very same one.

◀ Key Clinical Points ▶

- Twin studies show concordance rates for obsessive-compulsive disorder of 75%–90% for monozygotic twins and 10%–20% for dizygotic twins.
- OCD is present in 16%–18% of relatives of affected probands, compared to a prevalence of 2%–3% in the general population.
- The neurotransmitters most likely implicated in the pathophysiology of OCD include serotonin and dopamine.
- A specific corticostriatothalamocortical circuit that includes the orbitofrontal cortex, caudate nucleus, and thalamus is dysfunctional in subjects with OCD. This dysfunction has been repeatedly demonstrated in neuroimaging studies. Successful treatment attenuates this dysfunction.
- In terms of cognitive-behavioral factors, subjects with OCD typically demonstrate overestimation of the likelihood of unfavorable outcomes, an exaggerated sense of responsibility, overestimation of threat, perfectionism, perceived overimportance of thoughts, a need for control, and intolerance of ambiguity.
- Subjects with OCD perform as well as healthy control subjects on verbal and nonverbal memory tasks but underutilize organizational strategies.

References

Albin RL, Young AB, Penney JB: The functional anatomy of basal ganglia disorders. Trends Neurosci 12:366–375, 1989

Alexander GE, DeLong MR, Strick PL: Parallel organization of functionally segregated circuits linking basal ganglia and cortex. Ann Rev Neurosci 9:357–381, 1986

Alexander GE, Crutcher MD, DeLong MR: Basal ganglia-thalamocortical circuits: parallel substrates for motor, oculomotor, "prefrontal" and "limbic" functions. Prog Brain Res 85:119–146, 1990

Allen AJ, Leonard HL, Swedo SE: Case study: a new infection-triggered, autoimmune subtype of pediatric OCD and Tourette's syndrome. J Am Acad Child Adolesc Psychiatry 34:307–311, 1995

Alonso P, Menchón JM, Jiménez S, et al: Personality dimensions in obsessive-compulsive disorder: relation to clinical variables. Psychiatry Res 157:159–168, 2008

Alsobrook JP 2nd, Pauls DL: The genetics of Tourette syndrome. Neurol Clin 15:381–393, 1997

Alsobrook JP II, Pauls DL: A factor analysis of tic symptoms in Gilles de la Tourette's syndrome. Am J Psychiatry 159:291–296, 2002

Altemus M, Pigott T, Kalogeras KT, et al: Abnormalities in the regulation of vasopressin and corticotropin releasing factor secretion in obsessive-compulsive disorder. Arch Gen Psychiatry 49:9–20, 1992

American Psychiatric Association: Diagnostic and Statistical Manual of Mental Disorders, 4th Edition. Washington, DC, American Psychiatric Association, 1994

Arnold PD, Rosenberg DR, Mundo E, et al: Association of a glutamate (NMDA) subunit receptor gene (GRIN2B) with obsessive-compulsive disorder: a preliminary study. Psychopharmacology (Berl) 174:530–538, 2004

Arnold PD, Sicard T, Burroughs E, et al: Glutamate transporter gene SLC1A1 associated with obsessive-compulsive disorder. Arch Gen Psychiatry 63:769–776, 2006

Aylward EH, Harris GJ, Hoehn-Saric R, et al: Normal caudate nucleus in obsessive-compulsive disorder assessed by quantitative neuroimaging. Arch Gen Psychiatry 53:577–584, 1996

Ayoube EM, Wannemaker LW: Streptococcal antibody titers in Sydenham's chorea. Pediatrics 38:946–956, 1966

Baer L: Factor analysis of symptom subtypes of obsessive compulsive disorder and their relation to personality and tic disorders. J Clin Psychiatry 55(suppl):18–23, 1994

Baer L: Personality disorders in obsessive-compulsive disorder, in Obsessive-Compulsive Disorders: Practical Management, 3rd Edition. Edited by Jenike MA, Baer L, Minichiello WE. St Louis, MO, Mosby, 1998, pp 65–83

Bailly D, Servant D, Dewailly D, et al: Corticotropin releasing factor stimulation test in obsessive compulsive disorder. Biol Psychiatry 35:143–146, 1994

Barr LC, Goodman WK, Price LH, et al: The serotonin hypothesis of obsessive compulsive disorder: implications of pharmacologic challenge studies. J Clin Psychiatry 53(suppl):17–28, 1992

Baxter LR, Schwartz JM, Guze BH, et al: Neuroimaging in obsessive-compulsive disorder: seeking the mediating neuroanatomy, in Obsessive Compulsive Disorder: Theory and Management, 2nd Edition. Edited by Jenike MA, Baer L, Minichiello WE. Chicago, IL, Year Book Medical Publishers, 1990, pp 167–188

Baxter LR, Schwartz JM, Bergman KS, et al: Caudate glucose metabolic rate changes with both drug and behavior therapy for obsessive-compulsive disorder. Arch Gen Psychiatry 49:681–689, 1992

Beauclair L, Sultan S, Belanger MC, et al: Antianxiety and hypnotic effects of gabapentin in psychotic patients with comorbid anxiety related disorders. Paper presented at the American College of Neuropsychopharmacology annual meeting, San Juan, Puerto Rico, December 1996

Bejerot S, Schlette P, Ekselius L, et al: Personality disorders and relationship to personality dimensions measured by the Temperament and Character Inventory in patients with obsessive-compulsive disorder. Acta Psychiatr Scand 98:243–249, 1998

Bellodi L, Pasquali L, Diaferia G, et al: Do eating, mood and obsessive compulsive patients share a common personality profile? New Trends in Experimental and Clinical Psychiatry 8:87–94, 1992

Ben-Pazi A, Szechtman H, Eilam D: The morphogenesis of motor rituals in rats treated chronically with the dopamine agonist quinpirole. Behav Neurosci 115:1301–1317, 2001

Berrios X, Quesney F, Morales A, et al: Are all recurrences of "pure" Sydenham's chorea true recurrences of acute rheumatic fever? Pediatrics 10:867–872, 1985

Bienvenu OJ, Samuels JF, Riddle MA, et al: The relationship of obsessive-compulsive disorder to possible spectrum disorders: results from a family study. Biol Psychiatry 48:287–293, 2000

Billett EA, Richter MA, Sam F, et al: Investigation of dopamine system genes in obsessive-compulsive disorder. Psychiatr Genet 8:163–169, 1998

Black DW, Noyes R, Goldstein RB, et al: A family study of obsessive-compulsive disorder. Arch Gen Psychiatry 49:362–368, 1992

Blier P, Bouchard C: Modulation of 5HT release in the guinea pig brain following long-term administration of antidepressant drugs. Br J Pharmacol 113:485–495, 1994

Blier P, de Montigny C: Current advances and trends in the treatment of depression. Trends Pharmacol Sci 15:220–226, 1994

Blier P, Chaput Y, de Montigny C: Long-term 5HT reuptake blockade, but not monoamine oxidase inhibition, decreases the function of the terminal 5HT autoreceptors: an electrophysiological study in the rat brain. Naunyn Schmiedebergs Arch Pharmacol 337:246–254, 1988

Boone KB, Ananth J, Philpott L, et al: Neuropsychological characteristics of nondepressed adults with obsessive-compulsive disorder. Neuropsychiatry Neuropsychol Behav Neurol 4:96–109, 1991

Brett PM, Curtis D, Robertson MM, et al: Exclusion of the 5-HT-1A serotonin neuroreceptor and tryptophan oxygenase genes in a large British kindred multiply affected with Tourette's syndrome, chronic motor tics, and obsessive-compulsive behavior. Am J Psychiatry 152:437–440, 1995

Burke KC, Burke JD, Regier DA, et al: Age at onset of selected mental disorders in five community populations. Arch Gen Psychiatry 47:511–518, 1990

Camarena B, Rinetti G, Cruz C, et al: Association study of the serotonin transporter gene polymorphism in obsessive-compulsive disorder. Int J Neuropsychopharmacol 4:269–272, 2001

Campbell KM, de Lecea L, Severynse DM, et al: OCD-like behaviors caused by a neuropotentiating transgene targeted to cortical and limbic D1+ neurons. J Neurosci 19:5044–5053, 1999a

Campbell KM, McGrath MJ, Burton FH: Differential response of cortical-limbic neuropotentiated compulsive mice to dopamine D1 and D2 receptor antagonists. Eur J Pharmacol 371:103–111, 1999b

Campbell KM, Veldman MB, McGrath MJ, et al: TS+OCD-like neuropotentiated mice are supersensitive to seizure induction. Neuroreport 11:2335–2338, 2000

Capstick N, Seldrup J: Obsessional states: a study in the relationship between abnormalities occurring at the time of birth and the subsequent development of obsessional symptoms. Acta Psychiatr Scand 56:427–431, 1977

Carey G, Gottesman II: Twin and family studies of anxiety, phobic and obsessive compulsive disorders, in Anxiety: New Research and Changing Concepts. Edited by Klein DF, Rabkin JG. New York, Raven Press, 1981, pp 117–136

Carey RJ, Baer L, Jenike MA, et al: MMPI correlates of obsessive-compulsive disorder. J Clin Psychiatry 47:371–372, 1986

Carr AT: Compulsive neurosis: two psychological studies. Bull Br Psychol Soc 24:256–257, 1971

Carr AT: Compulsive neurosis: a review of the literature. Psychol Bull 81:311–318, 1974

Catapano F, Monteleone P, Maj M, et al: Dexamethasone suppression test in patients with primary obsessive-compulsive disorder and in healthy controls. Neuropsychobiology 23:53–56, 1990

Catapano F, Monteleone P, Fuschino A, et al: Melatonin and cortisol secretion in patients with primary obsessive-compulsive disorder. Psychiatry Res 44:217–225, 1992

Cavallini MC, Di Bella D, Pasquale L, et al: 5HT2C CYS23/SER23 polymorphism is not associated with obsessive-compulsive disorder. Psychiatry Res 77:97–104, 1998

Cavallini MC, Pasquale L, Bellodi L, et al: Complex segregation analysis for obsessive compulsive disorder and related disorders. Am J Med Genet 88:38–43, 1999

Chabane N, Delorme R, Millet B, et al: Early-onset obsessive-compulsive disorder: a subgroup with a specific clinical and familial pattern? J Child Psychol Psychiatry 46:881–887, 2005

Chappell P, Leckman J, Goodman W, et al: Elevated cerebrospinal fluid corticotropin-releasing factor in Tourette's syndrome: comparison to obsessive compulsive disorder and normal controls. Biol Psychiatry 39:776–783, 1996

Charney DS, Goodman WK, Price LH, et al: Serotonin function in obsessive-compulsive disorder: a comparison of the effects of tryptophan and m-chlorophenylpiperazine in patients and healthy subjects. Arch Gen Psychiatry 45:177–185, 1988

Christensen KJ, Kim SW, Dysken MW, et al: Neuropsychological performance in obsessive-compulsive disorder. Biol Psychiatry 31:4–18, 1992

Clark DA, Purdon C: New perspectives for a cognitive theory of obsessions. Aust Psychol 28:161–167, 1993

Cloninger CR: A systematic method for clinical description and classification of personality variants: a proposal. Arch Gen Psychiatry 44:573–588, 1987

Cloninger CR, Svrakic DM, Przybeck TR: A psychobiological model of temperament and character. Arch Gen Psychiatry 50:975–990, 1993

Coryell WH, Black DW, Kelly MW, et al: HPA axis disturbance in obsessive-compulsive disorder. Psychiatry Res 30:243–251, 1989

Cosgrove GR, Rauch SL: Psychosurgery. Neurosurg Clin North Am 6:167–176, 1995

Cottraux JA, Bouvard M, Claustrat B, et al: Abnormal dexamethasone suppression test in primary obsessive-compulsive patients: a confirmatory report. Psychiatry Res 13:157–165, 1984

Cruz C, Camarena B, King N, et al: Increased prevalence of the seven-repeat variant of the dopamine D4 receptor gene in patients' obsessive-compulsive disorder with tics. Neurosci Lett 231:1–4, 1997

Cummings JL: Frontal-subcortical circuits and human behavior. Arch Neurol 50:873–880, 1993

Cummings JL, Cunningham K: Obsessive-compulsive disorder in Huntington's disease. Biol Psychiatry 31:263–270, 1992

Deckersbach TO, Michael W, Savage CR, et al: The relationship between semantic organization and memory in obsessive-compulsive disorder. Psychother Psychosom 69:101–107, 2000a

Deckersbach T, Savage CR, Phillips KA, et al: Characteristics of memory dysfunction in body dysmorphic disorder. J Int Neuropsychol Soc 6:673–681, 2000b

Deckersbach T, Savage CR, Dougherty DD, et al: Spontaneous and directed application of verbal learning strategies in bipolar disorder and obsessive-compulsive disorder. Bipolar Disord 7:166–175, 2005

de Leeuw AS, Den Boer JA, Slaap BR, et al: Pentagastrin has panic-inducing properties in obsessive compulsive disorder. Psychopharmacology 126:339–344, 1996

Delmore R, Krebs M, Chabane F: Frequency and transmission of glutamate receptors GRIK2 and GRIK3 polymorphisms in patients with obsessive-compulsive disorder. Neuroreport 15:699–702, 2004

Delorme R, Golmard JL, Chabane N, et al: Admixture analysis of age at onset in obsessive-compulsive disorder. Psychol Med 35:237–243, 2005

Denys D, van der Wee N, Janssen J, et al: Low level of dopaminergic D/2 receptor binding in obsessive-compulsive disorder. Biol Psychiatry 55:1041–1045, 2004

Dickel DE, Veenstra-VanderWeele J, Cox NJ, et al: Association testing of the positional and functional candidate gene SLC1A1/EAAC1 in early-onset obsessive-compulsive disorder. Arch Gen Psychiatry 63:778–785, 2006

Dougherty DD, Rauch SL, Jenike MA: Pharmacological treatments for obsessive-compulsive disorder, in A Guide to Treatments That Work, 3rd Edition. Edited by Nathan PE, Gorman JM. New York, Oxford University Press, 2007, pp 447–473

Douglass HM, Moffitt TE, Dar R, et al: Obsessive-compulsive disorder in a birth cohort of 18-year-olds: prevalence and predictors. J Am Acad Child Adolesc Psychiatry 34:1424–1431, 1995

Eapen V, Pauls DL, Robertson MM: Evidence for autosomal dominant transmission in Gilles de la Tourette syndrome: United Kingdom Cohort Study. Br J Psychiatry 162:593–596, 1993

Eichstedt JA, Arnold SL: Childhood-onset obsessive-compulsive disorder: a tic-related subtype of OCD? Clin Psychol Rev 21:137–157, 2001

Einat H, Szechtman H: Perseveration without hyperlocomotion in a spontaneous alternation task in rats sensitized to the dopamine agonist quinpirole. Physiol Behav 57:55–59, 1995

Enoch M-A, Greenberg BD, Murphy DL, et al: Sexually dimorphic relationship of a 5-HT-sub(2A) promoter polymorphism with obsessive-compulsive disorder. Biol Psychiatry 49:385–388, 2001

Fernandez E, Lopez-Ibor J: Clomipramine in resistant psychiatric disorders and other treatments. Actas Luso Esp Neurol Psiquiatr Cienc Afines 26:119, 1967

Fineberg NA, Bullock T, Montgomery DB, et al: Serotonin reuptake inhibitors are the treatment of choice in obsessive-compulsive disorder. Int Clin Psychopharmacol 7(suppl):43–47, 1992

Fontanelle LF, Mendlowicz MV, Marques C, et al: Early- and late-onset obsessive-compulsive disorder in adult patients: an explanatory clinical and therapeutic study. J Psylchiatr Res 37:127–133, 2003

Frye PE, Arnold LE: Persistent amphetamine-induced compulsive rituals: response to pyridoxine (B6). Biol Psychiatry 16:583–587, 1981

Gehris TL, Kathol RG, Black DW, et al: Urinary free cortisol levels in obsessive-compulsive disorder. Psychiatry Res 32:151–158, 1990

Geller D, Biederman J, Jones J, et al: Is juvenile obsessive-compulsive disorder a developmental subtype of the disorder? A review of the pediatric literature. J Am Acad Child Adolesc Psychiatry 37:420–427, 1998

Geller DA, Biederman J, Faraone S, et al: Developmental aspects of obsessive compulsive disorder: findings in children, adolescents, and adults. J Nerv Ment Dis 189:471–477, 2001

Gellman RL, Aghajanian GK: Pyramidal cells in piriform cortex receive a convergence of inputs from monoamine activated GABAergic interneurons. Brain Res 600:63–73, 1993

Gerfen CR: The neostriatal mosaic: multiple levels of compartmental organization in the basal ganglia. Annu Rev Neurosci 15:285–320, 1992

Gibofsky A, Khanna A, Suh E, et al: The genetics of rheumatic fever: relationship to streptococcal infection and autoimmune disease. J Rheumatol Suppl 30:1–5, 1991

Giedd JN, Rapoport MD, Kruesi MD, et al: Sydenham's chorea: magnetic resonance imaging of the basal ganglia. Neurology 45:2199–2202, 1995

Goodman WK, McDougle CJ, Price LH, et al: m-Chlorophenylpiperazine in patients with obsessive-compulsive disorder: absence of symptom exacerbation. Biol Psychiatry 38:138–149, 1995

Gorman JM, Liebowitz MR, Fyer AJ, et al: Lactate infusions in obsessive-compulsive disorder. Am J Psychiatry 142:864–866, 1985

Grados M, Wilcox HC: Genetics of obsessive-compulsive disorder: a research update. Expert Rev Neurother 7:967–980, 2007

Grados MA, Mathews CA, Tourette Syndrome Association International Consortium for Genetics: Latent class analysis of Gilles de la Tourette syndrome using comorbidities: clinical and genetic implications. Biol Psychiatry 64:219–225, 2008

Graham JR: The MMPI: A Practical Guide. New York, Oxford University Press, 1977

Graybiel AM: Neurotransmitters and neuromodulators in the basal ganglia. Trends Neurosci 13:244–253, 1990

Graybiel AM: Building action repertoires: memory and learning functions of the basal ganglia. Curr Opin Neurobiol 5:733–741, 1995

Greenberg BD, Ziemann U, Corá-Locatelli G, et al: Altered cortical excitability in obsessive-compulsive disorder. Neurology 54:142–147, 2000

Greist JH, Jefferson JW, Kobak KA, et al: Efficacy and tolerability of serotonin transport inhibitors in obsessive-compulsive disorder: a meta-analysis. Arch Gen Psychiatry 52:53–60, 1995

Guidano V, Liotti G: Cognitive Processes and Emotional Disorders. New York, Guilford, 1983

Hanna GL, Himle JA, Curtis GC, et al: Serotonin transporter and seasonal variation in blood serotonin in families with obsessive-compulsive disorder. Neuropsychopharmacology 18:102–111, 1998

Hanna GL, Veenstra-VanderWelle J, Cox NJ, et al: Genome-wide linkage analysis of families with obsessive-compulsive disorder ascertained through pediatric probands. Am J Med Genet 114:541–552, 2002

Hanna GL, Himle JA, Curtis GC, et al: A family study of obsessive-compulsive disorder with pediatric probands. Am J Med Genet B Neuropsychiatr Genet 134:13–19, 2005

Hesse S, Muller U, Lincke T, et al: Serotonin and dopamine transporter imaging in patients with obsessive-compulsive disorder. Psychiatry Research: Neuroimaging 140:63–72, 2005

Hettema JM, Neale MC, Kendler KS: A review and meta-analysis of the genetic epidemiology of anxiety disorders. Am J Psychiatry 158:1568–1578, 2001

Hewlett WA: The use of benzodiazepines in obsessive compulsive disorder and Tourette's syndrome. Psychiatr Ann 23:309–316, 1993

Hollander E, DeCaria CM, Nitescu A, et al: Serotonergic function in obsessive-compulsive disorder: behavioral and neuroendocrine responses to oral m-chlorophenylpiperazine and fenfluramine in patients and healthy volunteers. Arch Gen Psychiatry 49:21–28, 1992

Ho Pian KL, Westenberg HG, den Boer JA, et al: Effects of meta-chlorophenylpiperazine on cerebral blood flow in obsessive-compulsive disorder and controls. Biol Psychiatry 44:367–370, 1998

Houk JC, Davis JL, Beiser DG (eds): Models of Information Processing in the Basal Ganglia. Cambridge, MA, MIT Press, 1995

Hoyer D, Clarke DE, Fozard JR, et al: International Union of Pharmacology classification of receptors for 5-hydroxytryptamine (serotonin). Pharmacol Rev 46:157–203, 1994

Hu XZ, Lipsky RH, Zhu G, et al: Serotonin transporter promoter gain-of-function genotypes are linked to obsessive-compulsive disorder. Am J Hum Genet 78:815–826, 2006

Husby G, Van de Rijn I, Zabriskie JB, et al: Antibodies reacting with cytoplasm of subthalamic and caudate nuclei neurons in chorea and acute rheumatic fever. J Exp Med 144:1094–1110, 1976

Insel TR: Toward a neuroanatomy of obsessive-compulsive disorder. Arch Gen Psychiatry 49:739–744, 1992

Insel TR, Murphy DL, Cohen RM, et al: Obsessive compulsive disorder: a double blind trial of clomipramine and clorgyline. Arch Gen Psychiatry 40:605–612, 1983

Inouye E: Similar and dissimilar manifestations of obsessive-compulsive neurosis in monozygotic twins. Am J Psychiatry 121:1171–1175, 1965

Iyo M, Sekine Y, Matsunaga T, et al: Methamphetamine-associated obsessional symptoms and effective risperidone treatment: a case report. J Clin Psychiatry 60:337–338, 1999

Jenike MA, Baer L, Brotman AW, et al: Obsessive-compulsive disorder and the dexamethasone suppression test. J Clin Psychopharmacol 7:182–184, 1987

Jenike MA, Breiter HC, Baer L, et al: Cerebral structural abnormalities in obsessive-compulsive disorder: a quantitative morphometric magnetic resonance imaging study. Arch Gen Psychiatry 53:625–632, 1996

Karayiorgou M, Sobin C, Blundell ML, et al: Family-based association studies support a sexually dimorphic effect of COMT and MAOA on genetic susceptibility to obsessive-compulsive disorder. Biol Psychiatry 45:1178–1189, 1999

Kettl PA, Marks IM: Neurological factors in obsessive compulsive disorder: two case reports and a review of the literature. Br J Psychiatry 149:315–319, 1986

Khanna S, John JP, Reddy LP: Neuroendocrine and behavioral responses to mCPP in obsessive-compulsive disorder. Psychoneuroendocrinology 26:209–223, 2001

Kim CH, Koo MS, Cheon KA, et al: Dopamine transporter density of basal ganglia assessed with [123I]IPT SPET in obsessive-compulsive disorder. Eur J Nucl Med Mol Imaging 30:1637–1643, 2003

Kim S-J, Veenstra-VanderWeele J, Hanna GL, et al: Mutation screening of human 5-HT2B receptor gene in early-onset obsessive-compulsive disorder. Mol Cell Probes 14:47–52, 2000

Kluge M, Schussler P, Kunzel HE, et al: Increased nocturnal secretion of ACTH and cortisol in obsessive compulsive disorder. J Psychiatr Res 41:928–933, 2007

Koizumi HM: Obsessive-compulsive symptoms following stimulants. Biol Psychiatry 20:1332–1333, 1985

Kotsopoulos S, Spivak M: Obsessive-compulsive symptoms secondary to methylphenidate treatment (letter). Can J Psychiatry 46:89, 2001

Kouris S: Methylphenidate-induced obsessive-compulsiveness (letter). J Am Acad Child Adolesc Psychiatry 37:135, 1998

Kusunoki K, Sato T, Taga C, et al: Low novelty-seeking differentiates obsessive-compulsive disorder from major depression. Acta Psychiatr Scand 101:403–405, 2000

Leckman JF, Pauls DL, Peterson BS, et al: Pathogenesis of Tourette syndrome: clues from the clinical phenotype and natural history. Adv Neurol 58:15–24, 1992

Leckman JF, Walker DE, Cohen DJ: Premonitory urges in Tourette's syndrome. Am J Psychiatry 150:98–102, 1993

Leckman JF, Grice DE, Boardman J, et al: Symptoms of obsessive-compulsive disorder. Am J Psychiatry 154:911–917, 1997

Lemus CZ, Robinson DG, Kronig M, et al: Behavioral responses to a dopaminergic challenge in obsessive-compulsive disorder. J Anxiety Disord 5:369–373, 1991

Lenane MC, Swedo SE, Leonard H, et al: Psychiatric disorders in first degree relatives of children and adolescents with obsessive compulsive disorder. J Am Acad Child Adolesc Psychiatry 29:407–412, 1990

Leonard HL, Swedo SE, Rapoport JL, et al: Treatment of obsessive-compulsive disorder with clomipramine and desipramine in children and adolescents: a double-blind crossover comparison. Arch Gen Psychiatry 46:1088–1092, 1989

Leonard HL, Lenane MC, Swedo SE, et al: Tics and Tourette's disorder: a 2- to 7-year follow-up of 54 obsessive-compulsive children. Am J Psychiatry 149:1244–1251, 1992

Lesch KP, Aulakh CS, Wolozin BL, et al: Regional brain expression of serotonin transporter mRNA and its regulation by reuptake inhibiting antidepressants. Brain Res Mol Brain Res 17:31–35, 1993

Lewis A: Problems of obsessional illness. Proc Roy Soc Med 29:325–336, 1935

Lieberman JA, Kane JM, Sarantakos S, et al: Dexamethasone suppression tests in patients with obsessive-compulsive disorder. Am J Psychiatry 142:747–751, 1985

Lucey JV, Barry S, Webb MG, et al: The desipramine-induced growth hormone response and the dexamethasone suppression test in obsessive-compulsive disorder. Acta Psychiatr Scand 86:367–370, 1992

Lyoo IK, Lee DW, Kim YS, et al: Patterns of temperament and character in subjects with obsessive-compulsive disorder. J Clin Psychiatry 62:637–641, 2001

Maj M, Gaebel W, Lopez-Ibor JJ, et al (eds): Psychiatric Diagnosis and Classification. New York, Wiley, 2002

Malison RT, McDougle CJ, van Dyck CH, et al: I-123-β-CIT SPECT imaging of striatal dopamine transporter binding in Tourette's disorder. Am J Psychiatry 152:1359–1361, 1995

Mansari ME, Bouchard C, Blier P: Alteration of serotonin release in the guinea pig orbitofrontal cortex by selective serotonin reuptake inhibitors: relevance to treatment of obsessive-compulsive disorder. Neuropsychopharmacology 13:117–127, 1995

Marazziti D, Zohar J, Cassano G: Biological Dissection of Obsessive Compulsive Disorder. Edited by Berend B, Hollander E, Marazziti D, et al. Chichester, UK, Wiley, 1994, pp 137–148

Martinot JL, Allilaire JF, Mazoyer BM, et al: Obsessive-compulsive disorder: a clinical, neuropsychological and positron emission tomography study. Acta Psychiatr Scand 82:233–242, 1990

McDougle CJ, Goodman WK, Delgado PL, et al: Pathophysiology of obsessive-compulsive disorder. Am J Psychiatry 146:1350–1351, 1989

McDougle CJ, Goodman WK, Leckman JF, et al: Haloperidol addition in fluvoxamine-refractory obsessive compulsive disorder: a double-blind, placebo-controlled study in patients with and without tics. Arch Gen Psychiatry 51:302–308, 1994a

McDougle CJ, Goodman WK, Price LH: Dopamine antagonists in tic-related and psychotic spectrum obsessive compulsive disorder. J Clin Psychiatry 55(suppl):24–31, 1994b

McFall ME, Wollersheim JP: Obsessive-compulsive neurosis: a cognitive-behavioral formulation and approach to treatment. Cognit Ther Res 3:333–348, 1979

McGrath MJ, Campbell KM, Parks CR III, et al: Glutamatergic drugs exacerbate symptomatic behavior in a transgenic model of comorbid Tourette's syndrome and obsessive-compulsive disorder. Brain Res 877:23–30, 2000

McKeon JP, McGuffin P, Robinson P: Obsessive-compulsive neurosis following head injury: a report of four cases. Br J Psychiatry 144:190–192, 1984

Mesulam M-M: Patterns in behavioral neuroanatomy: association areas, the limbic system, and hemispheric specialization, in Principles of Behavioral Neurology. Edited by Mesulam M-M. Philadelphia, PA, F.A. Davis, 1985, pp 1–70

Miguel EC, Coffey BJ, Baer L, et al: Phenomenology of intentional repetitive behaviors in obsessive-compulsive disorder and Tourette's syndrome. J Clin Psychiatry 56:246–255, 1995

Mindus P, Rauch SL, Nyman H, et al: Capsulotomy and cingulotomy as treatments for malignant obsessive-compulsive disorder: an update, in Current Insights in Obsessive-Compulsive Disorder. Edited by Berend B, Hollander E, Marazziti D, et al. Chichester, UK, Wiley, 1994, pp 245–276

Mishkin M, Petri HL: Memory and habits: some implications for the analysis of learning and retention, in Neuropsychology of Memory. Edited by Squire LR, Butters N. New York, Guilford, 1984, pp 287–296

Mishkin M, Malamut B, Bachevalier J: Memories and habits: two neural systems, in Neurobiology of Learning and Memory. Edited by Lynch G, McGaugh JL, Weinberger NM. New York, Guilford, 1984, pp 65–77

Modell J, Mountz J, Curtis G, et al: Neurophysiologic dysfunction in basal ganglia/limbic striatal and thalamocortical circuits as a pathogenetic mechanism of obsessive-compulsive disorder. J Neuropsychiatry Clin Neurosci 1:27–36, 1989

Monteleone P, Catapano F, Del Buono G, et al: Circadian rhythms of melatonin, cortisol and prolactin in patients with obsessive-compulsive disorder. Acta Psychiatr Scand 89:411–415, 1994

Muller N, Putz A, Kathmann N, et al: Characteristics of obsessive-compulsive symptoms in Tourette's syndrome, obsessive-compulsive disorder, and Parkinson's disease. Psychiatry Res 70:105–114, 1997

Mundo E, Richter MA, Zai G, et al: 5HT1Dbeta Receptor gene implicated in the pathogenesis of obsessive-compulsive disorder: further evidence from a family-based association study. Mol Psychiatry. 7:805–809, 2002

Murphy DL, Greenberg B, Altemus M, et al: The neuropharmacology and neurobiology of obsessive compulsive disorder: an update on the serotonin hypothesis, in Advances in the Neurobiology of Anxiety Disorders. Edited by Westenberg HGM, Murphy DL, Den Boer JA. New York, Wiley, 1996, pp 279–297

Murphy TK, Goodman WK, Fudge MW, et al: B lymphocyte antigen D8/17: a peripheral marker for childhood onset obsessive disorder and Tourette's syndrome? Am J Psychiatry 154:402, 1997

Nestadt G, Bienvenu OJ, Cai G, et al: Incidence of obsessive-compulsive disorder in adults. J Nerv Ment Dis 186:401–406, 1998

Nestadt G, Samuels J, Riddle M, et al: A family study of obsessive-compulsive disorder. Arch Gen Psychiatry 57:358–363, 2000

Nicolini N, Beatriz C, Carlos C, et al: Dopamine receptor gene polymorphism in OCD. Paper presented at the 149th Annual Meeting of the American Psychiatric Association, New York, May 1996

Novelli E, Nobile M, Diaferia G, et al: A molecular investigation suggests no relationship between obsessive-compulsive disorder and the dopamine D2 receptor. Neuropsychobiology 29:61–63, 1994

Olley A, Malhi G, Sachdev P: Memory and executive functioning in obsessive-compulsive disorder: a selective review. J Affect Disord 104:15–23, 2007

O'Sullivan R, Rauch SL, Breiter HC, et al: Reduced basal ganglia volumes in trichotillomania by morphometric MRI. Biol Psychiatry 42:39–45, 1997

Otto MW: Neuropsychological approaches to obsessive-compulsive disorder, in Obsessive Compulsive Disorder: Theory and Management, 2nd Edition. Edited by Jenike MA, Baer L, Minichiello WE. Chicago, IL, Year Book Medical, 1990, pp 132–148

Pauls DL: The genetics of obsessive compulsive disorder: a review of the evidence. Am J Med Genet C Semin Med Genet 148:133–139, 2008

Pauls DL, Leckman JF: The inheritance of Gilles de la Tourette's syndrome and associated behaviors. N Engl J Med 315:993–997, 1986

Pauls DL, Towbin KE, Leckman JF, et al: Gilles de la Tourette syndrome and obsessive compulsive disorder. Arch Gen Psychiatry 43:1180–1182, 1986

Pauls DL, Pakstis AJ, Kurlan R, et al: Segregation and linkage analysis of Tourette's syndrome and related disorders. J Am Acad Child Adolesc Psychiatry 29:195–203, 1990

Pauls DL, Alsobrook JP, Goodman W, et al: A family study of obsessive-compulsive disorder. Am J Psychiatry 152:76–84, 1995

Penades R, Catalan R, Andres S, et al: Executive function and nonverbal memory in obsessive-compulsive disorder. Psychiatry Res 133:81–90, 2005

Perna G, Bertani A, Arancio C, et al: Laboratory response of patients with panic and obsessive-compulsive disorders to 35% CO-sub-2 challenges. Am J Psychiatry 152:85–89, 1995

Peterson B, Riddle MA, Cohen DJ, et al: Reduced basal ganglia volumes in Tourette's syndrome using three-dimensional reconstruction techniques from magnetic resonance images. Neurology 43:941–949, 1993

Pfohl B, Black DW, Noyes R, et al: A test of the tridimensional personality theory: association with diagnosis and platelet imipramine binding in obsessive-compulsive disorder. Biol Psychiatry 28:41–46, 1990

Pigott TA, Zohar J, Hill JL, et al: Metergoline blocks the behavioral and neuroendocrine effects of orally administered m-chlorophenylpiperazine in patients with obsessive-compulsive disorder. Biol Psychiatry 29:418–426, 1991

Pineyro G, Blier P, Dennis T, et al: Desensitization of the neuronal 5-HT carrier following its long-term blockade. J Neurosci 14:3036–3047, 1994

Pogarell O, Hamann C, Popperl G, et al: Elevated brain serotonin transporter availability in patients with obsessive-compulsive disorder. Biol Psychiatry 54:1406–1413, 2003

Rachman S: Obsessions, responsibility and guilt. Behav Res Ther 31:149–154, 1993

Rapoport JL, Wise SP: Obsessive-compulsive disorder: is it a basal ganglia dysfunction? Psychopharmacol Bull 24:380–384, 1988

Rasmussen SA, Goodman WK, Woods SW, et al: Effects of yohimbine in obsessive compulsive disorder. Psychopharmacology (Berl) 93:308–313, 1987

Rauch SL, Baxter LR: Neuroimaging of OCD and related disorders, in Obsessive-Compulsive Disorders: Theory and Management, 3rd Edition. Edited by Jenike MA, Baer L, Minichiello WE. St Louis, MO, Mosby-Year Book, 1998, pp 2889–317

Rauch SL, Jenike MA: Neurobiological models of obsessive-compulsive disorder. Psychosomatics 34:20–32, 1993

Rauch SL, Jenike MA: Neural mechanisms of obsessive-compulsive disorder. Current Review of Mood and Anxiety Disorders 1:84–94, 1997

Rauch SL, Savage CR: Neuroimaging and neuropsychology of the striatum, in Neuropsychiatry of the Basal Ganglia. Edited by Miguel EC, Rauch SL, Leckman JF. Philadelphia, PA, WB Saunders, 1997, pp 741–768

Rauch SL, Savage CR: Investigating corticostriatal pathophysiology in obsessive compulsive disorders: procedural learning and imaging probes, in Obsessive-Compulsive Disorder: Contemporary Issues in Treatment. Edited by Goodman WK, Rudorfer MV, Maser JD. Mahwah, NJ, Erlbaum, 2000

Rauch SL, Shin LM: Functional neuroimaging studies in PTSD. Ann NY Acad Sci 821:83–98, 1997

Rauch SL, Jenike MA, Alpert NM, et al: Regional cerebral blood flow measured during symptom provocation in obsessive-compulsive disorder using ^{15}O-labeled CO_2 and positron emission tomography. Arch Gen Psychiatry 51:62–70, 1994

Rauch SL, Savage CR, Alpert NM, et al: A positron emission tomographic study of simple phobic symptom provocation. Arch Gen Psychiatry 52:20–28, 1995a

Rauch SL, Savage CR, Brown HD, et al: A PET investigation of implicit and explicit sequence learning. Hum Brain Mapp 3:271–286, 1995b

Rauch SL, van der Kolk BA, Fisler RE, et al: A symptom provocation study of posttraumatic stress disorder using positron emission tomography and script-driven imagery. Arch Gen Psychiatry 53:380–387, 1996

Rauch SL, Savage CR, Alpert NM, et al: The functional neuroanatomy of anxiety: a study of three disorders using PET and symptom provocation. Biol Psychiatry 42:446–452, 1997a

Rauch SL, Savage CR, Alpert NM, et al: Probing striatal function in obsessive compulsive disorder: a PET study of implicit sequence learning. J Neuropsychiatry 9:568–573, 1997b

Rauch SL, Dougherty DD, Shin LM, et al: Neural correlates of factor-analyzed OCD symptom dimensions: a PET study. CNS Spectr 3(3):37–43, 1998a

Rauch SL, Whalen PJ, Curran T, et al: Thalamic deactivation during early implicit sequence learning: a functional MRI study. Neuroreport 9:865–870, 1998b

Rauch SL, Whalen PJ, Dougherty DD, et al: Neurobiological models of obsessive compulsive disorders, in Obsessive-Compulsive Disorders: Theory and Management. Edited by Jenike MA, Baer L, Minichiello WE. St Louis, MO, Mosby-Year Book, 1998c, pp 222–253

Reber AS: Implicit learning and tacit knowledge. J Exp Psychol Gen 118:219–235, 1989

Reber AS: The cognitive unconscious: an evolutionary perspective. Conscious Cogn 1:93–133, 1992

Reber PJ, Squire LR: Parallel brain systems for learning with and without awareness. Learn Mem 1:217–229, 1994

Reddy PS, Reddy YC, Srinath S, et al: A family study of juvenile obsessive-compulsive disorder. Can J Psychiatry 46:346–351, 2001

Reimold M, Smolka MN, Zimmer A, et al: Reduced availability of serotonin transporters in obsessive-compulsive disorder correlates with symptom severity: a [11C]DASB PET study. J Neural Transm 114:1603–1609, 2007

Rettew DC, Swedo SE, Leonard HL, et al: Obsessions and compulsions across time in 79 children and adolescents with obsessive-compulsive disorder. J Am Acad Child Adolesc Psychiatry 31:1050–1056, 1992

Richter MA, Summerfeldt LJ, Joffe RT, et al: The Tridimensional Personality Questionnaire in obsessive-compulsive disorder. Psychiatry Res 65:185–188, 1996

Riddle MA, Scahill L, King R, et al: Obsessive compulsive disorder in children and adolescents: phenomenology and family history. J Am Acad Child Adolesc Psychiatry 29:766–772, 1990

Robinson D, Wu H, Munne RA, et al: Reduced caudate nucleus volume in obsessive-compulsive disorder. Arch Gen Psychiatry 52:393–398, 1995

Rosario-Campos MC, Leckman JF, Mercadante MT, et al: Adults with early-onset obsessive-compulsive disorder. Am J Psychiatry 158:1899–1903, 2001

Rosario-Campos MC, Leckman JF, Curi M, et al: A family study of early-onset obsessive-compulsive disorder. Am J Med Genet B Neuropsychiatr Genet 136B:92–97, 2005

Rosse RB, Fay-McCarthy M, Collins JP, et al: Transient compulsive foraging behavior associated with crack cocaine use. Am J Psychiatry 150:155–156, 1993

Rosse RB, McCarthy MF, Alim TN, et al: Saccadic distractibility in cocaine dependent patients: a preliminary laboratory exploration of the cocaine-OCD hypothesis. Drug Alcohol Depend 35:25–30, 1994

Rowe DC, Stever C, Gard JM, et al: The relation of the dopamine transporter gene (DAT1) to symptoms of internalizing disorders in children. Behav Genet 28:215–225, 1998

Salkovskis PM: Obsessional-compulsive problems: a cognitive-behavioural analysis. Behav Res Ther 23:571–583, 1985

Salloway S, Cummings JL: Subcortical structures and neuropsychiatric illness. Neuroscientist 2:66–75, 1996

Samuels J, Nestadt G: Epidemiology and genetics of obsessive-compulsive disorder. Int Rev Psychiatry 9:61–71, 1997

Samuels J, Shugart YY, Grados M, et al: Significant linkage to compulsive hoarding on chromosome 14 in families with obsessive-compulsive disorder: results from the OCD Collaborative Genetics Study. Am J Psychiatry 164:493–499, 2007

Satel SL, McDougle CJ: Obsessions and compulsions associated with cocaine abuse. Am J Psychiatry 148:947, 1991

Savage CR, Baer L, Keuthen NJ, et al: Organizational strategies mediate nonverbal memory impairment in obsessive-compulsive disorder. Biol Psychiatry 45:905–916, 1999

Savage CR, Deckersbach T, Wilhelm S, et al: Strategic processing and episodic memory impairment in obsessive compulsive disorder. Neuropsychology 14:141–151, 2000

Scarone S, Colombo C, Livian S, et al: Increased right caudate nucleus size in obsessive compulsive disorder: detection with magnetic resonance imaging. Psychiatry Research: Neuroimaging 45:115–121, 1992

Schacter DL, Tulving E (eds): Memory Systems 1994. Cambridge, MA, MIT Press, 1994

Schacter DL, Alpert NM, Savage CR, et al: Conscious recollection and the human hippocampal formation: evidence from positron emission tomography. Proc Natl Acad Sci USA 93:321–325, 1996

Shugart YY, Samuels J, Willour VL, et al: Genomewide linkage scan for linkage analysis of families with obsessive-compulsive disorder: evidence for susceptibility on chromosomes 3p, 7p, 1q, 15q, and 16q. Mol Psychiatry 11:763–770, 2006

Simpson HB, Lombardo I, Slifstein M, et al: Serotonin transporters in obsessive-compulsive disorder: a positron emission tomography study with [(11)C]McN 5652. Biol Psychiatry 54:1414–1421, 2003

Singer H, Hahn I, Moran T: Tourette's syndrome: abnormal dopamine uptake sites in postmortem striatum from patients with Tourette's syndrome. Ann Neurol 30:558–562, 1991

Singer HS, Reiss AL, Brown JE, et al: Volumetric MRI changes in basal ganglia of children with Tourette's syndrome. Neurology 43:950–956, 1993

Squire LR: Memory and the hippocampus: a synthesis from findings with rats, monkeys, and humans. Psychol Rev 99:195–231, 1992

Steketee G, Frost RO, Cohen I: Beliefs in obsessive-compulsive disorder. J Anxiety Disord 12:525–537, 1998

Stewart SE, Geller DA, Jenike M, et al: Long-term outcome of pediatric obsessive-compulsive disorder: a meta-analysis and qualitative review of the literature. Acta Psychiatr Scand 110:4–13, 2004

Stewart SE, Fagerness JA, Platko J, et al: Association of the SLC1A1 glutamate transporter gene and obsessive-compulsive disorder. Am J Med Genet B Neuropsychiatr Genet 144B:1027–1033, 2007a

Stewart SE, Platko J, Fagerness J, et al: A genetic family-based study of OLIG2 in obsessive-compulsive disorder. Arch Gen Psychiatry 64:209–214, 2007b

Swedo SE, Rapoport JL, Cheslow DL, et al: High prevalence of obsessive-compulsive symptoms in patients with Sydenham's chorea. Am J Psychiatry 146:246–249, 1989a

Swedo SE, Rapoport JL, Leonard HL, et al: Obsessive-compulsive disorder in children and adolescents: clinical phenomenology of 70 consecutive cases. Arch Gen Psychiatry 46:335–341, 1989b

Swedo SE, Leonard HL, Schapiro MB, et al: Sydenham's chorea: physical and psychological symptoms of St. Vitus' dance. Pediatrics 91:706–713, 1993

Swedo SE, Leonard HL, Kiessling LS: Speculation on antineuronal antibody-mediated neuropsychiatric disorders of childhood. Pediatrics 93:323–326, 1994

Swedo SE, Leonard HL, Mittleman BB, et al: Identification of children with pediatric autoimmune neuropsychiatric disorders associated with streptococcal infections by a marker associated with rheumatic fever. Am J Psychiatry 154:110–112, 1997

Swedo SE, Leonard HL, Garvey M, et al: Pediatric autoimmune neuropsychiatric disorders associated with streptococcal infections: clinical description of the first 50 cases. Am J Psychiatry 155:264–271, 1998

Szechtman H, Sulis W, Eilam D: Quinpirole induces compulsive checking behavior in rats: a potential animal model of obsessive-compulsive disorder (OCD). Behav Neurosci 112:1475–1485, 1998

Szechtman H, Eckert MJ, Tse WS, et al: Compulsive checking behavior of quinpirole-sensitized rats as an animal model of obsessive-compulsive disorder (OCD): form and control. BMC Neurosci 2:4 [Epub 2001 Apr 12], 2001

Thoren P, Asberg M, Cronholm B, et al: Clomipramine treatment of obsessive compulsive disorder, I: a controlled clinical trial. Arch Gen Psychiatry 37:1281–1285, 1980

Tonkonogy J, Barreira P: Obsessive-compulsive disorder and caudate-frontal lesion. Neuropsychiatry Neuropsychol Behav Neurol 2:203–209, 1989

Tukel R, Ertekin E, Batmaz S, et al: Influence of age of onset on clinical features in obsessive-compulsive disorder. Depress Anxiety 21:112–117, 2005

Ungerleider LG: Functional brain imaging studies of cortical mechanisms for memory. Science 270:769–775, 1995

Vallejo J, Olivares J, Marcos T, et al: Dexamethasone suppression test and primary obsessional compulsive disorder. Compr Psychiatry 29:498–502, 1988

van de Wetering BJM: The Gilles de la Tourette syndrome: a psychiatric-genetic study. (PhD Thesis.) Rotterdam, The Netherlands, Erasmus University, 1993

van der Wee NJ, Stevens H, Hardeman JA, et al: Enhanced dopamine transporter density in psychotropic-naive patients with obsessive-compulsive disorder shown by [123I]{beta}-CIT SPECT. Am J Psychiatry 161:2201–2206, 2004

van Grootheest DS, Cath DC, Beekman AT, et al: Twin studies on obsessive-compulsive disorder: a review. Twin Res Hum Genet 8:450–458, 2005

Walitza S, Renner TJ, Dempfle A, et al: Transmission disequilibrium of polymorphic variants in the tryptophan hydroxylase-2 gene in attention-deficit/hyperactivity disorder. Mol Psychiatry 10:1126–1132, 2005

Weilburg JB, Mesulam MM, Weintraub S, et al: Focal striatal abnormalities in a patient with obsessive-compulsive disorder. Arch Neurol 46:233–235, 1989

Weissman MM, Bland RC, Canino GJ, et al: The cross national epidemiology of obsessive compulsive disorder. The Cross National Collaborative Group. J Clin Psychiatry 55(suppl):5–10, 1994

Williams AC, Owen C, Heath DA: A compulsive movement disorder with cavitation of caudate nucleus. J Neurol Neurosurg Psychiatry 51:447–448, 1988

Wise SP, Murray EA, Gerfen CR: The frontal cortex-basal ganglia system in primates. Crit Rev Neurobiol 10:317–356, 1996

Wolf SS, Jones DW, Knable MB, et al: Tourette syndrome: prediction of phenotypic variation in monozygotic twins by caudate nucleus D2 receptor binding. Science 273:1225–1227, 1996

Zai G, Bezchilbnyk YB, Richter MA, et al: Myelin oligodendrocyte glycoprotein (MOG) gene is associated with obsessive-compulsive disorder. Am J Med Genet B Neuropsychiatr Genet 129B:64–68, 2004

Zald DH, Kim SW: Anatomy and function of the orbital frontal cortex, II: function and relevance to obsessive-compulsive disorder. J Neuropsychiatry 8:249–261, 1996

Zielinski CM, Taylor MA, Juzwin KR: Neuropsychological deficits in obsessive-compulsive disorder. Neuropsychiatry Neuropsychol Behav Neurol 4:110–126, 1991

Ziemann U, Paulus W, Rothenberger A: Decreased motor inhibition in Tourette's disorder: evidence from transcranial magnetic stimulation. Am J Psychiatry 154:1277–1284, 1997

Zitterl W, Aigner M, Stompe T, et al: [123I]-beta-CIT SPECT imaging shows reduced thalamus-hypothalamus serotonin transporter availability in 24 drug-free obsessive-compulsive checkers. Neuropsychopharmacology 32:1661–1668, 2007

Zohar J, Insel TR: Obsessive-compulsive disorder: psychobiological approaches to diagnosis, treatment, and pathophysiology. Biol Psychiatry 22:667–687, 1987

Zohar J, Mueller EA, Insel TR, et al: Serotonergic responsivity in obsessive-compulsive disorder: comparison of patients and healthy controls. Arch Gen Psychiatry 44:946–951, 1987

Recommended Readings

Dougherty DD, Rauch SL, Jenike MA: Pharmacological treatments for obsessive-compulsive disorder, in A Guide to Treatments That Work, 3rd Edition. Edited by Nathan PE, Gorman JM. New York, Oxford University press, 2007, pp 447–473

Geller DA, Biederman J, Faraone S, et al: Developmental aspects of obsessive compulsive disorder: findings in children, adolescents, and adults. J Nerv Ment Dis 189:471–477, 2001

Jenike MA, Baer L, Minichiello WD (eds): Obsessive-Compulsive Disorders: Practical Management, 3rd Edition. St Louis, MO, Mosby, 1998

Maia TV, Cooney RE, Peterson BS: The neural bases of obsessive-compulsive disorder in children and adults. Dev Psychopathol 20:1251–1283, 2008

Pauls DL: The genetics of obsessive compulsive disorder: a review of the evidence. Am J Med Genet C Semin Med Genet 148:133–139, 2008

Chapter 18

Pharmacotherapy for Obsessive-Compulsive Disorder

Naomi A. Fineberg, M.B.B.S., M.A., MRCPsych
Kevin J. Craig, M.B.B.Ch., M.Phil., MRCPsych

Obsessive-compulsive disorder (OCD) is a common, enduring, lifespan illness (Skoog and Skoog 1999; Wittchen and Jacobi 2005). Prior to the 1960s, OCD was considered untreatable. Since then, a relatively narrow range of pharmacotherapies have been adopted: clomipramine in the 1960s, selective serotonin reuptake inhibitors (SSRIs) in the 1980s, and antipsychotic augmentation in the 1990s (for a review, see Fineberg and Gale 2005). Nowadays, with good care and optimal drug treatment, most patients with OCD can look forward to substantial symptomatic improvement. The recognition and accurate diagnosis of OCD are the first steps in the proper treatment of this condition. If the diagnosis of OCD is overlooked, then inappropriate treatment may be prescribed. For example, patients with OCD often present with symptoms of depression or anxiety, but not all antidepressants and few, if any, anxiolytic medications are effective in the presence of OCD. The current standard of care in the United Kingdom is to offer either behavioral psychotherapy or medication as first-line treatment (National Institute for Health and Clinical Excellence [NICE] 2005). The form of behavior therapy that has been most effective in OCD is referred to as exposure and response prevention (see Chapter 19 in this volume, "Psychological Treatment for Obsessive-Compulsive Disorder," for a description of the use of behavior therapy in OCD). At present, the principal pharmacotherapy for OCD involves a trial of a serotonin reuptake inhibitor (SRI). Based on results from more than 100 randomized, controlled trials and several meta-analyses, good evidence is available to support the use of SRIs in treating OCD. A growing corpus of literature suggests that SRIs are effective in long-term treatment and relapse prevention and provides a detailed evaluation of side effects and tolerability. Although we recognize the importance of all aspects of management, in this chapter we focus on pharmacological approaches to treatment.

This chapter was adapted from Fineberg NA, Craig KJ: "Benefits and Limitations of Pharmacological Interventions in Obsessive Compulsive Disorder." *Clinical Neuropsychiatry* 3:345–363, 2006. The authors also gratefully acknowledge limited use of material from the chapter "Pharmacotherapy for Obsessive-Compulsive Disorder," by Wayne K. Goodman, M.D., that appeared in the previous edition of this volume.

Serotonin Reuptake Inhibitors

Modern pharmacotherapy for OCD began with the observation that clomipramine (the 3-chloro analogue of the tricyclic imipramine), but not other tricyclic antidepressants, relieved obsessive-compulsive symptoms. Clomipramine can be differentiated from other tricyclics by its marked potency for blocking serotonin reuptake. This distinctive psychopharmacological property led to the hypothesis that serotonin might be involved in the pathophysiology of OCD. The majority of evidence supporting a role for serotonin in OCD is based on drug response data (i.e., the preferential efficacy of SRIs) (Goodman et al. 1990). A number of early, small OCD studies demonstrated clomipramine's superiority relative to other tricyclic antidepressants, including desipramine (Insel et al. 1985; Leonard et al. 1988, 1991), imipramine (Foa et al. 1987; Volavka et al. 1985), nortriptyline (Thoren et al. 1980), and amitriptyline (Ananth et al. 1981). Although clomipramine is a powerful SRI, it has an active metabolite with strong noradrenergic properties. The "serotonin hypothesis" was given more weight by studies favorably comparing SSRIs to the noradrenergic tricyclic desipramine (Goodman et al. 1990; Hoehn-Saric et al. 2000) as well as monoamine oxidase inhibitors (MAOIs) such as phenelzine (Jenike et al. 1997). Although MAOIs are potent antidepressants, no study has convincingly demonstrated an advantage of these drugs over placebo. This might be due, in part, to their prodopaminergic action, which may exacerbate OCD symptoms. Although SRIs represent the cornerstone of pharmacological management for OCD, because clinical response is not always satisfactory, a major portion of this chapter is also devoted to biological approaches to SRI nonresponders.

Evaluation of Treatment Response in OCD

The 10-item Yale-Brown Obsessive Compulsive Scale (Y-BOCS; Goodman et al. 1989b) and the Clinical Global Impression Severity (CGI-S) and Improvement (CGI-I) scales (Guy 1976) represent the pivotal rating instruments for measuring OCD severity and treatment response. The magnitude of treatment response can be expressed as the mean change in baseline Y-BOCS scores for patients taking active drug (e.g., 8.2 in a recent meta-analysis of clomipramine; Ackerman and Greenland 2002) compared with placebo. Alternatively, results can be expressed as treatment responders versus nonresponders. Although no universally accepted definition of *treatment response* exists, a CGI-I rating of *improved* or *very much improved* and a decrease in Y-BOCS scores of 25% or 35% are widely used criteria and appear to separate active from inactive treatments (Simpson et al. 2006). This conservative level of Y-BOCS improvement contrasts with the standard 50% improvement required on Hamilton Rating Scale for Depression (Hamilton 1960) scores to consider treatment for major depressive disorder to be successful. Even using such a modest criterion, response rates in acute-phase OCD trials of SSRIs have rarely exceeded 60%, emphasizing the incomplete effect of these treatments in the short-term treatment of OCD (Table 18–1).

The concept of *remission* for OCD is also debatable, and no definition is universally accepted (Pallanti et al. 2002a). Remission has been described as a brief period during which sufficient improvement has occurred that the individual has minimal symptoms of OCD (Simpson et al. 2006). Study authors have chosen remission criteria ranging from Y-BOCS<16 to Y-BOCS≤ 7 (Cottraux et al. 2001; Eddy et al. 2004; Fineberg et al. 2006c; Hollander et al. 2003a; Simpson et al. 2006; Stein et al. 2007; van Oppen et al. 1995). A score of 16 on the Y-BOCS is generally considered too high to meaningfully represent true remission, and a score of 7 is considered too low to be achieved by all but a very few patients. In the analysis by Simpson et al. (2006), a Y-BOCS score of 7 did not discriminate between active and control treatments, whereas in two recent multicenter escitalopram studies, a score of 10 did discriminate (Fineberg et al. 2007b; Stein et al. 2007).

Clomipramine in Acute-Phase OCD Treatment Trials

According to Fineberg and Gale (2005), an early case report (Fernandez Cordoba and Lopez-Ibor Alino 1967) followed by a number of double-blind, placebo-controlled trials conclusively established clomipramine as an effective treatment for OCD. In a crossover study comparing clomipramine and desipramine (Insel et al. 1985), adult patients had a significant response to clomipramine, whereas desipramine was indistinguishable from placebo. These findings were replicated in children (Leonard et al. 1988, 1991). In placebo-controlled trials, efficacy has been demonstrated using as few as 14 patients (Greist et al. 1990), emphasizing the potency of the effect.

The introduction of large-scale controlled multicenter studies enabled the effects of drug interventions to be assessed and compared in reasonably heterogeneous groups of patients with OCD. Two large multi-

TABLE 18–1. OCD response rates in randomized, controlled trials of SRIs

Drug and daily dosage (duration in weeks)	CGI much or very much improved (A)	25% improvement on baseline Y-BOCS (B)	(A+B)	Study
Citalopram 20 mg (12)	57%	—	—	Montgomery et al. 2001
Citalopram 40 mg (12)	52%	—	—	Montgomery et al. 2001
Citalopram 60 mg (12)	65%	—	—	Montgomery et al. 2001
Clomipramine (12)	55%	—	—	Zohar and Judge 1996
Escitalopram 20 mg (24)	—	70%	—	Stein et al. 2007
Fluoxetine 20 mg (8)	—	—	36%	Montgomery et al. 1993
Fluoxetine 40 mg (8)	—	—	48%	Montgomery et al. 1993
Fluoxetine 60 mg (8)	—	—	47%	Montgomery et al. 1993
Fluoxetine 20 mg (8)	—	32%>35% improved	—	Tollefson et al. 1994
Fluoxetine 40 mg (8)	—	34%>35% improved	—	Tollefson et al. 1994
Fluoxetine 60 mg (8)	—	35%>35% improved	—	Tollefson et al. 1994
Fluoxetine (13)	55%	—	—	Geller et al. 2001
Fluoxetine (16)	57%	—	—	Liebowitz et al. 2002
Fluvoxamine (8)	43%	—	—	Goodman et al. 1989a
Fluvoxamine (10)	33%	—	—	Goodman et al. 1996
Fluvoxamine (10)	—	42%	—	Riddle et al. 2001
Fluvoxamine CR (12)	34%	63%	—	Hollander et al. 2003d
Fluvoxamine CR (12)	—	45%>35% improved	—	Hollander et al. 2003d
Paroxetine (12)	55%	—	—	Zohar and Judge 1996
Paroxetine (24)	—	67%	—	Stein et al. 2007
Sertraline (12)	39%	—	—	Greist et al. 1995a
Sertraline (12)	42%	—	—	March et al. 1998
Sertraline (12)	41%	—	—	Kronig et al. 1999

Note. CGI=Clinical Global Impression (Guy 1976); CR=continuous release; OCD=obsessive-compulsive disorder; SRIs=serotonin reuptake inhibitors; Y-BOCS=Yale-Brown Obsessive Compulsive Scale (Goodman et al. 1989b); —=data not reported.

center trials, comprising 238 and 263 cases, excluded comorbid depression (DeVeaugh-Geiss et al. 1989; Group CCS 1991). Clomipramine was flexibly dosed (up to 300 mg/day). In both studies, placebo response did not exceed 5% reduction on Y-BOCS scores over the course of 10 weeks. Significant differences for the clomipramine group began to emerge at weeks 1–2, and benefits for this group continued to accrue slowly and gradually up to the 10-week endpoint. The studies demonstrated a decrease in Y-BOCS scores by 38% and 44%, respectively, which was correlated with similar improvements in social and emotional well-being.

Clomipramine for OCD With Comorbid Mood Disorder

Studies of clinical OCD samples found that at least two-thirds of patients experienced depression at some point during their lifetime (Brawman-Mintzer et al. 1993). Moreover, the depression carried a substantial negative impact on individuals' quality of life (Richter et al. 2003). Few studies have specifically investigated OCD with comorbid depression, and most of these studies have used clomipramine as the active drug. In a 5-week study by Thoren et al. (1980), patients taking clomipramine showed significant improvement over those taking nortriptyline and placebo on the six-item obsessive-compulsive subscale of the Comprehensive

Psychopathologic Rating Scale. Similarly, Insel et al.'s (1983b) crossover study demonstrated clomipramine's superiority over clorgyline and placebo at 4 and 6 weeks. Other studies showed that clomipramine had similar positive effects for reducing obsessional symptoms (Jenike et al. 1989; Marks et al. 1980; Mavissakalian et al. 1985), although the studies did not report the effect of clomipramine on depression.

SSRIs in Acute-Phase OCD Treatment Trials

Fluvoxamine

Small studies with as few as 20 patients established efficacy for fluvoxamine compared with placebo by the 8- to 10-week endpoints (Cottraux et al. 1990; Goodman et al. 1989a; Perse et al. 1987), although a negative study was also reported (Jenike et al. 1990). Two multicenter trials of fluvoxamine involving 156 and 253 patients, respectively, and flexible dosing (100–300 mg/day) demonstrated improvement in Y-BOCS scores from weeks 2–4 onward (Goodman et al. 1996; Hollander et al. 2003d). In the study by Hollander et al. (2003d), the group treated with controlled-release fluvoxamine showed a 32% improvement in Y-BOCS scores at the 12-week endpoint compared with a 21% improvement in the placebo group. Remission (defined conservatively as a Y-BOCS score<16) was achieved in 44% of cases; however, a relatively large dropout rate occurred in the fluvoxamine group (19% vs. 6% in the placebo group), due mainly to side effects. Hoehn-Saric et al. (2000), in a study of depressed cases of OCD, reported superiority for fluvoxamine over desipramine for both Y-BOCS and Hamilton Rating Scale for Depression scores, highlighting the importance of treating comorbid OCD and depression with an SSRI.

In an open-label study, Rufer et al. (2005) followed, for 6–8 years, 30 inpatients with severe OCD who had been treated with fluvoxamine. The patients' initial treatment response of 41% remained stable at long-term follow-up. Response rates (defined as 35% Y-BOCS score reduction) of 60% were reported, and by the study end, 27% of patients had entered remission and no longer met criteria for OCD (Y-BOCS<7). However, the majority of patients had required further treatment—either medication or cognitive-behavioral therapy (CBT)—in the intervening years.

Fluoxetine

An 8-week multicenter trial by Montgomery et al. (1993) comparing three fixed dosages of fluoxetine (20 mg/day, *n*=52; 40 mg/day, *n*=52; 60 mg/day, *n*=54) showed no difference between 20-mg/day fluoxetine and placebo. The 40-mg/day dosage outperformed placebo on the responder analysis (>25% reduction in Y-BOCS scores, and CGI-I ratings of *improved* or *very much improved*), whereas the 60-mg/day dosage showed a further significant reduction in Y-BOCS scores compared with the other dosages as well as placebo. Importantly, no significant difference in reported side effects occurred between any of the groups. A similar but larger fixed-dosage, double-blind, randomized, controlled study by Tollefson et al. (1994) (*N*=355) also demonstrated that fluoxetine was an effective treatment for OCD. All fixed dosages were significantly better than placebo by 13 weeks, although there was a trend toward the higher-dosage treatment (60 mg/day) being more effective. Jenike et al. (1997) compared fixed-dosage fluoxetine 80 mg/day (*n*=23) and phenelzine 60 mg/day (*n*=20) to placebo (*n*=21) and showed efficacy for fluoxetine but not the MAOI.

Sertraline

An early small study that was arguably underpowered (*N*=19) produced a negative finding (Jenike et al. 1990). Subsequent studies demonstrated efficacy using accepted measures, such as the Y-BOCS, CGI, and National Institute of Mental Health Global Obsessive-Compulsive Scale (Chouinard et al. 1990; Kronig et al. 1999). A large study (*N*=325) by Greist et al. (1995c) demonstrated unusually high patient dropout rates in some of the fixed-dosage treatment arms over a 1-year treatment period. Pooled sertraline outperformed placebo, but there was only a 39% improvement in Y-BOCS scores in the sertraline group compared with 30% in the placebo group.

Paroxetine

A large multicenter study of paroxetine by Zohar and Judge (1996) included clomipramine as an active comparator agent. Paroxetine, given in dosages up to 60 mg/day (*n*=201), was significantly more effective than placebo (*n*=99) and was of comparable efficacy to clomipramine (50–250 mg/day; *n*=99). In another large trial (*N*=105), Hollander et al. (2003a) compared paroxetine in fixed dosages (20 mg/day, 40 mg/day, 60 mg/day) with placebo. Both higher paroxetine dosages significantly outperformed placebo and the 20-mg/day paroxetine dosage, which did not separate from placebo. These results suggested the minimum effective dosage of paroxetine to be 40 mg/day. A comparator study by Stein et al. (2007), which extended up to 24 weeks, included a 40-mg/day fixed-dosage arm (*n*=116), which showed efficacy against placebo at the 12- and 24-week rating points. Results from a small study by Kamijima et al. (2004) suggested that paroxetine is effective across different cultural settings.

Citalopram

A large fixed-dosage multinational study of citalopram (Montgomery et al. 2001) found an advantage for the pooled active drug over placebo for weeks 7–12, with the highest (60 mg/day) fixed-dosage treatment showing the earliest effect, by week 3. Citalopram was well tolerated, and only 4% of withdrew due to adverse events. In addition to improvement on Y-BOCS scores, the treatment groups showed significant improvement on psychosocial function, measured on the Sheehan Disability Scale (Sheehan et al. 1996).

Escitalopram

Escitalopram, an SSRI with dual actions on the serotonin transporter (Sanchez et al. 2004), was investigated in a large active-referenced multicenter study that extended for as long as 24 weeks (Stein et al. 2007). Patients were randomly assigned to receive escitalopram 10 mg/day (*n*=112), escitalopram 20 mg/day (*n*=114), paroxetine 40 mg/day (*n*=116), or placebo (*n*=113). After 12 weeks, both escitalopram 20 mg/day and paroxetine were superior to placebo, and by week 24, all three active treatments were superior, although escitalopram 20 mg/day was more effective than escitalopram 10 mg/day when compared with placebo. These results emphasize the importance of continuing treatment for long enough. They suggest that escitalopram (10–20 mg/day) is effective, with a faster onset of action for the 20-mg/day dosage.

Special Populations

Children and Adolescents

Clomipramine. OCD is a lifespan disorder, with many patients developing illness for the first time in childhood or early adolescence (Heyman et al. 2001). Flament et al. (1985) were the first to show efficacy for clomipramine in treating childhood OCD. Nineteen children with OCD, ages 6–18 years, entered a 5-week placebo-controlled crossover study. A significantly greater improvement in obsessional rating scores was observed in the clomipramine group. The largest study on childhood OCD, by DeVeaugh-Geiss et al. (1992), demonstrated a 37% improvement (measured by Children's Yale-Brown Obsessive Compulsive Scale [CY-BOCS; Scahill et al. 1997]) in the clomipramine group (*n*=31) compared with an 8% improvement in the placebo group (*n*=29). Leonard et al. (1989) reported a 10-week double-blind crossover trial of clomipramine and desipramine (*n*=48). Clomipramine was superior to desipramine in reducing obsessive-compulsive symptoms. Age at onset, duration and severity of illness, type of symptoms, and plasma drug concentrations did not predict clinical response to clomipramine. Sixty-four percent of patients who received clomipramine as their first active treatment showed at least some sign of relapse during desipramine treatment, supporting the efficacy of clomipramine and the lack of efficacy of desipramine.

Fluvoxamine. Riddle et al. (2001) studied fluvoxamine's effectiveness in a large randomized, controlled trial involving 120 children with OCD ages 8–17 years. Significant effects, as measured by the CY-BOCS, were noted as early as week 1 and continued to the trial endpoint at week 10. In contrast to the relatively large dropout rate in Hollander et al.'s (2003d) fluvoxamine group (reported earlier in chapter), only 3 young patients in Riddle et al.'s fluvoxamine group did not complete the trial due to side effects. This finding suggests satisfactory efficacy and tolerability for fluvoxamine in treating childhood OCD.

Fluoxetine. In all three studies that have examined fluoxetine in treating childhood OCD, fluoxetine has shown superiority over placebo. Riddle et al.'s (1992) crossover study used fixed dosages of 20 mg/day. Behavioral activation occurred as an adverse effect in a few children, and one child left the study early because of suicidal ideation. The authors considered these side effects to be dosage related and advocated initiating treatment at dosages lower than 20 mg/day. In a larger cohort (*N*=103), Geller et al. (2001) titrated dosages upward from 10 to 60 mg/day over 13 weeks. Fluoxetine was superior and well tolerated, and dropout rates from adverse events were similar for patients taking drug and those taking placebo. In the positive trial by Liebowitz et al. (2002), the maximum dosage was extended to 80 mg/day after the first 6 weeks. After 8 weeks, responders were allowed to continue double-blind treatment for a further 8 weeks. No patient withdrew due to adverse effects. These results suggest that fluoxetine is clinically effective across the full dosage range in children with OCD.

Sertraline. March et al. (1998) found that sertraline, titrated up to 200 mg/day, had a significant advantage over placebo in a cohort of children and adolescents with OCD. Cardiovascular parameters showed no clinically meaningful abnormalities. In a study by the Pediatric OCD Treatment Study (POTS) Team (2004), children and adolescents received CBT alone, sertraline alone, combined CBT and sertraline, or pill placebo. All three active treatments appeared acceptable and well tolerated, with no evidence of treatment-emergent harm to self or to others. The lack of a matched control treatment for CBT limited conclusions about relative efficacy. Sertraline alone and in combination with CBT was efficacious compared with pill placebo.

A pooled analysis of the childhood OCD studies comparing numbers needed to treat with those needed to harm revealed no suicidal actions and a positive risk ratio for the use of sertraline in children and adolescents with OCD (March et al. 2006).

Paroxetine. Geller et al. (2004) reported efficacy for paroxetine (10–50 mg/day) in a study of 204 children and adolescents from as young as age 7 years. Paroxetine was well tolerated: 10.2% of patients in the paroxetine group and 2.9% in the placebo group discontinued treatment because of adverse events. Interestingly, response rates decreased with increasing comorbidity.

Pregnant Women

Safety in prescribing medications during pregnancy can never be assured, and prospective parents need to be aware of the risks and benefits and be involved in prescribing decisions during pregnancy. Potential risks to the developing child include malformation (first trimester), toxicity (third trimester), and postnatal withdrawal symptoms. Balanced against these risks to the child is the risk of the mother's relapse if medication is discontinued, which may have a negative impact on both mother and child. Of the SSRIs, fluoxetine has the greatest amount of retrospective data.

Guidelines for prescribing for patients with OCD match general principles for prescribing medications during pregnancy:

- Aim for the minimum effective dosage.
- Be prepared to adjust dosages upward as pregnancy progresses, particularly in the third trimester when blood volume increases by up to 30%.
- Ensure good fetal screening during pregnancy.
- Communicate decisions and treatment plans to obstetricians and other health care teams involved.
- Monitor the neonate for discontinuation effects, which may include irritability, agitation, and (rarely) seizures, particularly when exposed to SSRIs that have a short half-life.

Breast-Fed Infants

Limited data have been published on the effects of psychotropic medications received by nursing mothers on breast-fed infants. The majority of publications are case reports or small studies. Little is known about long-term safety.

General principles include the following:

- Aim for the minimum effective dosage.
- Ensure that the child is monitored for specific adverse events from the medication as well as for normal development, feeding patterns, and behavior.

Elderly Patients

OCD is commonly a lifelong illness; however, compulsive symptoms may also occur for the first time in elderly individuals following a neurological insult. The pharmacokinetic and pharmacodynamic properties of most drugs differ in younger and older patients. Medication problems for older adults are complicated by the increased incidence of concomitant illness and polypharmacy. Adverse events are thus more common in elderly patients because of changes in drug metabolism and drug-drug interactions.

The following are guidelines for treating OCD in elderly patients:

- Use medication only when necessary.
- Begin with lower dosages and increase as needed, but do not undertreat.
- Avoid drugs that block α_1 or acetylcholine receptors because elderly patients are frequently more susceptible to the side effects from these medications.

SSRI Versus Clomipramine as First-Line Treatment

The clinical effectiveness of a medication depends on a balance between efficacy, safety, and tolerability. SSRIs are generally safe and well tolerated, according to placebo-referenced treatment trials (as listed in Table 18–1), which had adverse event–related withdrawal rates of around 5%–15%. As a group, SSRIs are associated with initially increased nausea, nervousness, insomnia, somnolence, dizziness, and diarrhea. Sexual side effects, which included reduced libido and delayed orgasm, affected up to 30% of individuals (Monteiro et al. 1987). Three controlled studies have compared the clinical effectiveness of different SSRIs, and the results were not strong enough to support the superior efficacy of any one compound (Bergeron et al. 2002; Mundo et al. 1997; Stein et al. 2007).

Pharmacokinetic variation is relevant in determining which SSRI to use. Fluoxetine, paroxetine, and to a much lesser extent sertraline all inhibit the P450 isoenzyme CYP2D6, which metabolizes tricyclic antidepressants, antipsychotics, antiarrhythmics, and betablockers. Fluvoxamine inhibits both CYP1A2 and CYP3A4, which eliminate warfarin, tricyclics, benzodiazepines, and some antiarrhythmics. Citalopram and escitalopram are relatively free from hepatic interactions and therefore may have an advantage in elderly and physically unwell patients. In addition to having fewer discontinuation effects, fluoxetine has a long half-life, which can be beneficial for patients who forget to take their medication. Fluoxetine has also been extensively used in pregnant patients and generally shown to be safe (Emslie and Judge 2000).

Most side effects of clomipramine can be predicted from its receptor binding profile. As with other tricyclic antidepressants, side effects typical of anticholinergic blockade (e.g., dry mouth and constipation) are common. Many patients complain of sedation and weight gain (Maina et al. 2004), likely resulting from antihistaminic (H_1) binding. Orthostatic hypotension is thought to be caused by α-adrenergic blockade. Nausea and tremor also are common with clomipramine, as with other SRIs. Impotence and anorgasmia occur with clomipramine, and sexual performance is impaired in up to 80% of patients. Compared with the SSRIs, clomipramine is associated with a greater risk of potentially dangerous side effects, including prolongation of the QT interval and seizures; the risk of seizures in patients taking clomipramine (up to 2%) increases significantly at dosages greater than 250 mg/day. The fact that intentional overdoses with clomipramine can be lethal needs to be kept in mind when prescribing for OCD, in view of the elevated suicide risk associated with the illness. Comorbidity rates of OCD and bipolar disorder have been cited to be as high as 30% (Kruger et al. 1995); SSRIs are considered less likely than clomipramine to precipitate mania, but mood-stabilizing medication is still advised to mitigate the risk (Kaplan and Hollander 2003).

The best way to determine the comparative efficacy of treatments is through a randomized, head-to-head, double-blind comparison. The results of several such studies comparing clomipramine with SSRIs have been published (Flament and Bisserbe 1997; Koran et al. 1996; Zohar and Judge 1996). By and large, these studies have failed to find evidence for the superior efficacy of any of the SRIs tested thus far; however, SSRIs are generally better tolerated and associated with fewer serious side effects than clomipramine (Table 18–2).

Meta-Analyses of SRIs

Meta-analyses cannot substitute for high-quality head-to-head comparator trials. By combining data from separate studies using specific rules, meta-analyses can provide more objective and quantifiable measures of treatment effect size than can narrative reviews. However, because they are subject to potential imbalances in populations studied and differing methodologies across studies, analyses of OCD trials, which spanned several decades, must be viewed with caution (Pigott and Seay 1999). Also, a significant difference reported in a large meta-analysis may reflect only a small difference between the treatments, which may not be clinically relevant. For these reasons, the evidence from meta-analyses is considered weaker than evidence from individual controlled studies.

Whereas most meta-analyses demonstrated similar significant advantages for all SRIs over placebo, some showed superiority for clomipramine over SSRIs, which were more or less comparable with each other (Abramowitz 1997; Ackerman and Greenland 2002; Greist et al. 1995b; Jenike et al. 1990; Kobak et al. 1998; Piccinelli et al. 1995; Stein et al. 1995). Variations across individual studies in factors such as year of publication, severity of OCD, length of single-blind prerandomization period, length of trial, unblinding by clomipramine-related adverse effects, and rising placebo response rates were recognized to have potentially biased the results in favor of clomipramine.

The United Kingdom's National Institute for Health and Clinical Excellence (NICE 2005) systematically accessed both unpublished and published randomized studies, which were included in the meta-analysis only if they met stringent methodological criteria, in order to develop an evidence-based treatment guideline. Clomipramine and SSRIs were indistinguishable in terms of efficacy in patients with OCD. However, limited evidence suggested that relative to SSRIs, clomipramine was associated with higher rates of premature, adverse events–related trial discontinuations.

Geller et al. (2003b) performed a meta-analysis on pharmacotherapy for childhood OCD. The results were

TABLE 18–2. Controlled studies comparing SSRIs with clomipramine in OCD treatment

Drug and study	*N*	Design (daily dosage)	Outcome	
			Tolerability	Efficacy
Citalopram				
Pidrman and Tuma 1998	24	CMI vs. CIT	CIT=CMI	CIT=CMI
Fluoxetine				
Piggott et al. 1990	11	CMI (50–250 mg) vs. FLX (20–80 mg)	FLX>CMI	CMI=FLX
Lopez-Ibor et al. 1996	30 vs. 24	CMI (150 mg) vs. FLX (40 mg)	FLX=CMI	CMI=FLX on primary criterion CMI> FLX on other criteria
Fluvoxamine				
Smeraldi et al. 1992	10	CMI (200 mg) vs. FLV (200 mg)	FLV=CMI	CMI=FLV
Freeman et al. 1994	30 vs. 34	CMI (150–250 mg) vs. FLV (150–250 mg)	FLV>CMI (on severe effects)	CMI=FLV
Koran et al. 1996	42 vs. 37	CMI (100–250 mg) vs. FLV (100–250 mg)	FLV=CMI	CMI=FLV
Milanfranchi et al. 1997	13 vs.13	CMI (50–300 mg) vs. FLV (50–300 mg)	FLV=CMI	CMI=FLV
Rouillon 1998	105 vs. 112	CMI (150–300 mg) vs. FLV (150–300 mg)	FLV>CMI	CMI=FLV
Paroxetine				
Zohar and Judge 1996	99 vs. 201 vs. 99	CMI (50–250 mg) vs. PAR (20–60 mg) vs. placebo	PAR>CMI	CMI> placebo PAR> placebo
Sertraline				
Bisserbe et al. 1997	82 vs. 86	CMI (50–200 mg) vs. SER (50–200 mg)	SER>CMI	SER=CMI

Note. CIT=citalopram; CMI=clomipramine; FLV=fluvoxamine; FLX=fluoxetine; OCD=obsessive-compulsive disorder; PAR=paroxetine; SER=sertraline; SSRIs=selective serotonin reuptake inhibitors.

consistent with those in the adult literature. In the absence of head-to-head studies, the authors recommended that clomipramine should not generally be used as a first-line treatment in children because of its more problematic side-effect profile. Fineberg et al. (2004) compared SRI treatment trials in childhood OCD with those in adult OCD. Effect sizes overlapped for children and adults to the extent that it was impossible to discriminate between the efficacy and tolerability of SRIs in adults and children with OCD. These results imply a similar treatment response for adults and children with OCD.

SRI Dose Selection

Clomipramine and fluvoxamine have not been investigated in OCD using fixed-dosage comparator groups. The study by Montgomery (1980) did show efficacy for clomipramine at a relatively low fixed dosage of 75 mg/day. Dosage-finding studies have suggested that higher dosages (60 mg/day) of fluoxetine (Ackerman et al. 1998) and paroxetine (Hollander et al. 2003a) are more effective than low dosages. In the case of paroxetine, 20 mg/day did not separate from placebo. The evidence for superiority of dosages of 60 mg/day of citalopram was less clear-cut and appeared only on some secondary analyses (Montgomery et al. 2001). The dosage-finding study by Greist et al. (1995a) may have lacked statistical power and was unable to distinguish a dose-response relationship for sertraline. In a fixed-dosage escitalopram study (Stein et al. 2007), findings indicated a clear superiority for the 20-mg/day dosage, which separated from placebo as early as week 6 and continued to effect greater placebo-referenced improvement up to week 24, whereas the 10-mg/day dosage only separated from placebo at week 16. These results argue persuasively for a dose-response relationship and further controlled exploration of higher SSRI dosages for OCD.

SRI Dose Titration

Although rapid upward titration of medications may produce earlier responses in patients with OCD, long-term benefits of this approach have not been established. In a double-blind study, pulse loading with intravenous (but not oral) clomipramine produced a large and rapid decrease in obsessive symptoms, but the early advantages were not sustained (Koran et al. 1997). A single-blind study compared rapid dosage escalation of oral sertraline to 150 mg/day over 5 days versus slower escalation over 15 days and found an early advantage (which disappeared after week 6) for the rapid titration group (Bogetto et al. 2002).

Early SSRI-related adverse effects, such as agitation and nausea, can be ameliorated by slowly titrating upward over weeks and months. The arguments for slower dosage increases are particularly persuasive for children and elderly patients. Special care with higher dosages is also required for patients with comorbidity. For example, OCD patients with comorbid panic disorder may be particularly sensitive to early anxiogenic effects of SSRIs, and lower-than-average dosages may be required for the first 1–2 weeks. OCD patients with comorbid bipolar affective disorder are susceptible to switching into mania and may require additional mood stabilizers (Kaplan and Hollander 2003). Longer-term side effects, such as sleep disturbance, headache, and sexual dysfunction, may be dosage related and are a common cause of drug discontinuation. Expert consensus currently favors beginning with moderated dosages, with upward dosage titrations to maximum should symptoms persist (NICE 2005).

Other Antidepressants

For first-line treatment of OCD, few rational alternatives to SRIs exist. Venlafaxine has generated some interest due to its predominantly serotonergic action at low dosages. Venlafaxine was not significantly better than placebo in a relatively short 8-week double-blind trial of 30 patients with OCD (Yaryura-Tobias and Neziroglu 1996). In a subsequent nonplacebo study by Denys et al. (2003), no significant differences were found between the group taking venlafaxine 300 mg/day (n=75) and the group taking paroxetine 60 mg/day (n=75), and the response rate was 40% in both groups. However, in a further study of nonresponders in the same group of patients, Denys et al. (2004b) investigated the effects of drug switching in resistant cases and found a more favorable response for venlafaxine-treated individuals switched to paroxetine than vice versa, casting further uncertainty on the efficacy of venlafaxine in treating OCD. Further investigation of venlafaxine seems worthwhile. Pallanti et al. (2004) compared two groups receiving citalopram with and without open-label mirtazapine. The group receiving two drugs achieved a significantly earlier treatment response, by week 4; however, no differences in efficacy between the groups were evident at weeks 8 and 12. Controlled studies are needed to properly evaluate a role for mirtazapine in OCD.

SRI Combinations

Combinations of SRIs have been found useful in some studies of OCD (Pallanti et al. 1999). However, caution is required if clomipramine is to be combined with SSRIs that potentially cross-react at the hepatic microsomes. Clomipramine plasma levels and electrocardiographic (ECG) monitoring are usually recommended. Citalopram, escitalopram, and to a lesser extent sertraline are unlikely to interfere with the clearance of clomipramine and are therefore preferred for this approach.

Maintenance SRI and Long-Term Trials

Patients with OCD should be warned, at the outset of SRI treatment, that the antiobsessional effect takes several weeks to develop fully. Sometimes progress seems remarkably slow, and patients may not recognize that changes are occurring. Recruiting family or friends to substantiate improvements is advisable. Side effects such as nausea and agitation tend to emerge early, before improvements are consolidated, but usually abate over time. Because placebo-referenced gains accrue for at least 6 months (Stein et al. 2007) and, according to open-label follow-up data, for at least 2 years (Rasmussen et al. 1997), patients need to allow time for the treatment effect to develop and should not discontinue or change the drug prematurely. A trial of at least 12 weeks at the maximum tolerated dosage and careful assessment are advisable before judging a medication's effectiveness.

Although the response to treatment with SRIs is characteristically partial, at least in the early stages, between 30% and 60% of patients with OCD reach a clinically relevant level of improvement within the limits of the acute treatment phase. According to results from the extended double-blind study by Stein et al. (2007), this figure increased to around 70% by 24 weeks (see Table 18–1). An important consideration is that the patients studied in randomized, controlled trials are often drawn from centers specializing in OCD, a situation that can result in lower response rates because more treatment-resistant patients are seen at such sites. Open-label studies, which more closely reflect typical clinical practice, are usually associated with higher rates of SRI response than are double-blind, placebo-controlled trials, partly because patients know they are receiving the active treatment. In a multicenter escitalopram relapse prevention trial, 320 of 468 (78%) patients taking open-label escitalopram (10 mg/day or 20 mg/day) achieved clinical response status by the 16-week endpoint (Fineberg et al. 2007b).

Remission rates represent a more exacting marker of treatment success and show greater sensitivity to change over time. In the study by Stein et al. (2007), patients with OCD continued to enter a state of remission across the full double-blind treatment period, so that by the 24-week endpoint, roughly 40% had achieved Y-BOCS scores<10. During 16 weeks of taking open-label escitalopram (10–20 mg/day), around 45% of patients achieved remission using the same criterion (Fineberg et al. 2007a). Based on findings from these studies, first-line treatments lead to remission or clinically meaningful improvement in around 45% and 75% of cases, respectively, in clinical trial populations.

Because OCD is a chronic illness, treatment needs to remain effective over a long term. Double-blind studies lasting up to 12 months have shown that patients who responded to acute treatment benefited from continuing with medication, with no evidence of tolerance developing. In a study by Tollefson et al. (1994), 76 patients taking all dosages of fluoxetine (20, 40, and 60 mg/day) continued to improve, but additional significant improvements were evident only for patients taking 60 mg/day, suggesting preferential benefit for remaining at the highest dosage level. In a larger extension study by Greist et al. (1995c), 118 patients who had responded to 12 weeks of treatment with sertraline or placebo continued under double-blind conditions for 40 weeks. Improvements were sustained for those who continued taking sertraline, and side effects improved over time. Fifty-nine completers were followed up for a second year while taking open-label sertraline and showed significant additional improvements in OCD symptoms and a reduced incidence of side effects (Rasmussen et al. 1997). These results suggest that treatment continues to be effective in the longer term and that further benefits accrue with ongoing treatment. They do not support dosage reduction.

Relapse Prevention

Studies examining the short-term effects of discontinuing clomipramine or SSRIs under double-blind, placebo-controlled conditions showed a rapid and incremental worsening of symptoms in most patients with OCD who switched from clomipramine to placebo (Flament et al. 1985; Leonard et al. 1988; Pato et al. 1988; Yaryura-Tobias and Neziroglu 1975), implying that treatment needs to be continued to remain effective. However, the results of relapse prevention studies to date have been mixed, largely owing to methodological differences. The conventional approach involves the random assignment of responders taking open-label drug to either continuation or placebo and measuring subsequent relapse rates. Definition of the relapse criterion is crucial in this regard (Fineberg et al. 2007a). In a small unpublished adulthood study that was peer reviewed for methodological adequacy by the NICE guideline group (NICE 2005) and that was undoubtedly underpowered, Bailer et al. (2005) selected 44 patients who had completed 12 weeks of double-blind paroxetine or placebo followed by 6 months of open-label paroxetine (20–60 mg/day). The results did not show efficacy for paroxetine (20–60 mg/day) on the selected relapse criterion, although a numerically greater percentage of relapses occurred in the patients who were randomized to placebo (63.6%) rather than paroxetine (42.1%) by the 24-week study endpoint. In a study of 193 children and adolescents with OCD (Geller et al. 2003a), the overall relapse rate was not significantly higher in the placebo group than in the paroxetine group (43.9% vs. 34.7%), possibly because the duration of follow-up was too short.

Table 18–3 shows the results of a meta-analysis of the published relapse prevention studies of adults with OCD (Fineberg et al. 2007a). In the study by Romano et al. (2001), patients continuing to take the highest dosage of fluoxetine (60 mg/day) showed significantly lower relapse rates than placebo, implying an ongoing advantage for staying at the higher dosage levels, but the study did not discriminate between continuation of pooled fluoxetine and discontinuation. In spite of its larger size and longer duration, the study by Koran et al. (2002) was unable to demonstrate a significant advantage for sertraline on the a priori criterion of preventing relapse, almost certainly because the study's criterion for relapse was too strictly defined. However, of those patients continuing to take sertraline, significantly fewer 1) were dropouts due to relapse or insufficient clinical response and 2) had acute exacerbation of symptoms. Also, ongoing sertraline was associated with continued improvement in Y-BOCS scores and quality of life measures. In contrast, the large-scale study of paroxetine by Hollander et al. (2003a) clearly demonstrated a significantly better outcome for those continuing to take the active drug over the 6-month double-blind discontinuation phase: 59% of patients randomly assigned to placebo relapsed, compared with 38% continuing to take paroxetine (20–60 mg/day), and paroxetine was well tolerated over the long term. In a large relapse prevention study using escitalopram (10–20 mg/day), patients randomly assigned to placebo relapsed significantly earlier. After 24 weeks, 52% of the placebo patients had relapsed, compared with 24% of patients taking escitalopram, and the risk of relapsing was 2.7 times higher for patients taking placebo than for those taking escitalopram (Fineberg et al. 2007b).

Taken together, these results support relapse prevention as a realistic target for OCD treatment and suggest that continuation of SSRI protects patients against relapse. These findings emphasize the importance of maintaining treatment with medication at an effective dosage level over the long term, and they argue against discontinuation of treatment even after 1 year. Protection is not complete, with roughly one-fourth of patients becoming unwell despite adherence to treatment over 24 weeks, indicating a clear need to devise even better relapse prevention strategies. The possibility that some patients may retain response at a lower dosage or following drug discontinuation must be weighed against the possibility that reinstatement of treatment after relapse may be associated with a poorer response.

Discontinuation Effects

Adverse events have been associated with abrupt discontinuation of clomipramine and SSRIs. The constellation of symptoms reported is variable but has most frequently included flulike symptoms, vertigo/dizziness, insomnia, vivid dreams, irritability, and headaches lasting from a few days to 3 weeks (Coupland et al. 1996). No medically significant events have been documented, but patients may describe marked discomfort. Relatively fewer reports of discontinuation effects following cessation of fluoxetine may reflect the long half-lives of the parent drug and its metabolite norfluoxetine. To reduce the risk of a discontinuation syndrome, a gradual taper is recommended for all SRIs except fluoxetine.

SRI Resistance

Research into SRI resistance has been hindered by lack of consensus on a definition of resistant OCD (Pallanti et al. 2002a; Simpson et al. 2006). In treatment trials, particularly those adding a second treatment to the first, patients responding partially but slowly to first-line treatments are likely to confound both treatment and placebo groups. On the other hand, if the criteria for resistance are too strictly applied, selected patients may be so refractory that they respond to no treatments whatsoever. Clear and universally accepted definitions of resistance are thus critical to any trial investigating augmentation strategies. Fineberg et al. (2006a) suggested that failure to improve baseline Y-BOCS scores by 25%

TABLE 18–3. Double-blind, placebo-controlled studies of relapse prevention in adult OCD

Drug and study	Duration of prior drug treatment	*N* in discontinuation phase	Weeks of follow-up after discontinuation	Outcome
Escitalopram Fineberg et al. 2007b	16 weeks	158	24	*Time to relapse on placebo> escitalopram* *Relapse rate on placebo> escitalopram*
Fluoxetine Romano et al. 2001	20 weeks	71	52	Relapse rate on placebo=pooled fluoxetine *Relapse rate on placebo>fluoxetine 60 mg*
Paroxetine Hollander et al. 2003a	12 weeks	105	24	*Relapse rate on placebo>paroxetine*
Sertraline Koran et al. 2002	52 weeks	223	28	Relapse rate on placebo=sertraline Acute exacerbation of OCD on placebo>sertraline Dropout due to relapse on placebo >sertraline

Note. Text in *italics* indicates positive outcomes on the a priori criterion for relapse. OCD=obsessive-compulsive disorder.

Source. Adapted from Fineberg NA, Pampaloni I, Pallanti S, et al: "Sustained Response Versus Relapse: The Pharmacotherapeutic Goal for Obsessive Compulsive Disorder." *International Clinical Psychopharmacology* 22:313–322, 2007.

after treatment with at least two SRIs given at maximally tolerated standard dosages for at least 12 weeks constitutes clinically meaningful SRI resistance.

Different factors may account for nonresponse to an adequate trial of an SRI. Some estimate of treatment adherence is helpful (e.g., using drug plasma levels or pill counts). Patients with OCD are generally compliant except when obsessive-compulsive symptoms interfere. Compulsive hoarding has been shown to respond poorly compared with other symptom dimensions in SSRI studies (Carey et al. 2008). According to meta-analysis, other factors linked with poor response to SRIs in adults with OCD include early onset, longer duration, more severe illness, and poor response to previous therapy. For childhood OCD, comorbidity with a number of other psychiatric conditions, including depression, tics, conduct disorder, and attention-deficit/hyperactivity disorder, has been linked to treatment resistance (Geller et al. 2003c; Mataix-Cols et al. 1999; Stein et al. 2001).

Dosing in SRI-Resistant OCD

Although SSRIs have been demonstrated to show a positive dose-response relationship and are generally well tolerated up to maximal standard dosage limits, few studies have addressed higher-dosage treatments for resistant OCD. Small positive open-label case studies have been reported for citalopram (160 mg/day) (Bejerot and Bodlund 1998) and sertraline (400 mg/day) (Byerly et al. 1996). A placebo-controlled study in patients with OCD who did not respond to normal dosages showed an improved response with high-dosage sertraline (250–400 mg/day), as measured on the Y-BOCS and CGI-I (Ninan et al. 2006). However, responder rates (decrease of ≥25% in Y-BOCS score and a CGI-I rating ≤3) were not significantly different for the 200-mg/day versus the high-dosage sertraline group, either on completer analysis (34% vs. 52%) or on endpoint analysis (33% vs. 40%). Risks are greater for increasing dosages of clomipramine owing to its inherent toxicity. Clomipramine has been systematically studied and found to be safe at dosages up to 300 mg/day (Group CCS 1991); however, the risks of cardiotoxicity and seizures (2%) make ECG and plasma monitoring advisable above this dosage level, and other strategies are usually preferable.

Intravenous SRI

Altering the mode of drug delivery may be another way to gain control of intractable OCD. Two double-blind trials (Fallon et al. 1998; Koran et al. 1997) supported the efficacy of intravenous clomipramine in treatment-refractory patients. Disadvantages of this experimental technique are its availability at only a few research settings and limited evidence on long-term benefits. Similar findings reported by Pallanti et al. (2002b), in a short open-label trial of intravenous citalopram, require substantiation under double-blind conditions.

Switching Antidepressants

According to the Expert Consensus Guidelines (March et al. 1997), clinicians should delay switching a patient's medication until an adequate trial (8–12 weeks at maximally tolerated dosage) has been attempted. Only limited evidence supports switching from one SSRI to another versus extending treatment with the same drug for longer. In one review, 11%–33% of patients not responding to the first SRI were reported to show clinically meaningful response to a second SRI, with decreasing likelihood of subsequent changes to other agents (Fineberg et al. 2006b). Two small open-label studies suggested that patients not responding to one or more SRIs might benefit from a change to venlafaxine (Hollander et al. 2002, 2003c). However, Denys et al. (2004b) found a more favorable response rate for venlafaxine-treated individuals switched to paroxetine (56%) than vice versa (19%).

Combination Strategies

The patient who has failed to show satisfactory improvement following two consecutive trials with different SRIs is eligible for combination treatment—that is, adding an agent from another class to an SRI.

SRI Plus Antipsychotic

Dopamine antagonists may have an indirect serotonergic effect by releasing neurons from dopaminergic inhibition; however, no positive trials have met today's clinical trial standards using antipsychotics as monotherapy in treatment of OCD. Clozapine, given as monotherapy to 12 adults with resistant OCD in an open-label design, showed no effect (McDougle et al. 1995). Aripiprazole (10–30 g/day) as monotherapy also did not show a clinical benefit in an open-label study of drug-naive and -resistant patients with OCD (Connor et al. 2005). However, growing evidence supports the use of antipsychotics as an add-on treatment with SRIs for resistant OCD. The balance of evidence from a growing number of small randomized, controlled studies suggests augmentation with haloperidol, risperidone, olanzapine, or quetiapine is beneficial. Two meta-analyses

TABLE 18–4. Responder rates for adjunctive antipsychotics in SRI-resistant OCD

Drug	≥25% improvement (Y-BOCS)	≥35% improvement (Y-BOCS)	≥25% improvement (Y-BOCS+CGI-I≤ 2)	≥35% improvement (Y-BOCS+CGI-I≤ 2)	Study
Haloperidol				64%+ Y-BOCS<16	McDougle et al. 1994
Olanzapine	46%				Bystritsky et al. 2004
	41%				Shapira et al. 2004
Quetiapine				40%	Denys et al. 2004a
			40%		Carey et al. 2005
	27%				Fineberg et al. 2005
Risperidone				50%	McDougle et al. 2000
			40%		Hollander et al. 2003b
		50%			Erzegovesi et al. 2005

Note. CGI-I=Clinical Global Impression Severity Improvement scale (Guy 1976); OCD=obsessive-compulsive disorder; SRI=serotonin reuptake inhibitor; Y-BOCS=Yale-Brown Obsessive Compulsive Scale (Goodman et al. 1989b).

of trials of adjunctive antipsychotic also suggested overall efficacy for this approach (Bloch et al. 2006; Skapinakis et al. 2007); in the analysis by Bloch et al., patients with comorbid tic disorders were particularly responsive to antipsychotics plus SRI. A single positive open-label study of the more selective dopamine antagonist amisulpride (200–600 mg/day) used as an adjunct to SRI in 20 patients with resistant OCD (Metin et al. 2003) merits replication under controlled conditions. Table 18–4 illustrates responder rates in double-blind studies, which varied from 27% to as high as 64%, depending on the chosen criterion.

First-generation antipsychotics have shown efficacy in combination with an SRI. In 17 patients with OCD who had not responded to fluvoxamine, McDougle et al. (1990) added open-label pimozide and reported some benefit, especially for individuals with comorbid chronic tics or schizotypal disorder. A subsequent double-blind, placebo-controlled study by the same authors (McDougle et al. 1994) showed significant Y-BOCS score improvement for patients with OCD taking haloperidol (2 mg/day) in addition to fluvoxamine. Mean Y-BOCS score reduction from baseline for patients taking haloperidol was 26%, and 11 of 17 (64%) patients receiving haloperidol achieved a strict responder status, compared with none of the patients taking placebo. Again, a stronger response was observed in patients with comorbid tics. The efficacy of haloperidol needs to be balanced against its side-effect profile. In the study by McDougle et al. (1994), 29% of patients experienced extrapyramidal side effects, including akathisia.

Second-generation antipsychotics affect a broader range of neurotransmitters, including serotonin. They are perceived to have a more benign profile of adverse effects and are being used increasingly for treatment-resistant OCD.

Risperidone. In a 12-week double-blind study of 33 patients with OCD who had been unresponsive to at least 12 weeks of prior treatment with an SRI, risperidone (2.2 mg/day) was found to be superior to placebo in reducing mean Y-BOCS scores to 31.8% of baseline, as well as improving anxiety and depressive symptoms (McDougle et al. 2000). Fifty percent of completers were nominated responders. However, the study lacked an intent-to-treat analysis. A small double-blind study by Hollander et al. (2003b) (N=16) was unable to demonstrate significance, although 4 of 10 patients randomly assigned to risperidone (0.5–3 mg/day) responded at the 8-week endpoint, compared with none of the 6 patients randomly assigned to placebo. A third trial enrolled 45 drug-naive subjects in a 12-week open-label fluvoxamine phase, after which 10 treatment nonresponders were randomly assigned to 6 weeks of low-dosage (0.5 mg/day) risperidone and 10 other nonresponders to placebo augmentation (Erzegovesi et al. 2005). The study authors did not report a between-group analysis, but 5 risperidone-treated patients responded compared with 2 taking placebo.

Quetiapine. In a negative study by Fineberg et al. (2005), 21 patients with OCD, diagnosed using DSM-IV criteria, who had no significant Axis I comorbidity and who had failed to respond to at least 6 months of SRI treatment were treated for 16 weeks with an SRI and quetiapine (≤400 mg/day) or an SRI and placebo. Of the quetiapine-treated cases, 27% were classified as responders, but no significant difference was found between groups in changes from baseline Y-BOCS scores at week 16 (14% for quetiapine vs. 6% for placebo).

Carey et al. (2005) showed that significant improvement occurs with adjunctive quetiapine in both treatment and placebo groups, with no significant difference between the two. In contrast, Denys et al. (2004a), in a double-blind, placebo-controlled study, reported efficacy for adjunctive quetiapine (<300 mg/day) in a sample of 40 patients who had previously failed to respond to at least two SRIs. An intent-to-treat analysis for the 20 quetiapine-treated patients showed a significant advantage over placebo from as early as 4 weeks on the Y-BOCS and a mean decrease of 31% on baseline Y-BOCS scores, compared with 6% in the placebo group at the 8-week endpoint.

A meta-analysis of the data from the studies mentioned above (N=102 cases) showed evidence of efficacy for adjunctive quetiapine (<400 mg/day) on changes from baseline on the Y-BOCS (P=0.008), although the analysis was limited by heterogeneity between studies (Fineberg et al. 2006c). A subsequent pooled analysis of the same trial data (Denys et al. 2007) also demonstrated superior response in the quetiapine addition group compared with the placebo group.

Olanzapine. A double-blind, placebo-controlled study by Bystritsky et al. (2004) included 26 patients with OCD who had been unresponsive to at least two 12-week trials of SRIs and one trial of behavior therapy. Olanzapine was well tolerated and, by intent-to-treat analysis, was significantly superior to placebo at the 6-week endpoint. Shapira et al. (2004) recruited a less treatment-refractory group of 44 patients with partial or no response to 8 weeks of treatment with open-label fluoxetine. Both the fluoxetine plus olanzapine (5–10 mg/day) and fluoxetine plus placebo groups improved over the 6-week randomization period, and no additional advantage was found for olanzapine augmentation.

Summary. Antipsychotics such as haloperidol and sulpiride are first-line treatments for Tourette syndrome, so efficacy in OCD supports a theoretical link between these disorders. Dose-ranging studies are required to test relative efficacy and tolerability. In view of potential adverse effects, treatment is usually started at low dosages and increased cautiously subject to tolerability (e.g., haloperidol 0.25–0.5 mg/day, titrated slowly to 2–4 mg/day; McDougle and Walsh 2001). Long-term studies are also required to test sustained efficacy, tolerability, and relapse prevention. One small study has reported a high level of relapse following open-label discontinuation (Maina et al. 2003).

Interestingly, some authors have reported emergent obsessions during treatment of schizophrenia with atypical antipsychotics, which may be related to their mixed receptor antagonist properties (Sareen et al. 2004). From a theoretical perspective, it is unclear why dopamine antagonists might have antiobsessional properties when added to SRIs but not when used alone or in OCD associated with schizophrenia.

SRI Plus Behavior Therapy

Although a combination of an SRI with exposure and response prevention is generally considered superior to either treatment given alone for the treatment of OCD, few controlled studies have addressed this possibility, and those that did either had methodological shortcomings or produced negative findings (Baldwin et al. 2005). Evidence for enhanced efficacy of exposure therapy with clomipramine remains inconsistent (Foa et al. 2005; Marks et al. 1988), but fluvoxamine has been shown to enhance the efficacy of exposure therapy (Cottraux et al. 1993) and multimodal CBT (Hohagen et al. 1998). Some studies have suggested that relapse rates are greater after initial treatment with a pharmacological rather than with a psychological intervention (Simpson et al. 2004).

Novel and Experimental Drug Treatments

A number of novel treatments have been proposed and tested in resistant OCD, but very few show promise. Table 18–5 lists those that so far have been shown *not* to be effective. Of those that have demonstrated positive results, many have been validated in small open-label trials. There have been a number of promising studies relating to the use of inositol. Dietary inositol is incorporated into neuronal cell membranes as inositol phospholipids, where it serves as a key metabolic precursor in G-protein-coupled receptors. Small studies have shown contradictory results for inositol in OCD and putative obsessive-compulsive spectrum disorders (Harvey et al. 2002; Levine 1997; Nemets et al. 2001).

Neuropeptides

Neuropeptides have important influences on many functions germane to OCD, such as memory, grooming, sexual and aggressive behavior, and stereotyped behavior. Neuropeptides also have a substantial interaction with the monoamine system. Furthermore, an increasing body of literature indicates that patients with OCD have neuropeptide abnormalities (for a review, see McDougle et al. 1999). Despite this evidence, few treatment trials have been attempted with neuropeptides, possibly due to difficulties in administering these compounds.

Oxytocin, known as the amnestic neuropeptide due to its attenuating effects on memory consolidation and retrieval, has had little success in treating OCD. In a case report, Ansseau et al. (1987) reported early improvement in symptoms, but side effects included psychosis, memory impairment, and hyponatremia. A number of small trials (Charles et al. 1989; den Boer and Westenberg 1992; Salzberg and Swedo 1992) and a randomized, placebo-controlled trial (Epperson et al. 1996) have also failed to show a discernable benefit. One possible explanation is that less than 0.003% of peripherally administered oxytocin crosses the blood-brain barrier (Mens et al. 1983).

Glutamatergic Modulation

A number of lines of research, from neuroimaging (Rosenberg et al. 2004) to genetics (Bloch et al. 2006), are converging to suggest that abnormal glutamatergic transmission may be important in OCD (for a review, see Pittenger et al. 2006). For example, a neuroimaging study found abnormally high glutamatergic concentrations in children with OCD (Rosenberg et al. 2000) that decreased in line with symptom severity during SSRI treatment. These findings have led to a number of trials involving drugs that modulate glutamate. To date, these are just at the stage of case reports and open-label series.

TABLE 18–5. Double-blind, placebo-controlled trials of agents with no proven effect in OCD

Drug	Clinical group	Study
Buspirone	Augmentation in refractory OCD	Grady et al. 1993
Buspirone	Augmentation in refractory OCD	McDougle et al. 1993
Buspirone	Augmentation in refractory OCD	Pigott et al. 1992
Clonazepam	Augmentation in refractory OCD	Crockett et al. 2004
Desipramine	Augmentation in refractory OCD	Barr et al. 1997
Lithium	Augmentation in refractory OCD	McDougle et al. 1991
Lithium	Augmentation in refractory OCD	Pigott et al. 1991
Naloxone	Monotherapy	Keuler et al. 1996
Oxytocin	Monotherapy	Epperson et al. 1996
Pindolol	Augmentation in refractory OCD	Dannon et al. 2000
St. John's wort	Augmentation in refractory OCD	Kobak et al. 2005

Note. OCD=obsessive-compulsive disorder.

Following a positive case study by Coric et al. (2003), the same authors reported an open-label trial of riluzole augmentation in patients with resistant OCD. By the 6-week endpoint, 7 of the 13 patients demonstrated a >35% reduction in Y-BOC scores, with 39% meeting criteria as treatment responders (Coric et al. 2005). A case report of topiramate leading to an improvement in resistant OCD (Hollander and Dell'Osso 2006) was followed by an open-label trial (mean dosage 253 mg/day) (Van Ameringen et al. 2006). Eleven of the 16 (68.8%) outpatients with OCD, who were partial responders or nonresponders to SRI monotherapy or SRI combination therapy (i.e., SRI plus an antipsychotic, other antidepressant, or benzodiazepine), were classed as responders (CGI-I<2). On the other hand, two cases have been reported of topiramate inducing obsessive-compulsive symptoms (Ozkara et al. 2005; Thuile et al. 2006), and the drug is associated with prominent amnestic effects at potentially therapeutic dosage levels. Some authors have reported on patients receiving other drugs that act on the glutamate system, including memantine (Pasquini and Biondi 2006; Poyurovsky et al. 2005) and *N*-acetylcysteine, a readily available amino acid compound that is thought to attenuate glutamatergic neurotransmission (Lafleur et al. 2006). Initial positive results for pregabalin and D-amphetamine (Insel et al. 1983a; Joffe et al. 1991) warrant further study.

Opiate Agonists and Antagonists

Oral morphine augmentation was shown to be effective in a double-blind crossover study of 23 patients with OCD who had failed two or more adequate SRI trials and had a Y-BOCS score of ≥20 (Koran et al. 2005). Subjects were randomly assigned to 2-week, random-order blocks of once-weekly morphine, lorazepam, and placebo. The median decrease in Y-BOCS score after morphine was 13%. Seven subjects (30%) were responders (Y-BOCS score decreases of ≥25%). The analysis showed significance for morphine versus placebo but not lorazepam versus placebo. In contrast, two randomized trials of naloxone found no significant effect (Keuler et al. 1996).

Immune Modulation

Some cases of childhood-onset OCD may be related to an infection-triggered autoimmune process similar to that of Sydenham's chorea. The acronym PANDAS describes cases of childhood-onset OCD resembling Sydenham's chorea with an acute onset following a group A beta-hemolytic streptococcal infection, neurological signs, and an episodic course (Swedo and Grant 2005). Although PANDAS remains a controversial diagnostic concept, it has stimulated new research into possible links among bacterial pathogens, autoimmune reactions, and neuropsychiatric symptoms. The proposed mediators are anti-basal ganglia antibodies (ABGA). Magnetic resonance imaging in PANDAS cases has supported the proposed pathology with evidence of inflammatory changes in basal ganglia. Dale et al. (2005) examined 50 children with idiopathic OCD. The mean ABGA binding was elevated in the patient cohort compared with the pediatric autoimmune (n=50), neurological (n=100), and streptococcal (n=40) control groups (P<0.005 in all comparisons), supporting the hypothesis that central nervous system autoimmunity may have a role in a significant subgroup of cases of OCD. Further study is required to examine whether the antibodies concerned are pathogenic. Various trials with immunomodulatory treatments (e.g., prednisone, plasmapheresis, intravenous immunoglobulins) or antimicrobial prophylaxis (e.g., penicillin) are under way (reviewed in Murphy et al. 2006).

Nonpharmacological Somatic Treatments

Despite isolated reports of its success in treatment-resistant cases (Husain et al. 1993; Khanna et al. 1988), electroconvulsive therapy has limited benefit in OCD. Its most useful role may be for treating depressive symptoms in treatment-refractory patients with OCD, particularly those at risk for suicide.

Repetitive transcranial magnetic stimulation (rTMS) has potential not only as a therapy but also as an instrument to help determine the neurocircuitry involved in disorders such as OCD. In rTMS, a pulsatile high-intensity electromagnetic field emitted from a coil placed against the scalp induces focal electrical currents in the underlying cerebral cortex, stimulating or disrupting cortical activity. Preliminary positive findings that rTMS applied to the right prefrontal cortex produced a transient reduction in compulsive urges (Greenberg et al. 1997) were not supported in two more recent negative controlled studies of sustained rTMS over the left dorsolateral prefrontal cortex (Prasko et al. 2006; Sachdev et al. 2007). Seizures have been reported in at least 6 of more than 250 subjects undergoing rTMS (Wasserman 1998). Local discomfort from activation of scalp musculature and nerves also occurs. Further evaluation of the procedure as an investigative and therapeutic tool in OCD seems justified.

Current ablative neurosurgical techniques for resistant cases of OCD interrupt connections between the frontal lobes and the subcortical structures (cingulotomy, capsulotomy). Modern stereotactic neurosurgical procedures should not be equated with the relatively crude surgical approaches of the past (Mindus et al. 1994). According to recent studies, stereotactic cingulotomy or capsulotomy may produce substantial clinical benefit in some patients with OCD without causing appreciable morbidity. However, in the absence of blinded comparator-controlled follow-up studies, we are unable to judge the true (placebo-corrected) efficacy of surgery, the optimal placement of lesions, and the longer-term outcome. Jenike et al. (1991) performed a retrospective follow-up study of 33 patients with OCD who underwent cingulotomy and found that 25%–30% experienced substantial benefit. In a more recent prospective study, Baer et al. (1995) evaluated 18 patients with OCD before and 6 months after bilateral cingulotomy. Five patients (28%) met criteria for treatment response. Given that neurosurgery is irreversible, stereotactic neurosurgery should be viewed as the option of last resort in the patient with severe OCD who has not responded at the very least to well-documented adequate trials of SRI pharmacotherapy (including clomipramine), exposure and response prevention, and combination strategies.

Deep brain stimulation is an alternative to traditional neurosurgery based on neuromodulation methods and has been used with success in the treatment of Parkinson's disease. Deep brain stimulation involves implanting electrodes that remain in situ and deliver an electric current into the neural structures considered to underpin OCD (Westenberg et al. 2007). It is reversible and is not intended to be ablative. In preliminary uncontrolled studies, stimulating targets including the anterior limb of the internal capsule, limbic part of the subthalamic nucleus (Wichmann and Delong 2006), and ventral capsule/ventral striatum (Greenberg et al. 2006) produced response rates of up to 50% in small groups of patients with highly resistant OCD. The study by Greenberg et al. (2006) openly followed up 8 of 10 cases to 36 months and found sustained advantages. However, deep brain stimulation was not without risks. Surgical adverse effects included an asymptomatic hemorrhage, a seizure, and a superficial infection. Psychiatric adverse effects included transient hypomanic symptoms and worsened depression and OCD when deep brain stimulation was interrupted by stimulator battery depletion. These results are nonetheless highly promising, given the treatment resistance of this patient group, and controlled studies to substantiate efficacy and to determine optimal electrode placement, stimulus parameters, and long-term effects are currently under way in several countries (Lipsman et al. 2007).

Case Study

Ms. Z was a 19-year-old female with a 6-year history of OCD. Fear of harming others and checking rituals took up more than 8 hours of her day. She lived with her parents and required significant support and prompting to keep her rituals from escalating further. On assessment she scored 32 on the Y-BOCS and did not meet criteria for major depression. She was initially opposed to pharmacological treatment due to fears and past experiences of side effects from medication. She had attempted CBT but found the exposure and response prevention too aversive. Following a discussion with her psychiatrist, she started taking citalopram drops (5 mg/day). The dosage was gradually increased over 6 weeks until she was tolerating 40 mg/day. She reported significant improvement, but after 12 weeks at this dosage, her Y-BOCS score was still 22. She was not able to tolerate a further dosage increase and was reluctant to change to another SSRI. Therefore, she started taking a low dose of adjunctive risperidone (1 mg each night). After an additional 12 weeks, her Y-BOCS score had decreased to 15. She reported substantial functional improvement and was able to return to complete her studies.

Conclusion

Figure 18–1 shows a suggested treatment pathway for patients with OCD. SRIs produce a rapid onset and a broad spectrum of actions and can be used to treat a wide range of conditions that occur comorbidly with OCD, including depression and anxiety. SSRIs offer advantages over clomipramine in terms of safety and tolerability and usually constitute first-line treatments. They have been shown to be cost-effective compared with other treatment options (NICE 2005). Higher dosages usually offer greater benefits, and gains continue to accrue gradually over weeks and months. For approximately 70% of patients, SSRIs effect a clinically meaningful response, and around 40% of patients enter remission after sustained treatment. Ongoing treatment protects against relapse for the majority of cases. For SRI-resistant cases, the strongest evidence supports the use of adjunctive antipsychotics, shown to be clinically effective in up to two-thirds of cases, with a particularly beneficial effect in those with comorbid tic disorders. Their long-term effects remain unclear, however, and trials in other diagnostic groups indicate that these effects may be significant. Rational alternatives include increasing the dosage of the SSRI or switching SRIs.

Improving the diagnosis and delivery of health care to patients with OCD must continue to be a high priority. Further research should be targeted at new therapeutic approaches and standardized methods to measure treatment response so that treatment choices can be guided by sound evidence. Novel techniques such as pharmaco-fMRI (functional magnetic resonance imaging) and pharmacogenomics may signal new candidate drugs with different and varied methods of action for future systematic exploration.

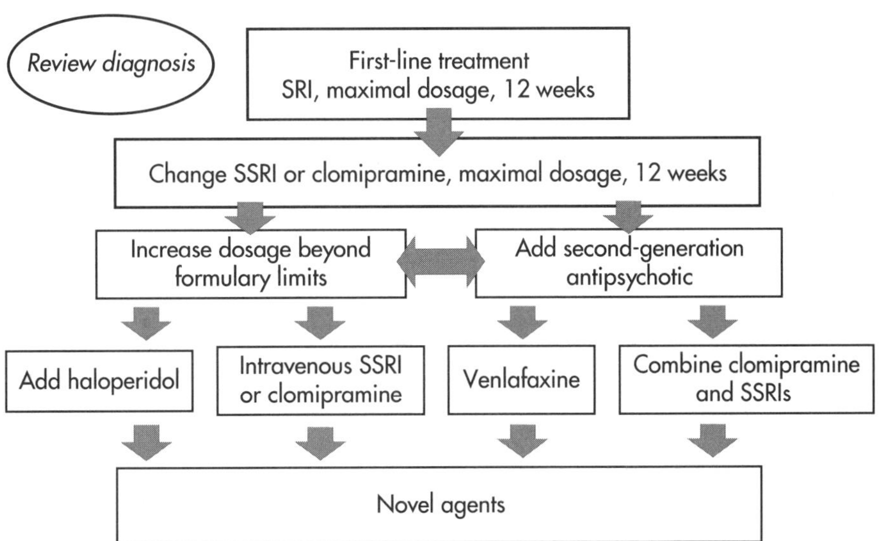

FIGURE 18–1. Obsessive-compulsive disorder: a pharmacological pathway.
SSRI=selective serotonin reuptake inhibitor.

Key Clinical Points

- Serotonin reuptake inhibitors remain the cornerstone of pharmacological treatment and lead to substantial clinical improvement, if continued for long enough, in the majority of patients with obsessive-compulsive disorder.
- Selective serotonin reuptake inhibitors are the preferred first-line treatment for OCD. Clomipramine is preferred for those who fail to respond to or cannot tolerate SSRIs.
- Gradual dosage titration upward within licensed limits, while measuring clinical response and side effects, is usually appropriate, although higher dosages may be more effective.
- An initial treatment period of at least 12 weeks at maximally tolerated dosage levels is advisable to properly judge effectiveness.
- Standardized rating scales (e.g., Y-BOCS, CGI-S, CGI-I) are helpful to objectify clinical response.
- For the majority of patients with OCD, symptoms respond only partially to SRIs, and in about one-third of cases, the response is poor.
- Maintenance treatment appears to protect against relapse.
- In treatment-resistant cases, combining pharmacotherapy with CBT, increasing dosages, or switching between SRIs are practical next steps.
- Growing evidence supports the efficacy of adding dopamine antagonists to first-line SRI medication at the lower end of their dosing range, but long-term data are lacking, and for many patients, the response remains unsatisfactory.

References

Abramowitz JS: Effectiveness of psychological and pharmacological treatments for obsessive-compulsive disorder: a quantitative review. J Consult Clin Psychol 65:44–52, 1997

Ackerman DL, Greenland S: Multivariate meta-analysis of controlled drug studies for obsessive-compulsive disorder. J Clin Psychopharmacol 22:309–317, 2002

Ackerman DL, Greenland S, Bystritsky A: Clinical characteristics of response to fluoxetine treatment of obsessive-compulsive disorder. J Clin Psychopharmacol 18:185–192, 1998

Ananth J, Pecknold JC, van den Steen N, et al: Double-blind comparative study of clomipramine and amitriptyline in obsessive neurosis. Prog Neuropsychopharmacol 5:257–262, 1981

Ansseau M, Legros JJ, Mormont C, et al: Intranasal oxytocin in obsessive-compulsive disorder. Psychoneuroendocrinology 12:231–236, 1987

Baer L, Rauch SL, Ballantin HT Jr, et al: Cingulotomy for intractable obsessive-compulsive disorder: prospective long-term follow-up of 18 patients. Arch Gen psychiatry 52:384–392, 1995

Bailer DC, Burnham D, Oakes R: Long-term treatment with paroxetine of outpatients with obsessive-compulsive disorder: an extension of the companion study. 1995, updated 2005. Available at http://www.gsk-clinicalstudyregister.com/files/pdf/2072.pdf [Study No.: MY-1053/BRL-029060/CPMS-127]. Accessed April 11, 2009.

Baldwin DS, Anderson IM, Nutt DJ, et al: Evidence-based guidelines for the pharmacological treatment of anxiety disorders: recommendations from the British Association for Psychopharmacology. J Psychopharmacol 19:567–596, 2005

Barr LC, Goodman WK, Anand A, et al: Addition of desipramine to serotonin reuptake inhibitors in treatment-resistant obsessive-compulsive disorder. Am J Psychiatry 154:1293–1295, 1997

Bejerot S, Bodlund O: Response to high doses of citalopram in treatment-resistant obsessive-compulsive disorder. Acta Psychiatr Scand 98:423–424, 1998

Bergeron R, Ravindran AV, Chaput Y, et al: Sertraline and fluoxetine treatment of obsessive-compulsive disorder: results of a double-blind, 6-month treatment study. J Clin Psychopharmacol 22:148–154, 2002

Bloch MH, Landeros-Weisenberger A, Kelmendi B, et al: A systematic review: antipsychotic augmentation with treatment refractory obsessive-compulsive disorder. Mol Psychiatry 11:622–632, 2006

Bogetto F, Albert U, Maina G: Sertraline treatment of obsessive-compulsive disorder: efficacy and tolerability of a rapid titration regimen. Eur Neuropsychopharmacol 12:181–186, 2002

Brawman-Mintzer O, Lydiard RB, Emmanuel N, et al: Psychiatric comorbidity in patients with generalized anxiety disorder. Am J Psychiatry 150:1216–1218, 1993

Byerly MJ, Goodman WK, Christensen R: High doses of sertraline for treatment-resistant obsessive-compulsive disorder. Am J Psychiatry 153:1232–1233, 1996

Bystritsky A, Ackerman DL, Rosen RM, et al: Augmentation of serotonin reuptake inhibitors in refractory obsessive-compulsive disorder using adjunctive olanzapine: a placebo-controlled trial. J Clin Psychiatry 65:565–568 2004

Carey PD, Vythilingum B, Seedat S, et al: Quetiapine augmentation of SRIs in treatment refractory obsessive-compulsive disorder: a double-blind, randomised, placebo-controlled study. BMC Psychiatry 5:5, 2005

Carey PD, Fineberg N, Lochner C, et al: Escitalopram in obsessive-compulsive disorder (OCD): response of symptom dimensions to pharmacotherapy. Poster presented at International Anxiety Disorders Symposium, Cape Town, South Africa, March 2008

Charles G, Guillaume R, Schittecatte M, et al: Oxytocin in the treatment of obsessive-compulsive disorder: a report of two cases. Psychiatry and Psychobiology 4:111–115, 1989

Chouinard G, Goodman W, Greist J, et al: Results of a double-blind placebo controlled trial of a new serotonin uptake inhibitor, sertraline, in the treatment of obsessive-compulsive disorder. Psychopharmacol Bull 26:279–284, 1990

Connor KM, Payne VM, Gadde KM, et al: The use of aripiprazole in obsessive-compulsive disorder: preliminary observations in 8 patients. J Clin Psychiatry 66:49–51, 2005

Coric V, Milanovic S, Wasylink S, et al: Beneficial effects of the antiglutamatergic agent riluzole in a patient diagnosed with obsessive-compulsive disorder and major depressive disorder. Psychopharmacology (Berl) 167:219–220, 2003

Coric V, Taskiran S, Pittenger C, et al: Riluzole augmentation in treatment-resistant obsessive-compulsive disorder: an open-label trial. Biol Psychiatry 58:424–428, 2005

Cottraux J, Mollard E, Bouvard M, et al: A controlled study of fluvoxamine and exposure in obsessive-compulsive disorder. Int Clin Psychopharmacol 5:17–30, 1990

Cottraux J, Mollard E, Bouvard M, et al: Exposure therapy, fluvoxamine, or combination treatment in obsessive-compulsive disorder: one-year follow-up. Psychiatry Res 49:63–75, 1993

Cottraux J, Note I, Yao SN, et al: A randomized controlled trial of cognitive therapy versus intensive behavior therapy in obsessive compulsive disorder. Psychother Psychosom 70:288–297, 2001

Coupland N, Bell C, Potokar J: Serotonin reuptake inhibitor withdrawal. J Clin Psychopharmacol 16:356–362, 1996

Crockett BA, Churchill E, Davidson JR: A double-blind combination study of clonazepam with sertraline in obsessive-compulsive disorder. Ann Clin Psychiatry 16:127–132, 2004

Dale RC, Heyman I, Giovannoni G, et al: Incidence of anti-brain antibodies in children with obsessive-compulsive disorder. Br J Psychiatry 187:314–319, 2005

Dannon PN, Sasson Y, Hirschmann S, et al: Pindolol augmentation in treatment-resistant obsessive compulsive disorder: a double-blind placebo-controlled trial. Eur Neuropsychopharmacol 10:165–169, 2000

den Boer JA, Westenberg HG: Oxytocin in obsessive compulsive disorder. Peptides 13:1083–1085, 1992

Denys D, van der Wee N, van Megen HJ, et al: A double blind comparison of venlafaxine and paroxetine in obsessive-compulsive disorder. J Clin Psychopharmacol 23:568–575, 2003

Denys D, de Geus F, van Megen HJ, et al: A double-blind, randomized, placebo-controlled trial of quetiapine addition in patients with obsessive-compulsive disorder refractory to serotonin reuptake inhibitors. J Clin Psychiatry 65:1040–1048, 2004a

Denys D, van Megen HJ, van der Wee N, et al: A double-blind switch study of paroxetine and venlafaxine in obsessive-compulsive disorder. J Clin Psychiatry 65:37–43, 2004b

Denys D, Fineberg N, Carey PD, et al: Quetiapine addition in obsessive-compulsive disorder: is treatment outcome affected by type and dose of serotonin reuptake inhibitors? Biol Psychiatry 61:412–414, 2007

DeVeaugh-Geiss J, Landau P, Katz R: Preliminary results from a multicenter trial of clomipramine in obsessive-compulsive disorder. Psychopharmacol Bull 25:36–40, 1989

DeVeaugh-Geiss J, Moroz G, Biederman J, et al: Clomipramine hydrochloride in childhood and adolescent obsessive-compulsive disorder: a multicenter trial. J Am Acad Child Adolesc Psychiatry 31:45–49, 1992

Eddy KT, Dutra L, Bradley R, et al: A multidimensional meta-analysis of psychotherapy and pharmacotherapy for obsessive-compulsive disorder. Clin Psychol Rev 24:1011–1030, 2004

Emslie G, Judge R: Tricyclic antidepressants and selective serotonin reuptake inhibitors: use during pregnancy, in children/adolescents and in the elderly. Acta Psychiatr Scand Suppl 403:26–34, 2000

Epperson CN, McDougle CJ, Price LH: Intranasal oxytocin in obsessive-compulsive disorder. Biol Psychiatry 40:547–549, 1996

Erzegovesi S, Guglielmo E, Siliprandi F, et al: Low-dose risperidone augmentation of fluvoxamine treatment in obsessive-compulsive disorder: a double-blind, placebo-controlled study. Eur Neuropsychopharmacol 15:69–74, 2005

Fallon BA, Liebowitz MR, Campeas R, et al: Intravenous clomipramine for obsessive-compulsive disorder refractory to oral clomipramine: a placebo-controlled study. Arch Gen Psychiatry 55:918–924, 1998

Fernandez Cordoba E, Lopez-Ibor Alino J: Use of monochlorimipramine in psychiatric patients who are resistant to other therapy (in Spanish). Actas Luso Esp Neurol Psiquiatr 26:119–147, 1967

Fineberg NA, Gale TM: Evidence-based pharmacotherapy of obsessive-compulsive disorder. Int J Neuropsychopharmacol 8:107–129, 2005

Fineberg N, Heyman I, Jenkins R, et al: Does childhood and adult obsessive compulsive disorder (OCD) respond the same way to treatment with serotonin reuptake inhibitors (SRIs)? Eur Neuropsychopharmacol 14 (suppl 3):S191, 2004

Fineberg NA, Sivakumaran T, Roberts A, et al: Adding quetiapine to SRI in treatment-resistant obsessive-compulsive disorder: a randomized controlled treatment study. Int Clin Psychopharmacol 20:223–226, 2005

Fineberg NA, Gale TM, Sivakumaran T: A review of antipsychotics in the treatment of obsessive compulsive disorder. J Psychopharmacol 20:97–103, 2006a

Fineberg NA, Nigam N, Sivakumaran T: Pharmacological strategies for treatment-resistant obsessive compulsive disorder. Psychiatr Ann 36:464–474, 2006b

Fineberg NA, Stein DJ, Premkumar P, et al: Adjunctive quetiapine for serotonin reuptake inhibitor–resistant obsessive-compulsive disorder: a meta-analysis of randomized controlled treatment trials. Int Clin Psychopharmacol 21:337–343, 2006c

Fineberg NA, Pampaloni I, Pallanti S, et al: Sustained response versus relapse: the pharmacotherapeutic goal for obsessive compulsive disorder. Int Clin Psychopharmacol 22:313–322, 2007a

Fineberg NA, Tonnoire B, Lemming O, et al: Escitalopram prevents relapse of obsessive-compulsive disorder. Eur Neuropsychopharmacol 17:430–439, 2007b

Flament MF, Bisserbe JC: Pharmacologic treatment of obsessive-compulsive disorder: comparative studies. J Clin Psychiatry 58 (suppl 12):18–22, 1997

Flament MF, Rapoport JL, Berg CJ, et al: Clomipramine treatment of childhood obsessive-compulsive disorder: a double-blind controlled study. Arch Gen Psychiatry 42:977–983, 1985

Foa EB, Steketee G, Kozak MJ, et al: Imipramine and placebo in the treatment of obsessive-compulsives: their effect on depression and on obsessional symptoms. Psychopharmacol Bull 23:8–11, 1987

Foa EB, Liebowitz MR, Kozak MJ, et al: Randomized, placebo-controlled trial of exposure and ritual prevention, clomipramine, and their combination in the treatment of obsessive-compulsive disorder. Am J Psychiatry 162:151–161, 2005

Geller DA, Hoog SL, Heiligenstein JH, et al: Fluoxetine treatment for obsessive-compulsive disorder in children and adolescents: a placebo-controlled clinical trial. J Am Acad Child Adolesc Psychiatry 40:773–779, 2001

Geller DA, Biederman J, Stewart SE, et al: Impact of comorbidity on treatment response to paroxetine in pediatric obsessive-compulsive disorder: is the use of exclusion criteria empirically supported in randomized clinical trials? J Child Adolesc Psychopharmacol 13 (suppl 1):S19–S29, 2003a

Geller DA, Biederman J, Stewart SE, et al: Which SSRI? A meta-analysis of pharmacotherapy trials in pediatric obsessive-compulsive disorder. Am J Psychiatry 160:1919–1928, 2003b

Geller DA, Coffey B, Faraone S, et al: Does comorbid attention-deficit/hyperactivity disorder impact the clinical expression of pediatric obsessive-compulsive disorder? CNS Spectr 8:259–264, 2003c

Geller DA, Wagner KD, Emslie G, et al: Paroxetine treatment in children and adolescents with obsessive-compulsive disorder: a randomized, multicenter, double-blind, placebo-controlled trial. J Am Acad Child Adolesc Psychiatry 43:1387–1396, 2004

Goodman WK, Price LH, Rasmussen SA, et al: Efficacy of fluvoxamine in obsessive-compulsive disorder: a double-blind comparison with placebo. Arch Gen Psychiatry 46:36–44, 1989a

Goodman WK, Price LH, Rasmussen SA, et al: The Yale-Brown Obsessive Compulsive Scale, II: validity. Arch Gen Psychiatry 46:1012–1016, 1989b

Goodman WK, Price LH, Delgado PL, et al: Specificity of serotonin reuptake inhibitors in the treatment of obsessive-compulsive disorder: comparison of fluvoxamine and desipramine. Arch Gen Psychiatry 47:577–585, 1990

Goodman WK, Kozak MJ, Liebowitz M, et al: Treatment of obsessive-compulsive disorder with fluvoxamine: a multicentre, double-blind, placebo-controlled trial. Int Clin Psychopharmacol 11:21–29, 1996

Grady TA, Pigott TA, L'Heureux F, et al: Double-blind study of adjuvant buspirone for fluoxetine-treated patients with obsessive-compulsive disorder. Am J Psychiatry 150:819–821, 1993

Greenberg BD, George MS, Martin JD, et al: Effect of prefrontal repetitive transcranial magnetic stimulation in obsessive-compulsive disorder: a preliminary study. Am J Psychiatry 154:867–869, 1997

Greenberg BD, Malone DA, Friehs GM, et al: Three-year outcomes in deep brain stimulation for highly resistant obsessive-compulsive disorder. Neuropsychopharmacology 31:2384–2893, 2006

Greist JH, Jefferson JW, Rosenfeld R, et al: Clomipramine and obsessive compulsive disorder: a placebo-controlled double-blind study of 32 patients. J Clin Psychiatry 51:292–297, 1990

Greist J, Chouinard G, DuBoff E, et al: Double-blind parallel comparison of three dosages of sertraline and placebo in outpatients with obsessive-compulsive disorder. Arch Gen Psychiatry 52:289–295, 1995a

Greist JH, Jefferson JW, Kobak KA, et al: Efficacy and tolerability of serotonin transport inhibitors in obsessive-compulsive disorder: a meta-analysis. Arch Gen Psychiatry 52:53–60, 1995b

Greist JH, Jefferson JW, Kobak KA, et al: A 1-year double-blind placebo-controlled fixed dose study of sertraline in the treatment of obsessive-compulsive disorder. Int Clin Psychopharmacol 10:57–65, 1995c

Group CCS: Clomipramine in the treatment of patients with obsessive-compulsive disorder. Clomipramine Collaborative Study Group. Arch Gen Psychiatry 48:730–738, 1991

Guy W: ECDEU Assessment Manual for Psychopharmacology, Revised. Bethesda, MD, U.S. Department of Health, Education and Welfare, 1976

Hamilton M: A rating scale for depression. J Neurol Neurosurg Psychiatry 23:56–62, 1960

Harvey BH, Brink CB, Seedat S, et al: Defining the neuromolecular action of myo-inositol: application to obsessive-compulsive disorder. Prog Neuropsychopharmacol Biol Psychiatry 26:21–32, 2002

Heyman I, Fombonne E, Simmons H, et al: Prevalence of obsessive-compulsive disorder in the British nationwide survey of child mental health. Br J Psychiatry 179:324–329, 2001

Hoehn-Saric R, Ninan P, Black DW, et al: Multicenter double-blind comparison of sertraline and desipramine for concurrent obsessive-compulsive and major depressive disorders. Arch Gen Psychiatry 57:76–82, 2000

Hohagen F, Winkelmann G, Rasche-Ruchle H, et al: Combination of behaviour therapy with fluvoxamine in comparison with behaviour therapy and placebo: results of a multicentre study. Br J Psychiatry Suppl (35):71–78, 1998

Hollander E, Dell'Osso B: Topiramate plus paroxetine in treatment-resistant obsessive-compulsive disorder. Int Clin Psychopharmacol 21:189–191, 2006

Hollander E, Bienstock CA, Koran LM, et al: Refractory obsessive-compulsive disorder: state-of-the-art treatment. J Clin Psychiatry 63 (suppl 6):20–29, 2002

Hollander E, Allen A, Steiner M, et al: Acute and long-term treatment and prevention of relapse of obsessive-compulsive disorder with paroxetine. J Clin Psychiatry 64:1113–1121, 2003a

Hollander E, Baldini Rossi N, Sood E, et al: Risperidone augmentation in treatment-resistant obsessive-compulsive disorder: a double-blind, placebo-controlled study. Int J Neuropsychopharmacol 6:397–401, 2003b

Hollander E, Friedberg J, Wasserman S, et al: Venlafaxine in treatment-resistant obsessive-compulsive disorder. J Clin Psychiatry 64:546–550, 2003c

Hollander E, Koran LM, Goodman WK, et al: A double-blind, placebo-controlled study of the efficacy and safety of controlled-release fluvoxamine in patients with obsessive-compulsive disorder. J Clin Psychiatry 64:640–647, 2003d

Husain MM, Lewis SF, Thornton WL: Maintenance ECT for refractory obsessive-compulsive disorder. Am J Psychiatry 150:1899–1900, 1993

Insel TR, Hamilton JA, Guttmacher LB, et al: D-amphetamine in obsessive-compulsive disorder. Psychopharmacology (Berl) 80:231–235, 1983a

Insel TR, Murphy DL, Cohen RM, et al: Obsessive-compulsive disorder: a double-blind trial of clomipramine and clorgyline. Arch Gen Psychiatry 40:605–612, 1983b

Insel TR, Mueller EA, Alterman I, et al: Obsessive-compulsive disorder and serotonin: is there a connection? Biol Psychiatry 20:1174–1188, 1985

Jenike MA, Baer L, Summergrad P, et al: Obsessive-compulsive disorder: a double-blind, placebo-controlled trial of clomipramine in 27 patients. Am J Psychiatry 146:1328–1330, 1989

Jenike MA, Hyman S, Baer L, et al: A controlled trial of fluvoxamine in obsessive-compulsive disorder: implications for a serotonergic theory. Am J Psychiatry 147:1209–1215, 1990

Jenike MA, Baer L, Ballantine T, et al: Cingulotomy for refractory obsessive-compulsive disorder: a long-term follow-up of 33 patients. Arch Gen Psychiatry 48:548–555, 1991

Jenike MA, Baer L, Minichiello WE, et al: Placebo-controlled trial of fluoxetine and phenelzine for obsessive-compulsive disorder. Am J Psychiatry 154:1261–1264, 1997

Joffe RT, Swinson RP, Levitt AJ: Acute psychostimulant challenge in primary obsessive-compulsive disorder. J Clin Psychopharmacol 11:237–241, 1991

Kamijima K, Murasaki M, Asai M, et al: Paroxetine in the treatment of obsessive-compulsive disorder: randomized, double-blind, placebo-controlled study in Japanese patients. Psychiatry Clin Neurosci 58:427–433, 2004

Kaplan A, Hollander E: A review of pharmacologic treatments for obsessive-compulsive disorder. Psychiatr Serv 54:1111–1118, 2003

Keuler DJ, Altemus M, Michelson D, et al: Behavioral effects of naloxone infusion in obsessive-compulsive disorder. Biol Psychiatry 40:154–156, 1996

Khanna S, Gangadhar BN, Sinha V, et al: Electroconvulsive therapy in obsessive-compulsive disorder. Convuls Ther 4:314–320, 1988

Kobak KA, Greist JH, Jefferson JW, et al: Behavioral versus pharmacological treatments of obsessive compulsive disorder: a meta-analysis. Psychopharmacology (Berl) 136: 205–216, 1998

Kobak KA, Taylor LV, Bystritsky A, et al: St John's wort versus placebo in obsessive-compulsive disorder: results from a double-blind study. Int Clin Psychopharmacol 20:299–304, 2005

Koran LM, McElroy SL, Davidson JR, et al: Fluvoxamine versus clomipramine for obsessive-compulsive disorder: a double-blind comparison. J Clin Psychopharmacol 16:121–129, 1996

Koran LM, Sallee FR, Pallanti S: Rapid benefit of intravenous pulse loading of clomipramine in obsessive-compulsive disorder. Am J Psychiatry 154:396–401, 1997

Koran LM, Hackett E, Rubin A, et al: Efficacy of sertraline in the long-term treatment of obsessive-compulsive disorder. Am J Psychiatry 159:88–95, 2002

Koran LM, Aboujaoude E, Bullock KD, et al: Double-blind treatment with oral morphine in treatment-resistant obsessive-compulsive disorder. J Clin Psychiatry 66:353–359, 2005

Kronig MH, Apter J, Asnis G, et al: Placebo-controlled, multicenter study of sertraline treatment for obsessive-compulsive disorder. J Clin Psychopharmacol 19:172–176, 1999

Kruger S, Cooke RG, Hasey GM, et al: Comorbidity of obsessive compulsive disorder in bipolar disorder. J Affect Disord 34:117–120, 1995

Lafleur DL, Pittenger C, Kelmendi B, et al: *N*-acetylcysteine augmentation in serotonin reuptake inhibitor refractory obsessive-compulsive disorder. Psychopharmacology (Berl) 184:254–256, 2006

Leonard H, Swedo S, Rapoport JL, et al: Treatment of childhood obsessive compulsive disorder with clomipramine and desmethylimipramine: a double-blind crossover comparison. Psychopharmacol Bull 24:93–95, 1988

Leonard HL, Swedo SE, Rapoport JL, et al: Treatment of obsessive-compulsive disorder with clomipramine and desipramine in children and adolescents: a double-blind crossover comparison. Arch Gen Psychiatry 46:1088–1092, 1989

Leonard HL, Swedo SE, Lenane MC, et al: A double-blind desipramine substitution during long-term clomipramine treatment in children and adolescents with obsessive-compulsive disorder. Arch Gen Psychiatry 48:922–927, 1991

Levine J: Controlled trials of inositol in psychiatry. Eur Neuropsychopharmacol 7:147–155, 1997

Liebowitz MR, Turner SM, Piacentini J, et al: Fluoxetine in children and adolescents with OCD: a placebo-controlled trial. J Am Acad Child Adolesc Psychiatry 41:1431–1438, 2002

Lipsman N, Neimat JS, Lozano AM: Deep brain stimulation for treatment-refractory obsessive-compulsive disorder: the search for a valid target. Neurosurgery 61:1–11; discussion 11–13, 2007

Maina G, Albert U, Ziero S, et al: Antipsychotic augmentation for treatment resistant obsessive-compulsive disorder: what if antipsychotic is discontinued? Int Clin Psychopharmacol 18:23–28, 2003

Maina G, Albert U, Salvi V, et al: Weight gain during long-term treatment of obsessive-compulsive disorder: a prospective comparison between serotonin reuptake inhibitors. J Clin Psychiatry 65:1365–1371, 2004

March JS, Frances A, Kahn DA, et al: The Expert Consensus Guideline Series: treatment of obsessive compulsive disorder. J Clin Psychiatry 58(suppl):1–72, 1997

March JS, Biederman J, Wolkow R, et al: Sertraline in children and adolescents with obsessive-compulsive disorder: a multicenter randomized controlled trial. JAMA 280:1752–1756, 1998

March JS, Klee BJ, Kremer CM: Treatment benefit and the risk of suicidality in multicenter, randomized, controlled trials of sertraline in children and adolescents. J Child Adolesc Psychopharmacol 16:91–102, 2006

Marks IM, Stern RS, Mawson D, et al: Clomipramine and exposure for obsessive-compulsive rituals, I. Br J Psychiatry 136:1–25, 1980

Marks IM, Lelliott P, Basoglu M, et al: Clomipramine, self-exposure and therapist-aided exposure for obsessive-compulsive rituals. Br J Psychiatry 152:522–534, 1988

Mataix-Cols D, Rauch SL, Manzo PA, et al: Use of factor-analyzed symptom dimensions to predict outcome with serotonin reuptake inhibitors and placebo in the treatment of obsessive-compulsive disorder. Am J Psychiatry 156:1409–1416, 1999

Mavissakalian M, Turner SM, Michelson L, et al: Tricyclic antidepressants in obsessive-compulsive disorder: antiobsessional or antidepressant agents? Am J Psychiatry 142:572–576, 1985

McDougle CJ, Walsh KH: Treatment of refractory OCD, in Obsessive Compulsive Disorder: A Practical Guide. Edited by Fineberg NA, Marazziti D, Stein D. London, Martin Dunitz, 2001, pp 135–152

McDougle CJ, Goodman WK, Price LH, et al: Neuroleptic addition in fluvoxamine-refractory obsessive-compulsive disorder. Am J Psychiatry 147:652–654, 1990

McDougle CJ, Price LH, Goodman WK, et al: A controlled trial of lithium augmentation in fluvoxamine-refractory obsessive-compulsive disorder: lack of efficacy. J Clin Psychopharmacol 11:175–184, 1991

McDougle CJ, Goodman WK, Leckman JF, et al: Limited therapeutic effect of addition of buspirone in fluvoxamine-refractory obsessive-compulsive disorder. Am J Psychiatry 150:647–649, 1993

McDougle CJ, Goodman WK, Leckman JF, et al: Haloperidol addition in fluvoxamine-refractory obsessive-compulsive disorder: a double-blind, placebo-controlled study in patients with and without tics. Arch Gen Psychiatry 51:302–308, 1994

McDougle CJ, Barr LC, Goodman WK, et al: Lack of efficacy of clozapine monotherapy in refractory obsessive-compulsive disorder. Am J Psychiatry 152:1812–1814, 1995

McDougle CJ, Barr LC, Goodman WK, et al: Possible role of neuropeptides in obsessive compulsive disorder. Psychoneuroendocrinology 24:1–24, 1999

McDougle CJ, Epperson CN, Pelton GH, et al: A double-blind, placebo-controlled study of risperidone addition in serotonin reuptake inhibitor–refractory obsessive-compulsive disorder. Arch Gen Psychiatry 57:794–801, 2000

Mens WB, Witter A, van Wimersma Greidanus TB: Penetration of neurohypophyseal hormones from plasma into cerebrospinal fluid (CSF): half-times of disappearance of these neuropeptides from CSF. Brain Res 262:143–149, 1983

Metin O, Yazici K, Tot S, et al: Amisulpiride augmentation in treatment resistant obsessive-compulsive disorder: an open trial. Hum Psychopharmacol 18:463–467, 2003

Mindus P, Rasmussen SA, Lindquist C: Neurosurgical treatment for refractory obsessive-compulsive disorder: implications for understanding frontal lobe function. J Neuropsychiatry Clin Neurosci 6:467–477, 1994

Monteiro WO, Noshirvani HF, Marks IM, et al: Anorgasmia from clomipramine in obsessive-compulsive disorder: a controlled trial. Br J Psychiatry 151:107–112, 1987

Montgomery SA: Clomipramine in obsessional neurosis: a placebo-controlled trial. Pharmacological Medicine 1:189–192, 1980

Montgomery SA, McIntyre A, Osterheider M, et al: A double-blind, placebo-controlled study of fluoxetine in patients with DSM-III-R obsessive-compulsive disorder. The Lilly European OCD Study Group. Eur Neuropsychopharmacol 3:143–152, 1993

Montgomery SA, Kasper S, Stein DJ, et al: Citalopram 20 mg, 40 mg and 60 mg are all effective and well tolerated compared with placebo in obsessive-compulsive disorder. Int Clin Psychopharmacol 16:75–86, 2001

Mundo E, Bianchi L, Bellodi L: Efficacy of fluvoxamine, paroxetine, and citalopram in the treatment of obsessive-compulsive disorder: a single-blind study. J Clin Psychopharmacol 17:267–271, 1997

Murphy TK, Sajid MW, Goodman WK: Immunology of obsessive-compulsive disorder. Psychiatr Clin North Am 29:445–469, 2006

National Institute for Health and Clinical Excellence: Obsessive-compulsive disorder: core interventions in the treatment of obsessive-compulsive disorder and body dysmorphic disorder. 2005. Available at http://www.nice.org.uk/Guidance/CG31. Accessed December 15, 2008.

Nemets B, Fux M, Levine J, et al: Combination of antidepressant drugs: the case of inositol. Hum Psychopharmacol 16:37–43, 2001

Ninan PT, Koran LM, Kiev A, et al: High-dose sertraline strategy for nonresponders to acute treatment for obsessive-compulsive disorder: a multicenter double-blind trial. J Clin Psychiatry 67:15–22, 2006

Ozkara C, Ozmen M, Erdogan A, et al: Topiramate related obsessive-compulsive disorder. Eur Psychiatry 20:78–79, 2005

Pallanti S, Quercioli L, Paiva RS, et al: Citalopram for treatment-resistant obsessive-compulsive disorder. Eur Psychiatry 14:101–106, 1999

Pallanti S, Hollander E, Bienstock C, et al: Treatment non-response in OCD: methodological issues and operational definitions. Int J Neuropsychopharmacol 5:181–191, 2002a

Pallanti S, Quercioli L, Koran LM: Citalopram intravenous infusion in resistant obsessive-compulsive disorder: an open trial. J Clin Psychiatry 63:796–801, 2002b

Pallanti S, Quercioli L, Bruscoli M: Response acceleration with mirtazapine augmentation of citalopram in obsessive-compulsive disorder patients without comorbid depression: a pilot study. J Clin Psychiatry 65:1394–1399, 2004

Pasquini M, Biondi M: Memantine augmentation for refractory obsessive-compulsive disorder. Prog Neuropsychopharmacol Biol Psychiatry 30:1173–1175, 2006

Pato MT, Zohar-Kadouch R, Zohar J, et al: Return of symptoms after discontinuation of clomipramine in patients with obsessive-compulsive disorder. Am J Psychiatry 145:1521–1525, 1988

Pediatric OCD Treatment Study (POTS) Team: Cognitive-behavior therapy, sertraline, and their combination for children and adolescents with obsessive-compulsive disorder: the Pediatric OCD Treatment Study (POTS) randomized controlled trial. JAMA 292:1969–1976, 2004

Perse TL, Greist JH, Jefferson JW, et al: Fluvoxamine treatment of obsessive-compulsive disorder. Am J Psychiatry 144:1543–1548, 1987

Piccinelli M, Pini S, Bellantuono C, et al: Efficacy of drug treatment in obsessive-compulsive disorder: a meta-analytic review. Br J Psychiatry 166:424–443, 1995

Pigott TA, Pato MT, L'Heureux F, et al: A controlled comparison of adjuvant lithium carbonate or thyroid hormone in clomipramine-treated patients with obsessive-compulsive disorder. J Clin Psychopharmacol 11:242–248, 1991

Pigott TA, L'Heureux F, Hill JL, et al: A double-blind study of adjuvant buspirone hydrochloride in clomipramine-treated patients with obsessive-compulsive disorder. J Clin Psychopharmacol 12:11–18, 1992

Pigott TA, Seay SM: A review of the efficacy of selective serotonin reuptake inhibitors in obsessive-compulsive disorder. J Clin Psychiatry 60:101–106, 1999

Pittenger C, Krystal JH, Coric V: Glutamate-modulating drugs as novel pharmacotherapeutic agents in the treatment of obsessive-compulsive disorder. NeuroRx 3:69–81, 2006

Poyurovsky M, Weizman R, Weizman A, et al: Memantine for treatment-resistant OCD. Am J Psychiatry 162:2191–2192, 2005

Prasko J, Pasková B, Záleský R, et al: The effect of repetitive transcranial magnetic stimulation (rTMS) on symptoms in obsessive compulsive disorder: a randomized, double blind, sham controlled study. Neuro Endocrinol Lett 27:327–332, 2006

Rasmussen S, Hackett E, DuBoff E, et al: A 2-year study of sertraline in the treatment of obsessive-compulsive disorder. Int Clin Psychopharmacol 12:309–316, 1997

Richter MA, Summerfeldt LJ, Antony MM, et al: Obsessive-compulsive spectrum conditions in obsessive-compulsive disorder and other anxiety disorders. Depress Anxiety 18:118–127, 2003

Riddle MA, Scahill L, King RA, et al: Double-blind, crossover trial of fluoxetine and placebo in children and adolescents with obsessive-compulsive disorder. J Am Acad Child Adolesc Psychiatry 31:1062–1069, 1992

Riddle MA, Reeve EA, Yaryura-Tobias JA, et al: Fluvoxamine for children and adolescents with obsessive-compulsive disorder: a randomized, controlled, multicenter trial. J Am Acad Child Adolesc Psychiatry 40:222–229, 2001

Romano S, Goodman W, Tamura R, et al: Long-term treatment of obsessive-compulsive disorder after an acute response: a comparison of fluoxetine versus placebo. J Clin Psychopharmacol 21:46–52, 2001

Rosenberg DR, MacMaster FP, Keshavan MS, et al: Decrease in caudate glutamatergic concentrations in pediatric obsessive-compulsive disorder patients taking paroxetine. J Am Acad Child Adolesc Psychiatry 39:1096–1103, 2000

Rosenberg DR, Mirza Y, Russell A, et al: Reduced anterior cingulate glutamatergic concentrations in childhood OCD and major depression versus healthy controls. J Am Acad Child Adolesc Psychiatry 43:1146–1153, 2004

Rufer M, Hand I, Alsleben H, et al: Long-term course and outcome of obsessive-compulsive patients after cognitive-behavioral therapy in combination with either fluvoxamine or placebo: a 7-year follow-up of a randomized double-blind trial. Eur Arch Psychiatry Clin Neurosci 255:121–128, 2005

Sachdev PS, Loo CK, Mitchell PB, et al: Repetitive transcranial magnetic stimulation for the treatment of obsessive compulsive disorder: a double-blind controlled investigation. Psychol Med 37:1645–1649, 2007

Salzberg AD, Swedo SE: Oxytocin and vasopressin in obsessive-compulsive disorder. Am J Psychiatry 149:713–714, 1992

Sanchez C, Bogeso KP, Ebert B, et al: Escitalopram versus citalopram: the surprising role of the R-enantiomer. Psychopharmacology (Berl) 174:163–176, 2004

Sareen J, Kirshner A, Lander M, et al: Do antipsychotics ameliorate or exacerbate obsessive compulsive disorder symptoms? A systematic review. J Affect Disord 82:167–174, 2004

Scahill L, Riddle MA, McSwiggin-Hardin M, et al: Children's Yale-Brown Obsessive Compulsive Scale: reliability and validity. J Am Acad Child Adolesc Psychiatry 36:844–852, 1997

Shapira NA, Ward HE, Mandoki M, et al: A double-blind, placebo-controlled trial of olanzapine addition in fluoxetine-refractory obsessive-compulsive disorder. Biol Psychiatry 55:553–555, 2004

Sheehan DV, Harnett-Sheehan K, Raj BA: The measurement of disability. Int Clin Psychopharmacol 11 (suppl 3):89–95, 1996

Simpson HB, Liebowitz MR, Foa EB, et al: Post-treatment effects of exposure therapy and clomipramine in obsessive-compulsive disorder. Depress Anxiety 19:225–233, 2004

Simpson HB, Huppert JD, Petkova E, et al: Response versus remission in obsessive-compulsive disorder. J Clin Psychiatry 67:269–276, 2006

Skapinakis P, Papatheodorou T, Mavreas V: Antipsychotic augmentation of serotonergic antidepressants in treatment-resistant obsessive-compulsive disorder: a meta-analysis of the randomized controlled trials. Eur Neuropsychopharmacol 17:79–93, 2007

Skoog G, Skoog I: A 40-year follow-up of patients with obsessive-compulsive disorder. Arch Gen Psychiatry 56:121–127, 1999

Stein DJ, Spadaccini E, Hollander E: Meta-analysis of pharmacotherapy trials for obsessive-compulsive disorder. Int Clin Psychopharmacol 10:11–18, 1995

Stein DJ, Montgomery SA, Kasper S, et al: Predictors of response to pharmacotherapy with citalopram in obsessive-compulsive disorder. Int Clin Psychopharmacol 16:357–361, 2001

Stein DJ, Andersen EW, Tonnoir B, et al: Escitalopram in obsessive-compulsive disorder: a randomized, placebo-controlled, fixed-dose, paroxetine-referenced, 24-week study. Curr Med Res Opin 23:701–711, 2007

Swedo S, Grant J: PANDAS: a model for human autoimmune disease. J Child Psychol Psychiatry 46:227–234, 2005

Thoren P, Åsberg M, Cronholm B, et al: Clomipramine treatment of obsessive-compulsive disorder, I: a controlled clinical trial. Arch Gen Psychiatry 37:1281–1285, 1980

Thuile J, Even C, Guelfi JD: Topiramate may induce obsessive-compulsive disorder. Psychiatry Clin Neurosci 60:394, 2006

Tollefson GD, Rampey AH Jr, Potvin JH, et al: A multicenter investigation of fixed-dose fluoxetine in the treatment of obsessive-compulsive disorder. Arch Gen Psychiatry 51:559–567, 1994

Van Ameringen M, Mancini C, Patterson B, et al: Topiramate augmentation in treatment-resistant obsessive-compulsive disorder: a retrospective, open-label case series. Depress Anxiety 23:1–5, 2006

van Oppen P, de Haan E, van Balkom AJ, et al: Cognitive therapy and exposure in vivo in the treatment of obsessive compulsive disorder. Behav Res Ther 33:379–390, 1995

Volavka J, Neziroglu F, Yaryura-Tobias JA: Clomipramine and imipramine in obsessive-compulsive disorder. Psychiatry Res 14:85–93, 1985

Wassermann EM: Risk and safety of repetitive transcranial magnetic stimulation: report and suggested guidelines from the International Workshop on the Safety of Repetitive Transcranial Magnetic Stimulation, June 5–7, 1996. Electroencephalogr Clin Neurophysiol 108:1–16, 1998

Westenberg HG: Obsessive-compulsive disorder revisited from a treatment perspective. Psychiatr Danub 19:375–377, 2007

Wichmann T, Delong MR: Deep brain stimulation for neurologic and neuropsychiatric disorders. Neuron 52:197–204, 2006

Wittchen HU, Jacobi F: Size and burden of mental disorders in Europe—a critical review and appraisal of 27 studies. Eur Neuropsychopharmacol 15:357–376, 2005

Yaryura-Tobias JA, Neziroglu F: The action of chlorimipramine in obsessive-compulsive neurosis: a pilot study. Curr Ther Res Clin Exp 17:111–116, 1975

Yaryaura-Tobias JA, Neziroglu FA: Venlafaxine in obsessive-compulsive disorder. Arch Gen Psychiatry 53:653–654, 1996

Zohar J, Judge R: Paroxetine versus clomipramine in the treatment of obsessive-compulsive disorder. OCD Paroxetine Study Investigators. Br J Psychiatry 169:468–474, 1996

Recommended Readings

Fineberg N, Marazitti D, Stein DJ (eds): Obsessive-Compulsive Disorder: A Practical Guide. London, Martin Dunitz, 2001

Heyman I, Mataix-Cols D, Fineberg NA: Obsessive-compulsive disorder. BMJ 333:424–429, 2006

Koran LM, Hanna GL, Hollander E, et al: Practice guideline for the treatment of patients with obsessive-compulsive disorder. Am J Psychiatry 164(suppl):5–53, 2007

National Institute for Health and Clinical Excellence: Obsessive-compulsive disorder: core interventions in the treatment of obsessive-compulsive disorder and body dysmorphic disorder. 2005. Available at http://www.nice.org.uk/Guidance/CG31. Accessed December 15, 2008.

Chapter 19

Psychological Treatment for Obsessive-Compulsive Disorder

Jonathan S. Abramowitz, Ph.D., ABPP

Obsessive-compulsive disorder (OCD) is an anxiety disorder characterized by recurrent, unwanted, and seemingly bizarre thoughts, images, impulses, or doubts that evoke distress (obsessions; e.g., persistent violent and morally repugnant ideas such as "Jesus is dead"); and repetitive behavioral or mental rituals performed to reduce this distress (compulsions; e.g., praying, confessing, and asking for assurances to prevent a feared consequence such as going to hell). Obsessional fears tend to involve issues related to uncertainty about personal safety or the safety of others. Compulsions are deliberately performed to reduce this uncertainty. Although not a diagnostic criterion, phobic-like avoidance is a cardinal feature of OCD. Most sufferers attempt to avoid situations and stimuli that trigger obsessional fear and urges to ritualize. For example, someone with obsessions about germs might avoid public washrooms, and someone with obsessions about causing fires might avoid using the oven.

Research consistently reveals that certain types of obsessions and compulsions co-occur within patients (e.g., Abramowitz et al. 2003b), including 1) obsessions about contamination, with decontamination (e.g., washing) rituals; 2) obsessions regarding responsibility for harm, with checking and reassurance-seeking rituals; 3) obsessions about order or symmetry, with arranging rituals; and 4) repugnant violent, sexual, or blasphemous obsessions, with covert rituals such as mental neutralizing rituals (e.g., praying, compulsive thought suppression). Some patients also have excessive concerns about numbers or their health.

Although many people with OCD recognize that their obsessional fears and rituals are senseless and excessive, others strongly believe their rituals serve to prevent the occurrence of disastrous consequences (i.e., they have "poor insight" [Foa et al. 1995]). For some patients, feared consequences include an identifiable disaster (e.g., "I will get AIDS if I touch a toilet"), whereas others fear that if rituals are not performed, anxiety will persist indefinitely or rise to unmanageable levels. Clinical observations suggest that a patient's degree of insight can vary over time as well as across symptom categories.

In this chapter, I begin with a historical overview of the development of effective psychological treatment techniques for OCD—namely, exposure and response prevention—with an emphasis on translational research that has bridged the gap from the animal behavior laboratory to the psychotherapy clinic. Next, I discuss the practical application and mechanisms of this treatment, before reviewing the empirical literature that establishes its efficacy and predictors of outcome. I turn then to cognitive therapy, a relatively new development in the treatment of OCD, and discuss its use in psychological treatment as guided by empirical research. Various formats for psychological treatment are reviewed next, followed by a focus on treatment-refractory groups. The chapter concludes with a discussion of recent advances in the treatment of a previously treatment-resistant group: OCD patients with purely cognitive (or covert) symptoms (sometimes referred to as "pure obsessionals").

Historical Overview

Development of Behavioral Treatment for OCD: A Translational Perspective

Prior to the 1970s and 1980s, treatment for OCD consisted largely of psychodynamic psychotherapy derived from psychoanalytic ideas of unconscious motivation. Although anecdotal reports exist (Freud 1909/1963), there are virtually no scientific studies assessing the efficacy of this approach. Nonetheless, the general consensus of clinicians of that era was that OCD was an unmanageable condition with a poor prognosis. This admission speaks to how much (or how *little*) confidence clinicians placed in such approaches. Indeed, available reports suggest that the effects of psychodynamically oriented therapies are neither robust nor durable for OCD.

By the last quarter of the twentieth century, however, the prognostic picture for OCD had improved dramatically. This was due in large part to the work of Victor Meyer (1966) and other behaviorally oriented clinicians and researchers (e.g., Jack Rachman, Issac Marks) who relied on animal models of obsessive-compulsive behavior established in the 1950s to guide the synthesis of behaviorally based therapies for humans. These historical developments provide us with one of the clearest and most compelling examples of translational research in the mental health field. Thus, I begin by placing contemporary psychological treatment for OCD in its historical context.

Early Laboratory Research

The early work of Richard Solomon and his colleagues (1953) provides an elegant, yet often overlooked, animal behavioral model of OCD. Solomon et al. studied dogs in shuttle boxes (small rooms divided in two by a hurdle over which the animal could jump). Each half of the shuttle box was separately furnished with an electric grate that could be independently electrified to give the dog an electric shock through its paws. In addition, there was a flickering light that served as a conditioned stimulus. The researchers produced a compulsive ritual-like behavior in the dogs by pairing the flickering light with an electric shock (the shock occurred 10 seconds after the light was turned on). The dog soon learned to terminate exposure to the shock by jumping into the other compartment of the shuttle box, which was not electrified. After several trials, the dog learned to altogether *avoid* the shock by jumping to the nonelectrified compartment in response to the flickering light (i.e., within 10 seconds). In other words, the experimenter had produced a conditioned "escape" response to the light, namely, jumping from one compartment of the box to the other.

Once this conditioned response was established, the electricity was disconnected and the dog never received another shock. Nevertheless, the animal continued to jump across the hurdle each time the conditioned stimulus (i.e., the light) was turned on. This continued for hundreds (and in some cases, thousands) of trials despite no actual risk of shock. Apparently, the dog had acquired an obsessive-compulsive behavior—jumping across the hurdle—which reduced its fear of shock and thus was maintained by negative reinforcement (the removal of an aversive stimulus such as emotional distress). This serves as an animal analogue to human OCD, in which, as described earlier, compulsive behavior is triggered by fear that is associated with situations or stimuli such as toilets, numbers, or obsessional thoughts (conditioned stimuli) that pose little or no actual risk of harm. This fear is then reduced by compulsive rituals (e.g., washing) and avoidance behaviors, which serve as an escape from distress and, in doing so, are negatively reinforced and thus become habitual.

Solomon and his colleagues also studied the reduction of the compulsive jumping behavior of their "obsessive-compulsive" dogs by using various techniques, the most effective of which involved a combination of procedures now known as *exposure and response prevention* (ERP). Specifically, the experimenter turned on the flickering light (analogous to in vivo exposure, as described later) and increased the height of the hurdle in the shuttle box so that the dog was unable to jump (analogous to response prevention, as described later). When this was done, the dog immediately showed signs of a strong fear response—yelping, running around the chamber, and defecating and urinating—because it expected to receive a shock. Gradually, however, this emotional reaction subsided (since the shock was never given) until finally, the dog displayed calmness without the slightest hint of distress. In behavioral terms, this experimental paradigm produced *extinction* of the fear. After several "extinction trials," the entire emotional and behavioral response was extinguished, so that even when the light was turned on and the height of the hurdle was lowered, the dog did not jump.

During the 1960s and 1970s, OCD researchers adapted similar research paradigms to human beings with OCD (Rachman and Hodgson 1980). Of course, no electric shocks were used, but the adaptation was as follows: patients with hand-washing rituals, after providing informed consent, were seated at a table with a container of dirt and miscellaneous garbage. The experimenter asked the patients to place their hands in the mixture and explained that no washing would be permitted for some length of time. When the patients began the procedure, an increase in anxiety, fear, and urges to wash were (of course) observed. This increase in distress was akin to the dogs' response once the light was turned on and the hurdle had been increased in height, making jumping (i.e., escape) impossible. Like Solomon's dogs, the OCD patients also evidenced a gradual reduction in distress and in urges to wash, thus demonstrating extinction. This procedure was repeated on subsequent days, the theory predicting that after some time, extinction would be complete and the OCD symptoms would be reduced.

From the Laboratory to the Clinic

Victor Meyer (1966) first reported the application of ERP treatment for OCD. He helped OCD inpatients deliberately confront, for 2 hours each day, situations and stimuli they usually avoided (e.g., floors, bathrooms). The purpose of the repeated and prolonged confrontation was to induce obsessional fears and urges to ritualize; yet the patients were also instructed to refrain from performing compulsive rituals after exposure. Of Meyer's 15 patients, 10 responded extremely well to this therapy and the remainder evidenced partial improvement. Follow-up studies conducted several years later found that only 2 of those who were successfully treated had relapsed (Meyer et al. 1974).

As in this original work, contemporary ERP entails therapist-guided, systematic, repeated, and prolonged exposure to situations that provoke obsessional fear, along with abstinence from compulsive behaviors. This might occur in the form of actual confrontation with feared low-risk situations (i.e., in vivo exposure) or in the form of imaginal confrontation with the feared disastrous consequences of confronting the low-risk situations (i.e., imaginal exposure). For example, an individual who fears causing bad luck if she steps on the cracks in the sidewalk would practice stepping on them and imagining being held responsible for harming others because she had stepped on the cracks.

Refraining from compulsive rituals (*response prevention*) is a vital component of treatment, because the performance of compulsive rituals would prematurely discontinue exposure and rob the patient of learning that 1) the obsessional situation is not truly dangerous, and 2) anxiety subsides on its own, even if the ritual is not performed. Thus, ERP requires that the patient remain in the exposure situation until the obsessional distress decreases spontaneously, without attempting to reduce the distress by withdrawing from the situation or by performing compulsive rituals or neutralizing strategies.

Cognitive-Behavioral Therapy for OCD

Assessment

A course of ERP begins with a thorough assessment of the patient's particular obsessional thoughts, ideas, and impulses; stimuli that trigger these obsessions; rituals and avoidance behavior; and the anticipated harmful consequences of confronting feared situations without performing rituals. Comorbid conditions that may complicate treatment are also identified, and plans for their management are established. Although the behavioral assessment focuses on obsessive-compulsive psychopathology, he or she also learns a great deal about the context in which OCD occurs, the complications it causes, and factors that precipitate symptomatic episodes (e.g., life stress), as well as those associated with fewer symptoms (e.g., vacations).

Some patients with OCD may be reluctant to disclose their obsessions and compulsions because they are embarrassed, or perhaps they have experienced their obsessions and carried out their rituals so often and for so long that they no longer recognize them as abnormal. The use of a checklist of common obsessions and compulsions, such as the symptom checklist that accompanies the Yale-Brown Obsessive Compulsive Scale (Y-BOCS; Goodman et al. 1989a, 1989b), often helps elicit this information more completely.

In addition, identifying all of the circumstances, both external (situations and stimuli) and internal (intrusive thoughts), that trigger obsessional distress and compulsive urges is crucial to designing an effective ERP program. This *functional assessment* should also elicit information about involvement of family, friends, and coworkers in the patient's rituals, because such involvement is quite common. Techniques have been developed to help people who have been accommodating the patient's OCD symptoms modify their own behavior so it is more consistent with the goals of treatment (as described below in the section "Managing Symptom

Accommodation by Others"). This change might include having the involved person serve as a cotherapist or coach.

Education and Treatment Planning

Before actual treatment commences, the therapist socializes the patient to a psychological model of OCD that is based on the behavioral model discussed earlier. The patient is also given a clear rationale for how ERP is expected to be helpful in reducing OCD. This educational component is an important step in therapy because it helps motivate the patient to tolerate the distress that typically accompanies exposure practice. A helpful rationale includes information about how ERP involves the provocation and reduction of distress during prolonged exposure. Information gathered during the assessment sessions is then used to plan, collaboratively with the patient, the specific exposure exercises that will be pursued.

In planning for ERP, the therapist must engineer experiences in which the patient confronts stimuli that evoke obsessional anxiety, but where the feared outcomes do not materialize and the only explanation is that the obsessional stimuli are not as dangerous as was thought. The exposure treatment plan, or *hierarchy*, is a list of specific situations, stimuli, and thoughts the patient will confront during therapy. The situations are put in order by the degree of *subjective units of distress* that exposure would provoke. Prolonged confrontation with each hierarchy item, one at a time, is conducted repeatedly (without rituals) until distress levels reduce to the point that the patient can manage adaptively within the situation. It is critical that hierarchy items match the patient's specific obsessional fears. For example, an individual with obsessional fears of germs must be exposed to the sources of feared germs. If she believes public bathrooms and public telephones are "contaminated," exposure must include confrontation with these things. An example of a hierarchy for such a patient appears in Table 19–1.

In addition to explaining and planning a hierarchy of exposure exercises, the educational stage of ERP must acquaint the patient with *response prevention* procedures. Importantly, the term "response prevention" does not imply that the therapist actively prevents the patient from performing rituals. Instead, the therapist must convince patients to resist urges to perform rituals on their own.

TABLE 19–1. Example of an exposure hierarchy

Exposure item	SUDS
Door handles and handrails	45
Images of "herpes germs"	55
Shaking hands with others	65
Public telephones	70
Garbage cans	75
Sweat from another person	80
Public bathrooms	85
Drops of urine	90
Paper towel with small smudge of feces	95

Note. SUDS=subjective units of distress.

Exposure Therapy Sessions

The exposure exercises typically begin with moderately distressing situations, stimuli, and images and escalate to the most distressing situations that must be confronted during treatment. Beginning with less anxiety-evoking exposure tasks increases the likelihood that the patient will learn to manage the distress and complete the exposure exercise successfully. Moreover, having success with initial exposures increases confidence in the treatment and helps motivate the patient to persevere during later, more difficult, exercises. At the end of each treatment session, for homework, the therapist instructs the patient to continue exposure for several hours and in different environmental contexts, without the therapist. Exposure to the most anxiety-evoking situations is not left to the end of the treatment, but rather is practiced about midway through the schedule of exposure tasks. This tactic allows the patient ample opportunity to repeat exposure to the most difficult situations in different contexts to allow generalization of treatment effects. During the later treatment sessions, the therapist emphasizes how important it is for the patient to continue to apply the ERP procedures learned during treatment. Depending on the patient's particular obsessions and compulsions, and on the practicality of confronting actual feared situations, treatment sessions might involve varying amounts of situational and imaginal exposure practice, sometimes necessitating that the patient and therapist leave the office or clinic to perform the exercises (Abramowitz 2006).

Compulsive rituals evolve to control discomfort after exposure to triggers, and response prevention removes this source of relief. At the beginning of therapy, therefore, short-term increases in obsessions and discomfort often occur as ritualistic urges are resisted. Strategies can be used to enable patients to continue exposure, without resorting to ritual behaviors, until habituation occurs. For example, patients can remind themselves that distress is uncomfortable but not unbearable and that it will eventually diminish if exposure is endured without giving in to rituals. A gradual approach to stopping rituals might be considered if patients have difficulty completely refraining, although complete abstinence from rituals should be upheld as a goal for therapy.

Although some clinicians teach patients relaxation techniques to help manage anxiety that accompanies ERP, this practice is counterproductive and should not be used. If exposure-induced anxiety is reduced or terminated via relaxation, this robs the patient of experiencing the natural decline in anxiety that occurs when exposure is prolonged and repeated. Such learning is crucial in overcoming OCD. Thus, relaxation techniques become as maladaptive as compulsive rituals. Moreover, the use of relaxation teaches patients that feelings of anxiety are something to be resisted, fought off, or escaped from. This is contrary to the idea of exposure therapy, which teaches patients to *endure* temporary anxiety—a common experience that does not have any serious consequences—until it naturally subsides. In short, despite the intuitive appeal of techniques for directly reducing anxiety, relaxation training has no place in the treatment of OCD. (In fact, as will be reviewed later, it is used as a placebo intervention in controlled treatment studies.) Durable improvement in OCD requires that the patient repeatedly experience the evocation of obsessional fear and subsequently observe that even when no rituals, escape, or avoidance behaviors are performed, anxiety subsides and feared disasters do not occur.

Managing Symptom Accommodation by Others

Many patients involve those around them in OCD symptoms, such as by asking a partner to carry out checking rituals or provide reassurance to decrease obsessive doubts, or demanding that family members take off their "contaminated" shoes as they enter the house. In many instances, such symptom accommodation becomes a way of life for the family or couple because it provides short-term relief from suffering for the patient. Over the long term, however, this behavior inadvertently maintains OCD symptoms, since it has the same effect as if the patient were personally performing the ritual or avoidance behavior. Because symptom accommodation is counterproductive to ERP, significant others must be educated about the nature and treatment of OCD and be taught more productive ways of managing the patient's obsessional distress and requests for help with rituals. Specifically, family members can be taught to respond to requests for rituals by saying things like, "I know you feel very anxious right now, but I'm not supposed to do that ritual for you anymore. How can I help you get through this without reinforcing your OCD symptoms?" (Abramowitz 2006).

Mechanisms of Action

Three mechanisms may be involved in the reduction of obsessions and compulsions during ERP. First, these treatment techniques provide opportunities for the extinction of conditioned fear responses, as discussed earlier. Repeated and uninterrupted exposure to feared stimuli produces *habituation*—an inevitable natural decrease in conditioned fear. Response prevention fosters habituation by blocking the performance of rituals that would immediately reduce anxiety and thereby foil the habituation process. Second, ERP corrects irrational fear-based beliefs and expectations associated with obsessions (e.g., the belief that one will get sick by using a public bathroom, or that certain thoughts automatically lead to doing bad things) by repeatedly presenting the patient with information that disconfirms these beliefs. Finally, ERP helps patients master their fears without having to rely on avoidance or compulsive rituals, which instills a sense of self-efficacy.

Foa and Kozak (1986) have drawn attention to three indicators of change during exposure-based treatment. First, physiological arousal and subjective fear must be evoked during exposure. Second, the fear responses gradually diminish *during* the exposure session (within-session habituation). Third, the initial fear response at the beginning of each exposure session declines *across* sessions (between-sessions habituation). Figure 19–1 shows a patient's pattern of anxious responding when exposed to sitting on a bathroom floor for 90 minutes on 4 consecutive days.

Efficacy and Effectiveness of ERP

Expert consensus treatment guidelines state that ERP is the first-line psychosocial intervention for OCD (March et al. 1997). In this section, I review empirical research on the outcome of ERP. Before turning to a review of individual treatment trials, let us first consider results from meta-analytic studies.

Meta-Analytic Findings

Data from a large number of controlled and uncontrolled outcome trials consistently indicate that ERP is

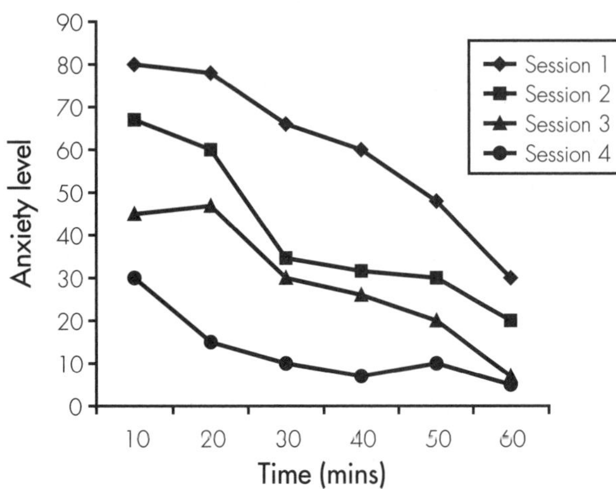

FIGURE 19–1. Pattern of a patient's anxiety reduction within and between exposure therapy sessions.

extremely helpful in reducing OCD symptoms. A meta-analysis of this literature (Abramowitz 1996) that included 24 studies conducted between 1975 and 1995 (involving more than 800 patients) revealed very large treatment effect sizes of 1.16 (on self-report measures) and 1.41 (interview measures) at posttest and 1.10 (for self-report measures) and 1.57 (for interview measures) at follow-up. Using a different meta-analytic approach, Foa and Kozak (1996) calculated the percentage of patients in each study who were "responders" (usually defined as achieving a pretreatment to posttreatment improvement of at least 30%). They found that across 13 ERP studies, 83% of patients were responders at posttreatment, and across 16 studies, 76% were responders at follow-up (mean follow-up period was 29 months). In concert, these findings suggest that the majority of OCD patients who undergo treatment with ERP evidence substantial short- and long-term benefit.

Randomized, Controlled Trials

The Yale-Brown Obsessive Compulsive Scale (Goodman et al. 1989a, 1989b), a 10-item semistructured clinical interview, is considered the gold standard as a measure of OCD severity. Because of its respectable psychometric properties (Taylor 1995), the Y-BOCS is widely utilized in OCD treatment outcome research and provides a useful measuring stick by which to compare results across studies. When administering the Y-BOCS, the interviewer rates the following five parameters for obsessions (items 1–5) and compulsions (items 6–10) on a scale from 0 (no symptoms) to 4 (extreme): time, interference with functioning, distress, resistance, and control. The total score is the sum of the 10 items and therefore ranges from 0 to 40. Y-BOCS scores of 0–7 tend to indicate subclinical OCD symptoms; scores of 8–15, mild symptoms; 16–25, moderate symptoms; 26–35, severe symptoms; and 36–40, extreme severity.

Table 19–2 summarizes the results of the five published randomized, controlled trials that examined the efficacy of ERP by using the Y-BOCS as an outcome measure. Two studies compared ERP with a credible psychotherapy control condition. Fals-Stewart et al. (1993) randomly assigned patients to individual ERP, group ERP, or a progressive relaxation control treatment. All treatments included 24 sessions delivered on a twice-weekly basis over 12 weeks. Although both ERP regimens were found to be superior to relaxation, there were no differences between group and individual ERP. Average improvement in the ERP groups was 41% on the Y-BOCS, and posttreatment scores fell within the mild range of severity.

In the second study, Lindsay et al. (1997) compared ERP to anxiety management training (AMT), a credible placebo treatment consisting of breathing retraining, relaxation, and problem-solving therapy. Both treatments were intensive: 15 daily sessions conducted over a 3-week period. On average, patients receiving ERP improved almost 62% from pretreatment to posttreatment on the Y-BOCS, with endpoint scores, again, in the mild range. In contrast, the AMT group showed no change in symptoms following treatment. The clear superiority of ERP over credible placebo therapies such as relaxation and AMT indicates that improvement in OCD symptoms can be attributed to the ERP procedures themselves, over and above any nonspecific factors such as time, attention, or expectancy of positive outcome.

Van Balkom et al. (1998) examined the relative efficacy of five treatment conditions: 1) ERP, 2) cognitive therapy (CT), 3) ERP plus fluvoxamine, 4) CT plus fluvoxamine, and 5) wait-list control. As Table 19–2 indicates, ERP fared somewhat less well in this study than in other randomized, controlled trials. A likely explanation for the 32% symptom reduction is that the ERP protocol was less than optimal. All exposure was conducted as homework assignments rather than in session under the therapist's supervision. Moreover, therapists did not discuss expectations of disastrous consequences with patients during the first 8 weeks of ERP, because this would have overlapped substantially with CT.

Foa et al. (2005) examined the relative efficacy of four treatment conditions: 1) intensive (15 daily sessions)

ERP (including in-session exposure), 2) clomipramine, 3) combined treatment (ERP plus clomipramine), and 4) pill placebo. ERP produced a 50% Y-BOCS score reduction, which was far superior to the effects of pill placebo. Moreover, endpoint Y-BOCS scores fell to within the mild range of OCD severity. In a similar study, Nakatani et al. (2005) randomly assigned patients to receive either weekly ERP sessions, fluvoxamine, or pill placebo. The ERP group evinced a mean Y-BOCS score reduction of nearly 60%, which was superior to that reported for the placebo group (7%). Moreover, at posttest, the ERP group's Y-BOCS scores were again within the mild range of symptoms. Overall, then, the findings from randomized, controlled trials suggest that ERP produces substantial and clinically meaningful improvement in OCD symptoms and that symptom reduction is attributable to the specific effects of these treatment procedures and not to nonspecific or "common" factors of psychotherapy.

Comparisons With Medication

Numerous double-blind randomized, placebo-controlled trials have established the efficacy of pharmacotherapy using serotonin reuptake inhibitors (SRIs; e.g., fluvoxamine) for OCD (e.g., Montgomery et al. 1993; see Chapter 18, "Pharmacotherapy for Obsessive-Compulsive Disorder," in this volume). Given that both are effective treatments, researchers have attempted to examine the relative efficacy of ERP and SRIs. For example, Foa et al.'s (2005) study included comparisons among 12 weeks of ERP, 12 weeks of clomipramine, and the combination of ERP plus clomipramine. Immediately following treatment, all active therapies showed superiority to placebo, yet ERP (mean 50% Y-BOCS reduction) was seen as superior to clomipramine (mean 35% Y-BOCS reduction). It is important to note that patients in this study received intensive ERP, meaning daily treatment sessions. Thus, this treatment regimen is not necessarily representative of typical clinical practice.

The study by Nakatani et al. (2005) also included a relevant comparison between ERP and fluvoxamine. The ERP program consisted of 12 weekly treatment sessions in which exposure exercises were planned for practice between sessions. Thus, most of the ERP work was conducted by the patient alone rather than as supervised by a therapist. Still, the 58% Y-BOCS reduction from ERP was significantly greater than the 29% reduction observed in the fluvoxamine group. These two studies indicate that ERP, even in patient-directed format, is a more effective treatment than pharmacotherapy by SRIs such as fluvoxamine. No recent studies have compared ERP to other forms of medication.

Combining ERP With Medication

Although the concurrent use of medication and psychological treatment seems intuitive and is commonly advocated in clinical practice, few studies have empirically examined whether this approach affords advantages over monotherapy. Three outcomes are possible with combination treatment for OCD. The desired outcome is a synergistic effect in which the effects of combined therapy are superior to either ERP or SRIs alone—for instance, if adding one treatment increases the magnitude of response to the other. A second possibility is that medication and ERP add little to each other—for instance, if either therapy is sufficiently powerful that the other has little room to contribute. The third scenario is that one treatment detracts from the efficacy of the other—for instance, if patients attribute their improvement to taking medication and subsequently fail to comply with ERP procedures. In this case, medication would *attenuate* the effects of ERP. To this end, the use of benzodiazepines is known to interfere with the effects of exposure therapy (for a review, see Deacon 2006). Specifically, because these medications reduce anxious arousal more quickly than would have occurred naturally, their use during exposure can serve as a safety signal and prevent the patient with OCD from learning that obsessional fear declines naturally even if the medication is not used. For this reason, benzodiazepines are contraindicated during ERP.

For the most part, the available studies suggest that simultaneous treatment with ERP and SRIs yields superior outcome compared with SRI monotherapy, but not compared with ERP alone (Cottraux et al. 1990; Foa et al. 2005; Hohagen et al. 1998; O'Connor et al. 1999; Van Balkom et al. 1998). One exception was reported by Hohagen et al. (1998), who found that combined ERP and fluvoxamine offered an advantage over ERP monotherapy; however, this finding was reported among severely depressed OCD patients. Importantly, many of the available studies have limitations, such as lack of statistical power and the exclusion of patients with comorbidity—perhaps the very patients who would show the greatest benefit from combined treatment.

Exposure and Response Prevention as an Adjunct to Medication

Because the typical pharmacotherapy trial leaves the average OCD patient clinically symptomatic (posttreat-

TABLE 19–2. Effects of exposure and response prevention in randomized, controlled trials

		Mean (SD) Y-BOCS total score					
		ERP group			Control group		
Study	**Control condition**	***n***	**Pre**	**Post**	***n***	**Pre**	**Post**
Fals-Stewart et al. 1993[a]	Relaxation	31	20.2	12.1	32	19.9	18.1
Lindsay et al. 1997	Anxiety management	9	28.7 (4.6)	11.0 (3.8)	9	24.4 (7.0)	25.9 (5.8)
Van Balkom et al. 1998	Waiting list	19	25.0 (7.9)	17.1 (8.4)	18	26.8 (6.4)	26.4 (6.8)
Foa et al. 2005	Pill placebo	29	24.6 (4.8)	11.0 (7.9)	26	25.0 (4.0)	22.2 (6.4)
Nakatani et al. 2005	Pill placebo	10	29.9 (3.1)	12.9 (4.9)	8	30.5 (3.7)	28.4 (5.5)

Note. ERP=exposure and response prevention; SD=standard deviation; Y-BOCS=Yale-Brown Obsessive Compulsive Scale.
[a]Standard deviation not reported in the study.

ment Y-BOCS scores in the 15–20 range are the norm; Greist et al. 1995), studies have examined whether adding ERP improves outcome following one or more adequate trials of SRIs. Simpson et al. (1999) offered ERP to 6 patients who had shown minimal response to adequate trials of SRIs. At the completion of ERP, scores on the Y-BOCS were substantially further reduced, indicating that ERP augments the effects of SRIs in patients with medication resistance. Similar results were reported by Kampman et al. (2002) who provided ERP to 14 patients who had shown less than 25% symptom reduction after 12 weeks on fluoxetine. Tolin et al. (2004) studied a sample of 20 patients with high rates of comorbid conditions who had not responded sufficiently to adequate medication trials. After a 1-month wait-list period, these patients received 15 sessions of ERP. Results indicated a statistically significant drop in OCD symptoms following ERP, and those who completed the study maintained their gains as long as 6 months after the end of treatment (follow-up mean Y-BOCS score=18.7).

In the largest and most well-controlled augmentation study to date, Tenneij et al. (2005) randomly assigned 96 OCD patients on adequate medication trials to receive 6 additional months of their medication or ERP. Patients who received ERP showed greater improvement on the Y-BOCS and were more likely to be in remission compared with those who continued on medication alone. Considered together, these studies indicate that ERP is recommended for OCD patients who have residual symptoms despite having tried SRI medications. Results of the Tenneij et al. (2005) study suggest that even medication *responders* can benefit further from adjunctive ERP. These data have substantial clinical implications, given that medication is the most widely available and most widely used form of treatment for OCD, yet it typically produces modest improvement.

Is Exposure and Response Prevention Effective in Nonresearch Settings?

Although randomized, controlled trials substantiate the efficacy of ERP, such studies are conducted under highly controlled research conditions. Thus, an important question concerns whether the beneficial effects of this treatment extend beyond the "ivory tower" to typical service delivery settings that serve less rarefied patient populations and where therapists do not receive supervision from top experts on ERP. Several studies have addressed this issue, reporting on outcomes in naturalistic settings (Franklin et al. 2000; Rothbaum and Shahar 2000; Warren and Thomas 2001). In the largest study, Franklin et al. (2000) examined outcome for 110 consecutively referred individuals with OCD who received 15 sessions of intensive ERP on an outpatient fee-for-service basis. Half of this sample had comorbid Axis I or Axis II diagnoses, and patients were only denied ERP if they were actively psychotic, abusing substances, or suicidal. Patients treated with ERP showed improvement as reflected by mean Y-BOCS scores that decreased from 26.8 to 11.8 (60% reduction in OCD symptoms). Moreover, only 10 patients dropped out of treatment prematurely.

In a multicultural naturalistic study, Friedman et al. (2003) found that although treatment was effective in reducing OCD and depressive symptoms, many patients reported significant residual symptoms after therapy: mean Y-BOCS scores for African American patients were 23.5 pretreatment and 17.2 posttreatment (27% reduction) and for Caucasians were 26.03 pretreatment and 17.65 posttreatment (23% reduction). There were no between-group differences in treatment outcome. Taken together, the findings from these naturalistic studies indicate that the effects of ERP for OCD are transportable from highly controlled research settings to typical clinical settings that serve more heterogeneous patient populations.

Predictors of Outcome With Exposure and Response Prevention

Although ERP is a highly effective intervention, up to 50% of patients drop out of treatment or show an unsatisfactory response. It would therefore be desirable to be able to predict whether a given patient is likely to respond. Research has identified several factors that predict outcome with ERP. These characteristics can be grouped into three broad categories: 1) treatment-related, 2) patient-related, and 3) environmental factors.

Characteristics of the Treatment

In two meta-analytic studies, Abramowitz (1996, 1997) examined the relationship between treatment outcome and the manner in which ERP is delivered. These results may be summarized as follows. First, ERP programs in which exposure exercises were conducted in-session and under the therapist's supervision produced greater short- and long-term improvements, compared with programs in which all exposure was performed by the patient as homework assignments. Second, combining situational (in vivo) and imaginal exposure was superior to situational exposure alone in reducing anxiety symptoms. Third, programs in which patients were helped to abstain from *all* compulsive rituals (i.e., complete response prevention) produced superior immediate and long-term effects compared with programs in which patients were instructed to refrain only partially from ritualistic behavior.

To determine the optimal exposure session frequency, Abramowitz et al. (2003a) compared 15 sessions of ERP delivered on an intensive basis (5 days per week for 3 weeks) to 15 sessions delivered twice-weekly over 8 weeks. Whereas intensive therapy was minimally superior to the twice-weekly regimen immediately following treatment (posttreatment Y-BOCS scores were 10.4 [intensive] and 12.7 [twice-weekly]), this difference disappeared at 3-month follow-up (Y-BOCS scores 13.13 [intensive] and 14.25 [twice-weekly]). Thus, a twice-weekly therapy schedule provides clinicians with a more pragmatic, yet equally effective, alternative to the highly demanding and often impractical intensive schedule.

Given the skills-based nature of ERP, it is not surprising that multiple studies report a relationship between outcome and adherence to treatment instructions (Abramowitz et al. 2002b; O'Sullivan et al. 1991). For example, Abramowitz et al. (2002b) found that better outcomes were associated with understanding the rationale for ERP techniques and adhering to the therapist's instructions for conducting in-session and homework exposure assignments. These findings suggest that it is important for clinicians to provide a compelling explanation for using ERP procedures and to elicit the patient's input when developing an exposure plan.

Characteristics of the Patient

A number of patient characteristics have been identified as predictors of poor response to ERP, including the presence of very poor insight into the senselessness of obsessions and compulsions (Foa 1979; Foa et al. 1999), severe depression (Abramowitz and Foa 2000; Abramowitz et al. 2000; Steketee et al. 2001), generalized anxiety disorder (Steketee et al. 2001), extreme emotional reactivity during exposure (Foa et al. 1983), and severe borderline personality traits (Steketee et al. 2001). Some studies have found that more severe OCD symptoms predict poor outcome (e.g., Franklin et al. 2000), although other investigations have not supported this finding (e.g., Foa et al. 1983). Consistent evidence, however, is emerging to suggest that patients who present with primarily hoarding symptoms respond less well to ERP than do patients with other presentations of OCD (Abramowitz et al. 2003b; Mataix-Cols et al. 2002).

Characteristics of the Patient's Environment

Results have been conflicting as to whether the patient's level of marital satisfaction affects the efficacy of ERP for OCD (Emmelkamp et al. 1990; Hafner 1982; Riggs et al. 1992). What is clearer is that hostility from relatives toward the patient is associated with poor response and premature dropout from ERP (Chambless and Steketee 1999). In contrast, when relatives express dissatisfaction with the patient's symptoms, but not personal rejection, such constructive criticism may have motivational properties that enhance treatment response. Our research team is currently developing a couples-based approach to the treatment of OCD that addresses these issues and important findings.

Other Psychosocial Approaches

Cognitive Therapy for OCD

Despite its efficacy, a problem with ERP is that some patients refuse or drop out of treatment, probably because of the distressing nature of exposure exercises. For example, in Foa et al.'s (2005) trial, 22% of patients withdrew upon learning they had been randomly assigned to this treatment condition, and 28% dropped out once ERP commenced. These issues prompted the application to OCD of cognitive treatment approaches—which have led to advances in the treatment of other anxiety disorders (Beck and Emery 1985). The basis of *cognitive therapy* is the rational and evidence-based challenging and correction of the irrational thoughts and beliefs that are thought to underlie obsessional fear (e.g., Clark 2004). Compared with ERP, cognitive approaches incorporate less prolonged exposure to fear cues. However, some authors champion *cognitive-behavioral therapy* (CBT), which entails CT combined with "behavioral experiments"—which are essentially mini-exposure exercises used to demonstrate erroneous beliefs and assumptions (e.g., using knives around a loved one to test beliefs about acting on unwanted urges to stab).

Cognitive interventions for OCD were derived from 1) cognitive formulations of OCD, which posit that particular sorts of dysfunctional beliefs play an important role in the psychopathology of this disorder, and 2) the assertion that modifying faulty thinking patterns could reduce OCD symptoms. Over the past 30 years, various cognitive models have been proposed, most of which represent variations of Salkovskis's (1996) formulation.

These models begin with the well-established finding that unwanted intrusive thoughts (such as those regarding sex, aggression, and harm) are universal experiences (e.g., Rachman and de Silva 1978). Clinical obsessions arise, however, when these intrusions are misinterpreted as having serious implications for which the person having the thoughts would be personally responsible (e.g., "Thinking about harming the baby means I'm a dangerous person who must take extra care to ensure that I don't lose control"). Such an appraisal evokes distress and motivates the person to try to suppress or remove the unwanted intrusion (e.g., by replacing it with a "good" thought) and to attempt to prevent harmful events associated with the thought (e.g., by avoiding the baby).

Compulsions and avoidance behaviors are conceptualized as instrumental for averting or undoing harm or for reducing the perceived responsibility for aversive outcomes. However, compulsions prevent the correction of mistaken beliefs by robbing the person of the opportunity to see that obsessional fears are unfounded. That is, when a compulsive ritual is performed and the feared event does not take place, the individual mistakenly attributes this to the ritual, rather than to the low probability of danger (e.g., "If I had not avoided bathing the infant, I would have drowned her").

Based on these models, CT for OCD focuses on modifying pathological interpretations of intrusive thoughts and correcting the associated dysfunctional beliefs (Clark 2004; Wilhelm and Steketee 2006). Treatment begins by educating the patient about the cognitive model and the rationale for CT. For example, patients are taught that their intrusive thoughts are not indicative of anything important, but that a problem arises if such thoughts are perceived as unacceptable or threatening. The patient is helped to understand that it is *the way that* he or she interprets the intrusive thoughts that is the source of the problem, leading to distress and to maladaptive behaviors such as compulsions. Once the unwanted intrusions are correctly perceived as non-threatening, then the obsessions and the associated compulsions can be eliminated.

Comparative Efficacy of Cognitive Interventions and Exposure and Response Prevention

How effective are cognitive treatments, compared with ERP? A meta-analysis by Abramowitz et al. (2002a) that included five studies directly comparing ERP and CT/CBT suggested no difference in the effectiveness of these treatment modalities. Closer examination, however, revealed that effect sizes for the cognitive treatments were larger when behavioral experiments were included in the cognitive protocols. In other words, ERP and CBT have similar treatment efficacy, yet CT that does not include exposure in any form appears to be less effective than ERP or CBT. Moreover, the efficacy of ERP was most likely to be greater than that of both CT and CBT when ERP involved therapist-assisted exposure rather than only homework-based exposure. (Properly implemented ERP involves both types of exposure.)

Long-Term Treatment

Hiss et al. (1994) reported encouraging results of a relapse prevention program following ERP treatment of OCD. For this study, 18 patients were treated with 3 weeks of intensive ERP and then randomly assigned to either a relapse prevention condition (consisting of four 90-minute sessions over 1 week) or a control condition (consisting of relaxation training and associative therapy). Based on a 50% improvement on the Y-BOCS as the criterion for treatment response, 75% of the patients assigned to the relapse prevention condition were responders after initial treatment and 75% were responders at 6-month follow-up. However, 70% of the patients assigned to the control condition were responders after initial treatment, but only 33% were responders at 6-month follow-up. Although there were few statistically significant results because of the small sample size, this study suggested that a brief relapse prevention program including brief telephone contacts may help prevent relapse, at least in cleaning and checking rituals.

Abramowitz (2006) described a follow-up program (outlined in this paragraph) that emphasizes practicing the ERP and cognitive skills learned during the active therapy period. Follow-up sessions can be initiated directly upon completion of an ERP trial (i.e., as a *maintenance* program) or incorporated into "booster sessions" for patients who begin to experience a return of symptoms at some later point after completing a course of ERP. In either instance, follow-up sessions should occur no more frequently than once per week (for 6 weeks) to allow ample time for the patient to practice between sessions. The follow-up program should incorporate the following components: 1) identifying high-risk situations and the relationship between OCD and stress; 2) practicing a lifestyle of confronting, rather than avoiding, obsessional stimuli; 3) preventing *lapses* from becoming *relapses*; 4) practicing evidence-based thinking; and 5) maintaining social support.

Special Populations

Mental Ritualizers

It was long thought that some individuals with OCD had obsessions without compulsive rituals ("pure obsessions"). Moreover, such patients were considered highly resistant to ERP (Baer 1994). More recently, however, clearer recognition of the frequency of mental rituals (often mistaken for obsessions because they are not visibly apparent behaviors) and covert neutralizing responses ("mini-rituals") has led to a reconceptualization of pure obsessions as "obsessions with covert rituals" (Abramowitz et al. 2003b; Clark and Guyitt 2008; Rachman 1993). This novel conceptualization has also led to the development of effective treatment for such patients. Specifically, Freeston et al. (1997) obtained excellent results with a treatment package that contains the following elements: 1) education about the cognitive and behavioral models of OCD; 2) ERP, consisting of in-session and homework exposure in which the patient repeatedly writes out the obsession, says it aloud, or records it on a continuous-loop audiotape and then plays it back repeatedly on a portable audiocassette player (Salkovskis and Westbrook 1989) while refraining from covert rituals and mental compulsions; and 3) CT, targeting exaggerated responsibility, inappropriate interpretations of intrusive thoughts, and inflated estimates of the probability and severity of negative outcomes. Compared with a wait-list control group, treated patients achieved substantial improvement: among all patients (n=28) Y-BOCS scores improved from 23.9 to 9.8 after an average of 25.7 sessions over 19.2 weeks. Moreover, patients retained their gains at 6-month follow-up (mean Y-BOCS score=10.8). This study demonstrated that ERP and CT can be successfully combined in the management of a presentation of OCD that had previously been considered resistant to psychological treatment.

Patients With Treatment-Refractory OCD

As mentioned earlier, patients with poor insight about their OCD symptoms improve less with ERP than those who have greater insight (Foa et al. 1999). Perhaps patients with poor insight have difficulty making changes as a result of exposure exercises. Alternatively, those with poor insight may be more reluctant to confront obsessional situations during therapy because of their fears. Although ERP is recommended even for patients with poor insight, those who struggle with this approach may benefit from the addition of cognitive techniques. A second augmentative approach in such cases is pharmacotherapy with selective serotonin reuptake inhibitors (SSRIs), and some psychiatrists will even prescribe antipsychotic medication for such patients.

As discussed in previous sections, some comorbid Axis I conditions can impede the effects of CBT for OCD. Major depressive disorder (Abramowitz and Foa 2000) and generalized anxiety disorder (Steketee et al. 2001) are particularly associated with poorer response to ERP. Perhaps seriously depressed patients become demoralized and experience difficulties in complying with CBT instructions. Strong negative affect may also exacerbate OCD symptoms and limit treatment gains. For generalized anxiety disorder patients, pervasive worry concerning other life issues is liable to detract from the time and emotional resources available for learning skills from ERP treatment (Steketee et al. 2001). Other Axis I conditions likely to interfere with ERP are those involving psychotic and manic symptoms that produce alterations in perception, cognition, and judgment. Active substance abuse or dependence also rules out the use of CBT. These problems presumably impede patients' ability to follow treatment instructions on their own or to attend to the cognitive changes that CBT aims to facilitate. It is therefore important for patients to receive treatment for these comorbid conditions before attempting ERP for OCD.

Practical Techniques

Cognitive and behavioral (i.e., ERP) treatments are time-limited, skills-based therapies in which the therapist takes a role akin to that of a coach or teacher, and the patient, that of a student. Treatment is typically provided on an individual basis and generally lasts from 12 to 20 sessions. Although each session has a more or less specific agenda, session time is generally spent helping the patient develop skills for reducing obsessions and compulsions. Homework practice is assigned for the patient to complete between sessions in order to gain mastery of these skills. As suggested in the previous literature review, treatment can take place on various schedules, including weekly or twice-weekly. A few specialty clinics offer treatment for OCD on an intensive basis, meaning 15 daily outpatient treatment sessions over a period of approximately 3 weeks. A practical advantage of the intensive approach over less intensive schedules is that massed sessions allow for regular therapist supervision, permitting rapid correction of subtle avoidance, rituals, or suboptimal exposure practice that might otherwise compromise outcome. As such, intensive therapy is recommended in cases of severe OCD and when the patient encounters extreme difficulty resisting compulsive urges. The primary disadvantage of intensive therapy is the obvious scheduling demands such a course entails, for both the clinician and the patient.

Group Cognitive-Behavioral Therapy

Group CBT programs that emphasize ERP and cognitive techniques have been found to be effective in reducing OCD symptoms (Anderson and Rees 2007; Cordioli et al. 2003; McLean et al. 2001). In one study, 12 weeks of group therapy emphasizing ERP was more effective than group therapy emphasizing CT techniques, although both programs were more effective than a wait-list control condition (McLean et al. 2001). In another investigation, group CBT resulted in significant improvement relative to results for the wait-list group, and patients continued to improve at 3-month follow-up (Cordioli et al. 2003). In the only study directly comparing individual and group CBT (involving CT and ERP techniques) for OCD, Anderson and Rees (2007) found that 10 weeks of either treatment was more effective than wait list but that there were no differences between group and individual treatment. Average posttest and follow-up Y-BOCS scores were in the 16–18 range (indicating mild symptom severity). Strengths of a group approach to the treatment of OCD include the support and cohesion that are nonspecific effects of group therapy. Potential disadvantages, however, include the relative lack of attention to each individual's particular symptom presentation, particularly given the heterogeneity of OCD.

Residential and Hospital-Based Treatment

Although most psychiatric hospitals are equipped to provide standard care for patients with OCD, programming in such facilities is often limited by the short duration of stay and lack of expertise in implementing ERP. Therefore, the initial focus in most hospitals is on stabilizing patients via medication and nonspecific psychotherapy (e.g., supportive counseling, stress management training). There are now, however, a handful of residential facilities in the United States that have specialized programs offering long-term inpatient treatment for severe OCD. These programs typically include individual and group ERP and cognitive interventions, medication management, and supportive therapy for comorbid psychiatric conditions. Length of stay may vary from a few weeks to a month or more. Two facilities that offer such services as of this writing are the Obsessive-Compulsive Disorders Institute at McLean Hospital (Belmont, Massachusetts) and the Obsessive-Compulsive Disorder Center at Rogers Memorial Hospital (Oconomowoc, Wisconsin).

One advantage of specialized residential OCD programs is that they provide constant supervision for patients requiring help with implementing treatment (i.e., conducting self-directed ERP). Moreover, such programs are ideal for individuals who lack family or friends to assist with treatment or have severe impairment in functioning, suicidal risk, or comorbid medical complications. A disadvantage, however, is that such programs are often costly. In addition, patients with obsessions and compulsions regarding specific places or stimuli (e.g., bathrooms at home) may have difficulty reproducing these feared situations within the hospital setting for the purposes of exposure. Thus, generalization of treatment effects must be considered. The only study to directly compare inpatient and outpatient ERP for OCD found that there were no differences in outcome between 20 sessions of outpatient and 5.4 months of inpatient treatment (van den Hout et al. 1988).

Conclusion

Few psychological disorders result in as much distress and functional impairment as OCD (Barlow 2002). In contrast to the lack of a definitive theory of the etiology of obsessions and compulsions, research has led to a very clear understanding of the processes that *maintain* these symptoms. ERP and CT, which are derived from this understanding, have received consistent empirical support, leading to a good prognosis for most sufferers. By far the most studied psychological intervention for OCD is ERP, which often produces substantial immediate and durable reductions in OCD symptoms. Evidence from effectiveness studies suggests that ERP is transportable to nonresearch settings and therefore should be a first-line treatment modality for OCD patients in general clinical settings (March et al. 1997). Moreover, ERP is quite helpful in further alleviating OCD symptoms that do not respond satisfactorily to pharmacotherapy. Even though these results are encouraging, full remission with psychological treatment is not the standard (Abramowitz 1998); response is, in fact, highly variable. We are beginning to uncover factors that reliably predict poor response to ERP, including severe depression and lack of insight into the senselessness of obsessional fears.

As we stand at the beginning of a new century, it is heartening to look back at how far we have come with respect to the psychological treatment of OCD. We can also look forward with hope that researchers will address a number of critical issues that require further study. For example, patient motivation to begin treatment, especially given the anxiety-provoking nature of ERP, is a problem. Readiness programs, in which patients read case histories or discuss treatment with former patients, might decrease refusal rates and increase treatment compliance. From the clinician's perspective, engineering and executing successful exposure-based therapy can often be a challenge. Indeed, the greatest barrier to successful treatment of OCD is that relatively few clinicians receive the kind of training needed to become proficient in these procedures. Therefore, research and development of programs for teaching service providers how to implement psychological treatments for OCD will have a major impact on improving access to these effective interventions.

◀ Key Clinical Points ▶

- Exposure and response prevention was derived as a treatment for obsessive-compulsive disorder from early laboratory research (with animals and humans) on the essential psychopathology of this disorder.
- ERP is the most effective treatment for OCD, as demonstrated in controlled comparisons with other forms of psychological treatment as well as with selective serotonin reuptake inhibitors.
- Whereas adding SSRIs does not enhance the efficacy of ERP, the effects of SSRIs can be augmented by adding ERP.
- ERP is also known to be effective in nonresearch clinical settings.
- Severe comorbid depression, generalized anxiety disorder, and poor insight into the senselessness of the obsessions and compulsions of OCD are predictors of poor outcome with ERP.
- Cognitive therapy is an efficacious treatment for OCD, but it is not as effective as ERP.

References

Abramowitz JS: Variants of exposure and response prevention in the treatment of obsessive-compulsive disorder: a meta-analysis. Behav Ther 27:583–600, 1996

Abramowitz JS: Does cognitive-behavioral therapy cure obsessive-compulsive disorder? A meta-analytic evaluation of clinical significance. Behav Ther 29:339–355, 1998

Abramowitz JS: Effectiveness of psychological and pharmacological treatments for obsessive-compulsive disorder: a quantitative review. J Consult Clin Psychol 65:44–52, 1997

Abramowitz JS: Understanding and Treating Obsessive-Compulsive Disorder: A Cognitive-Behavioral Approach. Mahwah, NJ, Lawrence Erlbaum, 2006

Abramowitz JS, Foa EB: Does comorbid major depressive disorder influence outcome of exposure and response prevention for OCD? Behav Ther 31:795–800, 2000

Abramowitz JS, Franklin ME, Street GP, et al: Effects of comorbid depression on response to treatment for obsessive-compulsive disorder. Behav Ther 31:517–528, 2000

Abramowitz JS, Franklin ME, Foa EB: Empirical status of cognitive-behavioral therapy for obsessive-compulsive disorder: a meta-analytic review. Romanian Journal of Cognitive and Behavioral Psychotherapy 2:89–104, 2002a

Abramowitz JS, Franklin ME, Zoellner LA, et al: Treatment compliance and outcome in obsessive-compulsive disorder. Behav Modif 26:447–463, 2002b

Abramowitz JS, Foa EB, Franklin ME: Exposure and ritual prevention for obsessive-compulsive disorder: effects of intensive versus twice-weekly sessions. J Consult Clin Psychol 71:394–398, 2003a

Abramowitz JS, Franklin ME, Schwartz S, et al: Symptom presentation and outcome of cognitive-behavioral therapy for obsessive-compulsive disorder. J Consult Clin Psychol 71:1049–1057, 2003b

Anderson RA, Rees CS: Group versus individual cognitive-behavioral treatment for obsessive-compulsive disorder: a controlled trial. Behav Res Ther 45:123–137, 2007

Baer L: Factor analysis of symptom subtypes of obsessive compulsive disorder and their relation to personality and tic disorders. J Clin Psychiatry 55:18–23, 1994

Barlow DH: Anxiety and Its Disorders. New York, Guilford, 2002

Beck AT, Emery G: Anxiety Disorders and Phobias: A Cognitive Perspective. New York, Basic Books, 1985

Chambless DL, Steketee G: Expressed emotion and behavior therapy outcome: a prospective study with obsessive-compulsive and agoraphobic outpatients. J Consult Clin Psychol 67:658–665, 1999

Clark DA: Cognitive-Behavioral Therapy for OCD. New York, Guilford, 2004

Clark DA, Guyitt B: Pure obsessions: conceptual misnomer or clinical anomaly? in Obsessive Compulsive Disorder: Subtypes and Spectrum Conditions. Edited by Abramowitz JS, McKay D, Taylor S. Amsterdam, The Netherlands, Elsevier, 2008, pp 53–75

Cordioloi A, Heldt A, Bochi D, et al: Cognitive-behavioral group therapy in obsessive-compulsive disorder: a randomized clinical trial. Psychother Psychosom 72:211–217, 2003

Cottraux J, Mollard E, Bouvard M, et al: A controlled study of fluvoxamine and exposure in obsessive-compulsive disorder. Int J Clin Psychopharmacol 5:17–30, 1990

Deacon BJ: The effect of pharmacotherapy on the effect of exposure therapy, in Handbook of Exposure Therapies. Edited by Richard D, Lauterbach D. Amsterdam, The Netherlands, Elsevier, 2006, pp 311–333

Emmelkamp PMG, de Haan E, Hoogduin CAL: Marital adjustment and obsessive-compulsive disorder. Br J Psychiatry 156:55–60, 1990

Fals-Stewart W, Marks AP, Schafer J: A comparison of behavioral group therapy and individual behavior therapy in treating obsessive-compulsive disorder. J Nerv Ment Dis 181:189–193, 1993

Foa EB: Failure in treating obsessive-compulsives. Behav Res Ther 17:169–176, 1979

Foa EB, Kozak MJ: Emotional processing of fear: exposure to corrective information. Psychol Bull 99:20–35, 1986

Foa EB, Kozak MJ: Psychological treatment for obsessive-compulsive disorder, in Long-Term Treatments of Anxiety Disorders. Edited by Mavissakalian MR, Prien RF. Washington, DC, American Psychiatric Press, 1996, pp 285–309

Foa EB, Grayson JB, Steketee GS, et al: Success and failure in the behavioral treatment of obsessive-compulsives. J Consult Clin Psychol 51:287–297, 1983

Foa EB, Kozak MJ, Goodman WK, et al: DSM-IV field trial: obsessive-compulsive disorder. Am J Psychiatry 152:90–96, 1995

Foa EB, Abramowitz JS, Franklin ME, et al: Feared consequences, fixity of belief, and treatment outcome in patients with obsessive-compulsive disorder. Behav Ther 30:717–724, 1999

Foa EB, Liebowitz MR, Kozak MJ, et al: Treatment of obsessive-compulsive disorder by exposure and ritual prevention, clomipramine, and their combination: a randomized, placebo controlled trial. Am J Psychiatry 162:151–161, 2005

Franklin ME, Abramowitz JS, Kozak MJ, et al: Effectiveness of exposure and ritual prevention for obsessive-compulsive disorder: randomized compared with nonrandomized samples. J Consult Clin Psychol 68:594–602, 2000

Freeston MH, Ladouceur R, Gagnon F, et al: Cognitive-behavioral treatment of obsessive thoughts: a controlled study. J Consult Clin Psychol 65:405–413, 1997

Freud S: Notes upon a case of obsessional neurosis (1909), in Three Case Histories. Edited by Rieff P. New York, Collier Books, 1963, pp 1–82

Friedman S, Smith LC, Halpern B, et al: Obsessive-compulsive disorder in a multi-ethnic urban outpatient clinic: initial presentation and treatment outcome with exposure and ritual prevention. Behav Ther 34:397–410, 2003

Goodman WK, Price LH, Rasmussen SA, et al: The Yale-Brown Obsessive Compulsive Scale, I: development, use, and reliability. Arch Gen Psychiatry 46:1006–1011, 1989a

Goodman WK, Price LH, Rasmussen SA, et al: The Yale-Brown Obsessive Compulsive Scale, II: validity. Arch Gen Psychiatry 46:1012–1016, 1989b

Greist J, Jefferson J, Kobak K, et al: Efficacy and tolerability of serotonin transporter inhibitors in obsessive-compulsive disorder. Arch Gen Psychiatry 52:53–60, 1995

Hafner RJ: Marital interaction in persisting obsessive-compulsive disorders. Aust N Z J Psychiatry 16:171–178, 1982

Hiss H, Foa EB, Kozak MJ: Relapse prevention program for treatment of obsessive-compulsive disorder. J Consult Clin Psychol 62:801–808, 1994

Hohagen F, Winkelmann G, Rasche-Rauchle H, et al: Combination of behaviour therapy with fluvoxamine in comparison with behaviour therapy and placebo. Br J Psychiatry 173:71–78, 1998

Kampman M, Keijsers GPJ, Hoogduin CAL, et al: Addition of cognitive-behavior therapy for obsessive-compulsive disorder patients non-responding to fluoxetine. Acta Psychiatr Scand 106:314–319, 2002

Lindsay M, Crino R, Andrews G: Controlled trial of exposure and response prevention in obsessive-compulsive disorder. Br J Psychiatry 171:135–139, 1997

March JS, Frances A, Carpenter D, et al: The Expert Consensus Guidelines Series: Treatment of Obsessive-Compulsive Disorder. J Clin Psychiatry 58(suppl), 1997

Mataix-Cols D, Marks IM, Greist JH, et al: Obsessive-compulsive symptom dimensions as predictors of compliance with and response to behaviour therapy: results from a controlled trial. Psychother Psychosom 71:255–262, 2002

Meyer V: Modification of expectations in cases with obsessional rituals. Behav Res Ther 4:273–280, 1966

Meyer V, Levy R, Schnurer A: The behavioral treatment of obsessive-compulsive disorders, in Obsessional States.

Edited by Beech H. London, Methuen, 1974, pp 233–258

McLean PD, Whittal ML, Thordarson DS, et al: Cognitive versus behavior therapy in the group treatment of obsessive-compulsive disorder. J Consult Clin Psychol 69:205–214, 2001

Montgomery SA, McIntyre A, Ostenheider M, et al: A double-blind placebo-controlled study of fluoxetine in patients with DSM-III-R obsessive-compulsive disorder. Eur Neuropsychopharmacol 3:142–152, 1993

Nakatani E, Nakagawa A, Nakao T, et al: A randomized trial of Japanese patients with obsessive-compulsive disorder: effectiveness of behavior therapy and fluvoxamine. Psychother Psychosom 74:269–276, 2005

O'Connor K, Todorov C, Robillard S, et al: Cognitive-behaviour therapy and medication in the treatment of obsessive-compulsive disorder: a controlled study. Can J Psychiatry 44:64–71, 1999

O'Sullivan G, Noshirvani H, Marks I, et al: Six-year follow-up after exposure and clomipramine therapy for obsessive compulsive disorder. J Clin Psychiatry 52:150–155, 1991

Rachman S: Obsessions, responsibility and guilt. Behav Res Ther 31:149–154, 1993

Rachman S, de Silva P: Abnormal and normal obsessions. Behav Res Ther 16:233–248, 1978

Rachman S, Hodgson R: Obsessions and Compulsions. Englewood Cliffs, NJ, Prentice Hall, 1980

Riggs DS, Hiss H, Foa EB: Marital distress and the treatment of obsessive compulsive disorder. Behav Ther 23:585–597, 1992

Rothbaum BO, Shahar F: Behavioral treatment of obsessive-compulsive disorder in a naturalistic setting. Cogn Behav Pract 7:262–270, 2000

Salkovskis PM: Cognitive-behavioral approaches to the understanding of obsessional problems, in Current Controversies in the Anxiety Disorders. Edited by Rapee R. New York, Guilford, 1996, pp 103–133

Salkovskis PM, Westbrook D: Behaviour therapy and obsessional ruminations: can failure be turned into success? Behav Res Ther 27:149–160, 1989

Simpson HB, Gorfinkle KS, Liebowitz MR: Cognitive-behavioral therapy as an adjunct to serotonin reuptake inhibitors in obsessive-compulsive disorder: an open trial. J Clin Psychiatry 60:584–590, 1999

Solomon RL, Kamin LJ, Wynne LC: Traumatic avoidance learning: the outcomes of several extinction procedures with dogs. J Abnorm Soc Psychol 48:291–302, 1953

Steketee GS, Chambless DL, Tran GQ: Effects of Axis I and II comorbidity on behavior therapy outcome for obsessive-compulsive disorder and agoraphobia. Compr Psychiatry 42:76–86, 2001

Taylor S: Assessment of obsessions and compulsions: reliability, validity, and sensitivity to treatment effects. Clin Psychol Rev 15:261–296, 1995

Tenneij NH, Van Megen HJ, Denys DA, et al: Behavior therapy augments response of patients with obsessive-compulsive disorder responding to drug treatment. J Clin Psychiatry 66:1169–1175, 2005

Tolin DF, Maltby N, Diefenbach GJ, et al: Cognitive-behavioral therapy for medication nonresponders with obsessive-compulsive disorder: a wait-list-controlled open trial. J Clin Psychiatry 65:922–931, 2004

Van Balkom AJ, de Haan E, Van Oppen P, et al: Cognitive and behavioral therapies alone versus in combination with fluvoxamine in the treatment of obsessive compulsive disorder. J Nerv Ment Dis 186:492–499, 1998

van den Hout M, Emmelkamp P, Kraaykamp H, et al: Behavioral treatment of obsessive-compulsives: inpatient vs outpatient. Behav Res Ther 26:331–332, 1988

Warren R, Thomas JC: Cognitive-behavior therapy of obsessive-compulsive disorder in private practice: an effectiveness study. J Anxiety Disord 15:277–285, 2001

Wilhelm S, Steketee G: Cognitive Therapy for Obsessive-Compulsive Disorder: A Guide for Practitioners. Oakland, CA, New Harbinger, 2006

Recommended Readings

Abramowitz JS: Obsessive-Compulsive Disorder: Advances in Psychotherapy—Evidence Based Practice. Cambridge, MA, Hogrefe and Huber, 2006

Abramowitz JS: Understanding and Treating Obsessive-Compulsive Disorder: A Cognitive-Behavioral Approach. Mahwah, NJ, Lawrence Erlbaum, 2006

Abramowitz JS, Taylor S, McKay D (eds): Clinical Handbook of Obsessive-Compulsive Disorder and Related Problems. Baltimore, MD, Johns Hopkins University Press, 2008

Antony MM, Purdon C, Summerfeldt L (eds): Psychological Treatment of Obsessive-Compulsive Disorder: Fundamentals and Beyond. Washington, DC, American Psychological Association Press, 2008

Kozak MJ, Foa EB: Mastery of Obsessive Compulsive Disorder: Therapist's Guide. San Antonio, TX, Psychological Corporation, 1997

Wilhelm S, Steketee G: Cognitive Therapy for Obsessive-Compulsive Disorder: A Practitioner's Guide. Oakland, CA, New Harbinger, 2006

Web Sites of Interest

Anxiety Disorders Association of America. http://www.adaa.org.

Association for Behavioral and Cognitive Therapies. http://www.abct.org.

Obsessive Compulsive Foundation. http://www.ocfoundation.org.

Chapter 20

The Obsessive-Compulsive Spectrum of Disorders

Sarah Ketay, Ph.D.
Dan J. Stein, M.D., Ph.D.
Eric Hollander, M.D.

The idea that obsessive-compulsive disorder (OCD) might share underlying pathogenic mechanisms with a range of other conditions (e.g., obsessive-compulsive personality, psychosis) has early roots, for example, in psychodynamic theory. The recognition that not only people with OCD but also individuals with a range of other disorders characterized by unwanted repetitive symptoms (e.g., trichotillomania, body dysmorphic disorder) respond selectively to serotonin reuptake inhibitors gave impetus to the modern concept of a psychobiologically based obsessive-compulsive (OC) spectrum of disorders. Although various descriptions of such a spectrum have been put forward, even a conservative definition would mean that OC spectrum disorders are highly prevalent. In this chapter, we outline different approaches to the concept of OC spectrum disorders and summarize current knowledge on psychobiology and management.

Disorders are posited to belong in the OC spectrum based on their similarities to OCD in various domains (Hollander 1993; Stein and Hollander 1993). However, there is no clear consensus about which disorders should be considered members of the OC spectrum. Some disorders have a great deal in common with OCD, whereas others may fall at the opposite end of a compulsive-impulsive spectrum of conditions (Hollander et al. 2008). There are shared and distinct neural correlates of OCD, and some neural correlates are shared with other related disorders in the OC spectrum (Mataix-Cols and van den Heuvel 2006). Furthermore, it is unlikely that OC spectrum disorders fall on a single dimension. For example, on the basis of a cluster analysis, Lochner and Stein (2006) suggested three clusters of OC spectrum disorders, namely those characterized by *reward deficiency* (e.g., pathological gambling), *impulsivity* (e.g., intermittent explosive disorder), and *somatic symptoms* (e.g., body dysmorphic disorder).

In this chapter we begin by emphasizing the close phenomenological and psychobiological relationships between OCD and Tourette syndrome (TS). We then discuss somatoform disorders putatively related to OCD, namely, body dysmorphic disorder (BDD) and hypochondriasis (HYP). Although trichotillomania (TTM) is currently classified as an impulse control disorder, there is evidence that hair-pulling and other body-focused repetitive behaviors may lie on an OC spectrum of disorders. Finally, we describe the concept of a compulsive-impulsive spectrum of disorders.

Tourette Syndrome, Neurological Conditions, and a Psychobiological Basis for the Obsessive-Compulsive Spectrum

Tourette syndrome is characterized by motor and vocal tics. TS differs from OCD in that tics are involuntary, whereas in OCD, compulsions are goal-directed. On the other hand, this kind of differentiation is not always easy to make, given that tics arise in response to sensory urges and are under partial control, and complex tics can appear as goal-directed as compulsions. Current nosology indicates that a tic-like compulsion, such as touching someone with one hand after touching them with the other, can be conceptualized as a complex motor tic but may also be conceptualized as a compulsion without an obsession (Shavitt et al. 2006). Furthermore, tics are common in OCD, and OCD is often found in patients with TS (Hebebrand et al. 1997). One group examined patients with comorbid OCD and TS and found that those patients had significantly more violent sexual and symmetrical obsessions and more touching, blinking, counting, and self-damaging compulsions than patients with either OCD or TS without comorbidity (George et al. 1993).

It seems clear from the results of family and twin studies that OCD and TS are genetically related (Shavitt et al. 2006). First-degree relatives of TS probands have higher frequencies of OC symptoms, OCD, and TS than seen in relatives of control subjects (Pauls and Leckman 1986). Conversely, there is a higher prevalence of tics and TS in the family members of probands with OCD than would be expected by chance. Early segregation analyses of family data indicated an autosomal dominant transmission in TS (Pauls et al. 1986). More recent studies suggest that the mode of inheritance is more complex (Keen-Kim and Freimer 2006). Some findings suggest that there are genes of major effect, with other genes acting as modifiers (Pauls 2001). Ongoing investigation of candidate genes is taking place (Keen-Kim and Freimer 2006). Numerous rare genetic variants have been found to be associated with penetrant familial subtypes, and on occasion, these may also be associated with OCD and other OC spectrum disorders (Abelson et al. 2005; Wendland et al. 2006; Zuchner et al. 2006).

TS and OCD may also share underlying neuronal circuitry. Neurological case reports have long suggested that striatal circuits are important in OCD (Cheyette and Cummings 1995). One voxel-level meta-analysis of functional magnetic resonance imaging (fMRI) findings on OCD (Menzies et al. 2008) revealed consistent abnormalities in orbitofrontal-striatal and other brain areas in this disorder.

Similarly, TS appears to be mediated by these circuits (Saka and Graybiel 2003). Using magnetic resonance imaging (MRI), Amat et al. (2006), for example, found a higher frequency of cerebral hyperintensities in the subcortex, primarily the basal ganglia and thalamus, in children and adolescents with TS, OCD, and attention-deficit/hyperactivity disorder (ADHD) compared with psychiatrically healthy control subjects. Using HMPAO single-photon emission tomographic imaging, one study demonstrated similar regional cerebral blood flow patterns in individuals with TS and their relatives who did not have TS but did exhibit OC behaviors (Moriarty et al. 1997). This study suggests that brain imaging results are comparable in individuals from families with TS even when phenotypes are different. A review concluded that there is evidence that both TS and OCD involve abnormalities in corticostriatothalamocortical pathways (Shavitt et al. 2006).

Pharmacological treatments of TS and OCD share some overlapping features. Selective serotonin reuptake inhibitors (SSRIs) are the first-line pharmacotherapy for OCD and are more effective than placebo in reducing symptoms of OCD (Soomro et al. 2008). Dopamine blockers are used as augmenting agents in patients with treatment-refractory OCD. In TS, on the other hand, dopamine blockers are useful for tics, but SSRIs may be useful for the treatment of comorbid OCD.

In summary, although OCD and TS seem to be clearly different disorders with divergent phenomenology, a good deal of work has emphasized similarities in underlying psychobiology. There are many advantages in reminding clinicians of this relationship. OCD patients should be screened for tics, and TS patients should be screened for OCD. However, the relationship between TS and OCD is not an exclusive one; for example, TS also has a close relationship with ADHD.

Body Dysmorphic Disorder and Hypochondriasis

Body dysmorphic disorder is a somatoform disorder that is characterized by preoccupation with imagined ugliness. There are similarities between OCD and BDD in symptomatology, psychobiology, and treatment.

BDD shares several clinical similarities with OCD. Preoccupations experienced by BDD patients are often described as obsessional, persistent, intrusive thoughts that are distressing and difficult to resist and control (Eisen et al. 2004). Patients with BDD may report repetitive behaviors such as mirror-checking or camouflaging, requests for reassurance, and skin-picking (Frare et al. 2004; Hollander and Phillips 1993; Phillips 1996), which resemble OCD compulsions. On the other hand, an important difference between the preoccupations experienced in BDD and those experienced in OCD is the focus of concern. In BDD, the concern is appearance and imagined ugliness, such as a large nose or ugly skin. In OCD, there may be a broad range of different preoccupations, only some of which are somatic in nature.

Clinical similarities between BDD and OCD include comparable prevalence in both sexes, onset during adolescence, and chronic course (Phillips 1991). In addition, BDD and OCD often appear to be comorbid with one another. Phillips et al. (2007) specifically compared the clinical features of patients with OCD, with BDD, and with comorbid BDD/OCD. When comparing clinical features for OCD and BDD, the two disorders did not significantly differ in terms of demographic features, age at onset, illness duration, most measures of functioning, and most comorbid illnesses. Several clinically important differences between OCD and BDD have also been noted (Phillips et al. 2007). Specifically, subjects with BDD were more likely to be delusional than those with OCD and were also more likely to have lifetime suicidal ideation, lifetime major depressive disorder, and lifetime substance use disorder. Poor insight has been positively correlated with more severe symptoms in BDD, but not necessarily in OCD (Eisen et al. 2004). In sum, it can be argued that despite showing some differences between BDD and OCD, comparative work has revealed a number of similarities.

The psychobiology of BDD has begun to be investigated, although relatively few neuroimaging studies have been conducted in this area. A number of studies indicate a role for frontostriatal and temporal-parietal regions in the neurobiology of BDD (Carey et al. 2004; Gabbay et al. 2003; Rauch et al. 2003). As discussed earlier, frontostriatal dysfunction has also been posited to play a role in OCD (Menzies et al. 2008; Tallis 1997; van den Heuvel et al. 2005).

In a review, Castle et al. (2006) noted there have been few cognitive investigations of patients with BDD. The authors were aware of only nine published studies investigating cognitive functioning in patients with BDD, with results indicating a range of cognitive deficits, including impairment in executive function, memory, facial emotion perception, and attributional bias. Cognitive deficits in executive function and memory have also been suggested in OCD patients (Olley et al. 2007). The authors conducted a systematic review of the neuropsychological literature in OCD and found that patients with OCD exhibited problems in organizational strategies during encoding in various neuropsychological tasks (Olley et al. 2007). Hanes (1998) assessed the neuropsychological functioning of patients with BDD compared to that of patients with OCD and schizophrenia. Results showed normal performance for BDD patients for mnestic and motor function but found a deficit in tests of executive functions. This deficit is consistent with frontal system involvement in BDD. The BDD and OCD groups performed similarly on neuropsychological measures, whereas subjects with schizophrenia had wider deficits in this area.

Further evidence for a link between OCD and BDD is their similarities in treatment response. First-line treatments of BDD are the SSRIs, and these medicines are effective irrespective of the patient's degree of insight (Hadley et al. 2002; Phillips et al. 2006). There is some evidence that, as in the case of OCD, BDD patients may require higher doses and longer treatments (Grant and Phillips 2005). There is a superior response to clomipramine over desipramine in both BDD (Hollander et al. 1999) and OCD. In addition, cognitive-behavioral therapy, using principles of exposure and response prevention (Veale et al. 1996), is effective for both OCD and BDD (Foa and Kozak 1996; Freeston et al. 1997; Rosen et al. 1995).

Hypochondriasis is characterized by preoccupation with a fear of having, or the idea that one has, a serious disease. Like OCD, HYP is characterized by intrusive anxiety-provoking thoughts and repetitive behaviors to allay this anxiety. Patients with HYP are also likely to receive a lifetime diagnosis of OCD. However, the prevalence of HYP in OCD is unknown, and data are too limited to make a definitive link between the two conditions (Barsky 1992). HYP differs from OCD insofar as the patient's disease concerns may not be experienced as an intrusive mental event (Barsky 1992). If the ideation is not resisted, there is often medical help-seeking.

If HYP is related to OCD, one might expect to see a similar neurobiology in terms of imaging and challenge studies. Unfortunately, only limited studies on the neurobiology of HYP and few comparative studies have been performed to date. There is robust evidence that OCD has a strong familial link, but the same has not been shown in HYP (Fallon et al. 2000). Noyes et al. (1997) performed a family study and found that the frequency of HYP and OCD was not increased among first-degree relatives of patients with HYP. More definitive studies with larger samples and more complete assessments of the psychopathology among first-degree relatives of individuals with HYP are necessary before definitive conclusions can be reached.

Again, there is some overlap in the pharmacotherapy and psychotherapy of HYP and OCD. A small database of open-label trials has suggested efficacy of SSRIs in patients with HYP (Fallon et al. 1996; Greeven et al. 2007). In addition to SSRI treatment, cognitive-behavioral therapy and techniques, including exposure and response prevention, may be effective in the treatment of HYP (Visser and Bouman 2001).

In summary, there are clear overlaps in the phenomenology of OCD, BDD, and HYP. There are relatively few studies of the psychobiology of these conditions, and family studies have not suggested a particularly close link. Nevertheless, important similarities in treatment approach to OCD, BDD, and HYP support the value of including these conditions on the OC spectrum.

Body-Focused Repetitive Behaviors

Trichotillomania is classified in DSM-IV as an impulse-control disorder. TTM is characterized by the repeated urge to pull out hair. Patients pull out scalp hair, eyelashes, facial hair, nose hair, pubic hair, eyebrows, or other body hair, resulting in noticeable bald patches (Stein et al. 1999).

The urge to hair-pull resembles a compulsion similar to that experienced in OCD in that, according to the DSM-IV definition, the individual experiences an increasing level of tension that occurs immediately before hair-pulling or during attempts to avoid pulling. The patient feels a sensation of relief, pleasure, or gratification during hair-pulling. However, TTM and OCD differ in that there are no preceding obsessions in hair-pulling.

Lochner et al. (2005) specifically compared OCD with TTM. Important differences were found between the two disorders, with OCD patients reporting significantly more lifetime disability than TTM patients, as well as higher comorbidity, more maladaptive beliefs, more sexual abuse, more harm avoidance, and less novelty seeking. However, fewer TTM patients responded to treatment.

A small number of studies in which the neurobiology of TTM was researched yielded results indicating a potential neurostructural and neurofunctional deficit in patients with TTM (Woods et al. 2006). As with OCD, there is some evidence of basal ganglia involvement in TTM. Stein et al. (2002) demonstrated that TTM patients who experience more severe hair-pulling have a greater decrease in activity in the frontal and parietal regions and left caudate. Consistent with similarities in underlying neurocircuitry, there may be some overlapping neuropsychological deficits that occur in both OCD and TTM (Bohne et al. 2005).

In contrast to OCD, there may be cerebellar involvement in TTM. Keuthen et al. (2007) used MRI to examine the cerebellum volumes of patients with TTM compared with psychiatrically healthy control subjects. The cerebellum has been thought of as the neuroanatomic locus of control for complex, coordinated motor sequences. The investigators found significantly reduced cerebellar volumes in patients with TTM. Bohne et al. (2005) compared cognitive inhibition in TTM and OCD. Results indicated that deficits in cognitive inhibition seemed to be specific to OCD. Together, results of these studies suggest an underlying neurobiological cause of TTM that shares some similarities with OCD but also indicates that a separate system may be involved with TTM.

A genetic basis for TTM has been suggested, although a specific gene has not been identified (Lenane et al. 1992; Stemberger et al. 2000). Hemmings et al. (2006) report data supporting the hypothesis that 5-HT_{2A} plays a role in mediating impulse control problems in TTM. It is possible that mutations in *SLITRK1* may on occasion play a role in the genetics of TTM (Zuchner et al. 2006). A range of other genes also deserve exploration; for example, the gene *HOXB8* has been found to be necessary for normal grooming behavior in mice, and mice with disruptions in *HOXB8* display excessive grooming that leads to lesions (Greer and Capecchi 2002).

Relatively few controlled pharmacotherapy or psychotherapy treatment studies of TTM have been performed (Woods et al. 2006). In a systematic review (Bloch et al. 2007), three main treatment modalities for TTM were examined, including pharmacotherapy with an SSRI; pharmacotherapy with clomipramine, a tricyclic antidepressant; and habit-reversal therapy. In contrast to OCD, which often responds to SSRIs, SSRIs were not shown to be more efficacious than placebo in the treatment of TTM. Clomipramine, however, was found to be more successful than placebo in reducing symptoms in TTM. Habit-reversal therapy reduced the severity of hair-pulling and associated impairment more than both clomipramine and placebo.

Despite the conclusions of this meta-analysis, it is possible that some patients with TTM respond to SSRIs. In addition, as in the case of patients with OCD, some may respond to dopamine D_2 receptor blockers. Some outcome studies have demonstrated a positive response to SSRIs and D_2 blockers in TTM, which has led to the hypothesis that dysregulation of the serotonin and dopamine systems is functionally related to the severity of hair-pulling (Stein and Hollander 1992; Swedo et al. 1989).

Others have hypothesized that endogenous opiate activity is implicated in TTM (Christenson et al. 1994a) because of the efficacy of naltrexone (an opiate antagonist) in reducing hair-pulling. One possible prediction of the opioid hypothesis is that patients with TTM are characterized by a decrease in pain sensitivity. However, these results have not been supported (Christenson et al. 1994b; Frecska and Arato 2002).

Skin-picking, a body-focused repetitive behavior, has also been included in the OC spectrum (Bartz and Hollander 2006). Body-focused behaviors other than hair-pulling may currently be diagnosed according to DSM-IV as a stereotypic movement disorder. Nevertheless, TTM and skin-picking share similar phenomenology, in that they both feature repetitive, self-injurious, stereotypic behaviors. Indeed, TTM and pathological skin-picking were found to have similar demographic features, psychiatric comorbidity rates, and personality dimensions (Lochner et al. 2005). It is also notable that the most common impulse control disorder in OCD is skin-picking (Grant et al. 2006b) and that a range of other body-focused behaviors, such as nose-picking and lip-chewing, are common in TTM (Christenson and Crow 1996).

In summary, there are important similarities as well as differences in the phenomenology of OCD, TTM, and body-focused repetitive behaviors. Studies of underlying psychobiology suggest that there may be some overlap in underlying mechanisms, with possible involvement in striatal circuitry. Although clomipramine has been found to be effective in treating TTM, several studies investigating pharmacotherapy with SSRIs have been disappointing. Habit-reversal therapy employs somewhat different principles from those used in the psychotherapy of OCD. Nevertheless, there may be some heuristic value in suggesting that body-focused repetitive behaviors lie on an obsessive-compulsive spectrum, in order to encourage their diagnosis and treatment.

The Compulsive-Impulsive Spectrum

Impulsive disorders such as pathological gambling and sexual disorders (i.e., obsessions, compulsions, and paraphilias) have been posited to lie on the impulsive end of a compulsive-impulsive spectrum of disorders (Bartz and Hollander 2006; Phillips 2002). Although these disorders are characterized as impulsive, there may be a compulsive element to them in that they function to reduce anxiety and are characterized by repetitive thoughts and behaviors (Hollander and Wong 1995). The concept of "behavioral addiction" may also be useful for describing these conditions. However, there are also important differences in the phenomenology of such disorders and that of OCD.

There may be some overlaps in the neurobiology of OCD and behavioral addictions insofar as both are characterized by dopaminergic dysfunction in frontostriatal circuits and impaired behavioral inhibition (Hollander et al. 2007). Nevertheless, results from studies of the neural underpinnings of behavioral addictions such as pathological gambling suggest differences from findings in OCD (Grant et al. 2006a). One fMRI study of males with pathological gambling, for example, found relatively decreased activation within cortical, basal ganglionic, and thalamic brain regions in subjects with pathological gambling addiction compared with psychiatrically healthy control subjects (Potenza et al. 2003). Thus, there may be increased frontal activity in OCD (Menzies et al. 2008) but decreased frontal activity in impulsivity (Berlin et al. 2005; Torregrossa et al. 2008).

Treatment of behavioral addictions also differs from that used for OCD. For example, data on the efficacy of SSRIs in the treatment of pathological gambling are inconclusive (Grant et al. 2003a). Some studies show a significant advantage of SSRIs over placebo; others do not (Blanco et al. 2002; Grant et al. 2003b; Kim et al. 2002). Some evidence shows that individuals with pathological gambling respond to opioid antagonists (Grant et al. 2006c; Kim et al. 2001), agents that have not been effective in treating OCD. Cognitive therapy has been found to be effective in treating pathological gambling (Hodgins and Petry 2004). Nevertheless, the specific focus of the cognitive therapy differs from the exposure and response prevention treatment used for OCD (Simpson and Fallon 2000). During the treatment of pathological gambling, for example, cognitive therapy aims to show that ritualistic behavior does not control the outcome of gambling (Ladouceur et al. 2001; Sylvain et al. 1997).

Relatively few studies have been conducted of the phenomenology, psychobiology, and pharmacotherapy of a range of other putative behavioral addictions such as excessive exercise, Internet addiction, and sexual addictions. However, from a phenomenological perspective, these differ from OCD in a number of ways, and it seems likely that there will also be important differences in psychobiology and management.

In summary, although behavioral addictions such as pathological gambling and Internet, sexual, and exercise addictions may share some phenomenological and psychobiological features with OCD, there are marked dissimilarities across these constructs.

Conditions Related to the Obsessive-Compulsive Spectrum

Several other conditions have also been considered as potentially belonging in the OCD spectrum, including autism and eating disorders. There are clearly important differences between OCD and these conditions. At the same time, exploration of the relationships between these disorders and OCD has led to some interesting findings. For instance, patients with autistic disorder have shown some symptomatic response to SSRIs (Kolevzon et al. 2006). In particular, a reduction was seen in social and communication deficits (Kolevzon et al. 2006). There may also be a genetic component to the obsessive-compulsive symptoms in autism. Thus, first-degree family members of autistic patients have high rates of OCD and may have subtle social deficits and language problems (Hollander et al. 2003).

Eating disorders are often comorbid with OCD and share some similar phenomenology (Phillips and Kaye 2007). Some studies have suggested that many individuals with anorexia nervosa and bulimia nervosa exhibit childhood perfectionism and obsessive-compulsive personality patterns, and these symptoms predate the onset of the eating disorder (Anderluh et al. 2003). Nevertheless, eating disorders differ from OCD in psychobiology and treatment. Studies on the effectiveness of SSRIs in eating disorders, for example, have yielded mixed results (Mayer and Walsh 1998; Vaswani et al. 2003).

Several other conditions may be related to OCD on the basis of phenomenology, psychobiology, or treatment response. In addition to TS, other neurologic conditions with compulsive symptoms and basal ganglia dysfunction include Sydenham's chorea and pediatric autoimmune neuropsychiatric disorders associated with streptococcal infection (PANDAS) (Swedo et al. 2001). Further exploration of the psychobiology and treatment of these conditions may ultimately lead to new ways of approaching the management of OCD.

Conclusion

Recent advances, particularly in neurogenetics and brain imaging, have contributed to our understanding of OCD, and thus to our understanding of putative OCD spectrum disorders. Nevertheless, data from psychobiological studies comparing OCD with putative spectrum disorders have yielded mixed findings. The concept of an OC spectrum disorder may be clinically valuable insofar as it encourages appropriate diagnosis and treatment of a number of disorders that are often overlooked. On the other hand, it is important to be aware of significant differences in putative OC spectrum disorders and to avoid being overly inclusive. Additional studies are needed to delineate the psychobiology of OCD and putative OCD spectrum disorders and to determine the optimal response of these conditions to treatment.

◀ Key Clinical Points ▶

- There is controversy about the extent to which different disorders are related to OCD, but certain obsessive-compulsive spectrum disorders have clear overlaps in phenomenology and psychobiology.
- The construct of an OCD spectrum has heuristic value insofar as it encourages diagnosis and treatment of a range of disorders that are often overlooked by clinicians and researchers.
- Like OCD, some putative obsessive-compulsive spectrum disorders respond selectively to SSRIs and to cognitive-behavioral therapy.

References

Abelson JF, Kwan KY, O'Roak BJ, et al: Sequence variants in SLITRK1 are associated with Tourette's syndrome. Science 310:317–320, 2005

Amat JA, Bronen RA, Saluja S, et al: Increased number of subcortical hyperintensities on MRI in children and adolescents with Tourette's syndrome, obsessive-compulsive disorder, and attention deficit hyperactivity disorder. Am J Psychiatry 1636:1106–1108, 2006

Anderluh MB, Tchanturia K, Rabe-Hesketh S, et al: Childhood obsessive-compulsive personality traits in adult women with eating disorders: defining a broader eating disorder phenotype. Am J Psychiatry 160:242–247, 2003

Barsky AJ: Hypochondriasis and obsessive-compulsive disorder. Psychiatr Clin North Am 15:791–801, 1992

Bartz JA, Hollander E: Is obsessive-compulsive disorder an anxiety disorder? Prog Neuropsychopharmacol Biol Psychiatry 303:338–352, 2006

Berlin HA, Rolls ET, Iverson SD: Borderline personality disorder, impulsivity disorder, impulsivity, and the orbitofrontal cortex. Am J Psychiatry 162:2360–2373, 2005

Blanco C, Petkova E, Ibanez A, et al: A pilot placebo-controlled study of fluvoxamine for pathological gambling. Ann Clin Psychiatry 14:9–15, 2002

Bloch MH, Landeros-Weisenberger A, Dombrowski P, et al: Systematic review: pharmacological and behavioral treatment for trichotillomania. Biol Psychiatry 62:839–846, 2007

Bohne A, Keithen NJ, Tuschen-Caffier B, et al: Cognitive inhibition in trichotillomania and obsessive-compulsive disorder. Behav Res Ther 437:923–942, 2005

Carey P, Seedat S, Warwick J, et al: SPECT imaging of body dysmorphic disorder. J Neuropsychiatry Clin Neurosci 16:357–359, 2004

Castle D, Rossel S, Kyrios M: Body dysmorphic disorder. Psychiatr Clin North Am 292:521–538, 2006

Cheyette SR, Cummings JL: Encephalitis lethargica: lessons for contemporary neuropsychiatry. J Neuropsychiatry Clin Neurosci 7:125–135, 1995

Christenson GA, Crow SJ: The characterization and treatment of trichotillomania. J Clin Psychiatry 57:42–49, 1996

Christenson GA, Crow SJ, MacKenzie TB, et al: A placebo controlled double-blind study of naltrexone for trichotillomania (abstract), in New Research Program and Abstracts of the 150th Annual Meeting of the American Psychiatric Association, Philadelphia, PA, May 1994a

Christenson GA, Raymond NC, Faris PL, et al: Pain thresholds are not elevated in trichotillomania. Biol Psychiatry 36:347–349, 1994b

Eisen JL, Phillips KA, Coles ME, et al: Insight in obsessive compulsive disorder and body dysmorphic disorder. Compr Psychiatry 451:10–15, 2004

Fallon BA, Schneier FR, Marshall R, et al: The pharmacotherapy of hypochondriasis. Psychopharmacol Bull 32:607–611, 1996

Fallon BA, Qureshi AI, Laje G, et al: Hypochondriasis and its relationship to obsessive-compulsive disorder. Psychiatr Clin North Am 23:605–616, 2000

Foa EB, Kozak MJ: Psychological treatment for obsessive-compulsive disorder, in Long-Term Treatments of Anxiety Disorders. Edited by Mavisssakalian MR, Prien RF. Washington, DC, American Psychiatric Press, 1996, pp 285–309

Frare F, Perugi G, Ruffolo G, et al: Obsessive-compulsive disorder and body dysmorphic disorder: a comparison of clinical features. Eur Psychiatry 19:292–298, 2004

Frecska E, Arato M: Opiate sensitivity test in patients with stereotypic movement disorder and trichotillomania. Prog Neuropsychopharmacol Biol Psychiatry 26:909–912, 2002

Freeston MH, Ladouceur R, Rheaume J, et al: Cognitive-behavior treatment of obsessive thoughts. J Consult Clin Psychiatry 65:405–413, 1997

Gabbay V, Asnis GM, Bello JA, et al: New onset of body dysmorphic disorder following frontotemporal lesion. Neurology 61:123–125, 2003

George MS, Trimble MR, Ring HA, et al: Obsessions in obsessive-compulsive disorder with and without Gilles de la Tourette's syndrome. Am J Psychiatry 150:93–97, 1993

Grant JE, Phillips KA: Recognizing and treating body dysmorphic disorder. Ann Clin Psychiatry 174:205–210, 2005

Grant JE, Kim SW, Potenza MN: Advances in the pharmacological treatment of pathological gambling. J Gamb Stud 191:85–109, 2003a

Grant JE, Kim SW, Potenza MN, et al: Paroxetine treatment of pathological gambling: a multi-center randomized controlled trial. Int Clin Psychopharmacol 18:243–249, 2003b

Grant JE, Brewer JA, Potenza MN: The neurobiology of substance and behavioral addictions. CNS Spectr 11:924–930, 2006a

Grant JE, Mancebo MC, Pinto A, et al: Impulse control disorders in adults with obsessive compulsive disorder. J Psychiatr Res 406:494–501, 2006b

Grant JE, Potenza MN, Hollander E, et al: A multicenter investigation of the opioid antagonist nalmefene in the treatment of pathological gambling. Am J Psychiatry 163:303–312, 2006c

Greer JM, Capecchi MR: Hoxb8 is required for normal grooming behavior in mice. Neuron 331:23–34, 2002

Greeven A, Van Balkom AJ, Visser S, et al: Cognitive behavior therapy and paroxetine in the treatment of hypochondriasis: a randomized controlled trial. Am J Psychiatry 164:91–99, 2007

Hadley SJ, Greenberg J, Hollander E: Diagnosis and treatment of body dysmorphic disorder in adolescents. Curr Psychiatry Rep 42:108–113, 2002

Hanes KR: Neuropsychological performance in body dysmorphic disorder. J Int Neuropsychol Soc 42:167–171, 1998

Hebebrand J, Klug B, Fimmers R, et al: Rates for tic disorders and obsessive compulsive symptomatology in families of children and adolescents with Gilles de la Tourette syndrome. J Psychiatr Res 31:519–530, 1997

Hemmings SM, Kinnear CJ, Lochner C, et al: Genetic correlates in trichotillomania: a case-control association study in the South African Caucasian population. Isr J Psychiatry Relat Sci 432:93–101, 2006

Hodgins DC, Petry NM: Cognitive and behavioral treatments in pathological gambling: a clinical guide to treatment. Edited by Grant JE, Potenza MN. Washington, DC, American Psychiatric Publishing, 2004, pp 169–187

Hollander E: Obsessive-Compulsive Related Disorders. Washington, DC, American Psychiatric Press, 1993, pp 1–16

Hollander E, Phillips KA: Body image and experience disorders: body dysmorphic and depersonalization disorders, in Obsessive-Compulsive Related Disorders. Edited by Hollander E. Washington, DC, American Psychiatric Press, 1993, pp 17–48

Hollander E, Wong CM: Body dysmorphic disorder, pathological gambling and sexual compulsions. J Clin Psychiatry 564:7–12, 1995

Hollander E, Allen A, Kwon J, et al: Clomipramine vs desipramine crossover trial in body dysmorphic disorder: selective efficacy of a serotonin reuptake inhibitor in imagined ugliness. Arch Gen Psychiatry 56:1033–1039, 1999

Hollander E, King A, Delaney K, et al: Obsessive-compulsive behaviors in parents of multiplex autism families. Psychiatry Res 1171:11–16, 2003

Hollander E, Kim S, Zohar J: OCSDs in the forthcoming DSM-V. CNS Spectr 125:320–323, 2007

Hollander E, Braun A, Simeon D: Should OCD leave the anxiety disorders in DSM-V? The case for obsessive compulsive-related disorders. Depress Anxiety 25:317–329, 2008

Jenike MA, Breiter HC, Baer L, et al: Cerebral structural abnormalities in obsessive-compulsive disorder: a quantitative morphometric magnetic resonance imaging study. Arch Gen Psychiatry 53:625–632, 1996

Keen-Kim D, Freimer NB: Genetics and epidemiology of Tourette syndrome. J Child Neurol 218:665–671, 2006

Keuthen NJ, Makris N, Schlerf JE, et al: Evidence for reduced cerebellar volumes in trichotillomania. Biol Psychiatry 61:374–381, 2007

Kim SW, Grant JE, Adson DE, et al: Double-blind naltrexone and placebo comparison study in the treatment of pathological gambling. Biol Psychiatry 49:914–921, 2001

Kim SW, Grant JE, Adson DE, et al: A double-blind placebo-controlled study of the efficacy and safety of paroxetine in the treatment of pathological gambling. J Clin Psychiatry 63:501–507, 2002

Kolevzon A, Mathewson KA, Hollander E: Selective serotonin reuptake inhibitors in autism: a review of efficacy and tolerability. J Clin Psychiatry 673:407–414, 2006

Ladouceur R, Sylvain C, Boutin C, et al: Cognitive treatment of pathological gambling. J Nerv Ment Dis 189:774–780, 2001

Lenane MC, Swedo SE, Rapoport JL, et al: Rates of obsessive compulsive disorder in first degree relatives of patients with trichotillomania: a research note. J Child Psychol Psychiatry 335:925–933, 1992

Lochner C, Stein DJ: Does work on obsessive-compulsive spectrum disorders contribute to understanding the heterogeneity of obsessive-compulsive disorder? Prog Neuropsychopharmacol Biol Psychiatry 30:353–361, 2006

Lochner C, Seedat S, du Toit PL, et al: Obsessive-compulsive disorder and trichotillomania: a phenomenological comparison. BMC Psychiatry 5:2, 2005

Mataix-Cols D, van den Heuvel OA: Common and distinct neural correlates of obsessive-compulsive and related disorders. Psychiatr Clin North Am 29:391–410, 2006

Mayer LE, Walsh BT: The use of selective serotonin reuptake inhibitors in eating disorders. J Clin Psychiatry 59:28–34, 1998

Menzies L, Chamberlain SR, Lairdd AR, et al: Integrating evidence from neuroimaging and neuropsychological studies of obsessive-compulsive disorder: the orbito-fronto-striatal model revisited. Neurosci Biobehav Rev 32:525–549, 2008

Moriarty J, Eapen V, Costa DC, et al: HMPAO SPET does not distinguish obsessive-compulsive and tic syndromes in families multiply affected with Gilles de la Tourette's syndrome. Psychol Med 27:737–740, 1997

Noyes R, Holt CS, Hsappel RL, et al: A family study of hypochondriasis. J Nerv Ment Dis 185:223–232, 1997

Olley A, Malhi G, Sachdev P: Memory and executive functioning in obsessive compulsive disorder: a selective review. J Affect Disord 104:15–23, 2007

Pauls DL: The genetics of Tourette syndrome. Curr Psychiatry Rep 32:152–157, 2001

Pauls DL, Leckman JF: The inheritance of Gilles de la Tourette's syndrome and associated behaviors: evidence for autosomal dominant. N Engl J Med 315:993–997, 1986

Pauls DL, Towbin KE, Leckman JF, et al: Gilles de la Tourette's syndrome and obsessive compulsive disorder: evidence supporting a genetic relationship. Arch Gen Psychiatry 43:1180–1182, 1986

Phillips KA: Body dysmorphic disorder: the distress of imagined ugliness. Am J Psychiatry 1489:1138–1149, 1991

Phillips KA: The Broken Mirror: Understanding and Treating Body Dysmorphic Disorder. New York, Oxford University Press, 1996

Phillips KA: The obsessive-compulsive spectrums. Psychiatr Clin North Am 254:791–809, 2002

Phillips KA, Kaye WH: The relationship of body dysmorphic disorder and eating disorders to obsessive-compulsive disorder. CNS Spectr 125:347–358, 2007

Phillips KA, Pagano ME, Menard W: Pharmacotherapy for body dysmorphic disorder: treatment received and illness severity. Ann Clinical Psychiatry 184:251–257, 2006

Phillips KA, Pinto A, Menard W, et al: Obsessive-compulsive disorder versus body dysmorphic disorder: a comparison study of two possibly related disorders. Depress Anxiety 24:399–409, 2007

Potenza MN, Leung HC, Blumberg HP, et al: An fMRI Stroop task study of ventromedial prefrontal cortical function in pathological gamblers. Am J Psychiatry 160:1990–1994, 2003

Rauch SL, Phillips KA, Segal E, et al: A preliminary morphometric magnetic resonance imaging study of regional brain volumes in body dysmorphic disorder. Psychiatry Res 122:13–19, 2003

Robinson D, Wu H, Munne RA, et al: Reduced caudate nucleus volume in obsessive-compulsive disorder. Arch Gen Psychiatry 52:393–398, 1995

Rosen JC, Reiter J, Orosan P: Cognitive behavioral body image therapy for body dysmorphic disorder. J Consult Clin Psychol 63:263–269, 1995

Saka E, Graybiel AM: Pathophysiology of Tourette's syndrome: striatal pathways revisited. Brain Dev 25 (suppl 1):S15–S19, 2003

Shavitt RG, Houni AG, Campos MCR, et al: Tourette's syndrome. Psychiatr Clin North Am 29:471–486, 2006

Simpson HB, Fallon BA: Obsessive-compulsive disorder: an overview. J Psychiatr Pract 6:3–17, 2000

Soomro GM, Altman D, Rajagopal S, et al: Selective serotonin re-uptake inhibitors (SSRIs) versus placebo for obsessive compulsive disorder (OCD). Cochrane Database Syst Rev Jan 23; (1):CD001765, 2008

Stein DJ, Hollander E: Low-dose pimozide augmentation of serotonin reuptake blockers in the treatment of trichotillomania. J Clin Psychiatry 53:123–126, 1992

Stein DJ, Hollander E: The spectrum of obsessive-compulsive related disorders, in Obsessive-Compulsive Related Disorders. Edited by Hollander E. Washington, DC, American Psychiatric Press, 1993, pp 241-271

Stein DJ, Christenson GA, Hollander EH (eds): Trichotillomania. Washington, DC, American Psychiatric Press, 1999

Stein DJ, van Heerden B, Hugo C, et al: Functional brain imaging and pharmacotherapy in trichotillomania single photon emission computed tomography before and after treatment with the selective serotonin reuptake inhibitor citalopram. Prog Neuropsychopharmacol Biol Psychiatry 26:885–890, 2002

Stemberger RM, Thomas AM, Mansueto CS, et al: Personal toll of trichotillomania: behavioral and interpersonal sequelae. J Anxiety Disord 141:97–104, 2000

Swedo SE, Leonard HL, Rapoport JL, et al: A double-blind comparison of clomipramine and desipramine in the treatment of trichotillomania hairpulling. N Engl J Med 321:497–501, 1989

Swedo SE, Garvey M, Snider L, et al: The PANDAS subgroup: recognition and treatment. CNS Spectr 65:419–422, 425–426, 2001

Sylvain C, Ladouceur R, Boisvert JM: Cognitive and behavioral treatment of pathological gambling: a controlled study. J Consult Clin Psychol 65:727–732, 1997

Tallis F: The neuropsychology of obsessive-compulsive disorder: a review and consideration of clinical implications. Br J Clin Psychol 36 (pt 1):3–20, 1997

Torregrossa MM, Quinn JJ, Taylor JR: Impulsivity, compulsivity, and habit: the role of orbitofrontal cortex revisited. Biol Psychiatry 633:253–255, 2008

van den Heuvel OA, Veltman DJ, Groenewegen HJ, et al: Frontal-striatal dysfunction during planning in obsessive-compulsive disorder. Arch Gen Psychiatry 623:301–309, 2005

Vaswani M, Linda FK, Ramesh S: Role of selective serotonin reuptake inhibitors in psychiatric disorders: a comprehensive review. Prog Neuropsychopharmacol Biol Psychiatry 271:85–102, 2003

Veale D, Grounay K, Dryden W, et al: Body dysmorphic disorder: a cognitive behavioral model and pilot randomized controlled trial. Behav Res Ther 34:717–729, 1996

Visser S, Bouman TK: The treatment of hypochondriasis: exposure plus response prevention vs cognitive therapy. Behav Res Ther 394:423–442, 2001

Wendland JR, Kruse MR, Murphy DL: Functional SLITRK1 var321, varCDfs and SLC6A4 G56A variants and susceptibility to obsessive-compulsive disorder. Mol Psychiatry 11:802–804, 2006

Woods DW, Wetterneck CT, Flessner CA: Understanding and treating trichotillomania: what we know and what we don't know. Psychiatr Clin North Am 292:487–501, 2006

Zuchner S, Cuccaro ML, Tran-Viet KN, et al: SLITRK1 mutations in trichotillomania. Mol Psychiatry 1110:887–889, 2006

Recommended Readings

Bloch MH, Landeros-Weisenberger A, Dombrowski P, et al: Systematic review: pharmacological and behavioral treatment for trichotillomania. Biol Psychiatry 62:839–846, 2007

Grant JE, Phillips KA: Recognizing and treating body dysmorphic disorder. Ann Clin Psychiatry 17:205–210, 2005

Leckman JF, Cohen DJ: Tourette's Syndrome: Tics, Obsessions, Compulsions: Developmental Psychopathology and Clinical Care. New York, Wiley, 1998

Marcus DK, Gurley JR, Marchi MM, et al: Cognitive and perceptual variables in hypochondriasis and health anxiety: a systematic review. Clin Psychol Rev 27:127–139, 2007

Phillips K: The Broken Mirror: Understanding and Treating Body Dysmorphic Disorder. New York, Oxford University Press, 1996

Shavitt RG, Houni AG, Campos MCR, et al: Tourette's syndrome. Psychiatr Clin North Am 29:471–486, 2006

Stein DJ, Christenson GA, Hollander EH (Eds): Trichotillomania. Washington, DC, American Psychiatric Press, 1999

Woods DW, Wetterneck CT, Flessner CA: Understanding and treating trichotillomania: what we know and what we don't know. Psychiatr Clin North Am 292:487–501, 2006

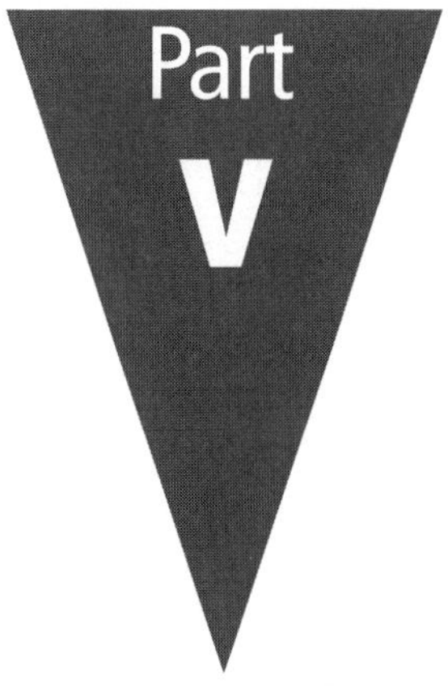

Panic Disorder/Agoraphobia

Chapter 21

Phenomenology of Panic Disorder

Mark H. Pollack, M.D.
Jordan W. Smoller, M.D., Sc.D.
Michael W. Otto, Ph.D.
Elizabeth Hoge, M.D.
Naomi Simon, M.D., M.Sc.

Epidemiology

Panic disorder was not defined as a discrete disorder until the publication of DSM-III (American Psychiatric Association 1980); therefore, few, if any, specific data are available on its epidemiology before that point. The lifetime prevalence rates of panic attacks and panic disorder have been estimated through a series of epidemiological studies: the Epidemiologic Catchment Area (ECA) study, the more recent National Comorbidity Survey (NCS) and National Comorbidity Survey Replication (NCS-R), and the National Epidemiologic Survey on Alcohol and Related Conditions (NESARC).

These four epidemiological studies used slightly different diagnostic criteria. The ECA study was conducted from 1980 to 1983 and thus depended on the DSM-III criteria in use at that time, as determined by the Diagnostic Interview Schedule (Robins et al. 1985). The NCS, conducted from 1990 to 1992, and its revision, conducted from 2001 to 2003, used the more recently developed DSM-III-R and DSM-IV criteria, respectively, as diagnosed by the Composite International Diagnostic Interview (Wittchen et al. 1991; World Mental Health Survey Initiative-CIDI, in Kessler and Ustün 2004). The NESARC also used the DSM-IV criteria, and face-to-face interviews were conducted with a representative sample of 43,093 Americans from 2001 to 2002. The NCS surveys were both nationwide and based on a probability sample of the continental United States. The NCS surveyed men and women between ages 15 and 54 years, whereas the ECA, the later NCS-R, and the NESARC studies interviewed patients 18 years and older (Eaton et al. 1994; Grant et al. 2006; Kessler et al. 2003a).

The lifetime prevalence of panic attacks in the ECA study, as defined with DSM-III criteria (including four or more psychophysiological symptoms), was 9.7%. The NCS estimate, as defined with similar criteria, was 15.6%; however, when the definition of panic attack was more narrowly defined with DSM-III-R criteria, its prevalence decreased to 7.3%. The ECA study determined that approximately 1.7% of the general population experience panic disorder in their lifetimes; the NCS estimated the lifetime prevalence at 3.5%. The 1-month prevalence of panic disorder was 0.5% in the ECA study and 1.5% in the NCS. In the NCS-R, the lifetime prevalence of panic attacks (without panic disorder) was 22%, although the lifetime prevalence of panic disorder (with and without agoraphobia) was 4.7% (Kessler et al. 2006).

Panic disorder is more commonly diagnosed in women than in men; the female-to-male ratio is approximately 3 to 1 in patients with agoraphobia and 2 to 1 in patients without agoraphobia. Although the onset of panic disorder occurs, on average, in the third decade, approximately half of adult patients with panic disorder report experiencing significant difficulties with anxiety during childhood, in the form of overanxious disorder, social phobia, or separation anxiety disorder (Pollack et al. 1996). Although early reports posited a specific link between separation anxiety in childhood and adult panic disorder (Klein 1964), this conceptualization has been broadened to include a more general link between childhood and adult anxiety difficulties (Aronson and Logue 1987; Berg 1976; Berg et al. 1974; Otto et al. 1994). The onset of panic disorder has also been reported to occur spontaneously (Biederman et al. 1997), but most individuals with panic disorder are able to identify a life stressor occurring within the year prior to onset of panic, which may be associated with its onset (Manfro et al. 1996; Roy-Byrne et al. 1986). It is unclear whether patients with panic disorder actually experience more life stressors than other individuals or whether they are more sensitive to the aversive effects of life events because of genetic endowment, temperamental predisposition, or conditioning.

Diagnostic Considerations

Panic disorder is a common, distressing, and often disabling condition in which patients experience recurrent unexpected panic attacks followed by at least 1 month of persistent concerns about having additional attacks (i.e., anticipatory anxiety), worry about the implications of the attack, or a significant change in behavior (e.g., avoidance) related to the attacks (Table 21–1) (American Psychiatric Association 2000). In order for the diagnosis of panic disorder to be made, the panic attacks cannot be due to the physiological effects of a substance or a medical condition or be better accounted for by anxiety episodes occurring in conjunction with other psychiatric disorders such as social phobia, specific phobia, posttraumatic stress disorder, or depression.

Panic attacks are periods of intense fear, apprehension, or discomfort that develop suddenly and reach a peak of intensity within 10 minutes of the initiation of symptoms. The DSM-IV-TR (American Psychiatric Association 2000) criteria require that 4 of 13 symptoms be present to diagnose a panic attack (Table 21–2). Notably, most of the symptoms (i.e., 11 of 13) of a panic attack are physical rather than emotional; this may contribute to the frequent presentation of patients with panic disorder in general medical settings and increased rates of use of medical services among affected patients (Katon 1984; Katon et al. 1986; Margraf et al. 1987; G.E. Simon and VonKorff 1991). The sudden onset of panic attacks and their episodic nature distinguish them

TABLE 21–1. DSM-IV-TR diagnostic criteria for panic disorder without agoraphobia

A. Both (1) and (2):

(1) recurrent unexpected panic attacks

(2) at least one of the attacks has been followed by 1 month (or more) of one (or more) of the following:

(a) persistent concern about having additional attacks

(b) worry about the implications of the attack or its consequences (e.g., losing control, having a heart attack, "going crazy")

(c) a significant change in behavior related to the attacks

B. Absence of agoraphobia

C. The panic attacks are not due to the direct physiological effects of a substance (e.g., a drug of abuse, a medication) or a general medical condition (e.g., hyperthyroidism).

D. The panic attacks are not better accounted for by another mental disorder, such as social phobia (e.g., occurring on exposure to feared social situations), specific phobia (e.g., on exposure to a specific phobic situation), obsessive-compulsive disorder (e.g., on exposure to dirt in someone with an obsession about contamination), posttraumatic stress disorder (e.g., in response to stimuli associated with a severe stressor), or separation anxiety disorder (e.g., in response to being away from home or close relatives).

TABLE 21–2. DSM-IV-TR criteria for panic attack

A discrete period of intense fear or discomfort, in which four (or more) of the following symptoms developed abruptly and reached a peak within 10 minutes:

(1) palpitations, pounding heart, or accelerated heart rate

(2) sweating

(3) trembling or shaking

(4) sensations of shortness of breath or smothering

(5) feeling of choking

(6) chest pain or discomfort

(7) nausea or abdominal distress

(8) feeling dizzy, unsteady, lightheaded, or faint

(9) derealization (feelings of unreality) or depersonalization (being detached from oneself)

(10) fear of losing control or going crazy

(11) fear of dying

(12) paresthesias (numbness or tingling sensations)

(13) chills or hot flushes

from the more diffuse symptoms characterizing anticipatory or generalized anxiety.

Panic attacks are not unique to panic disorder and may occur on exposure to feared events in any of the anxiety disorders (Barlow et al. 1985). Moreover, panic episodes are reported, albeit infrequently, in individuals without anxiety disorders. As compared with panic attacks occurring in the context of panic disorder, these nonclinical panic episodes are less likely to involve fears of dying, having a heart attack, and losing control, and they tend to occur during stressful situations such as public speaking and interpersonal conflicts and before tests and examinations (Norton et al. 1985, 1986, 1992).

Given the ubiquity of panic attacks, differential diagnosis is aided by diagnostic revisions made in DSM-IV (American Psychiatric Association 1994) that emphasize fears of recurrent panic attacks as a core feature of panic disorder. In DSM-III-R (American Psychiatric Association 1987), panic disorder was defined, in part, by the number of attacks (i.e., four) occurring over a 4-week period. In DSM-IV, this criterion was changed to emphasize fears of panic attacks as defined by 1 month or more of persistent concerns about having additional attacks, worry about the implications of attacks, and/or a significant change in behavior (e.g., avoidance) associated with the attacks. This diagnostic change placed central attention on a patient's phobic responses to the panic attacks themselves and their perceived consequences (e.g., "I'm having a heart attack," "I may lose control," "I may faint"). In contrast, other disorders may be characterized by panic responses that accompany feared responses to other phobic events, such as exposure to a social situation in social phobia, to a trauma cue in posttraumatic stress disorder, or to an obsessional concern (e.g., contamination) in obsessive-compulsive disorder.

Panic attacks that occur with fewer than 4 of the 13 panic symptoms specified by DSM-IV-TR are referred to as *limited-symptom attacks*. Many patients with panic disorder have a combination of full- and limited-symptom attacks. For some individuals, the early phases of treatment may be characterized by a decrease in full-symptom attacks with a transient increase in limited-symptom attacks, as treatment begins to become effective. Although limited-symptom attacks are associated with fewer symptoms, they may still be quite distressing and associated with significant impairment and increased treatment-seeking behavior (Klerman et al. 1991).

The severity and frequency of panic attacks vary; some patients experience episodes once or twice a week, others experience multiple attacks on a daily basis. The frequency of panic attacks may be a misleading indicator of the true severity of the condition, because some patients may reduce the frequency of attacks by avoiding situations that trigger them (e.g., agoraphobic avoidance). Thus, a consensus conference on the assessment of panic disorder recommended broadening the domain of symptoms evaluated to include not only panic attack frequency and severity but also phobic anxiety, avoidance, and interference with function (Shear and Maser 1994). The Panic Disorder Severity Scale (Shear et al. 1997) is a validated instrument used to assess these aspects of the panic disorder syndrome and their change with treatment.

The presence of agoraphobia frequently complicates panic disorder (Table 21–3). In clinical settings, more than three-quarters of patients with panic disorder report at least mild agoraphobic avoidance (Breier et al. 1986). The diagnosis of agoraphobia refers to a patient's fear or avoidance of situations from which escape might be difficult or embarrassing or in which help may not be readily available in the event of a panic attack. Agoraphobic situations may include being alone; traveling in public transportation; going over bridges; being in ele-

TABLE 21–3. DSM-IV-TR diagnostic criteria for panic disorder with agoraphobia

A. Both (1) and (2):
   (1) recurrent unexpected panic attacks
   (2) at least one of the attacks has been followed by 1 month (or more) of one (or more) of the following:
      (a) persistent concern about having additional attacks
      (b) worry about the implications of the attack or its consequences (e.g., losing control, having a heart attack, "going crazy")
      (c) a significant change in behavior related to the attacks

B. The presence of agoraphobia

C. The panic attacks are not due to the direct physiological effects of a substance (e.g., a drug of abuse, a medication) or a general medical condition (e.g., hyperthyroidism).

D. The panic attacks are not better accounted for by another mental disorder, such as social phobia (e.g., occurring on exposure to feared social situations), specific phobia (e.g., on exposure to a specific phobic situation), obsessive-compulsive disorder (e.g., on exposure to dirt in someone with an obsession about contamination), posttraumatic stress disorder (e.g., in response to stimuli associated with a severe stressor), or separation anxiety disorder (e.g., in response to being away from home or close relatives).

vators, tunnels, or grocery stores; and standing in long lines. Agoraphobia also may occur in any situation in which the patient previously experienced a panic attack. Despite their fear, some patients may push themselves through the agoraphobic situation, whereas others avoid the situations or can face them only in the presence of a trusted companion. Some patients become literally homebound, unable to venture beyond their doorstep, for fear of having a panic attack outside the perceived relative safety of their home. For some patients, the avoidance behavior may be cued by interoceptive or internal stimuli, such as rapid heart rate, which may occur in the context of physical exercise or sexual arousal. Through conditioning, these stimuli may trigger a cognitive cascade of alarm and result in patients' avoidance of physical exertion or other situations that cause autonomic arousal.

Relation Between Panic Disorder and Agoraphobia

In DSM-IV-TR, agoraphobia is a condition that may occur in the context of two disorders: panic disorder with agoraphobia and agoraphobia without history of panic disorder. In both disorders, however, agoraphobia is described as occurring in response to panic attacks (panic disorder with agoraphobia) or panic-like symptoms (agoraphobia without history of panic disorder). This view of agoraphobia as a consequence of panic has evolved from both theoretical considerations and clinical observations (Klein 1981). However, it is not universally held and remains the subject of one of the more interesting controversies in psychiatric nosology (Ballenger and Fyer 1996).

Broadly speaking, two descriptions of the panic disorder–agoraphobia connection have been most prominent. The prevailing view in American psychiatry, as reflected in DSM-IV-TR, has been that agoraphobia is almost always a complication of panic disorder. Klein and Klein (1989) reviewed evidence that agoraphobia usually develops after the onset of spontaneous panic attacks and represents the fear and avoidance of situations in which help may not be readily available should a panic attack recur. An alternative view, more closely allied with European psychiatry and reflected in ICD-10 (World Health Organization 1992), is that agoraphobia is a distinct disorder that may or may not follow the onset of panic attacks (Marks 1987). In ICD-10, the diagnosis of panic disorder with agoraphobia is given only if a primary diagnosis of agoraphobia has been excluded. Which view is better supported by the available data? Three types of studies—epidemiological, clinical, and family and genetic studies—bear on this question, but the answers they provide are inconclusive.

Epidemiological Studies

The common comorbidity of panic disorder and agoraphobia has been well documented in community surveys around the world, in which the lifetime prevalence of agoraphobia among those with panic disorder has ranged from 22.5% to 58.2% (Weissman et al. 1997). Agoraphobia is up to 20 times more common among individuals with panic disorder than among those without it (Weissman et al. 1997). However, data from the largest epidemiological surveys of psychiatric disorders in the United States seem to provide strong evidence that agoraphobia is not typically a consequence of panic disorder.

In the National Institute of Mental Health ECA study of approximately 15,000 individuals examined at five centers in the United States, the overall lifetime prevalence of agoraphobia without panic disorder was 5.6%, whereas the lifetime prevalence of panic disorder was only 1.6% (Eaton 1995; Regier et al. 1988). In the NCS conducted by Kessler et al. (1994), the lifetime prevalence of agoraphobia was 6.7%, whereas the lifetime prevalence of panic disorder was 3.5%, and only a minority (36%) of those diagnosed with agoraphobia reported ever having had an unexpected panic attack (Eaton et al. 1994; Magee et al. 1996). These frequencies were confirmed with the NCS replication, which showed a lifetime prevalence of panic without agoraphobia of 3.7% and panic with agoraphobia of 1.1% (Kessler et al. 2006). A more recent large-scale (N=43,093) U.S. epidemiological study, the NESARC, found lifetime prevalence of 4.0% for panic disorder without agoraphobia of only 1.1% for panic disorder with agoraphobia (Grant et al. 2006). In this survey, agoraphobia without a history of panic disorder was measured as 0.17% lifetime prevalence. These prevalence rates, however, were based on lifetime diagnoses made at the time of a cross-sectional community survey and, as such, could be subject to recall biases. However, Eaton and Keyl (1990) also found that the incidence of agoraphobia without panic disorder was higher than the incidence of agoraphobia following panic disorder in a prospective study of the ECA sample. Their study included the 11,756 individuals who were interviewed in wave 1 of the ECA and again 1 year later and who reported no history of any agoraphobia-related fear at the initial interview. The 1-year incidence of agoraphobia was 2.2%, and at least two-thirds of the new patients reported no history of a panic attack. In community studies, then, agoraphobia occurs commonly in those with panic disorder, but most individuals with agoraphobia do not have panic disorder.

Clinical Studies

Evidence from clinical investigations paints a very different picture. These studies indicate the diagnosis of agoraphobia without a history of panic is quite rare, and in several studies it was nonexistent (Goisman et al. 1995; Lelliott et al. 1989; Noyes et al. 1987; Pollard et al. 1989; Thyer and Himle 1985). For example, in one series of 55 patients with agoraphobia, 54 (98%) reported onset of agoraphobia following the onset of panic attacks (Breier et al. 1986). Other investigators who compared patients with panic disorder and those with panic disorder plus agoraphobia found few differences in terms of clinical or demographic variables, concluding that panic disorder and agoraphobia are manifestations of a single underlying disorder (Noyes et al. 1987; Thyer et al. 1985). Because the presence of agoraphobia was associated with earlier age at onset, greater symptom severity, and more chronicity, these studies have suggested that panic disorder with agoraphobia is a more severe variant of panic disorder (Noyes et al. 1987).

Although most clinical studies have supported the hypothesis that agoraphobia is a sequela of panic, this finding has not been universal. In one study of patients with panic disorder with agoraphobia, Fava et al. (1988) reported that 18 of 20 patients (90%) reported the onset of phobic avoidance before their first panic attack. In a clinical sample of 472 children and adolescents, Biederman et al. (1997) found that agoraphobia had a higher prevalence than panic disorder (15% vs. 6%) and an earlier mean age at onset.

Family and Genetic Studies

Family and genetic studies can provide powerful methods for delineating boundaries between disorders (Smoller and Tsuang 1998). For example, if relatives of probands with either panic disorder or agoraphobia are at elevated risk for both disorders, then this would lend support to the hypothesis that these disorders can be expressions of a common genetic diathesis. In one study (Noyes et al. 1986), familial risk of panic disorder was elevated in relatives of probands who had either panic disorder or agoraphobia with panic attacks; however, the risk of agoraphobia was elevated only among relatives of probands with agoraphobia. These results were interpreted as indicating that agoraphobia is a more severe variant of panic disorder, although they are not inconsistent with the possibility that agoraphobia is separately transmitted. In another study, however, relatives of probands with agoraphobia did show an elevated risk of agoraphobia without panic disorder (Horwath et al. 1995). Data from twin studies have largely indicated that genetic influences on panic disorder and agoraphobia overlap. In a population-based twin study of more than 5,000 twins, Hettema et al. (2005) found that the structure of genetic and environmental influences on the anxiety disorders was not isomorphic with the clinically defined categories. Using structural equation modeling, they identified two genetic factors underlying the disorders: one factor primarily predisposing to panic disorder, agoraphobia, and generalized anxiety disorder, and the second primarily influencing specific phobias. Genetic linkage analyses have also provided evidence that genetic effects on panic and phobic disorders transcend diagnostic boundaries (Kaabi et al. 2006; Smoller et al. 2001). The results of these studies provide some support for the position that panic disorder and agoraphobia are expressions of a single underlying disorder (Smoller et al. 2008). Because DSM-IV-TR defines agoraphobia as a response to panic or panic-like symptoms, the phenotypes of panic and agoraphobia have become linked by definition, so that future family and genetic studies may have difficulty testing whether they can be independent.

Discussion

Unfortunately, the causal and clinical relation between panic disorder and agoraphobia has not been conclusively resolved. Several explanations have been offered for the striking discrepancy between the results of epidemiological and clinical investigations, including differences in diagnostic criteria, methods of assessment, and sampling techniques. With the exception of the prospective ECA study, almost all available data are based on retrospective reports, which can be subject to recall bias. When asked to provide a retrospective account of the development of agoraphobia, patients, like clinicians, may seek an explanation for these symptoms. The experience of an initial panic attack is so salient that it may dominate an individual's memory of anxiety symptomatology (Lelliott et al. 1989). Clinical studies also may overestimate the association between agoraphobia and panic disorder because of the phenomenon of Berkson's bias (Berkson 1946). If both panic attacks and agoraphobia independently contribute to treatment seeking, then individuals with both features will be overrepresented in clinical settings.

Alternatively, epidemiological studies may have underestimated the presence of panic symptoms or panic disorder among individuals with agoraphobia. In large studies, such as the ECA and NCS, diagnoses were obtained via fully structured interviews administered by lay interviewers. Some have argued that these methods may have misclassified respondents with respect to panic disorder and/or agoraphobia. As a test of this hypothesis, Horwath et al. (1993) studied 22 subjects from the ECA study who had been given diagnoses of agoraphobia without panic disorder or panic attacks. These subjects were reinterviewed with a semistructured clinical interview (Schedule for Affective Disorders and Schizophrenia–Lifetime Anxiety Version) by master's-level social workers or psychologists who were blind to the ECA diagnoses. This clinical interview allowed a diagnosis of simple phobia to be made for individuals who fear crowds, tunnels, bridges, public transportation, or going out of the house alone. After clinical reappraisal, only one case of agoraphobia without panic remained. The other subjects were rediagnosed as having agoraphobia with panic (2 subjects), simple or social phobia (12 subjects), or no phobia or panic (7 subjects). Although based on a small sample, these results are consistent with the hypothesis that the ECA study overestimated the prevalence of agoraphobia without panic.

Although areas of uncertainty remain, the available evidence does support a few inferences: 1) in clinical settings, agoraphobia most often appears to be associated with panic, and most patients who present clinically report that initial panic attacks preceded or coincided with the onset of agoraphobia; 2) panic attacks are a strong risk factor for the development of agoraphobia, and panic generally precedes agoraphobia in patients who have panic disorder with agoraphobia; 3) community studies and a clinical study of children provided consistent evidence, however, that agoraphobia does not always arise as a consequence of panic attacks or panic disorder; and 4) the presence of both panic disorder and agoraphobia is associated with a more severe and chronic course of anxiety symptoms than is seen in panic disorder alone. The remaining ambiguities may succumb to further epidemiological, clinical, and genetic investigation. Of particular interest clinically is determining why some patients with panic disorder develop agoraphobia but others do not. The identification of factors involved in the vulnerability to agoraphobia could provide an important focus for preventive efforts.

Impairment Associated With Panic Disorder

The effects of psychiatric disorders, in general, on both physical and emotional health have received increasing empirical attention. For example, a large medical outcome study (Wells et al. 1989) documented the deleterious effects of depression on physical and emotional function, finding the effects to be as bad as or worse than those of other chronic medical conditions. Examination of the health and social consequences of panic disorder has also shown significant impairment and disability. For example, research has shown that panic disorder results in impairment of quality of life and well-being that is equal to that of major depression or a medical illness such as diabetes (Cramer et al. 2005; Markowitz et al. 1989; Rubin et al. 2000). In another study, examination of quality of life in a group of panic disorder patients evaluated before initiating treatment in a clinical setting documented significant disruption in patients with panic disorder, including significant impairment in physical and mental functioning comparable to and sometimes worse than that in patients with chronic medical conditions and depression (Candilis et al. 1999). Panic has been associated with high rates of vocational dysfunction and financial dependence as well as excessive use of medical services (Klerman et al. 1991; Roy-Byrne et al. 1999). A European study examining the economic costs of panic disorder, including medical costs and nonmedical costs such as lost productivity, found an annual per capita cost of 10,269 euros (Batelaan et al. 2007). Patients with panic disorder are at an increased risk for substance abuse and suicide attempts (Goodwin and Roy-Byrne 2006).

Panic disorder is common in the general medical setting (range 2%–13%; median prevalence 4%–6% [Roy-Byrne et al. 1999]) and is associated with increased health care use in affected individuals. In one survey of 250 primary care physicians, anxiety was cited as the most common psychiatric problem seen in their patients (Orleans et al. 1985), with up to 13% of primary care patients having panic disorder alone or in combination with depression (Katon et al. 1986). Like other psychiatric conditions, panic disorder often is unrecognized and untreated in primary care settings; a World Health Organization primary care study documented that the diagnosis of panic was overlooked in half the affected patients in primary care (Lecrubier and Ustün 1998; Ormel et al. 1994; Sartorius et al. 1993). Underrecognition may, in part, be attributable to the typical presentation of panic patients with predominantly somatic symptoms (chest pain, dizziness, shortness of breath, irritable bowel) rather than psychological symptoms (Bridges and Goldberg 1985; Katon 1984). Analysis of data from the ECA study indicated that patients with panic disorder were five to eight times more likely than nonaffected individuals to be high users of medical services (G.E. Simon and VonKorff 1991). Even the presence of panic attacks not meeting full criteria for panic disorder may be associated with significant impairment in functioning and treatment seeking (Klerman et al. 1991). Recognition and treatment of panic disorder in general medical settings is critical, given the association of the disorder with adverse effects across multiple domains of functioning and the demonstration that treatment results in symptomatic relief, improvement in role functioning, decreased use of medical resources, and reduction in overall costs (Salvador-Carulla et al. 1995). In addition, men with panic disorder may be at premature risk for death from cardiovascular causes (Coryell et al. 1982; Kawachi et al. 1994a). Additional recent research has also found that women who experience panic attacks are at greater risk for cardiovascular and cerebrovascular events (Smoller et al. 2007). One study (Tucker et al. 1997) reported that selective serotonin reuptake inhibitor treatment of panic disorder normalized the decreased heart rate variability that has been hypothesized to contribute to excessive cardiac mortality associated with panic.

Comorbidity

Panic disorder may be complicated by the presence of comorbid conditions, including other anxiety disorders (social anxiety disorder, generalized anxiety disorder, specific phobia, posttraumatic stress disorder, obsessive-compulsive disorder) as well as depression and alcohol abuse.

Social anxiety disorder may occur in up to one-third (Stein et al. 1990) of patients with panic disorder. The differential diagnosis between panic and social anxiety disorder may sometimes be difficult, particularly when panic attacks occur in social situations. Focus on the core fears of the patient may help in making the diagnosis. In panic disorder, the patient's central fear is of having a panic attack and may manifest in situations outside of social ones. Patients with social anxiety disorder, who panic on exposure to social scrutiny, focus primarily on the possibility of humiliation or embarrassment in social situations. For many patients, both types of fears may be present, and the diagnosis of both conditions is warranted.

Generalized anxiety disorder is also frequently comorbid with panic disorder. To receive the diagnosis of generalized anxiety disorder, patients must be excessively worried about life activities or stressors, with the anxiety focused not just on anticipation of recurrent panic attacks. The episodic and crescendo nature of panic attacks as compared with the more persistent, but often less intense, anxiety associated with generalized anxiety disorder is another distinguishing element.

Patients with specific phobias, posttraumatic stress disorder, and obsessive-compulsive disorder may also experience panic attacks, but these are typically cued by exposure to or anticipation of specific phobic situations (e.g., heights or other phobic situations in the case of specific phobias, situations evocative of traumatic events associated with trauma in the case of posttraumatic stress disorder, and contamination in patients with obsessive-compulsive disorder). For individuals affected with these conditions, panic attacks are cued by specific situations and would not be expected to occur spontaneously unless panic disorder also was present.

Among the most common conditions comorbid with panic disorder is depression, with a lifetime prevalence of major depressive disorder of 38% in epidemiological samples (Kessler et al. 2006), and possibly higher in clinical samples (Ball et al. 1994; Breier et al. 1984; Kessler et al. 1998; Stein et al. 1990). Depression may either predate or emerge after the onset of panic disorder and reflect a reactive demoralization to the negative effects of panic or the emergence of an independent condition. As is true with other comorbid conditions, the presence of comorbid depression may complicate treatment and increase the overall severity of the patient's distress; the presence of panic attacks in patients with major depression is associated with an increased risk of suicide (Fawcett et al. 1990), and the presence of comorbid depression in individuals with panic disorder appears to confer increased risk for suicide (Cox et al. 1994). Although data from the ECA study (Weissman et al. 1989) and a more recent study (Sareen et al. 2005a) suggest an increased risk for suicide associated with panic disorder alone, other studies of this issue have suggested that the risk is elevated predominantly in those panic disorder patients with comorbid disorders, such as depression and/or personality dysfunction (Beck et al. 1991; Cox et al. 1994; Friedman et al. 1992; Hornig and McNally 1995; Vickers and McNally 2004). It is worth noting, however, that the incidence of comorbidity with panic disorder is very high. Thus, clinically, panic may be considered a marker of increased risk of suicide, and assessment of suicidality is warranted.

More recently, panic disorder comorbidity with bipolar disorder has been examined in several studies. Data from a treatment-seeking population of individuals with bipolar disorder suggest lifetime rates of panic with or without agoraphobia of approximately 18% in bipolar I and 14% in bipolar II disorder (N.M. Simon et al. 2004b). Moreover, panic has been associated with earlier age at onset of bipolar disorder, shorter euthymic periods, poorer quality of life, greater substance abuse comorbidity, higher levels of suicidality, and poorer response to treatment, both prospectively and retrospectively (Bauer et al. 2005; Frank et al. 2002; Gaudiano and Miller 2005; McElroy et al. 2001; Otto et al. 2006; N.M. Simon et al. 2004b).

Unfortunately, there remains a paucity of data to guide treatment of patients with panic and bipolar comorbidity, although the presence of bipolar disorder has important implications for treatment selection for panic disorder, such as avoiding monotherapy with antidepressants and prioritizing mood stabilization (N.M. Simon et al. 2004a).

Alcohol abuse and dependence may also be present in a significant subset of individuals with panic disorder, with a recent study suggesting approximately 34% of those with panic disorder with agoraphobia meet criteria for at least one lifetime substance use disorder (Conway et al. 2006). Some individuals report that their abuse of alcohol developed in the context of an attempt to self-medicate their anxiety. However, the temporal relation between alcohol abuse and panic disorder tends to follow diagnostic values, with the mean age at onset of alcohol abuse in the late teens and early 20s and panic disorder in the late 20s (Otto et al. 1992). One study found that approximately half of individuals with panic and substance use disorders had an earlier onset of the substance use disorder (Sareen et al. 2006). It is of note that individuals with anxiety disorders who attempt to self-medicate do appear to be at increased risk for substance use comorbidity, as well as mood disorders and suicidality (Bolton et al. 2006). Clinically, the presence of alcohol and other substance use disorders may be associated with poor outcome and should be considered in all individuals presenting with panic and other anxiety disorders. Alcohol and substance use disorders represent a relative contraindication to the use of benzodiazepines. Patients abusing alcohol or drugs require focused substance abuse treatment, in addition to the treatment directed at the panic disorder, to facilitate comprehensive recovery.

Medical disorders have also been shown to occur more commonly and are associated with increased impairment in individuals with panic disorder (Kessler et al. 2003b; Sareen et al. 2005b). In particular, panic has been associated with respiratory conditions, including asthma (Goodwin et al. 2003) and chronic obstructive pulmonary disease (Karajgi et al. 1990). Another report combining prior panic studies that examined both thyroid history and test results also supports significantly elevated rates of thyroid dysfunction (6.5%), suggesting patients with panic disorder should be screened at least once for thyroid disease (N.M. Simon et al. 2002). Comorbidity of panic disorder with vertigo due to vestibular dysfunction may also occur, with some symptom overlap and the development of agoraphobic avoidance that includes environmental factors that may heighten dizziness; some preliminary open-label data suggest treatment with a selective serotonin reuptake inhibitor (SSRI) may result in symptomatic improvement of the dizziness and associated distress (Staab et al. 2004). Cardiac symptoms and disease are another important area of medical overlap with panic disorder. Many somatic symptoms such as heart palpitations or chest pain that occur during panic attacks may not be easily differentiated from those due to a primary cardiac disorder—and many patients seek care initially complaining of cardiac symptoms. Although the precise etiology of these associations remains to be elucidated, panic disorder may have implications for cardiac health and mortality, with a number of studies supporting increased risk for fatal coronary heart disease, changes in QT and heart rate variability, and sudden death in both men and women (Albert et al. 2005; Kawachi et al. 1994a, 1994b; Yeragani et al. 2000). In contrast to tricyclic antidepressants, treatment of panic disorder with SSRIs has been associated with a significant improvement in heart rate variability, which theoretically may decrease risk for mortality due to sudden cardiac death and may be due to alterations in autonomic activity (Pohl et al. 2000; Tucker et al. 1997).

Conclusion

Panic disorder is a common, distressing, and disabling condition. It is frequently complicated by the presence of agoraphobia and other anxiety disorders, mood disorders, and alcohol and substance abuse. It is often present in the general medical setting and is associated with increased use of medical services, underscoring the need for timely recognition and treatment.

◀ Key Clinical Points ▶

- Recent epidemiological data suggest a lifetime prevalence of over 5% for panic disorder with and without associated agoraphobia.
- Panic disorder is two to three times more commonly diagnosed in women than men, with a typical age at onset in the third decade, though many patients report a history of anxiety difficulties beginning in childhood.
- Although panic attacks are often the most dramatic feature of panic disorder, comprehensive evaluation of affected individuals should include not only panic attack frequency and severity but also phobic anxiety, avoidance, and functional capacity.
- Panic disorder is associated with significant distress and dysfunction, as well as increased utilization of medical resources, greater risk for adverse cardiovascular events, and overall reduced quality of life.
- Panic disorder is often complicated by the presence of comorbid conditions, including other anxiety disorders, mood disorders (both unipolar and bipolar), alcohol and other substance abuse, and medical disorders.

References

Albert CM, Chae CU, Rexrode KM, et al: Phobic anxiety and risk of coronary heart disease and sudden cardiac death among women. Circulation 111:480–487, 2005

American Psychiatric Association: Diagnostic and Statistical Manual of Mental Disorders, 3rd Edition. Washington, DC, American Psychiatric Association, 1980

American Psychiatric Association: Diagnostic and Statistical Manual of Mental Disorders, 3rd Edition, Revised. Washington, DC, American Psychiatric Association, 1987

American Psychiatric Association: Diagnostic and Statistical Manual of Mental Disorders, 4th Edition. Washington, DC, American Psychiatric Association, 1994

American Psychiatric Association: Diagnostic and Statistical Manual of Mental Disorders, 4th Edition, Text Revision. Washington, DC, American Psychiatric Association, 2000

Aronson T, Logue C: On the longitudinal course of panic disorder: developmental history and predictors of phobic complications. Compr Psychiatry 28:344–355, 1987

Ball SG, Otto MW, Pollack MH, et al: Predicting prospective episodes of depression in patients with panic disorder: a longitudinal study. J Consult Clin Psychol 62:359–365, 1994

Ballenger JC, Fyer AJ: Panic disorder and agoraphobia, in DSM-IV Sourcebook, Vol 2. Edited by Widiger TA, Frances AJ, Pincus HA, et al. Washington, DC, American Psychiatric Association, 1996, pp 411–471

Barlow DH, Vermilyea J, Blanchard EB, et al: The phenomenon of panic. J Abnorm Psychol 94:320–328, 1985

Batelaan N, Smit F, de Graaf R, et al: Economic costs of full-blown and subthreshold panic disorder. J Affect Disord 104:127–136, 2007

Bauer MS, Altshuler L, Evans DR, et al: Prevalence and distinct correlates of anxiety, substance, and combined comorbidity in a multi-site public sector sample with bipolar disorder. J Affect Disord 85:301–315, 2005

Beck AT, Steer RA, Sanderson WC, et al: Panic disorder and suicidal ideation and behavior: discrepant findings in psychiatric outpatients. Am J Psychiatry 148:1195–1199, 1991

Berg I: School phobia in the children of agoraphobic women. Br J Psychiatry 128:86–89, 1976

Berg I, Marks I, McGuire R, et al: School phobia and agoraphobia. Psychol Med 4:428–434, 1974

Berkson S: Limitations of the application of fourfold table analysis to hospital data. Biometrics Bulletin 2:47–53, 1946

Biederman J, Faraone S, Marrs A, et al: Panic disorder and agoraphobia in consecutively referred children and adolescents. J Am Acad Child Adolesc Psychiatry 36:214–223, 1997

Bolton J, Cox B, Clara I, et al: Use of alcohol and drugs to self-medicate anxiety disorders in a nationally representative sample. J Nerv Ment 194:818–825, 2006

Breier A, Charney DS, Heninger GR: Major depression in patients with agoraphobia and panic disorder. Arch Gen Psychiatry 41:1129–1135, 1984

Breier A, Charney DS, Heninger GR: Agoraphobia with panic attacks: development, diagnostic stability, and course of illness. Arch Gen Psychiatry 43:1029–1036, 1986

Bridges KW, Goldberg BP: Somatic presentation of DSM-III psychiatric disorders in primary care. J Psychsom Res 29:563–569, 1985

Candilis PJ, McLean RY, Otto MW, et al: Quality of life in patients with panic disorder. J Nerv Ment Dis 187:429–434, 1999

Conway KP, Compton W, Stinson FS, et al: Lifetime comorbidity of DSM-IV mood and anxiety disorders and specific drug use disorders: results from the National Epidemiologic Survey on Alcohol and Related Conditions. J Clin Psychiatry 67:247–257, 2006

Coryell W, Noyes R, Clancy J: Excess mortality in panic disorder. Arch Gen Psychiatry 39:701–703, 1982

Cox BJ, Direnfeld DM, Swinson RP, et al: Suicidal ideation and suicide attempts in panic disorder and social phobia. Am J Psychiatry 151:882–887, 1994

Cramer V, Torgersen S, Kringlen E: Quality of life and anxiety disorders: a population study. J Nerv Ment Dis 193:196–202, 2005

Eaton WW: Progress in the epidemiology of anxiety disorders. Epidemiol Rev 17:32–38, 1995

Eaton WW, Keyl P: Risk factors for the onset of Diagnostic Interview Schedule/DSM III agoraphobia in a prospective population-based study. Arch Gen Psychiatry 47:819–824, 1990

Eaton WW, Kessler RC, Wittchen HU, et al: Panic and panic disorder in the United States. Am J Psychiatry 151:413–420, 1994

Fava G, Grandi S, Canestrari R: Prodromal symptoms in panic disorder with agoraphobia. Am J Psychiatry 145:1564–1567, 1988

Fawcett J, Scheftner WA, Fogg L, et al: Time-related predictors of suicide in major affective disorder. Am J Psychiatry 147:1189–1194, 1990

Frank E, Cyranowski JM, Rucci P, et al: Clinical significance of lifetime panic spectrum symptoms in the treatment of patients with Bipolar 1 disorder. Arch Gen Psychiatry 59:905–911, 2002

Friedman S, Jones JC, Chernen L, et al: Suicidal ideation and suicide attempts among patients with panic disorder: a survey of two outpatient clinics. Am J Psychiatry 149:680–685, 1992

Gaudiano BA, Miller IW: Anxiety disorder comorbidity in bipolar I disorder: relationship to depression severity and treatment outcome. Depress Anxiety 21:71–77, 2005

Goisman R, Warshaw M, Steketee G, et al: DSM-IV and the disappearance of agoraphobia without a history of panic disorder: new data on a controversial diagnosis. Am J Psychiatry 152:1438–1443, 1995

Goodwin RD, Roy-Byrne PP: Panic and suicidal ideation and suicide attempts: results from the National Comorbidity Survey. Depress Anxiety 23:124–132, 2006

Goodwin RD, Jacobi F, Thefeld W: Mental disorders and asthma in the community. Arch Gen Psychiatry 60:1125–1130, 2003

Grant BF, Hasin DS, Stinson FS, et al: The epidemiology of DSM-IV panic disorder and agoraphobia in the United States: results from the National Epidemiologic Survey on Alcohol and Related Conditions. J Clin Psychiatry 67:363–374, 2006

Hettema JM, Prescott CA, Myers JM, et al: The structure of genetic and environmental risk factors for anxiety disorders in men and women. Arch Gen Psychiatry 62:182–189, 2005

Hornig CD, McNally RJ: Panic disorder and suicide attempt. A reanalysis of data from the Epidemiologic Catchment Area Study. Br J Psychiatry 167:76–79, 1995

Horwath E, Lish J, Johnson J, et al: Agoraphobia without panic: clinical reappraisal of an epidemiologic finding. Am J Psychiatry 150:1496–1501, 1993

Horwath E, Wolk SI, Goldstein RB, et al: Is the comorbidity between social phobia and panic disorder due to familial cotransmission or other factors? Arch Gen Psychiatry 52:574–582, 1995

Kaabi B, Gelernter J, Woods SW, et al: Genome scan for loci predisposing to anxiety disorders using a novel multivariate approach strong evidence for a chromosome 4 risk locus. Am J Hum Genet 78:543–553, 2006

Karajgi B, Rifkin A, Doddi S, et al: The prevalence of anxiety disorders in patients with chronic obstructive pulmonary disease. Am J Psychiatry 147:200–201, 1990

Katon W: Panic disorder and somatization: a review of 55 cases. Am J Med 77:101–106, 1984

Katon W, Vitaliano PP, Russo J, et al: Panic disorder: epidemiology in primary care. J Fam Pract 23:233–239, 1986

Kawachi I, Colditz GA, Ascherio A, et al: Prospective study of phobic anxiety and risk of coronary heart disease in men. Circulation 89:1992–1997, 1994a

Kawachi I, Sparrow D, Vokonas PS: Symptoms of anxiety and risk of coronary heart disease. The Normative Aging Study. Circulation 90:2225–2229, 1994b

Kessler RC, Ustün TB: The World Mental Health (WMH) Survey Initiative Version of the World Health Organization (WHO) Composite International Diagnostic Interview (CIDI). Int J Methods Psychiatr Res 13:93–121, 2004

Kessler RC, McGonagle KA, Zhao S, et al: Lifetime and 12-month prevalence of DSM-III-R psychiatric disorders in the United States: results from the National Comorbidity Survey. Arch Gen Psychiatry 51:8–19, 1994

Kessler RC, Stang PE, Wittchen HU, et al: Lifetime panic-depression comorbidity in the National Comorbidity Survey. Arch Gen Psychiatry 55:801–808, 1998

Kessler RC, Berglund P, Demler O, et al: The epidemiology of major depressive disorder: results from the National Comorbidity Survey Replication (NCS-R). JAMA 289:3095–3105, 2003a

Kessler RC, Ormel J, Demler O, et al: Comorbid mental disorders account for the role impairment of commonly occurring chronic physical disorders: results from the National Comorbidity Survey. J Occup Environ Med 45:1257–1266, 2003b

Kessler RC, Chiu WT, Jin R, et al: The epidemiology of panic attacks, panic disorder, and agoraphobia in the National Comorbidity Survey Replication. Arch Gen Psychiatry 63:415–424, 2006

Klein DF: Delineation of two drug responsive anxiety syndromes. Psychopharmacologia 5:397–408, 1964

Klein DF: Anxiety reconceptualized, in Anxiety: New Research and Changing Concepts. Edited by Klein DF, Rabkin JG. New York, Raven, 1981, pp 235–264

Klein DF, Klein H: The nosology, genetics, and theory of spontaneous panic and phobia, in Psychopharmacology of Anxiety. Edited by Tyrer P. Oxford, England, Oxford University Press, 1989, pp 163–195

Klerman GL, Weissman MM, Ouellette R, et al: Panic attacks in the community: social morbidity and health care utilization. JAMA 265:742–746, 1991

Lecrubier Y, Ustün TB: Panic and depression: a worldwide primary care perspective. Int Clin Psychopharmacol 13(suppl):S7–S11, 1998

Lelliott P, Marks I, McNamee G, et al: Onset of panic disorder with agoraphobia: toward an integrated model. Arch Gen Psychiatry 46:1000–1004, 1989

Magee WJ, Eaton WW, Wittchen H-U, et al: Agoraphobia, simple phobia, and social phobia in the National Comorbidity Survey. Arch Gen Psychiatry 53:159–168, 1996

Manfro GG, Otto MW, McArdle ET, et al: Relationship of antecedent stressful life events to childhood and family history of anxiety and the course of panic disorder. J Affect Disord 41:135–139, 1996

Margraf J, Taylor CB, Ehlers A, et al: Panic attacks in the natural environment. J Nerv Ment Dis 175:558–565, 1987

Markowitz JS, Weissman MM, Ouellette R, et al: Quality of life in panic disorder. Arch Gen Psychiatry 46:984–992, 1989

Marks IM: Fears, Phobias, and Rituals: Panic, Anxiety, and Their Disorders. New York, Oxford University Press, 1987

McElroy SL, Keck PE, Nolen WA, et al: Axis I psychiatric comorbidity and its relationship to historical illness variables in 288 patients with bipolar disorder. Am J Psychiatry 158:420–426, 2001

Norton GR, Harrison B, Hauch J, et al: Characteristics of people with infrequent panic attacks. J Abnorm Psychol 94:216–221, 1985

Norton GR, Dorward J, Cox BJ: Factors associated with panic attacks in nonclinical subjects. Behav Ther 17:239–252, 1986

Norton GR, Cox BJ, Malan J: Nonclinical panickers: a critical review. Clin Psychol Rev 12:121–139, 1992

Noyes R, Crowe RR, Harris EL, et al: Relationship between panic disorder and agoraphobia: a family study. Arch Gen Psychiatry 43:227–232, 1986

Noyes R, Clancy J, Garvey M: Is agoraphobia a variant of panic disorder or a separate illness? J Anxiety Disord 1:3–13, 1987

Orleans CT, George LK, Houpt JL, et al: How primary care physicians treat psychiatric disorders: a national survey of family practitioners. Am J Psychiatry 142:52–57, 1985

Ormel J, VonKorff M, Ustun TB, et al: Common mental disorders and disability across cultures. JAMA 272:1741–1748, 1994

Otto MW, Pollack MH, Sachs GS, et al: Alcohol dependence in panic disorder patients. J Psychiatr Res 26:29–38, 1992

Otto MW, Gould R, Pollack MH: Cognitive-behavioral treatment of panic disorder: considerations of the treatment of patients over the long term. Psychiatr Ann 24:299–306, 1994

Otto MW, Simon NM, Wisniewski SR, et al: Prospective 12-month course of bipolar disorder in outpatients with and without anxiety comorbidity. Br J Psychiatry 189:20–25, 2006

Pohl R, Jampala V, Balon R, et al: Effects of nortriptyline and paroxetine on QT variability in patients with panic disorder. Depress Anxiety 11:126–130, 2000

Pollack MH, Otto MW, Majcher D, et al: Relationship of childhood anxiety to adult panic disorder: correlates and influence on course. Am J Psychiatry 153:376–381, 1996

Pollard C, Bronson S, Kenney M: Prevalence of agoraphobia without panic in clinical settings (letter). Am J Psychiatry 146:559, 1989

Regier DA, Boyd JH, Burke JD, et al: One-month prevalence of mental disorders in the United States. Arch Gen Psychiatry 45:977–986, 1988

Robins LN, Helzer JE, Orvaschel H, et al: The Diagnostic Interview Schedule, in Epidemiologic Field Methods in Psychiatry: The NIMH Epidemiologic Catchment Area Program. Edited by Eaton WW, Kessler LG. New York, Academic Press, 1985, pp 143–170

Roy-Byrne PP, Geraci M, Uhde TW: Life events and course of illness in patients with panic disorder. Am J Psychiatry 143:1033–1035, 1986

Roy-Byrne PP, Stein MB, Russo J, et al: Panic disorder in the primary care setting: comorbidity, disability, service utilization, and treatment. J Clin Psychiatry 60:492–499, 1999

Rubin HC, Rapaport MH, Levine B, et al: Quality of well being in panic disorder: the assessment of psychiatric and general disability. J Affect Disord 57:217–221, 2000

Salvador-Carulla L, Segui J, Fernandez-Cano P, et al: Costs and offset effect in panic disorders. Br J Psychiatry 166(suppl):23–28, 1995

Sareen J, Cox BJ, Afifi TO, et al: Anxiety disorders and risk for suicidal ideation and suicide attempts: a population-based longitudinal study of adults. Arch Gen Psychiatry 62:1249–1257, 2005a

Sarren J, Cox BJ, Clara I, et al: The relationship between anxiety disorders and physical disorders in the U.S. National Comorbidity Survey. Depress Anxiety 21:193–202, 2005b

Sareen J, Chartier M, Paulus MP, et al: Illicit drug use and anxiety disorders: findings from two community surveys. Psychiatry Res 142:11–17, 2006

Sartorius N, Ustün TB, Costa e Silva JA, et al: An international study of psychological problems in primary care: preliminary report from the World Health Organization Collaborative Project on "Psychological problems in general health care." Arch Gen Psychiatry 50:819–824, 1993

Shear MK, Maser JD: Standardized assessment for panic disorder research: a conference report. Arch Gen Psychiatry 51:346–354, 1994

Shear MK, Brown TA, Barlow DH, et al: Multicenter Collaborative Panic Disorder Severity Scale. Am J Psychiatry 154:1571–1575, 1997

Simon GE, VonKorff M: Somatization and psychiatric disorders in the NIMH Epidemiologic Catchment Area study. Am J Psychiatry 148:1494–1500, 1991

Simon NM, Blacker D, Korbly NB, et al: Hypothyroidism and hyperthyroidism in anxiety disorders revisited: new data and literature review. J Affect Disord 69:209–217, 2002

Simon NM, Otto MW, Weiss RD, et al: Pharmacotherapy for bipolar disorder and comorbid conditions: Baseline data from the STEP-BD. J Clin Psychopharmacol 24:512–520, 2004a

Simon NM, Otto MW, Wisniewski SR, et al: Anxiety disorder comorbidity in bipolar disorder patients: data from the first 500 participants in the Systematic Treatment Enhancement Program for Bipolar Disorder (STEP-BD). Am J Psychiatry 161:2222–2229, 2004b

Smoller JW, Tsuang MT: Panic and phobic anxiety: defining phenotypes for genetic studies. Am J Psychiatry 155:1152–1162, 1998

Smoller JW, Acierno JS Jr, Rosenbaum JF, et al: Targeted genome screen of panic disorder and anxiety disorder proneness using homology to murine QTL regions. Am J Med Genet 105:195–206, 2001

Smoller JW, Pollack MH, Wassertheil-Smoller S, et al: Panic attacks and risk of incident cardiovascular events among postmenopausal women in the Women's Health Initiative Observational Study. Arch Gen Psychiatry 64:1153–1160, 2007

Smoller JW, Gardner-Schuster E, Covino J: The genetic basis of panic and phobic anxiety disorders. Am J Med Genet C Semin Med Genet 148:118–126, 2008

Staab JP, Ruckenstein MJ, Amsterdam JD: A prospective trial of sertraline for chronic subjective dizziness. Larygoscope 114:1637–1641, 2004

Stein MB, Tancer ME, Uhde TW: Major depression in patients with panic disorder: factors associated with course and recurrence. J Affect Disord 19:287–296, 1990

Thyer B, Himle J: Temporal relationship between panic attack onset and phobic avoidance in agoraphobia. Behav Res Ther 23:607–608, 1985

Thyer B, Himle J, Curtis G, et al: A comparison of panic disorder and agoraphobia with panic attacks. Compr Psychiatry 26:208–214, 1985

Tucker P, Adamson P, Miranda R Jr, et al: Paroxetine increases heart rate variability in panic disorder. J Clin Psychopharmacol 17:370–376, 1997

Vickers K, McNally RJ: Panic Disorder and suicide attempt in the National Comorbidity Survey. J Abnorm Psychol 113:582–591, 2004

Weissman MM, Klerman GL, Markowitz JS, et al: Suicidal ideation and suicide attempts in panic disorder and attacks. N Engl J Med 321:1209–1214, 1989

Weissman MM, Bland RC, Canino GJ, et al: The cross-national epidemiology of panic disorder. Arch Gen Psychiatry 54:305–309, 1997

Wells KB, Stewart A, Hays RD, et al: The functioning and well-being of depressed patients: results from the Medical Outcomes Study. JAMA 262:914–919, 1989

Wittchen HU, Robins LN, Cottler LB, et al: Cross-cultural feasibility, reliability and sources of variance of the Composite International Diagnostic Interview (CIDI). Br J Psychiatry 159:645–653, 1991

World Health Organization: The ICD-10 Classification of Mental and Behavioural Disorders: Clinical Descriptions and Diagnostic Guidelines. Geneva, Switzerland, World Health Organization, 1992

Yeragani VK, Pohl R, Jampala VC, et al: Increased QT variability in patients with panic disorder and depression. Psychiatry Res 93:225–235, 2000

Recommended Readings

Craske MG, Waters AM: Panic disorder, phobias, and generalized anxiety disorder. Annu Rev Clin Psychol 1:197–225, 2005

Katon WJ: Panic disorder. N Engl J Med 354:2360–2367, 2006

Pollack MH, Otto MW (eds): Longitudinal Perspectives on Anxiety Disorders. Psychiatric Clinics of North America, Vol 18. Philadelphia, PA, WB Saunders, 1995

Rosenbaum JF, Pollack MH (eds): Panic Disorder and Its Treatment. New York, Marcel Dekker, 1998

Smoller JW, Sheidley BR, Tsuang MT (eds): Psychiatric Genetics: Applications in Clinical Practice. Washington, DC, American Psychiatric Publishing, 2008

Web Sites of Interest

Anxiety Disorders Association of America. http://www.adaa.org

Center for Anxiety and Traumatic Stress Disorders, Massachusetts General Hospital. http://www.mghanxiety.org

National Institute of Mental Health: Panic Disorder. http://www.nimh.nih.gov/health/topics/panic-disorder/index.shtml

Chapter 22

Pathogenesis of Panic Disorder

Ranjeeb Shrestha, M.D.
Navin Natarajan, M.D.
Jeremy D. Coplan, M.D.

Panic disorder is a chronic illness characterized by progression through three symptom domains: 1) the initial unexpected panic attacks, 2) the subsequent persistent concern for future attacks, and 3) avoidance of perceived environmental triggers of the panic attack (American Psychiatric Association 2000). Despite the significant progress made in the arena of effective drug treatments and the beneficial utility of cognitive-behavioral therapy (CBT), the etiology of panic disorder and the precise mechanisms underlying effective treatment remain unclear.

In this chapter, the pathogenesis of panic disorder is reviewed using an integrated overview of the many theories and recent developments in this rapidly advancing field. The innovative concepts that have emerged in psychiatric genetics and the progress that has been made in understanding gene-by-environment interactions are elaborated. In addition to the neurobiology of panic disorder, other theories of pathogenesis, including dynamic, cognitive-behavioral, and hyperventilation models, are also reviewed. Finally, the possible directions of future research in this dynamic field will be discussed.

Historical Background

The symptoms of panic disorder have long been recognized under various guises: soldier's heart, DaCosta's syndrome, and cardiac neurosis all referred to a symptomatology reminiscent of modern-day panic disorder (Demitrack and Abbey 1996). Presumably, the disorder has also been subsumed under other sundry diagnoses such as hypochondriacal neurosis, hyperventilatory syndrome, and neurocirculatory anesthesia (Block and Szidon 1994).

One of the critical factors in spurring the notion that panic disorder may have a "chemical" basis was the discovery by Klein and Fink (1962) that the tricyclic antidepressant imipramine effectively blocked the panic attacks often observed in patients with anxiety neurosis. The spontaneous panic attack was viewed as the core pathology of panic disorder, with subsequent development of anticipatory anxiety and phobic avoidance as secondary symptoms (Klein 1964). Those patients with anxiety neurosis without panic attacks were subsequently categorized as having generalized anxiety disorder. Twenty-five years following Klein's seminal observations, Dr. Gorman and colleagues in 1989 proposed their first neuroanatomical model for panic disorder, which was modified in 2000. Gorman's neuroanatomical models continue to remain important catalysts for research in the biological model of panic disorder. In tandem with the development of biological models, theories based on respiration, such as the hyperventilation model by Ley (1985) and the false suffocation alarm model by Klein (1993), have been proposed.

Different schools of psychology, from psychodynamic to cognitive-behavioral theories, have been described to advance understanding of the pathogenesis of panic disorder. Contemporary models incorporating biological vulnerabilities along with dynamic, cognitive, and learned behavior have yielded rich perspectives in understanding and treating panic disorder. In this chapter, the relationship between the seemingly disparate biological, respiratory, and psychological theories will be explored.

Biological Theories of Panic

Evidence for a biological basis of panic disorder was provided by the observation that a range of psychotropic medications, in addition to imipramine, eliminated or at least significantly ameliorated panic disorder symptoms. Currently accepted medications for panic disorder include the selective serotonin reuptake inhibitors (SSRIs), the tricyclic antidepressants, the high-potency benzodiazepines, and the reversible and irreversible monoamine oxidase inhibitors (MAOIs) (Coplan et al. 1996b).

The acute pharmacological effects of psychotropic medications prompted speculation that specific neurotransmitter systems may be directly implicated in the onset, maintenance, and/or progression of the illness. Biological theories therefore include noradrenergic (a component of acute tricyclic antidepressant effects), serotonergic (SSRI and tricyclic antidepressant mechanism of action), and GABAergic (high-potency benzodiazepine mechanism of action) systems.

Noradrenergic Theory

Redmond (1981) conducted seminal studies in chair-restrained rhesus monkeys, demonstrating that direct electrical stimulation of the locus coeruleus, a collection of noradrenalin-producing neurons located bilaterally in the pons area, produced fear responses reminiscent of animals being threatened by a predator. Additional evidence was provided for the view that noradrenergic stimulation was implicated in fear and anxiety responses by the observation that administration of the α_2 antagonists yohimbine and piperoxane produced behavioral effects analogous to those of direct electrical stimulation. These important preclinical studies led investigators to study the noradrenergic system in panic disorder.

When considering a single individual noradrenergic neuron, three important synaptic junctions are emphasized. The first concerns the α_2 autoreceptor mechanism, which regulates firing of the neuron by mediating negative feedback inhibition. α_2 Antagonists interrupt this negative feedback, whereas α_2 agonists, such as the centrally acting antihypertensive agent clonidine, enhance negative feedback. The latter therefore reduces noradrenergic firing and diminishes anxiety, at least on a temporary basis. The second synaptic junction of importance concerns afferent projections that synapse on noradrenergic neurons. These include inhibitory (serotonergic and GABAergic) and excitatory (glutamatergic) inputs. Thus, the three neurotransmitter systems affected by antipanic drugs intersect at the noradrenergic neuron. The final synaptic junction is between noradrenergic axonal efferents and an extensive range of projection sites ranging from the prefrontal cortex to the spinal cord. Efferent axons of locus coeruleus that project to the hypothalamus are of special significance to panic disorder (Charney and Heninger 1986). In the hypothalamus, norepinephrine terminals synapse onto two important neuroendocrine systems, leading to the release of corticotropin-releasing factor (CRF) and growth hormone–releasing factor into the portal circulation. The release of these two peptide-releasing factors produces activation of the hypothalamic-pituitary-adrenal (HPA) axis and the hypothalamic-pituitary-somatotropin (HPS) axis, respectively.

Several groups of investigators (Abelson et al. 1992; Charney and Heninger 1986; Nutt 1989; Uhde et al. 1992) have conducted important studies of the noradrenergic system in panic disorder. In keeping with the notion that noradrenergic stimulation would increase anxiety, they showed that yohimbine administration produced panic attacks in patients with panic disorder. Studies that used clonidine, which stimulates release of growth hormone-releasing factor through α_2 agonism in the hypothalamus, indicated that the growth hormone response to clonidine was blunted in patients with panic disorder. The same blunting has been observed in major depressive disorder and generalized anxiety disorder. In panic disorder, the blunting of the growth hormone response to clonidine was thought to reflect downmodulation of postsynaptic α_2 receptors following chronic noradrenergic discharge. In addition, studies indicated that the degree of blood pressure decrease, cortisol secretion, and noradrenergic turnover regularly induced by clonidine administration was exaggerated in panic disorder. Coplan and colleagues (1997a, 1997b) have speculated that the noradrenergic system may be dysregulated in panic disorder. Dysregulation may be viewed as an inability of the usual homeostatic mechanisms to contain perturbations of a neurotransmitter system from either excessive activation or inhibition. For example, in comparison with psychiatrically healthy control subjects, panic disorder patients exhibit markedly elevated within-subject volatility of plasma levels of the noradrenergic metabolite 3-methoxy-4-hydroxy-phenylglycol (MHPG), despite the tonic inhibition induced by clonidine administration.

In cognitively healthy subjects, under both baseline and stressful conditions, the noradrenergic system and the HPA axis appear to work in synchrony. Elevations or reductions of activity within the one system are accompanied by parallel changes in the other system. The coordinated interaction between these two systems has been cited by Chrousos and Gold (1992) as crucial for the mammalian organism's stress response. If noradrenergic function is hyperactive in panic disorder, as has been documented, the question is raised as to how the HPA axis responds and whether healthy synchronization of the two systems remains intact. Thus, there is evidence that the two systems become "desynchronized" in panic disorder in order to protect against noradrenergic-driven activation of the HPA axis (Coplan et al. 1995). However, moderate HPA axis activation in panic disorder suggests that the desynchronization is not completely successful (Coplan et al. 1995).

Serotonergic Theory

The serotonergic system has long been a major area of focus not only for panic disorder but also for psychiatry as a whole. The rostral nuclei appear most relevant to psychiatry, with prominent projections to neocortex. A range of more caudal nuclei modulate autonomic responses and have received less attention. The two major rostral nuclei are 1) the dorsal raphe, which provides projections to the cerebral cortex (primarily the prefrontal) and to the basal ganglia and the nucleus locus coeruleus; and 2) the median raphe, which likewise projects to the cerebral cortex, but also projects strongly to limbic structures such as the hippocampus.

Although approximately 15 serotonin receptor subtypes have now been discovered, neurotransmission through 5-HT_{1A} receptors located on pyramidal neurons of the hippocampus has been viewed as crucial by Deakin (1996) in engendering a sense of resilience to the organism. If neurotransmission at this site is inadequate, anxiety and avoidant behavior may ensue. Serotonergic neurotransmission via the 5-HT_{1A} receptor is also an important stimulus for expression of brain-derived neurotrophic factor in the hippocampus. Brain-derived neurotrophic factor is a potent promoter of dentate gyrus neurogenesis, which has been associated with antidepressant response. Activation of the HPA axis, which occurs phasically in panic disorder (Coplan et al. 1998a), may contribute to disruption of hippocampal 5-HT_{1A} neurotransmission by uncoupling the 5-HT_{1A} receptor from its intracellular G-protein messenger system (Lesch and Lerer 1991) and may therefore suppress neurogenesis.

A potential role in panic disorder for aberrant noradrenergic-serotonergic function has been posited. Investigation of the impact of serotonin on noradrenergic function was prompted by the uniform and superior antipanic effects of the SSRIs (Boyer 1995). Supporting a stabilizing effect of serotonin on the locus coeruleus, noradrenergic volatility levels declined to control levels when challenged with clonidine. Not all studies support such a clear inhibitory or stabilizing role of SSRIs on noradrenergic function. Goddard and colleagues (1993) reported that although fluvoxamine attenuated the anxiogenic effects of yohimbine in patients with panic disorder, it failed to block the yohimbine-induced MHPG increase.

Hyperventilation is one of the cardinal physiological correlates of panic anxiety. Some researchers have suggested a link between the serotonergic system and hyperventilation derived from the clinical observation that serotonin exerts clinical benefit through enhancement of serotonin neurotransmission, and a normalization of ventilatory overdrive accompanies clinical improvement of panic disorder. In animal studies, deficient serotonin neurotransmission, through administration of the noncompetitive serotonin antagonist parachlorophenylalanine, produced hyperventilation and carbon dioxide sensitivity (Olson et al. 1979). Conversely, increasing serotonin neurotransmission in rats with the serotonin precursor 5-hydroxytryptophan depressed ventilation and reduced carbon dioxide sensitivity (Lundberg et al. 1980). Kent et al. (1996) depleted serotonin using a tryptophan-free highly concentrated amino acid mixture, which resulted in a reduction in serotonin neurotransmission along with an increase in minute ventilation in panic disorder patients. However, control subjects' ventilatory function remained unaltered despite depletion. Evidence therefore indicates that serotonin does play a role in human ventilation and that patients with panic disorder are particularly sensitive to serotonin depletion. Enhancement of serotonin neurotransmission by an SSRI thus may exert therapeutic effects by normalizing aberrant ventilatory patterns, in addition to normalizing noradrenergic dysregulation.

It is a common clinical observation that patients who are started on SSRI initially complain of increased anxiety, but over the course of a few weeks the anxiety actually decreases. Investigators have found an association between the short arm of the serotonin transporter gene and the jitteriness syndrome (Perlis et al. 2003). One plausible hypothesis is based on knockout mice, whereby knockout of the serotonin transporter results in an increase in dorsal raphe serotonin, hyperpolarization of serotonin neurons via the 5-HT_{1A} presynaptic autoreceptor, and a deficit in postsynaptic 5-HT, with anxiogenic effects. The role of the serotonin transporter gene will be elaborated in greater details later in this chapter.

GABAergic Theory

In the brain, γ-aminobutyric acid (GABA) is the most important and ubiquitous inhibitory neurotransmitter, whereas glutamate is the most prominent excitatory neurotransmitter. The balance between GABA and glutamate activities is critical. If the GABA activity overwhelms the glutamate activity, then sedation, ataxia, and amnesia result. On the other hand, if the GABA activity is attenuated, then an increase in arousal, restlessness, insomnia, and, more importantly, anxiety may result (Nutt and Malizia 2001). The $GABA_A$–benzodiazepine receptor complex consists of five protein subunits that are arranged like a rosette with a central core permeable to chloride and other ions (Nayeem et al. 1994; Schofield et al. 1987). When GABA binds with this complex, it induces conformational change, which increases the permeability of the chloride ions. The resulting chloride flux hyperpolarizes the neuron, reducing the excitability of the neurons and producing a generalized inhibitory effect in neuronal activities (Nutt and Malizia 2001).

Benzodiazepine allosterically changes the receptor complex to increase the efficiency of GABA, enabling the GABAergic circuits to produce a larger inhibitory effect.

Various regions of the brain known to be associated with panic symptoms have been identified neuroradiologically to have abnormalities in the binding of benzodiazepine-$GABA_A$ receptor complexes. In a study by Malizia and colleagues (1998), positron emission tomography (PET) scanning was used to detect benzodiazepine binding sites on the $GABA_A$ receptor complexes using radioligand ^{11}C-labeled flumazenil in both panic disorder patients and controls. Patients with panic disorder were found to have a global decrease in benzodiazepine binding, with the peak decrease occurring in the orbitofrontal complex and the insula. These regions are believed to have crucial roles in panic disorder. In a follow-up study by Cameron and colleagues (2006) using the same flumazenil–^{11}C ligand, benzodiazepine binding was found to be decreased in the insular cortex in patients with panic disorder, suggesting attenuated inhibitory effect of GABA on that region. The insula is related to visceral-somatic afferent and efferent functions. Its overactivation due to the decreased inhibition from GABA could lead to some of the visceral-somatic symptoms that are seen in panic disorder. Other studies using single-photon emission computed tomography (SPECT) and iomazenil as the radioligand have also shown decreases in benzodiazepine receptor complexes, particularly in the temporal cortex, the hippocampus, and the precuneus (Bremner et al. 2000; Kaschka et al. 1995). Similarly, Goddard et al. (2001) demonstrated that there was a decrease in GABA binding in the occipital regions of brain using ^{1}H magnetic resonance spectroscopic technique.

Several preclinical studies have shed significant light on the relationship between GABA-glutamate and panic disorder. In a study on rodents by researchers at Indiana University, $GABA_A$ neurotransmissions were blocked in the dorsomedial hypothalamus (DMH), an area believed to be associated with panic disorder, using L–allylglycine (L-AG). When that cohort of rats as well as controls were injected with sodium lactate, a known panicogen, panic-like responses were seen only in the $GABA_A$-blocked rats (Shekhar et al. 1996). In a follow-up study by Johnson and Shekhar (2006), glutamate-mediated *N*-methyl-D-aspartate (NMDA) excitatory receptors were also blocked in the rats with chronic inhibition of GABA synthesis. When this cohort of rats was injected with sodium lactate, there was no panic like response, demonstrating the role of GABA-glutamate imbalance in the genesis of panic symptoms.

Glutamic acid decarboxylase (GAD) is an enzyme that converts the amino acid glutamate into GABA. Studies conducted on *GAD65*, which is one of the genes coding for GAD, have shed light on the role of abnormalities in the synthesis of GABA in panic disorder. In mice whose *GAD65* gene was knocked out, there were higher levels of spontaneous fear behavior, increase in fear conditioning, and a blunting in the behavioral sensitivity to benzodiazepines, even though there was no alteration in the density of postsynaptic $GABA_A$ receptors (Stork et al. 2000).

Role of Panicogens in Panic Disorder

Pitts and McClure (1967) were the first researchers to demonstrate that panic attacks could be induced in the laboratory by sodium lactate injection. Since then, a plethora of panicogens have been and continue to be discovered. Panicogens can be broadly classified into two groups. The first group of panicogens may work by activating the HPA axis and other specific neurotransmitter systems. They include, among others, cholecystokinin (CCK), yohimbine, caffeine, *m*-chlorophenylpiperazine (m-CPP) and *N*-methyl-β-carboline-3-carboxamide. Among the first group of panicogens, CCK, which is found both in the gastrointestinal regions and in the brain, has been extensively studied and appears to act through central CCK-4 receptors in the brain, possibly leading to release of adrenocorticotropic hormone (ACTH) from the pituitary (Strohle et al. 2000). However, the significance of CCK in the pathophysiology of panic disorder is in doubt, because studies using CCK-4 antagonists have not uniformly prevented panic attacks (Netto and Guimaraes 2003; Pande et al. 1999). As we have discussed earlier, yohimbine is an α_2-adrenergic receptor antagonist that causes a surge in the release of norepinephrine. Caffeine is known to induce panic attack in some susceptible individuals through antagonism at the adenosine receptors, especially the adenosine 2A receptor (Hamilton et al. 2004). Notably, adenosine is the second most common inhibitory neurotransmitter in the central nervous system, after GABA. m-CPP acts as a nonspecific serotonergic agonist, while *N*-methyl-β-carboline-3-carboxamide acts as a benzodiazepine inverse agonist.

The second group of panicogens includes carbon dioxide, sodium bicarbonate, and sodium lactate, among others. It is likely this group of panicogens share a mechanism of action that involves lactate metabolism as a common pathway. The mechanism of action of lactate in panic disorder has been a matter of significant controversy. Researchers using rodents have demonstrated that lactate via osmosensitive periventricular pathways such as the organum vasculosom of lamina terminalis activates the GABA-deficient dorsomedial hypothalamic nucleus/perifornical regions, crucial areas of brain known to trigger a cascade of responses leading to panic-like symptoms (Johnson et al. 2007; Shekhar and Keim 1997). The latter observations may help explain why panic is associated with ventilatory dysregulation, given that respiratory alkalosis leads to an increase in blood and brain lactate concentrations. Interestingly, voluntary hyperventilation is not a potent panicogenic procedure, suggesting inhibitory modulation or top-down governance by the prefrontal cortex (Gorman et al. 1994).

Although Gorman et al. (1989) originally proposed that panicogens activate brain stem sites, a subsequent view based on an extended database posits that panicogens induce panic through nonspecific activation of a frontolimbic fear network (Gorman et al. 2000). The topic of fear networks will be explored in greater detail later in this chapter.

Role of Genetics in the Pathogenesis of Panic Disorder

In recent years there have been significant advances in our knowledge of the role of genetics in the pathogenesis of panic disorder. As in all psychiatric disorders, the role of genetics in panic disorder is complex, with multiple genes likely conferring vulnerability to the disorder by still-unknown mechanisms. Two twin studies have attributed 30%–40% of the variance for the liability to develop panic disorder to genetic factors (Kendler et al. 2001; Scherrer et al. 2000). In a meta-analysis of five family studies on panic disorder, researchers from the Medical College of Virginia reported a highly significant association between panic disorder diagnosis in probands and panic disorder diagnosis in first-degree relatives. The odds ratio average across the five studies was 5.0, strongly suggesting a familial component to panic disorder liability (Hettema et al. 2001).

There are three major approaches to psychiatric genetic studies. The first approach involves searching for a direct linear relationship between genes and behavior and includes processes such as linkage analysis and association analysis; the second involves identification of panic disorder endophenotypes; and the third involves studying gene-by-environment interactions.

The search for a direct gene-behavior relationship has concentrated on genes deemed functionally significant in the pathophysiology of panic disorder. The central CCK system has received considerable scrutiny. However, evidence regarding the role of CCK-related genes in panic disorder is conflicting. Although the role of CCK-4 as panicogen is well established (Netto and Guimaraes 2004; Rehfeld 2000), studies linking CCK genes to panic attacks have yielded conflicting results (Hosing et al. 2004; Wang et al. 1998). Another biological system that has been implicated in panic disorder is that of adenosine, a purine nucleoside. An association study by Deckert and his group (1998) and a linkage study by Hamilton et al. (2004) both found significant associations between the adenosine 2A coding region and panic disorder. This successful replication is considered among the first for genetic studies of panic disorder.

Monoamine oxidase type A (MAO A) is an enzyme that acts as a catalyst in the oxidation of monoamines such as 5-HT and norepinephrine, thus leading to their inactivation. Several genetic studies have shown association between MAO A genes and panic disorder, especially in female patients (Deckert et al. 1999; Maron et al. 2005b; Samochowiec et. al. 2004). However, a study by Hamilton et al. (2000) in twins did not support this association.

The gene coding for the enzyme cathechol-*O*-methyltransferase (COMT), which is involved in the inactivation of catecholamines, has also been implicated in panic disorder. Two alleles encoding for this gene include the H and L alleles. The L allele is associated with low activity and encodes for methionine, whereas the H allele is associated with higher activity and encodes for valine. A Korean study with 54 panic disorder patients reported higher proportions of the L/L genotype in patients with panic disorder as well as poorer treatment response in comparison with other genotypes such as H/H or H/L (Woo et al. 2002). A Canadian study showed the valine allele *Val158Met* COMT polymorphism, or a nearby locus, was involved in the pathogenesis of panic disorder (Rothe et al. 2006).

There has been considerable interest in the role of the serotonin transporter gene in panic disorder. The serotonin transporter is a protein critical to the regulation of serotonin function in the brain, because it terminates the action of serotonin in the synapse via reuptake. The variant site is commonly known as *5HTTLPR* (serotonin-transporter-linked promoter region). There are two common functional alleles of *5HTTLPR*: the short ("s") allele and the long ("l") allele. These "s" alleles encode an attenuated promoter segment and are associated with reduced transcription and functional capacity of the serotonin transporter relative to the "l" allele. Researchers in Italy (Perna et al. 2005) have shown that functional polymorphisms within the promoter region of *5HTT* gene in females lead to differing efficacy of an SSRI in panic disorder. The homozygotes for the long variant (l/l) of the *5HTTLPR* and heterozygotes, having both the long and the short variant (l/s), showed a better response to paroxetine than the homozygotes for the short variant (s/s). Furthermore, the presence of the long allelic variant was associated with positive response for treating panic attacks but showed no effect in treating anticipatory anxiety or phobic avoidance. Lesch et al. (1996) also found the short allele of *5HTTLPR* to be associated with anxiety-related personality. However, not all studies have supported the role of the s/s allele of *5HTTLPR* in panic disorder. For example, a study by Maron and colleagues (2005a) showed the l/l genotype to be associated with panic. In addition, other studies done in the United States as well as in Japan have failed to show any association between the *5HTTLPR* and panic disorder (Deckert et al. 1997; Hamilton et al. 1999; Inada et al. 2003; Ishiguro et al. 1997; Sand et al. 2000). Notably, Inada and colleagues (2003) did find genes coding for serotonin 2A receptors to be associated with panic disorder.

Another approach to understanding the role of genes in panic disorder is through identifying certain endophenotypes. Here, panic disorder is studied in the context of medical conditions with which it is frequently comorbid. Several different studies have shown the joint hypermobility syndrome, an inherited connective tissue condition, to occur at a rate of approximately 70% in patients with panic disorder, as opposed to about 15% in psychiatrically healthy control subjects (Bulbena et al. 1993; Martin-Santos et al. 1998). In those studies, the connective tissue laxity appeared to extend to the mitral valve. Rates of mitral valve prolapse were elevated in the panic disorder patients with joint hypermobility, in comparison with nonhypermobile control subjects with anxiety disorder. However, more recent studies have shown no association between panic disorder and joint hypermobility syndrome (Gulpek et al. 2004).

Panic disorder has been associated with interstitial cystitis that is linked to locus q32–33 on chromosome 13 (Hamilton et al. 2003). Chromosome 13 has also been linked to a syndrome consisting of interstitial cystitis, thyroid disorders, and panic disorder (Weissman et al. 2004). Other frequent associations with panic disorder include fibromyalgia, chronic fatigue syndrome, irritable bowel syndrome, hypothyroidism, asthma, allergic rhinitis, sinusitis and migraine, depression, bipolarity, and antidepressant medication "poop-out" (loss of effectiveness). The possibility is therefore raised that a certain familial form of the disorder exists that shares psychiatric, connective tissue, aberrant pain perception, and autoimmune features (Coplan et al. 2004).

Role of Environment in Panic Disorder

The role of environment in the development of panic disorder has been studied using animal models. Certain animal models rely heavily on classical and operant conditioning in inducing anxiety-like states. However, it is significant to note that except for posttraumatic stress disorder (PTSD), in which there is a clear antecedent "conditioning" event in the form of severe trauma, no study has shown any definitive proof of environmental conditioning in any other anxiety disorder. This said, it is common clinical experience that patients often present with panic disorder after a major loss, separation or illness of a significant other, or sexual or physical assault. Also, occupational and financial problems seem to trigger the onset, and so do drug/alcohol withdrawal and intoxication.

Coplan and colleagues (1998b, 2001, 2005) have conducted several studies that have examined the role of adverse life events in the behavior and neurobiological functioning of groups of nonhuman primates. In a series of experiments by Rosenblum and Paully (1984), macaque monkeys were raised in three different experimental foraging conditions: low foraging demand (LFD), high foraging demand (HFD), and variable foraging demand (VFD). In the LFD paradigm, a group of nursing mothers of the infant monkeys was exposed to conditions where food was always easily available. In the HFD paradigm, another group of mothers was exposed to a condition where food was always difficult to find. Although enough food was always available even in the HFD paradigm, the mothers had to search for it. And in the VFD paradigm, the nursing mothers of the infant-mother dyads were exposed for a 2-week period to conditions where food was readily available, followed by a 2-week period when food was difficult to find. The major finding of the study was that the infants whose mothers underwent the VFD paradigm were noticed to be more anxious, less social, and more subordinate than their LFD and HFD peers. It was also identified that the infants of the VFD primates, when faced with a novel environment, clung to their mothers like children with separation anxiety. Klein (1993) viewed separation-induced distress, or separation anxiety, as the developmental precursor most akin to adult panic disorder. Thus, the VFD model provides an interesting primate phenocopy of a childhood anxiety disorder whose phenotypic expression in all likelihood represents a combination of environmental and genetic influences. The VFD monkeys also manifested increased cerebrospinal fluid (CSF) CRF and decreased CSF cortisol (Coplan et al. 1996a). CSF CRF is believed to be reflective of extrahypothalamic CRF from the amygdala, the closely related bed nucleus of the stria terminalis, and the prefrontal cortex (Plotsky et al. 1995). Thus, a relatively brief period of disturbance of maternal-infant interaction may lead to persistent elevations of CRF, with implications for a long-standing template engendering susceptibility to anxiety and affective-related disturbances. CSF cortisol levels, however, were low. The combination of high CRF and low cortisol is most similar to the findings observed in PTSD rather than panic disorder (Yehuda et al. 1995). Thus, adverse early rearing may lead to a PTSD-like neurobiology. Yehuda and colleagues (2000) observed aberrant patterns of cortisol regulation in grown children whose parents were Holocaust survivors with diagnoses of PTSD. Panic attacks are quite frequent in PTSD patients and in patients with borderline personality disorder who have increased rates of traumatic experiences. Thus, the aberrant neurobiology of the VFD cohorts may bear relevance to an environmentally induced form of separation anxiety, with potential relevance to panic disorder in humans.

Gene-Environment Interaction

A gene-environment interaction is said to have occurred if the genotype variation alters the effect of exposure to an environmental pathogen on the individual's health (Caspi and Moffitt 2006). As mentioned earlier, this is another approach to studying the relative impact of gene and environment in the pathogenesis of disorders. This model has been best investigated in human twin studies and in animal models where the environmental conditions can be manipulated.

In a study by Coplan and colleagues (2007) on macaque monkeys, serotonin transporter genotyping was done on infant male subjects who were studied while undergoing 16 weeks of the VFD procedure. During the final LFD/HFD cycle, behavioral observations were performed repeatedly that were designed to study the extent of infant attachment to its mother. Aggregate measures of infant proximity to mother were separately evaluated for the final LFD and final VFD period, assigning values from 1 to 5, where 1 indicated the greatest degree of infant proximity and 5 indicated the greatest magnitude of distance possible of infant from mother. Results indicated that during the final LFD period, infants with the short allele of the *5HTTLPR* exhibited a significantly greater degree of proximity to their mothers than their long-allele counterparts. For the corresponding HFD period, no effect of genotype was noted. In conclusion, these preliminary data suggest an influence of serotonin transporter genotype on infant behavior within the context of the VFD paradigm. Moreover, the findings were in the predicted direction, with VFD-reared infants possessing the s/s allele exhibiting greater degrees of "reactive attachment," a putative measure of infant anxiety, than their l/l counterparts. Thus, the VFD-rearing experience appears to interact at a behavioral level with the allelic variant of the *5HTT*.

A different study involving macaque monkeys was conducted by Barr and colleagues (2004). Monkeys were raised in two experimental paradigms: by their own mothers and among their peers. Furthermore, the two groups were divided into two subgroups: one with s/l arm of *5HTTLPR* and another with l/l arm of *5HTTLPR*. These animals were separated at age 6 months to induce separation stress. It was found that the peer-raised cohort of monkeys with s/l arm of *5HTTLPR* had higher levels of ACTH than the l/l groups in response to separation stress. The elevated levels of ACTH in primates with s/l arm suggested increased activity of limbic-hypothalamic-pituitary-adrenal axis in response to separation stress, with its potential implication in anxiety and panic disorder.

As discussed earlier, GAD synthesizes GABA from glutamate. Studies have shown the variation in GAD enzyme gene to be associated with panic symptoms. In a study by Hettema and colleagues (2006), two genes—*GAD1* and *GAD2*—were studied in twins for association with risk for internalizing disorders, including panic disorder. Results suggested that variations in *GAD1* contributed to the individual differences in a range of anxiety disorders, including panic and depression, whereas variations in *GAD2* did not yield any correlation.

Psychological Theories of Panic

Dynamic Model

Psychodynamic theory addresses panic attacks as the expression of an intense unconscious conflict that serves a specific psychological purpose (Busch et al. 1999). During childhood, individuals with panic disorder struggle with a core conflict of dependency and inadequacy that arises from an inborn fear of unfamiliar situations, augmented by traumatic developmental experiences such as frightening or overcontrolling parents (Shear et al. 1993). The perception of inadequate protection from a caregiver results in feelings of anger in the child. This anger, in turn, elicits fear that the expression of the anger may result in further abandonment by and separation from the caregiver (Busch et al. 1999). The ego uses multiple immature and neurotic defenses to protect against anxiety and awareness of internal conflicts (Kipper et al. 2005). During adulthood, this underlying conflict becomes activated when the individual experiences a life stressor that symbolizes a disruption in attachments (Busch et al. 1999).

Contemporary models, such as those proposed by the Cornell Panic-Anxiety Study Group, integrate both biological and developmental stressors in the pathogenesis of panic disorder (Milrod et al. 2004; Shear et al. 1993). Individuals at risk for panic disorder are described to possess innate neurophysiological vulnerability, and the experience of trauma, such as poor parenting, leads to the development of conflicts regarding separation and independence, as well as difficulty in modulating angry emotions (Taylor et al. 2007). This concept is particularly evident in the relationship between the phenomena of separation anxiety and panic disorder. In a study analyzing the dreams and early memories of patients with panic disorder, Free et al. (1993) found a higher affective undercurrent of separation anxiety and higher covert hostility. Retrospective studies have found that childhood separation anxiety disorder may predispose to development of panic disorder as adults; however, the evidence is far from being conclusive (Biederman et al. 2006, 2007; Silove 1996).

Cognitive-Behavioral Models

In 1986, Clark described the concept of *catastrophic misinterpretation*, whereby an individual misinterprets benign internal bodily sensations or external stimuli as potentially harmful, triggering a bodily state of imminent disaster. This dysfunctional catastrophic misinterpretation leads to anxiety, which in turn stimulates further bodily sensations, triggering more misinterpretations (Taylor et al. 2007). For example, a person who experiences a headache can respond to it with a catastrophic thought, "I have brain cancer." This exaggerated response leads to increased apprehension and additional physical sensations such as palpitations, which, in turn, drive catastrophic misinterpretations (Bouton et al. 2001). Figure 22–1 depicts the conceptualization of panic disorder based on the cognitive-behavioral theories.

Barlow (1988) proposed the alarm theory based on classical conditioning, which encompasses three disparate "alarms"—true, false, and learned—each eliciting anxiety. The true alarm describes actual life-threatening danger, such as when a person on the edge of a cliff may experience panic-like symptoms, a ubiquitous phenomenon common to all individuals. False alarm occurs

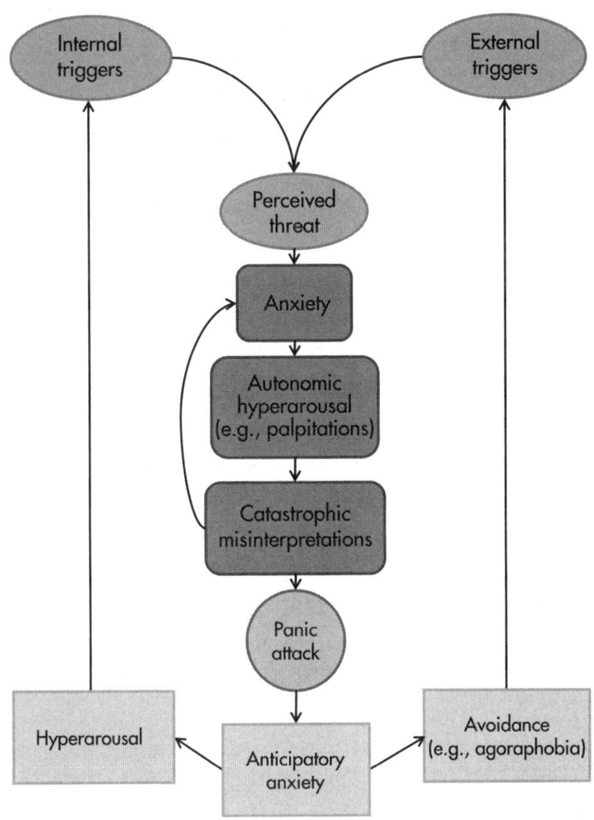

FIGURE 22–1. Cognitive-behavioral model of panic disorder.

when there is the spontaneous onset of fear symptoms with no known danger stimuli. This describes a panic *attack* and, although not ubiquitous, is experienced by many individuals. A panic *disorder* develops when an individual associates such a false alarm to a benign bodily sensation (an interoceptive cue) or an external (exteroceptive) cue, leading to the formation of a learned alarm (Bouton et al. 2001). This form of pairing may occur in human beings randomly, and those who are vulnerable develop anticipatory apprehension of what were once benign stimuli. Individuals typically experience panic in stimulating environments, such as crowded places, leading to agoraphobia as a learned avoidance when they experience a decrease in anxiety each time they avoid a situation (Taylor et al. 2007). CBT incorporates elements from both cognitive and behavioral models in the treatment of panic disorder by identifying and challenging cognitive distortions and providing exposure to stimuli and feared situations.

As mentioned earlier, many individuals experience panic attacks, but those who are vulnerable develop panic disorder. Bouton and colleagues (2001) described vulnerability factors that may influence the development of panic disorder. Innate genetic factors can predispose an individual to respond with exaggerated anxiety to physiological arousal. Other vulnerabilities include prior inability to experience mastery and control, experiences with unpredictability, and learning through childhood and familial experiences (Bouton et al. 2001).

Anxiety Sensitivity

Reiss and McNally (1985) developed a model of anxiety sensitivity wherein individuals with panic disorder are described as possessing a core fear toward anxiety and its associated somatic symptoms. Though this is similar to cognitive misinterpretation, anxiety sensitivity theorists differentiate it as the *fear* of anxiety/arousal sensations, not the misinterpretation of the sensations (McNally 1994). The propensity to respond with fear to innocuous stimuli can be measured by using the Anxiety Sensitivity Index (Reiss et al. 1986). For example, a person who has a headache and high anxiety sensitivity may fear that he or she may have a brain tumor, whereas a person with low sensitivity may dismiss the symptom as simply bothersome (McNally 2002). The Anxiety Sensitivity Index has been shown to be a significant predictor of the onset of panic in different patient populations (Ehlers 1995; Hayward et al. 2000; Maller and Reiss 1992).

Hyperventilation and Respiratory Theories

Hyperventilation has been historically associated with psychiatric conditions, although the relationship to panic disorder appears particularly prominent (Hardonk and Beumer 1979). There are two models that explore the importance of hyperventilation and the physiological response to CO_2 levels in the etiology of panic attacks. Ley (1985) proposed the hyperventilation theory, which states that when an individual hyperventilates, he or she produces a host of compensatory symptoms that can elicit symptoms of panic disorder, including shortness of breath, dizziness, palpitations, and tingling. These somatic symptoms can in turn elicit fear, which leads to further hyperventilation, producing a cycle that elicits a panic attack (Meuret et al. 2005). An alternative theory postulated by Klein (1993) described the fundamental disturbance as physiological oversensitivity to CO_2 levels, leading to triggering of a false suffocation alarm. High CO_2 levels serve as an innate alarm system that informs an individual of suffocation. Hence, people with such high sensitivity hyperventilate to achieve a persistent hypocapnic state to prevent stimulating the false suffocation alarm (Klein 1993). In contrast to the hyperventilation theory, the false suffocation alarm model proposes that the individual hyperventilates to avoid panic attacks, whereas the former states that hyperventilation causes panic attacks.

Neuroanatomical Hypothesis of Panic Disorder

The neuroanatomical hypothesis proposed by Gorman and colleagues is considered seminal, given that it incorporates various clinical and preclinical findings into an integrated model to explain how different modalities of treatments seem to be beneficial in panic disorder (Gorman et al. 1989, 2000). The central theme of their hypothesis is that panic originates from an abnormally sensitive fear network that involves the prefrontal cortex, insula, thalamus, and amygdala and projections to the hippocampus, brain stem, and hypothalamus. In this section, current research findings have been added to support and further integrate this model with other contemporary theories. Figure 22–2 gives an overview of the neuroanatomical hypothesis delineating the various neuroanatomical and neurochemical pathways involved in panic disorder.

The role of the amygdala is thought to be central in the etiology of panic disorder. Two nuclei of the amygdala are of great significance in the anxiety circuitry. The lateral nucleus is the main input nucleus, and the central nucleus is the main output nucleus. The lateral nucleus of the amygdala has been conceptualized as the interface with several sensory systems. The central nucleus of the amygdala receives input from the anterior thalamus via the lateral nucleus of the amygdala. Significantly, the thalamus receives efferents from the brain stem and many other sensory modalities. Thus, the sensory information that is channeled to the amygdala is from widespread regions of the brain, including the cerebral cortex. Conditioned fear memory is processed and stored in amygdala, whereas contextual memory is stored in the hippocampus, which relays the information to the amygdala (Phillips and LeDoux 1992). Although earlier studies had shown the lateral nucleus of the amygdala as primarily being involved in the learning and consolidation of fear conditioning (LeDoux et al. 1990), more recent studies have shown involvement of both central and lateral nuclei (Wilensky et al. 2006). NMDA receptors in the amygdala are involved in the acquisition as well as the retention of fear extinction learning (Sotres-Bayon et al. 2006). Antituberculosis medication D-cylcoserine, which is a partial agonist of NMDA receptors, has been shown to be associated with improved extinction of fear learning in both preclinical and clinical studies (Davis et al. 2006a, 2006b; Ressler et al. 2004).

The efferents from the central nucleus of the amygdala project to the parabrachial nucleus, the lateral nucleus of the hypothalamus, the locus coeruleus, the paraventricular nucleus of the hypothalamus, and periaqueductal gray matter. The efferent to the parabrachial nucleus is responsible for increasing respiratory rate (Takeuchi et al. 1982); the efferent to the lateral nucleus of the hypothalamus activates the sympathetic nervous system, which leads to further arousal (Price and Amaral 1981). Locus coeruleus efferents increase norepinephrine, leading to autonomic responses such as increased blood pressure, increased heart rate, and fear responses (Cedarbaum and Aghajanian 1978). Paraventricular nucleus efferents activate the HPA axis. Efferents to periaqueductal gray lead to increases in defensive behavior and postural freezing (Amorapanth et al. 1999).

The frontal cortex is involved in processing and evaluation of sensory information. Studies have shown the amygdala receives afferents from the prefrontal cortex, which modulates its activities by conscious evaluation and appraisal of the environment (Hariri et al. 2003). Some studies have shown decreased cortical blood flow during or prior to panic attacks, which could account for reduced inhibitory activity and consequent overactivation of the amygdala (Kent et al. 2005; Ponto et al. 2002). Restoring control over the amygdala by the prefrontal cortex may be a mechanism underlying the decreased response to the fear stimuli seen in extinction and habituation (Phelps et al. 2004). In conclusion, problems in relay and coordination of upstream (cortical) and downstream (brain stem) sensory information result in the heightened amygdalar activity causing behavioral, autonomic, and neuroendocrine activation.

Gorman et al. (2000) proposes that the many varieties of panicogens act by producing nonspecific physiological responses that trigger the sensitized brain fear network. The cortical processing is defective and misinterprets the physiological triggers, which leads to activation of the amygdala and the fear network, which have been conditioned to respond to the noxious stimuli. This concept is very similar to the concept of catastrophic misinterpretation and anxiety sensitivity, as

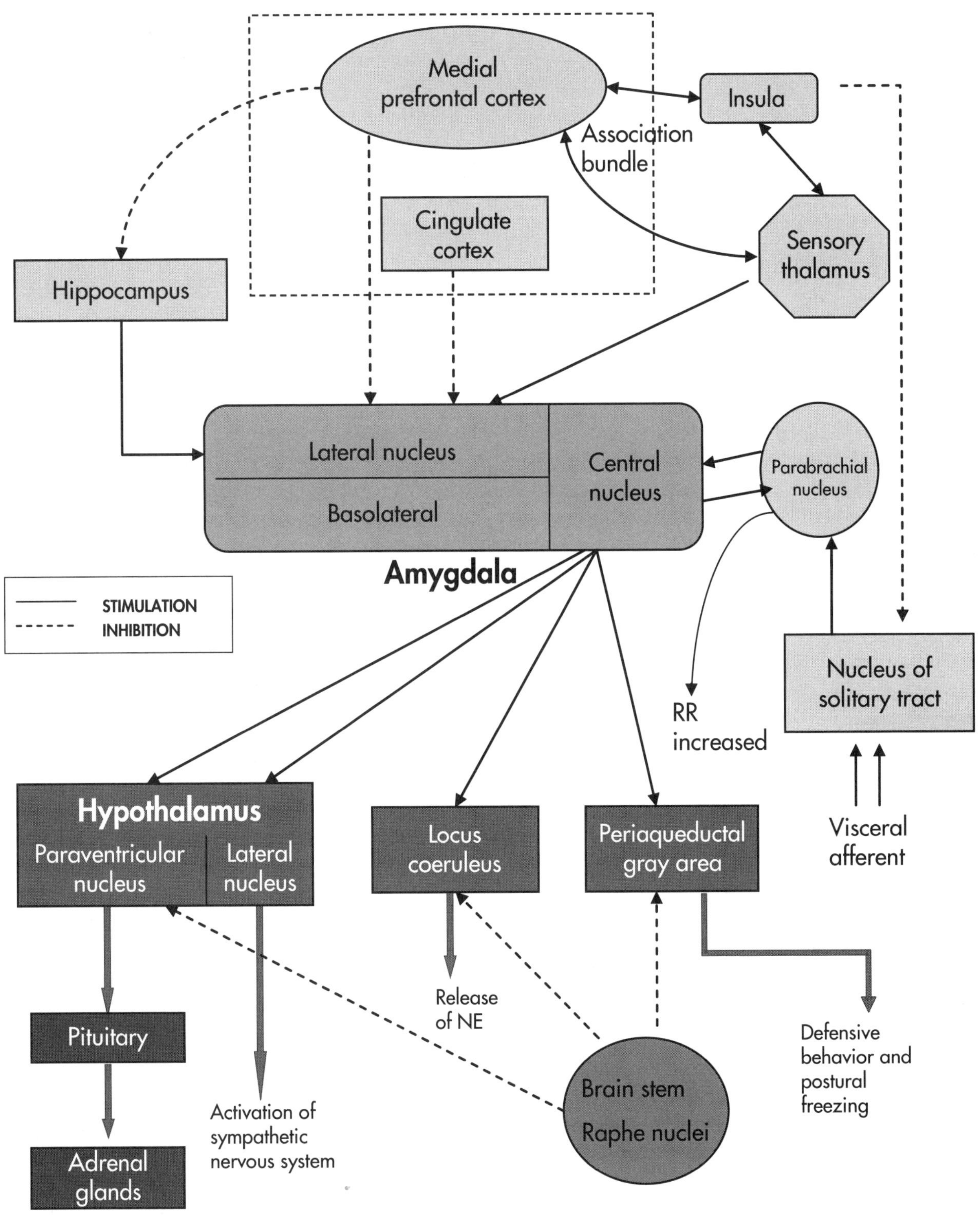

FIGURE 22–2. Panic disorder circuitry.
NE=norepinephrine; RR=relative risk.

discussed earlier. An experiment by Gutman and colleagues (2005) underscores the hypothesis of a sensitized fear network. Panic disorder patients and control subjects were subjected to doxapram, a known panicogen. Although similar physiological responses were observed in both groups, panic disorder patients panicked, whereas the control subjects did not. This observation supports Gorman and colleagues' view that it is not the physiological response per se but the interaction of the physiological response with a sensitized fear network that leads to panic.

Based on this model for panic disorder, the mechanism of action of different medications and psychotherapies can also be postulated. SSRIs act by enhancing serotonin neurotransmission in the synapses. Serotonergic neurons originating in the raphe nuclei project to the locus coeruleus, the periaqueductal gray, and the hypothalamus. These projections are generally inhibitory (Coplan et al. 1998b), and their functions have been described in detail in the earlier "Serotonergic Theory" section of this chapter.

SSRIs block the downstream manifestation of anxiety by diminishing arousal and defense escape behavior, decreasing the level of CRF, and correcting chaotic ventilatory patterns, in addition to stabilizing the locus coeruleus. As the patient realizes that symptoms that were once experienced as life-threatening have been blocked, a desensitization of the fear network occurs, which may explain the long-term benefits from SSRIs (Gorman et al. 2000).

Benzodiazepines have been found effective in ameliorating panic symptoms through their effect on potentiating GABA. Several studies have revealed, as previously detailed, that deficits of $GABA_A$–benzodiazepine receptor binding in areas including the medial prefrontal cortex, insula, and amygdala are associated with panic disorder. The prefrontal cortex has an inhibitory impact on the amygdala and the whole fear network (Grace and Rosenkranz 2002). A diminished level of GABA in the prefrontal cortex could lead to decreased inhibition of the amygdala. In addition, it may also lead to the loss of the delicate balance between GABA and glutamate, with consequent overexcitement of the amygdala secondary to enhanced glutamate actions. Johnson et al. (2007) demonstrated that lactate acts directly on GABA-deficient DMH, leading to the cascade of responses producing panic attacks. Thus, benzodiazepine acts by improving the inhibitory effect of prefrontal cortex, as well as by correcting the imbalance between GABA and glutamate. A study by Sibille et al. (2000) showed that the inactivation of 5-HT_{1A} receptor in mice resulted in downregulation of a major subunit of GABA receptor and a decrease in GABA binding and benzodiazepine-resistant anxiety. This outcome suggests possible links between the GABAergic and serotonergic systems.

The effectiveness of other treatment modalities such as CBT can also be understood using this model. Gorman and colleagues (2000) suggested that any effective psychological therapies involve some reduction in contextual fear (hippocampus) and catastrophic misinterpretation (prefrontal cortex). LeDoux (1996) proposed that psychotherapy could play a role in strengthening the ability of the cortex to better control the automatic behavior and response of the amygdala. CBT may decrease panic attacks by improving the patient's ability to handle phobic avoidance and catastrophic thinking, both of which are cortical processes (Gorman et al. 2000). A study done in Japan (Sakai et al. 2006) showed differences in the PET scans of pre- and post-CBT patients. In patients who were successfully treated with CBT, PET scan showed decreased glucose utilization in the right hippocampus, left anterior cingulate, left cerebellum, and pons, with an increase in glucose utilization in the medial prefrontal cortices.

Conclusion

Understanding of the neurobiological pathogenesis of panic disorder will likely advance as new findings from animal models and clinical sciences emerge. Rapid development in neuroradiology may make it finally possible to study brain structure and brain processes previously only imagined. Newer methods of genetic testing might bring light to the current obscure situation. Furthermore, although our current diagnostic classifications are clinically helpful, it is unlikely that the biological and genetic studies will yield results that conform to these narrow boundaries—requiring a much broader approach to diagnosis.

Key Clinical Points

- Panic disorder has been recognized in various forms for centuries. Explanations of its causation have varied widely, from being viewed as a purely physical condition to being viewed as a completely psychological one.
- Psychological theories provide understanding from dynamic and cognitive-behavioral perspectives. Dynamic theorists describe panic symptoms as an expression of undesirable psychic conflicts regarding fear of abandonment and anger. Cognitive behaviorists formulate that through misinterpretation and conditioning of normal physiological sensations, an individual triggers a vicious cycle, culminating in a full-blown panic attack. By cognitive restructuring and behavioral modification, an individual unlearns and is able to prevent panic attacks.
- Hyperventilation theorists postulate that hyperventilation produces physiological arousal that can be misinterpreted, leading to a panic attack. Others propose that hyperventilation occurs secondary to an abnormal sensitivity to CO_2, leading to triggering of a false suffocation alarm.
- A range of drugs is now widely accepted to be effective in panic disorder and provides support for the biological basis of panic disorder, specifically implicating noradrenergic, serotonergic, and GABAergic systems.
- Noradrenergic dysregulation is well documented in panic disorder, but drugs that augment serotonin neurotransmission also reduce noradrenergic volatility, suggesting a stabilizing and perhaps more primary role for serotonin.
- SSRIs may act in panic disorder by blocking the downstream manifestation of anxiety, diminishing arousal and defense escape behavior by stabilizing the locus coeruleus, decreasing levels of corticotropin-releasing factor, and correcting ventilatory patterns associated with panic disorder.
- The GABA-glutamate imbalance plays a pivotal role in the pathogenesis of panic disorder. Panic disorder patients have been found to have deficient GABA–benzodiazepine receptors in key sites of the fear network, including the prefrontal cortex, insula, and amygdala.
- Some panicogens, such as cholecystokinin and adenosine, act by directly modulating neurotransmitter systems. Others like CO_2 and sodium lactate cause panic, possibly by increasing lactate in the brain. Lactate may have a direct effect on the dorsomedial hypothalamus/perifornical and other regions of brain, which could explain how hyperventilation leads to panic.
- Several different genes have been implicated in panic disorder, including the cholecystokinin, adenosine 2A, MAO A, and COMT genes. Endophenotypal studies have revealed several systemic illnesses to be associated with the presence of panic disorder. Gene-environment analyses have shown association between environmental stressors and the s/s alleles of the *5HTTLPR*, producing anxiety states in some animal and clinical studies.
- Gorman's neuroanatomical hypothesis incorporates findings from different clinical and preclinical studies and describes a comprehensive fear network. He posits that the many varieties of panicogens act by producing nonspecific physiological responses that trigger a sensitized brain fear network.
- Psychological therapies may work by modifying the top-down regulatory measures. In patients whose panic symptoms responded positively to cognitive-behavioral therapy, neuroimaging evidence suggests a positive impact in some of the brain regions that Gorman, in his neuroanatomical hypothesis, described as malfunctional in panic disorder.

References

Abelson JL, Glitz D, Cameron OG, et al: Endocrine, cardiovascular, and behavioral responses to clonidine in patients with panic disorder. Biol Psychiatry 32:18–25, 1992

American Psychiatric Association: Diagnostic and Statistical Manual of Mental Disorders, 4th Edition, Text Revision. Washington, DC, American Psychiatric Association, 2000

Amorapanth P, Nader K, LeDoux JE: Lesions of periaqueductal gray dissociate-conditioned freezing from conditioned suppression behavior in rats. Learn Mem 6:491–499, 1999

Barlow DH: Anxiety and Its Disorders: The Nature and Treatment of Anxiety and Panic. New York, Guilford, 1988

Barr CS, Newman TK, Shannon C, et al: Rearing condition and rh5-HTTLPR interact to influence limbic-hypothalamic-pituitary-adrenal axis response to stress in infant macaques. Biol Psychiatry 55:733–738, 2004

Bouton ME, Mineka S, Barlow DH: A modern learning theory perspective on the etiology of panic disorder. Psychol Rev 108:4–32, 2001

Biederman J, Petty CR, Faraone SV, et al: Antecedents to panic disorder in nonreferred adults. J Clin Psychiatry 67:1179–1186, 2006

Biederman J, Petty CR, Hirshfeld-Becker DR, et al: Developmental trajectories of anxiety disorders in offspring at high risk for panic disorder and major depression. Psychiatry Res 153:245–252, 2007

Block M, Szidon P: Hyperventilation syndromes. Compr Ther 20:306–311, 1994

Boyer W: Serotonin uptake inhibitors are superior to imipramine and alprazolam in alleviating panic attacks: a meta-analysis. Int Clin Psychopharmacol 10:45–49, 1995

Bremner JD, Innis RB, White T, et al: SPECT [I-123]iomazenil measurement of the benzodiazepine receptor in panic disorder. Biol Psychiatry 47:96–106, 2000

Bulbena A, Duro JC, Porta M, et al: Anxiety disorders in the joint hypermobility syndrome. Psychiatry Res 46:59–68, 1993

Busch FN, Milrod BL, Singer MB: Theory and technique in psychodynamic treatment of panic disorder. J Psychother Pract Res 8:234–242, 1999

Cameron OG, Huang GC, Nichols T: Reduced gamma-aminobutyric acid(A)-benzodiazepine binding sites in insular cortex of individuals with panic disorder. Arch Gen Psychiatry 64:793–800, 2007

Caspi A, Moffitt TE: Gene-environment interactions in psychiatry: joining forces with neuroscience. Nat Rev Neurosci 7:583–590, 2006

Cedarbaum JM, Aghajanian GK: Afferent projections to the rat locus coeruleus as determined by a retrograde tracing technique. J Comp Neurol 178:1–16, 1978

Charney DS, Heninger GR: Abnormal regulation of noradrenergic function in panic disorders: effects of clonidine in healthy subjects and patients with agoraphobia and panic disorder. Arch Gen Psychiatry 43:1042–1054, 1986

Chrousos GP, Gold PW: The concepts of stress and stress system disorders: overview of physical and behavioral homeostasis. JAMA 267:1244–1252, 1992

Clark DM: A cognitive approach to panic. Behav Res Ther 24:461–470, 1986

Coplan JD, Pine D, Papp L, et al: Uncoupling of the noradrenergic-hypothalamic-pituitary-adrenal axis in panic disorder patients. Neuropsychopharmacology 13:65–73, 1995

Coplan JD, Andrews MW, Rosenblum LA, et al: Persistent elevations of cerebrospinal fluid concentrations of corticotropin-releasing factor in adult nonhuman primates exposed to early life stressors: implications for the pathophysiology of mood and anxiety disorders. Proc Natl Acad Sci U S A 93:1619–1623, 1996a

Coplan J, Pine D, Papp L: An algorithm approach to the treatment of panic disorder. Psychiatric Annals 26:192–201, 1996b

Coplan JD, Papp LA, Pine D, et al: Clinical improvement with fluoxetine therapy and noradrenergic function in patients with panic disorder. Arch Gen Psychiatry 54:643–648 1997a

Coplan JD, Pine DS, Papp LA, et al: A view on noradrenergic, hypothalamic-pituitary-adrenal axis and extrahypothalamic corticotrophin-releasing factor function in anxiety and affective disorders: the reduced growth hormone response to clonidine. Psychopharmacol Bull 33:193–204, 1997b

Coplan JD, Goetz R, Klein DF, et al: Plasma cortisol concentrations preceding lactate-induced panic: psychological, biochemical, and physiological correlates. Arch Gen Psychiatry 55:130–136, 1998a

Coplan JD, Trost RC, Owens MJ: Cerebrospinal fluid concentrations of somatostatin and biogenic amines in grown primates reared by mothers exposed to manipulated foraging conditions. Arch Gen Psychiatry 55:473–477, 1998b

Coplan JD, Smith EL, Altemus M, et al: Variable foraging demand rearing: sustained elevations in cisternal cerebrospinal fluid corticotropin-releasing factor concentrations in adult primates. Biol Psychiatry 50:200–204, 2001

Coplan JD, Reddy D, Bulbena A: The Alpim Syndrome: Anxiety of the Mind and Body, 24th National Conference of the Anxiety Disorders Association of America, Miami, FL, March 2004

Coplan JD, Altemus M, Mathew SJ, et al: Synchronized maternal-infant elevations of primate CSF CRF concentrations in response to variable foraging demand. CNS Spectr 10:530–536, 2005

Coplan J, Tang C, Martinez J: Freshest data: vulnerable genes, early life stress and impairment of adult white matter: implications for affective disorders. Paper presented at Society of Biological Psychiatry 62nd Annual Scientific Program and Convention, San Diego, CA, May 17–19, 2007

Davis M, Myers KM, Chhatwal J, et al: Pharmacological treatments that facilitate extinction of fear: relevance to psychotherapy. NeuroRx 3:82–96, 2006a

Davis M, Ressler K, Rothbaum BO, et al: Effects of D-cycloserine on extinction: translation from preclinical to clinical work. Biol Psychiatry 60:369–375, 2006b

Deakin J: Antidepressant drugs and the psychosocial origins of depression. J Psychopharmacol 10:31–38, 1996

Deckert J, Catalano M, Heils A, et al: Functional promoter polymorphism of the human serotonin transporter: lack of association with panic disorder. Psychiatr Genet 7:45–47, 1997

Deckert J, Nothen MM, Franke P, et al: Systematic mutation screening and association study of the A1 and A2a adenosine receptor genes in panic disorder suggest a contribution of the A2a gene to the development of disease. Mol Psychiatry 3:81–85, 1998

Deckert J, Catalano M, Syagailo Y, et al: Excess of high activity monoamine oxidase A gene promoter alleles in female patients with panic disorder. Hum Mol Genet 8:621–624, 1999

Demitrack M, Abbey S: Historical Overview and Evolution of Contemporary Definitions of Chronic Fatigue States in Chronic Fatigue Syndrome: An Integrative Approach to Evaluation and Treatment. Guilford, New York, 1996, pp 3–35

Ehlers A: A 1-year prospective study of panic attacks: clinical course and factors associated with maintenance. J Abnorm Psychol 104:164–172, 1995

Free NK, Winget CN, Whitman RM: Separation anxiety in panic disorder. Am J Psychiatry 150:595–599, 1993

Goddard AW, Woods SW, Sholomskas DE, et al: Effects of the serotonin reuptake inhibitor fluvoxamine on yohimbine-induced anxiety in panic disorder. Psychiatry Res 48:119–133, 1993

Goddard AW, Mason GF, Almai A, et al: Reductions in occipital cortex GABA levels in panic disorder detected with 1h-magnetic resonance spectroscopy. Arch Gen Psychiatry 58:556–561, 2001

Gorman JM, Liebowitz MR, Fyer AJ, et al: A neuroanatomical hypothesis for panic disorder. Am J Psychiatry 146:148–161, 1989

Gorman JM, Papp LA, Coplan JD, et al: Anxiogenic effects of CO2 and hyperventilation in patients with panic disorder. Am J Psychiatry 151:547–553, 1994

Gorman JM, Kent JM, Sullivan GM, et al: Neuroanatomical hypothesis of panic disorder, revised. Am J Psychiatry 157:493–505, 2000

Grace AA, Rosenkranz JA: Regulation of conditioned responses of basolateral amygdala neurons. Physiol Behav 77:489–493, 2002

Gulpek D, Bayraktar E, Akbay SP, et al: Joint hypermobility syndrome and mitral valve prolapse in panic disorder. Prog Neuropsychopharmacol Biol Psychiatry 28:969–973, 2004

Gutman DA, Coplan J, Papp L, et al: Doxapram-induced panic attacks and cortisol elevation. Psychiatry Res 133:253–261, 2005

Hamilton SP, Heiman GA, Haghighi F, et al: Lack of genetic linkage or association between a functional serotonin transporter polymorphism and panic disorder. Psychiatr Genet 9:1–6, 1999

Hamilton SP, Slager SL, Heiman GA, et al: No genetic linkage or association between a functional promoter polymorphism in the monoamine oxidase-A gene and panic disorder. Mol Psychiatry 5:465–466, 2000

Hamilton SP, Fyer AJ, Durner M, et al: Further genetic evidence for a panic disorder syndrome mapping to chromosome 13q. Proc Natl Acad Sci USA 100:2550–2555, 2003

Hamilton SP, Slager SL, De Leon AB, et al: Evidence for genetic linkage between a polymorphism in the adenosine 2A receptor and panic disorder. Neuropsychopharmacology 29:558–565, 2004

Hardonk HJ, Beumer HM: Hyperventilation Syndrome, in Handbook of Clinical Neurology. Edited by Vinken PJ, Bruyn GW. Amsterdam, North-Holland, 1979, pp 309–360

Hariri AR, Mattay VS, Tessitore A, et al: Neocortical modulation of the amygdala response to fearful stimuli. Biol Psychiatry 53:494–501, 2003

Hayward C, Killen JD, Kraemer HC, et al: Predictors of panic attacks in adolescents. J Am Acad Child Adolesc Psychiatry 39:207–214, 2000

Hettema JM, Neale MC, Kendler KS: A review and meta-analysis of the genetic epidemiology of anxiety disorders. Am J Psychiatry 158:1568–1578, 2001

Hettema JM, An SS, Neale MC, et al: Association between glutamic acid decarboxylase genes and anxiety disorders, major depression, and neuroticism. Mol Psychiatry 11:752–762, 2006

Hosing VG, Schirmacher A, Kuhlenbaumer G, et al: Cholecystokinin- and cholecystokinin-B-receptor gene polymorphisms in panic disorder. J Neural Transm Suppl 68:147–156, 2004

Inada Y, Yoneda H, Koh J, et al: Positive association between panic disorder and polymorphism of the serotonin 2A receptor gene. Psychiatry Res 118:25–31, 2003

Ishiguro H, Arinami T, Yamada K, et al: An association study between a transcriptional polymorphism in the serotonin transporter gene and panic disorder in a Japanese population. Psychiatry Clin Neurosci 51:333–335, 1997

Johnson PL, Shekhar A: Panic-prone state induced in rats with GABA dysfunction in the dorsomedial hypothalamus is mediated by NMDA receptors. J Neurosci 26:7093–7104, 2006

Johnson PL, Truitt WA, Fitz SD, et al: Neural pathways underlying lactate-induced panic. Neuropsychopharmacology 33:2093–2107, 2007

Kaschka W, Feistel H, Ebert D: Reduced benzodiazepine receptor binding in panic disorders measured by iomazenil SPECT. J Psychiatr Res 29:427–434, 1995

Kendler KS, Gardner CO, Prescott CA: Panic syndromes in a population-based sample of male and female twins. Psychol Med 31:989–1000, 2001

Kent JM, Coplan JD, Martinez J, et al: Ventilatory effects of tryptophan depletion in panic disorder: a preliminary report. Psychiatry Res 64:83–90, 1996

Kent JM, Coplan JD, Mawlawi O, et al: Prediction of panic response to a respiratory stimulant by reduced orbitofrontal cerebral blood flow in panic disorder. Am J Psychiatry 162:1379–1381, 2005

Kipper L, Blaya C, Teruchkin B, et al: Evaluation of defense mechanisms in adult patients with panic disorder: before and after treatment. J Nerv Ment Dis 193:619–624, 2005

Klein DF: Delineation of two drug-responsive anxiety syndromes. Psychopharmacologia 5:397–408, 1964

Klein DF: False suffocation alarms, spontaneous panics, and related conditions: an integrative hypothesis. Arch Gen Psychiatry 50:306–317, 1993

Klein DF, Fink M: Psychiatric reaction patterns to imipramine. Am J Psychiatry 119:432–438, 1962

LeDoux J: The Emotional Brain: The Mysterious Underpinning of Emotional life. New York, Simon and Schuster, 1996

LeDoux JE, Cicchetti P, Xagoraris A, et al: The lateral amygdaloid nucleus: sensory interface of the amygdala in fear conditioning. J Neurosci 10:1062–1069, 1990

Lesch KP, Lerer B: The 5-HT receptor–G-protein–effector system complex in depression, I: effect of glucocorticoids. J Neural Transm Gen Sect 84:3–18, 1991

Lesch KP, Bengel D, Heils A, et al: Association of anxiety-related traits with a polymorphism in the serotonin transporter gene regulatory region. Science 274:1527–1531, 1996

Ley R: Blood, breath, and fears: a hyperventilation theory of panic attacks and agoraphobia. Clin Psychol Rev 5:271–285, 1985

Lundberg DB, Mueller RA, Breese GR: An evaluation of the mechanism by which serotonergic activation depresses respiration. J Pharmacol Exp Ther 212:397–404, 1980

Malizia AL, Cunningham VJ, Bell CJ, et al: Decreased brain GABA(A)-benzodiazepine receptor binding in panic disorder: preliminary results from a quantitative PET study. Arch Gen Psychiatry 55:715–720, 1998

Maller R, Reiss S: Anxiety sensitivity in 1984 and panic attacks in 1987. J Anxiety Disord 6:241–247, 1992

Maron E, Lang A, Tasa G, et al: Associations between serotonin-related gene polymorphisms and panic disorder. Int J Neuropsychopharmacol 8:261–266, 2005a

Maron E, Nikopensius T, Koks S, et al: Association study of 90 candidate gene polymorphisms in panic disorder. Psychiatr Genet 15:17–24, 2005b

Martin-Santos R, Bulbena A, Porta M, et al: Association between joint hypermobility syndrome and panic disorder. Am J Psychiatry 155:1578–1583, 1998

McNally RJ: Panic Disorder: A Critical Analysis. New York, Guilford, 1994

McNally RJ: Anxiety sensitivity and panic disorder. Biol Psychiatry 52:938–946, 2002

Meuret AE, Ritz T, Wilhelm FH, et al: Voluntary hyperventilation in the treatment of panic disorder—functions of hyperventilation, their implications for breathing training, and recommendations for standardization. Clin Psychol Rev 25:285–306, 2005

Milrod B, Busch F, Shapiro T: Psychodynamic Approaches to the Adolescent With Panic Disorder. Melbourne, FL, Krieger, 2004

Nayeem N, Green TP, Martin IL, et al: Quaternary structure of the native GABAA receptor determined by electron microscopic image analysis. J Neurochem 62:815–818, 1994

Netto CF, Guimaraes FS: Anxiogenic effect of cholecystokinin in the dorsal periaqueductal gray. Neuropsychopharmacology 29:101–107, 2004

Nutt DJ: Altered central alpha 2-adrenoceptor sensitivity in panic disorder. Arch Gen Psychiatry 46:165–169, 1989

Nutt DJ, Malizia AL: New insights into the role of the GABA(A)-benzodiazepine receptor in psychiatric disorder. Br J Psychiatry 179:390–396, 2001

Olson EB Jr, Dempsey JA, McCrimmon DR: Serotonin and the control of ventilation in awake rats. J Clin Invest 64:689–693, 1979

Pande AC, Greiner M, Adams JB, et al: Placebo-controlled trial of the CCK-B antagonist, CI-988, in panic disorder. Biol Psychiatry 46:860–862, 1999

Perlis RH, Mischoulon D, Smoller JW, et al: Serotonin transporter polymorphisms and adverse effects with fluoxetine treatment. Biol Psychiatry 54:879–883, 2003

Perna G, Favaron E, Di Bella D, et al: Antipanic efficacy of paroxetine and polymorphism within the promoter of the serotonin transporter gene. Neuropsychopharmacology 30:2230–2235, 2005

Phelps EA, Delgado MR, Nearing KI, et al: Extinction learning in humans: role of the amygdala and vmPFC. Neuron 43:897–905, 2004

Phillips RG, LeDoux JE: Differential contribution of amygdala and hippocampus to cued and contextual fear conditioning. Behav Neurosci 106:274–285, 1992

Pitts FN Jr, McClure JN Jr: Lactate metabolism in anxiety neurosis. N Engl J Med 277:1329–1336, 1967

Plotsky P, Owens M, Nemeroff C: Neuropeptide alteration in mood disorders, in Psychopharmacology: The Fourth Generation of Progress. Edited by Bloom F, Kupfer D. New York, Raven, 1995, pp. 971–981

Ponto LL, Kathol RG, Kettelkamp R, et al: Global cerebral blood flow after CO2 inhalation in normal subjects and patients with panic disorder determined with [15O]water and PET. J Anxiety Disord 16:247–258, 2002

Price JL, Amaral DG: An autoradiographic study of the projections of the central nucleus of the monkey amygdala. J Neurosci 1:1242–1259, 1981

Redmond DE Jr: Clonidine and the primate locus coeruleus: evidence suggesting anxiolytic and anti-withdrawal effects. Prog Clin Biol Res 71:147–163, 1981

Rehfeld JF: Cholecystokinin and panic disorder—three unsettled questions. Regul Pept 93:79–83, 2000

Reiss S, McNally R: Expectancy model of fear, in Theoretical Issues in Behavior Therapy. Edited by Reiss S, Bootzin R. New York, Academic Press, 1985, pp 107–121

Reiss S, Peterson RA, Gursky DM, et al: Anxiety sensitivity, anxiety frequency and the prediction of fearfulness. Behav Res Ther 24:1–8, 1986

Ressler KJ, Rothbaum BO, Tannenbaum L, et al: Cognitive enhancers as adjuncts to psychotherapy: use of D-cycloserine in phobic individuals to facilitate extinction of fear. Arch Gen Psychiatry 61:1136–1144, 2004

Rosenblum LA, Paully GS: The effects of varying environmental demands on maternal and infant behavior. Child Dev 55:305–314, 1984

Rothe C, Koszycki D, Bradwejn J, et al: Association of the Val158Met catechol O-methyltransferase genetic polymorphism with panic disorder. Neuropsychopharmacology 31:2237–2242, 2006

Sakai Y, Kumano H, Nishikawa M, et al: Changes in cerebral glucose utilization in patients with panic disorder treated with cognitive-behavioral therapy. Neuroimage 33:218–226, 2006

Samochowiec J, Hajduk A, Samochowiec A, et al: Association studies of MAO-A, COMT, and 5-HTT genes polymorphisms in patients with anxiety disorders of the phobic spectrum. Psychiatry Res 128:21–26, 2004

Sand P, Lesch KP, Catalano M, et al: Polymorphic MAO-A and 5-HT-transporter genes: analysis of interactions in panic disorder. World J Biol Psychiatry 1:147–150, 2000

Scherrer JF, True WR, Xian H, et al: Evidence for genetic influences common and specific to symptoms of generalized anxiety and panic. J Affect Disord 57:25–35, 2000

Schofield PR, Darlison MG, Fujita N, et al: Sequence and functional expression of the GABA A receptor shows a ligand-gated receptor super-family. Nature 328:221–227, 1987

Shear MK, Cooper AM, Klerman GL, et al: A psychodynamic model of panic disorder. Am J Psychiatry 150:859–866, 1993

Shekhar A, Keim SR: The circumventricular organs form a potential neural pathway for lactate sensitivity: implications for panic disorder. J Neurosci 17:9726–9735, 1997

Shekhar A, Keim SR, Simon JR, et al: Dorsomedial hypothalamic GABA dysfunction produces physiological arousal following sodium lactate infusions. Pharmacol Biochem Behav 55:249–256, 1996

Sibille E, Pavlides C, Benke D, et al: Genetic inactivation of the Serotonin (1A) receptor in mice results in downregulation of major GABA(A) receptor alpha subunits, reduction of GABA(A) receptor binding, and benzodiazepine-resistant anxiety. J Neurosci 20:2758–2765, 2000

Silove D, Manicavasagar V, Curtis J, et al: Is early separation anxiety a risk factor for adult panic disorder? A critical review. Compr Psychiatry 37:167–179, 1996

Sotres-Bayon F, Cain CK, LeDoux JE: Brain mechanisms of fear extinction: historical perspectives on the contribution of prefrontal cortex. Biol Psychiatry 60:329–336, 2006

Stork O, Ji FY, Kaneko K, et al: Postnatal development of a GABA deficit and disturbance of neural functions in mice lacking GAD65. Brain Res 865:45–58, 2000

Strohle A, Holsboer F, Rupprecht R: Increased ACTH concentrations associated with cholecystokinin tetrapeptide-induced panic attacks in patients with panic disorder. Neuropsychopharmacology 22:251–256, 2000

Takeuchi Y, McLean JH, Hopkins DA: Reciprocal connections between the amygdala and parabrachial nuclei: ultrastructural demonstration by degeneration and axonal transport of horseradish peroxidase in the cat. Brain Res 239:583–588, 1982

Taylor S, Wald J, Asmundson J: Psychopathology of panic disorder. Psychiatry 5:188–192, 2007

Uhde TW, Tancer ME, Rubinow DR, et al: Evidence for hypothalamo-growth hormone dysfunction in panic disorder: profile of growth hormone (GH) responses to clonidine, yohimbine, caffeine, glucose, GRF and TRH in panic disorder patients versus healthy volunteers. Neuropsychopharmacology 6:101–118, 1992

Wang Z, Valdes J, Noyes R, et al: Possible association of a cholecystokinin promotor polymorphism (CCK-36CT) with panic disorder. Am J Med Genet 81:228–234, 1998

Weissman MM, Gross R, Fyer A, et al: Interstitial cystitis and panic disorder: a potential genetic syndrome. Arch Gen Psychiatry 61:273–279, 2004

Wilensky AE, Schafe GE, Kristensen MP, et al: Rethinking the fear circuit: the central nucleus of the amygdala is required for the acquisition, consolidation, and expression of Pavlovian fear conditioning. J Neurosci 26:12387–12396, 2006

Woo JM, Yoon KS, Yu BH: Catechol O-methyltransferase genetic polymorphism in panic disorder. Am J Psychiatry 159:1785–1787, 2002

Yehuda R, Boisoneau D, Lowy MT, et al: Dose-response changes in plasma cortisol and lymphocyte glucocorticoid receptors following dexamethasone administration in combat veterans with and without posttraumatic stress disorder. Arch Gen Psychiatry 52:583–593, 1995

Yehuda R, Bierer LM, Schmeidler J, et al: Low cortisol and risk for PTSD in adult offspring of holocaust survivors. Am J Psychiatry 157:1252–1259, 2000

Recommended Readings

Bouton ME, Mineka S, Barlow DH: A modern learning theory perspective on the etiology of panic disorder. Psychol Rev 108:4–32, 2001

Busch FN, Milrod BL, Singer MB: Theory and technique in psychodynamic treatment of panic disorder. J Psychother Pract Res 8:234–242, 1999

Caspi A, Moffitt TE: Gene-environment interactions in psychiatry: joining forces with neuroscience. Nat Rev Neurosci 7:583–590, 2006

Coplan JD, Andrews MW, Rosenblum LA, et al: Persistent elevations of cerebrospinal fluid concentrations of corticotropin-releasing factor in adult nonhuman primates exposed to early life stressors: implications for the pathophysiology of mood and anxiety disorders. Proc Natl Acad Sci USA 93:1619–1623, 1996

Gorman JM, Kent JM, Sullivan GM, et al: Neuroanatomical hypothesis of panic disorder, revised. Am J Psychiatry 157:493–505, 2000

Hettema JM, Neale MC, Kendler KS: A review and meta-analysis of the genetic epidemiology of anxiety disorders. Am J Psychiatry 158:1568–1578, 2001

Johnson PL, Truitt WA, Fitz SD, et al: Neural pathways underlying lactate-induced panic. Neuropsychopharmacology 33:2093–2107, 2007

Klein DF: False suffocation alarms, spontaneous panics, and related conditions: an integrative hypothesis. Arch Gen Psychiatry 50:306–317, 1993

LeDoux J: The Emotional Brain: The Mysterious Underpinning of Emotional Life. New York, Simon and Schuster, 1996

Chapter 23

Pharmacotherapy for Panic Disorder

Borwin Bandelow, M.D., Ph.D.
David S. Baldwin, M.D.

Panic disorder is a severe and often disabling condition with a lifetime prevalence rate of 3.1%–4.5% (Wittchen and Jacobi 2005). The treatment of panic disorder with antidepressants goes back to the year 1959, when Donald F. Klein established the tricyclic antidepressant (TCA) imipramine for the treatment of this anxiety disorder (Klein and Fink 1962). In 1960, the first benzodiazepine, chlordiazepoxide, was introduced. Since the mid-1980s (den Boer and Westenberg 1988; Evans et al. 1986), the selective serotonin reuptake inhibitors (SSRIs) have been used in patients with panic disorder, followed by the dual reuptake inhibitor venlafaxine in 1993.

The effectiveness of pharmacotherapy for panic disorder has been established in many randomized, controlled studies. As a result of increased efforts in the systematic clinical evaluation of psychopharmacological agents for the treatment of anxiety in recent years, a comprehensive database has been collected so that precise recommendations can be provided for treating panic disorder.

According to the principles of evidence-based medicine, the present overview of pharmacotherapy of this anxiety disorder is based on results from randomized, controlled trials (Baldwin et al. 2005; Bandelow et al. 2008).

Psychological treatments play an important role in the treatment of panic disorder and are discussed elsewhere in this volume (Chapter 24, "Psychotherapy for Panic Disorder"). In this chapter, we focus on psychopharmacological treatment.

Although there is no evidence for superiority of a certain medication class in terms of efficacy, some of the available drugs have advantages regarding their side-effect profiles. Drugs available for the treatment of panic disorder are listed in Table 23–1.

Medication Treatments

First-Line Treatments

Selective Serotonin Reuptake Inhibitors

The efficacy of SSRIs in panic disorder has been demonstrated in many controlled studies, and they are considered to be the first-line drugs for this disorder. Efficacy has been shown for the following SSRIs:

- *Citalopram* was effective in a placebo- and comparator-controlled trial (Wade et al. 1997) and in one comparison with fluoxetine (Amore et al. 1999b).
- *Escitalopram* was effective in a citalopram- and placebo-controlled trial (Bandelow et al. 2007b; Stahl et al. 2003).
- *Fluoxetine* was effective in double-blind, placebo-controlled (Michelson et al. 1998, 2001), and com-

TABLE 23–1. Recommendations for drug treatment of panic disorder

Treatment	Examples	Recommended daily dose for adults
Treatment of acute panic attacks		
Benzodiazepines	Alprazolam	0.5–2 mg
	Lorazepam melting tablets	1–2.5 mg
Standard treatment		
SSRIs	Citalopram	20–60 mg
	Escitalopram	10–20 mg
	Fluoxetine	20–40 mg
	Fluvoxamine	100–300 mg
	Paroxetine	20–60 mg
	Sertraline	50–200 mg
SNRI	Venlafaxine	75–300 mg
TCAs	Clomipramine	75–250 mg
	Imipramine	75–250 mg
Examples of agents to be tried when other treatment strategies are not effective or not tolerated		
Benzodiazepines	Alprazolam	1.5–8 mg
	Clonazepam	1–4 mg
MAOI	Phenelzine	45–90 mg
NRI	Reboxetine	4–8 mg
NASSA	Mirtazapine	45 mg
RIMA	Moclobemide	300–600 mg

Note. These recommendations are based on randomized, double-blind clinical studies published in peer-reviewed journals. Not all of the recommended drugs are licensed for these indications in every country. MAOI=monoamine oxidase inhibitor; NASSA=noradrenergic and specific serotonergic antidepressant; RIMA=reversible inhibitor of monoamine oxidase; NRI=norepinephrine reuptake inhibitor; SSRIs=selective serotonin reuptake inhibitors; TCAs=tricyclic antidepressants.

parator-controlled (Amore et al. 1999a, 1999b; Bystritsky et al. 1994) trials.

- *Fluvoxamine* showed efficacy in a number of double-blind, placebo-controlled studies (Asnis et al. 2001; Black et al. 1993; de Beurs et al. 1995; den Boer and Westenberg 1990; Hoehn-Saric et al. 1993; Pols et al. 1993). In one study, fluvoxamine and the comparator imipramine were both more effective than placebo and equally effective (Bakish et al. 1996). One small study did not show superiority to placebo on the main efficacy measure, but did on some other instruments (Sandmann et al. 1998). Another study did not show efficacy for fluvoxamine, but did show a strong effect for imipramine in comparison to placebo (Nair et al. 1996).
- *Paroxetine* showed efficacy in double-blind, placebo-controlled (Ballenger et al. 1998; Oehrberg et al. 1995; Pollack and Doyle 2003; Sheehan et al. 2005), and comparator-controlled (Bakker et al. 1999; Bandelow et al. 2004; Lecrubier et al. 1997; Oehrberg et al. 1995; Pollack et al. 2007) studies.
- *Sertraline* was also effective in double-blind, placebo-controlled studies (Londborg et al. 1998; Pohl et al. 1998; Pollack et al. 1998) and one comparator trial (Bandelow et al. 2004).
- *Zimeldine* was effective in a single double-blind, placebo-controlled trial in "agoraphobia with panic attacks" with imipramine as a comparator; however, the drug was withdrawn from the market (Evans et al. 1986)

Usually, treatment with SSRIs is well tolerated. Restlessness, jitteriness, an increase in anxiety symptoms, and insomnia in the first days or weeks of treatment may hamper compliance with treatment. Lowering the starting dose of SSRIs may reduce this overstimulation. Other side effects include fatigue, dizziness, nausea, anorexia, or weight gain. Sexual dysfunctions (decreased libido, impotence, or ejaculatory disturbances) may be a problem in long-term treatment (Baldwin 2004), and discontinuation syndromes have been observed (Price et al. 1996; Stahl et al. 1997).

The anxiolytic effect may start with a latency of 2–4 weeks (in some cases, as long as 6–8 weeks). To avoid overstimulation and insomnia, doses should be given in the morning and at midday, except in patients reporting daytime sedation.

Serotonin-Norepinephrine Reuptake Inhibitors

The efficacy of the antidepressant venlafaxine, a selective serotonin-norepinephrine reuptake inhibitor (SNRI), was demonstrated in double-blind, placebo-controlled studies (Bradwejn et al. 2005; Pollack et al. 1996) and a placebo-controlled study that used paroxetine as comparator (Pollack et al. 2007). The side-effect profile of venlafaxine is similar to that of the SSRIs. When using higher doses (300 mg/day or more), blood pressure should be monitored.

Second-Line Treatments

Tricyclic Antidepressants

Treatment with TCAs has been shown to improve the symptoms of panic disorder. Efficacy was shown for the following agents:

- *Clomipramine* in double-blind, placebo-controlled (Bandelow et al. 2000; Johnston et al. 1988) and comparator-controlled (Cassano et al. 1988; Lecrubier et al. 1997; Modigh et al. 1992; Wade et al. 1997) studies
- *Imipramine* in double-blind, placebo-controlled (Klein 1964; Zitrin et al. 1980, 1983) and comparator-controlled (Cross-National Collaborative Panic Study 1992; Nair et al. 1996; Sheehan et al. 1990; Uhlenhuth et al. 1989) studies
- *Lofepramine* in a double-blind, placebo-controlled study with clomipramine as an active comparator (Fahy et al. 1992)

Especially at the beginning of treatment, compliance with TCA treatment may be hampered by adverse effects such as initially increased anxiety, dry mouth, postural hypotension, tachycardia, sedation, sexual dysfunctions, and impaired psychomotor function and car driving safety. Weight gain may be a problem in long-term treatment. In general, the frequency of adverse events is higher for TCAs than for newer antidepressants such as the SSRIs (Amore et al. 1999a; Bakish et al. 1996; Bakker et al. 1999; Bystritsky et al. 1994; Lecrubier and Judge 1997; Wade et al. 1997). For example, in one SSRI-TCA comparison, adverse events occurred in 73.2% of paroxetine-treated and 89.2% of clomipramine-treated patients (Lecrubier and Judge 1997). Thus, the SSRIs should be tried first before TCAs are used.

The dosage should be titrated up slowly until dosage levels as high as in the treatment of depression are reached. Patients should be informed that the onset of the anxiolytic effect of the drug may have a latency of 2–4 weeks (in some cases, up to 6–8 weeks).

Third-Line Treatments

Benzodiazepines

The efficacy of benzodiazepines in panic disorder has been shown in some controlled clinical studies:

- *Alprazolam* was superior to placebo and as effective as comparator drugs in a number of studies (Andersch et al. 1991; Ballenger et al. 1988; Cross-National Collaborative Panic Study 1992; Lydiard et al. 1992; Noyes et al. 1996; Uhlenhuth et al. 1989).
- *Clonazepam* was investigated in double-blind, placebo-controlled studies (Beauclair et al. 1994; Dyukova et al. 1992; Moroz and Rosenbaum 1999; Rosenbaum et al. 1997) and one placebo- and comparator-controlled trial (Tesar et al. 1991).
- *Diazepam* was evaluated in a placebo- and comparator-controlled (Noyes et al. 1996) and in a comparator-controlled (Dunner et al. 1986) trial.
- *Lorazepam* was as effective as alprazolam in two studies (Charney and Woods 1989; Schweizer et al. 1990a).

The anxiolytic effects start immediately after oral ingestion or parenteral application. In contrast to antidepressants, benzodiazepines do not lead to initially increased nervousness. In general, they have a good record of safety. Because of central nervous system depression, benzodiazepine treatment may be associated with sedation, dizziness, prolonged reaction time, and other side effects. Cognitive functions and driving skills may be affected. After long-term treatment with benzodiazepines (e.g., over 4–8 months), dependency may occur in some patients (Bradwejn 1993; Livingston 1994; Nelson and Chouinard 1999; Rickels et al. 1990; Schweizer et al. 1990b; Shader and Greenblatt 1993; Smith and Landry 1990), especially in predisposed patients (Schweizer et al. 1998). Withdrawal reactions have their peak severity at 2 days for short half-life and 4–7 days for long half-life benzodiazepines (Rickels et al. 1990). It is claimed that prolonged withdrawal reactions may occasionally occur. However, tolerance seems to be rare (Rickels 1982). Thus, treatment with benzodiazepines requires a careful weighing of risks and benefits. There is some controversy in the field as to whether benzodiazepines can be used as first-line agents in anxiety disorders. In patients for whom other treatment modalities were not effective or were not tolerated due to side effects, year-long treatment with benzodiazepines may be justified. However, patients with a history of benzodiazepine abuse should be excluded from treatment. Cognitive-behavioral interventions may facilitate benzodiazepine discontinuation (Otto et al. 1993; Spiegel 1999). Benzodiazepines may also be used in combination with antidepressants during the first weeks before the onset of efficacy of the antidepressants (Goddard et al. 2001).

When treating comorbid panic disorder, clinicians should be aware that in contrast to antidepressants, benzodiazepines do not treat comorbid conditions such as depression or obsessive-compulsive disorder.

Monoamine Oxidase Inhibitors

Phenelzine. Despite the widespread use of phenelzine in panic disorder, evidence of its efficacy is based on only one study (Sheehan et al. 1980). In this study, phenelzine, a monoamine oxidase inhibitor (MAOI), was superior to placebo and equal or even superior to imipramine on some measures. Because of the possibility of severe side effects and interactions of other drugs or food components with MAOIs, phenelzine is not considered a first-line drug and should only be used by experienced psychiatrists when other treatment modalities have been unsuccessful or have not been tolerated. To avoid overstimulation and insomnia, doses should be given in the morning and at midday.

Other Medications

Some available drugs have shown preliminary evidence of efficacy or mixed results. These drugs may be used off-label in patients with nonresponse to standard treatments:

- *Moclobemide.* Results with the reversible inhibitor of monoamine oxidase moclobemide were inconsistent. Moclobemide was as effective as fluoxetine (Tiller et al. 1999) or clomipramine (Krüger and Dahl 1999). However, it was not superior to placebo in a double-blind study (Loerch et al. 1999). In another study, superiority to placebo could only be established for the more severely ill patients, but not for the whole group (Uhlenhuth et al. 2002). Thus, the drug may be a treatment option for otherwise unresponsive patients. It is not available in the United States but is available in Canada and many other countries. Side effects include restlessness, insomnia, dry mouth, and headache. To avoid overstimulation and insomnia, doses should be given in the morning and at midday.
- *Reboxetine.* The efficacy of the norepinephrine reuptake inhibitor (NRI) reboxetine was shown in a double-blind, placebo-controlled study (Versiani et al. 2002). In single-blind studies the drug was as effective as fluvoxamine (Seedat et al. 2003) but less effective than paroxetine (Bertani et al. 2004). The drug is not available in the United States but is available in many other countries.
- *Mirtazapine.* In a small double-blind comparison of the α_2/5-HT_2/5-HT_3 blocker mirtazapine and fluvoxamine, no differences were found between the two drugs (Ribeiro et al. 2001). In an open trial, mirtazapine showed efficacy in panic disorder (Carpenter et al. 1999).
- *Buspirone.* The 5-HT_{1A} agonist buspirone is effective in generalized anxiety disorder. However, in panic disorder, buspirone was not superior to placebo (Sheehan et al. 1990, 1993) and was less effective than imipramine (Sheehan et al. 1990), clorazepate (Schweizer and Rickels 1988), and alprazolam (Sheehan et al. 1993).
- *Bupropion.* The norepinephrine-dopamine reuptake inhibitor bupropion was not effective in a small controlled study (Sheehan et al. 1983) but showed some effect in a small open-label trial (Simon et al. 2003).
- *Propranolol.* Because beta-blockers may influence autonomic anxiety symptoms such as palpitations and tremor, they have been used in the treatment of panic disorder. However, the beta-blocker propranolol was not superior to placebo (Munjack et al. 1989) and was less effective than comparator drugs (Munjack et al. 1989; Noyes et al. 1984). In another double-blind, placebo-controlled study with small sample size, the effects of propranolol were not different from those of alprazolam, although alpraz-

olam showed a more rapid onset of efficacy (Ravaris et al. 1991).

- *Valproate.* The anticonvulsant valproate (valproic acid) was effective in one very small double-blind, placebo-controlled crossover study (Lum et al. 1990) and in open studies (Keck et al. 1993; Primeau et al. 1990; Woodman and Noyes 1994).
- *Tiagabine.* The γ-aminobutyric acid (GABA) reuptake inhibitor tiagabine, used as an anticonvulsant, showed efficacy in a case series (Zwanzger et al. 2001b).
- *Vigabatrin.* An irreversible inhibitor of GABA transaminase, vigabatrin is an antiepileptic drug that was also used successfully in a series of three patients (Zwanzger et al. 2001a).
- *Gabapentin.* In a double-blind, placebo-controlled study, the anticonvulsant gabapentin was only superior to placebo in more severely ill panic patients (Pande et al. 2000).
- *Inositol.* The intracellular second-messenger precursor inositol showed superiority to placebo in a small double-blind, placebo-controlled study (Benjamin et al. 1995) and was equally as effective as the SSRI fluvoxamine (Palatnik et al. 2001).
- *Ondansetron.* The 5-HT_3 antagonist ondansetron and the anticonvulsant valproate were also effective in open trials (Schneier et al. 1996).

Although herbal preparations are often offered to patients with panic disorder in primary care (Bandelow et al. 1995), there are no controlled studies showing efficacy for any herbal treatment.

Long-Term Treatment

Mostly, panic disorder has a waxing and waning course. After remission, treatment should continue for at least several months in order to prevent relapses. A number of studies have investigated the long-term value of SSRI and TCA treatment (Table 23–2). Some of these trials are long-term studies comparing a drug and placebo for a longer period (i.e., 26–60 weeks). The other trials are relapse prevention studies, in which patients usually receive open-label treatment with the study drug for a shorter period, after which responders are randomly assigned to receive ongoing active drug treatment or placebo. In summary, SSRIs, the SNRI venlafaxine, TCAs, and moclobemide showed long-term efficacy in these studies.

Data on how long maintenance treatment should be continued are scarce. In one study, patients who had 18 months of maintenance treatment with imipramine had fewer relapses after discontinuation than patients who were discontinued after only 6 months of treatment. The results support the hypothesis that successful imipramine maintenance treatment of patients with panic and agoraphobia can have protective effects against relapse, at least in the first 6 months after the maintenance treatment period (Mavissakalian and Perel 1992b). Expert consensus conferences generally recommend duration of pharmacotherapy of at least 12–24 months (American Psychiatric Association 1998).

Regarding SSRIs, the same doses are usually prescribed in the maintenance treatment of panic disorder as in the acute treatment phase. To our knowledge, there are no studies examining reduced doses of SSRIs in maintenance treatment. In an open study on the TCA imipramine, patients who were stabilized on imipramine and received further treatment with half their previous dose of imipramine did not show relapse or sustained worsening (Mavissakalian and Perel 1992a).

Comparisons of Antipanic Drugs

In studies comparing the efficacy of TCAs and SSRIs, no differences in terms of efficacy could be found between the two classes of drugs (Amore et al. 1999a; Bakish et al. 1996; Bakker et al. 1999; Bystritsky et al. 1994; Cavaljuga et al. 2003; Lecrubier and Judge 1997; Wade et al. 1997), with the exception of maprotiline, which had no effect, in contrast to the SSRI fluvoxamine (den Boer and Westenberg 1988). However, in most of these studies, SSRIs were better tolerated than TCAs. Also, in patients with comorbid panic disorder and major depressive disorder, sertraline and imipramine were equally effective, but sertraline showed significantly greater tolerability and compliance than imipramine (Lepola et al. 2003). Comparisons among the SSRIs did not reveal differences with regard to efficacy (Bandelow et al. 2004; Perna et al. 2001), although escitalopram showed evidence of superiority over citalopram on some outcome measures (Bandelow et al. 2007b).

There are no direct comparisons between SSRIs and benzodiazepines in the treatment of panic disorder. According to a meta-analysis, the effect sizes for SSRIs were higher than for the benzodiazepine alprazolam (Boyer 1995).

In a number of studies, alprazolam was compared with the TCA imipramine (Andersch et al. 1991; Charney et al. 1986; Cross-National Collaborative Panic Study 1992; Lepola et al. 1990; Rizley et al. 1986; Taylor et al. 1990; Uhlenhuth et al. 1989). No differences

TABLE 23–2. Randomized, controlled trials for the long-term treatment of panic disorder: double-blind, placebo-controlled (DBPC) design

Study	Weeks	Design	Efficacy
Ferguson et al. 2007	12 open+26 DBPC	Relapse prevention	Venlafaxine>placebo
Kamijima et al. 2005	8 DBPC+8 DBPC	Relapse prevention	Sertraline>placebo on most measures except the primary efficacy measure (relapse)
Lepola et al. 2003	26 DBPC	Long-term (patients with panic disorder and major depression)	Sertraline=imipramine (sertraline better tolerated)
Rapaport et al. 2001	52 open+26 DBPC	Relapse prevention	Sertraline>placebo
Amore et al. 1999a	26 DBPC	Long-term	Fluoxetine=imipramine (fluoxetine better tolerated)
Amore et al. 1999b	24 DBPC+26 open	Long-term	Citalopram=fluoxetine
Tiller et al. 1999	8 DBPC+52 DBPC	Long-term	Moclobemide=fluoxetine (moclobemide better tolerated)
Lepola et al. 1998	8 DBPC+52 DBPC	Relapse prevention	Citalopram=clomipramine>placebo
Rickels and Schweizer 1998	8 DBPC+26 DBPC	Long-term	8 weeks: alprazolam=imipramine 26 weeks: alprazolam>imipramine (alprazolam better tolerated, but discontinuation problems)
Lecrubier and Judge 1997	12 DBPC+36 DBPC	Relapse prevention	Paroxetine=clomipramine>placebo
Curtis et al. 1993	8 DBPC+up to 35 DBPC	Relapse prevention	Alprazolam=imipramine>placebo

could be found between the two drugs in terms of global improvement.

The advantages and disadvantages of antipanic drugs are summarized in Table 23–3.

Practical Guidelines for Treatment

Recommended dosages are indicated in Table 23–1. SSRIs have a flat response curve; that is, approximately 75% of patients respond to the initial (low) dose. However, for paroxetine, a dosage of 40 mg/day was more effective than 20 mg/day.

In some patients, treatment may be started with half the recommended dose in the first days or weeks. Patients with panic disorder are sensitive to antidepressants and may easily discontinue treatment because of initial jitteriness and nervousness.

For TCAs, it is recommended that the drug be initiated at a low dose and that the dose be increased every 3–5 days. The antidepressant dose should be increased to the highest recommended level when initial treatment with a low or medium dose fails. In order to increase compliance, it may be feasible to give all the antidepressant medication in a single dose, depending on the patient's tolerance. Benzodiazepine doses should be as low as possible but as high as necessary to achieve a complete treatment result.

A treatment algorithm is provided in Table 23–4. Some frequently asked questions for the treatment of panic disorder are addressed in Table 23–5.

Special Populations

Pregnant Women

The risks of drug treatment during pregnancy must be weighed against the risk of withholding treatment for panic disorder. According to the majority of studies, the use of SSRIs and TCAs in pregnancy imposes no increased risk for fetal malformations (Altshuler et al. 2001; Alwan et al. 2007; Austin and Mitchell 1998; Emslie and Judge 2000; Ericson et al. 1999; Hogberg and Wang 2005; Kallen and Otterblad Olausson 2007; Koren et al. 2005; Lattimore et al. 2005; Malm et al. 2005; Misri et al. 2000a, 2000b; Nordeng and Spigset

TABLE 23–3. Advantages and disadvantages of antianxiety drugs

Medication class	Advantages	Disadvantages
SSRIs	No dependency Sufficient evidence from clinical studies Favorable side-effect profile Relatively safe in overdose	Latency of effect 2–6 weeks Initial jitteriness, nausea, restlessness, sexual dysfunctions, and other side effects
SNRI: venlafaxine	No dependency Sufficient evidence from clinical studies Favorable side effect profile Relatively safe in overdose	Latency of effect 2–6 weeks Initial jitteriness, nausea, restlessness, sexual dysfunctions, increase of blood pressure in high doses, and other side effects
TCAs	No dependency Sufficient evidence from clinical studies	Latency of effect 2–6 weeks Anticholinergic effects, cardiovascular side effects, weight gain, sexual dysfunctions, and other side effects May be lethal in overdose
MAOI: phenelzine	No dependency	Latency of effect 2–6 weeks Dietary restrictions Activation, insomnia, weight gain, orthostatic hypotension, sexual dysfunctions, gastrointestinal symptoms, and other side effects Multiple daily dosing needed May be lethal in overdose
Benzodiazepines	Rapid onset of action Sufficient evidence from clinical studies Favorable side-effect profile (with the exception of addiction potential) Relatively safe in overdose	Dependency possible Sedation, slow reaction time, and other side effects

Note. MAOI=monoamine oxidase inhibitor; SNRI=serotonin-norepinephrine reuptake inhibitor; SSRIs=selective serotonin reuptake inhibitors; TCAs=tricyclic antidepressants.

TABLE 23–4. Treatment algorithm for panic disorder

What are the first-line treatments?	SSRIs and the SNRI venlafaxine Cognitive-behavioral therapy
When should treatment be stopped because of lack of efficacy?	After 4–6 weeks
What if partial response occurs after 4–6 weeks?	Treat another 4–6 weeks with increased dose before changing the treatment strategy
What are the treatment options for treatment-resistant cases?	Switching from one SSRI to another Switching from venlafaxine to an SSRI or vice versa Switching to tricyclic antidepressants Switching to benzodiazepines, reboxetine,[a] phenelzine, or moclobemide[a] Switching to drugs that have been effective in preliminary open studies or case reports: mirtazapine, valproate, inositol, ondansetron, gabapentin, tiagabine, vigabatrin Switching to drugs that were effective in other anxiety disorders in double-blind, placebo-controlled studies: pregabalin, duloxetine, quetiapine, buspirone
Can antipanic drugs be combined?	Usually, monotherapy is the better option. Combinations of drugs may be used in treatment-resistant cases. These combinations are supported by studies: –Benzodiazepines may be used in combination in the first weeks, before onset of efficacy of the antidepressants –Augmentation of fluoxetine with pindolol –Augmentation of clomipramine with lithium –Augmentation with olanzapine

Note. SNRI = serotonin-norepinephrine-serotonin reuptake inhibitor; SSRIs = selective serotonin reuptake inhibitors.
[a]Not available in the United States.

2005), although some reports have raised concerns about fetal cardiac effects, newborn persistent pulmonary hypertension, and other effects (American College of Obstetricians and Gynecologists 2006). Preschool-age children exposed to fluoxetine in utero show no significant neurobehavioral changes (Goldstein and Sundell 1999). The findings of a prospective controlled study suggest that long-term prenatal exposure to TCAs or fluoxetine does not adversely affect cognition, language development, or temperament (Nulman et al. 2002).

An association between the use of benzodiazepines and congenital malformations has been reported (Laegreid et al. 1990). However, there has been no consistent proof that benzodiazepines may be hazardous. The available literature indicates that it is safe to take diazepam or chlordiazepoxide during pregnancy. It has been suggested that it would be prudent to avoid alprazolam during pregnancy (Iqbal et al. 2002). To avoid the potential risk of congenital defects, physicians should prescribe the benzodiazepines that have long safety records.

Breastfeeding Women

SSRIs and TCAs are excreted into breast milk, and low levels have been found in infant serum (Misri et al. 2000b; Simpson and Noble 2000; Spigset and Hagg 1998). In mothers receiving TCAs (with the exception of doxepine), it seems unwarranted to recommend that breastfeeding should be discontinued. Fluoxetine, however, should probably be avoided during lactation (Spigset and Hagg 1998). Treatment with other SSRIs (citalopram, fluvoxamine, paroxetine, or sertraline) seems to be compatible with breastfeeding, although this view should be considered preliminary, given the lack of available relevant data (Gentile et al. 2007; Spigset and Hagg 1998).

Regarding anxiolytic benzodiazepines, adverse drug reactions in infants have been described during maternal treatment with diazepam. During maternal treatment with all anxiolytic benzodiazepines, the infant should be observed for signs of sedation, lethargy, poor suckling, and weight loss, and if high doses have to be used and long-term administration is required, breastfeeding should probably be discontinued (Iqbal et al. 2002; Spigset and Hagg 1998).

Children and Adolescents

In the majority of studies, the average age at onset of panic disorder was found to be between 23 and 28 years (Bandelow 2003). Therefore, panic disorder in children and adolescents is relatively rare. There are no double-

TABLE 23–5. Treatment of panic disorder: frequently asked questions

How can compliance be improved?	Inform the patient about late onset of action and possible side effects that might occur in the first weeks of treatment (such as insomnia or restlessness with SSRIs/SNRIs).
Can medication be stopped after onset of efficacy?	Expert conferences recommend extension of treatment for at least 1 year to avoid relapses.
Will drug treatment be lifelong?	In most patients, symptoms of panic disorder usually lessen after age 40–45; the disorder has a waxing and waning course. Therefore, only a few patients may require long-term treatment over a few years.
Is there a possibility of irreversible side effects after year-long treatment?	There is no evidence of irreversible side effects with SSRIs, SNRIs, or TCAs.
What dosages are used in maintenance treatment?	SSRIs should be used in the same dosages as in acute treatment, whereas TCAs may be used in half the dosage recommended for acute treatment.
Should medication be stopped before starting cognitive-behavioral therapy?	There is no evidence that drugs may weaken the effects of cognitive-behavioral therapy; in contrast, meta-analyses have shown that a combination of both treatment modalities is more effective than both monotherapies.

Note. SNRIs = serotonin-norepinephrine reuptake inhibitors; SSRIs = selective serotonin reuptake inhibitors; TCAs = tricyclic antidepressants.

blind treatment studies for this age group. Experiences with the pharmacological treatment of anxiety disorders in children and adolescents derive mainly from the controlled clinical studies conducted in patients with obsessive-compulsive disorder. These data suggest that SSRIs should be first-line treatment in children and adolescents (see also Emslie and Judge 2000). However, treatment with SSRIs and SNRIs has been associated with suicidal ideation (not suicide attempts) in adolescents with depression and anxiety disorders. Therefore, the risks and benefits of drug treatment should be weighed carefully in this population, and it may be preferable to reserve pharmacological treatments for patients who do not respond to evidence-based psychological approaches.

The Elderly

The symptoms of panic disorder tend to decrease after age 45–50 years. Therefore, panic disorder is relatively rare in elderly patients. However, panic attacks may occur in elderly patients with major depression. Few studies exist that investigate the treatment of anxiety disorders in the elderly, although escitalopram and citalopram appeared effective in reducing panic attack frequency in a small sample of elderly patients with recurrent panic attacks associated with a range of anxiety disorders (Rampello et al. 2006).

Factors to be regarded in the treatment of the elderly include an increased sensitivity for anticholinergic properties of drugs, an increased sensitivity for extrapyramidal symptoms, an increased risk for orthostatic hypotension and electrocardiographic changes, and possible paradoxical reactions to benzodiazepines. Thus, treatment with TCAs or benzodiazepines is less favorable, whereas SSRIs and SNRIs appear to be safe.

Management of Treatment-Resistant Panic Disorder

Many patients continue to experience recurrent panic attacks, agoraphobic avoidance, or continuing distress and impairment, even after standard treatment. According to clinical studies, about 20%–40% of patients treated with standard treatments remain symptomatic (Bandelow et al. 2004; Black et al. 1993). In naturalistic settings, this percentage may be even higher, because the patients selected in clinical studies are often less severely ill, are younger, and have less comorbid conditions than the general patient population.

Several risk factors predicting poorer outcome of treatment have been identified, including the following:

- Long duration of illness (Shinoda et al. 1999; Slaap and den Boer 2001)
- High baseline illness severity (Pollack et al. 2000)
- Severe agoraphobic avoidance (Lotufo-Neto et al. 2001; Slaap and den Boer 2001)
- Strong hypochondriacal fears (Shinoda et al. 1999)
- Frequent emergency room visits (Roy-Byrne et al. 2003)
- Comorbidity with other anxiety disorders (Baillie and Rapee 2004; Berger et al. 2004; Scheibe and Albus 1997), depression (Heldt et al. 2003; Lotufo-

Neto et al. 2001), or personality disorders (Berger et al. 2004; Prasko et al. 2005; Steketee et al. 2001)

- Reduced general mental health (Baillie and Rapee 2004)
- Unemployment (Roy-Byrne et al. 2003)
- Delayed response to medication (Pollack et al. 2002)
- Low treatment compliance with a regimen of cognitive-behavioral therapy (CBT) (Schmidt and Woolaway-Bickel 2000).

It should be ascertained that the diagnosis is correct, the patient is compliant with therapy, the dosage prescribed is therapeutic, and there has been an adequate trial period. Concurrent prescription drugs may interfere with efficacy—for example, metabolic enhancers or inhibitors. Some patients metabolize drugs very fast. Although the determination of plasma levels is not used routinely due to the low correlations between oral dose and plasma levels or between plasma levels and clinical effect, this method might be helpful in identifying patients who do not take their medication at all or are fast metabolizers. Psychosocial factors may affect response, and depression, borderline personality disorder, and substance abuse are especially likely to complicate panic disorder.

Few studies are available to guide selection of treatment for patients with treatment-resistant panic disorder. Data from controlled clinical studies of patients with treatment-responsive panic disorder are not easily transferable to treatment-resistant cases. In the only existing preliminary double-blind, placebo-controlled study with treatment-resistant cases, it was demonstrated that *pindolol* has an augmenting effect on fluoxetine (Hirschmann et al. 2000), but this strategy is rarely used in practice. In a small single-blind crossover design, nonresponders to the SSRI citalopram were switched to the NRI *reboxetine* and vice versa, showing that a trial of agents targeted to other receptors is worthwhile in nonresponders (Seedat et al. 2003).

In a small open study, an augmentation strategy in which patients receiving a TCA had fluoxetine added, and those receiving fluoxetine had a TCA added, was very successful (Tiffon et al. 1994).

Sodium valproate and *clonazepam* were combined in the treatment of four patients with panic disorder who were resistant to several antipanic drug treatments (Ontiveros and Fontaine 1992).

In a single case, the addition of *lithium* to clomipramine treatment was successful (Cournoyer 1986). In some cases, the addition of 5–12.5 mg *olanzapine* to various drug combinations led to a relief of panic attacks (Etxebeste et al. 2000; Khaldi et al. 2003).

Some drugs that have been investigated and shown to be useful in the treatment of other anxiety disorders may also work in panic disorder. These include drugs that have shown efficacy in generalized anxiety disorder, such as the azapirone *buspirone*, the SNRI *duloxetine,* the calcium channel modulator *pregabalin* (Baldwin and Ajel 2007; Bandelow et al. 2007c), and the atypical antipsychotic *quetiapine* (Bandelow et al., in press).

Psychological treatments such as CBT have to be considered in all patients, regardless of whether they are nonresponders or not. The addition of group CBT to pharmacotherapy may be beneficial in nonresponders to pharmacological approaches (Heldt et al. 2003; Otto et al. 1999; Pollack et al. 1994).

Novel Treatment Approaches

Many novel treatment approaches are currently under investigation to improve treatment for anxiety disorders. Antipanic drugs are needed that would have a faster onset, higher response rates, no addiction potential, and fewer side effects than currently available antidepressants.

New targets for anxiolytic drugs include the neurokinin receptors, but *onasetant,* a neurokinin-3 (NK3) receptor antagonist, did not show efficacy in panic disorder (Kronenberg et al. 2005). Preclinical studies with metabotropic glutamate (mGlu) type 2 receptor agonists have shown promising results in the treatment of anxiety. However, in a small trial, the effects of mGlu receptor agonist *LY354740* did not differ from placebo (Bergink and Westenberg 2005).

For a number of putative anxiolytic compounds currently under development, only preclinical or preliminary data exist. These include serotonin receptor agonists and antagonists, sigma ligands, neuropeptide Y agonists, adenosine A1 and A2 receptor agonists, corticotropin-releasing hormone receptor antagonists, natriuretic peptide, and nitroflavonoids. Moreover, these compounds have not yet been investigated in large-scale clinical studies.

Nonpharmacological Treatment

All patients with panic disorder require supportive interviews and attention to emotional states. Also, psychoeducative methods, including information about the nature and etiology of panic disorder and agoraphobia and the mechanism of action of psychological and drug treatments, are essential. Many patients may require specific psychological treatment interventions (see Chapter 24, "Psychotherapy for Panic Disorder," in this volume).

Psychological and pharmacological treatment modalities must be seen as partners, not alternatives, in the treatment of panic disorder. In a meta-analysis of studies that included both CBT and drug treatment, a combination of both modalities was found to be more effective than CBT or drug treatment alone (Bandelow et al. 2007a).

Exercise has been proposed as a remedy for all kinds of psychiatric disorders; however, only a few controlled studies have been performed to assess its usefulness. In the first study examining the role of exercise in an anxiety disorder, patients with panic disorder were randomly assigned to one of three treatment modalities: running, clomipramine, or placebo. Both exercise and clomipramine led to a significant decrease of symptoms in comparison with placebo; however, exercise was still found to be significantly less effective than clomipramine (Bandelow et al. 2000). In a subsequent study, a combination of drug treatment and exercise was investigated. Patients received paroxetine or placebo in a double-blind manner. Additionally, patients in both groups were randomly allocated to exercise, and a control group received relaxation training. Whereas paroxetine was found to be superior to placebo, outcome for subjects who exercised did not differ from outcome for the control group—perhaps due to the high effect sizes obtained in the latter treatment modality. In evaluating the results of both studies together, exercise seems to have some effect on panic disorder; however, this effect seems to be less pronounced than the effect of medication (Wedekind D, Broocks A, Weiss P, Rotter-Glattkowski K, et al.: "A Randomized, Controlled Trial on the Effects of Paroxetine Versus Placebo in Combination With Aerobic Exercise or Relaxation Training in the Treatment of Panic Disorder," manuscript submitted for publication).

The following example represents a typical case of panic disorder with agoraphobia.

Clinical Example

Mrs. Sandra S, age 36 years, started to have panic attacks after giving birth to her child 5 years previously. During the attacks, which would last for about half an hour, she experienced fast and irregular heartbeat, trembling, dizziness, the feeling that she could faint at any moment, numb feelings in her face and on the left side of her body, and fear of dying. She was referred several times to emergency treatments in a hospital, where a complete checkup did not reveal any irregularities. She was on sick leave frequently because of her anxiety attacks. About 6 months after her first attacks, she developed agoraphobia in crowded spaces. As a consequence, she tended to avoid going to parties, restaurants, shopping malls, or cinemas.

Her general practitioner began treating Mrs. S with St. John's wort tablets and homoeopathic formulations, which did not change the course of illness. She was referred to a psychosomatic hospital, where she received individual and group psychotherapy for 3 months. Soon after she was discharged, her symptoms reappeared.

After 2 years of severe panic disorder, Mrs. S was referred to the university department for anxiety disorders. She received treatment with an SSRI, which showed efficacy after 3 weeks. Initial jitteriness disappeared after 10 days. The patient was also treated with individual ambulatory CBT, which involved therapist-guided exposure to crowded places. Mrs. S continued in stable remission and was able to resume her work.

Conclusion

Panic disorder is a common and disabling disorder. Due to increased efforts in recent years in the systematic clinical evaluation of psychopharmacological agents for the treatment of anxiety, a comprehensive database has been collected so that precise recommendations can be provided for treating panic disorder.

The drugs recommended as the first-line treatment for panic disorder are the SSRIs or the SNRI venlafaxine. TCAs such as imipramine or clomipramine are also effective in panic disorder. However, because of their more unfavorable side-effect profile as compared with SSRIs or SNRIs, these drugs stay second in line. In treatment-resistant cases, benzodiazepines such as alprazolam may be used when the patient does not have a history of dependency and tolerance. Benzodiazepines can be combined with antidepressants temporarily during the first weeks of treatment, until the onset of efficacy of the antidepressants. The irreversible MAOI phenelzine is also effective in treating panic disorder, but its use should be restricted to otherwise treatment-resistant cases because of possible dangerous side effects and interactions.

A number of treatment options exist for patients who are nonresponsive to standard treatments. In most cases, drug treatment and CBT may substantially improve quality of life in panic disorder patients.

◀ Key Clinical Points ▶

- Panic disorder is a chronic and disabling condition that often requires longstanding treatment. As a rule, pharmacotherapy should be applied for at least 1 year.
- Pharmacotherapy and cognitive-behavioral therapy seem to have synergistic effects.
- Selective serotonin reuptake inhibitors or the serotonin-norepinephrine reuptake inhibitor venlafaxine are first-line treatments for panic disorder. Tricyclic antidepressants may be used as second-line treatments. Benzodiazepines and monoamine oxidase inhibitors are third-line treatments.

References

Altshuler LL, Cohen LS, Moline ML, et al: The Expert Consensus Guideline Series: treatment of depression in women. Postgrad Med Mar:1–107, 2001

Alwan S, Reefhuis J, Rasmussen SA, et al: Use of selective serotonin-reuptake inhibitors in pregnancy and the risk of birth defects. N Engl J Med 356:2684–2692, 2007

American College of Obstetricians and Gynecologists: ACOG Committee Opinion No. 354: treatment with selective serotonin reuptake inhibitors during pregnancy. Obstet Gynecol 108:1601–1603, 2006

American Psychiatric Association: Practice guideline for the treatment of patients with panic disorder. Work Group on Panic Disorder. Am J Psychiatry 155:1–34, 1998

Amore M, Magnani K, Cerisoli M, et al: Panic disorder: a long-term treatment study: fluoxetine vs imipramine. Hum Psychopharmacol Clin Exp 14:429–434, 1999a

Amore M, Magnani K, Cerisoli M, et al: Short-term and long-term evaluation of selective serotonin reuptake inhibitors in the treatment of panic disorder: fluoxetine vs citalopram. Hum Psychopharmacol Clin Exp 14:435–440, 1999b

Andersch S, Rosenberg NK, Kullingsjo H, et al: Efficacy and safety of alprazolam, imipramine and placebo in treating panic disorder: a Scandinavian multicenter study. Acta Psychiatr Scand Suppl 365:18–27, 1991

Asnis GM, Hameedi FA, Goddard AW, et al: Fluvoxamine in the treatment of panic disorder: a multi-center, double-blind, placebo-controlled study in outpatients. Psychiatry Res 103:1–14, 2001

Austin MPV, Mitchell PB: Psychotropic medications in pregnant women: treatment dilemmas. Med J Aust 169:428–431, 1998

Baillie AJ, Rapee RM: Predicting who benefits from psychoeducation and self help for panic attacks. Behav Res Ther 42:513–527, 2004

Bakish D, Hooper CL, Filteau MJ, et al: A double-blind placebo-controlled trial comparing fluvoxamine and imipramine in the treatment of panic disorder with or without agoraphobia. Psychopharmacol Bull 32:135–141, 1996

Bakker A, van Dyck R, Spinhoven P, et al: Paroxetine, clomipramine, and cognitive therapy in the treatment of panic disorder. J Clin Psychiatry 60:831–838, 1999

Baldwin DS: Sexual dysfunction associated with antidepressant drugs. Expert Opin Drug Saf 3:457–470, 2004

Baldwin DS, Ajel K: The role of pregabalin in the treatment of generalized anxiety disorder. Neuropsychiatr Dis Treat 3:185–191, 2007

Baldwin DS, Anderson IM, Nutt DJ, et al: Evidence-based guidelines for the pharmacological treatment of anxiety disorders: recommendations from the British Association for Psychopharmacology. J Psychopharmacol 19:567–596, 2005

Ballenger JC, Burrows GD, DuPont RL Jr, et al: Alprazolam in panic disorder and agoraphobia: results from a multicenter trial, I: efficacy in short-term treatment. Arch Gen Psychiatry 45:413–422, 1988

Ballenger JC, Wheadon DE, Steiner M, et al: Double-blind, fixed-dose, placebo-controlled study of paroxetine in the treatment of panic disorder. Am J Psychiatry 155:36–42, 1998

Bandelow B: Epidemiology of depression and anxiety, in Handbook on Depression and Anxiety. Edited by Kasper S, den Boer JA, Sitsen AJM. New York, Marcel Dekker, 2003, pp 49–68

Bandelow B, Sievert K, Röthemeyer M, et al: What treatments do patients with panic disorder and agoraphobia get? Eur Arch Psychiatry Clin Neurosci 245:165–171, 1995

Bandelow B, Broocks A, Pekrun G, et al: The use of the Panic and Agoraphobia Scale (P and A) in a controlled clinical trial. Pharmacopsychiatry 33:174–181, 2000

Bandelow B, Behnke K, Lenoir S, et al: Sertraline versus paroxetine in the treatment of panic disorder: an acute, double-blind noninferiority comparison. J Clin Psychiatry 65:405–413, 2004

Bandelow B, Seidler-Brandler U, Becker A, et al: Meta-analysis of randomized controlled comparisons of psychopharmacological and psychological treatments for anxiety disorders. World J Biol Psychiatry 8:175–187, 2007a

Bandelow B, Stein DJ, Dolberg OT, et al: Improvement of quality of life in panic disorder with escitalopram, citalopram, or placebo. Pharmacopsychiatry 40:152–156, 2007b

Bandelow B, Wedekind D, Leon T: Pregabalin for the treatment of generalized anxiety disorder: a novel pharmacologic intervention. Expert Rev Neurother 7:769–781, 2007c

Bandelow B, Zohar J, Hollander E, et al: World Federation of Societies of Biological Psychiatry (WFSBP) guidelines for the pharmacological treatment of anxiety, obsessive-compulsive and post-traumatic stress disorders: first revision. World J Biol Psychiatry 9:248–312, 2008

Bandelow B, Chouinard G, Bobes J, et al: Once-daily extended-release quetiapine fumarate (quetiapine XR) monotherapy in generalized anxiety disorder: a phase III, randomized, double-blind, placebo- and active (paroxetine)-controlled study. Int J Neuropsychopharmacol (in press)

Beauclair L, Fontaine R, Annable L, et al: Clonazepam in the treatment of panic disorder: a double-blind, placebo-controlled trial investigating the correlation between clonazepam concentrations in plasma and clinical response. J Clin Psychopharmacol 14:111–118, 1994

Benjamin J, Levine J, Fux M, et al: Double-blind, placebo-controlled, crossover trial of inositol treatment for panic disorder. Am J Psychiatry 152:1084–1086, 1995

Berger P, Sachs G, Amering M, et al: Personality disorder and social anxiety predict delayed response in drug and behavioral treatment of panic disorder. J Affect Disord 80:75–78, 2004

Bergink V, Westenberg HG: Metabotropic glutamate II receptor agonists in panic disorder: a double blind clinical trial with LY354740. Int Clin Psychopharmacol 20:291–293, 2005

Bertani A, Perna G, Migliarese G, et al: Comparison of the treatment with paroxetine and reboxetine in panic disorder: a randomized, single-blind study. Pharmacopsychiatry 37:206–210, 2004

Black DW, Wesner R, Bowers W, et al: A comparison of fluvoxamine, cognitive therapy, and placebo in the treatment of panic disorder. Arch Gen Psychiatry 50:44–50, 1993

Boyer W: Serotonin uptake inhibitors are superior to imipramine and alprazolam in alleviating panic attacks: a meta-analysis. Int Clin Psychopharmacol 10:45–49, 1995

Bradwejn J: Benzodiazepines for the treatment of panic disorder and generalized anxiety disorder: clinical issues and future directions. Can J Psychiatry 384:S109–113, 1993

Bradwejn J, Ahokas A, Stein DJ, et al: Venlafaxine extended-release capsules in panic disorder: flexible-dose, double-blind, placebo-controlled study. Br J Psychiatry 187:352–359, 2005

Bystritsky A, Rosen RM, Murphy KJ, et al: Double-blind pilot trial of desipramine versus fluoxetine in panic patients. Anxiety 1:287–290, 1994

Carpenter LL, Leon Z, Yasmin S, et al: Clinical experience with mirtazapine in the treatment of panic disorder. Ann Clin Psychiatry 11:81–86, 1999

Cassano GB, Petracca A, Perugi G, et al: Clomipramine for panic disorder, I: the first 10 weeks of a long-term comparison with imipramine. J Affect Disord 14:123–127, 1988

Cavaljuga S, Licanin I, Kapic E, et al: Clomipramine and fluoxetine effects in the treatment of panic disorder. Bosn J Basic Med Sci 3:27–31, 2003

Charney DS, Woods SW: Benzodiazepine treatment of panic disorder: a comparison of alprazolam and lorazepam. J Clin Psychiatry 50:418–423, 1989

Charney DS, Woods SW, Goodman WK, et al: Drug treatment of panic disorder: the comparative efficacy of imipramine, alprazolam, and trazodone. J Clin Psychiatry 47:580–586, 1986

Cournoyer J: Reponse rapide a l'addition du carbonate de lithium d'un trouble: panique resistant aux antidépresseurs tricycliques [Rapid response of a disorder to the addition of lithium carbonate: panic resistant to tricyclic antidepressants]. Can J Psychiatry 31:335–338, 1986

Cross-National Collaborative Panic Study: Drug treatment of panic disorder: comparative efficacy of alprazolam, imipramine, and placebo. Br J Psychiatry 160:191–202, 1992

Curtis GC, Massana J, Udina C, et al: Maintenance drug therapy of panic disorder. J Psychiatr Res 27 (suppl 1):127–142, 1993

de Beurs E, van Balkom AJ, Lange A, et al: Treatment of panic disorder with agoraphobia: comparison of fluvoxamine, placebo, and psychological panic management combined with exposure and of exposure in vivo alone. Am J Psychiatry 152:683–691, 1995

den Boer JA, Westenberg HG: Effect of a serotonin and noradrenaline uptake inhibitor in panic disorder: a double-blind comparative study with fluvoxamine and maprotiline. Int Clin Psychopharmacol 3:59–74, 1988

den Boer JA, Westenberg HG: Serotonin function in panic disorder: a double blind placebo controlled study with fluvoxamine and ritanserin. Psychopharmacology (Berl) 102:85–94, 1990

Dunner DL, Ishiki D, Avery DH, et al: Effect of alprazolam and diazepam on anxiety and panic attacks in panic disorder: a controlled study. J Clin Psychiatry 47:458–460, 1986

Dyukova GM, Shepeleva IP, Vorob'eva OV: Treatment of negative crises (panic attacks). Neurosci Behav Physiol 22:343–345, 1992

Emslie G, Judge R: Tricyclic antidepressants and selective serotonin reuptake inhibitors: use during pregnancy, in children/adolescents and in the elderly. Acta Psychiatrica Scandinavica 101:26–34, 2000

Ericson A, Kallen B, Wiholm BE: Delivery outcome after the use of antidepressants in early pregnancy. Eur J Clin Pharmacol 55:503–508, 1999

Etxebeste M, Aragüés E, Malo P, et al: Olanzapine and panic attacks. Am J Psychiatry 157:659–660, 2000

Evans L, Kenardy J, Schneider P, et al: Effect of a selective serotonin uptake inhibitor in agoraphobia with panic attacks: a double-blind comparison of zimeldine, imipramine and placebo. Acta Psychiatr Scand 73:49–53, 1986

Fahy TJ, O'Rourke D, Brophy J, et al: The Galway Study of Panic Disorder, I: clomipramine and lofepramine in DSM III-R panic disorder: a placebo controlled trial. J Affect Disord 25:63–75, 1992

Ferguson JM, Khan A, Mangano R, et al: Relapse prevention of panic disorder in adult outpatient responders to treatment with venlafaxine extended release. J Clin Psychiatry 68:58–68, 2007

Gentile S, Rossi A, Bellantuono C: SSRIs during breastfeeding: spotlight on milk-to-plasma ratio. Arch Womens Ment Health 10:39–51, 2007

Goddard AW, Brouette T, Almai A, et al: Early coadministration of clonazepam with sertraline for panic disorder. Arch Gen Psychiatry 58:681–686, 2001

Goldstein DJ, Sundell K: A review of the safety of selective serotonin reuptake inhibitors during pregnancy. Hum Psychopharmacol Clin Exp 14:319–324, 1999

Heldt E, Manfro GG, Kipper L, et al: Treating medication-resistant panic disorder: predictors and outcome of cognitive-behavior therapy in a Brazilian public hospital. Psychother Psychosom 72:43–48, 2003

Hirschmann S, Dannon PN, Iancu I, et al: Pindolol augmentation in patients with treatment-resistant panic disorder: A double-blind, placebo-controlled trial. J Clin Psychopharmacol 20:556–559, 2000

Hoehn-Saric R, McLeod DR, Hipsley PA: Effect of fluvoxamine on panic disorder. J Clin Psychopharmacol 13:321–326, 1993

Hogberg U, Wang M: Depression and pregnancy: may selective serotonin reuptake inhibitors be associated to behavioural teratogenicity? (Comment on "The obstetrician and depression during pregnancy" by Campagne DM [Eur J Obstet Gynecol Reprod Biol 116(2):125–130, 2004]). Eur J Obstet Gynecol Reprod Biol 120:123–124, 2005

Iqbal MM, Sobhan T, Ryals T: Effects of commonly used benzodiazepines on the fetus, the neonate, and the nursing infant. Psychiatr Serv 53:39–49, 2002

Johnston D, Troyer I, Whitsett S: Clomipramine treatment of agoraphobic women: an eight-week controlled trial. Arch Gen Psychiatry 45:453–459, 1988

Kallen BA, Otterblad Olausson P: Maternal use of selective serotonin re-uptake inhibitors in early pregnancy and infant congenital malformations. Birth Defects Res A Clin Mol Teratol 79:301–308, 2007

Kamijima K, Kuboki T, Kumano H, et al: A placebo-controlled, randomized withdrawal study of sertraline for panic disorder in Japan. Int Clin Psychopharmacol 20:265–273, 2005

Keck PE Jr, Taylor VE, Tugrul KC, et al: Valproate treatment of panic disorder and lactate-induced panic attacks. Biol Psychiatry 33:542–546, 1993

Khaldi S, Kornreich C, Dan B, et al: Usefulness of olanzapine in refractory panic attacks. J Clin Psychopharmacol 23:100–101, 2003

Klein D: Delineation of two drug-responsive anxiety syndromes. Psychopharmacology 5:397–408, 1964

Klein D, Fink M: Psychiatric reaction patterns to imipramine. Am J Psychiatry 119:432–438, 1962

Koren G, Matsui D, Einarson A, et al: Is maternal use of selective serotonin reuptake inhibitors in the third trimester of pregnancy harmful to neonates? CMAJ 172:1457–1459, 2005

Kronenberg G, Berger P, Tauber RF, et al: Randomized, double blind study of SR142801 (onasetant): a novel neurokinin-3 (NK3) receptor antagonist in panic disorder with pre- and posttreatment cholecystokinin tetrapeptide (CCK-4) challenges. Pharmacopsychiatry 38:24–29, 2005

Krüger MB, Dahl AA: The efficacy and safety of moclobemide compared to clomipramine in the treatment of panic disorder. Eur Arch Psychiatry Clin Neurosci 249 (suppl 1):S19–S24, 1999

Laegreid L, Olegard R, Conradi N, et al: Congenital malformations and maternal consumption of benzodiazepines: a case-control study. Dev Med Child Neurol 32:432–441, 1990

Lattimore KA, Donn SM, Kaciroti N, et al: Selective serotonin reuptake inhibitor (SSRI) use during pregnancy and effects on the fetus and newborn: a meta-analysis. J Perinatol 25:595–604, 2005

Lecrubier Y, Judge R: Long-term evaluation of paroxetine, clomipramine and placebo in panic disorder. Collaborative Paroxetine Panic Study Investigators. Acta Psychiatr Scand 95:153–160, 1997

Lecrubier Y, Bakker A, Dunbar G, et al: A comparison of paroxetine, clomipramine and placebo in the treatment of panic disorder. Collaborative Paroxetine Panic Study Investigators. Acta Psychiatr Scand 95:145–152, 1997

Lepola U, Heikkinen H, Rimon R, et al: Clinical evaluation of alprazolam in patients with panic disorder a double-blind comparison with imipramine. Hum Psychopharmacol 5:159–163, 1990

Lepola UM, Wade AG, Leinonen EV, et al: A controlled, prospective, 1-year trial of citalopram in the treatment of panic disorder. J Clin Psychiatry 59:528–534, 1998

Lepola U, Arato M, Zhu Y, et al: Sertraline versus imipramine treatment of comorbid panic disorder and major depressive disorder. J Clin Psychiatry 64:654–662, 2003

Livingston MG: Benzodiazepine dependence. Br J Hosp Med 51:281–286, 1994

Loerch B, Graf-Morgenstern M, Hautzinger M, et al: Randomised placebo-controlled trial of moclobemide, cognitive-behavioural therapy and their combination in panic disorder with agoraphobia. Br J Psychiatry 174:205–212, 1999

Londborg PD, Wolkow R, Smith WT, et al: Sertraline in the treatment of panic disorder: a multi-site, double-blind, placebo-controlled, fixed-dose investigation. Br J Psychiatry 173:54–60, 1998

Lotufo-Neto F, Bernik M, Ramos RT, et al: A dose-finding and discontinuation study of clomipramine in panic disorder. J Psychopharmacol 15:13–17, 2001

Lum M, Fontaine R, Elie R, et al: Divalproex sodium's antipanic effect in panic disorder: a placebo-controlled study. Biol Psychiatry 27:164A–165A, 1990

Lydiard RB, Lesser IM, Ballenger JC, et al: A fixed-dose study of alprazolam 2 mg, alprazolam 6 mg, and placebo in panic disorder. J Clin Psychopharmacol 12:96–103, 1992

Malm H, Klaukka T, Neuvonen PJ: Risks associated with selective serotonin reuptake inhibitors in pregnancy. Obstet Gynecol 106:1289–1296, 2005

Mavissakalian M, Perel JM: Clinical experiments in maintenance and discontinuation of imipramine therapy in panic disorder with agoraphobia. Arch Gen Psychiatry 49:318–323, 1992a

Mavissakalian M, Perel JM: Protective effects of imipramine maintenance treatment in panic disorder with agoraphobia. Am J Psychiatry 149:1053–1057, 1992b

Michelson D, Lydiard RB, Pollack MH, et al: Outcome assessment and clinical improvement in panic disorder: evidence from a randomized controlled trial of fluoxetine and placebo. The Fluoxetine Panic Disorder Study Group. Am J Psychiatry 155:1570–1577, 1998

Michelson D, Allgulander C, Dantendorfer K, et al: Efficacy of usual antidepressant dosing regimens of fluoxetine in panic disorder: randomised, placebo-controlled trial. Br J Psychiatry 179:514–518, 2001

Misri S, Burgmann A, Kostaras D: Are SSRIs safe for pregnant and breastfeeding women? Can Fam Physician 46:626–628, 2000a

Misri S, Kostaras D, Kostaras X: The use of selective serotonin reuptake inhibitors during pregnancy and lactation: current knowledge. Can J Psychiatry 45:285–287, 2000b

Modigh K, Westberg P, Eriksson E: Superiority of clomipramine over imipramine in the treatment of panic disorder: a placebo-controlled trial. J Clin Psychopharmacol 12:251–261, 1992

Moroz G, Rosenbaum JF: Efficacy, safety, and gradual discontinuation of clonazepam in panic disorder: a placebo-controlled, multicenter study using optimized dosages. J Clin Psychiatry 60:604–612, 1999

Munjack DJ, Crocker B, Cabe D, et al: Alprazolam, propranolol, and placebo in the treatment of panic disorder and agoraphobia with panic attacks. J Clin Psychopharmacol 9:22–27, 1989

Nair NP, Bakish D, Saxena B, et al: Comparison of fluvoxamine, imipramine, and placebo in the treatment of outpatients with panic disorder. Anxiety 2:192–198, 1996

Nelson J, Chouinard G: Guidelines for the clinical use of benzodiazepines: pharmacokinetics, dependency, rebound and withdrawal. Canadian Society for Clinical Pharmacology. Can J Clin Pharmacol 6:69–83, 1999

Nordeng H, Spigset O: Treatment with selective serotonin reuptake inhibitors in the third trimester of pregnancy: effects on the infant. Drug Saf 28:565–581, 2005

Noyes R Jr, Anderson DJ, Clancy J, et al: Diazepam and propranolol in panic disorder and agoraphobia. Arch Gen Psychiatry 41:287–292, 1984

Noyes R Jr, Burrows GD, Reich JH, et al: Diazepam versus alprazolam for the treatment of panic disorder. J Clin Psychiatry 57:349–355, 1996

Nulman I, Rovet J, Stewart DE, et al: Child development following exposure to tricyclic antidepressants or fluoxetine throughout fetal life: a prospective, controlled study. Am J Psychiatry 159:1889–1895, 2002

Oehrberg S, Christiansen PE, Behnke K, et al: Paroxetine in the treatment of panic disorder: a randomised, double-blind, placebo-controlled study. Br J Psychiatry 167:374–379, 1995

Ontiveros A, Fontaine R: Sodium valproate and clonazepam for treatment-resistant panic disorder. J Psychiatry Neurosci 17:78–80, 1992

Otto MW, Pollack MH, Sachs GS, et al: Discontinuation of benzodiazepine treatment: efficacy of cognitive-behavioral therapy for patients with panic disorder. Am J Psychiatry 150:1485–1490, 1993

Otto MW, Pollack MH, Penava SJ, et al: Group cognitive-behavior therapy for patients failing to respond to pharmacotherapy for panic disorder: a clinical case series. Behav Res Ther 37:763–770, 1999

Palatnik A, Frolov K, Fux M, et al: Double-blind, controlled, crossover trial of inositol versus fluvoxamine for the treatment of panic disorder. J Clin Psychopharmacol 21:335–339, 2001

Pande AC, Pollack MH, Crockatt J, et al: Placebo-controlled study of gabapentin treatment of panic disorder. J Clin Psychopharmacol 20:467–471, 2000

Perna G, Bertani A, Caldirola D, et al: A comparison of citalopram and paroxetine in the treatment of panic disorder: a randomized, single-blind study. Pharmacopsychiatry 34:85–90, 2001

Pohl RB, Wolkow RM, Clary CM: Sertraline in the treatment of panic disorder: a double-blind multicenter trial. Am J Psychiatry 155:1189–1195, 1998

Pollack MH, Doyle AC: Treatment of panic disorder: focus on paroxetine. Psychopharmacol Bull 37 (suppl 1):53–63, 2003

Pollack MH, Otto MW, Kaspi SP, et al: Cognitive behavior therapy for treatment-refractory panic disorder. J Clin Psychiatry 55:200–205, 1994

Pollack MH, Worthington JJ 3rd, Otto MW, et al: Venlafaxine for panic disorder: results from a double-blind, placebo-controlled study. Psychopharmacol Bull 32:667–670, 1996

Pollack MH, Otto MW, Worthington JJ, et al: Sertraline in the treatment of panic disorder: a flexible-dose multicenter trial. Arch Gen Psychiatry 55:1010–1016, 1998

Pollack MH, Rapaport MH, Clary CM, et al: Sertraline treatment of panic disorder: response in patients at risk for poor outcome. J Clin Psychiatry 61:922–927, 2000

Pollack MH, Rapaport MH, Fayyad R, et al: Early improvement predicts endpoint remission status in sertraline and placebo treatments of panic disorder. J Psychiatr Res 36:229–236, 2002

Pollack MH, Lepola U, Koponen H, et al: A double-blind study of the efficacy of venlafaxine extended-release, paroxetine, and placebo in the treatment of panic disorder. Depress Anxiety 24:1–14, 2007

Pols H, Zandergen J, de Loof C, et al: Clinical effects of fluvoxamine on panic symptomatology. Acta Psychiatr Belg 93:169–177, 1993

Prasko J, Houbova P, Novak T, et al: Influence of personality disorder on the treatment of panic disorder: comparison study. Neuro Endocrinol Lett 26:667–674, 2005

Price JS, Waller PC, Wood SM, et al: A comparison of the post-marketing safety of four selective serotonin reuptake inhibitors including the investigation of symptoms occurring on withdrawal. Br J Clin Pharmacol 42:757–763, 1996

Primeau F, Fontaine R, Beauclair L: Valproic acid and panic disorder. Can J Psychiatry 35:248–250, 1990

Rampello L, Alvano A, Raffaele R, et al: New possibilities of treatment for panic attacks in elderly patients: escitalopram versus citalopram. J Clin Psychopharmacol 26:67–70, 2006

Rapaport MH, Wolkow R, Rubin A, et al: Sertraline treatment of panic disorder: results of a long-term study. Acta Psychiatr Scand 104:289–298, 2001

Ravaris CL, Friedman MJ, Hauri PJ, et al: A controlled study of alprazolam and propranolol in panic-disordered and agoraphobic outpatients. J Clin Psychopharmacol 11:344–350, 1991

Ribeiro L, Busnello JV, Kauer-Sant'Anna M, et al: Mirtazapine versus fluoxetine in the treatment of panic disorder. Braz J Med Biol Res 34:1303–1307, 2001

Rickels K: Benzodiazepines in the treatment of anxiety. Am J Psychother 36:358–370, 1982

Rickels K, Schweizer E: Panic disorder: long-term pharmacotherapy and discontinuation. J Clin Psychopharmacol 18:12S–18S, 1998

Rickels K, Schweizer E, Case WG, et al: Long-term therapeutic use of benzodiazepines, I: effects of abrupt discontinuation [published erratum appears in Arch Gen Psychiatry 48:51, 1991]. Arch Gen Psychiatry 47:899–907, 1990

Rizley R, Kahn RJ, McNair DM, et al: A comparison of alprazolam and imipramine in the treatment of agoraphobia and panic disorder. Psychopharmacol Bull 22:167–172, 1986

Rosenbaum JF, Moroz G, Bowden CL: Clonazepam in the treatment of panic disorder with or without agoraphobia: a dose-response study of efficacy, safety, and discontinuance. Clonazepam Panic Disorder Dose-Response Study Group. J Clin Psychopharmacol 17:390–400, 1997

Roy-Byrne PP, Russo J, Cowley DS, Katon WJ: Unemployment and emergency room visits predict poor treatment outcome in primary care panic disorder. J Clin Psychiatry 64:383–389, 2003

Sandmann J, Lorch B, Bandelow B, et al: Fluvoxamine or placebo in the treatment of panic disorder and relationship to blood concentrations of fluvoxamine. Pharmacopsychiatry 31:117–121, 1998

Scheibe G, Albus M: Predictors and outcome in panic disorder: a 2-year prospective follow-up study. Psychopathology 30:177–184, 1997

Schmidt NB, Woolaway-Bickel K: The effects of treatment compliance on outcome in cognitive-behavioral therapy for panic disorder: quality versus quantity. J Consult Clin Psychol 68:13–18, 2000

Schneier FR, Garfinkel R, Kennedy B, et al: Ondansetron in the treatment of panic disorder. Anxiety 2:199–202, 1996

Schweizer E, Rickels K: Buspirone in the treatment of panic disorder: a controlled pilot comparison with clorazepate (letter). J Clin Psychopharmacol 8:303, 1988

Schweizer E, Pohl R, Balon R, et al: Lorazepam vs alprazolam in the treatment of panic disorder. Pharmacopsychiatry 23:90–93, 1990a

Schweizer E, Rickels K, Case WG, et al: Long-term therapeutic use of benzodiazepines, II: effects of gradual taper. Arch Gen Psychiatry 47:908–915, 1990b

Schweizer E, Rickels K, De Martinis N, et al: The effect of personality on withdrawal severity and taper outcome in benzodiazepine dependent patients. Psychol Med 28:713–720, 1998

Seedat S, van Rheede van Oudtshoorn E, Muller JE, et al: Reboxetine and citalopram in panic disorder: a single-blind, cross-over, flexible-dose pilot study. Int Clin Psychopharmacol 18:279–284, 2003

Shader RI, Greenblatt DJ: Use of benzodiazepines in anxiety disorders. N Engl J Med 13:1398–1405, 1993

Sheehan DV, Ballenger J, Jacobsen G: Treatment of endogenous anxiety with phobic, hysterical, and hypochondriacal symptoms. Arch Gen Psychiatry 37:51–59, 1980

Sheehan DV, Davidson J, Manschreck T, et al: Lack of efficacy of a new antidepressant (bupropion) in the treatment of panic disorder with phobias. J Clin Psychopharmacol 3:28–31, 1983

Sheehan DV, Raj AB, Sheehan KH, et al: Is buspirone effective for panic disorder? J Clin Psychopharmacol 10:3–11, 1990

Sheehan DV, Raj AB, Harnett Sheehan K, et al: The relative efficacy of high-dose buspirone and alprazolam in the treatment of panic disorder: a double-blind placebo-controlled study. Acta Psychiatr Scand 88:1–11, 1993

Sheehan DV, Burnham DB, Iyengar MK, et al: Efficacy and tolerability of controlled-release paroxetine in the treatment of panic disorder. J Clin Psychiatry 66:34–40, 2005

Shinoda N, Kodama K, Sakamoto T, et al: Predictors of 1-year outcome for patients with panic disorder. Compr Psychiatry 40:39–43, 1999

Simon NM, Emmanuel N, Ballenger J, et al: Bupropion sustained release for panic disorder. Psychopharmacol Bull 37:66–72, 2003

Simpson K, Noble S: Fluoxetine: a review of its use in women's health. CNS Drugs 14:301–328, 2000

Slaap BR, den Boer JA: The prediction of nonresponse to pharmacotherapy in panic disorder: a review. Depress Anxiety 14:112–122, 2001

Smith DE, Landry MJ: Benzodiazepine dependency discontinuation: focus on the chemical dependency detoxification setting and benzodiazepine-polydrug abuse. J Psychiatr Res 24 (suppl 2):145–156, 1990

Spiegel DA: Psychological strategies for discontinuing benzodiazepine treatment. J Clin Psychopharmacol 19:17S–22S, 1999

Spigset O, Hagg S: Excretion of psychotropic drugs into breast milk: pharmacokinetic overview and therapeutic implications. CNS Drugs 9:111–134, 1998

Stahl MM, Lindquist M, Pettersson M, et al: Withdrawal reactions with selective serotonin re-uptake inhibitors as reported to the WHO system. Eur J Clin Pharmacol 53:163–169, 1997

Stahl SM, Gergel I, Li D: Escitalopram in the treatment of panic disorder: a randomized, double-blind, placebo-controlled trial. J Clin Psychiatry 64:1322–1327, 2003

Steketee G, Chambless DL, Tran GQ: Effects of Axis I and II comorbidity on behavior therapy outcome for obsessive-compulsive disorder and agoraphobia. Compr Psychiatry 42:76–86, 2001

Taylor CB, Hayward C, King R, et al: Cardiovascular and symptomatic reduction effects of alprazolam and imipramine in patients with panic disorder: results of a double-blind, placebo-controlled trial. J Clin Psychopharmacol 10:112–118, 1990

Tesar GE, Rosenbaum JF, Pollack MH, et al: Double-blind, placebo-controlled comparison of clonazepam and alprazolam for panic disorder. J Clin Psychiatry 52:69–76, 1991

Tiffon L, Coplan JD, Papp LA, et al: Augmentation strategies with tricyclic or fluoxetine treatment in seven partially responsive panic disorder patients. J Clin Psychiatry 55:66–69, 1994

Tiller JW, Bouwer C, Behnke K: Moclobemide and fluoxetine for panic disorder. International Panic Disorder Study Group. Eur Arch Psychiatry Clin Neurosci 249 (suppl 1):S7–S10, 1999

Uhlenhuth EH, Matuzas W, Glass RM, et al: Response of panic disorder to fixed doses of alprazolam or imipramine. J Affect Disord 17:261–270, 1989

Uhlenhuth EH, Warner TD, Matuzas W: Interactive model of therapeutic response in panic disorder: moclobemide, a case in point. J Clin Psychopharmacol 22:275–284, 2002

Versiani M, Cassano G, Perugi G, et al: Reboxetine, a selective norepinephrine reuptake inhibitor, is an effective and well-tolerated treatment for panic disorder. J Clin Psychiatry 63:31–37, 2002

Wade AG, Lepola U, Koponen HJ, et al: The effect of citalopram in panic disorder. Br J Psychiatry 170:549–553, 1997

Wittchen HU, Jacobi F: Size and burden of mental disorders in Europe: a critical review and appraisal of 27 studies. Eur Neuropsychopharmacol 15:357–376, 2005

Woodman CL, Noyes R Jr: Panic disorder: treatment with valproate. J Clin Psychiatry 55:134–136, 1994

Zitrin CM, Klein DF, Woerner MG: Treatment of agoraphobia with group exposure in vivo and imipramine. Arch Gen Psychiatry 37:63–72, 1980

Zitrin CM, Klein DF, Woerner MG, et al: Treatment of phobias, I: Comparison of imipramine hydrochloride and placebo. Arch Gen Psychiatry 40:125–138, 1983

Zwanzger P, Baghai T, Boerner RJ, et al: Anxiolytic effects of vigabatrin in panic disorder. J Clin Psychopharmacol 21:539–540, 2001a

Zwanzger P, Baghai TC, Schule C, et al: Tiagabine improves panic and agoraphobia in panic disorder patients. J Clin Psychiatry 62:656–657, 2001b

Recommended Readings

Review Articles

Baldwin DS, Anderson IM, Nutt DJ, et al: Evidence-based guidelines for the pharmacological treatment of anxiety disorders: recommendations from the British Association for Psychopharmacology. J Psychopharmacol 19:567–596, 2005

Bandelow B, Zohar J, Hollander E, et al: World Federation of Societies of Biological Psychiatry (WFSBP) guidelines for the pharmacological treatment of anxiety, obsessive-compulsive and post-traumatic stress disorders: first revision. World J Biol Psychiatry 9:248–312, 2008

Books

Antony MA, Stein MB (eds): Handbook of Anxiety and the Anxiety Disorders. New York, Oxford University Press, 2008

Stein DJ (ed): Clinical Manual of Anxiety Disorders. Washington, DC, American Psychiatric Press, 2004

Web Sites of Interest

Anxiety Disorders Associations of America. Getting help. (n.d.). http://www.adaa.org/GettingHelp/AboutAnxietyDisorders.asp

Mental Health America: Factsheet: panic disorder. 2008. http://www.nmha.org/go/panic-disorder

National Institute of Mental Health: Panic disorder. 2009. http://www.nimh.nih.gov/health/topics/panic-disorder

Chapter 24

Psychotherapy for Panic Disorder

Stefan G. Hofmann, Ph.D.
Winfried Rief, Ph.D.
David A. Spiegel, M.D.

Before panic disorder was identified as a distinct type of anxiety in DSM-III (American Psychiatric Association 1980), psychosocial therapies tended to focus primarily on the behavioral pattern of situational avoidance that frequently occurs in patients with panic attacks. During the 1960s and 1970s, systematic desensitization, consisting of imaginal exposure to feared situations paired with muscle relaxation, was the principal form of treatment. That approach was used in preference to in vivo exposure because it was thought that the latter might engender too much anxiety for patients to manage. However, studies evaluating systematic desensitization for agoraphobia found that it was largely ineffective (Gelder and Marks 1966; Marks 1971). During the 1980s, in parallel with the increasing recognition of the importance of fear of panic attacks as a factor in the development and progression of panic disorder, investigators began to experiment with treatments aimed more specifically at patients' experiences of anxiety related to panic and somatic sensations rather than at avoidance behavior.

Contemporary treatments for panic disorder typically combine exposure instructions with cognitive interventions. These treatments have been referred to as cognitive therapy, behavioral therapy, cognitive-behavioral therapy (CBT), and exposure therapy. All of these treatments are based on the same basic premise: that panic disorder is in part maintained by cognitive and behavioral factors and that it can be treated by targeting these factors through cognitive and behavioral interventions. Another common element of all effective interventions for panic disorder and agoraphobia is in vivo exposure practices. As currently administered, in vivo exposure typically includes the construction of a hierarchy of feared situations that the patient is encouraged to enter repeatedly, starting with easier ones and continuing until anxiety diminishes. Sometimes, the therapist accompanies the patient initially, but ultimately the patient is expected to do the task alone.

Reviews and meta-analyses of treatment studies in which in vivo situational exposure was used found that 60%–75% of treatment completers experienced clinical improvement (Barlow 2002; Gould et al. 1995; Jacobson et al. 1988; Jansson and Ost 1982; Mitte 2005; Munby and Johnson 1980; Trull et al. 1988), and follow-up studies have found maintenance of gains in most cases (Burns et al. 1986; Fava et al. 1995; Jansson et al. 1986; Munby and Johnson 1980). However, a meta-analysis of well-controlled placebo-controlled CBT trials suggests that panic disorder with or without agoraphobia is one of the least responsive anxiety disorders (Hofmann and Smits 2009). Moreover, many patients refuse or drop out of treatment. Although study findings on dropout rates vary, a reasonable estimate is that approximately one in four patients who initiates treatment drops out (Clum 1989; Fava et al. 1995; Hofmann and Smits 2008; Marks 1978).

Cognitive-Behavioral Therapy

Underlying Theoretical Model

A widely cited description of the cognitive model was presented by Clark (1986). According to this model, panic attacks result from the catastrophic misinterpretation of certain bodily sensations, such as palpitations, breathlessness, and dizziness. An example of such a catastrophic misinterpretation is a healthy individual perceiving palpitations as evidence of an impending heart attack. The cognitive model states that various external stimuli (e.g., the feeling of being trapped in a supermarket) or internal stimuli (bodily sensations, thoughts, or images) trigger a state of apprehension if these stimuli are perceived as a threat. This state is accompanied by fearful bodily sensations that, if interpreted catastrophically, further increase the apprehension and the intensity of bodily sensations, thus forming a vicious cycle. This model states that the attacks appear to come from "out of the blue" because patients fail to distinguish between the triggering body sensations and the subsequent panic attack and the general beliefs about the meaning of an attack. The cognitive model does not rule out any biological factors in panic. In contrast, it is assumed that biological variables contribute to an attack by triggering benign bodily fluctuations or intensifying fearful bodily sensations. Therefore, pharmacological treatments can be effective in reducing the frequency of panic attacks if they reduce the frequency of bodily fluctuations that can trigger panic or if they block the bodily sensations that accompany anxiety. However, if the patient's tendency to interpret bodily sensations in a catastrophic fashion is not changed, discontinuation of drug treatment is likely to be associated with a high rate of relapse.

Other popular models of panic include the hyperventilation theory (Ley 1985), the suffocation alarm theory (Klein 1993), the fear-of-fear model (Goldstein and Chambless 1978), the expectancy model (Reiss and McNally 1985), and the modern learning theory of panic (Bouton et al. 2001). A critical comparison of these models is provided by Roth et al. (2005). Aside from the cognitive model, the models most relevant for the contemporary treatment approaches are the expectancy model, the fear-of-fear model, and the modern learning theory of panic. The fear-of-fear model posits that certain internal bodily sensations become the conditioned stimuli for the conditioned response of a panic attack, which then results in the development of fear of fear, a process also known as interoceptive conditioning. However, the fear-of-fear concept in panic disorder is difficult to describe in terms of interoceptive conditioning because it is unclear how to identify and separate the conditioned stimulus from the conditioned response and the unconditioned stimulus from the unconditioned response. An elaboration of this and other critical issues is given by McNally (1994). In contrast to the fear-of-fear model, the expectancy model suggests that panic patients fear anxiety symptoms because of greater anxiety sensitivity, which is conceptualized as a dispositional construct that determines the tendency to respond fearfully to anxiety symptoms. Finally, an elaboration on the learning principles underlying panic disorder was provided by Bouton et al. (2001). This model distinguishes between *anxiety*, an anticipatory emotional state that functions to prepare the individual for a threatening event, and *panic*, an emotional state that exists to deal with a threatening event that is already in progress. The model assumes that panic disorder develops because exposure to panic attacks causes the conditioning of anxiety to exteroceptive and interoceptive cues. The presence of conditioned anxiety then potentiates the next panic attack, making anxiety a precursor of panic. The model further considers a number of general and specific vulnerability factors that might influence the person's susceptibility to conditioning, such as early experiences with uncontrollable and unpredictable events, and vicarious learning events that focus on certain bodily sensations.

Review of Principal Short-Term Trials

Fava et al. (1995) reported the results of exposure therapy on a cohort of 110 patients with a primary diagnosis of panic disorder with agoraphobia who received 12 biweekly 30-minute sessions of in vivo exposure therapy emphasizing self-directed practice. In that study, 81 subjects achieved remission, defined as being panic-free for the past month and "much better" on a global rating of improvement. Survival analyses estimated the likelihood of staying in remission at 2, 5, and 7 years posttreatment to be 96%, 77%, and 67%, respectively. For the intent-to-treat (ITT) sample of 110 patients who entered therapy, those numbers translate into projected remission rates of 71% at 2 years, 57% at 5 years, and 49% at 7 years. Interestingly, in the Fava et al. study, the intention-to-treat sample was a consecutive series of patients meeting DSM-III-R (American Psychiatric Association 1987) criteria for panic disorder with agoraphobia, which included all levels of agoraphobic avoidance. Although many patients improved sufficiently to be classified as responders at the posttreatment assessment, they continued to have some degree of agoraphobic fear and avoidance, which, when present, is a poor prognostic sign. Among the 81 patients who responded to treatment, two-thirds of those who had residual agoraphobia at posttreatment relapsed within 5 years. It is also noteworthy that benzodiazepine use was permitted during the study, and a sizable proportion of the patients (one-fourth at the conclusion of treatment) were taking benzodiazepines.

Whether an optimal intensity for exposure therapy exists is not clear. A few studies have compared massed with spaced exposure sessions. In general, massed exposure has not shown better results than more gradual procedures (Chambless 1990), and some investigators (e.g., Hafner and Marks 1976; Jansson and Ost 1982) have found higher treatment dropout rates with massed exposure. However, investigators at the Christoph-Dornier Foundation in Germany reported excellent results with a highly intensive protocol (Ehlers et al. 1995; Fiegenbaum 1988; Hahlweg et al. 2001; Schroeder et al. 1996). In that treatment, agoraphobic patients underwent 8–10 days of intensive, therapist-accompanied, ungraded exposure in which tasks were selected based on convenience of grouping rather than their positions on a fear hierarchy. The program began with a 2- to 4-hour session in which the treatment rationale was explained, after which patients were given a week to decide whether they were prepared to commit to treatment. In a preliminary study, Fiegenbaum (1988) compared that approach with graded, massed exposure in which patients gradually worked up to greater levels of fear in a hierarchy of feared situations. The two treatments were equally effective at posttreatment and at 8-month follow-up, but ungraded exposure was superior to graded exposure at 5-year follow-up. Subsequently, Ehlers et al. (1995) reported on a sample of 150 patients treated with ungraded exposure. Attrition was surprisingly low; 7% dropped out after the treatment rationale had been explained, and only 2% dropped out during treatment. Among those who completed the treatment, 85% described themselves as "much" or "very much" improved at posttreatment, and 77% did so at 1-year follow-up. The average therapist time per patient was 28 hours.

As impressive as those results are, they do not necessarily indicate a superiority of Fiegenbaum's (1988) approach over other, more gradual forms of exposure therapy. Among the intention-to-treat subjects, the response rate for Fiegenbaum's treatment in the Ehlers et al. (1995) trial was approximately 77% at posttreatment and 70% at 1-year follow-up, comparable to the 2-year remission rate of 71% reported by Fava et al. (1995). Like the latter study, the Ehlers et al. trial enrolled patients with all levels of agoraphobic avoidance. We do not know how many subjects had residual agoraphobia posttreatment and whether, as in the Fava et al. study, residual agoraphobia was associated with a poorer long-term outcome. Furthermore, more recent data suggest that the dropout rate reported by Ehlers et al. may have been lower than that which usually occurs with Fiegenbaum's approach. A review of 253 patients, of whom 222 had agoraphobia treated with ungraded, massed exposure, found an overall dropout rate of 27% (8% after pretreatment assessment, 15% after explanation of the treatment, and 4% during exposure; Schroeder et al. 1996).

One of the most well-studied and comprehensive CBT protocols is panic control treatment (PCT; Craske et al. 2000; Hofmann and Spiegel 1999). PCT consists of the following components: education about the nature of anxiety and panic, identification and correction of maladaptive thoughts about anxiety and its consequences, training in arousal reduction techniques such as slow breathing, and graded exposure to bodily sensations that resemble those experienced during anxiety and panic (interoceptive exposure). Treatment is usually delivered in 11 or 12 sessions over a period of 3–4 months.

The efficacy of PCT has been reported in numerous studies. In one (Barlow et al. 1989), an early form of PCT (consisting of cognitive restructuring and interoceptive exposure) was compared with applied relaxation therapy (Ost 1987), a combination of PCT and applied relaxation therapy, and a wait-list control condition. All three active treatments were judged to be superior to the wait-list control condition on a variety of measures at posttreatment. Approximately 86% of the patients in the PCT alone and PCT plus applied relaxation therapy groups and 60% in the applied relaxation therapy alone group were panic-free by the end of treatment. At follow-up 2 years later, 81% of the patients in the PCT group were panic-free, compared with only 43% and 36% in the other two groups, respectively (Craske et al. 1991).

In a later study, Klosko et al. (1990, 1995) compared PCT with alprazolam, a drug placebo, and a wait-list control condition. Again, 87% of the patients in the PCT group were panic-free by the end of treatment, compared with 50% in the alprazolam group, 36% in the placebo group, and 33% in the wait-list group. PCT was found to be superior to all three other conditions. Subsequently, Telch et al. (1993) found that PCT was effective when administered in an 8-week group format. At posttreatment, 85% of the PCT patients were panic-free, compared with 30% in a wait-list control condition. When a more stringent outcome measure was used (including measures of panic frequency, general anxiety, and agoraphobic avoidance), 63% of the PCT patients and only 9% of the wait-list subjects were classified as improved.

More recently, PCT was compared with imipramine, a pill placebo, and combinations of PCT with imipramine or a pill placebo in a large, multicenter trial (Barlow et al. 2000). PCT alone was comparable to imipramine alone on nearly all measures during acute and continuation treatment, with better maintenance of gains after treatment discontinuation. We discuss this study further later in this chapter.

Similar good results have been reported with treatments that focus more exclusively on cognitive restructuring (e.g., Beck et al. 1992; Clark 1989). These therapies involve approximately the same amount of therapist time as PCT and appear to be comparably efficacious, although they have not been compared directly with PCT. For example, Clark et al. (1994) compared cognitive therapy, applied relaxation therapy, imipramine, and a wait-list control condition. At posttreatment, 75% of the cognitive therapy patients were panic-free, compared with 70% in the imipramine condition, 40% in the applied relaxation therapy condition, and 7% in the wait-list condition. Cognitive therapy was determined to be superior to the wait-list control condition on all panic and anxiety measures, whereas imipramine and applied relaxation therapy were gauged as better than the wait-list control condition on approximately half of the measures. At 9-month follow-up, after imipramine had been discontinued, the panic-free rates were 85% for cognitive therapy, 60% for imipramine, and 47% for applied relaxation therapy.

Abbreviated, Computer-Assisted, and Self-Directed CBT

A few studies have investigated the efficacy of abbreviated or self-directed forms of CBT for panic disorder. In one such study, Coté et al. (1994) found that 10 hours of in-person and telephone therapy were as effective as 20 hours of standard face-to-face CBT administered over the same period. More recently, Craske et al. (1995) found that a four-session CBT protocol was more effective than an equivalent amount of nondirective supportive therapy. The short treatment was not compared with alternative effective therapy.

Clark et al. (1999) compared 12 sessions of standard cognitive therapy to a 5-session version of the same treatment combined with self-study modules and a wait-list control condition (n=14 per condition). The two active treatments, which were administered over a 3-month period, were superior to the wait-list condition on all measures and did not differ significantly from each other. As in previous CBT studies, the great majority (78%) of the patients in the Clark et al. study had no more than mild agoraphobia; however, 22% had moderate agoraphobia. Promising results have also been reported with self-help treatments involving minimal (e.g., 3 hours) therapist contact (Gould and Clum 1995; Gould et al. 1993; Hecker et al. 1996; Lidren et al. 1994). In most of these trials, the self-directed treatments were not compared with clinician-administered therapies. An exception is the Hecker et al. (1996) study, which compared a 12-week self-help program that was based on PCT with 12 weekly sessions of therapist-conducted PCT that covered the same material (eight subjects per condition). Patients in the self-help condition met with a therapist three times during the 12-week period to receive reading assignments and answers to their questions. Although three patients in the self-help group (38%) dropped out, those who completed treatment in both conditions improved significantly and maintained their gains at 6-month follow-up, with no differences between groups.

The data are somewhat more mixed regarding self-help treatments for moderate to severe agoraphobia. In a small early study, Holden et al. (1983) found that a self-help manual incorporating cognitive restructuring and graded in vivo exposure was ineffective for patients with severe agoraphobia. However, subjects in that study were described as experiencing "motivational difficulties" (p. 545) in that they did not comply with the in vivo practice instructions. In contrast, Ghosh and Marks (1987) found that exposure therapy administered by either a self-help book or a computer program based on the book was as effective for agoraphobia as therapist-administered treatment. Since the Ghosh and Marks (1987) report, there has been increasing interest in the use of computer technologies, including interactive voice response and virtual reality systems, in the treatment of mental health problems (for a review, see

Marks et al. 1998). These technologies offer the promises of greater consistency, cost-effectiveness, convenience, and accessibility of treatment.

Newman et al. (1996, 1997) used a handheld computer to ask patients about panic and anxiety symptoms and provided coping and exposure instructions. In a small trial (N=18), the use of the computer plus 4 sessions of CBT proved as effective as 11 sessions of CBT alone. More recently, Calbring et al. (2006) evaluated a 10-week Internet-based bibliotherapy self-help program with short weekly telephone calls for panic disorder with or without agoraphobia. A total of 60 patients were randomly assigned to either a wait-list control group or a multimodal treatment package based on CBT plus minimal therapist contact via e-mail. The results showed that all treated participants improved significantly on bodily interpretations, maladaptive cognitions, avoidance, general anxiety and depression levels, and quality of life. Treatment gains on self-report measures were maintained at the 9-month follow-up. A blind telephone interview after the end of treatment showed that 77% of the treated patients no longer fulfilled the criteria for panic disorder, whereas all of the wait-list subjects still met the criteria. The study findings provide further support for a new generation of self-help interventions.

Review of Comparator Trials

Given the variety of available treatments for panic disorder and the multidimensional nature of the disorder, it is logical that clinicians would seek to improve treatment outcome by combining different therapeutic modalities. Two common approaches have involved the coadministration of psychosocial treatments and pharmacotherapy and the combination of various elements of CBT with situational exposure therapy for agoraphobia.

Several investigators have combined exposure therapy with other psychosocial treatment interventions, including relaxation therapy (Michelson et al. 1988, 1996; Ost et al. 1984), cognitive therapy (de Beurs et al. 1995; Emmelkamp and Mersch 1982; Emmelkamp et al. 1986; Michelson et al. 1988; Ost 1989; van den Hout et al. 1994; Williams and Rappaport 1983), and breathing retraining (Bonn et al. 1984; deRuiter et al. 1989). In most instances in which comparisons were made, the combined therapies were not found to be significantly superior to exposure alone. A notable exception to this rule was revealed in the study reported by Michelson et al. (1996), which compared graded in vivo situational exposure alone with the same procedure combined with the addition of cognitive therapy or relaxation training in patients with moderate to severe panic disorder with agoraphobia. Of the three treatments, exposure plus cognitive therapy was found to be most effective. At posttreatment, 44% of the subjects who had received that treatment achieved high end-state functioning, compared with 22% in the exposure plus relaxation condition and 22% who received exposure alone. Those differences were maintained at 1-year follow-up, when the corresponding numbers were 71%, 33%, and 38%, respectively. Analyses showed that catastrophic cognitions related to anxiety and panic were important factors affecting short- and long-term outcomes.

Telch et al. (1994) compared the singular and combined effects of CBT and in vivo exposure therapy instructions for panic disorder with agoraphobia. In that study, all treatments were administered in a group format in twelve 90-minute sessions over an 8-week period. Results reportedly showed little evidence of treatment specificity. However, on a composite index of treatment response, patients who had received the combined treatment showed the greatest improvement at posttreatment and 6-month follow-up. The advantage appears to have been lost by 12-month follow-up because of delayed improvement in subjects who had received the single treatments. More promising results were found in a treatment combining 2 days of individually administered, ungraded, massed exposure with 6 sessions of group CBT plus a self-study workbook in 29 patients who had moderate to severe agoraphobia (Heinrichs et al. 2000). The findings showed that patients exhibited marked improvements on measures of agoraphobia, social anxiety, fear of anxiety sensations, general anxiety, depression, and disability.

In 1994, Wolfe and Maser observed that the modal clinical treatment for panic disorder was a combination of psychosocial therapy and medication, "although the psychosocial treatment most often coadministered with medication is not the empirically tested cognitive-behavior therapies" (p. 12). The high prevalence of combined treatment approaches reflects a prevailing belief by both physicians and patients that those regimens are superior to drugs or psychotherapy alone. Rapaport et al. (1996) and Waikar et al. (1994/1995) found that approximately three-fourths of patients seeking specialist treatment for anxiety disorders held that view. In contrast to those opinions, clinical studies of combined treatments have not consistently found significant advantages over single treatments. Considering the added cost and risks of combination therapies, it would seem important to show a benefit.

One of the earliest rationales for combining psychosocial treatments and pharmacotherapy for panic disorder was Klein's (1980) suggestion that drugs might work preferentially to suppress panic attacks, whereas exposure therapy more specifically addressed agoraphobic avoidance. In accordance with that suggestion, several studies have been conducted in which the effects of combined drug and exposure treatments were compared with those of one or both treatments alone (for reviews, see Mavissakalian 1993; Telch and Lucas 1994). Most of those studies involved tricyclic antidepressants (de Beurs et al. 1995; Marks et al. 1983; Mavissakalian and Michelson 1986a, 1986b; Mavissakalian and Perel 1985; Mavissakalian et al. 1983; Telch et al. 1985; Zitrin et al. 1980, 1983), but combined treatment studies have also been done with monoamine oxidase inhibitors (Solyom et al. 1981) and benzodiazepines (Hafner and Marks 1976; Marks et al. 1993; Wardle et al. 1994).

Overall, these studies showed modest short-term advantages across assessment domains for the combination of an antidepressant drug and exposure therapy over either treatment alone. The limited available data on combinations of a benzodiazepine and exposure therapy were less positive. In the Hafner and Marks (1976) and Wardle et al. (1994) studies, the administration of low-dose diazepam prior to exposure sessions or on a daily basis throughout exposure therapy had no significant effect, either positive or negative, on treatment outcome, although patients were somewhat less anxious during treatment. In the Marks et al. (1993) study, high-dose alprazolam plus exposure was marginally better than exposure plus a pill placebo during acute treatment, but relapse was substantially greater in the former cell when treatment was discontinued.

Few studies of combinations of pharmacotherapy with CBT have been published. A review of the literature on benzodiazepines and CBT found little evidence that the combination is superior to CBT alone for most patients (Spiegel and Bruce 1997), and some studies have found poorer long-term outcomes for the combination than for CBT alone (Brown and Barlow 1995; Otto et al. 1996). This potential detrimental effect of benzodiazepines on the outcome of CBT appears to be minimized if the drugs are discontinued before the conclusion of CBT (Bruce et al. 1999; Otto et al. 1993; Spiegel et al. 1994). Cottraux et al. (1995) compared the combination of buspirone and CBT with a pill placebo plus CBT in a sample of panic disorder patients with agoraphobia. The combined treatment was superior to CBT plus placebo at posttreatment (16 weeks) on measures of generalized anxiety and agoraphobic avoidance, but the differences disappeared by 1-year follow-up. Data relating to the combination of antidepressants with full CBT for panic disorder come from a multicenter study referred to earlier in this chapter (Barlow et al. 2000). In that study, the combination of CBT (specifically, PCT) plus imipramine was compared with each treatment alone, with a pill placebo, and with the combination of CBT and a pill placebo. After 3 months of treatment, CBT plus imipramine showed marginally better results than CBT alone but did not differ from imipramine alone or CBT plus placebo. After 9 months of treatment, the combination was reported to be better than both single treatments and CBT plus placebo; however, these advantages were lost when all treatments were discontinued. At follow-up 6 months after treatment discontinuation, only CBT alone and CBT plus placebo continued to show superiority to placebo. Interestingly, most patients refused to participate in the trial because of the prospect of receiving the medication pill but not CBT (Hofmann et al. 1998a).

On the basis of these studies, it would appear that the routine administration of pharmacotherapy with CBT is not warranted in most instances, because combining effective psychological treatment with conventional anxiolytic medication is typically not more effective than unimodal therapy. However, recent advances in the neuroscience of fear reduction have led to novel approaches for combining psychological therapy and pharmacological agents. Exposure-based treatments in humans partly rely on extinction to reduce the fear response in anxiety disorders. Animal studies have shown that D-cycloserine (DCS), partial agonist at the glycine recognition site of the glutamatergic *N*-methyl-D-aspartate receptor, facilitates extinction learning. Similarly, recent human trials have shown that DCS enhances fear reduction during exposure therapy of specific phobias (Ressler et al. 2004) and social anxiety disorder (Hofmann et al. 2006). A recently completed study also points to the potential value of DCS as an augmentation strategy of CBT for panic disorder (Hofmann 2007; Tolin et al. 2006). This study recruited 25 patients with panic disorder and mild to moderate agoraphobia. Patients were randomly assigned to five weekly sessions of individual exposure therapy for panic disorder plus 50 mg of DCS or the CBT plus pill placebo. During the exposure practices, patients were repeatedly exposed to fearful somatic sensations of anxiety. Clinical interview data by blind raters examining improvement with the Clinical Global Impression Scale (CGI; Guy 1976) showed that at posttreatment, 62% of patients receiving DCS were considered to be in remission, as compared with 21% of the patients in the placebo group. At follow-up, 75% of DCS patients but only 31% of patients in the placebo condition were in remission. The between-group effect sizes (Cohen's *d*) on change scores from baseline to posttreatment and from baseline to 1-month follow-up were large, favoring greater change in the DCS group than in the placebo group. These results, if they can be replicated in larger clinical trials, have the potential to revolutionize the field of psychiatric treatments for anxiety disorders.

Factors Affecting Outcome

The presence of agoraphobia has been consistently shown to be associated with a lower recovery rate (Fava et al. 1995; Keller et al. 1994; Williams and Falbo 1996). For example, in the study by Williams and Falbo (1996), panic-free rates at posttreatment and at a 1-to 2-year follow-up were 94% and 88%, respectively, among patients with low baseline agoraphobia, but only 52% and 30% among those with high agoraphobia.

The presence of personality disorders has also been discussed as a possible treatment moderator. Although panic disorder and agoraphobia are highly comorbid with personality disorders, panic patients with Axis II diagnoses show the same degree of improvement in anxiety symptoms as patients without personality disorders after cognitive-behavioral treatment for panic disorder (Dreessen et al. 1994). Moreover, CBT for panic disorder was accompanied by a reduction in personality disorder traits (Hofmann et al. 1998b). Other studies suggest that pretreatment scores on the Anxiety Sensitivity Index (e.g., Clark et al. 1994; Michelson et al. 1996) and pretreatment depressive symptoms (Barlow et al. 2000) are associated with poor treatment outcome. However, these findings should be considered preliminary.

Treatment Mechanism and Active Treatment Ingredients

Another open question is the issue of treatment mediation and the active ingredient of CBT. A reanalysis of the Barlow et al. (2000) study suggests that fears of social catastrophes before and following treatment with CBT or pharmacotherapy predict poor outcome (Hicks et al. 2005). Moreover, changes in panic-related cognitions mediate changes in panic severity only in treatments that include CBT (Hofmann et al. 2007). Similar results were reported by Smits et al. (2004), which showed that the effects of CBT on agoraphobia and panic symptoms were partially mediated by reductions of fear of fear. Although these data are encouraging and partially support the cognitive model of panic, none of these early mediation studies has been designed to test whether treatment-induced changes in cognitions temporally precede changes in panic symptoms. This is an important area for future research.

In addition to mediation analyses, other investigators have attempted to identify the active treatment components of CBT. Although good results have been reported for treatments that differ considerably in their emphasis on specific CBT interventions (Clark et al. 1985, 1994; Margraf et al. 1993), it remains unclear which component is particularly important or essential. Relaxation practices are a treatment component that is frequently included in CBT protocols. Relaxation therapies, such as progressive muscle relaxation (PMR) in which patients learn to discriminate tense from relaxed muscles and systematically relax specific muscle groups, have long been used in the treatment of generalized anxiety and tension. However, as traditionally administered, these therapies generally have been regarded as weak treatments for panic disorder and agoraphobia. PMR, for example, often has been chosen as a nonspecific or placebo psychological control in clinical trials of panic disorder treatments (Marks et al. 1993). Indeed, relaxation procedures have been reported to *precipitate* panic attacks in some individuals with panic disorder (e.g., Barlow 2002). Nevertheless, some evidence indicates that certain modifications of relaxation techniques may be beneficial for panic disorder (e.g., Barlow et al. 1989; Beck et al. 1994; Ost 1988).

Of particular note is a treatment developed by Ost (1987) known as *applied relaxation therapy*. Applied relaxation therapy begins with training in traditional PMR, after which patients are taught to relax rapidly and selectively during normal activities whenever they experience early signs of panic. Ost (1988) found that applied relaxation therapy was superior to standard PMR in a group of panic disorder patients without significant agoraphobia. All patients in the applied relaxation group were panic-free at both posttreatment and follow-up, compared with 71% at posttreatment and 57% at follow-up in the PMR group. Subsequently, Ost et al. (1993) found that applied relaxation therapy was as effective as standard in vivo exposure therapy or cognitive therapy in patients with panic disorder with agoraphobia, although the investigators suggested that the lack of differences among the treatments may have been the result of self-directed exposure by patients in the applied relaxation and cognitive therapy groups.

Other studies have found more mixed results with applied relaxation therapy. An example is the Barlow et al. (1989) study mentioned earlier in this chapter, in which a comparison was made of an early version of PCT with applied relaxation therapy, a combination of those two treatments, and a wait-list control condition. In that study, all three active treatments showed superiority to the wait-list condition on a variety of measures at posttreatment. Applied relaxation therapy tended to have a greater effect than PCT on generalized anxiety related to panic attacks, but a smaller proportion of the participants in the applied relaxation condition were panic-free at posttreatment (60% vs. 85% and 87% in the other two treatments), and attrition was higher in the applied relaxation group (33% vs. 6% in the CBT group and 17% in the combined treatment group). The 2-year follow-up of participants in the trial by Barlow and colleagues indicated that those who had received applied relaxation therapy, either alone or in combination with PCT, were doing less well than those who had received PCT alone (Craske et al. 1991). Whereas 81% of the patients in the latter group were panic-free at follow-up, only 43% and 36%, respectively, of those in the combined treatment and applied relaxation only groups were panic-free. The implications of these findings are unclear. On the surface, it appears that the addition of applied relaxation therapy to PCT had a detrimental effect on the long-term outcome of PCT. However, it seems more likely that it simply took time away from PCT, with the result that subjects in the combined treatment condition received less instruction and practice in PCT skills than those in the PCT alone condition.

Similar results were reported by Clark et al. (1994). In this study, cognitive therapy, applied relaxation therapy, and imipramine were compared in a sample of patients with panic disorder with up to moderate agoraphobic avoidance. All three treatments were shown to be more effective than a wait-list control condition at posttreatment, but cognitive therapy was reported to be superior to applied relaxation therapy and imipramine on most measures at 3-month follow-up, and both cognitive therapy and imipramine were seen as superior to applied relaxation therapy at 6-month follow-up.

Relaxation techniques for the treatment of panic disorder often include instruction in slow, diaphragmatic breathing. It has been suggested that panic attacks are closely related to hyperventilation in some panic patients (e.g., Ley 1993). In fact, some uncontrolled studies have revealed that respiratory control strategies along with education about hyperventilatory sensations led to a significant reduction in panic attack frequency (Bonn et al. 1984; Clark et al. 1985; Salkovskis et al. 1986). However, other findings suggest that supplementing in vivo exposure with respiratory control strategies or CBT did not improve overall treatment effectiveness (deRuiter et al. 1989; Rijken et al. 1992). Breathing retraining is rarely used as a single treatment modality for panic disorder.

In one dismantling study, the investigators questioned the utility of the breathing retraining component (Schmidt et al. 2000). However, another study showed that changes in respiration mediate changes in panic symptoms (Meuret et al. 2009). Some indirect comparative data are available from a meta-analysis by Gould et al. (1995). In that analysis, among studies involving psychosocial treatments for panic disorder, therapies incorporating both cognitive restructuring and interoceptive exposure had the highest overall mean effect size (0.88; N=7 studies). This finding is consistent with those of other studies, thus providing preliminary evidence for the efficacy of repeated exposure to panic-provocation procedures (Hofmann et al. 1999).

In sum, there are no clear patient characteristics and treatment components that predict treatment outcome. Earlier CBT protocols vary considerably in the specific treatment techniques and components that were included. For example, the meta-analysis by Gould et al. (1995) identified only three studies that involved cognitive therapy alone as treatment, and the results were markedly varied (effect size range −0.95 to +1.10). The authors concluded that "the effectiveness of cognitive therapy alone appears to be highly variable and may depend on the specific interventions used" (Gould et al. 1995, p. 832). A more recent meta-analysis of well-designed placebo-controlled CBT trials of panic disorder (Hofmann and Smits 2008) showed a controlled pre-post effect size of 0.35 (95% confidence interval: 0.04–0.65) for treatment completers. Although the finding indicates significantly more improvement among those receiving treatment than among subjects in the placebo group, there is clearly much room for improvement.

Other Psychosocial Approaches

Psychodynamic Psychotherapies

Although little empirical research has shown the efficacy of psychodynamic therapies for panic disorder (Coté and Barlow 1993), such interventions are frequently used for panic disorder (Goisman et al. 1994). Like cognitive theories of panic disorder, psychodynamic theories hypothesize that anxiety is generated when danger situations are activated. However, unlike cognitive theories, most dynamic theories propose that these danger situations are unconscious and include the threatened emergence of prohibited instinctual urges or the impending disruption of self-representation or object representations (Shear 1991). Accordingly, psychodynamic treatments for panic disorder typically focus on the elucidation of unconscious sources of anxiety and associated, characterologically based maladaptive behaviors. The presumed curative components of treatment typically involve the establishment of a transference relationship and the demonstration and acknowledgment of troublesome or angry feelings held by the patient that are associated with panic attacks (Milrod and Shear 1991b). Through recognition and expression of those feelings, and of intense affects in general, patients can relieve anxiety that would otherwise emerge as panic.

Preliminary studies and case reports indicate that psychodynamic psychotherapies can be efficacious for the treatment of panic disorder (Fewtrell 1984; Malan 1976; Milrod 1995; Milrod and Shear 1991a; Milrod et al. 2007; Sifneos 1972; Silber 1984; see also, Chapter 8, "Psychodynamic Concepts of Anxiety," in this volume). In one study, Wilborg and Dahl (1996) investigated the effect of adding psychodynamic psychotherapy to a pharmacological intervention. Patients received either 9 months of clomipramine therapy (up to 150 mg/day) or the same medication treatment plus 15 weekly sessions of psychodynamic therapy. The psychotherapy included all the main components of dynamic psychotherapy, including clarification, confrontation, and interpretation of resistance, defensive styles, and associated isolated affects. At posttreatment, all patients who had received the combined therapy were panic-free, compared with 75% of those who had received only the medication. More important, at follow-up, 18 patients who had received clomipramine alone had relapsed, compared with only 20% of those who had received the combined treatment. Moreover, patients from the combined condition group showed greater global improvement on outcome measures than patients who received clomipramine alone. Although these results are promising, their interpretation is limited by the lack of a psychotherapy control condition in the study.

Emotion-Focused Psychotherapy

A treatment related to psychodynamic psychotherapy for panic disorder is emotion-focused therapy (EFT), which was developed by Shear and colleagues (Shear and Weiner 1997; Shear et al. 1995). EFT specifically targets emotion regulation as it relates to interpersonal control and to fears of being abandoned or trapped. EFT differs from traditional psychodynamic therapy in that it does not emphasize the interpretation of unconscious material or focus on linking early experiences with present symptoms. Instead, the treatment strategies used during EFT target fear and avoidance of negative affect and their triggers. Several case reports and studies comparing nondirective and empathetic supportive therapy with CBT have offered some early support for this approach (Borkovec and Mathews 1988; Klein et al. 1983; Shear et al. 1994; Sifneos 1972).

Long-Term Treatment

As discussed earlier, patients who receive pharmacotherapy are at high risk for deterioration. A review of the literature suggests that only about 30%-45% of patients remain well following medication discontinuation (Ballenger 1992). Long-term outcome following CBT is better than with pharmacotherapy. For example, in a meta-analysis of long-term outcome studies for panic disorder, Gould et al. (1995) reported that treatment effect sizes for CBT were maintained from posttreatment to follow-up, whereas those for pharmacological treatment slipped considerably. CBT follow-up studies typically report panic-free rates in excess of 80% at 1–2 years posttreatment (Beck et al. 1992; Clark et al. 1994; Craske et al. 1991). However, as encouraging as these data are, cross-sectional follow-up assessments necessarily underestimate the presence of infrequent panic attacks and other fluctuating panic disorder symptoms. For example, Brown and Barlow (1995) studied symptom change in a group of treated patients with panic disorder and no or mild agoraphobia. The authors found that that although 75% of patients were panic-free at 24-month follow-up, only 21% met criteria for high end-state functioning at both 3 and 24 months posttreatment and were panic-free for the year preceding the 24-month assessment. These findings suggest that panic disorder is a chronic illness with intermittent periods of symptom exacerbations. Current acute treatment regimens seem to be insufficient to substantially alter its course and produce lasting improvement. Future studies must be specifically focused on strategies to improve the long-term outcome.

Special Populations

Individuals with panic disorder vary greatly in age, demographic characteristics, and comorbid diagnoses. For example, retrospective reports on adults suggest that panic disorder often begins during adolescence or young adulthood (e.g., Bernstein et al. 1996). However, there is no evidence to suggest that these characteristics moderate response to CBT.

Similarly, as mentioned previously, there is little evidence to suggest that specific comorbid diagnoses predict poor outcome of CBT (with the exception of agoraphobia and depression). For example, even severe mental disorders, such as schizophrenia, do not predict poor outcome of CBT. The significant association between panic and schizophrenia remains unclear. It might be possible that the schizophrenic thought disorder is directly associated with the misinterpretation of bodily sensations or that panic and schizophrenia are connected via certain biochemical substances that are important factors in both domains of psychopathology (Hofmann 1999). Despite this high level of comorbidity and chronicity of schizophrenia, preliminary studies suggest that panic disorder can be effectively treated with a modified version of CBT in patients with schizophrenia (Hofmann et al. 2000).

Treatment-Refractory Panic Disorder

Although CBT is a generally effective intervention, a substantial number of patients remain symptomatic or show no improvement at all, especially in the long term. Unfortunately, this seems to be the rule, not the exception. For example, the largest CBT trial on panic disorder to date (Barlow et al. 2000) showed that the acute response rate for the combined treatment was approximately 60% for all active treatment groups (CBT, imipramine, and the combination of both). At 6 months after treatment discontinuation, the ITT response rates were 41.0% for CBT plus placebo, 31.9% for CBT alone, 19.7% for imipramine alone, 13% for placebo, and 26.3% for CBT combined with imipramine. These findings suggest that combining imipramine with CBT has limited advantage acutely, but greater advantage by the end of maintenance. Each treatment worked well immediately following treatment and during maintenance, and CBT was more durable in follow-up than imipramine. Nevertheless, a large proportion of patients did not improve, and the majority of patients did not remain improved. There is a paucity of research in the literature on the factors that predict nonresponse or relapse. Clearly, this is an important area for future research.

Practical Techniques and Experimental Approaches

As discussed previously, there are many different CBT protocols that differ in their specific treatment techniques and components. The best-validated protocol is PCT (e.g., Barlow et al. 2000; see Hofmann and Spiegel 1999, for an overview). The protocol is specifically designed to treat panic disorder with no or mild agoraphobia. An optional agoraphobia supplement was developed later, for use with patients who have significant situational avoidance (Craske et al. 2000).

The general goal of PCT is to foster within patients the ability to identify and correct maladaptive thoughts and behaviors that initiate, sustain, or exacerbate anxiety and panic attacks. In service of that goal, the treatment combines education, cognitive interventions, relaxation and controlled breathing procedures, and exposure techniques. The original PCT protocol is usually delivered in 11 or 12 weekly sessions, either individually to patients or in a small-group format. The treatment includes a variety of information and skill-building components, as follows: 1) psychoeducation, 2) cognitive restructuring, 3) breathing retraining, 4) interoceptive exposure, and 5) situational exposure.

In early sessions, patients are taught about the nature and function of fear and its nervous system substrates. The fear response is presented as a normal and generally protective state that enhances our ability to survive and compete in life. Panic attacks are conceptualized as inappropriate fear reactions arising from spurious but otherwise normal activation of the body's fight-or-flight nervous system. Like other fear reactions, they are portrayed as alarms that stimulate us to take immediate defensive action. Because we normally associate fight-or-flight responses with the presence of danger, panic attacks typically motivate a frantic search for the source of threat. When none is found, the individual may look inward and interpret the symptoms as signs that something is seriously wrong with him or her (e.g., "I'm dying of a heart attack," "I'm losing my mind").

In addition to normalizing and demystifying panic attacks, the educational component of PCT provides patients with a model of anxiety that emphasizes the interaction between the mind and body and provides a rationale and framework for the skills to be taught during treatment. A three-component model is utilized, in which the dimensions of anxiety are grouped into physical, cognitive, and behavioral categories. The physical component includes bodily changes (e.g., neurological, hormonal, cardiovascular) and their associated somatic sensations (e.g., shortness of breath, palpitations, lightheadedness). The cognitive component consists of the rational and irrational thoughts, images, and impulses that accompany anxiety or fear (e.g., thoughts of dying, images of losing control, impulses to run). The behavioral component contains the things people do when they are anxious or afraid (e.g., pacing, leaving, avoiding a situation, carrying a safety object). Most importantly, these three components are described as interacting with each other, often with the result of heightened anxiety. Having laid this foundation, the individual receiving PCT is then taught skills for controlling each of the three components of anxiety. To manage some of the physical aspects of anxiety, such as sensations caused by hyperventilation (e.g., lightheadedness, tingling sensations) or muscle tension (e.g., trembling, dyspnea), patients are taught how to use slow, diaphragmatic breathing or progressive muscle relaxation. To reduce anxiety-exacerbating thoughts and images, patients are taught to critically examine, based on past experience and logical reasoning, their estimations of the likelihood that a feared event will occur, the probable consequences if it should occur, and their ability to cope with it. In addition, they are assisted in designing and conducting behavioral experiments to test their predictions.

To change maladaptive anxiety and fear behaviors, patients are taught to engage in graded therapeutic exposure to cues they associate with panic attacks. The exposure component of standard PCT (called *interoceptive exposure*) focuses primarily on internal cues—specifically, frightening bodily sensations. During exposure, patients deliberately provoke physical sensations such as smothering, dizziness, or tachycardia by means of exercises such as breathing through a straw, spinning, or doing vigorous exercise. These exercises are done initially during treatment sessions, with therapist modeling, and subsequently by patients at home. As patients become less afraid of the sensations, more naturalistic activities are assigned, such as drinking caffeinated beverages, having sexual intercourse, or watching scary movies.

Recent experimental approaches include the development of a unified treatment protocol for all emotional disorders, including panic disorder (Barlow et al. 2004). Following a standard psychoeducational phase common to all psychotherapeutic approaches, the treatment includes the following three components: 1) altering antecedent cognitive reappraisals, an intensive emotional regulation procedure that directly facilitates the next two steps in treatment; 2) preventing emotional avoidance, a broad-based effort that goes well beyond traditional attempts to prevent behavioral avoidance in phobic disorders by targeting cognitive, behavioral, and somatic experiential avoidance; and 3) facilitating action tendencies not associated with the emotion that is disordered. This treatment takes place in the context of provoking emotional expression (emotion exposure) through situational, internal, and somatic (interoceptive) cues as well as through standard mood induction exercises, and it differs from patient to patient only in the situational cues and exercises utilized. This treatment is currently in development (Barlow et al. 2004).

Limitations of Existing Studies

Several limitations of existing studies of panic disorder treatments warrant caution in interpreting and comparing published efficacy data. First, studies of exposure therapy typically have involved more highly agoraphobic patient samples than have studies of cognitive therapy or CBT. When the latter therapies were initially developed, panic disorder was defined by the occurrence of a certain number of panic attacks within a specified period of time (DSM-III, DSM-III-R). The psychosocial treatments prevailing at the time (e.g., relaxation therapies and situational exposure) tended to focus on general arousal or behavioral avoidance. As noted earlier, CBT differed in that it focused directly on patients' experiences of panic attacks and associated anxiety.

Accordingly, clinical trials of CBT were conducted with patients for whom panic attacks were the primary problem—that is, patients with little or no agoraphobic avoidance. In contrast, exposure therapy trials enrolled subjects with moderate or severe avoidance. Furthermore, until recently, the measures used to assess treatment efficacy with the two approaches have also differed. CBT (and pharmacotherapy) studies have typically used response criteria based on panic attack frequency (e.g., panic-free status), whereas exposure therapy trials have emphasized measures of agoraphobic avoidance. Panic frequency and agoraphobic avoidance have been found to vary relatively independently of each other (Basoglu et al. 1994; Craske and Barlow 1988). In general, the question of how to best assess treatment efficacy for panic disorder is far from settled. It is clear that traditional measures of panic attacks are insufficient; generally, these bear little relation to other dimensions of the disorder. Because of that, some studies have used global or composite measures (e.g., high end-state functioning) to evaluate treatment response (Barlow et al. 1989; Brown and Barlow 1995; Bruce et al. 1999; Clark et al. 1994; Mavissakalian and Perel 1992). However, those measures have been idiosyncratically defined and have varied from study to study. In response to this problem, in 1992 the National Institute of Mental Health convened an expert panel to recommend standardized measures for panic disorder research (Shear and Maser 1994). The panel recommended assessment of a range of symptom and performance measures but stopped short of proposing a measure of overall treatment efficacy. Finally, long-term efficacy data in nearly all studies (psychosocial and pharmacological) have been based on cross-sectional assessments of improvement. As Brown and Barlow (1995) pointed out, such assessments fail to consider the course of symptoms over time. In the few instances when individual panic disorder patients have been followed up longitudinally after treatment, many have shown fluctuating courses, with periods of symptom recrudescence. For example, Brown and Barlow (1995) followed up 63 patients treated with variations of CBT and found that although 40% met criteria for high end-state functioning at 3 months posttreatment and 57% at 24 months posttreatment, only 27% met the criteria at both 3 and 24 months after treatment. Fluctuating courses have also been observed in patients treated with exposure therapy (Burns et al. 1986). Moreover, very little is known about effective maintenance treatment strategies for panic disorder and agoraphobia (Ost 1989).

Conclusion

Naturalistic studies indicate that despite the availability of proven treatments, many patients with panic disorder or panic disorder with agoraphobia do not receive effective treatment in the community. For example, the Harvard/Brown Anxiety Disorders Research Program assessed recovery and relapse in 323 panic disorder patients with agoraphobia and 73 without agoraphobia who were treated naturalistically (Keller et al. 1994). In the first 22 months after onset of an episode, only 43% of the patients without agoraphobia and 18% of those with agoraphobia had recovered. Moreover, among recovered patients, 40% of those without agoraphobia and 60% of those with agoraphobia relapsed within 18 months. High relapse rates were also found in a naturalistic study at Massachusetts General Hospital (Pollack et al. 1990). Consistent with those dismal statistics, surveys have shown that only a small number of patients treated in clinical settings receive an empirically validated psychosocial treatment (Breier et al. 1986; Goisman et al. 1993; Taylor et al. 1989). As Barlow and Hofmann (1997) noted, that situation is caused by, at least in part, a lack of availability, especially in primary care settings, of clinicians who have been trained in those therapies. Lack of information about the efficacy of psychosocial treatments and a misguided belief that pharmacotherapy is less expensive also may be factors. Clearly, if the outlook for patients is to improve, greater efforts must be made to educate health care practitioners and managers about the effectiveness and favorable cost of psychological treatments for panic disorder and to ensure that such treatments are accessible to patients.

◀ Key Clinical Points ▶

- Cognitive-behavioral therapy (CBT) is effective for treating panic disorder with or without agoraphobia. The treatment is based on Clark's model of panic, which provides an alternative psychological explanation to biological theories of panic disorder.
- CBT is more effective than pharmacotherapy in the long term. Interestingly, combining pharmacotherapy and CBT is not more effective than monotherapy.
- Panic control therapy is one of the best-researched treatment protocols. This therapy combines CBT and psychoeducation with interoceptive and situational exposure practices and breathing retraining. The efficacy of exposure techniques and cognitive-behavioral interventions is well established, whereas the efficacy of breathing-retraining strategies is still controversial.

- **On the basis of the existing data, CBT should be considered as a first-line treatment for panic disorder and agoraphobia. It appears that exposure to feared situations or bodily symptoms is a particularly efficacious component of CBT. If the patient does not respond, pharmacotherapy should be considered as the second-line treatment, either alone or in combination with the CBT.**

References

American Psychiatric Association: Diagnostic and Statistical Manual of Mental Disorders, 3rd Edition. Washington, DC, American Psychiatric Association, 1980

American Psychiatric Association: Diagnostic and Statistical Manual of Mental Disorders, 3rd Edition, Revised. Washington, DC, American Psychiatric Association, 1987

Ballenger JC: Medication discontinuation in panic disorder. J Clin Psychiatry 53:26–31, 1992

Barlow DH: Anxiety and Its Disorders: The Nature and Treatment of Anxiety and Panic, 2nd Edition. New York, Guilford, 2002

Barlow DH, Hofmann SG: Efficacy and dissemination of psychosocial treatment expertise, in Science and Practice of Cognitive Behaviour Therapy. Edited by Clark DF, Fairburn CG. Oxford, England, Oxford University Press, 1997, pp 95–117

Barlow DH, Craske MG, Cerny JA, et al: Behavioral treatment of panic disorder. Behav Ther 20:261–282, 1989

Barlow DH, Gorman JM, Shear MK, et al: Cognitive-behavioral therapy, imipramine, or their combination for panic disorder: a randomized controlled trial. JAMA 283:2529–2536, 2000

Barlow DH, Allen LB, Choate ML: Toward a unified treatment for emotional disorders. Behav Ther 35:205–230, 2004

Basoglu M, Marks IM, Kiliç C, et al: Relationship of panic, anticipatory anxiety, agoraphobia and global improvement in panic disorder with agoraphobia treated with alprazolam and exposure. Br J Psychiatry 164:647–652, 1994

Beck AT, Sokol L, Clark DA, et al: A crossover study of focused cognitive therapy for panic disorder. Am J Psychiatry 149:778–783, 1992

Beck AT, Stanley MA, Baldwin LE, et al: Comparison of cognitive therapy and relaxation training for panic disorder. J Consult Clin Psychol 62:818–826, 1994

Bernstein GA, Borchardt CM, Perwien AR: Anxiety disorders in children and adolescents: a review of the past 10 years. J Am Acad Child Adolesc Psychiatry 35:1110–1119, 1996

Bonn JA, Readhead CPA, Timmons BH: Enhanced adaptive behavioral response in agoraphobic patients pretreated with breathing retraining. Lancet 2:665–669, 1984

Borkovec TD, Mathews AM: Treatment of nonphobic anxiety disorders: a comparison of nondirective, cognitive, and coping desensitization therapy. J Consult Clin Psychol 56:877–884, 1988

Bouton ME, Mineka S, Barlow DH: A modern learning theory perspective on the etiology of panic disorder. Psychol Rev 108:4–32, 2001

Breier A, Charney DS, Heninger GR: Agoraphobia with panic attacks: development, diagnostic stability, and course of illness. Arch Gen Psychiatry 43:1029–1036, 1986

Brown TA, Barlow DH: Long-term outcome of cognitive-behavioral treatment of panic disorder: clinical predictors and alternative strategies for assessment. J Consult Clin Psychol 63:754–765, 1995

Bruce TJ, Spiegel DA, Hegel MT: Cognitive behavior therapy helps prevent relapse and recurrence of panic disorder following alprazolam discontinuation: a long-term follow-up of the Peoria and Dartmouth studies. J Consult Clin Psychol 67:151–156, 1999

Burns LE, Thorpe GL, Cavallaro LA: Agoraphobia 8 years after behavioral treatment: a follow-up study with interview, self-report, and behavioral data. Behav Ther 17:580–591, 1986

Calbring P, Bohman S, Brunt S, et al: Remote treatment of panic disorder: a randomized trial of internet-based cognitive-behavior therapy supplemented with telephone calls. Am J Psychiatry 163:2119–2125, 2006

Chambless DL: Spacing of exposure sessions in treatment of agoraphobia and simple phobia. Behav Ther 21:217–229, 1990

Clark DM: A cognitive approach to panic. Behav Res Ther 24:461–470, 1986

Clark DM: Anxiety states: panic and generalized anxiety, in Cognitive Behaviour Therapy for Psychiatric Problems: A Practical Guide. Edited by Hawton K, Salkovskis PM, Kirk J, et al. Oxford, England, Oxford University Press, 1989, pp 52–96

Clark DM, Salkovskis PM, Chalkley AJ: Respiratory control as a treatment for panic attacks. J Behav Ther Exp Psychiatry 16:23–30, 1985

Clark DM, Salkovskis PM, Hackman A, et al: A comparison of cognitive therapy, applied relaxation, and imipramine in the treatment of panic disorder. Br J Psychiatry 164:759–769, 1994

Clark DM, Salkovskis PM, Hackmann A, et al: Brief cognitive therapy for panic disorder: a randomized controlled trial. J Consult Clin Psychol 67:583–589, 1999

Clum GA: Psychological interventions vs drugs in the treatment of panic. Behav Ther 20:429–457, 1989

Coté G, Barlow DH: Effective psychological treatment of panic disorder, in Handbook of Effective Psychotherapy. Edited by Giles TR. New York, Plenum, 1993, pp 151–169

Coté G, Gauthier JG, Laberge B, et al: Reduced therapist contact in the cognitive behavioral treatment of panic disorder. Behav Ther 25:123–145, 1994

Cottraux J, Note I-D, Cungi C, et al: A controlled study of cognitive behaviour therapy with buspirone or placebo in panic disorder with agoraphobia. Br J Psychiatry 167:635–641, 1995

Craske MG, Barlow DH: A review of the relationship between panic and avoidance. Clin Psychol Rev 8:667–685, 1988

Craske MG, Brown TA, Barlow DH: Behavioral treatment of panic disorder: a two-year follow-up. Behav Ther 22:289–304, 1991

Craske MG, Maidenberg E, Bystritsky A: Brief cognitive-behavioral versus non-directive therapy for panic disorder. J Behav Ther Exp Psychiatry 26:113–120, 1995

Craske MG, Barlow DH, Meadows EA: Mastery of Your Anxiety and Panic (MAP-3): Therapist Guide for Anxiety, Panic, and Agoraphobia, 3rd Edition. New York, Harcourt, 2000

de Beurs E, van Balkom AJ, Lange A, et al: Treatment of panic disorder with agoraphobia: comparison of fluvoxamine, placebo, and psychological panic management combined with exposure and of exposure in vivo alone. Am J Psychiatry 152:683–691, 1995

deRuiter C, Rijken H, Garssen B, et al: Breathing retraining, exposure and a combination of both, in the treatment of panic disorder with agoraphobia. Behav Res Ther 27:647–655, 1989

Dreessen L, Arntz A, Luttels C, et al: Personality disorders do not influence the results of cognitive-behavior therapies for anxiety disorders. Compr Psychiatry 35:265–274, 1994

Ehlers A, Feigenbaum W, Florin I, et al: Efficacy of exposure in vivo in panic disorder with agoraphobia in a clinical setting. Paper presented at the World Congress of Behavioural and Cognitive Therapies, Copenhagen, July 1995

Emmelkamp PMG, Mersch PP: Cognition and exposure in vivo in the treatment of agoraphobia: short-term and delayed effects. Cogn Ther Res 6:77–90, 1982

Emmelkamp PMG, Brilman E, Kuiper H, et al: The treatment of agoraphobia: a comparison of self-instructional training, rational emotive therapy, and exposure in vivo. Behav Modif 10:37–53, 1986

Fava GA, Zielezny M, Savron G, et al: Long-term effects of behavioural treatment for panic disorder with agoraphobia. Br J Psychiatry 166:87–92, 1995

Feigenbaum W: Long-term efficacy of ungraded versus graded massed exposure in agoraphobics, in Panic and Phobias: Treatments and Variables Affecting Course and Outcome. Edited by Hand I, Wittchen H. Berlin, Springer-Verlag, 1988, pp 83–88

Fewtrell WD: Psychological approaches to panic attack: some recent developments. British Journal of Experimental and Clinical Hypnosis 1:21–24, 1984

Gelder MG, Marks IM: Severe agoraphobia: a controlled prospective trial of behavior therapy. Br J Psychiatry 112:309–319, 1966

Ghosh A, Marks IM: Self-treatment of agoraphobia by exposure. Behav Ther 18:3–16, 1987

Goisman RM, Rogers MP, Steketee GS, et al: Utilization of behavioral methods in a multicenter anxiety disorders study. J Clin Psychiatry 54:213–218, 1993

Goisman RM, Warshaw MG, Peterson LG: Panic, agoraphobia, and panic disorder with agoraphobia: data from a multicenter anxiety disorders study. J Nerv Ment Dis 182:72–79, 1994

Goldstein A, Chambless D: A reanalysis of agoraphobia. Behav Ther 9:47–59, 1978

Gould RA, Clum GA: Self-help plus minimal therapist contact in the treatment of panic disorder: a replication and extension. Behav Ther 26:533–546, 1995

Gould RA, Clum GA, Shapiro D: The use of bibliotherapy in the treatment of panic: a preliminary investigation. Behav Ther 26:241–252, 1993

Gould RA, Otto MW, Pollack MH: A meta-analysis of treatment outcome for panic disorder. Clin Psychol Rev 15:819–844, 1995

Guy W: ECDEU Assessment Manual for Psychopharmacology. Publication (ADM) 76-338. Washington, DC, U.S. Department of Health, Education and Welfare, 1976, pp 217–222

Hafner J, Marks IM: Exposure in vivo of agoraphobics: contributions of diazepam, group exposure, and anxiety evocation. Psychol Med 6:71–88, 1976

Hahlweg K, Feigenbaum W, Frank M: Short- and long-term effectiveness of an empirically supported treatment for agoraphobia. J Consult Clin Psychol 69:375–382, 2001

Hecker JE, Losee MC, Fritzler BK, et al: Self-directed versus therapist-directed cognitive behavioral treatment for panic disorder. J Anxiety Disord 10:253–265, 1996

Heinrichs N, Spiegel DA, Hofmann SG: Panic disorder with agoraphobia, in Handbook of Brief Cognitive Behaviour Therapy. Edited by Bond F, Dryden W. Chichester, England, Wiley, 2000

Hicks TV, Leitenberg H, Barlow DH, et al: Physical, mental, and social catastrophic cognitions as prognostic factors in cognitive-behavioral and pharmacological treatments for panic disorder. J Consult Clin Psychol 73:506–514, 2005

Hofmann SG: Relationship between panic and schizophrenia. Depress Anxiety 9:101–106, 1999

Hofmann SG: Enhancing exposure-based therapy from a translational research perspective. Behav Res Ther 45:1987–2001, 2007

Hofmann SG, Smits JAJ: Cognitive behavioral therapy for adult anxiety disorders: a meta-analysis of randomized placebo-controlled trials. J Clin Psychiatry 43:634–641, 2009

Hofmann SG, Spiegel DA: Panic control treatment and its applications. J Psychother Pract Res 8:3–11, 1999

Hofmann SG, Barlow DH, Papp LA, et al: Pretreatment attrition in a comparative treatment outcome study on panic disorder. Am J Psychiatry 155:43–47, 1998a

Hofmann SG, Shear MK, Barlow DH, et al: Effects of panic disorder treatments on personality disorder characteristics. Depress Anxiety 8:14–20, 1998b

Hofmann SG, Bufka L, Barlow DH: Panic provocation procedures in the treatment of panic disorder: early perspectives and case studies. Behav Ther 30:307–319, 1999

Hofmann SG, Bufka LF, Brady SM, et al: Cognitive-behavioral treatment of panic in patients with schizophrenia: preliminary findings. Journal of Cognitive Psychotherapy 14:27–37, 2000

Hofmann SG, Meuret AE, Smith JA, et al: Augmentation of exposure therapy for social anxiety disorder with D-cycloserine. Arch Gen Psychiatry 63:298–304, 2006

Hofmann SG, Meuret AE, Rosenfield D, et al: Preliminary evidence for cognitive mediation during cognitive behavioral therapy of panic disorder. J Consult Clin Psychol 75:374–379, 2007

Holden AE, O'Brian GT, Barlow DH, et al: Self-help manual for agoraphobia: a preliminary report on effectiveness. Behav Res Ther 14:545–556, 1983

Jacobson NS, Wilson L, Tupper C: The clinical significance of treatment gains resulting from exposure-based interventions for agoraphobia: a re-analysis of outcome data. Behav Ther 19:539–554, 1988

Jansson L, Ost LG: Behavioral treatments for agoraphobia: an evaluative review. Clin Psychol Rev 2:311–336, 1982

Jansson L, Jerremalm A, Ost LG: Follow-up of agoraphobic patients treated with exposure in vivo or applied relaxation. Br J Psychiatry 149:486–490, 1986

Keller MB, Yonkers KA, Warshaw MG, et al: Remission and relapse in subjects with panic disorder and agoraphobia. J Nerv Ment Dis 182:290–296, 1994

Klein DF: Anxiety reconceptualized. Compr Psychiatry 21:411–427, 1980

Klein DF: False suffocation alarms, spontaneous panics, and related conditions: an integrative hypothesis. Arch Gen Psychiatry 50:306–317, 1993

Klein DF, Zitrin CM, Woerner MG, et al: Treatment of phobias, II: behavioral therapy and supportive psychotherapy—are there any specific ingredients? Arch Gen Psychiatry 40:139–145, 1983

Klosko JS, Barlow DH, Tassinari R, et al: A comparison of alprazolam and behavior therapy in treatment of panic disorder. J Consult Clin Psychol 58:77–84, 1990

Klosko JS, Barlow DH, Tassinari R, et al: "A comparison of alprazolam and behavior therapy in treatment of panic disorder": correction. J Consult Clin Psychol 63:830, 1995

Ley R: Blood, breath, and fears: a hyperventilation theory of panic attacks and agoraphobia. Clin Psychol Rev 5:271–285, 1985

Ley R: Breathing retraining in the treatment of hyperventilatory panic attacks. Clin Psychol Rev 13:393–408, 1993

Lidren DM, Watkins PL, Gould RA, et al: A comparison of bibliotherapy and group therapy in the treatment of panic disorder. J Consult Clin Psychol 62:865–869, 1994

Malan D: The Frontier of Brief Psychotherapy. New York, Plenum, 1976

Margraf J, Barlow DH, Clark DM, et al: Psychological treatment of panic: work in progress on outcome, active ingredients, and follow-up. Behav Res Ther 1:1–8, 1993

Marks IM: Phobic disorders four years after treatment: a prospective follow-up. Br J Psychiatry 129:362–371, 1971

Marks IM: Living With Fear: Understanding and Coping With Anxiety. New York, McGraw-Hill, 1978

Marks IM, Gray S, Cohen D, et al: Imipramine and brief therapist-aided exposure in agoraphobics having self-exposure homework. Arch Gen Psychiatry 40:153–162, 1983

Marks IM, Swinson RP, Basoglu M, et al: Alprazolam and exposure alone and combined in panic disorder with agoraphobia: a controlled study in London and Toronto. Br J Psychiatry 162:776–787, 1993

Marks I, Shaw S, Parkin R: Computer-aided treatments of mental health problems. Clin Psychol Sci Pract 5:151–170, 1998

Mavissakalian M: Combined behavioral therapy and pharmacotherapy of agoraphobia. J Psychiatr Res 27(suppl):179–191, 1993

Mavissakalian M, Michelson L: Agoraphobia: relative and combined effectiveness of therapist-assisted in vivo exposure and imipramine. J Clin Psychiatry 47:117–122, 1986a

Mavissakalian M, Michelson L: Two-year follow-up of exposure and imipramine treatment of agoraphobia. Am J Psychiatry 143:1106–1112, 1986b

Mavissakalian M, Perel J: Imipramine in the treatment of agoraphobia: dose-response relationships. Am J Psychiatry 142:1032–1036, 1985

Mavissakalian M, Perel JM: Clinical experiments in maintenance and discontinuation of imipramine therapy in panic disorder with agoraphobia. Arch Gen Psychiatry 49:318–323, 1992

Mavissakalian M, Michelson L, Dealy RD: Pharmacological treatment of agoraphobia: imipramine vs imipramine with programmed practice. Br J Psychiatry 143:348–355, 1983
McNally RJ: Panic Disorder: A Critical Analysis. New York, Guilford, 1994
Meuret AE, Rosenfeld D, Hofmann SG, et al: Changes in respiration mediate changes in fear of bodily sensations in panic disorder. J Psychiatr Res 43:634–643, 2009
Michelson L, Mavissakalian M, Marchione K: Cognitive, behavioral, and psychophysiological treatments of agoraphobia: a comparative outcome investigation. Behav Ther 19:97–120, 1988
Michelson LK, Marchione KE, Greenwald M, et al: A comparative outcome and follow-up investigation of panic disorder with agoraphobia: the relative and combined efficacy of cognitive therapy, relaxation training, and therapist-assisted exposure. J Anxiety Disord 10:297–330, 1996
Milrod B: The continued usefulness of psychoanalysis in the treatment armamentarium for panic disorder. J Am Psychoanal Assoc 43:151–162, 1995
Milrod B, Shear MK: Dynamic treatment of panic disorder: a review. J Nerv Ment Dis 179:741–743, 1991a
Milrod B, Shear MK: Psychodynamic treatment of panic: three case histories. Hosp Community Psychiatry 42:311–312, 1991b
Milrod B, Leon AC, Busch F, et al: A randomized controlled clinical trial of psychoanalytic psychotherapy for panic disorder. Am J Psychiatry 164:265–272, 2007
Mitte K: A meta-analysis of the efficacy of psycho-and pharmacotherapy in panic disorder with and without agoraphobia. J Affect Disord 88:27–45, 2005
Munby J, Johnson DW: Agoraphobia: the long-term follow-up of behavioral treatment. Br J Psychiatry 137:418–427, 1980
Newman MG, Kennardy J, Herman S, et al: The use of handheld computers as an adjunct to CBT. Comput Human Behav 12:135–143, 1996
Newman MG, Kennardy J, Herman S, et al: Comparison of cognitive-behavioral treatment of panic disorder with computer assisted brief cognitive behavioral treatment. J Consult Clin Psychol 65:178–183, 1997
Ost LG: Applied relaxation: description of a coping technique and review of controlled studies. Behav Res Ther 25:397–409, 1987
Ost LG: Applied relaxation vs progressive relaxation in the treatment of panic disorder. Behav Res Ther 26:13–22, 1988
Ost LG: A maintenance program for behavioral treatment of anxiety disorders. Behav Res Ther 27:123–130, 1989
Ost LG, Jerremalm A, Jansson L: Individual response patterns and the effects of different behavioral methods in the treatment of agoraphobia. Behav Res Ther 22:697–707, 1984
Ost LG, Westling BE, Hellstrom K: Applied relaxation, exposure in vivo, and cognitive methods in the treatment of panic disorder with agoraphobia. Behav Res Ther 31:383–394, 1993
Otto MW, Pollack MH, Sachs GS, et al: Discontinuation of benzodiazepine treatment: efficacy of cognitive-behavioral therapy for patients with panic disorder. Am J Psychiatry 150:1485–1490, 1993
Otto MW, Pollack MH, Sabatino SA: Maintenance and remission following cognitive behavior therapy for panic disorder: possible deleterious effects of concurrent medication treatment. Behav Ther 27:473–482, 1996
Pollack MH, Otto MW, Rosenbaum JF, et al: Longitudinal course of panic disorder: findings from the Massachusetts General Hospital Naturalistic Study. J Clin Psychiatry 12(suppl):12–16, 1990
Rapaport MH, Frevert T, Babior S, et al: Comparison of descriptive variables for symptomatic volunteers and clinical patients with anxiety disorders. Anxiety 2:117–122, 1996
Reiss S, McNally RJ: Expectancy model of fear, in Theoretical Issues in Behavior Therapy. Edited by Reiss S, Bootzin RR. San Diego, CA, Academic Press, 1985, pp 107–121
Ressler KJ, Rothbaum BO, Tannenbaum L, et al: Cognitive enhancers as adjuncts to psychotherapy: use of D-cycloserine in phobic individuals to facilitate extinction of fear. Arch Gen Psychiatry 61:1136–1144, 2004
Rijken H, Kraimaat F, deRuiter C, et al: A follow-up study on short term treatment of agoraphobia. Behav Res Ther 30:63–66, 1992
Roth WT, Wilhelm FH, Pettit D: Are current theories of panic falsifiable? Psychol Bull 131:171–192, 2005
Salkovskis PM, Jones DRO, Clark DM: Respiratory control in the treatment of panic attacks: replication and extension with concurrent measurement of behaviour and pCO_2. Br J Psychiatry 148:526–532, 1986
Schmidt NB, Woolaway-Bickel K, Trakowski J, et al: Dismantling cognitive-behavioral treatment for panic disorder: questioning the utility of breathing retraining. J Consult Clin Psychol 68:417–424, 2000
Schroeder B, Frank M, Funfstuck G, et al: Exposure in vivo in anxiety disorders: the impact of marital quality on drop-out and treatment effectiveness. Poster presented at the annual meeting of the Association for Advancement of Behavior Therapy, New York, NY, November 1996
Shear MK: The psychodynamic approach in the treatment of panic disorder, in Panic Disorder and Agoraphobia: A Comprehensive Guide for the Practitioner. Edited by Walker JR, Norton GR, Ross CA. Pacific Grove, CA, Brooks/Cole, 1991, pp 335–351
Shear MK, Maser JD: Standardized assessment for panic disorder research: a conference report. Arch Gen Psychiatry 51:346–354, 1994

Shear MK, Weiner K: Psychotherapy for panic disorder. J Clin Psychiatry 58:38–45, 1997

Shear MK, Plikonis PA, Cloitre M, et al: Cognitive behavioral treatment compared with nonprescriptive treatment of panic disorder. Arch Gen Psychiatry 51:395–401, 1994

Shear MK, Cloitre M, Heckelman L: Emotion-focused treatment for panic disorder: a brief, dynamically informed therapy, in Dynamic Therapies for Psychiatric Disorders (Axis I). Edited by Barber JP, Crits-Christoph P. New York, Basic Books, 1995, pp 267–293

Sifneos PE: Short-Term Psychotherapy and Emotional Crisis. Cambridge, MA, Harvard University Press, 1972

Silber A: Temporary disorganization facilitating recall and mastery: an analysis of a symptom. Psychoanal Q 53:498–501, 1984

Smits JA, Powers MB, Cho Y, et al: Mechanism of change in cognitive-behavioral treatment of panic disorder: evidence for the fear of fear mediational hypothesis. J Consult Clin Psychol 72:646–652, 2004

Solyom C, Solyom L, LaPierre Y, et al: Phenelzine and exposure in the treatment of phobias. Biol Psychiatry 16:239–247, 1981

Spiegel DA, Bruce TJ: Benzodiazepines and exposure-based cognitive behavior therapies for panic disorder: conclusions from combined treatment trials. Am J Psychiatry 154:773–780, 1997

Spiegel DA, Bruce TJ, Gregg SF, et al: Does cognitive behavior therapy assist slow-taper alprazolam discontinuation in panic disorder? Am J Psychiatry 151:876–881, 1994

Taylor CB, King R, Margraf J, et al: Use of medication and in vivo exposure in volunteers for panic disorder research. Am J Psychiatry 146:1423–1426, 1989

Telch MJ, Lucas RA: Combined pharmacological and psychological treatment of panic disorder: current status and future directions, in Treatment of Panic Disorder: A Consensus Development Conference. Edited by Wolfe BE, Maser JD. Washington, DC, American Psychiatric Press, 1994, pp 177–197

Telch MJ, Agras WS, Taylor CB, et al: Combined pharmacological and behavioral treatment for agoraphobia. Behav Res Ther 23:325–335, 1985

Telch MJ, Lucas RA, Schmidt NB, et al: Group cognitive-behavioral treatment of panic disorder. Behav Res Ther 31: 279–287, 1993

Telch MJ, Schmidt NB, Jaimez L, et al: Singular and combined efficacy of in vivo exposure and CBT in the treatment of panic disorder with agoraphobia: interim results. Paper presented at the annual meeting of the Association for Advancement of Behavior Therapy, San Diego, CA, November 1994

Tolin DF, Pearlson GD, Krystal JH, et al: A controlled trial of D-cycloserine with brief CBT for panic disorder. Paper presented at the 40th annual convention of the Association for Behavioral and Cognitive Therapies, Chicago, IL, November 2006

Trull TJ, Nietzel MT, Main A: The use of meta-analysis to assess the clinical significance of behavior therapy for agoraphobia. Behav Ther 19:527–538, 1988

van den Hout M, Arntz A, Hoekstra R: Exposure reduced agoraphobia but not panic, and cognitive therapy reduced panic but not agoraphobia. Behav Res Ther 32:447–451, 1994

Waikar SV, Bystritsky A, Craske MG, et al: Etiological beliefs and treatment preferences in anxiety-disordered patients. Anxiety 1:134–137, 1994/1995

Wardle J, Hayward P, Higgitt A, et al: Effects of concurrent diazepam treatment on the outcome of exposure therapy in agoraphobia. Behav Res Ther 32:203–215, 1994

Wilborg IM, Dahl AA: Does brief dynamic psychotherapy reduce the relapse rate of panic disorder? Arch Gen Psychiatry 53:689–694, 1996

Williams SL, Falbo J: Cognitive and performance-based treatment for panic attacks in people with varying degrees of agoraphobic disability. Behav Res Ther 34:253–264, 1996

Williams SL, Rappaport A: Cognitive treatment in the natural environment for agoraphobics. Behav Ther 14:299–313, 1983

Wolfe BE, Maser JD: Origins and overview of the consensus development conference on the treatment of panic disorder, in Treatment of Panic Disorder: A Consensus Development Conference. Edited by Wolfe BE, Maser JD. Washington, DC, American Psychiatric Press, 1994, pp 3–16

Zitrin CM, Klein DF, Woerner MG: Treatment of agoraphobia with group exposure in vivo and imipramine. Arch Gen Psychiatry 37:63–72, 1980

Zitrin CM, Klein DF, Woerner MG, et al: Treatment of phobias, I: comparison of imipramine hydrochloride and placebo. Arch Gen Psychiatry 40:125–138, 1983

Recommended Readings

Barlow DH: Anxiety and Its disorders: The Nature and Treatment of Anxiety and Panic, 2nd Edition. New York, Guilford, 2002

Bouton ME, Mineka S, Barlow DH: A modern learning theory perspective on the etiology of panic disorder. Psychol Rev 108:4–32, 2001

Clark DM: A cognitive approach to panic. Behav Res Ther 24:461–470, 1986

Hofmann SG, Spiegel DA: Panic control treatment and its applications. J Psychother Pract Res 8:3–11, 1999

McNally RJ: Panic Disorder. New York, Guilford, 1994

Roth WT, Wilhelm FH, Pettit D: Are current theories of panic falsifiable? Psychol Bull 131:171–192, 2005

Social Anxiety Disorder (Social Phobia)

Chapter 25

Phenomenology of Social Anxiety Disorder

Holly J. Ramsawh, Ph.D.
Denise A. Chavira, Ph.D.
Murray B. Stein, M.D., M.P.H.

DSM Social Phobia: Past to Present

The history of social phobia (social anxiety disorder) as a diagnostic category is relatively brief. Although the term *social phobia* was coined in the early 1900s to describe individuals with performance-related anxieties (Janet 1903), it was not included in the first two versions of the DSM nomenclature (American Psychiatric Association 1952, 1968). Instead, symptoms resembling social phobia were subsumed under the rubric of phobic disorders. It was not until the advent of DSM-III (American Psychiatric Association 1980) and findings suggesting that certain phobias were qualitatively distinct (Marks and Gelder 1966) that social phobia was given its own diagnostic category.

In its first appearance in DSM-III, social phobia was defined as an excessive fear of observation or scrutiny in performance-related situations (e.g., public speaking, eating in front or others, writing in front of others). Exposure to these situations typically resulted in paniclike symptoms (e.g., heart palpitations, tremors, blushing, sweating), leading many individuals to avoid these social situations or to endure them with a great deal of distress. DSM-III criteria also specified that individuals experiencing these symptoms recognize their fears as unreasonable or excessive. If multiple social situations were avoided, an Axis II diagnosis of avoidant personality disorder was to supersede a social phobia diagnosis. As a result, many individuals received a diagnosis of avoidant personality disorder rather than social phobia. Although the diagnostic criteria for these two disorders overlapped considerably, avoidant personality disorder was to be differentiated by its pervasiveness, the intense feelings of inferiority it produced, and its earlier age of onset.

The differential diagnosis between social phobia and avoidant personality disorder was not without its consequences and inadequacies. Most importantly, it had profound treatment implications; for example, an individual with a personality disorder was less likely to receive pharmacological therapy than someone with social phobia (Liebowitz et al. 1985). In fact, it is probable that the assignment of an Axis II diagnosis reduced the chances that any form of therapy would be applied, perhaps resulting in a neglected patient population.

In DSM-III-R (American Psychiatric Association 1987), an attempt was made to improve the classification criteria by expanding the social phobia category to include individuals who feared many social situations. With this revision, avoidant personality disorder was dropped as an exclusionary criterion. Such inclusiveness resulted in a very heterogeneous diagnostic group; for example, an individual who feared only public speaking situations was given the same diagnosis as one who feared most social interactions. Consequently, DSM-III-R created a generalized subtype for persons who feared "most" social situations, including both performance (e.g., giving speeches, speaking at a meeting) and interactional situations (e.g., talking to strangers, interacting at a party). Those who did not fit this subtype were informally termed "nongeneralized"; however, labels such as "circumscribed," "discrete," "limited," and "specific" were also applied.

Despite these revisions, DSM-III-R did not escape criticism. Heckelman and Schneier (1995) noted three main problems. 1) There was ambiguity surrounding what constituted "most" social situations, a methodological issue that has profound research implications. 2) It was unclear whether the subtypes were quantitatively or qualitatively distinct entities. 3) A central flaw seemed to be the absence of an intermediate subtype that could be used to describe persons with the fear of several—but fewer than "most"—interpersonal situations. Another difficulty that quickly became apparent was how to adequately distinguish the generalized social phobia subtype from avoidant personality disorder (Herbert et al. 1992; Holt et al. 1992; Turner et al. 1992).

To address these issues, the American Psychiatric Task Force on DSM-IV (1991) examined the reliability and validity of alternative subtyping systems. A proposed alternative classification was a tripartite system consisting of 1) individuals who had circumscribed social fears (e.g., public speaking anxiety, fear of writing in front of others), 2) individuals who had "limited" interactional fears (i.e., fear of "some" but not "most" social situations), and 3) individuals who feared "most" social situations (Heimberg et al. 1993). Although this subtyping system appeared to have clinical validity, empirical studies were unable to support the presence of qualitative distinctions between the limited interactional and the circumscribed subtypes. It was decided that more research was necessary before changes to the current subtyping system were applied.

Overall, the DSM-IV diagnostic criteria for social phobia (social anxiety disorder) (American Psychiatric Association 1994, 2000; Table 25–1) remained largely consistent with those put forth in DSM-III-R. With regard to the subtyping system, the generalized subtype was once again included to distinguish individuals with fears of "most" social situations from those with specific fears. DSM-IV also advised its users to consider the comorbid diagnosis of avoidant personality disorder when diagnosing social phobia. Perhaps the area of greatest revision involved modification of the social phobia criteria to include children. Previously, children who had symptoms resembling social phobia were given diagnoses of avoidant disorder of childhood or overanxious disorder. Empirical data, however, suggested that these disorders were not readily distinguishable from social phobia (Beidel 1991; Francis et al. 1992). This diagnostic challenge was further complicated by the proposition that such comorbidity would inevitably obscure an accurate understanding of the lifetime course of social phobia (Heckelman and Schneier 1995). As a result, avoidant and overanxious disorder diagnoses in children were deleted from DSM and the criteria for social phobia were expanded to apply to children. Specifically, DSM-IV advised that anxiety might be expressed differently in children (e.g., by children's crying, tantrums, freezing, or withdrawal) than in adults. It was also noted that children, unlike adults, might not perceive their reactions to social situations as being unreasonable or excessive.

Diagnostic Issues

Distinctions Between Subtypes

Any discussion of clear-cut distinctions between social phobia subtypes is muddled by the fact that subtypes are not consistently defined in the literature. Some authors have defined subtypes by the *number* of situations feared (Heimberg et al. 1993; Hofmann and Roth 1996), whereas other investigators make distinctions based on *type* of feared situation (e.g., anxiety limited to public speaking versus generalized social interaction anxiety) (Kessler et al. 1998; Stemberger et al. 1995; Turner et al. 1992). Despite varying definitions, most findings suggest that the generalized subtype is more severe and causes greater impairment than the nongeneralized or circumscribed subtype. Specifically, empirical findings suggest that individuals with generalized social phobia report greater symptom severity, impairment, comorbid anxiety and depression, social skills deficits, and self-criticism than individuals with circumscribed or nongeneralized social phobia (Boone et al. 1999; Cox et al. 2004, 2005; Eng et al. 2000; Heimberg et al. 1990; Herbert et al. 1992; Holt et al. 1992; Tillfors and Furmark 2007; Tran and Chambless 1995). Recent findings also suggest that generalized social phobia may be associated with elevated serotonin synthesis in several brain regions, providing neurobiological support for greater severity of the generalized subtype (Furmark et al. 2007). Regarding treatment findings, some studies have found that patients with generalized social phobia respond less

TABLE 25–1. DSM-IV-TR diagnostic criteria for social phobia (social anxiety disorder)

A. A marked and persistent fear of one or more social or performance situations in which the person is exposed to unfamiliar people or to possible scrutiny by others. The individual fears that he or she will act in a way (or show anxiety symptoms) that will be humiliating or embarrassing. **Note:** In children, there must be evidence of the capacity for age-appropriate social relationships with familiar people and the anxiety must occur in peer settings, not just in interactions with adults.

B. Exposure to the feared social situation almost invariably provokes anxiety, which may take the form of a situationally bound or situationally predisposed panic attack. **Note:** In children, the anxiety may be expressed by crying, tantrums, freezing, or shrinking from social situations with unfamiliar people.

C. The person recognizes that the fear is excessive or unreasonable. **Note:** In children, this feature may be absent.

D. The feared social or performance situations are avoided or else are endured with intense anxiety or distress.

E. The avoidance, anxious anticipation, or distress in the feared social or performance situation(s) interferes significantly with the person's normal routine, occupational (academic) functioning, or social activities or relationships, or there is marked distress about having the phobia.

F. In individuals under age 18 years, the duration is at least 6 months.

G. The fear or avoidance is not due to the direct physiological effects of a substance (e.g., a drug of abuse, a medication) or a general medical condition and is not better accounted for by another mental disorder (e.g., panic disorder with or without agoraphobia, separation anxiety disorder, body dysmorphic disorder, a pervasive developmental disorder, or schizoid personality disorder).

H. If a general medical condition or another mental disorder is present, the fear in Criterion A is unrelated to it, e.g., the fear is not of stuttering, trembling in Parkinson's disease, or exhibiting abnormal eating behavior in anorexia nervosa or bulimia nervosa.

Specify if:

Generalized: if the fears include most social situations (also consider the additional diagnosis of avoidant personality disorder)

well to typical cognitive-behavioral therapies (Brown et al. 1995; Heimberg et al. 1985; Lincoln et al. 2005; Turner et al. 1994).

Some authors have suggested that any differentiation into subtypes is arbitrary, given that no clear demarcations between subtypes have been found and that many of the reported differences are related to severity and do not constitute categorical distinctions. Instead, they propose that social phobia exists along a continuum—the greater the number of feared situations, the greater the severity tends to be (Furmark et al. 2000; Kollman et al. 2006; Stein et al. 2000; Vriends et al. 2007b). For example, a study using National Comorbidity Survey Replication data revealed that both performance and interaction fears loaded onto a single latent factor (Ruscio et al. 2008). However, other evidence supports the categorical subtype system, particularly in the case of public speaking anxiety, as a distinct subtype.

Differences have been found between discrete public speaking anxiety and more generalized social fears. It has been observed that when social phobia exists in only one or two limited situations, it is typically of the public speaking variant (Eng et al. 2000; Furmark et al. 2000; Kessler et al. 1998; Tillfors and Furmark 2007; Turner et al. 1992). Physiological differences have also been noted—patients with circumscribed (public speaking or other performance) social phobia exhibit greater cardiac reactivity than those with generalized social phobia during public speaking tasks (Boone et al. 1999; Heimberg et al. 1990; Hofmann et al. 1995; Levin et al. 1993). In a related study with psychiatrically healthy control subjects, trait social anxiety predicted startle response during anticipation of a speech task, also suggesting a relationship between public speaking anxiety and physiological responsiveness (Cornwell et al. 2006). Using an information-processing paradigm (i.e., the Stroop task), McNeil et al. (1995) found subtype differences: individuals with circumscribed social phobia had longer latencies of response to public speaking stimuli than individuals with generalized social phobia. With regard to etiological variables, some authors have found that generalized social phobia was more frequently associated with a history of childhood shyness (Cox et al. 2005; Stemberger et al. 1995), whereas "specific" social phobia was more commonly associated with traumatic conditioning experiences (Stemberger et al. 1995). In contrast with the findings of Ruscio et al. (2008), other investigations examining the latent structure of social anxiety support categorical distinctions. In one such study, social interaction anxiety evidenced a stronger relationship with low positive affect, whereas performance anxiety showed a stronger association with physiological hyperarousal (Hughes et al. 2006). Similarly, Norton et al. (1997) found that generalized social fears were most strongly related to neuroticism, whereas performance fears were most strongly linked to anxiety sensitivity, a construct typically associated with panic disorder. Finally, a few behavioral and pharmacological studies suggest that specific social phobia can be treated using either different modalities or less elaborate interventions, compared with generalized social phobia. For example, Ost et al. (1981) found that individuals with social phobia characterized by high levels of physiological reactivity (apparently corresponding to the specific or circumscribed subtype) responded more favorably to applied relaxation, whereas those with social skills deficits (corresponding to the generalized subtype) had better outcome with social skills training. Regarding pharmacological treatment, some studies support the use of beta-blockers in treatment of public speaking or performance anxiety (Brantigan et al. 1982; Gorman et al. 1985; James and Savage 1984), although beta-blockers have generally not been found to be effective in generalized social phobia (Liebowitz et al. 1992).

Given the distinct physiological, etiological, and treatment characteristics found to be associated with circumscribed public speaking and performance fears, along with generally lower distress levels and comorbidity, some authors have suggested that the public speaking subtype of social phobia is closely related to the specific phobias (Hook and Valentiner 2002). Notable similarities include the presence of acute autonomic arousal upon exposure to the feared stimulus, the underrepresention of individuals with discrete public speaking fears in clinical settings (Kessler et al. 1998), and the frequent association with traumatic conditioning experiences (Hofmann et al. 1995; Ost and Hugdahl 1981). However, given the variable definitions of circumscribed social phobia, it is unclear whether these data are most applicable to public speaking fears alone, or to anxiety in performance situations in general.

Thus far, the validity of subtyping systems is far from conclusive. Although there is some evidence for categorical distinctions between generalized social phobia and circumscribed or discrete phobias (e.g., public speaking), the difference between the more vaguely defined "nongeneralized" category and other subtypes is unclear. At this point, social phobia subtypes may have some clinical utility; however, their validity as separate and qualitatively distinct subgroups requires further research.

Comorbidity With Avoidant Personality Disorder

Considerable overlap exists between generalized social phobia and avoidant personality disorder; comorbidity rates range from 22% to 89% (Fahlen 1995; Grant et al. 2005b; Herbert et al. 1992; Holt et al. 1992; Lampe et al. 2003; Marteinsdottir et al. 2001; Schneier et al. 1991). Whereas both categorical and quantitative differences have been found between social phobia subtypes, most studies suggest that avoidant personality disorder is not distinct from generalized social phobia, but is instead a more severe variant of the disorder. Study designs comparing generalized social phobia subjects with and without avoidant personality disorder have found that the presence of avoidant personality disorder was associated with greater symptom severity, trait anxiety, and functional impairment (Furmark et al. 2007; Herbert et al. 1992; Marteinsdottir et al. 2001; Tillfors et al. 2004). However, other studies have not found avoidant personality disorder to be associated with greater severity on variables that include subjective reports of distress, heart rate, speech length or quality, negative thoughts recounted during the behavioral tasks, or information processing tasks (Herbert et al. 1992; Hofmann et al. 1995; Holt et al. 1992; McNeil et al. 1995; Turner et al. 1992). In a study of individuals with avoidant personality disorder, the authors reported that those with and without comorbid social phobia did not evidence meaningful differences on demographic or clinical characteristics (Ralevski et al. 2005). Further supporting the hypothesis that the two conditions may be variations of the same construct, Stein et al. (1998) found similar rates of these two disorders in first-degree relatives of generalized social phobia probands. Another family study of social phobia and avoidant personality disorder found that having a family member with significant social anxiety symptoms was associated with a two- to threefold increase in risk of both diagnoses, suggesting that they "load" similarly in families (Tillfors et al. 2001). With respect to treatment, research findings do not support the hypothesis that a comorbid avoidant personality disorder diagnosis is a significant predictor of treatment outcome among individuals with generalized social phobia (Brown et al. 1995; Hope et al. 1995; Oosterbaan et al. 2002; van Velzen et al. 1997).

In addition to differences related to severity, a few investigators have noted qualitative differences between avoidant personality disorder and social phobia. Worthy of note is a study by Tran and Chambless (1995), who found a trend for social skills deficits to be associated with avoidant personality disorder. In addition, a study conducted in 2007 found that avoidant personality disorder without comorbid social phobia was more strongly associated with eating disorders than was social phobia without avoidant personality disorder; in turn, social phobia alone was more associated with panic disorder than was avoidant personality disorder alone (Hummelen et al. 2007). However, the authors did not specify subtype in their social phobia group, leaving open the possibility that these individuals may have been diagnosed with circumscribed social phobia (which may have a stronger relationship with panic disorder than the generalized subtype). Although additional investigation of qualitative markers is ongoing, the bulk of the current evidence suggests that generalized social phobia and avoidant personality disorder are quantitatively related; that is, the latter may be seen as a severe variant of the former.

Epidemiological Findings

In the United States, epidemiological and community-based studies have reported lifetime prevalence rates of social phobia ranging from 2.4% to 13.0% (Kessler et al. 1994, 2005; Magee et al. 1996; Ruscio et al. 2008; Schneier et al. 1992), making it the third most common psychiatric disorder (after major depressive disorder and alcohol dependence). Variations in diagnostic rates can be attributed to changes in diagnostic criteria, required level of impairment, and differing methodologies. For example, structured interviews, such as the Diagnostic Interview Schedule (DIS; Robins et al. 1981), query three types of social fears, whereas other interview schedules, such as the Composite International Diagnostic Interview (CIDI; World Health Organization 1990), assess six types of social fears. Use of the DIS has elicited lifetime prevalence rates of social phobia ranging from 0.5% to 3.0%. The CIDI and other interview schedules that probe more social fears have tended to yield higher lifetime prevalence rates (4.7% to 16%) (Furmark et al. 1999; Kessler et al. 2005; Magee et al. 1996; Ruscio et al. 2008; Stein et al. 2000) (Table 25–2).

Cross-National and Cultural Findings

As shown in Table 25–2, relatively similar rates of social phobia are found in the United States, Canada, and Europe, and lower rates are reported in non-Western countries, such as Nigeria and Korea. These lower prevalence rates are perplexing in light of research that has documented the presence of a putative Asian pattern of social anxiety called *taijin-kyofu-sho* (TKS) in countries such as Japan and Korea (Murphy 1982). Unlike the traditional conceptualization of social phobia in Western nations, which involves the fear of humiliating oneself, TKS involves the fear of offending others by embarrassing them or by making them uncomfortable through a personal flaw or shortcoming (e.g., blushing in front of others, emitting an unpleasant body odor, or exposing an unsightly body part). There is not yet consensus on a definition of TKS, and it may be a somewhat broader construct than social phobia (Nagata et al. 2003; Suzuki et al. 2003); however, there appears to be significant overlap between TKS and both social phobia and avoidant personality disorder (Kleinknecht et al. 1997; Nagata et al. 2006; Ono et al. 1996). Some authors have suggested that fear of causing discomfort to others, a core symptom in TKS, can be subsumed under fear of negative evaluation and, thus, may not be a separate construct from social phobia (Chang 1997; Magee et al. 2006). Case reports of TKS in the United States also call into question its status as an Asian culture-bound syndrome separate from social phobia (Clarvit et al. 1996; McNally et al. 1990). Studies suggest that pharmacotherapeutic interventions used for treatment of social phobia are also effective for TKS (Matsunaga et al. 2001; Nagata et al. 2003, 2006).

Epidemiological findings presenting prevalence rates of social phobia across ethnic groups within the United States have been scant. Comparable rates of social phobia are present among Caucasians, African Americans, and Hispanics (Canino et al. 1987; Magee et al. 1996), although more recent data suggest that both African Americans and Hispanics have a lower lifetime prevalence compared with their Caucasian counterparts (Breslau et al. 2006; Grant et al. 2005a; Ruscio et al. 2008). Differences have also been found between Asian Americans and Caucasians: in a college student sample, Asian Americans scored higher than Caucasians on measures of social anxiety and depression (Okazaki 1997). Findings from this study also revealed that self-construal variables were important predictors of social anxiety; that is, interdependent self-construals (e.g., emphasis on self as part of a group) were better predictors of social anxiety than independent self-construals (e.g., emphasis on self as being autonomous). Furthermore, less acculturated Asian Americans reported higher avoidance and distress in social situations. Additional research is necessary to understand the variables (e.g., language, social

TABLE 25–2. Social phobia lifetime prevalence rates, based on the CIDI and alternative structured interviews such as the DIS

		Lifetime prevalence rates (%)	
Location	**Reference**	**CIDI**	**Other interviews**
United States	Schneier et al. 1992		2.4
	Magee et al. 1996	13.3	
	Stein et al. 2000	7.2	
	Grant et al. 2005a		5.0
	Kessler et al. 2005	12.1	
	Ruscio et al. 2008	12.1	
Canada	Bland et al. 1988		1.7
	Stein et al. 2000	13.0	
Brazil	Andrade et al. 2002	3.5	
China	Lee et al. 2007	0.5	
France	Lépine et al. 2005	4.7	
Iran	Mohammadi et al. 2006		0.8
New Zealand	Browne et al. 2006	9.4	
Nigeria	Gureje et al. 2006	0.3	
Puerto Rico	Canino et al. 1987		1.6
Taiwan	Hwu et al. 1989		0.6
Korea	Cho et al. 2007	0.2	
Switzerland	Wacker et al. 1992	16.0	
Sweden	Furmark et al. 1999	15.6	

Note. CIDI=Composite International Diagnostic Interview; DIS=Diagnostic Interview Schedule.

ideals, child-rearing practices, and social affiliation) that may mediate the expression of social anxiety.

In attempts to explain the presence or absence of cross-cultural differences, methodological factors should also be considered. For example, translation of interview schedules developed in English into other languages may affect the sensitivity of the instruments. In addition, instruments that have a Western psychiatric focus may not be sensitive to patterns of symptomatology found in non-Western countries (Chapman et al. 1995; Guarnaccia et al. 1989). Finally, it has been suggested that members of some cultures are less willing to disclose information in the structured interviews used by research studies (Gureje et al. 2006).

Demographic Characteristics

Epidemiological studies have also found that individuals with social phobia are more likely to be female, single, and unemployed and to have lower income and education compared with those without the disorder (Grant et al. 2005a; Ruscio et al. 2008; Schneier et al. 1992; Wells et al. 1994). In patient samples, however, social phobia seems to be equally distributed among males and females (Boyd et al. 1990; Degonda and Angst 1993; Turk et al. 1998). Overall, social phobia and simple phobias typically have an earlier age at onset than other anxiety disorders (Grant et al. 2005a; Kessler et al. 2005; Scheibe and Albus 1992). Epidemiological and patient sample studies suggest that the typical age at onset of social phobia is early to mid-adolescence and that onset after age 25 is relatively uncommon (Kessler et al. 2005; Magee et al. 1996). There is some evidence that the nongeneralized or specific subtype has a slightly later age of onset (Kessler et al. 1999; Mannuzza et al. 1995; Wittchen et al. 1999).

Course

There have been few studies examining the longitudinal course of social phobia. Data from the Harvard/Brown

Anxiety Research Project (HARP), a naturalistic longitudinal study of anxiety disorders, suggests that social phobia has a chronic and unremitting course (Ramsawh et al. 2009; Yonkers et al. 2001, 2003). A study from the HARP group found that in comparison with generalized anxiety disorder and panic disorder, individuals with social phobia had the smallest probability of recovery over 12 years (Bruce et al. 2005). Somewhat higher rates of recovery have been suggested in a 1.5-year follow-up study of social phobia in a community sample (Vriends et al. 2007a); however, another community study found substantial stability of symptoms over 15 years of follow-up (Merikangas et al. 2002). Social phobia has been found to be most likely to remit during the first 2 years of follow-up, after which recovery rate decreases (Yonkers et al. 2003).

Comorbidity

Numerous studies suggest that most individuals with social phobia have one or more comorbid conditions (Lépine and Pelissolo 1996; Merikangas and Angst 1995; Ruscio et al. 2008; Schneier et al. 1992) and that the presence of psychiatric comorbidity is associated with a poorer prognosis (Davidson et al. 1993; Vriends et al. 2007a). Axis I disorders that are most frequently comorbid with social phobia are major depression (Faravelli et al. 2000; Kessler et al. 1999; Reich et al. 1993; Stein et al. 1999; Van Ameringen et al. 1991), panic disorder (Angst 1993; Stein et al. 1989), agoraphobia (Goisman et al. 1995), specific phobias (Chartier et al. 2003; Mohammadi et al. 2006), generalized anxiety disorder (Borkovec et al. 1995; Grant et al. 2005a; Mennin et al. 2000; Turner et al. 1991), substance use disorders (Crum and Pratt 2001; Dilsaver et al. 1992; Page and Andrews 1996), sexual dysfunction (Bodinger et al. 2002; Corretti et al. 2006; Figueira et al. 2001), and eating disorders (Hummelen et al. 2007; Kaye et al. 2004).

Studies investigating the longitudinal course of comorbid conditions have found that social phobia generally precedes mood, substance use, and eating disorders (Alpert et al. 1994; Brewerton et al. 1993; Bulik et al. 1997; Kessler et al. 1999). Furthermore, the presence of social anxiety in nondepressed persons is associated with an increased likelihood of subsequent depressive disorder (Bittner et al. 2004; Stein et al. 2001). In a clinical sample, comorbid generalized anxiety disorder exacerbated the 12-year course of social phobia by further decreasing likelihood of recovery, whereas comorbid major depression increased likelihood of relapse of social phobia in those who had previously recovered (Bruce et al. 2005). In another study from the Keller group, comorbid avoidant personality disorder was associated with a 41% decrease in the likelihood of recovery (Massion et al. 2002).

Impairment

Even in the absence of comorbidity, social phobia has been associated with significant distress, as manifested by financial problems, work impairment and days missed from work, impaired school performance and dropout, weakened social support systems, increased use of psychotropic medication, and more help-seeking from medical and mental health professionals (Davidson et al. 1993; Merikangas et al. 2007; Schneier et al. 1992, 1994; Van Ameringen et al. 2003). Although increased suicidal thoughts have been reported, actual suicide attempts were associated with increased comorbidity (Cox et al. 1994; Sareen et al. 2005a; Schneier et al. 1992). Patients with social phobia also reported reduced quality of life compared with community norms (Cramer et al. 2005; Safren et al. 1996–1997; Simon et al. 2002; Stein and Kean 2000). On a construct closely related to quality of life (illness intrusiveness; the extent to which an illness interferes with everyday functioning), patients with social phobia appeared as impaired as persons with chronic medical conditions such as end-stage renal disease or multiple sclerosis (Antony et al. 1998). The relationship between quality of life and social phobia appears to be even more pronounced in the generalized subtype (Kessler et al. 1998; van Velzen et al. 2000).

Social Phobia in Primary Care Settings

Several studies have shown that anxiety disorders are highly prevalent among general medical clinic attendees (Fifer et al. 1994; Schonfeld et al. 1997; Sherbourne et al. 1996). In studies of social phobia in primary care, investigators have found somewhat lower current prevalence rates than have reported in the general population (i.e., in the range of 5%–6%) (Gross et al. 2005; Kroenke et al. 2007), although the finding that individuals with social phobia make fewer annual visits to primary care clinics may partially explain this discrepancy (Gross et al. 2005). Social phobia is associated with poor recognition on the part of primary care practitioners (Kashdan et al. 2006; Stein et al. 1999; Weiller et al. 1996) and often goes untreated or is treated inadequately (Harman et al. 2002; Stein et al. 2004; Weisberg et al. 2007; Young et al. 2001). Social phobia in primary care settings is associated with meaningfully reduced role functioning, increased number of sick days, and reduced quality of life (Schonfeld et al. 1997; Stein et al. 2005).

Social Phobia and Medical Illness

Epidemiological studies suggest an association between anxiety disorders and medical illness (Demyttenaere et al. 2007; Ormel et al. 2007; Sareen et al. 2005b, 2006). Although few studies have examined the relationship between medical illness and social phobia in particular, it has been linked to heart disease and associated risk factors (Landen et al. 2004; Sareen et al. 2005b), autoimmune disorders (Lindal et al. 1995; Sareen et al. 2005b), and Parkinson's disease (de Rijk and Bijl 1998; Stein et al. 1990). With regard to Parkinson's disease, some reports suggest social phobia estimates as high as 29% among individuals with Parkinson's disease, if DSM hierarchy rules are ignored (i.e., typically, social phobia is not diagnosed if the social anxiety is exclusively about symptoms of a medical condition, such as tremor) (Stein et al. 1990). Given that most surveys adhere to DSM hierarchy rules, the true prevalence of clinically significant social phobia symptoms in Parkinson's disease and other medical conditions is likely underdiagnosed.

Genetic Factors

Familial Associations in Social Phobia

Findings from family studies (Chapman et al. 1995; Fyer et al. 1993; Reich and Yates 1988) and twin studies (Hettema et al. 2005; Kendler et al. 1992; Middeldorp et al. 2005; Warren et al. 1999) suggest that social phobia has a heritable component. Specifically, family studies have found that relatives of social phobia probands have an increased risk for social phobia compared with rates for relatives of control subjects (16% vs. 5%, respectively). Similarly, studies of offspring of adults with social phobia in clinical samples have found increased rates of social phobia (Mancini et al. 1996; Merikangas et al. 1999).

Although a familial component appears to be present in social phobia, few studies have explored this relationship in social phobia subtypes. Stein et al. (1998) investigated this question and found that the incidence of generalized social phobia was far higher among first-degree relatives of people with generalized social phobia (25%) than among relatives of control subjects without social phobia (less than 5%), although the percentage of first-degree relatives who had nongeneralized social phobia did not differ significantly between the groups. Moreover, avoidant personality disorder occurred at a greatly increased rate (20%) among the relatives of people with generalized social phobia, but it was absent from the control group. Such findings are consistent with those of Mannuzza et al. (1995), who similarly found that the rate of social phobia was elevated only in the relatives of subjects with generalized social phobia. Tillfors et al. (2001) also found an elevated rate of avoidant personality disorder in relatives of individuals with social phobia. Taken together, these findings indicate that generalized social phobia is highly familial; they also provide support for the hypothesis that avoidant personality disorder may represent one extreme of the spectrum of social phobia.

Temperament and Social Phobia

A possibly heritable dimension of personality that shares some clinical features with social anxiety is behavioral inhibition. Behavioral inhibition, which has been described as a tendency to react aversively to the presence of unfamiliar situations and novel stimuli, has been observed in children as young as 21 months (Garcia-Coll et al. 1984; Kagan et al. 1988b). Behaviorally, children showing this tendency are more likely to withdraw, cry, freeze, or cling to their attachment figure in unfamiliar situations. Biological measures suggest that children with an inhibited temperament have higher levels of cortisol in their saliva and higher heart rates in stressful situations (Garcia-Coll et al. 1984). Some investigators have postulated that the threshold of responsivity in limbic and hypothalamic structures to unfamiliarity and challenge is lower for inhibited than for uninhibited children (Kagan et al. 1987, 1993). Consequently, inhibited children show increases in muscle tension, heightened cardiac arousal, pupillary dilation, and/or increased cortisol in response to minimally unfamiliar or challenging events. Follow-up studies have found that approximately 75% of inhibited children retain this classification through age 7½ years (Kagan 1989; Kagan et al. 1988b).

Studies using the Kagan et al. (1988a) longitudinal cohort found that inhibited children were at elevated risk for anxiety disorders such as avoidant disorder, which is very similar to social phobia (Biederman et al. 1990). Inhibited children also had parents with significantly greater risks for more than two anxiety disorders, anxiety disorders from childhood continuing into adulthood, social phobia, and childhood avoidant and overanxious disorders (Rosenbaum et al. 1991). In addition, Rosenbaum et al. (1992) found that the prevalence of social phobia in the parents of children with behavioral inhibition (10%) was higher than in the parents of children without behavioral inhibition (0%).

More recent studies also support an association between behavioral inhibition and social phobia. Biederman et al. (2001) found that 17% of behaviorally inhibited children had a current diagnosis of social phobia, versus 5% of children who were not inhibited. Similarly, in follow-up studies of children who had been classified as inhibited or uninhibited at baseline, 28% to 61% originally classified as inhibited had social phobia at follow-up, compared with 14% to 27% of those originally labeled as uninhibited (Hirshfeld-Becker et al. 2007; Kagan et al. 1988b; Schwartz et al. 1999). Studies have also found that behavioral inhibition early in life is associated with increased odds of receiving a social phobia diagnosis in adolescence and adulthood (Hayward et al. 1998; Wittchen et al. 1999). In a neuroimaging study of adults previously classified as inhibited or uninhibited during the second year of life, past inhibition was associated with a greater amygdala response to novel as opposed to familiar faces (Schwartz et al. 2003). This study finding suggests that the effects of behavioral inhibition can last into adulthood and appear to be related to social phobia–related patterns of neural activation.

In addition, findings suggest that behavioral inhibition may be differentially related to social anxiety. For example, Mick and Telch (1998) found higher levels of retrospectively reported childhood behavioral inhibition in college students with symptoms of social phobia (assessed with self-report questionnaires) than in participants with symptoms of generalized anxiety disorder or subjects in the control group. In a longitudinal study, Hirshfeld-Becker et al. (2007) found that the presence of behavioral inhibition in preschool-age children predicted the onset of social phobia, but not other anxiety disorders, at 5-year follow-up.

Social Phobia as a Spectrum Disorder

Social Phobia and Shyness

Reviews of the literature have found that social phobia and shyness have many symptoms in common (Henderson and Zimbardo 2001; Turner et al. 1990). Individuals who are shy cannot be differentiated from individuals with social phobia on the basis of physical symptoms (e.g., somatic arousal and heart rate activity) (Amies et al. 1983; Kagan et al. 1988b; Ludwig and Lazarus 1983). In addition, cognitions reflecting fear of negative evaluation are common to both constructs. According to Turner et al. (1990), areas that may differentiate the two symptom patterns include severity of avoidance, degree of impairment, and course. Compared with shyness, social phobia is associated with more avoidance and greater functional impairment, and it is seen as more chronic.

Self-reported rates of shyness from college samples range from 40% to 50% (Carducci and Zimbardo 1995; Zimbardo 1977). In a study using National Comorbidity Survey data, 26% of females and 19% of males reported a childhood history of shyness (Cox et al. 2005). In comparison, lifetime rates of social phobia range from 3% to 16% in epidemiological studies (Furmark et al. 1999; Grant et al. 2005a; Kessler et al. 2005). In addition, Cox et al. (2005) found that childhood shyness was robustly associated with adult social phobia, even when current social phobia was excluded, which underscores the robustness of the relationship; the association was particularly strong for generalized social phobia.

According to Johnson et al. (1996), only a portion of individuals who describe themselves as shy actually exhibit clinical or subclinical social phobia. Surprisingly, however, few data are available to support this hypothesis. At present, only a few studies have assessed the distribution of social phobia among highly shy individuals. St. Lorant et al. (2000) retrospectively reviewed charts of 114 patients presenting for treatment at a shyness clinic and reported that 97% of the sample had a generalized social phobia diagnosis. In a different study that used a nonclinical (college student) sample, 49% of those who were highly shy (i.e., in the upper tenth percentile of the distribution of shyness) received a diagnosis of social phobia, whereas only 18% of those who were normatively shy (i.e., in the fortieth to sixtieth percentile) received that diagnosis (Chavira et al. 2002). When subtypes were examined, approximately 36% of highly shy young adults met DSM-IV criteria for the generalized type of social phobia, compared with only 4% of normatively shy young adults; equal rates of highly versus normatively shy individuals were found in the nongeneralized social phobia group. There were also more individuals who met criteria for avoidant personality disorder in the highly shy group than in the comparison group. In another study using a college sample, 18% of shy individuals were diagnosed with social phobia, whereas only 3% of non-shy participants received a social phobia diagnosis (Heiser et al. 2003). In addition, shy individuals with comorbid social phobia were shyer, had higher neuroticism, were more introverted, and had greater psychiatric comorbidity than those in the "pure" shyness group.

On the basis of these findings, it is possible that shyness is a trait that, at its extreme, becomes impairing and thereupon assumes the characteristics of a disorder, namely social phobia. Furthermore, extreme shyness seems to be more related to the interactional fears that characterize generalized social phobia than to the performance-oriented fears that frequently typify nongeneralized social phobia and more circumscribed social phobias (e.g., public speaking phobias). This relationship is further demonstrated by the disproportionately higher rates of avoidant personality disorder in highly shy individuals. Overall, such findings partially support a spectrum model, in which higher shyness levels are indicative of more problematic degrees of social anxiety, merging at the upper extreme into clinical disorders such as generalized social phobia and avoidant personality disorder. Additional research is necessary to evaluate this relationship further and to more fully understand the variables that distinguish extreme shyness from social phobia.

◀ Key Clinical Points ▶

- Social phobia (social anxiety disorder) has been shown to be a highly prevalent disorder in epidemiological studies. Although discrete public speaking fears are more common in the general population, individuals with the generalized subtype of social phobia are more likely to present for treatment. Generalized social phobia is associated with greater severity, impairment, and comorbidity relative to "nongeneralized" social fears.
- Social phobia typically first appears in early to mid-adolescence, and it has been shown to have a chronic and unremitting course. Psychiatric comorbidity further worsens prognosis.
- Generalized social phobia may have a heritable component. Traits including behavioral inhibition and shyness may contribute to this heritability. Behaviorally inhibited children are at increased risk for onset of social phobia later in life.

References

Alpert JE, Maddocks A, Rosenbaum JF, et al: Childhood psychopathology retrospectively assessed among adults with early onset major depression. J Affect Disord 31:165–171, 1994

American Psychiatric Association: Diagnostic and Statistical Manual: Mental Disorders. Washington, DC, American Psychiatric Association, 1952

American Psychiatric Association: Diagnostic and Statistical Manual of Mental Disorders, 2nd Edition. Washington, DC, American Psychiatric Association, 1968

American Psychiatric Association: Diagnostic and Statistical Manual of Mental Disorders, 3rd Edition. Washington, DC, American Psychiatric Association, 1980

American Psychiatric Association: Diagnostic and Statistical Manual of Mental Disorders, 3rd Edition, Revised. Washington, DC, American Psychiatric Association, 1987

American Psychiatric Association: Diagnostic and Statistical Manual of Mental Disorders, 4th Edition. Washington, DC, American Psychiatric Association, 1994

American Psychiatric Association: Diagnostic and Statistical Manual of Mental Disorders, 4th Edition, Text Revision. Washington, DC, American Psychiatric Association, 2000

American Psychiatric Association Task Force on DSM-IV: DSM-IV Options Book: Work in Progress 9/1/91. Washington, DC, American Psychiatric Association, 1991

Amies PL, Gleder MG, Shaw PM: Social phobia: a comparative clinical study. Br J Psychiatry 142:174–179, 1983

Andrade L, Walters EE, Gentil V, et al: Prevalence of ICD-10 mental disorders in a catchment area in the city of Sao Paulo, Brazil. Soc Psychiatry Psychiatr Epidemiol 37:316–325, 2002

Angst J: Comorbidity of anxiety, phobia, compulsion and depression. Int Clin Psychopharmacol 8:21–25, 1993

Antony MM, Roth D, Swinson RP, et al: Illness intrusiveness in individuals with panic disorder, obsessive-compulsive disorder, or social phobia. J Nerv Ment Dis 186:311–315, 1998

Beidel DC: Social phobia and overanxious disorder in school-age children. J Am Acad Child Adolesc Psychiatry 30:545–552, 1991

Biederman J, Rosenbaum JF, Hirshfeld DR, et al: Psychiatric correlates of behavioral inhibition in young children of parents with and without psychiatric disorders. Arch Gen Psychiatry 47:21–26, 1990

Biederman J, Hirshfeld-Becker DR, Rosenbaum JF, et al: Further evidence of association between behavioral inhibition and social anxiety in children. Am J Psychiatry 158:1673–1679, 2001

Bittner A, Goodwin RD, Wittchen HU, et al: What characteristics of primary anxiety disorders predict subsequent major depressive disorder? J Clin Psychiatry 65:618–626, 2004

Bland RC, Orn H, Newman SC: Lifetime prevalence of psychiatric disorders in Edmonton. Acta Psychiatr Scand Suppl 338:24–32, 1988

Bodinger L, Hermesh H, Aizenberg D, et al: Sexual function and behavior in social phobia. J Clin Psychiatry 63:874–879, 2002

Boone ML, McNeil W, Masia CL, et al: Multimodal comparisons of social phobia subtypes and avoidant personality disorder. J Anxiety Disord 13:271–292, 1999

Borkovec TD, Abel JL, Newman H: Effects of psychotherapy on comorbid conditions in generalized anxiety disorder. J Consult Clin Psychol 63:479–483, 1995

Boyd JH, Rae DS, Thompson JW, et al: Phobia: prevalence and risk factors. Soc Psychiatry Psychiatr Epidemiol 25:314–323, 1990

Brantigan CO, Brantigan TA, Joseph N: Effect of beta-blockade and beta-stimulation on stage fright. Am J Med 72:88–94, 1982

Breslau J, Aguilar-Gaxiola S, Kendler KS, et al: Specifying race-ethnic differences in risk for psychiatric disorder in a USA national sample. Psychol Med 36:57–68, 2006

Brewerton TD, Lydiard RB, Ballenger JC, et al: Eating disorders and social phobia (letter). Arch Gen Psychiatry 50:70, 1993

Brown EJ, Heimberg RG, Juster HR: Social phobia subtype and avoidant personality disorder: effect on severity of social phobia, impairment, and outcome of cognitive-behavioral treatment. Behav Ther 26:467–486, 1995

Browne MAO, Wells JE, Scott KM, et al: Lifetime prevalence and projected lifetime risk of DSM-IV disorders in Te Rau Hinengaro: The New Zealand Mental Health Survey. Aust N Z J Psychiatry 40:865–874, 2006

Bruce SE, Yonkers KA, Otto MW, et al: Influence of psychiatric comorbidity on recovery and recurrence in generalized anxiety disorder, social phobia, and panic disorder: a 12-year prospective study. Am J Psychiatry 162:1179–1187, 2005

Bulik CM, Sullivan PF, Fear JL, et al: Eating disorders and antecedent anxiety disorders: a controlled study. Acta Psychiatr Scand 96:101–107, 1997

Canino GJ, Bird HR, Shrout PE, et al: The prevalence of specific psychiatric disorder in Puerto Rico. Arch Gen Psychiatry 44:727–735, 1987

Carducci BJ, Zimbardo PG: Are you shy? Psychol Today 28:34–40, 1995

Chang SC: Social anxiety (phobia) and east Asian culture. Depress Anxiety 5:115–120, 1997

Chapman TF, Mannuzza S, Fyer AJ: Epidemiology and family studies of social phobia, in Social Phobia: Diagnosis, Assessment, and Treatment. Edited by Heimberg RG, Liebowitz MR, Hope DA, et al. New York, Guilford, 1995, pp 21–40

Chartier MJ, Walker JR, Stein MB: Considering comorbidity in social phobia. Soc Psychiatry Psychiatr Epidemiol 38:728–734, 2003

Chavira DA, Stein MB, Malcarne VL: Scrutinizing the relationship between shyness and social phobia. J Anxiety Disord 16:585–598, 2002

Cho MJ, Kim JK, Jeon HJ, et al: Lifetime and 12-month prevalence of DSM-IV psychiatric disorders among Korean adults. J Nerv Ment Dis 195:203–210, 2007

Clarvit SR, Schneier FR, Liebowitz MR: The offensive subtype of taijin-kyofu-sho in New York City: the phenomenology and treatment of a social anxiety disorder. J Clin Psychiatry 57:523–527, 1996

Cornwell BR, Johnson L, Berardi L, et al: Anticipation of public speaking in virtual reality reveals a relationship between trait social anxiety and startle reactivity. Biol Psychiatry 59:664–666, 2006

Corretti G, Pierucci S, De Scisciolo M, et al: Comorbidity between social phobia and premature ejaculation: study on 242 males affected by sexual disorders. J Sex Marital Ther 32:183–187, 2006

Cox BJ, Direnfeld DM, Swinson RP, et al: Suicidal ideation and suicide attempts in panic disorder and social phobia. Am J Psychiatry 151:882–887, 1994

Cox BJ, Fleet C, Stein MB: Self-criticism and social phobia in the U.S. National Comorbidity Survey. J Affect Disord 82:227–234, 2004

Cox BJ, MacPherson PSR, Enns MW: Psychiatric correlates of childhood shyness in a nationally representative sample. Behav Res Ther 43:1019–1027, 2005

Cramer V, Torgersen S, Kringlen E: Quality of life and anxiety disorders: a population study. J Nerv Ment Dis 193:196–202, 2005

Crum RM, Pratt LA: Risk of heavy drinking and alcohol use disorders in social phobia: a prospective analysis. Am J Psychiatry 158:1693–1700, 2001

Davidson JRT, Hughes DL, George LK, et al: The epidemiology of social phobia: findings from the Duke Epidemiological Catchment Area Study. Psychol Med 23:709–718, 1993

de Rijk C, Bijl RV: Prevalence of mental disorders in persons with Parkinson's disease. Ned Tijdschr Geneeskd 142:27–31, 1998

Degonda M, Angst J: The Zurich study, XX: social phobia and agoraphobia. Eur Arch Psychiatry Clin Neurosci 243:95–102, 1993

Demyttenaere K, Bruffaerts R, Lee S, et al: Mental disorders among persons with chronic back or neck pain: results from the world mental health surveys. Pain 129:332–342, 2007

Dilsaver SC, Qamar AB, Del Medico VJ: Secondary social phobia in patients with major depression. Psychiatry Res 44:33–40, 1992

Eng W, Heimberg RG, Coles ME, et al: An empirical approach to subtype identification in individuals with social phobia. Psychol Med 30:1345–1357, 2000

Fahlen T: Personality traits in social phobia, I: comparisons with healthy controls. J Clin Psychiatry 56:560–568, 1995

Faravelli C, Zucchi T, Viviani B, et al: Epidemiology of social phobia: a clinical approach. Eur Psychiatry 15:17–24, 2000

Fifer SK, Mathias SD, Patrick DL, et al: Untreated anxiety among adult primary care patients in a health maintenance organization. Arch Gen Psychiatry 51:740–750, 1994

Figueira I, Possidente E, Marques C, et al: Sexual dysfunction: a neglected complication of panic disorder and social phobia. Arch Sex Behavior 30:369–377, 2001

Francis G, Last CG, Strauss CC: Avoidant disorder and social phobia in children and adolescents. J Am Acad Child Adolesc Psychiatry 31:1086–1089, 1992

Furmark T, Tillfors M, Everz P, et al: Social phobia in the general population: prevalence and sociodemographic profile. Soc Psychiatry Psychiatr Epidemiol 34:416–424, 1999

Furmark T, Tillfors M, Stattin H, et al: Social phobia subtypes in the general population revealed by cluster analysis. Psychol Med 30:1335–1344, 2000

Furmark T, Marteinsdottir I, Heurling K, et al: Presynaptic serotonin synthesis in different social phobia subtypes assessed with PET and [11C] 5-hydroxytryptophan. Biol Psychiatry 61:50S, 2007

Fyer AJ, Mannuzza S, Chapman TF, et al: A direct interview family study of social phobia. Arch Gen Psychiatry 50:286–293, 1993

Garcia-Coll C, Kagan J, Reznick JS: Behavioral inhibition in young children. Child Dev 55:1005–1019, 1984

Goisman RM, Goldenberg I, Vasile RG, et al: Comorbidity of anxiety disorders in a multicenter anxiety study. Compr Psychiatry 36:303–311, 1995

Gorman JM, Liebowitz MR, Fyer AJ, et al: Treatment of social phobia with atenolol. J Clin Psychopharmacol 5:298–301, 1985

Grant BF, Hasin DS, Blanco C, et al: The epidemiology of social anxiety disorder in the United States: results from the national epidemiologic survey on alcohol and related conditions. J Clin Psychiatry 66:1351–1361, 2005a

Grant BF, Hasin DS, Stinson FS, et al: Co-occurrence of 12-month mood and anxiety disorders and personality disorders in the US: results from the national epidemiologic survey on alcohol and related conditions. J Psychiatr Res 39:1–9, 2005b

Gross R, Olfson M, Gameroff MJ, et al: Social anxiety disorder in primary care. Gen Hosp Psychiatry 27:161–168, 2005

Guarnaccia PJ, Rubio-Stipec M, Canino G: Ataques de nervios in the Puerto Rican Diagnostic Interview Schedule: the impact of cultural categories on psychiatric epidemiology. Cult Med Psychiatry 13:275–295, 1989

Gureje O, Lasebikan VO, Kola L, et al: Lifetime and 12-month prevalence of mental disorders in the Nigerian Survey of Mental Health and Well-Being. Br J Psychiatry 188:465–471, 2006

Harman JS, Rollman BL, Hanusa BH, et al: Physician office visits of adults for anxiety disorders in the United States, 1985–1998. J Gen Intern Med 17:165–172, 2002

Hayward C, Killen JD, Kraemer HC, et al: Linking self-reported childhood behavioral inhibition to adolescent social phobia. J Am Acad Child Adolesc Psychiatry 37:1308–1316, 1998

Heckelman LR, Schneier FR: Diagnostic issues, in Social Phobia: Diagnosis, Assessment, and Treatment. Edited by Heimberg RG, Liebowitz MR, Hope DA, et al. New York, Guilford, 1995, pp 3–20

Heimberg RG, Becker RE, Goldfinger K, et al: Treatment of social phobia by exposure, cognitive restructuring, and homework assignments. J Nerv Ment Dis 173:236–245, 1985

Heimberg RG, Hope DA, Dodge CS, et al: DSM-III-R subtypes of social phobia: comparison of generalized social phobics and public speaking phobics. J Nerv Ment Dis 178:172–179, 1990

Heimberg RG, Holt CS, Schneier FR, et al: The issue of subtypes in the diagnosis of social phobia. J Anxiety Disord 7:249–269, 1993

Heiser NA, Turner SM, Beidel DC: Shyness: relationship to social phobia and other psychiatric disorders. Behav Res Ther 41:209–221, 2003

Henderson L, Zimbardo P: Shyness, social anxiety, and social phobia, in From Social Anxiety to Social Phobia. Edited by Hofmann SG, DiBartolo PM. Boston, MA, Allyn and Bacon, 2001, pp 46–64

Herbert JD, Hope DA, Bellack AS: Validity of the distinction between generalized social phobia and avoidant personality disorder. J Abnorm Psychol 101:332–339, 1992

Hettema JM, Prescott CA, Myers JM, et al: The structure of genetic and environmental risk factors for anxiety disorders in men and women. Arch Gen Psychiatry 62:182–189, 2005

Hirshfeld-Becker DR, Biederman J, Henin A, et al: Behavioral inhibition in preschool children at risk is a specific predictor of middle childhood social anxiety: a five-year follow-up. J Dev Behav Pediatr 28:225–233, 2007

Hofmann SG, Roth WT: Issues related to social anxiety among controls in social phobia research. Behav Ther 27:79–91, 1996

Hofmann SG, Newman MG, Ehlers A, et al: Psychophysiological differences between subgroups of social phobia. J Abnorm Psychol 104:224–231, 1995

Holt CS, Heimberg RG, Hope DA: Avoidant personality disorder and the generalized subtype of social phobia. J Abnorm Psychol 101:318–325, 1992

Hook JN, Valentiner DP: Are specific and generalized social phobias qualitatively distinct? Clinical Psychology Science and Practice 9:379–395, 2002

Hope DA, Herbert JD, White C: Diagnostic subtype, avoidant personality disorder, and efficacy of cognitive-behavioral group therapy for social phobia. Cognit Ther Res 19:399–417, 1995

Hughes AA, Heimberg RG, Coles ME, et al: Relations of the factors of the tripartite model of anxiety and depression to types of social anxiety. Behav Res Ther 44:1629–1641, 2006

Hummelen B, Wilberg T, Pedersen G, et al: The relationship between avoidant personality disorder and social phobia. Compr Psychiatry 48:348–356, 2007

Hwu HG, Yeh EK, Chang LY: Prevalence of psychiatric disorders in Taiwan defined by the Chinese Diagnostic Interview Schedule. Acta Psychiatr Scand 79:136–147, 1989

James I, Savage I: Beneficial effect of nadolol on anxiety-induced disturbances of performance in musicians: a comparison with diazepam and placebo. Am Heart J 108:1150–1155, 1984

Janet P: Les Obsessions et la Psychasthenie. Paris, France, Felix Alcan, 1903

Johnson MR, Turner SM, Beidel DC, et al: Personality function, in Social Phobia: Clinical and Research Perspectives. Edited by Stein MB. Washington, DC, American Psychiatric Press, 1996, pp 77–117

Kagan J: Temperamental contributions to social behavior. Am Psychol 22:668–674, 1989

Kagan J, Reznick JS, Snidman N: The physiology and psychology of behavioral inhibition in children. Child Dev 58:1459–1473, 1987

Kagan J, Reznick JS, Snidman N: Biological bases of childhood shyness. Science 240:167–171, 1988a

Kagan J, Reznick JS, Snidman N, et al: Childhood derivatives of inhibition and lack of inhibition to the unfamiliar. Child Dev 59:1580–1589, 1988b

Kagan J, Snidman N, Arcus D: On the temperamental categories of inhibited and uninhibited children, in Social Withdrawal, Inhibition, and Shyness in Childhood. Edited by Rubin KH, Asendorpf JB. Hillsdale, NJ, Lawrence Erlbaum, 1993, pp 19–28

Kashdan TB, Frueh BC, Knapp RG, et al: Social anxiety disorder in veterans affairs primary care clinics. Behav Res Ther 44:233–247, 2006

Kaye WH, Bulik CM, Thornton L, et al: Comorbidity of anxiety disorders with anorexia and bulimia nervosa. Am J Psychiatry 161:2215–2221, 2004

Kendler KS, Neale MC, Kessler RC, et al: The genetic epidemiology of phobias in women: the interrelationship of agoraphobia, social phobia, situational phobia, and simple phobia. Arch Gen Psychiatry 49:273–281, 1992

Kessler RC, McGonagle KA, Zhao S, et al: Lifetime and 12-month prevalence of DSM-III-R psychiatric disorders in the United States: results from the National Comorbidity Survey. Arch Gen Psychiatry 51:8–19, 1994

Kessler RC, Stein MB, Berglund P: Social phobia subtypes in the National Comorbidity Survey. Am J Psychiatry 155: 613–619, 1998

Kessler RC, Stang P, Wittchen HU, et al: Lifetime comorbidities between social phobia and mood disorders in the US National Comorbidity Survey. Psychol Med 29:555–567, 1999

Kessler RC, Berglund P, Demler O, et al: Lifetime prevalence and age-of-onset distributions' of DSM-IV disorders in the national comorbidity survey replication. Arch Gen Psychiatry 62:593–602, 2005

Kleinknecht RA, Dinnel DL, Kleinknecht EE, et al: Cultural factors in social anxiety: a comparison of social phobia symptoms and taijin kyofusho. J Anxiety Disord 11:157–177, 1997

Kollman DM, Brown TA, Liverant GI, et al: A taxometric investigation of the latent structure of social anxiety disorder in outpatients with anxiety and mood disorders. Depress Anxiety 23:190–199, 2006

Kroenke K, Spitzer RL, Williams JBW, et al: Anxiety disorders in primary care: prevalence, impairment, comorbidity, and detection. Ann Intern Med 146:317–325, 2007

Lampe L, Slade T, Issakidis C, et al: Social phobia in the Australian National Survey of Mental Health and Well-Being (NSMHWB). Psychol Med 33:637–646, 2003

Landen M, Baghaei F, Rosmond R, et al: Dystipiclemia and high waist-hip ratio in women with self-reported social anxiety. Psychoneuroendocrinology 29:1037–1046, 2004

Lee S, Tsang A, Zhang MY, et al: Lifetime prevalence and inter-cohort variation in DSM-IV disorders in metropolitan China. Psychol Med 37:61–71, 2007

Lépine JP, Pelissolo A: Comorbidity and social phobia: clinical and epidemiological issues. Int Clin Psychopharmacol 11:35–41, 1996

Lépine JP, Gasquet I, Kovess V, et al: Prevalence and comorbidity of psychiatric disorders in the French general population. Encephale 31:182–194, 2005

Levin AP, Saoud JB, Strauman T, et al: Responses of "generalized" and "discrete" social phobics during public speaking. J Anxiety Disord 7:207–221, 1993

Liebowitz MR, Gorman JM, Fyer AJ, et al: Social phobia: a review of a neglected anxiety disorder. Arch Gen Psychiatry 42:729–736, 1985

Liebowitz MR, Schneier F, Campeas R, et al: Phenelzine vs. atenolol in social phobia: a placebo-controlled comparison. Arch Gen Psychiatry 49:290–300, 1992

Lincoln TM, Rief W, Hahlweg K, et al: Who comes, who stays, who profits? Predicting refusal, dropout, success, and relapse in a short intervention for social phobia. Psychother Res 15:210–225, 2005

Lindal E, Thorlacius S, Steinsson K, et al: Psychiatric disorders among subjects with systemic lupus erythematosus in an unselected population. Scand J Rheumatol 24:346–351, 1995

Ludwig R, Lazarus P: Relationship between shyness in children and constricted cognitive control as measured by the Stroop Color-Word Test. J Consult Clin Psychol 51:386–389, 1983

Magee WJ, Eaton WW, Wittchen HU, et al: Agoraphobia, simple phobia, and social phobia in the National Comorbidity Survey. Arch Gen Psychiatry 53:159–168, 1996

Magee L, Rodebaugh TL, Heimberg RG: Negative evaluation is the feared consequence of making others uncomfortable: a response to Rector, Kocovski, and Ryder. J Soc Clin Psychol 25:929–936, 2006

Mancini C, Van Ameringen M, Szatmari P, et al: A high-risk pilot study of the children of adults with social phobia. J Am Acad Child Adolesc Psychiatry 35:1511–1517, 1996

Mannuzza S, Schneier FR, Chapman TF, et al: Generalized social phobia: reliability and validity. Arch Gen Psychiatry 52:230–237, 1995

Marks IM, Gelder MG: Different ages of onset in varieties of phobias. Am J Psychiatry 123:218–221, 1966

Marteinsdottir I, Furmark T, Tillfors M, et al: Personality traits in social phobia. Eur Psychiatry 16:143–150, 2001

Massion AO, Dyck IR, Shea T, et al: Personality disorders and time to remission in generalized anxiety disorder, social phobia, and panic disorder. Arch Gen Psychiatry 59:434–440, 2002

Matsunaga H, Kiriike N, Matsui T, et al: Taijin kyofusho: a form of social anxiety disorder that responds to serotonin reuptake inhibitors. Int J Neuropsychopharmacol 4:231–237, 2001

McNally RJ, Cassiday KL, Calamari JE: Taijin-kyofu-sho in a Black American woman: behavioral treatment of a culture-bound anxiety disorder. J Anxiety Disord 4:83–87, 1990

McNeil DW, Ries BJ, Taylor LJ, et al: Comparison of social phobia subtypes using Stroop tests. J Anxiety Disord 9:47–57, 1995

Mennin DS, Heimberg RG, Jack MS: Comorbid generalized anxiety disorder in primary social phobia: symptom severity, functional impairment, and treatment response. J Anxiety Disord 14:325–343, 2000

Merikangas KR, Angst J: Comorbidity and social phobia: evidence from clinical, epidemiologic, and genetic studies. Eur Arch Psychiatry Clin Neurosci 244:297–303, 1995

Merikangas KR, Avenevoli S, Dierker L, et al: Vulnerability factors among children at risk for anxiety disorders. Biol Psychiatry 46:1523–1535, 1999

Merikangas KR, Avenevoli S, Acharyya S, et al: The spectrum of social phobia in the Zurich cohort study of young adults. Biol Psychiatry 51:81–91, 2002

Merikangas KR, Ames M, Cui L, et al: The impact of comorbidity of mental and physical conditions on role disability in the US adult household population. Arch Gen Psychiatry 64:1180–1188, 2007

Mick MA, Telch MJ: Social anxiety and history of behavioral inhibition in young adults. J Anxiety Disord 12:1–20, 1998

Middeldorp CM, Birley AJ, Cath DC, et al: Familial clustering of major depression and anxiety disorders in Australian and Dutch twins and siblings. Twin Res Hum Genet 8:609–615, 2005

Mohammadi MR, Ghanizadeh A, Mohammadi M, et al: Prevalence of social phobia and its comorbidity with psychiatric disorders in Iran. Depress Anxiety 23:405–411, 2006

Murphy HBM: Comparative Psychiatry. Berlin, Germany, Springer-Verlag, 1982

Nagata T, Oshima J, Wada A, et al: Open trial of milnacipran for taijin-kyofusho in Japanese patients with social anxiety disorder. Int J Psychiatry Clin Pract 7:107–112, 2003

Nagata T, van Vliet I, Yamada H, et al: An open trial of paroxetine for the "offensive subtype" of taijin kyofusho and social anxiety disorder. Depress Anxiety 23:168–174, 2006

Norton GR, Cox BJ, Hewitt PL, et al: Personality factors associated with generalized and non-generalized social anxiety. Pers Individ Dif 22:655–660, 1997

Okazaki S: Sources of ethnic differences between Asian American and white American college students on measures of depression and social anxiety. J Abnorm Psychol 186:52–60, 1997

Ono Y, Yoshimura K, Sueoka R, et al: Avoidant personality disorder and taijin kyoufu: social-cultural implications of the WHO/ADAMHA International Study of Personality Disorders in Japan. Acta Psychiatr Scand 93:172–176, 1996

Oosterbaan DB, van Balkom A, Spinhoven P, et al: The influence on treatment gain of comorbid avoidant personality disorder in patients with social phobia. J Nerv Ment Dis 190:41–43, 2002

Ormel J, Von Korff M, Burger H, et al: Mental disorders among persons with heart disease: results from World Mental Health Surveys. Gen Hosp Psychiatry 29:325–334, 2007

Ost LG, Hugdahl K: Acquisition of phobias and anxiety response patterns in clinical patients. Behav Res Ther 19:439–447, 1981

Ost LG, Jerremalm A, Johansson J: Individual response patterns and the effects of different behavioral methods in the treatment of social phobia. Behav Res Ther 19:1–16, 1981

Page AC, Andrews G: Do specific anxiety disorders show specific drug problems? Aust N Z J Psychiatry 30:410–414, 1996

Ralevski E, Sanislow CA, Grilo CM, et al: Avoidant personality disorder and social phobia: distinct enough to be separate disorders? Acta Psychiatr Scand 112:208–214, 2005

Ramsawh HJ, Raffa SD, Edelen MO, et al: Anxiety in middle adulthood: effects of age and time on the 14-year course of panic disorder, social phobia, and generalized anxiety disorder. Psychol Med 39:615–624, 2009

Reich JH, Yates W: Family history of psychiatric disorder in social phobia. Compr Psychiatry 29:72–75, 1988

Reich J, Warshaw M, Peterson LG, et al: Comorbidity of panic and major depressive disorder. J Psychiatr Res 27:23–33, 1993

Robins LN, Helzer JE, Croughan J, et al: National Institute of Mental Health Diagnostic Interview Schedule: its history, characteristics and validity. Arch Gen Psychiatry 38:381–389, 1981

Rosenbaum JF, Biederman J, Hirshfeld DR, et al: Further evidence of an association between behavioral inhibition and anxiety disorders: results from a family study of children from a non-clinical sample. J Psychiatr Res 25:49–65, 1991

Rosenbaum JF, Biederman J, Bolduc EA, et al: Comorbidity of parental anxiety disorders as risk for childhood-onset anxiety in inhibited children. Am J Psychiatry 149:475–481, 1992

Ruscio AM, Brown TA, Chiu WT, et al: Social fears and social phobia in the USA: results from the National Comorbidity Survey Replication. Psychol Med 38:15–28, 2008

Safren SA, Heimberg RG, Brown EJ, et al: Quality of life in social phobia. Depress Anxiety 4:126–133, 1996–1997

Sareen J, Cox BJ, Afifi TO, et al: Anxiety disorders and risk for suicidal ideation and suicide attempts: a population-based longitudinal study of adults. Arch Gen Psychiatry 62:1249–1257, 2005a

Sareen J, Cox BJ, Clara I, et al: The relationship between anxiety disorders and physical disorders in the US National Comorbidity Survey. Depress Anxiety 21:193–202, 2005b

Sareen J, Jacobi F, Cox BJ, et al: Disability and poor quality of life associated with comorbid anxiety disorders and physical conditions. Arch Intern Med 166:2109–2116, 2006

Scheibe G, Albus M: Age at onset, precipitating events, sex distribution, and co-occurrence of anxiety disorders. Psychopathology 25:11–18, 1992

Schneier FR, Spitzer RL, Gibbon M, et al: The relationship of social phobia subtypes and avoidant personality disorder. Compr Psychiatry 32:496–502, 1991

Schneier FR, Johnson J, Hornig CD, et al: Social phobia: comorbidity and morbidity in an epidemiologic sample. Arch Gen Psychiatry 49:282–288, 1992

Schneier FR, Heckelman LR, Garfinkel R, et al: Functional impairment in social phobia. J Clin Psychiatry 55:322–329, 1994

Schonfeld WH, Verboncoeur CJ, Fifer SK, et al: The functioning and well-being of patients with unrecognized anxiety disorders and major depressive disorder. J Affect Disord 43:105–119, 1997

Schwartz CE, Snidman N, Kagan J: Adolescent social anxiety as an outcome of inhibited temperament in childhood. J Am Acad Child Adolesc Psychiatry 38:1008–1016, 1999

Schwartz CE, Wright CI, Shin LM, et al: Inhibited and uninhibited infants "grown up": adult amygdalar response to novelty. Science 300:1952–1953, 2003

Sherbourne CD, Jackson CA, Meredith LS, et al: Prevalence of comorbid anxiety disorders in primary care outpatients. Arch Fam Med 5:27–34, 1996

Simon NM, Otto MW, Korbly NB, et al: Quality of life in social anxiety disorder compared with panic disorder and the general population. Psychiatr Serv 53:714–718, 2002

St. Lorant T, Henderson L, Zimbardo PG: Comorbidity in chronic shyness. Depress Anxiety 12:232–237, 2000

Stein MB, Kean Y: Disability and quality of life in social phobia. Am J Psychiatry 157:1606–1613, 2000

Stein MB, Shea CA, Uhde TW: Social phobic symptoms in patients with panic disorder: practical and theoretical implications. Am J Psychiatry 146:235–238, 1989

Stein MB, Heuser IJ, Juncos JL, et al: Anxiety disorders in patients with Parkinson's disease. Am J Psychiatry 147:217–220, 1990

Stein MB, Chartier MJ, Hazen AL, et al: A direct-interview family study of generalized social phobia. Am J Psychiatry 155:90–97, 1998

Stein MB, McQuaid JR, Laffaye C, et al: Social phobia in the primary care medical setting. J Fam Pract 48:514–519, 1999

Stein MB, Torgrud LJ, Walker JR: Social phobia symptoms, subtypes, and severity: findings from a community survey. Arch Gen Psychiatry 57:1046–1052, 2000

Stein MB, Fuetsch M, Muller N, et al: Social anxiety disorder and the risk of depression: a prospective community study of adolescents and young adults. Arch Gen Psychiatry 58:251–256, 2001

Stein MB, Sherbourne CD, Craske MG, et al: Quality of care for primary care patients with anxiety disorders. Am J Psychiatry 161:2230–2237, 2004

Stein MB, Roy-Byrne PP, Craske MG, et al: Functional impact and health utility of anxiety disorders in primary care outpatients. Med Care 43:1164–1170, 2005

Stemberger RT, Turner SM, Beidel DC, et al: Social phobia: an analysis of possible developmental factors. J Abnorm Psychol 104:526–531, 1995

Suzuki K, Takei N, Kawai M, et al: Is taijin kyofusho a culture-bound syndrome? Am J Psychiatry 160:1358, 2003

Tillfors M, Furmark T: Social phobia in Swedish university students: prevalence, subgroups and avoidant behavior. Soc Psychiatry Psychiatr Epidemiol 42:79–86, 2007

Tillfors M, Furmark T, Ekselius L, et al: Social phobia and avoidant personality disorder as related to parental history of social anxiety: a general population study. Behav Res Ther 39:289–298, 2001

Tillfors M, Furmark T, Ekselius L, et al: Social phobia and avoidant personality disorder: one spectrum disorder? Nord J Psychiatry 58:147–152, 2004

Tran GQ, Chambless DL: Psychopathology of social phobia: effects of subtype and of avoidant personality disorder. J Anxiety Disord 9:489–501, 1995

Turk CL, Heimberg RG, Orsillo SM, et al: An investigation of gender differences in social phobia. J Anxiety Disord 12:209–223, 1998

Turner SM, Beidel DC, Townsley RM: Social phobia: relationship to shyness. Behav Res Ther 28:297–305, 1990

Turner SM, Beidel DC, Borden JW, et al: Social phobia: Axis I and II correlates. J Abnorm Psychol 100:102–106, 1991

Turner SM, Beidel DC, Townsley RM: Social phobia: a comparison of specific and generalized subtypes and avoidant personality disorder. J Abnorm Psychol 101:326–331, 1992

Turner SM, Beidel DC, Jacob RG: Social phobia: a comparison of behavior therapy and atenolol. J Consult Clin Psychol 62:350–358, 1994

Van Ameringen M, Mancini C, Styan G, et al: Relationship of social phobia with other psychiatric illness. J Affect Disord 21:93–99, 1991

Van Ameringen M, Mancini C, Farvolden P: The impact of anxiety disorders on educational achievement. J Anxiety Disord 17:561–571, 2003

van Velzen CJM, Emmelkamp PMJ, Scholing A: The impact of personality disorders on behavioral treatment outcome for social phobia. Behav Res Ther 35:889–900, 1997

van Velzen CJM, Emmelkamp PMJ, Scholing A: Generalized social phobia versus avoidant personality disorder: differences in psychopathology, personality traits, and social and occupational functioning. J Anxiety Disord 14: 395–411, 2000

Vriends N, Becker ES, Meyer A, et al: Recovery from social phobia in the community and its predictors: data from a longitudinal epidemiological study. J Anxiety Disord 21:320–337, 2007a

Vriends N, Becker ES, Meyer A, et al: Subtypes of social phobia: are they of any use? J Anxiety Disord 21:59–75, 2007b

Wacker HR, Mullegans R, Klein KH, et al: Identification of cases of anxiety disorders and affective disorders in the community according to ICD-10 and DSM-III-R by using the Composite International Diagnostic Interview (CIDI). Int J Methods Psychiatr Res 2:91–100, 1992

Warren SL, Schmitz S, Emde RN: Behavioral genetic analyses of self-reported anxiety at 7 years of age. J Am Acad Child Adolesc Psychiatry 38:1403–1408, 1999

Weiller E, Bisserbe JC, Boyer P, et al: Social phobia in general health care: an unrecognized undertreated disabling disorder. Br J Psychiatry 168:169–174, 1996

Weisberg RB, Dyck I, Culpepper L, et al: Psychiatric treatment in primary care patients with anxiety disorders: a comparison of care received from primary care providers and psychiatrists. Am J Psychiatry 164:276–282, 2007

Wells JC, Tien AY, Garrison R, et al: Risk factors for the incidence of social phobia as determined by the Diagnostic Interview Schedule in a population-based study. Acta Psychiatr Scand 90:84–90, 1994

Wittchen HU, Stein MB, Kessler RC: Social fears and social phobia in a community sample of adolescents and young adults: prevalence, risk factors and co-morbidity. Psychol Med 29:309–323, 1999

World Health Organization: The Composite International Diagnostic Interview (CIDI). Geneva, Switzerland, World Health Organization, 1990

Yonkers KA, Dyck IR, Keller MB: An eight-year longitudinal comparison of clinical course and characteristics of social phobia among men and women. Psychiatr Serv 52:637–643, 2001

Yonkers KA, Bruce SE, Dyck IR, et al: Chronicity, relapse, and illness: course of panic disorder, social phobia, and generalized anxiety disorder: findings in men and women from 8 years of follow-up. Depress Anxiety 17:173–179, 2003

Young AS, Klap R, Sherbourne CD, et al: The quality of care for depressive and anxiety disorders in the United States. Arch Gen Psychiatry 58:55–61, 2001

Zimbardo PG: Shyness: What It Is, What to Do About It. Reading, MA, Addison-Wesley, 1977

Recommended Readings

Bandelow B, Stein DJ: Social Anxiety Disorder. New York, Marcel Dekker, 2004

Beidel DC, Turner SM: Shy Children, Phobic Adults: Nature and Treatment of Social Anxiety. Washington, DC, American Psychological Association, 2007

Keller MB: Social anxiety disorder clinical course and outcome: review of Harvard/Brown Anxiety Research Project (HARP) findings. J Clin Psychiatry 67(suppl):14–19, 2006

Mathew SJ, Coplan JD, Gorman JM: Neurobiological mechanisms of social anxiety disorder. Am J Psychiatry 158:1558–1567, 2001

Rapee RM, Heimberg RG: A cognitive-behavioral model of anxiety in social phobia. Behav Res Ther 35:741–756, 1997

Schmidt LA, Schulkin J: Extreme Fear, Shyness and Social Phobia: Origins, Biological Mechanisms, and Clinical Outcomes. New York, Oxford University Press, 1999

Stein MB: An epidemiologic perspective on social anxiety disorder. J Clin Psychiatry 67(suppl):3–8, 2006

Chapter 26

Pathogenesis of Social Anxiety Disorder

Mary Morreale, M.D.
Manuel E. Tancer, M.D.
Thomas W. Uhde, M.D.

As with other psychiatric disorders, the pathogenesis of social phobia (social anxiety disorder) is not fully understood. Nevertheless, over the past decade there has been an explosion of research devoted to delineating the pathophysiology of social fears, social anxiety, and social phobia. In this chapter, we summarize available research and outline future directions for the field.

Part of what has made understanding the pathogenesis of social phobia difficult is the heterogeneity of the populations that have been studied. Many studies have been conducted in undergraduate psychology students, who score above or below the median split on a given psychometric instrument. Other studies have involved community samples that have not received treatment for an anxiety problem. A third study population has been treatment-seeking individuals, who probably differ in important ways from community samples. In addition to the heterogeneity of the populations studied, another obstacle is the likelihood that multiple pathways lead to the clinical manifestation of social phobia. It is unlikely that a single gene, neurobiological abnormality, or difference in environmental condition will explain all cases. Instead, social phobia is likely the result of complex interactions among inherited traits, environment, temperament, personal experience, and neurobiological vulnerability.

The relationships among social fears, social anxiety, and social phobia have not been precisely defined, and this complicates the review and integration of existing studies. For example, "social anxiety" is a widely used psychological construct and is the focus of many reports in the literature. These reports, as noted above, often describe undergraduates who score high or low on a median split of a particular rating scale. "Shyness" is another psychological construct. Research indicates that among "shy" individuals, 53% of women and 40% of men develop a lifetime diagnosis of an anxiety disorder, the most prominent being social phobia. Thus, more than half of those who perceive themselves as shy do not go on to meet criteria for any anxiety disorder. In this chapter, the term *social phobia* is used to refer to individuals meeting DSM-IV-TR (American Psychiatric Association 2000) criteria. The terms *social fears, social anxiety*, and *shy* are used to describe nonclinical, subclinical, or analog populations. The following material will focus on biological and psychological factors that contribute to the development of social phobia.

Biological Factors

A wide range of neurobiological measures have been examined in patients with social phobia. Brain systems implicated in social phobia include the noradrenergic (M.B. Stein et al. 1992; Tancer et al. 1993a, but see Tancer et al. 1994/1995a), dopaminergic (Liebowitz et al. 1987, but see Tancer et al. 1994/1995a), glutamatergic (Phan et al. 2005), and serotonergic (Tancer et al. 1994/1995a) systems; gamma-aminobutyric acid (GABA) (Condren 2003); and activity of the peptide neurotransmitter substance P (Furmark et al. 2005).

For the sake of clarity, this section is subdivided into sections on genetics, family and twin studies, chemical challenge paradigms, peripheral markers, psychoneuroendocrine assessments, immunological studies, neuroimaging studies, electroencephalography, sleep studies, and autonomic reactivity assessments. The neurobiology of social phobia has been reviewed by Miner and Davidson (1995) and Tancer et al. (1995). In this section, we briefly refer to earlier studies but focus mostly on data reported since those reviews.

Genetics

Available data suggest a heritable contribution to social phobia. Several large direct-interview family studies with social phobia probands have been reported. Fyer et al. (1993) compared the rates of social phobia in 83 first-degree relatives of 30 probands with social phobia and no other lifetime anxiety disorder diagnosis, with rates of social phobia in 231 first-degree relatives of 77 probands with no lifetime mental disorder diagnosis. They reported that 16% of the relatives of the probands with social phobia met diagnostic criteria for social phobia, compared with 5% of the relatives of the control probands (relative risk=3.12, *P*<0.005). In another investigation, M.B. Stein et al. (1998) reported on a direct-interview family study with two important methodological differences. First, to be included, the probands with social phobia had to have the generalized subtype of social phobia. Second, the inclusion criteria allowed for comorbid anxiety disorder in the probands with social phobia and allowed for lifetime mental illness diagnosis, with the exception of social phobia, in the control probands. The investigators compared 106 first-degree relatives of 23 probands with social phobia and 74 relatives of 24 probands without social phobia. Generalized social phobia was found in 26.4% of the relatives of the probands with social phobia, compared with 2.7% of the relatives of the probands without social phobia (relative risk=9.7, 95% confidence interval 2.5–38.1). Interestingly, the rate of performance-only social phobia was similar in the relatives of the probands with generalized social phobia and in the relatives of the probands without social phobia (14.2% vs. 14.9%). This suggests that generalized, but not discrete, social phobia runs in families. Similarly, studies by both Biederman et al. (2006) and Cooper et al. (2006) have found evidence of intergenerational specificity for social phobia and separation anxiety, but not for other anxiety disorders.

Although family studies can determine whether disorders aggregate in families at a rate greater than would occur by chance alone, they cannot separate genetic from environmental contributions. Twin and adoption studies can, however, help investigators make this distinction. Two early twin studies examined the heritability of DSM-III-R (American Psychiatric Association 1987) anxiety disorders and reached different conclusions regarding social phobia. Kendler et al. (1992) examined data from 2,163 directly-interviewed female twins. They concluded that 30%–40% of the development of social phobia is genetic and the remainder is caused by individual-specific environmental experiences. In the examination of 20 monozygotic and 29 dizygotic twin pairs with a variety of anxiety diagnoses versus 12 monozygotic and 20 dizygotic twin pairs with other nonpsychotic mental disorders, Skre et al. (1993) reported no difference between social phobia concordance rates in monozygotic and dizygotic twin pairs. In a study of subclinical social fears, Skre et al. (2000) discovered a heritability of 47%. More recently, Ogliari et al. (2006) examined 378 twin pairs, ages 8–17 years, using a questionnaire based on DSM-IV (American Psychiatric Association 1994) nosology. An approximate heritability of 60% was discovered in social phobia, which is higher than the rates elucidated in other studies. No shared environmental influences emerged; however, the authors questioned the statistical significance of this finding in light of results from the previously mentioned studies. They concluded that shared environmental factors seem to have a "marginally" causal role. Taken together, these twin studies suggest that although social phobia itself is not inherited, susceptibility to the disorder may be. Given the diverse findings reported across these studies, however, it is clear that additional research is needed.

Only one genetic linkage study specifically examining social phobia has been published. In 2004, Gelernter et al. tested 163 subjects, all of them relatives of individuals diagnosed with panic disorder. From this genome-wide scan, a "suggestive" linkage was identified between the norepinephrine transporter protein (SLC6A2) and social phobia risk.

A range of association studies have focused on specific genes. Two studies have examined the association of catechol-*O*-methyltransferase (COMT) polymorphisms in patients with social phobia. Because prefrontal dopamine levels have been associated with the etiology and expression of anxiety, COMT, which catalyzes the degradation of dopamine, is an important enzyme to evaluate. Lachman et al. (1996) elucidated a functional polymorphism in the COMT gene (Met allele) that has decreased activity. The alternate high-activity Val allele increases dopamine catabolism, therefore theoretically increasing anxiety symptoms. McGrath et al. (2004) examined 1,234 women, genotyping them for the Val allele polymorphism and evaluating phobic symptoms using the Crown-Crisp Experimental Index. Although their study did not specifically target a diagnosis of social phobia, results suggest that the Val/Val allele genotype was associated with an increased risk of phobic anxiety. These results were not replicated in a Japanese study that found increased Met allele in patients with panic disorder, which McGrath and associates attributed to ethnic differences (Ohara et al. 1998). McGrath and associates suggested that estrogen's inhibition of COMT transcription might have a role in the increased incidence of anxiety disorders in women. Another study focusing on COMT polymorphisms examined monoamine oxidase A (MAO-A) and 5-hydroxytryptamine (5-HTT) gene polymorphisms as well. Samochowiec et al. (2004) examined 101 patients with various phobic spectrum disorders. They found no significant differences in the allele and genotype frequencies of the COMT and 5-HTT polymorphisms between phobic subjects and 202 psychiatrically healthy control subjects. Although they did find an association between an MAO-A polymorphism leading to a more active enzyme in females with generalized anxiety disorder and specific phobia, they did not find a role for this polymorphism in females with social phobia. In summary, there is no significant association between social phobia and this functional singular nucleotide polymorphism in the COMT gene.

Kennedy et al. (2001) examined 26 patients who met DSM-IV criteria for either generalized or specific social phobia, 13 with generalized social phobia, and 37 with avoidant personality disorder (which the authors believe has overlap with generalized social phobia). The authors studied polymorphisms in the dopamine D_2, D_3, and D_4 receptor genes, as well as the dopamine transporter gene. Their results indicated a lack of major effect for each of the four dopamine gene markers under the broad diagnosis of social phobia. Major effect does not, however, rule out a contribution to the development of social phobia. Rowe et al. (1998) did find a relationship between the dopamine transporter gene and symptoms of internalizing disorders in children, including, but not specific to, social phobia.

Lochner et al. (2007) examined 63 patients with a DSM-IV diagnosis of generalized social phobia. The subjects' DNA was genotyped to evaluate components of serotonergic and dopaminergic pathways. The authors found a possible role for the T-containing genotypes of the 5-HT_{2A} T102C polymorphism in the development of social phobia. The function of T102C may lead to increased expression of 5-HT_{2A}. These results would be consistent with other studies linking serotonergic involvement in social phobia. In a study by M.B. Stein et al. (1998), however, a connection between social phobia and 5-HT_{2A} was not elucidated.

In a study discussed in more depth in the section of this chapter on neuroimaging, Furmark et al. (2004) genotyped 17 subjects with social phobia for a 5-HTT promoter polymorphism. The short variant of the allele, which is associated with less serotonin transporter expression and reduced uptake, has been associated with anxiety in many, but not all, studies. Subjects in this study were asked to complete an anxiogenic public speaking task while undergoing positron emission tomography (PET) scans. Trait anxiety, state anxiety, and depression were increased in subjects who had the short variant of the allele, which also predicted increased amygdalar activation. Similar data from Hariri et al. (2002) found increased amygdalar response to angry or fearful faces in carriers of the S allele. Schultz et al. (2005) examined the same polymorphism in 64 community-dwelling adults over age 55 years. Their results indicated a nonsignificant trend toward possession of the short variant of the allele and phobic anxiety. Not all studies, however, have confirmed an association between the S allele and anxiety traits, and attempts to link this polymorphism specifically to social phobia have failed.

Smoller et al. (2003, 2005) found an association between single nucleotide polymorphisms in the corticotropin-releasing factor gene in children with behavioral inhibition, a condition that will be discussed later as a potential etiological precursor to social phobia.

In summary, there have been multiple studies related to genetic vulnerabilities associated with social phobia. Although no single gene appears responsible for the etiology of social phobia, multiple genetic variants might contribute partially to its development

Neurochemistry

Challenge Paradigms

A variety of chemical challenge studies have been conducted in patients with social phobia. In the earliest studies, investigators found that epinephrine challenge was unable to replicate social phobia symptoms (Papp et al. 1988), lactate challenge was unable to induce panic attacks in individuals with social phobia (Liebowitz et al. 1985), and caffeine was able to cause panic attacks in approximately 25% of the patients with social phobia, but the anxiety it produced was quite different from their spontaneous social anxiety (Tancer et al. 1994/1995b).

McCann et al. (1997) combined an intravenous pentagastrin challenge with a social interaction task in patients with social phobia, patients with panic disorder, and psychiatrically healthy volunteers. Pentagastrin, an analog of cholecystokinin tetrapeptide, has been found to provoke panic attacks in patients with panic disorder and in patients without panic disorder, in a dose-dependent fashion (Abelson and Nesse 1994; van Megen et al. 1994). McCann and associates found that the social interaction test plus placebo infusion was anxiogenic in both anxiety groups and in the volunteers, whereas the social interaction test plus intravenous pentagastrin (0.6 mg/kg over 60 seconds) caused panic attacks in 47% (8 of 17) of the patients with social phobia, 64% (7 of 11) of the patients with panic disorder, and 11% (2 of 19) of the psychiatrically healthy control subjects. Interestingly, in the context of a social interaction test, neither the patients with social phobia nor the patients with panic disorder described the panic attacks as similar to their naturally occurring symptoms. The authors concluded that the ability of pentagastrin to induce panic attacks in both patients with social phobia and patients with panic disorder at rates greater than in psychiatrically healthy volunteers is evidence of a "shared neurobiological substrate" between the two anxiety disorders.

Van Vliet et al. (1997) reported a second pentagastrin challenge study in seven patients meeting DSM-IV criteria for social phobia versus seven psychiatrically healthy control subjects. Under double-blind conditions, subjects underwent two infusions. Unlike in the McCann et al. (1997) study, no social interaction test was given. Van Vliet's group also administered pentagastrin (0.6 mg/kg) over the course of 10 seconds instead of 60 seconds. Five of the seven (71%) patients with social phobia, compared with two of the seven (29%) control subjects, met strict criteria for a panic attack following pentagastrin administration. No subject had a panic attack following the placebo administration. As in the McCann report, patients with social phobia in the van Vliet group described the panic attacks caused by pentagastrin as different from their typical phobic anxiety. These two studies represent the only concordant replication studies in social phobia, but the fact that the induced panic was different from the patients' typical anxiety symptoms suggests that pentagastrin fails a required component of an ideal chemical challenge (symptom convergence, specificity, clinical validation, and replicability) (Gorman et al. 1987; Guttmacher et al. 1983; Uhde and Tancer 1989).

Inhalation of various concentrations of carbon dioxide (CO_2) has been used to induce anxiety (Gorman et al. 1990; Holt and Andrews 1989b). Gorman et al. (1990) reported that 35% CO_2, administered as a "double-breath," induced panic attacks in patients with social phobia at a rate greater than room air inhalation. In contrast, psychiatrically healthy volunteers had no increased rate of panic following CO_2 administration compared with room air inhalation. Caldirola et al. (1997) conducted a study in which patients with social phobia, patients with panic disorder, and psychiatrically healthy volunteers inhaled one vital capacity of 35% CO_2 and 65% O_2, or compressed air. Both patients with social phobia and patients with panic disorder had greater anxiogenic responses to CO_2 than to compressed air, and both reported greater distress than volunteers.

Room air hyperventilation also has been used as a mechanism to induce symptoms of anxiety (Holt and Andrews 1989a; Maddock and Carter 1991; Spinhoven et al. 1992). Holt and Andrews (1989a) reported that patients with panic disorder and/or agoraphobia had higher symptom ratings following room air hyperventilation when compared with patients with social phobia or generalized anxiety disorder. The latter populations had more symptoms when compared with psychiatrically healthy volunteers. Interestingly, the patient groups did not differ in end-expiratory pCO_2 levels. Finally, Asmundson and Stein (1994) examined the physiological and anxiogenic effects of respiratory manipulations in 15 patients with social phobia compared with 15 patients with panic disorder and 15 psychiatrically healthy control subjects. As in the study by Holt and Andrews (1989a), there were no group differences in the physiological response to hypoventilation, normoventilation, or hyperventilation. Two (13%) of the 15 patients with social phobia, 2 (13%) of the 15 patients with panic disorder, and none of the volunteers experienced a panic attack during hyperventilation.

Tancer et al. (1994/1995a) reported an exaggerated cortisol response and a trend toward increased prolactin levels in the patient group following a *d,l*-fenfluramine (5-HT releasing agent) challenge in 21 patients with generalized social phobia and 22 psychiatrically healthy volunteers. Supporting Tancer's work, Hollander et al. (1998) challenged 18 patients with generalized social phobia with the serotonergic probe *m*-chlorophenylpiperazine (m-CPP). The authors observed a normal prolactin response and increased cortisol levels, which were particularly robust in the female cohort. More recently, Shlik et al. (2004) administered citalopram (20 mg intravenously over 30 minutes) to 18 patients diagnosed with generalized social phobia and 18 psychiatrically healthy control subjects. Although the citalopram challenge led to increased prolactin and cortisol levels, there were no significant differences in levels between patients and control subjects. The authors concluded that patients with social phobia did not have major alterations in 5-HT receptor function. Interestingly, the authors did suggest that the increase in headaches experienced in patients with social phobia could be secondary to hypersensitivity of some subtypes of 5-HT.

Tancer et al. (1994/1995a) did not find abnormalities of dopaminergic function after challenging patients with social phobia with an L-dopa probe but suggested that more selective dopamine probes may be needed to detect dysfunction.

Tancer et al. (1993b) observed a reduced growth hormone response after administration of intravenous, but not oral, clonidine in patients diagnosed with social phobia. A blunted growth hormone response to clonidine has also been observed in patients with panic disorder, with generalized anxiety disorder, and with major depressive disorder. This finding may indicate reduced postsynaptic α_2-adrenergic receptor function secondary to norepinephrine hyperactivity.

Condren et al. (2003) administered baclofen injections ($GABA_B$ receptor agonist) to assess GABA abnormalities in patients with social phobia. The authors compared 15 patients with generalized social phobia with 15 psychiatrically healthy control subjects. Results showed a blunted growth hormone response in patients with social phobia. The authors concluded that subsensitive hypothalamic $GABA_B$ receptors may be involved in the development of this disorder.

In summary, a variety of anxiogenic stimuli have been used in patients with social phobia. To date, none of the symptoms provoked are similar to the individual's typical phobic symptomatology. The fact that patients with social phobia appear to be more sensitive than psychiatrically healthy volunteers to the anxiogenic effects of pentagastrin, CO_2 inhalation, or hyperventilation may be a function of basal arousal rather than a specific clue to the etiology of social phobia. Challenge studies examining neurotransmitter and hormonal differences must be replicated before solid conclusions can be drawn.

Peripheral Markers

Another commonly used research procedure involves measuring receptor density, and/or affinities on platelets and/or lymphocytes, as surrogate markers of central neurotransmitter activity.

M.B. Stein and his collaborators examined a variety of peripheral markers and found no evidence of peripheral abnormalities in patients with generalized social phobia. Specifically, M.B. Stein et al. (1993a) reported no differences in lymphocyte β-receptor density or binding affinity in 17 patients with generalized social phobia compared with 17 age- and sex-matched psychiatrically healthy volunteers when iodinated pindolol was used as the ligand. M.B. Stein et al. (1995) examined platelet serotonin transporter capacity by using [^{3}H] paroxetine binding in 18 patients with generalized social phobia compared with 15 patients with panic disorder and 23 psychiatrically healthy volunteers. The patient groups were medication-free. The density and binding affinity of the serotonin transporter did not differ between groups. More recently, Barkan et al. (2006) measured the activity of the serotonin transporter (5-HTT) via the uptake of [^{3}H]5-HT to blood lymphocytes in 15 unmedicated patients diagnosed with generalized social phobia versus 18 psychiatrically healthy control subjects. The authors discovered no differences in maximum uptake velocity and similar affinities between the two groups, indicating that the function of lymphocyte 5-HTT is not dysfunctional in patients with social phobia. Laufer et al. (2005) assessed platelet vesicular monoamine transporter density in 20 unmedicated patients diagnosed with generalized social phobia versus 15 psychiatrically healthy control subjects. This transporter is important in the storage and release of monoamines, and untreated depressed patients have been found to have increased densities. Their study showed no differences in platelet VMAT2 density between patients and control subjects. Given the findings of no abnormalities in VMAT2 and the information elucidated in the two aforementioned studies examining the serotonin transporter, Laufer concluded that a presynaptic dysfunction in social phobia seems unlikely.

Johnson et al. (1998) examined the density of peripheral benzodiazepine receptors in the platelets of patients with generalized social phobia. Low peripheral benzodiazepine receptor densities have been reported previously in patients with panic disorder, posttraumatic stress disorder, and generalized anxiety disorder, but not in patients with obsessive-compulsive disorder or major depressive disorder. A group of 53 patients with generalized social phobia were compared with another group of 53 psychiatrically healthy volunteers. The mean receptor density in the generalized social phobia group was 2,744±1,242 fmol/mg protein, compared with 4,327±1,850 fmol/mg protein in the control subjects.

Possible abnormalities in signal transduction and/or second messenger systems have been examined by quantifying G-protein subunit levels from platelets and leukocytes in 10 untreated patients with social phobia, 13 untreated patients with panic disorder, and 12 psychiatrically healthy subjects (M.B. Stein et al. 1996). None of the G-protein subunit levels examined differed across the three groups.

In summary, platelet benzodiazepine receptor density is the only peripheral marker study that has differentiated patients with social phobia from control subjects. Unfortunately, these results should be considered preliminary, given that no replication studies are available.

Neuroendocrinology

Stress of any etiology hypothetically results in hypothalamic-pituitary-adrenal (HPA) activation and subsequent increases in cortisol. Conflicting data have emerged regarding HPA axis excitability in social phobia. Uhde et al. (1994) studied 54 patients with social phobia and found that mean urinary cortisol levels over 3 days did not differ from those of 16 psychiatrically healthy control subjects. Potts et al. (1991) reported similar results. Using a subtler marker of HPA axis dysfunction, the dexamethasone suppression test, Uhde's group discovered neither differing levels of cortisol nor differing rates of cortisol nonsuppression in patients with social phobia versus psychiatrically healthy control subjects. Martel et al. (1999) found no differences in measured salivary cortisol levels between adolescent girls with social phobia and control subjects after an anxiogenic task. The results of all four studies imply a lack of global HPA axis dysfunction in patients with social phobia.

Contradicting these findings, children with behavioral inhibition, a proposed precursor to social phobia, have been found to have elevated cortisol levels. Granger et al. (1994) discovered an increase in cortisol levels in socially anxious children in response to a parent-child conflict task. More recently, Condren et al. (2003) evaluated 15 patients with generalized social phobia and 15 psychiatrically healthy control subjects before and after a mental arithmetic and short-term memory task performed in front of an audience. Baseline cortisol levels did not differ between groups, but the anxiogenic task did result in a significantly increased cortisol response in the subjects with social phobia. As noted previously, cortisol levels did increase with serotonin-based chemical challenges in patients with social phobia.

To complicate matters even further, Levin et al. (1993) discovered a decrease in cortisol levels in both subjects with social phobia and control subjects after a public speaking task. Clearly, the data show that large studies must be conducted in which the connection between social phobia and cortisol response is evaluated.

Tancer et al. (1990) conducted a TSH (thyrotropin-stimulating hormone) test in 13 patients with social phobia and 22 psychiatrically healthy control subjects. No significant differences between patients and control subjects were found in plasma T_3, T_4, free T_4, TSH, and antithyroid antibody levels. The authors concluded that hypothalamic-pituitary-thyroid dysfunction is not a requisite neuroendocrine correlate of social phobia.

In summary, no clear differences have emerged regarding psychoneuroendocrine data in social phobia.

Immunology

There are limited data reflecting the relationship between immunological dysfunction and social phobia. Following up on reports of psychoneuroimmunological abnormalities in depression and schizophrenia, Rapaport and Stein (1994) examined serum levels of interleukin-2 (an immune modulator) and soluble interleukin-2 receptor levels (a marker of T-cell activation) in 15 patients with generalized social phobia and 15 psychiatrically healthy volunteers. The groups had similar mean interleukin-2 and soluble interleukin-2 receptor levels. Covelli et al. (2005) found deficits in phagocytosis and killing exerted by polymononuclear cells and monocytes in subjects with phobic disorders. The investigators also discovered an increased release of interleukin-1*B* in subjects with phobia. Further studies are necessary to elucidate details related to immune function in patients with social phobia.

Brain Imaging

Structure

Potts et al. (1994) conducted a volumetric magnetic resonance imaging study in 22 patients with social phobia compared with 22 age- and sex-matched volunteers. No differences in caudate, putamen, thalamus, or cerebral volumes were found between the groups. The investigators did report an age-dependent reduction in putamen volumes only in the patients with social phobia; the volume change was not correlated with illness severity. There have been no replications of this study.

Functional Activity

M.B. Stein and Leslie (1996) evaluated regional cerebral blood flow (rCBF) patterns with technetium-99m hexamethylpropyleneamine oxime (HMPAO) single-photon emission computed tomography (SPECT) in 11 patients with social phobia and 11 psychiatrically healthy volunteers and reported no group differences.

Van der Linden et al. (2000) examined rCBF in 15 patients with social phobia using HMPAO SPECT before and after treatment with the selective serotonin reuptake inhibitor (SSRI) citalopram. Treatment led to blood flow reductions (from baseline) in the anterior and lateral parts of the left temporal cortex; the anterior, lateral, and posterior parts of the left midfrontal cortex; and the left cingulum. Unfortunately, there was no psychiatrically healthy comparison group in the study.

Additional PET studies have been published. Nutt et al. (1998) measured rCBF using the oxygen 15-H_2O PET method. They found that social anxiety induced by exposure in imagination to autobiographical data resulted in increased blood flow in the left superior anterior cingulate, medial frontal cortex, and parietal cortex and decreased blood flow in the temporal-occipital cortex, temporal pole, pons, and left amygdala. Tillfors et al. (2001) compared 18 subjects with social phobia with 6 psychiatrically healthy control subjects. Utilizing PET, the group measured rCBF while both groups spoke privately and then in front of a group. Increased anxiety experienced by subjects with social phobia was associated with increased blood flow in the amygdala. Patients with social phobia were found to have decreased flow in the orbitofrontal and insular cortices, as well as the temporal pole. Additionally, subjects with social phobia had a diminished increase in flow in the parietal and secondary visual cortices when compared with control subjects. The authors concluded that the pattern of increased subcortical activation in subjects with social phobia, compared with the increased cortical activation in psychiatrically healthy control subjects, indicated that those with social phobia were activating a "phylogenetically older danger-recognition system."

As mentioned in the section on genetic contributions to social phobia, Furmark et al.'s (2004) study of subjects with social phobia reported no difference in amygdala rCBF between long and short allele subjects at baseline, but right amygdala activation did increase in short allele subjects during an anxiogenic task. In a later study, Furmark et al. (2005) treated 36 patients with social phobia with the neurokinin-1 antagonist GR205171, citalopram, or placebo and evaluated cerebral blood flow via PET during an anxiogenic public speaking task. Results indicated that patients improved with both treatments, compared with subjects in the placebo group, and that this improvement was paralleled by a significantly reduced rCBF response to public speaking in the rhinal cortex, amygdala, and parahippocampal-hippocampal regions. Interestingly, in a previous study utilizing similar methodology, Furmark et al. (2002) discovered that cognitive-behavioral therapy was roughly equal to citalopram in symptom reduction and rCBF changes.

There have been multiple new studies utilizing functional magnetic resonance imaging (fMRI) in individuals with social phobia. The majority of these studies evaluate brain response to different facial expressions. These studies will be discussed chronologically. Amir et al. (2005) compared 11 subjects with generalized social phobia with 11 psychiatrically healthy control subjects. Participants viewed disgust and neutral faces and were rated on reaction time to facial expression and perception of emotional valence. Subjects with social phobia were found to have a significant increase in right anterior cingulate activity when processing disgust versus neutral faces. Although there were no differences in ratings related to the emotional valence of negative facial expressions, subjects with social phobia did rate disgust faces more quickly. The authors suggested that subjects with social phobia have difficulties inhibiting negative emotional responses.

Straube et al. (2004) exposed 10 subjects with social phobia and 10 psychiatrically healthy control subjects to photographic and schematic faces with either angry or neutral expressions. Subjects were asked to determine whether the face was a photograph or schematic drawing (the implicit task) and which emotion was depicted (the explicit task). After fMRI, the subjects were also asked to rate emotional valence and arousal. Reaction times and accuracy were analyzed as well. Results indicated that subjects with social phobia had greater insular responses to photographic angry versus neutral faces, regardless of task, suggesting that angry expressions were more intensively processed even when it was not required. Subjects with social phobia also showed amygdalar activation to angry versus neutral faces during both tasks, whereas psychiatrically healthy control subjects showed amygdalar activation in the explicit task only. Subjects with social phobia also demonstrated activation in the parahippocampal gyrus and extrastriate cortex. Those subjects with social phobia consistently rated valence of emotional expression as more unpleasant.

Phan et al. (2006) asked 10 subjects with generalized social phobia to view and identify the emotional expression of angry, fearful, disgusted, sad, neutral, and happy photographic faces. When compared with control subjects, patients with social phobia did not differ in accuracy of identification or response time. They did, however, have greater right amygdala activation to harsh versus happy and neutral faces. This activation was associated with intensity of social anxiety symptoms, indicating a relationship between severity of symptoms and amygdalar activity.

In 2005, Straube and colleagues again examined fMRI activity in patients with social phobia. Nine patients with generalized social phobia were exposed to pictures expressing angry, happy, and neutral expressions. Subjects rated the faces for valence (very unpleasant to very pleasant) and arousal (not arousing to very arousing). When compared with control subjects, patients with social phobia were found to have significantly greater amygdala activation to angry as well as happy faces. Threatening (angry) faces were associated with increased activation in the insula. The authors suggested that whereas the amygdala processes information related to social threat, safety, and acceptance, the insula appears to be responsible for the threat relevance of incoming information.

Sareen et al. (2007) asked 10 participants with generalized social phobia to complete an implicit sequence learning task while undergoing fMRI. When compared with control subjects, subjects with social phobia did not differ on behavioral performance but did have significantly decreased neural activation in the left caudate head, left inferior parietal lobe, and insula. The authors suggested that this evidence of striatal dysfunction could be secondary to a dysfunction in dopamine neurotransmission, and they noted that left caudate dysfunction could contribute to information processing biases.

Cooney et al. (2006) evaluated 10 subjects with social phobia, 9 of whom were diagnosed with the generalized subtype, versus 10 psychiatrically healthy control subjects. Participants viewed varying emotional expressions and made valence ratings (positive, negative, and neutral). An oval with a crosshair in the center was included as a schematic neutral. Results of this study indicate that neutral faces elicit affective appraisals in both groups of subjects. However, patients with social phobia activate the right amygdala while viewing neutral faces and schematic ovals, whereas psychiatrically healthy control subjects activate the left amygdala. In the group with social phobia, a significant correlation was found between state and trait anxiety and right amygdalar activation. The authors postulated that left amygdalar activation in psychiatrically healthy control subjects could indicate more sustained cognitive appraisal versus a rapid attention to expression in those with social phobia.

Yoon et al. (2007) examined 11 patients with generalized social phobia and 11 psychiatrically healthy control subjects. Subjects viewed varying facial expressions by type and intensity of expressed emotion. Subjects with social phobia had significantly greater bilateral amygdalar activation to high- versus low-intensity expressions when compared with control subjects, indicating that amygdalar activation can be modulated by strength of affect.

Finally, Campbell et al. (2007) examined the ability of subjects to identify various emotional expressions. In 14 female subjects with generalized social phobia, the peak amygdalar response for both positive and negative facial expressions occurred later than the peak response of psychiatrically healthy women. The authors concluded that patients with social phobia demonstrate deficits in emotional facial processing and are internally centered, attending less to the task than control subjects.

Neurochemical Activity

Tiihonen et al. (1997) measured striatal dopamine reuptake site density with ^{123}I-2β-carbomethoxy-3β-(4-iodophenyl) tropane (^{123}I-β-CIT), a SPECT cocaine analog, in 11 patients with social phobia and age- and gender-matched volunteers. The authors reported that patients with social phobia had markedly lower dopamine reuptake site densities in the striatum. They concluded that social phobia may be associated with dopamine dysfunction. Interestingly, high rates of social phobia have been found in patients with Parkinson's disease (Stein et al. 1990).

Schneier et al. (2000) used ^{123}I-iodobenzamide (^{123}I-IBZM) SPECT to examine dopamine D_2 receptor-binding potential in 10 unmedicated patients with social phobia. They found that the patients had lower striatal D_2 binding potential than age- and gender-matched psychiatrically healthy volunteers. Although these two studies are not a replication, they are consistent with Liebowitz et al.'s (1987) proposal of dopaminergic dysfunction in patients with social phobia. Unfortunately, the findings are inconsistent with a negative levodopa challenge conducted by Tancer et al. (1994/1995a).

Lanzenberger et al. (2007) found significantly lower 5-HT_{1A} in subjects with social phobia versus control subjects, particularly in the amygdala but also in the insula, anterior cingulate cortex, and dorsal raphe nucleus. No differences were found within the hippocampus.

Tupler et al. (1997) used proton magnetic resonance spectroscopy (^{1}H-MRS) to measure concentrations of putative neuronal markers *N*-acetylaspartate, creatine, choline, and myoinositol. At baseline, 19 patients with social phobia had significantly lower *N*-acetylaspartate-to-choline and higher choline-to-creatine and myoinositol-to-creatine ratios in cortical gray matter compared with 10 control subjects. White matter regions of interest did not differ between groups. Following 8 weeks of clinically effective treatment with clonazepam, the ratios did not change. This exciting finding has yet to be replicated.

Phan et al. (2005) examined 10 medication-naïve patients diagnosed with generalized social phobia with ^{1}H-MRS as well. Compared with psychiatrically healthy control subjects, the patients with social phobia had elevated levels of glutamate in the anterior cingulate cortex. These levels were associated with symptom severity.

In summary, several differences between patients with social phobia and psychiatrically healthy control subjects have been reported. Anxiety provocation leads to increased activation of the amygdala in patients diagnosed with social phobia and those carrying the short allele of the 5-HTT promoter. Two studies in which patients with social phobia were treated with citalopram demonstrated decreased blood flow in the amygdala and other brain regions following treatment. Interestingly, research indicates that cognitive-behavioral therapy may have the same effect. Finally, the results of several imaging studies suggest dopaminergic receptor dysfunction.

Electroencephalography

There is growing evidence that both children and adults who are shy, anxious, or depressed exhibit greater relative right frontal electroencephalographic (EEG) activity at rest and increased overall frontal EEG activity. Although only a small sample size was used (n=6), Campbell et al. (2007) compared the children of parents who had received the diagnosis of social phobia with children of psychiatrically healthy control subjects (n=7). The authors discovered that subject children with social phobia had greater overall EEG activation in the frontal region, specifically in the midfrontal site. The authors attribute this finding to a predisposition to experience emotion with greater intensity. Bruder et al. (2004) found that when they were given fused-words syllable-and-tone tests, patients with social phobia had a smaller left hemisphere advantage compared with control subjects. They attribute this dysfunction specifically to anxiety, not comorbid conditions. The authors suggested that these results support a dysfunction in mediation of verbal processing, which may contribute to stress during social encounters. These findings are consistent with previous studies demonstrating left hemisphere dysfunction on laterality tests.

Sleep Studies

Subjective complaints of insomnia and idiosyncratic sleep disturbances are common in some patients with social phobia (M.B. Stein et al. 1993b). Utilizing a sleep questionnaire, Stein and colleagues reported that patients with social phobia complained of decreased sleep quality and increased sleep latency. Interestingly, in a group of patients with social phobia who did not report major subjective sleep difficulties, polysomnography data were mostly normal (Brown et al. 1994).

In a study examining sleep-related problems in children ages 6–17 years diagnosed with a variety of anxiety disorders, Alfano et al. (2007) found evidence of significantly greater sleep-related problems in children diagnosed with social phobia when compared with youth without social phobia. Among children with social phobia, 90% had at least one sleep-related problem. Considering that sleep disturbances among children are common and encompass a wide range of presentations, these results should be interpreted cautiously.

Autonomic Reactivity

The palpitations, sweating, and flushing symptoms characteristic of patients with social phobia have led to a variety of studies focusing on autonomic function. Levin et al. (1993) found similar increases in heart rate and blood pressure in patients with social phobia and psychiatrically healthy control subjects during a public speaking task. Supporting these data, Mauss et al. (2003) examined 35 subjects with high-trait social anxiety and 35 subjects with low-trait social anxiety before, during, and after two anxiogenic impromptu speeches. Although patients with high levels of anxiety reported greater subjective anxiety during speech and recovery periods, minimal autonomic differences were found between the groups. Naftolowitz et al. (1994) reported no differences in physiological parameters, plasma cortisol, and norepinephrine elevations between volunteers and patients with social phobia. Interestingly, in both the Naftolowitz et al. (1994) and Heimberg et al. (1990) studies, patients with the specific subtype of social phobia had greater heart rate increases before and during anxiogenic challenges.

M.B. Stein et al. (1992) reported increased norepinephrine responses to postural challenge in a sample of patients with mixed social phobia. M.B. Stein et al. (1994) failed to replicate this finding in a larger (15 vs. 10) sample of patients with generalized social phobia. They did note an exaggerated blood pressure elevation following Valsalva maneuver, suggesting impaired parasympathetic activity.

In summary, autonomic studies suggest differential responses between patients with generalized versus specific subtypes of social phobia.

Psychological Factors

Several psychological models have been proposed for the development of social phobia. Models based on development, personality, and cultural factors as well as cognitive-behavioral theory have been discussed. These have been previously reviewed, and the reader is urged to consult the following references for details: Barlow 1988; Bruch and Cheek 1995; Mineka and Zinbarg 1995. We briefly discuss these models and highlight some of their limitations in this chapter.

Childhood/Developmental Factors

Behavioral Inhibition Model

Behavioral inhibition, a psychological construct developed by Kagan et al. (1988), refers to a stable temperament, recognizable in early childhood (see Chapter 5, "Anxious Traits and Temperaments," in this volume). Operationally, it defines a subset of children who behave in a fearful manner when exposed to a novel test environment. Compared with noninhibited children, behaviorally inhibited children have increased latency to speak, decreased exploratory behavior, increased heart rate, and elevated cortisol and catecholamine levels. Behavioral inhibition can lead to decreased and/or uncomfortable social interactions, which may eventually lead to social fears and social anxiety. Theoretically, these traits may lead to social phobia. A 21-year longitudinal study of 1,265 children revealed that those children who were inhibited at age 8 years had significantly higher rates of social phobia at ages16 to 21 years (Goodwin 2004). Supporting this finding, Hirshfeld-Becker et al. (2007) followed behaviorally inhibited toddlers to age 6 years and discovered that inhibited children had significantly higher rates of social anxiety, but not other anxiety disorders, when compared with noninhibited children (17% vs. 5%). When this cohort was examined in middle to late childhood, the authors found that behavioral inhibition in the earliest examination was specifically associated with social phobia. Kagan's group reported that, as adults, children with behavioral inhibition had greater amygdalar reactivity to novel versus familiar situations.

Biederman et al. (1990) reported that children of adults with agoraphobia or panic disorder have markedly increased rates of behavioral inhibition compared with children of depressed parents. Unfortunately, the prevalence of behavioral inhibition in the children of parents with social phobia has not been determined. Mancini et al. (1996) evaluated children of parents with social phobia and reported high rates of overanxious disorder and social phobia. Because a comparison group was not included, it is difficult to ascertain whether these increased rates are specific to children whose parents have been diagnosed with social phobia.

Family Environment

Compared with adults with agoraphobia, adults with social phobia retrospectively report that their parental figures emphasized concern regarding the opinions of others and de-emphasized familial sociability. In retrospective studies, socially anxious subjects described their parents as more overprotective and less affectionate than did psychiatrically healthy control subjects and subjects with agoraphobia.

A study by DeWit et al. (2003) noted gender differences in the effects of family environment. The absence of a parent or close adult confidant was associated with increased risk of social phobia in male subjects. Parental conflict, childhood physical abuse by a father figure, and maternal mania determined increased risk in females.

Given the retrospective nature of these materials and the possibility that social anxiety distorts the subjects' perception of early experience, causality is difficult to infer.

Attachment Theory and Psychodynamic Contributions

Attachment theory indicates that in times of heightened danger, our earliest internal working models are mobilized. As individuals may "unconsciously seek out objects who resonate with early attachment figures and patterns of relating that provided the only felt security" (Eagle 1997), patients with social phobia whose early attachment figures were threatening may be unconsciously repeating early experiences.

Although selected from poverty-stricken populations at risk for developmental issues, Warren et al. (1997) reported that infants with early ambivalent attachment were significantly more likely to develop anxiety disorders than those with secure or avoidant attachment patterns. A study of 136 eleven-year-olds by Bar-Haim et al. (2007) examined early attachment and the development of social phobia. The authors discovered a significant attachment effect in the prediction of social phobia, which, interestingly, differed between males and females. Compared with males who were securely attached at age 12 months, those who were ambivalently attached had higher scores of social phobia at age 11 years. These results did not replicate with female subjects. Notably, within all attachment types, overall levels of anxiety were within normal ranges. Unfortunately, formal diagnostic interviews were not used to assess diagnosis.

Early-Childhood Language Impairment

Voci et al. (2006) looked at 202 young adults ages 18–20 years who had been diagnosed with language impairment at age 5 years. They found that compared with control subjects (children with appropriate language abilities), children with language impairments showed significantly greater risk for developing social phobia during late adolescence. The 1-year prevalence rate for social phobia in the language-impaired population was 16%, one of the highest rates of this disorder in community epidemiological literature. The authors postulated that experiences of rejection in these children promoted a hypersensitivity to negative feedback or expectations of negative social interactions. Interestingly, rates of generalized versus specific type of social phobia did not differ. Unfortunately, the study authors were unable to determine whether language impairment continued to predict social phobia after controlling for other childhood risk factors.

Personality Factors

Shyness is a personality trait that begins early in life in most people (Buss 1980). Shyness has a genetic component; monozygotic twins are more closely concordant in shyness than are dizygotic twins. Bruch and Cheek (1995) described two types of shyness: a "fearful" shyness, which develops at a very early age, and a "self-conscious" shyness, which develops around the time of adolescence. The notion is that shyness leads to discomfort in particular social situations, which can lead to worry about such situations and arousal or avoidance. Although many individuals with social phobia describe themselves as shy, this is not a universal finding. Conversely, many shy individuals do not meet the criteria for social phobia.

Cognitive and Behavioral Models

Two models related to the cognitive development of social phobia have been postulated. The Clark and Wells (1995) model indicates that patients with social phobia have negative perceptions of both themselves and their social environment based on early experience. These assumptions cause them to judge social situations as dangerous, producing anxiety. Patients become highly self-focused and project their own negative assumptions of themselves on others. Such a cognitive model is consistent with psychometric data on rating scales (Shea Gelernter et al. 1991). Rapee and Heimberg's (1997) model suggests that during social situations, those diagnosed with social phobia focus on negative aspects of themselves and negative appraisals from the environment. A study by Mattia et al. (1993) validated an attentional bias toward self. Utilizing the Stroop task, these authors found that patients with social phobia demonstrated a delay in color naming for words related to social scrutiny and rejection. Mattia and colleagues' results indicate that patients with social phobia ruminate on social scrutiny, are self-focused, and are less capable of attending to the primary task than matched community controls.

Chavira and Stein (2005) discussed behavioral models of social phobia, which indicate that impairments in social skills lead to poor performance and subsequent avoidance of social situations. As a result, realistic negative appraisals of social competence are formed.

Cultural Factors

Breslau et al. (2006) utilized the National Comorbidity Survey Replication to investigate variations in race-ethnic differences among several DSM-IV diagnoses, including social phobia. Their paper examined 5,424 subjects who were Hispanic, non-Hispanic black, or non-Hispanic white. Compared to non-Hispanic whites, Hispanics had a significantly lower lifetime prevalence rate for social phobia. Non-Hispanic blacks had a nonsignificant decrease in lifetime prevalence of social phobia. The authors suggested that ethnic identification and religious participation might be protective factors. The fact that race-ethnic differences in psychiatric disorders emerge in childhood suggests that this period is an important one to study.

Interestingly, cultural biases may have an impact on the maintenance of behavioral inhibition. Chen et al. (1998) noted increased inhibition in Chinese versus Canadian children and discovered that Chinese children with inhibited behaviors had an associated positive adjustment in adolescence, including increased academic leadership and achievement (Chen et al. 1997).

Other Theories

Conditioning Model

The conditioning model is based on the theory that a conditioned aversive situation can lead to the development of phobias (Barlow 1988). The available empirical data are not consistent; some reports support such a model (Stemberger et al. 1995), but others do not (Hofmann et al. 1995). Retrospective data from research on adults suggest that approximately 40%–60% recall a traumatic incident leading to the development of their phobia. It is important to note that there is often a delay of more than 10 years between the onset of symptoms and elicitation of help for the symptoms, and by then, many traumatic events may have been forgotten. On the contrary, a patient may have identified a traumatic event well into the course of the disorder as the causative trauma. Detailed evaluation of traumatic experiences in monozygotic twins discordant for social phobia may help identify the role of conditioning in the development of social phobia.

Ethological Model

Ohman (1986) initially formulated the ethological model that later was more completely articulated by Mineka and Zinbarg (1995) and Stein and Bouwer (1997). This model posits an evolutionary wariness of being stared at. Averting eye contact may be viewed as a sign of submissiveness, which would have an evolutionary advantage in individuals with low societal status. The mean age at onset of social phobia roughly coincides with puberty, unlike that of other anxiety disorders. Interestingly, pubertal onset is the developmental period when social hierarchies begin to emerge (Hermans and vanHonk 2006).

In summary, various models have been proposed to explain the development and persistence of social phobia. For the most part, the models are not mutually exclusive, and data supporting one do not negatively affect the rest. The models should be tested by following groups of youth at high risk for the development of social phobia in a longitudinal fashion.

Conclusion

Multiple biological and psychological factors have been implicated in the pathogenesis of social phobia. Dysfunction of dopaminergic, serotonergic, noradrenergic, and glutamatergic systems, GABA, and substance P have all been suggested, but further work is needed before definitive conclusions can be drawn. Although genetic research is at an early stage, direct-interview family studies have shown a role for genetic transmission. The first linkage scan has appeared, and a number of promising candidate genes have been studied. Brain imaging research has helped define distinguishing characteristics in the structure, functional activity, and mediating neurocircuitry of subjects with social phobia.

As far as psychological factors are concerned, several mechanisms likely contribute to the etiology of social phobia. A clear association between behavioral inhibition and the development of social phobia has been elucidated. Cognitive and behavioral models indicate that patients with social phobia are self-focused and falsely perceive the environment as negative. Given the limitations of retrospective reporting of both family environment and aversive causative events, additional prospective research is needed in this area.

An integration of biological and psychological contributions to social phobia is suggested in research related to behavioral inhibition, genetic transmission, and brain imaging. Smoller et al. (2003) found an association between behavioral inhibition and a polymorphism in the gene responsible for corticotropin-releasing factor. Kagan et al. (1988) speculated, and neuroimaging studies confirm, that inhibited children have a reduced threshold for limbic arousal. Future work should lead to a more detailed and better integrated view of pathogenesis.

◀ Key Clinical Points ▶

- The etiology of social phobia (social anxiety disorder) is multifactorial.
- Although no single gene appears responsible for the etiology of social phobia, multiple genetic variants might partially contribute to its development.
- Studies utilizing anxiogenic stimuli have failed to provoke symptoms typical of patients' individual phobic symptomatology. Although patients with social phobia appear to be more sensitive than healthy volunteers to the anxiogenic effects of various substances and circumstances, the reason for this is unclear.
- Regarding the psychoneuroendocrine axis, no clear differences exist between patients with social phobia and healthy control subjects.
- In patients diagnosed with social phobia, anxiety provocation leads to increased amygdalar activation. Both pharmacotherapy and psychotherapy have been shown to reverse this effect.
- Several imaging studies in patients diagnosed with social phobia suggest dopaminergic receptor dysfunction.
- Although patients with social phobia may complain of sleep difficulties, results of polysomnographic studies have been normal.
- Studies suggest a differential autonomic response in patients diagnosed with the generalized versus specific subtype of social phobia.
- Children who exhibit behavioral inhibition have an increased risk of developing social phobia.
- Patients with social phobia have negative cognitions, including negative perceptions of themselves and their environments.
- When compared to Caucasians and African Americans, Hispanics have a significantly lower lifetime prevalence rate for social phobia.

References

Abelson JL, Nesse RM: Pentagastrin infusions in patients with panic disorder, I: symptoms and cardiovascular responses. Biol Psychiatry 36:73–83, 1994

Alfano CA, Ginsburg GS, Kingery JN: Sleep-related problems among children and adolescents with anxiety disorders. J Am Acad Child Adolesc Psychiatry 46:224–232, 2007

American Psychiatric Association: Diagnostic and Statistical Manual of Mental Disorders, 3rd Edition, Revised. Washington, DC, American Psychiatric Association, 1987

American Psychiatric Association: Diagnostic and Statistical Manual of Mental Disorders, 4th Edition. Washington, DC, American Psychiatric Association, 1994

American Psychiatric Association: Diagnostic and Statistical Manual of Mental Disorders, 4th Edition, Text Revision. Washington, DC, American Psychiatric Association, 2000

Amir N, Klumpp H, Elias J, et al: Increased activation of the anterior cingulate cortex during processing of disgust faces in individuals with social phobia. Biol Psychiatry 57:975–981, 2005

Asmundson GJG, Stein MB: Vagal attenuation in panic disorder: an assessment of parasympathetic nervous system function and subjective reactivity to respiratory manipulations. Psychosom Med 56:187–193, 1994

Bar-Haim Y, Dan O, Eshel Y, et al: Predicting children's anxiety from early attachment relationships. J Anxiety Disord 21:1061–1068, 2007

Barkan T, Hermesh H, Marom S, et al: Serotonin uptake to lymphocytes of patients with social phobia compared to normal individuals. Eur Neuropsychopharmacol 16:19–23, 2006

Barlow D: Anxiety and Its Disorders: The Nature and Treatment of Anxiety and Panic. New York, Guilford, 1988

Biederman J, Rosenbaum JF, Hirshfeld DR, et al: Psychiatric correlates of behavioral inhibition in young children of parents with and without psychiatric disorders. Arch Gen Psychiatry 47:21–26, 1990

Biederman J, Petty C, Faraone SV, et al: Effects of parental anxiety disorders in children at high risk for panic disorders: a controlled study. J Affect Disord 94:191–197, 2006

Breslau J, Aguilar-Gaxiola S, Kendler KS, et al: Specifying race-ethnic differences in risk for psychiatric disorder in a USA national sample. Psychol Med 36:57–68, 2006

Brown TM, Black B, Uhde TW: The sleep architecture of social phobia. Biol Psychiatry 35:420–421, 1994

Bruch MA, Cheek JM: Developmental factors in childhood and adolescent shyness, in Social Phobia: Diagnosis, Assessment, and Treatment. Edited by Heimberg RG, Liebowitz MR, Hope DA, et al. New York, Guilford, 1995, pp 163–182

Bruder GE, Schneier FR, Stewart JW, et al: Left hemisphere dysfunction during verbal dichotic listening tests in patients who have social phobia with or without comorbid depressive disorder. Am J Psychiatry 161:72–78, 2004

Buss AH: Self-Consciousness and Social Anxiety. San Francisco, CA, WH Freeman, 1980

Caldirola D, Perna G, Arancio C, et al: The 35% CO2 challenge test in patients with social phobia. Psychiatry Res 71:41–48, 1997

Campbell DW, Sareen J, Paulus MP, et al: Time-varying amygdala response to emotional faces in generalized social phobia. Biol Psychiatry 62:455–463, 2007

Chavira DA, Stein MA: Childhood social anxiety disorder: from understanding to treatment. Child Adolesc Psychiatric Clin North Am 14:797–818, 2005

Chen X, Rubin KH, Li D: Relation between academic achievement and social adjustment: evidence from Chinese children. Dev Psychol 33:518–525, 1997

Chen X, Hastings PD, Rubin KH, et al: Child-rearing attitudes and behavioral inhibition in Chinese and Canadian toddlers: a cross-cultural study. Dev Psychol 34:677–686, 1998

Clark DM, Wells A: A cognitive model of social phobia, in Social Phobia: Diagnosis, Assessment, and Treatment. Edited by Heimberg RG, Liebowitz MR, Hope DA, et al. New York, Guilford, 1995, pp 69–93

Condren RM, Lucey JV, Thakore JH: A preliminary study of baclofen-induced growth hormone release in generalised social phobia. Hum Psychopharmacol 18:125–130, 2003

Cooney RE, Atlas LY, Joormann J, et al: Amygdala activation in the processing of neutral faces in social anxiety disorder: is neutral really neutral? Psychiatry Research: Neuroimaging 148:35–39, 2006

Cooper PJ, Fearn V, Willetts L, et al: Affective disorder in the parents of a clinical sample of children with anxiety disorder. J Affect Disord 93:205–212, 2006

Covelli V, Passeri ME, Leogrande D, et al: Drug targets in stress-related disorders. Curr Med Chem 12:1801–1809, 2005

DeWit DJ, Chandler-Coutts M, Offord DR, et al: Gender differences in the effects of family adversity on the risk of onset of DSM-III-R social phobia. Anxiety Disord 19:479–502, 2003

Eagle M: Attachment and psychoanalysis. Br J Med Psychol 70 (pt 3):217–229, 1997

Furmark T, Tillfors M, Marteinsdottir I, et al: Common changes in cerebral blood flow in patients with social phobia treated with citalopram or cognitive-behavioral therapy. Arch Gen Psychiatry 59:425–433, 2002

Furmark T, Tillfors M, Garpenstrand H, et al: Serotonin transporter polymorphism related to amygdala excitability and symptom severity in patients with social phobia. Neurosci Lett 362:189–192, 2004

Furmark T, Appel L, Michelgard A, et al: Cerebral blood flow changes after treatment of social phobia with the neurokinin-1 antagonist GR2051671, citalopram, or placebo. Biol Psychiatry 58:132–142, 2005

Fyer AJ, Mannuzza S, Chapman TF, et al: A direct interview family study of social phobia. Arch Gen Psychiatry 50:286–293, 1993

Gelernter J, Grier PP, Stein MB, et al: Genome-wide linkage scan for loci predisposing to social phobia: evidence for a chromosome 16 risk locus. Am J Psychiatry 161:59–66, 2004

Goodwin RD, Fergusson DM, Horwood LJ: Early anxious/withdrawn behaviours predict later internalising disorders. J Child Psychol Psychiatry 45:874–883, 2004

Gorman JM, Fyer MR, Liebowitz MR, et al: Pharmacologic provocation of panic attacks, in Psychopharmacology: The Third Generation of Progress. Edited by Meltzer HY. New York, Raven, 1987, pp 985–998

Gorman JM, Papp LA, Martinez J, et al: High-dose carbon dioxide challenge test in anxiety disorder patients. Biol Psychiatry 28:743–757, 1990

Granger DA, Weisz JR, Kauneckis D: Neuroendocrine reactivity, internalizing behavior problems, and control-related cognitions in clinic-referred children and adolescents. J Abnorm Psychol 103:267–276, 1994

Guttmacher LB, Murphy DL, Insel TR: Pharmacological models of anxiety states. Compr Psychiatry 24:312–326, 1983

Hariri AR, Mattay VS, Tessitore A, et al: Serotonin transporter genetic variation and the response of the human amygdala. Science 297:400–403, 2002

Heimberg RG, Hope DA, Dodge CS, et al: DSM-III-R subtypes of social phobia: comparison of generalized social phobics and public speaking phobics. J Nerv Ment Dis 178:172–179, 1990

Hermans EJ, vanHonk J: Toward a framework for defective emotion processing in social phobia. Cognit Neuropsychiatry 11:307–331, 2006

Hirshfeld-Becker DR, Biederman J, Henin A, et al: Behavioral inhibition in preschool children at risk is a specific predictor of middle childhood social anxiety: a five-year follow-up. J Dev Behav Pediatr 28:225–233, 2007

Hofmann SG, Ehlers A, Roth RT: Conditioning theory: a model for the etiology of public speaking anxiety? Behav Res Ther 33:567–571, 1995

Hollander E, Kwon J, Weiller F, et al: Serotonergic function in social phobia: comparison to normal control and obsessive-compulsive disorder subjects. Psychiatry Res 79:213–217, 1998

Holt PE, Andrews G: Hyperventilation and anxiety in panic disorder, social phobia, GAD and normal controls. Behav Res Ther 27:453–460, 1989a

Holt PE, Andrews G: Provocation of panic: three elements of the panic reaction in four anxiety disorders. Behav Res Ther 27:253–261, 1989b

Johnson MR, Marazziti D, Brawman-Mintzer O, et al: Abnormal peripheral benzodiazepine receptor density associated with generalized social phobia. Biol Psychiatry 43:306–309, 1998

Kagan J, Reznick JS, Snidman N: Biological bases of childhood shyness. Science 240:167–171, 1988

Kendler KS, Neale MC, Kessler RC, et al: The genetic epidemiology of phobias in women: the interrelationship of agoraphobia, social phobia, situational phobia, and simple phobia. Arch Gen Psychiatry 49:273–281, 1992

Kennedy JL, Neves-Pereira M, King N, et al: Dopamine system genes not linked to social phobia. Psychiatr Genet 11:213–217, 2001

Lachman HM, Papolos DF, Saito T, et al: Human catechol-O-methyltransferase pharmacogenetics: description of a functional polymorphism and its potential application to neuropsychiatric disorders. Pharmacogenetics 6:243–245, 1996

Lanzenberger RR, Mitterhauser M, Sprindelegger C, et al: Reduced serotonin-1A receptor binding in social anxiety disorders. Biol Psychiatry 61:1081–1089, 2007

Laufer N, Zucker M, Hermesh H, et al: Platelet vesicular monoamine transporter density in untreated patients diagnosed with social phobia. Psychiatry Res 136:247–250, 2005

Levin AP, Saoud JB, Gorman JM, et al: Responses of generalized and discrete social phobias during public speaking challenge. J Anxiety Disord 7:207–221, 1993

Liebowitz MR, Fyer AJ, Gorman JM, et al: Specificity of lactate infusions in social phobia versus panic disorder. Am J Psychiatry 142:947–950, 1985

Liebowitz MR, Campeas R, Hollander E: MAOIs: impact on social behavior (letter to the editor). Psychiatry Res 22:89–90, 1987

Lochner C, Hemmings S, Seedat S, et al: Genetics and personality traits in patients with social anxiety disorder: a case-control study in South Africa. Eur Neuropsychopharmacol 17:321–327, 2007

Maddock RJ, Carter CS: Hyperventilation-induced panic attacks in panic disorder with agoraphobia. Biol Psychiatry 29:843–854, 1991

Mancini C, van Ameringen M, Szatmari P, et al: A high-risk pilot study of the children of adults with social phobia. J Am Acad Child Adolesc Psychiatry 35:1511–1517, 1996

Martel FL, Hayward C, Lyons DM, et al: Salivary cortisol levels in socially phobic adolescent girls. Depress Anxiety 10:25–27, 1999

Mattia JI, Heimberg RG, Hope DA: The revised Stroop color-naming task in social phobics. Behav Res Ther 31:305–313, 1993

Mauss IB, Wilhelm FH, Gross JJ: Autonomic recovery and habituation in social anxiety. Psychophysiology 40:548–653, 2003

McCann UD, Slate SO, Geraci M, et al: A comparison of the effects of intravenous pentagastrin on patients with social phobia, panic disorder and healthy controls. Neuropsychopharmacology 16:229–237, 1997

McGrath M, Kawachi I, Ascherio A, et al: Association between catechol-O-methyltransferase and phobic anxiety. Am J Psychiatry 161:1703–1705, 2004

Mineka S, Zinbarg R: Conditioning and ethological models of social phobia, in Social Phobia: Diagnosis, Assessment, and Treatment. Edited by Heimberg RG, Liebowitz MR, Hope DA, et al. New York, Guilford, 1995, pp 134–162

Miner CM, Davidson JR: Biological characterization of social phobia. Eur Arch Psychiatry Clin Neurosci 244:304–308, 1995

Naftolowitz DF, Vaughn BV, Ranc J, et al: Response to alcohol in social phobia. Anxiety 1:96–99, 1994

Nutt DJ, Bell CJ, Malizia AL: Brain mechanisms of social anxiety disorder. J Clin Psychiatry 59(suppl):4–11, 1998

Ogliari A, Citterio A, Zanoni A, et al: Genetic and environmental influences on anxiety dimensions in Italian twins evaluated with the SCARED questionnaire. Anxiety Disord 20:760–777, 2006

Ohara K, Nagai M, Suzuki Y, et al: No association between anxiety disorders and catechol-O-methyltransferase polymorphism. Psychiatry Res 80:145–148, 1998

Ohman A: Face the beast and fear the face: animal and social fears as prototypes for evolutionary analyses of emotion. Psychophysiology 23:123–145, 1986

Papp LA, Gorman JM, Liebowitz MR, et al: Epinephrine infusions in patients with social phobia. Am J Psychiatry 145:733–736, 1988

Phan KL, Fitzgerald DA, Cortese BM, et al: Anterior cingulate neurochemistry in social anxiety disorder: 1H-MRS at 4 tesla. Brain Imaging 16:183–186, 2005

Phan KL, Fitzgerald DA, Nathan PJ, et al: Association between amygdala hyperactivity to harsh faces and severity of social anxiety in generalized social phobia. Biol Psychiatry 59:424–429, 2006

Potts NL, Davidson JR, Krishnan KR, et al: Levels of urinary free cortisol in social phobia. J Clin Psychiatry 52(suppl): 41–42, 1991

Potts NL, Davidson JR, Krishnan KR, et al: Magnetic resonance imaging in social phobia. Psychiatry Res 52:35–42, 1994

Rapaport MH, Stein MB: Serum interleukin-2 and soluble interleukin-2 receptor levels in generalized social phobia. Anxiety 1:50–53, 1994

Rapee RM, Heimberg RG: A cognitive-behavioral model of anxiety in social phobia. Behav Res Ther 35:741–756, 1997

Rowe DC, Stever C, Gard JM, et al: The relation of the dopamine transporter gene (DAT1) to symptoms of internalizing disorders in children. Behav Genet 28:215–225, 1998

Samochowiec J, Hajduk A, Samochowiec A, et al: Association studies of MAO-A, COMT, and 5-HTT genes polymorphisms in patients with anxiety disorders of the phobic spectrum. Psychiatry Res 128:21–26, 2004

Sareen J, Campbell DW, Leslie WD, et al: Striatal function in generalized social phobia: a functional magnetic resonance imaging study. Biol Psychiatry 61:396–404, 2007

Schneier FR, Liebowitz MR, Abi-Dargham A, et al: Low dopamine D(2) receptor binding potential in social phobia. Am J Psychiatry 157:457–459, 2000

Schultz SK, Moser DJ, Bishop JR, et al: Phobic anxiety in late-life in relationship to cognitive and 5HTTLPR polymorphism. Psychiatr Genet 15:305–306, 2005

Shea Gelernter CA, Uhde TW, Cimbolic P, et al: Comparison of cognitive therapy versus pharmacotherapy in social phobia. Arch Gen Psychiatry 48:938–945, 1991

Shlik J, Maron E, Tru I, et al: Citalopram challenge in social anxiety disorder. Int J Neuropsychopharmacol 7:177–182, 2004

Skre I, Onstad S, Torgersen S, et al: A twin study of DSM-III-R anxiety disorders. Acta Psychiatr Scand 88:85–92, 1993

Skre I, Onstad S, Torgersen S, et al: The heritability of common phobic fear: a twin study of a clinical sample. J Anxiety Disord 14:549–562, 2000

Smoller JW, Rosenbaum JF, Biederman J, et al: Association of a genetic marker at the corticotropin-releasing hormone locus with behavioral inhibition. Biol Psychiatry 54:1376–1381, 2003

Smoller JW, Yamaki LH, Fagerness JA, et al: The corticotropin-releasing hormone gene and behavioral inhibition in children at risk for panic disorder. Biol Psychiatry 57:1485–1489, 2005

Spinhoven P, Onstein EJ, Sterk PJ, et al: The hyperventilation provocation test in panic disorder. Behav Res Ther 30:453–461, 1992

Stein DJ, Bouwer C: Blushing and social phobia: a neuroethological speculation. Med Hypotheses 49:101–108, 1997

Stein MB, Leslie WD: A brain single-photon emission computed tomography (SPECT) study of generalized social phobia. Biol Psychiatry 39:825–828, 1996

Stein MB, Heuser IJ, Juncos JL, et al: Anxiety disorders in patients with Parkinson's disease. Am J Psychiatry 147:217–220, 1990

Stein MB, Tancer ME, Uhde TW: Heart rate and plasma norepinephrine responsivity to orthostatic challenge in anxiety disorders: comparison of patients with panic disorder and social phobia and normal control subjects. Arch Gen Psychiatry 49:311–317, 1992

Stein MB, Huzel LL, Delaney SM: Lymphocyte beta-adrenoceptors in social phobia. Biol Psychiatry 34:45–50, 1993a

Stein MB, Kroft CDL, Walker JR: Sleep impairment in patients with social phobia. Psychiatry Res 49:251–256, 1993b

Stein MB, Asmundson GJG, Chartier M: Autonomic responsivity in generalized social phobia. J Affect Disord 31: 211–221, 1994

Stein MB, Delaney SM, Chartier MJ, et al: [3H]Paroxetine binding to platelets of patients with social phobia: comparison to patients with panic disorder and healthy volunteers. Biol Psychiatry 37:224–228, 1995

Stein MB, Chen G, Potter WZ, et al: G-protein level quantification in platelets and leukocytes from patients with panic disorder. Neuropsychopharmacology 15:180–186, 1996

Stein MB, Chartier MJ, Hazen AL, et al: A direct-interview family study of generalized social phobia. Am J Psychiatry 155:90–97, 1998

Stemberger RT, Turner SM, Beidel DC, et al: Social phobia: an analysis of possible developmental factors. J Abnorm Psychol 104:526–531, 1995

Straube T, Kolassa IT, Glauer M, et al: Effect of task conditions on brain response to threatening faces in social phobics: an event-related functional magnetic resonance imaging study. Biol Psychiatry 56:921–930, 2004

Straube T, Mentzel HJ, Miltner WHR: Common and distinct brain activation to threat and safety signals in social phobia. Neuropsychobiology 52:163–168, 2005

Tancer ME, Stein MB, Gelernter CS, et al: The hypothalamic-pituitary-thyroid axis in social phobia. Am J Psychiatry 147:929–933, 1990

Tancer ME, Stein MB, Black B, et al: Blunted growth hormone responses to both growth hormone releasing factor and clonidine in panic disorder. Am J Psychiatry 150:336–337, 1993a

Tancer ME, Stein MB, Uhde TW: Growth hormone response to intravenous clonidine in social phobia: comparison to patients with panic disorder and healthy volunteers. Biol Psychiatry 34:591–595, 1993b

Tancer ME, Mailman RB, Stein MB, et al: Neuroendocrine responsivity to monoaminergic system probes in generalized social phobia. Anxiety 1:216–223, 1994/1995a

Tancer ME, Stein MB, Uhde TW: Lactic acid response to caffeine in panic disorder: comparison with social phobics and normal controls. Anxiety 1:138–140, 1994/1995b

Tancer ME, Lewis MH, Stein MB: Neurobiology of social phobia, in Social Phobia. Edited by Stein MB. Washington, DC, American Psychiatric Press, 1995, pp 229–257

Tiihonen J, Kuikka J, Bergstrom K, et al: Dopamine reuptake site densities in patients with social phobia. Am J Psychiatry 154:239–242, 1997

Tillfors M, Furmark T, Marteinsdottir I, et al: Cerebral blood flow in subjects with social phobia during stressful speaking tasks: a PET study. Am J Psychiatry 158:1220–1226, 2001

Tupler LA, Davidson JR, Smith RD, et al: A repeat proton magnetic resonance spectroscopy study in social phobia. Biol Psychiatry 42:419–424, 1997

Uhde TW, Tancer ME: Chemical models of panic: a review and critique, in Psychopharmacology of Anxiety. Edited by Tyrer P. Oxford, England, Oxford University Press, 1989, pp 109–131

Uhde TW, Tancer ME, Gelernter CS, et al: Normal urinary free cortisol and postdexamethasone cortisol in social phobia: comparison to normal volunteers. J Affect Disord 30:155–161, 1994

Van der Linden G, van Heerden B, Warwick J, et al: Functional brain imaging and pharmacotherapy in social phobia: single photon emission computed tomography before and after treatment with the selective serotonin reuptake inhibitor citalopram. Prog Neuropsychopharmacol Biol Psychiatry 24:419–438, 2000

van Megen HJGM, Westenberg HGM, den Boer JA, et al: Pentagastrin induced panic attacks: enhanced sensitivity in panic disorder patients. Psychopharmacology 114:449–455, 1994

van Vliet IM, Westenberg HG, Slaap BR, et al: Anxiogenic effects of pentagastrin in patients with social phobia and healthy controls. Biol Psychiatry 42:76–78, 1997

Voci SC, Beitchman JH, Brownlie EB, et al: Social anxiety in late adolescence: the importance of early childhood language impairment. Anxiety Disord 20:915–930, 2006

Warren SL, Huston L, Egeland B, et al: Child and adolescent anxiety disorders and early attachment. J Am Acad Child Adolesc Psychiatry 36:637–644, 1997

Yoon KL, Fitzgerald DA, Angstadt M, et al: Amygdala reactivity to emotional faces at high and low intensity in generalized social phobia: a 4-tesla functional MRI study. Psychiatry Research: Neuroimaging 154:93–98, 2007

Recommended Readings

Albano AM: Cognitive Behavioral Therapy for Social Phobia in Adolescents: Stand Up, Speak Out Therapist Guide. New York, Oxford University Press, 2007

Markway BG: Dying of Embarrassment: Help for Social Anxiety and Phobia. Oakland, CA, New Harbinger Publications, 1992

Chapter 27

Pharmacotherapy for Social Anxiety Disorder

Carlos Blanco, M.D., Ph.D.
Franklin R. Schneier, M.D.
Oriana Vesga-López, M.D.
Michael R. Liebowitz, M.D.

Over the past two decades, the growing recognition of social anxiety disorder as a highly prevalent and disabling condition has brought attention to its treatment. The two best-established treatments for social anxiety disorder are cognitive-behavioral therapy (CBT) and pharmacotherapy, and each has been shown to substantially reduce avoidance and discomfort, greatly benefiting affected patients. Earlier onset of action, more potent short-term effects, and widespread availability of treatment have favored pharmacotherapy, and medications have become safer and more tolerable. On the other hand, the effects of CBT may persist for longer periods of time after treatment is discontinued and do not carry risks of side effects (see Chapter 28, "Psychotherapy for Social Anxiety Disorder," in this volume).

Most trials of treatments for social anxiety disorder have included only adult patients with the generalized subtype and have excluded patients with major Axis I and II disorders, serious suicide risk, or substance abuse and those in psychotherapy. Most of the trials have used the Liebowitz Social Anxiety Scale (LSAS; Liebowitz 1987) as a primary outcome measure. It includes 24 situations: 13 about social interactions (social) and 11 about being observed in public (performance). Each of the situations is rated independently for "fear" ranging from 0 to 3: 0 (none), 1 (mild), 2 (moderate), or 3 (severe); and for "avoidance" ranging from 0 to 3: 0 (never), 1 (occasionally, 1%–33% of the time), 2 (often, 34%–66% of the time), or 3 (usually, 67%–100% of the time). Total scores thus range from 0 to 144. Scores above 30 are suggestive of social anxiety disorder. Scores above 60 are almost always seen in individuals with the generalized subtype. Among patients seeking treatment, scores are often in the 80s or higher. Scores between 30 and 60 may represent either the nongeneralized type of social anxiety disorder with symptoms limited to specific performance situations; mild generalized social fears; or partial remission of the generalized subtype in patients who have been treated. Accordingly, an individual with a severe circumscribed disorder and low anxiety levels in other situations may score fairly low on the scale.

In this chapter, we present a review of the latest research literature on pharmacotherapy for social anxiety disorder and offer some practical guidelines for its implementation. We focus mainly on controlled trials. Selected open-label trials are also included to provide necessary historical background or when double-blind trials of a particular medication have not been conducted.

Medication Treatments

Selective Serotonin Reuptake Inhibitors

Numerous placebo-controlled trials have shown that selective serotonin reuptake inhibitors (SSRIs) are highly efficacious in the treatment of social anxiety disorder, and six meta-analyses (Blanco et al. 2003; Fedoroff and Taylor 2001; Gould et al. 1997; Hedges et al. 2007; D.J. Stein et al. 2004a; van der Linden et al. 2000) have supported their efficacy. In conjunction with their favorable side-effect profile and their ability to treat comorbid depression, SSRIs have been established as a first-line medication for social anxiety disorder. Although controlled trials have been reported for all the SSRIs except citalopram, at present paroxetine, sertraline, and fluvoxamine CR (controlled-release formulation) are the only SSRIs approved by the U.S. Food and Drug Administration (FDA) for the treatment of social anxiety disorder.

Paroxetine

M.B. Stein et al. (1996) conducted an 11-week open-label study of paroxetine in the treatment of generalized social anxiety disorder in 36 patients. The target dosage was 50 mg/day, and patients were withdrawn from the study if they were unable to tolerate a minimum of 20 mg/day. At a mean dosage of 47.9 mg/day (SD=6.2), 23 of the 30 patients who completed the study were considered responders on the basis of a clinician rating of much or very much improved on the Clinical Global Impression (CGI) scale. LSAS scores decreased from 75.1 (SD=25.4) at baseline to 37.2 (SD=32.5) at the end of the open-label phase. Sixteen responders were randomly assigned to receive paroxetine for an additional 12 weeks (with no change in dosage) or placebo for 12 weeks (after a 1-week tapering period with paroxetine 20 mg/day) on a double-blind basis. One of the eight patients taking paroxetine relapsed, compared with five of the eight taking placebo.

This study was followed by a 12-week randomized clinical trial of 187 patients with generalized social anxiety disorder (M.B. Stein et al. 1996). The initial paroxetine dosage was 20 mg/day, with weekly increases of 10 mg/day permitted after the second week of treatment, up to a maximum of 50 mg/day. Response was defined as a score of 1 or 2 on the CGI scale. Fifty-five percent of the patients receiving paroxetine and 24% of those receiving placebo were classified as responders. Patients taking paroxetine (n=94) had greater mean improvement from baseline than did those taking placebo (n=93) on the LSAS (30.6 vs. 14.4) and the Sheehan Disability Scale social life (2.7 vs. 1.4) and work (1.4 vs. 0.7) items.

These findings were confirmed by a larger 12-week multicenter trial (N=323). In this double-blind, placebo-controlled study, Baldwin et al. (1999) found a response rate of 66% in the paroxetine group and 32% in the placebo group.

In a fourth controlled study, conducted in Sweden by Allgulander (1999), 92 patients were randomly assigned to receive paroxetine or placebo for 3 months. Patients began with a paroxetine dosage of 20 mg/day or placebo, and the dosage was increased by 10 mg/day every week. At the end of the study, 70% of the patients receiving paroxetine and 8% of the patients receiving placebo had a CGI score of much or very much improved and were considered responders.

A fifth study (Liebowitz et al. 2002) was set to determine the efficacy and safety of various daily dosages of paroxetine during 12 weeks of treatment. Three hundred eighty-four subjects were randomly assigned under double-blind conditions to receive paroxetine 20 mg/day (n=97), 40 mg/day (n=95), or 60 mg/day (n=97) or placebo (n=95). Patients treated with paroxetine at any dosage had significantly greater improvement on mean LSAS total scores compared with those receiving placebo (although the authors, adopting a very conservative statistical approach, only considered the 20-mg/day dosage to be superior to placebo). Patients treated with paroxetine 20 mg/day and 60 mg/day also had significantly better responses on the social item of the Sheehan Disability Scale than did patients treated with placebo.

D.J. Stein et al. (2002b), in a reanalysis of three randomized, controlled trials, studied the time course of response to paroxetine in subjects with social anxiety disorder. Of 132 responders at week 4 (as determined by a CGI score of 1 or 2), 111 (84%) remained responders at week 12. In the placebo group, of 56 responders by week 4, 40 (71%) remained responders at week 12. Furthermore, of 166 patients classified as paroxetine nonresponders at week 8, 46 (28%) became responders at week 12 after continuing treatment with paroxetine, suggesting that the length of treatment should be prolonged for more than 8 weeks to be optimal. In the placebo group, only 15 (8.2%) who were nonresponders at week 8 became responders at week 12.

Sertraline

In the first controlled trial of sertraline for social anxiety disorder, Katzelnick et al. (1995) randomly assigned 12 patients to receive sertraline or placebo using a crossover study design. The patients were randomly assigned to initially receive either sertraline (n=6) (50–200 mg/day, flexible dosing) or placebo (n=6) for 10 weeks, followed by dosage tapering and no treatment for 2 weeks. The patients were subsequently crossed over to the other treatment group for another 10 weeks. Sertraline dosage was initially 50 mg/day and increased by 50 mg/day every 2 weeks if no treatment response was seen, unless the patient was unable to tolerate it. The mean daily dosage at the end of sertraline treatment was 133.5 mg (SD=68.5; range 50–200 mg/day). The main outcome measure was the LSAS score. A statistically significant improvement on the LSAS was found with sertraline but not with placebo. The mean change in total score with sertraline was 22.0 (SD=17.3), compared with 5.5 (SD=15.8) with placebo.

In a larger double-blind controlled trial, Van Ameringen et al. (2001) randomly assigned 204 patients to receive sertraline (n=135) or placebo (n=69) for 20 weeks. The starting dosage was 50 mg/day and the maximum allowed dosage was 200 mg/day. The mean dosage at endpoint was 146.7 mg/day (SD=57). Sertraline was found to be superior to placebo, with response rates of 53% (71 of 134) versus 29% (20 of 69) in the intent-to-treat sample at the end of 20 weeks, with response defined as a score of 1 or 2 on the CGI-Improvement (CGI-I) subscale. All secondary efficacy measures showed significantly greater improvement in patients in the sertraline group.

In order to evaluate the ability of sertraline to prevent relapse, the study included a continuation phase (Walker et al. 2000). Patients who were considered responders at the end of week 20 and had been receiving sertraline (n=50) were randomly assigned, again in a double-blind fashion, to either continue taking sertraline or switch to placebo, and patients (n=15) who were considered responders and had been receiving placebo continued to receive placebo under double-blind conditions for an additional 24 weeks. In the intent-to-treat analyses, 1 (4%) of the 25 patients in the sertraline-continuation group and 9 (36%) of the 25 patients in the placebo-switch group relapsed at study endpoint, a statistically significant difference. Overall, the risk for relapse in the placebo group was 10-fold the risk for relapse in the sertraline group. The sertraline group had larger improvements in CGI–Severity of Illness (CGI-S) subscale, Marks Fears Questionnaire–Social Phobia subscale, and Brief Social Phobia Scale (BSPS) scores.

A study by Blomhoff et al. (2001) compared the efficacy of sertraline, exposure therapy, or their combination in a general practice setting. A total of 387 patients received sertraline at a dose that ranged from 50 to 150 mg/day or placebo for a 24-week period. Patients were further randomly assigned to receive either exposure therapy or general medical care. Response was defined as a reduction of at least 50% of SPS (Social Phobia Scale) symptom burden compared to baseline, a CGI-SP score <3, and a CGI-SP overall improvement score <2. Combined use of sertraline and exposure therapy and the use of sertraline alone were significantly superior to placebo. No differences were found between patients in the exposure therapy and nonexposure therapy groups. Sertraline with exposure did not differ from sertraline alone. No difference was found between exposure alone and placebo.

A more recent study conducted by Liebowitz et al. (2003) randomly assigned 211 patients to receive sertraline (flexible dosing, ≤200 mg/day) or placebo. The study found that at week 12 sertraline was associated with a significantly greater reduction in the LSAS score than placebo. Using a score of 1or 2 in the CGI scale as the criterion, 47% of subjects in the sertraline group were considered responders versus 26% in the placebo group.

Citalopram and Escitalopram

To date, only one small open-label trial of citalopram for the treatment of social anxiety disorder has been published. It consisted of 10 patients with generalized social anxiety disorder, 6 of whom had not responded to or had not tolerated prior treatment with a medication. The mean dosage was 55 mg/day (SD=12.7). Citalopram was well tolerated, and patients improved significantly on all outcome measures (Simon et al. 2002).

More information is available on escitalopram for the treatment of social anxiety disorder. A 12-week placebo-controlled trial conducted by Kasper et al. (2005) evaluated the efficacy of escitalopram in treating generalized social anxiety disorder. A total of 358 patients were randomly assigned to receive escitalopram at a dosage of 10–20 mg/day (n=181) or placebo (n=177). The study found a 54% response rate (defined as CGI-I score of 1 or 2) with escitalopram versus a 39% response rate in the placebo group (P<0.01) and a significant reduction in the work and social items of the Sheehan Disability Scale in the escitalopram group. The LSAS total score decreased from 96.3 (SD=17.4) at baseline to 62.2 (SD=30.7) by the end of week 12 in the escitalopram group compared with a decrease from 95.4 (SD=16.4) to 68.8 (SD=29.7) in the placebo group.

This treatment difference in week-12 change from baseline favoring escitalopram was statistically significant. The mean dosage at week 12 was 17.6 mg/day. Escitalopram was well tolerated in general, with headache as the most common side effect.

A smaller trial (Pallanti and Quercioli 2006) was conducted with 29 subjects in whom at least one previous treatment with paroxetine (≥60 mg/day for ≥12 weeks) had failed; in this study subjects received escitalopram in an open-label fashion for 12 weeks. Patients with a concurrent diagnosis of major depressive episode or marked depressive symptoms were excluded, as were patients meeting criteria for other Axis I disorders. Low-dose benzodiazepine medication for the control of sleep disorders was permitted. Of the 29 patients, 24 (82.8%) completed the trial. Three patients dropped out due to noncompliance without experiencing significant side effects, and the other two withdrew due to increased anxiety/agitation during the first week. The mean dosage of escitalopram in the patients completing the trial was 18.5 mg/day. At the end of week 12, 14 of the 29 subjects (48.3%) were considered responders on the basis of the CGI-I score (much or very much improved) and the LSAS score (>35% reduction from baseline).

With regard to long-term treatment, Lader et al. (2004) conducted a randomized, double-blind, placebo-controlled, fixed-dose trial that compared placebo (n=166), escitalopram 5 mg (n=167), escitalopram 10 mg (n=167), escitalopram 20 mg (n=170), and paroxetine 20 mg (n=169). The trial had a 24-week duration and included patients who had generalized social anxiety disorder. At week 12, both the 5-mg and 20-mg doses of escitalopram and the paroxetine 20-mg dose were significantly more efficacious than placebo. Escitalopram efficacy at the 10-mg dose nearly reached significance compared with placebo (P=0.059). Response to treatment, defined as a CGI-I of 2 or less, was significantly superior in all active treatment groups compared with placebo at week 12. At week 24, escitalopram was superior to placebo at all doses, and escitalopram 20 mg was significantly superior to paroxetine from week 16 onward based on the change from baseline in mean LSAS score.

A study by Montgomery et al. (2005) examined the ability of escitalopram to decrease rates of relapse after acute treatment of social anxiety disorder. The study was divided into two phases. In the first phase of this study, 517 patients with a long duration of generalized anxiety disorder entered a 12-week open-label trial with a flexible dosage of escitalopram (10–20 mg/day). Patients who responded (n=371) (with response defined as having a CGI-I score of ≤2) were then allocated to a 24-week double-blind, randomized study with either escitalopram (continuing the dosage level administered at the end of the open-label trial) (n=190) or placebo (n=181). Relapse was defined as either an increase in LSAS total score of at least 10 compared with the score at randomization or withdrawal due to lack of efficacy. Using survival analysis estimates, investigators found a 22% relapse rate in the escitalopram group compared with a 50% relapse rate in patients receiving placebo (log-rank test, P<0.001). The study found the relapse risk was 2.8 times higher for placebo-treated patients than for escitalopram-treated patients. The estimated median time to relapse was 407 days in the escitalopram group versus 144 days in the placebo group.

Some of these studies were used for further analysis of the effect of escitalopram on different patient subgroups and symptom dimensions. In an exploratory factor analysis of the LSAS, D.J. Stein et al. (2004b) defined six symptom dimensions: social interaction, eating/drinking in public, speaking in public, assertiveness, observation fear, and partying. The analysis gathered data from the three randomized, controlled trials mentioned above (Kasper et al. 2005; Lader et al. 2004; Montgomery et al. 2005), which included patients with a severe level of symptoms and no comorbid disorders. Escitalopram was found to be significantly superior to placebo in terms of all six factors. The analysis also found escitalopram to be efficacious in both genders, in patients with both more severe and less severe symptoms, in patients with both chronic and less chronic forms of the disorder, and in patients with or without comorbid depressive symptoms. In a similar analysis, D.J. Stein et al. (2006) found escitalopram 20 mg to be more efficacious than paroxetine 20 mg for five of the six symptom dimensions in the 24-week Lader et al. (2004) trial.

Fluvoxamine

Van Vliet et al. (1994) conducted a 12-week placebo-controlled study of fluvoxamine in 30 patients with social anxiety disorder. Fluvoxamine dosages were initially 50 mg/day and gradually increased to 150 mg/day, depending on tolerance to side effects. Efficacy was measured with the LSAS, Hopkins Symptom Checklist–90, Hamilton Anxiety Scale, and State-Trait Anxiety Inventory. One patient taking fluvoxamine dropped out because of nausea, and one patient taking placebo dropped out because of lack of efficacy. At the end of the study, patients taking fluvoxamine showed statistically significant improvement on all scales compared with the placebo recipients. A 50% reduction in the LSAS score was used as the criterion for response; 7 of the 15 patients (47%) taking fluvoxamine and 1 of the 15 (7%) taking placebo were classified as responders to treatment. Fourteen of the 15 patients (93%) taking fluvoxamine chose to enter a 12-week continuation phase of the study. Further improvement was seen in general anxiety and in scores on both the fear and avoidance subscales of the LSAS.

Fluvoxamine also was superior to placebo in the treatment of social anxiety disorder in a multicenter randomized trial (N=92) conducted by M.B. Stein et al. (1999). In this 12-week trial, subjects were assigned to receive either fluvoxamine (50–300 mg/day) (n=48) or placebo (n=44). Almost all patients (91.3%) had generalized social anxiety disorder. The mean dosage of fluvoxamine at study endpoint was 202 mg/day (SD=86). Significantly more patients responded to fluvoxamine (42.9%) than to placebo (22.7%) as defined by a CGI-I score of 1 or 2. Fluvoxamine was separated statistically from placebo on all social anxiety disorder rating scales at week 8 and beyond. It was statistically superior to placebo on all three social anxiety disorder dimensions (i.e., fear, avoidance, and physiological symptoms) measured by the BSPS. Fluvoxamine also resulted in significantly greater decreases in measures of psychosocial disability than did placebo.

The controlled-release form of fluvoxamine has also been investigated for treatment of the generalized subtype of social anxiety disorder (Westenberg et al. 2004). Fluvoxamine CR at flexible doses ranging from 100 to 300 mg/day (n=146) was compared to placebo (n=148) in a randomized, controlled trial lasting 12 weeks. The mean dosage at study endpoint was 209 mg/day. There was a statistically significant improvement compared with placebo in the mean change from baseline in LSAS total score from week 4 onward. CGI-S, Sheehan Disability Scale, and CGI-I scores also showed statistically significant improvements in the fluvoxamine group compared with the placebo group. Response rates (with response defined as a CGI-I of ≤2) were not statistically different among fluvoxamine CR and placebo recipients.

In another trial of fluvoxamine CR (Davidson et al. 2004b), 279 patients with social anxiety disorder were randomly assigned to receive fluvoxamine CR (100–300 mg/day) or placebo for 12 weeks. Treatment with fluvoxamine CR resulted in statistically and clinically significant improvements in symptoms associated with generalized social anxiety disorder as early as week 4, which continued through week 12, as shown on LSAS and CGI-I scores, and from week 6 to week 12 on the Sheehan Disability Scale, CGI-S, and Patient Global Impression–Improvement scores. Fluvoxamine CR was also statistically superior to placebo with regard to the LSAS fear and avoidance subscales from week 4 onward. Reported side effects were similar to the ones in previous studies.

Fluoxetine

Initial uncontrolled studies of fluoxetine (Black et al. 1992; Schneier et al. 1992; Sternbach 1990; Van Ameringen et al. 1993) also suggested that fluoxetine could be efficacious in the treatment of social anxiety disorder. There have been three placebo-controlled studies of fluoxetine for social anxiety disorder. Kobak et al. (2002) randomly assigned 60 patients to 14 weeks of treatment with either fluoxetine, at doses ranging between 20 and 60 mg/day, or placebo. At the end of the study, no significant differences were found between fluoxetine and placebo recipients.

In the second trial, D.M. Clark et al. (2003) randomly assigned 60 patients meeting the criteria for generalized social anxiety disorder to receive cognitive therapy, fluoxetine plus self-exposure, or placebo plus self-exposure for 16 weeks. After 16 weeks, the medication blind was broken and patients in the fluoxetine plus self-exposure group continued their medication for 3 months and had up to three treatment sessions during a "booster period." Patients in the CT group had the same number of booster sessions. Patients initially allocated to placebo were withdrawn from the trial at 16 weeks and offered their choice of CT, fluoxetine plus self-exposure, or a combination of both treatments. The study found significant improvements on most measures in all three treatment groups. On measures of social anxiety disorder, CT was superior to fluoxetine plus self-exposure and placebo plus self-exposure at midtreatment and posttreatment. The efficacy of fluoxetine plus self-exposure was not different from that of placebo plus self-exposure. CT remained superior to fluoxetine plus self-exposure at the end of the booster period and at 12-month follow-up. Additionally, there were few differences between the treatments with regard to general mood measures.

The third randomized, controlled trial (Davidson et al. 2004a) compared fluoxetine, comprehensive group CBT, placebo, and the combinations of comprehensive CBT (CCBT) plus fluoxetine and CCBT plus placebo in a 14-week randomized, double-blind, placebo-controlled trial. Two hundred ninety-five patients were randomly assigned to the treatment groups and were included in the intent-to-treat analysis. Response rates (CGI-I≤2) in the intent-to-treat sample were 50.9% (n=29) in the fluoxetine group, 31 51.7% (n=31) in the CCBT group, 54.2% (n=32) in the CCBT plus fluoxetine group, 50.8% (n=30) in the CCBT plus placebo group, and 31.7% (n=19) in the placebo group, with all treatments being significantly better than placebo. On the BSPS, all active treatments were superior to placebo. In the linear mixed-effects models analysis, all active treatments were superior to placebo but did not differ from each other.

Overall, these findings suggest that fluoxetine may have some efficacy in the treatment of social anxiety disorder, but the results appear less robust than the results with other SSRIs.

Summary

In summary, several randomized, controlled trials have established the efficacy of both SSRIs and serotonin-norepinephrine reuptake inhibitors (SNRIs; see "Serotonin-Norepinephrine Reuptake Inhibitors" section below) in the treatment of generalized social anxiety disorder. The fact that SSRIs and SNRIs share similar pharmacological properties and safety profiles has supported their role as the first-line pharmacological agents. None of these medications has been established as superior to another in efficacy or acceptability, although fluoxetine is the only SSRI with two published randomized, controlled trials that failed to demonstrate efficacy superior to that of placebo (D.M. Clark et al. 2003; Kobak et al. 2002) and one showing some effect (Davidson et al. 2004a). Fluvoxamine (M.B. Stein et al. 1999; van Vliet et al. 1994) and escitalopram (Kasper et al. 2005; Lader et al. 2004) have randomized, controlled trial support for efficacy but have not received FDA approval for the specific indication of generalized social anxiety disorder. Paroxetine in its immediate-release and controlled-release forms is one of the SSRIs most studied in randomized, controlled trials for the treatment of social anxiety disorder, and it was the first drug to receive FDA approval for this indication. It is the only SSRI, however, to be classified in pregnancy risk class D, a disadvantage for the substantial population of women of childbearing potential with social anxiety disorder, and in some studies paroxetine has manifested higher rates of adverse effects, such as weight gain and withdrawal symptoms (e.g., Aberg-Wistedt et al. 2000). As discussed in the next section, venlafaxine has also proved to be efficacious, with some trials suggesting its efficacy is similar to that of paroxetine. Less information is available on duloxetine; larger studies will help clarify its role.

Dose-response curves with SSRIs have been shown to be relatively flat in patients with this disorder. Although most patients can tolerate regular starting doses without experiencing the hyperstimulation common in panic disorder patients, medication is frequently initiated at half the usual effective dose, with dose increases after the first week of treatment. Because some patients appear to benefit from higher doses, it is a common practice to increase the dosage as tolerated in those who have no response after 4 weeks of treatment.

Serotonin-Norepinephrine Reuptake Inhibitors

Venlafaxine

A preliminary open-label trial (Emmanuel et al. 1995) on the efficacy of venlafaxine has been followed by larger randomized, controlled trials. Rickels et al. (2004) randomly assigned 272 patients to receive venlafaxine ER (the extended-release formulation) at flexible dosages (75–225 mg/day) or placebo for 12 weeks. Venlafaxine ER was superior to placebo on total LSAS scores from week 4 onward. Scores on the CGI-S, CGI-I, and Sheehan Disability Scale also showed venlafaxine ER to be more efficacious than placebo after week 4. A higher percentage of patients in the venlafaxine ER group than in the placebo group discontinued the study because of adverse effects. Adverse effects and failure to return were the main reasons for discontinuation in the venlafaxine ER group, whereas unsatisfactory response was the predominant reason among patients in the placebo group.

In a second trial, Liebowitz et al. (2005b) randomly assigned 279 subjects to receive either venlafaxine ER or placebo. Venlafaxine ER was significantly better than placebo on the LSAS, CGI-I, and Social Phobia Inventory (SPIN) scores. Response (defined as a 1 or 2 on the CGI scale) and remission (defined as an LSAS score of ≤30) rates were significantly greater in the venlafaxine ER group than in the placebo group, with response rates of 44% versus 30% and remission rates of 20% versus 7%. Adverse effects that led to withdrawal included nausea, dizziness, and insomnia. There were no reports of serious adverse events.

In addition, a double-blind, controlled trial conducted by M.B. Stein et al. (2005) randomly assigned 395 subjects with generalized social anxiety disorder to receive either venlafaxine ER at a fixed low dosage (75 mg/day) (n=131), venlafaxine ER at a higher flexible dosage (150–225 mg/day) (n=130), or placebo (n=134) for 28 weeks. A greater and sustained improvement (decrease in LSAS total score) occurred in both of the venlafaxine ER groups compared with the placebo group. By the end of the 28 weeks, 33% of placebo-treated patients were considered responders (defined as CGI scores of ≤2) compared with 58% of venlafaxine ER–treated patients (combining the high- and low-dosage groups; P<0.001 vs. placebo), with no significant differences in response rates between the low- and higher-dosage venlafaxine groups. The same was observed regarding remission (defined as an LSAS score of ≤30), with a 16% remission rate in the placebo group and a 31% rate in venlafaxine ER recipients (combining the high- and low-dosage groups; P<0.01 vs. placebo) and no significant difference between the two venlafaxine groups.

Two randomized trials of venlafaxine have included paroxetine as an active comparator in addition to placebo (Allgulander et al. 2004; Liebowitz et al. 2005a). In the first trial (Allgulander et al. 2004), patients with generalized social anxiety disorder (N=434) were randomly assigned to receive venlafaxine ER (75–225 mg/day), paroxetine (20–50 mg/day), or placebo for 12 weeks. Whereas response rates (with response defined as CGI-I scores of ≤2) for both active treatment groups were significantly greater than those for the placebo group as early as week 3, remission emerged earlier with venlafaxine (week 4) than with paroxetine (week 8). Remission rates (with remission defined as an LSAS total score of <30) were 38% in the venlafaxine ER group, 29% in the paroxetine group, and 13% in the placebo group (P<0.001 for venlafaxine ER vs. placebo; P=0.002 for paroxetine vs. placebo).

In the second trial (Liebowitz et al. 2005a), 440 patients with generalized social anxiety disorder were randomly assigned to receive venlafaxine ER (n=146), paroxetine (n=147), or placebo (n=147) for 12 weeks. The reduction in LSAS mean score was significantly greater in the venlafaxine ER and paroxetine groups than in the placebo group. Response rates were significantly greater (P<0.001) with both venlafaxine ER and paroxetine (58.6% and 62.5%, respectively) than with placebo (36.1%).

Duloxetine

This new antidepressant belonging to the SNRI class has been shown to be effective at dosages of 60–120 mg/day in the treatment of depression and generalized anxiety disorder. Crippa et al. (2007) have described two case reports of patients with generalized social anxiety disorder treated with duloxetine. Neither of them had any Axis I comorbid disorders. Patients started taking duloxetine at a dosage of 60 mg/day for 4 weeks, which then increased to 120 mg/day; in the case of the second patient, the dosage had to be reduced back to 60 mg/day. The first patient's BSPS score decreased from 64 at baseline to 31 at week 4 and decreased to 17 after week 8. CGI-S scores decreased from 7 to 2 by week 8. For the second patient, the BSPS score decreased from 60 at baseline to 38 and 24—and CGI-S scores decreased from 6 to 5 and 2—after 4 and 8 weeks of treatment, respectively. A 6-month follow-up of both patients showed no relapse of their social anxiety symptoms. Randomized, controlled trials evaluating duloxetine's efficacy in the short- and long-term treatment of social anxiety disorder are currently ongoing.

Monoamine Oxidase Inhibitors

Irreversible, Nonselective Monoamine Oxidase Inhibitors

Monoamine oxidase inhibitors (MAOIs) were the first antidepressants to be widely studied as a treatment for social anxiety disorder. The suggestion that MAOIs might have efficacy in the treatment of social anxiety disorder first came from two different sources. One line of evidence consisted of placebo-controlled studies of phenelzine in mixed phobic populations (Sheehan et al. 1980; Solyom et al. 1981). Although those studies had important methodological problems, such as the lack of operationalized diagnostic criteria, small sample sizes, and the use of low doses of medication, all of them reported a significant improvement in symptom measures related to social anxiety disorder. The second line of evidence came from studies on the use of phenelzine in patients with atypical depression. Two studies in the early 1980s found that phenelzine ameliorated interpersonal sensitivity (Liebowitz et al. 1984; Paykel et al. 1982). Because interpersonal sensitivity may be common to both social anxiety disorder and atypical depression, the findings suggested that MAOIs may be useful in the treatment of social anxiety disorder.

Phenelzine. Four double-blind, placebo-controlled trials have studied the efficacy of phenelzine in social anxiety disorder. Liebowitz et al. (1992) randomly assigned 85 patients to 8-week treatment with phenelzine, atenolol, or placebo. Mean medication dosages were as follows: phenelzine, 75.7 mg/day (SD=16; range 45–90 mg/day); atenolol, 97.6 mg/day (SD=10.9; range 50–100 mg/day). Only patients who completed at least 4 weeks of treatment, with 2 weeks at therapeutic dosages (phenelzine 45 mg/day or atenolol 50 mg/day), were included in the statistical analysis (n=74). A CGI scale rating of 1–2 was used to define responders, and the response rates were as follows: phenelzine, 64%; atenolol, 30%; and placebo, 23%. Both social and performance anxiety were reduced, and social and work functioning improved. Improvements were greater as assessed by the clinician's scales than by self-ratings. Responders were enrolled for an additional 8 weeks to study the durability of the improvement and the possibility of further gains, but no additional improvements in clinical status were detected.

In a second study, Gelernter and colleagues (1991) randomly assigned 65 patients to one of four treatment groups: 1) group CBT, 2) phenelzine, 3) alprazolam, or 4) placebo. All pharmacotherapy and placebo recipients were also given exposure instructions. Duration of the trial was 12 weeks for all treatments. Clinician raters were blind to the particular medication groups but not to medication versus group therapy. Medication dosages were increased until all social phobic symptoms had disappeared, until side effects precluded further increases, or until the maximum medication dosage was reached (i.e., phenelzine 90 mg/day, alprazolam 6.3 mg/day). Actual mean dosages were phenelzine 55 mg/day (SD=16; range 30–90 mg/day) and alprazolam 4.2 mg/day (SD=1.3; range 2.1–6.3 mg/day). At 12 weeks, phenelzine and alprazolam both were associated with superior ratings on the physician-rated Work and Disability Scale compared with placebo. CBT recipients were not rated on this scale. Phenelzine also was superior to all the other treatments on the State-Trait Anxiety Inventory (Spielberger 1983). At 2-month follow-up, those gains were maintained. Patients were considered responders if their final social anxiety disorder scores on the Fear Questionnaire (Marks and Mathews 1979) were equal to or below those of normative samples. According to that criterion, 69% of the patients taking phenelzine were responders, compared with 38% of those taking alprazolam, 24% of those receiving CBT, and 20% of those taking placebo.

The third study, conducted by Versiani and colleagues (1992), was a comparison of phenelzine, moclobemide, and placebo. It included 78 patients and consisted of three 8-week phases. Nonresponders (according to CGI scores) in each 8-week phase were withdrawn from the study. Responders in each 8-week phase were randomly assigned to either active treatment or placebo. In the acute phase, patients given phenelzine had their dosages titrated up to 90 mg/day or the highest tolerated dosage, whereas patients given moclobemide had dosages titrated up to 600 mg/day or the highest tolerated dosage. The actual mean dosage of phenelzine was 67.5 mg/day (SD=15.0), and the actual mean dosage of moclobemide was 570.7 mg/day (SD=55.6). At week 8, phenelzine was superior to placebo on all global and social anxiety disorder measures. Additionally, phenelzine was superior to moclobemide on the social avoidance subscale of the LSAS (Liebowitz 1987). Responders were defined as patients with a CGI score of 1 or 2, as well as at least a 70% decline on the LSAS. Of the patients taking phenelzine who completed 16 weeks of treatment, 91% were classified as responders. Those patients within the active treatment groups who were switched to placebo in the third phase of the study had an increase in the mean scores of all parameters at week 24, indicating that some patients relapse when treatment is discontinued. Although 59% of the patients had met criteria for avoidant personality disorder at baseline, at week 8 only 3 of the patients taking active drugs—compared with 14 of 16 in the placebo group—continued to meet those criteria. Moclobemide was also superior to placebo in this study (see "Moclobemide" section).

In the fourth study, Heimberg et al. (1998) recruited 133 patients for a study comparing phenelzine, placebo, an educational supportive group, and group CBT for 12 weeks. Phenelzine and CBT were superior to the other treatments, and phenelzine also was superior to CBT on some measures. Patients with generalized social anxiety disorder were more impaired at the initiation of the study and remained more impaired at the end of the trial than patients with nongeneralized social anxiety disorder, but there were no differences in the degree of change in the two groups.

Tranylcypromine. Tranylcypromine, another MAOI, has been studied in only two published open-label trials. In the first one (Versiani et al. 1988), 32 patients with social anxiety disorder were followed for 1 year. The treatment phase lasted 1 year; after that, the drug was discontinued gradually during 1 week. Three dropped out in the first month of treatment, did not achieve a minimum dosage of 40 mg/day for 2 weeks, and were not included in the analyses. Of the remaining 29 patients, 62% showed marked improvement, 17% showed moderate improvement, and 21% showed no improvement. In all responders, improvement was maintained throughout the year. In some instances, initial improvement waned temporarily but was restored by increasing the dosage. When tranylcypromine was discontinued, 62% of the patients relapsed to baseline within 3 months, and an additional 22% had a partial return of their symptoms.

In a second tranylcypromine study, an 8-week open-label trial including 81 patients, Versiani et al. (1989) found statistically significant reductions in both CGI-S and LSAS scores. CGI-S scores decreased from 5.2 (SD=0.9) to 1.5 (SD=1.0). LSAS scores changed from 90.4 (SD=18.7) to 28.2 (SD=17.9).

Summary. Substantial evidence shows that phenelzine is highly efficacious in the treatment of many patients with social anxiety disorder. However, the side-effect profile of irreversible, nonselective MAOIs such as phenelzine and tranylcypromine—particularly the risk of hypertensive crisis if a low-tyramine diet and related precautions are not strictly followed—has led to the preference for using SSRIs and venlafaxine in clinical practice.

Reversible Inhibitors of Monoamine Oxidase A

The limitations of standard nonreversible MAOIs led to the development of the reversible inhibitors of monoamine oxidase A (RIMAs), which have a significantly lesser ability to potentiate the pressor effect of tyramine. This allows for relaxation or total elimination of dietary restrictions. Other MAOI side effects such as fatigue and hypotension also seem to be much less common with RIMAs. Unfortunately, their efficacy in treating social anxiety disorder appears inferior to that of phenelzine. No RIMAs are currently marketed in the United States. Two RIMAs have been studied: moclobemide and brofaromine (which is an SSRI in addition to a RIMA).

Moclobemide. Five double-blind, placebo-controlled studies of moclobemide have been published, with mixed results. In the aforementioned study by Versiani and coworkers (1992) (see the "Phenelzine" section), moclobemide was superior to placebo as measured on the LSAS, CGI scale, Social Avoidance and Distress Scale (Watson and Friend 1969), and Willoughby Personality Inventory (Willoughby 1932), an index of social anxiety, at the end of week 8. Moclobemide was as efficacious as phenelzine on all measures, except on the social avoidance subscale of the LSAS. Among the 21 week-8 responders who entered a continuation phase, 14 (67%) were classified as responders at the end of week 16. Moclobemide was much better tolerated than phenelzine, with rates of side effects similar to those in placebo recipients, especially in the second phase of the study.

A larger double-blind, multicenter study (International Multicenter Clinical Trial Group on Moclobemide in Social Phobia 1997) compared two dosages of moclobemide (300 and 600 mg/day) with placebo over a 12-week period. The 600-mg dosage was superior to placebo on all measures of social anxiety disorder, general anxiety, and disability. The 300-mg dosage was superior to placebo as measured on the LSAS and Patient Impression of Change–Social Phobia scale. However, the magnitude of drug-versus-placebo differences on both dosages was smaller than those seen in the Versiani et al. (1992) study or studies of other active compounds such as phenelzine, clonazepam, or the SSRIs.

Noyes et al. (1997) compared five dosages of moclobemide (75, 150, 300, 600, and 900 mg/day) versus placebo in a 12-week double-blind study. Those assigned to the 75- and 150-mg/day groups received the full dosage from the time of randomization, and those assigned to the 300-, 600-, and 900-mg/day groups received 150 mg/day initially followed by increases in increments of 150 mg/day every 4 days until the full dosage was reached. None of the moclobemide dosages was superior to placebo. At the end of 12 weeks, 35% of the subjects who received 900 mg/day and 33% of those who received placebo were rated as at least much improved on the CGI scale.

Schneier et al. (1998) administered moclobemide or placebo to 77 patients with social anxiety disorder in a double-blind study with a flexible-dose design. Moclobemide was initiated at 100 mg twice a day and dosages were increased over 2 weeks to a maximum of 400 mg twice a day, adjusted as clinically indicated. The mean dosage was 728 mg/day in the moclobemide group. At the end of the eighth week, 7 (18%) of the 40 moclobemide recipients and 5 (14%) of the 37 placebo recipients were rated as much or very much improved on the CGI scale (responders). Moclobemide was superior to placebo on only 2 of 10 outcome measures. Patients who were rated by an independent evaluator to be at least minimally improved on the CGI scale after 8 weeks (n=21) were offered an additional 8 weeks of the same treatment. Among the nine moclobemide and seven placebo recipients who agreed to continue, some further improvement occurred on the CGI scale in the moclobemide group, but neither group showed significant changes on any continuous measures.

D.J. Stein et al. (2002a) randomly assigned 309 subjects with social anxiety disorder to treatment with moclobemide or placebo for 12 weeks. At the end of week 12, 43% of patients in the moclobemide group and 31% in the placebo group were considered responders ($P<0.01$) as defined by a CGI-S score of 1 or 2. Exploratory analyses showed that the presence of a comorbid anxiety disorder was predictive of response and that those with current dysthymia tended to have a somewhat lower response rate ($P=0.07$). Subjects were offered the option to continue for an additional 6 months of treatment. This phase included 50 patients taking moclobemide and 40 taking placebo. Patients in the moclobemide group continued to improve while some patients in the placebo group relapsed. At the end of month 9, 43 of 50 (86%) were considered responders in the moclobemide group, compared with 23 of 40 (58%) in the placebo group.

In summary, published placebo-controlled studies of moclobemide have shown mixed results. Overall, moclobemide is probably better tolerated but less efficacious than phenelzine in the treatment of social anxiety disorder.

Brofaromine. Even though brofaromine is classified as a reversible and selective, type A MAOI, this antidepressant also has serotonin reuptake inhibitory properties. Van Vliet et al. (1992) studied brofaromine in a 12-week placebo-controlled trial with 30 patients with social anxiety disorder. The brofaromine dosage was gradually increased from 50 mg/day to 150 mg/day (75 mg twice daily) over 3 weeks and then maintained at 150 mg/day for the rest of the study. Brofaromine was superior to placebo as measured on the LSAS, general (or anticipatory) anxiety, interpersonal sensitivity, obsessive-compulsive, and phobic avoidance subscales. Eighty percent of the patients taking brofaromine and 14% of those taking placebo judged themselves responders, although criteria for response were not provided. Based on a final Hamilton Anxiety Scale score of less than 10 as a criterion for response, 73% of the patients taking brofaromine were classified as responders, compared with 0% of the placebo group. The subjects taking brofaromine had an increase in plasma serotonin and melatonin levels and a decrease in 5-hydroxyindoleacetic acid, homovanillic acid, and 3-methoxy-4-hydroxyphenylglycol (MHPG) levels, suggesting that the drug was active. However, no data on the correlation between clinical and biochemical measures were provided. Twelve patients entered a follow-up phase of 12 additional weeks. Eleven patients (10 taking brofaromine and 1 taking placebo) completed that phase. In the patients taking brofaromine and the patient taking placebo, improvement in general anxiety and on the avoidance subscale, but not the anxiety subscale, of the LSAS was noted. Four months after discontinuing brofaromine, three patients had relapsed.

In a second double-blind trial, Fahlén et al. (1995) randomly assigned 77 patients to receive brofaromine ($n=37$) or placebo ($n=40$) for 12 weeks. Patients were given a fixed dosage of 150 mg/day or a matching placebo after a 2-week titration phase. A much or very much improved outcome on the CGI scale was used as the criterion for response; 78% of the patients taking brofaromine and 23% of those in the placebo group were classified as responders. Changes in LSAS scores also were significantly greater in the brofaromine group than in the placebo group. LSAS scores for the brofaromine and placebo groups were 67.2 and 65.3 at baseline, respectively. The corresponding endpoint mean scores were 34.4 and 53.3. The clinical effects were not correlated with blood levels of brofaromine. Further improvement was achieved by the brofaromine group during a 9-month follow-up period, whereas 60% of the placebo responders who continued long-term treatment relapsed.

In a third study, Lott et al. (1997) treated patients with brofaromine ($n=52$) or placebo ($n=50$) for 10 weeks. Brofaromine dosages were started at 50 mg/day and titrated up to 150 mg/day depending on tolerance and treatment response. The actual mean dosage of brofaromine was 107.2 mg/day (SD=27.9). Patients taking brofaromine had a significantly greater change from baseline on the LSAS than did patients taking placebo. A significantly greater percentage of the brofaromine recipients (50%) than placebo recipients (19%) were rated much or very much improved at study endpoint on the CGI scale. Mean LSAS scores decreased from 81.8 at baseline to 62.6 at endpoint in the brofaromine group and from 79.8 to 70.7 in the placebo group. The superiority of brofaromine over placebo in this trial could be characterized as modest because the endpoint LSAS score of 62.6 is still within the clinical range for social anxiety disorder. However, it is also important to take into account the small placebo response, suggesting either a difficult sample to treat or the use of very stringent ratings.

Summary. RIMAs were initially seen as promising alternatives to phenelzine and tranylcypromine. They seem to be safer and better tolerated than nonreversible MAOIs because they allow the dietary restrictions that are required with nonreversible MAOIs to be greatly relaxed or even eliminated. However, the evidence at hand suggests that RIMAs are also less effective. Moclobemide is not marketed in the United States, and brofaromine development was stopped by the manufacturer during the treatment trials for reasons unrelated to the efficacy or safety of the drug in social anxiety disorder.

Monoamine Oxidase B Inhibitors

Selegiline. Simpson et al. (1998b) conducted an open-label trial of selegiline, a selective MAO B inhibitor, in 16 patients with social anxiety disorder. The oral dosage of selegiline was fixed at 5 mg twice a day. Nine patients completed the trial. Two patients dropped out because of side effects, and one had to stop taking selegiline because of the need to take other medications that could cause toxic interactions with selegiline. Four patients were lost to follow-up. Only three patients were considered responders, with an average improvement of 33% in the LSAS score, suggesting only moderate efficacy with low-dose selegiline. Further research is needed to establish whether selegiline is more efficacious at higher doses.

Other Antidepressants

Tricyclic Antidepressants

Based on its efficacy in the treatment of panic disorder, imipramine has been studied in patients with social anxiety disorder, but these trials have failed to demonstrate its efficacy in the treatment of this disorder. Zitrin et al. (1983) found no improvement in patients with social anxiety disorder treated with imipramine. Benca et al. (1986) reported on two patients with social anxiety disorder who showed a rapid resolution of symptoms after treatment with imipramine (250 mg/day). Both patients had panic attacks and mitral valve prolapse, rendering them atypical. An open-label trial by Simpson et al. (1998a) did not find imipramine to be efficacious in social anxiety disorder. The authors treated 15 patients with imipramine at a mean dosage of 176.4 mg/day. Nine patients completed the study; six dropped out because of side effects. The mean change in the LSAS score was 15%. The response rate, defined as much or very much improved on the CGI scale, was 20%.

In two studies, clomipramine was used to treat social anxiety disorder. Beaumont (1977) treated a mixed population of patients with social anxiety disorder and agoraphobia, but only modest improvement was seen. The heterogeneity of the sample and the use of non-DSM-III (American Psychiatric Association 1980) criteria made interpretation of the data difficult. In a later study, Pecknold et al. (1982) combined clomipramine with L-tryptophan and compared it with the use of clomipramine plus placebo. No additional benefit was found from the addition of L-tryptophan.

Bupropion

Bupropion is a weak dopamine and norepinephrine reuptake inhibitor. Emmanuel et al. (1991) successfully treated one patient with bupropion (300 mg/day). Assessment of this case was complicated by the presence of comorbid depression in the patient. Others have reported negative results in a limited number of patients (Potts and Davidson 1995).

In a 12-week open-label trial with bupropion SR (sustained release) in patients with generalized social anxiety disorder, 5 of the 10 patients who completed the study were considered to be responders. Dosages at study endpoint ranged between 200 and 400 mg/day, with the medication being generally well tolerated (Emmanuel et al. 2000).

Nefazodone

Nefazodone appears to have both 5-hydroxytryptamine (5-HT; serotonin) reuptake and 5-HT type 2A (5-HT_{2A}) receptor blockade properties. To date, there has been only one randomized, placebo-controlled trial on the efficacy of nefazodone (Van Ameringen et al. 2007). A total of 105 patients were randomly assigned to receive nefazodone (n=52) or placebo (n=53) for 14 weeks. Dosages ranged from 300 to 600 mg/day. Patients with comorbid secondary major depressive disorder were permitted to take part in the study if their baseline score on the Montgomery-Åsberg Depression Rating Scale (MADRS) was 19 or less and no risk of suicide was evident. Mean dosage at endpoint was 493.9 (SD=128.1) mg/day. Patients in both groups improved, but there was no differential improvement with nefazodone versus placebo. Three patients who were randomly assigned to treatment did not take at least one dose of the study medication. Of 51 subjects in the nefazodone group, 16 (31.4%) were classified as responders (much or very much improved score on CGI-I at endpoint) compared with 12 of 51 (23.5%) in the placebo group, a nonsignificant difference. Using a decrease in LSAS score of at least 50% as the criterion for response and an LSAS score of 30 or less as the criterion for remission, the study also failed to find differences between the two treatment groups.

Reboxetine

Although not currently marketed in the United States, reboxetine is classified as an antidepressant with selective norepinephrine reuptake properties. There is only one open-label study (Atmaca et al. 2003) of its efficacy, involving 23 patients with social anxiety disorder. Of those, 20 had the generalized form of the disorder and 3 had the nongeneralized subtype. The dosage range was 4–8 mg/day. Of the 23 patients, 22 completed the 8-week trial. Reductions in the mean Hamilton Anxiety Scale scores and total LSAS scores from baseline to the last assessment were statistically significant. At week 8, 14 of the patients (63.6%) were considered responders with a 50% or greater reduction in LSAS total score and a score of 1 or 2 on the CGI-I. Reboxetine was well tolerated in general.

Mirtazapine

Mirtazapine has been on the market in the United States since 1996. Its mechanism of action is thought to be mediated by the blockade of several serotonin and α_2-adrenergic receptors. In an early open-label trial, Van Veen et al. (2002) treated 14 patients with generalized social anxiety disorder with mirtazapine (30 mg/day) for 12 weeks. Patients had no comorbid depression. Twelve patients completed the study. Two patients (14.3%) dropped out because of side effects, but mirtazapine was generally well tolerated. Five of the 12 patients who completed the study (41.7%) were classified as responders based on a CGI score of 1 or 2 and a 40% reduction in the LSAS score. The mean total score on the LSAS, as well as the anxiety and avoidance subscores, decreased significantly.

In a subsequent placebo-controlled study of mirtazapine, 66 female subjects were randomly assigned to a fixed 30 mg/day dosage of mirtazapine (n=33) or placebo (n=33) for 10 weeks (Muehlbacher et al. 2005). Primary outcome measures were self-reported changes on the SPIN, LSAS, and Short Form of the Medical Outcomes Study (SF-36). Mirtazapine was significantly superior to placebo on the SPIN and LSAS as well as on five of eight scales of the SF-36 (general health perceptions, vitality, social functioning, role-emotional, and mental health subscales). All patients tolerated mirtazapine relatively well. The most common side effects included dry mouth, drowsiness, sedation, increased appetite, and weight gain.

Benzodiazepines

Since the development of chlordiazepoxide several decades ago, benzodiazepines have been known to have anxiolytic properties. Benzodiazepines have been shown to be useful in the treatment of generalized anxiety disorder and panic disorder; a logical extension was to assess their usefulness in social anxiety disorder. However, the first reports of the efficacy of benzodiazepines for social anxiety disorder only appeared in the literature in the late 1980s (Deltito and Stam 1989; Lydiard et al. 1988). Even though clinical experience suggests that benzodiazepines may be effective when used on an as-needed basis for performance fears, systematic studies (i.e., clinical trials) have been conducted only for standing-dose treatment.

The most widely studied benzodiazepines for the treatment of social anxiety disorder are clonazepam and alprazolam. Several open-label trials with clonazepam have reported positive results. Versiani et al. (1989) treated 40 patients with social anxiety disorder for 8 weeks. Statistically significant decreases in the CGI-S and LSAS scores were noted between baseline and posttreatment assessment. Munjack and colleagues (1990) compared 10 patients treated with clonazepam and 10 patients who received no treatment, matching them for baseline severity of illness. Of the clonazepam recipients, three were rated as very much improved on the CGI scale, three much improved, three minimally improved, and one unchanged. In the no-treatment group, one patient was rated as markedly improved and one mildly improved. The clonazepam group also was superior to the no-treatment group on the LSAS and self-ratings of social anxiety. However, scores of social disability did not change.

Ontiveros and Fontaine (1990) treated five patients with clonazepam at an average dosage of 3 mg/day; all patients improved. Reiter et al. (1990) treated 11 patients with clonazepam. Six were very much improved, one was much improved, and two were minimally improved.

Following those results, clonazepam showed efficacy in a 10-week placebo-controlled study of 75 patients (Davidson et al. 1993). The mean dosage of clonazepam at endpoint was 2.4 mg/day (range 0.5–3 mg/day). At the end of the treatment, 78% of the patients taking clonazepam were classified as responders according to the CGI scale, compared with 20% of patients taking placebo. Drug effects were evident on measures of performance and generalized social anxiety, fear and phobic avoidance, interpersonal sensitivity, fears of negative evaluation, and disability. Prior to this double-blind study, Davidson and coworkers (1991) had conducted an open-label trial with 26 patients treated for an average of 11.3 months (range 1–20 months). At the end of the trial, 42% of the patients were very much improved, 42% were much improved, and 15% were minimally or not improved.

Two open-label trials and one double-blind study of alprazolam in social anxiety disorder have been performed. In the first open-label trial, Lydiard and colleagues (1988) administered alprazolam, in dosages ranging from 3 to 8 mg/day, to four patients. All four patients had moderate to marked reduction of their symptoms. One of the patients who initially had a partial response had a full response when phenelzine was added. The duration of treatment was not reported. In the second open-label trial, Reich and Yates (1988) treated 14 patients for 8 weeks. The mean dosage of alprazolam was 2.9 mg/day (range 1–7 mg/day). Ten patients were very much improved and four were much improved on the CGI scale. One week after drug discontinuation, however, symptoms returned to baseline. It was unclear whether that was due, at least in part, to alprazolam withdrawal. In the only double-blind study of alprazolam, Gelernter et al. (1991) compared phenelzine, alprazolam, placebo, and CBT. The mean alprazolam dosage was 4.2 mg/day (SD=1.3). Response was defined as a posttreatment Fear Questionnaire score equal to or below the scores of a normative sample of individuals without social anxiety disorder. Only 38% of the patients taking alprazolam were considered responders at 12 weeks. Patients were reassessed 2 months after discontinuation of alprazolam. In most cases, symptoms had returned, suggesting the low durability of already limited gains. Given the time lapse since discontinuation of the drug, it is unlikely that those symptoms represented benzodiazepine withdrawal.

The use of bromazepam to treat social anxiety disorder has also been reported. Versiani et al. (1989) treated 10 patients in an 8-week open-label trial. The mean dosage was 26.4 mg/day (SD=4.9). CGI-S scores decreased from a baseline of 5.0 (SD=0.8) to 1.3 (SD=0.5) at the end of treatment. The LSAS score improved from a baseline of 69.3 (SD=20.5) to 15.8 (SD=9.1) at week 8. In a subsequent study, Versiani et al. (1997) randomly assigned 30 patients to receive bromazepam (dosages ≤36 mg/day) or placebo for 12 weeks. Bromazepam was superior to placebo on the LSAS, CGI, and Sheehan Disability Scale scores and other secondary measures.

In summary, all open-label trials suggest that benzodiazepines are useful in the treatment of social anxiety disorder. In double-blind studies, clonazepam and bromazepam, but not alprazolam, have been superior to placebo. Whether those differences are due to true differential efficacy or are related to study design and sampling requires further examination. Benzodiazepines also may be helpful used on an as-needed basis for performance anxiety. The benefit of decreased anxiety must be balanced with the risk of sedation interfering with the quality of performance. It must be taken into account that patients with social anxiety disorder can present with other comorbid psychiatric disorders, such as depression. Benzodiazepines are not recommended as monotherapy for patients with concomitant major depression and must be used with caution in patients with a history of substance use disorders.

β-Adrenergic Blockers

β-Adrenergic blockers came into use initially as a treatment for cardiac conditions and subsequently showed efficacy in the treatment of essential tremor. Later studies showed a connection between anxiety, signs and symptoms of peripheral arousal, and increased plasma levels of norepinephrine. This led to beta-blocker trials in nonclinical samples of performers with high levels of anxiety (it is likely that those individuals currently would receive diagnoses of social anxiety disorder, nongeneralized subtype). The results of those trials seemed to indicate that beta-blockers are successful in decreasing the autonomic manifestations of anxiety. Beta-blockers are currently used on an as-needed basis for nongeneralized social anxiety disorder, based on anecdotal evidence from performers with social anxiety disorder. The controlled trials of beta-blockers to treat social anxiety disorder (described in this section) have used standing doses and have combined patients with generalized and nongeneralized social anxiety disorder. Although the results suggested that beta-blockers are not effective in treating the generalized subtype of the disorder, the subsamples of patients with the nongeneralized subtype have been too small to perform meaningful analyses.

Falloon et al. (1981) conducted a study of social skills training combined with either propranolol or placebo for patients with generalized social anxiety disorder. No treatment differences were found between the groups. However, results were difficult to interpret because of a small sample size and lack of a drug-only group.

Gorman et al. (1985) conducted an open-label trial of atenolol in 10 patients with social anxiety disorder. The number of patients with nongeneralized versus generalized social anxiety disorder was not reported.

Five patients had a marked reduction in social anxiety disorder symptoms and four reported a moderate reduction, as assessed by clinicians and patients. Medication generally was well tolerated.

However, in the aforementioned double-blind study of phenelzine (Liebowitz et al. 1992; see the "Phenelzine" section), the difference in response rates between patients taking atenolol versus placebo was nonsignificant (30% vs. 23%). The mean dosage of atenolol was 97.6 mg/day (SD=10.9). Some further improvement occurred in the 8-week continuation phase but still was not significantly different from results in the placebo group. The nongeneralized social anxiety disorder subgroup was too small to perform meaningful separate analyses.

Similarly, Turner at al. (1994) included 72 patients in a 12-week study of atenolol (25–100 mg/day) versus flooding versus placebo. Twenty-five patients were given atenolol, 26 were assigned to flooding (a type of exposure therapy), and 21 were given placebo. Patients who received behavior therapy were seen for 90 minutes twice a week for the first 2 months and once a week for the last month, for a total of 20 sessions. Flooding was superior to atenolol, which was not superior to placebo. On a composite index of improvement, 89% of patients in the flooding group improved, compared with 47% of patients in the atenolol group and 44% of the placebo group. Six months posttreatment, 9 of the 25 atenolol recipients and 6 of the 26 flooding recipients were lost to follow-up. However, those who were assessed had maintained most of their gains.

Beta-blockers have not been proven superior to placebo in controlled clinical trials for the treatment of social anxiety disorder. However, anecdotal experience and studies of samples of anxious performers suggest that they are effective in treating specific and circumscribed performance anxiety, especially for patients with prominent symptoms of sympathetic hyperarousal such as palpitations and tremor. Beta-blockers have the advantage over benzodiazepines of rarely impairing concentration or coordination. Nonselective beta-blockers (affecting both β_1 receptors in the heart and β_2 receptors that mediate tremor), such as propranolol or nadolol, may in theory be more effective than those that are selective for the β_1 receptor, such as atenolol or metoprolol, although this remains to be empirically tested (Schneier 1995). Patients may be instructed to try a test dose at home, to ensure that the degree of β-blockade is sufficient and that untoward side effects will not develop during a performance. Most healthy individuals tolerate propranolol quite well, especially because the sympathetic arousal of anxiety partly compensates for the hypotensive effects. Propranolol (10–40 mg) taken 45–60 minutes before the performance is sufficient for most patients.

Other Medications

Buspirone

Some studies have shown that the anxiolytic effects of buspirone can be as efficacious as those of benzodiazepines in the treatment of generalized anxiety disorder, with less addiction liability. Buspirone is an azaspirone that acts as a full agonist on the serotonin type 1A (5-HT_{1A}) autoreceptor and as a partial agonist on the postsynaptic 5-HT_{1A} receptor. Positive results of the trials with SSRIs for social anxiety disorder stimulated further research with drugs that have a serotonergic effect.

Munjack et al. (1991) conducted a 12-week open-label trial of buspirone in 17 patients with generalized social anxiety disorder. Eleven patients completed the trial, receiving an average dosage of 48 mg/day. Of those who completed the trial, 4 (36%) reported marked improvement, 5 (45%) reported moderate improvement, and 2 (18%) reported minimal improvement. The overall response rate (defined as marked or moderate improvement) was 53% of the original sample.

Schneier et al. (1993) conducted another 12-week open-label trial with 21 patients. Seventeen completed at least 2 weeks of treatment and were included in the analysis. The response rate in this study (47%) was similar to that in Munjack and colleagues' (1991) study. Interestingly, responders received a higher average dosage of buspirone than did nonresponders (56.9 vs. 38.3 mg/day).

D.B. Clark and Agras (1991) treated 34 musicians with social anxiety disorder. Subjects received 6 weeks of buspirone treatment, 6 weeks of placebo treatment, five sessions of group CBT plus buspirone, or five sessions of CBT plus placebo. The average dosage of buspirone was 32 mg/day. Buspirone was not superior to placebo, but CBT was superior to both buspirone without psychotherapy and placebo without psychotherapy.

Van Vliet et al. (1997) investigated the efficacy of buspirone in a 12-week placebo-controlled study. Thirty patients with social anxiety disorder were treated with fixed-dosage buspirone (30 mg/day) or placebo. Efficacy was measured with the LSAS and Hamilton Anxiety Scale. Response was defined as a 50% or greater reduction in LSAS scores. Only one patient receiving buspirone and another taking placebo were classified as responders. A subjective and clinically relevant improvement was reported by four patients taking buspirone and two taking placebo. There were no statistically significant differences between the two treatment groups on any of the outcome measures. Notably, the fixed dosage of buspirone was lower than the mean dosage taken by nonresponders in Schneier and associates' (1993) open-label trial. No correlations were found between baseline MHPG level and any of the outcome measures.

Neither of the two double-blind trials of buspirone was able to show efficacy with buspirone as monotherapy for social anxiety disorder, in contrast with the promising results of the open-label trials. Additionally, the dosage of buspirone needed seems to be near the upper end of its recommended dosage range (60 mg/day) for other, approved indications, which may limit its usefulness on the basis of side effects such as nausea or headache. Buspirone may, however, augment partial responses to SSRIs.

Pergolide

The postulated theory of dopamine dysregulation in social anxiety disorder has suggested a possible therapeutic role for this dopamine type 1 (D_1) and type 2 (D_2) receptor agonist used in the treatment of Parkinson's disease. Villarreal et al. (2000) treated four subjects openly with pergolide (25–600 μg/day). Two subjects completed the 12-week study. Two subjects dropped out after 4 weeks; one dropped out due to side effects/lack of efficacy, and one was lost to follow-up. Conclusions could not be drawn from such a small sample.

Anticonvulsants

Topiramate. This glutamatergic and γ-aminobutyric acid (GABA)–ergic anticonvulsant has been used for a variety of psychiatric disorders, ranging from bipolar disorder (Vasudev et al. 2006) to refractory depression (Dursun and Devarajan 2001), cocaine/alcohol dependence (Johnson 2005), and binge eating (Tata and Kockler 2006). Recently, Van Ameringen et al. (2004a) conducted a 16-week open-label trial to investigate its efficacy in treating social anxiety disorder, the generalized subtype. The trial included 23 outpatients, who could have comorbid anxiety disorders, major depressive disorder (with an MADRS score of ≤19 and onset at least 5 years after the onset of social anxiety disorder), or attention-deficit/hyperactivity disorder. The mean dosage at endpoint was 222.8±141.8 mg/day, with a dosage range of 25–400 mg/day. Twelve subjects completed the trial, and 11 discontinued it because of lack of efficacy, adverse effects, scheduling conflicts, loss to follow-up, or reoccurrence of depressive symptoms. Efficacy measures included the CGI-I at the end of week 16 and the change from baseline to endpoint in the LSAS. Among the 12 completers, 9 (75%) were considered responders with a CGI-I score of 1 or 2 at 16 weeks; however, in the intent-to-treat analysis, only 11 of the 23 (48%) were considered responders. The mean percentage drop in LSAS score was 45.1% among completers but 29.4% in the intent-to-treat group. In the intent-to-treat group, the disorder remitted in 8 of 23 (35%) patients when remission was defined as a CGI-I score of ≤2 and in 6 of 23 (26%) when it was defined as an LSAS score of ≤30. All patients experienced adverse effects, which included weight loss, paresthesias, headache, cognitive impairment, anorexia, gastrointestinal upset, tiredness, lightheadedness, agitation, and metallic taste. Five patients withdrew from the study due to side effects. Based on these results, the evidence of the efficacy of topiramate for social anxiety disorder remains inconclusive. Larger randomized and controlled trials are needed to establish its role in treating social anxiety disorder.

Levetiracetam. Levetiracetam is a novel anticonvulsant that modulates voltage-gated calcium channels in the central nervous system. It has shown efficacy in the treatment of refractory seizure disorders and has also shown positive effects in animal models of mania. In a first open-label, flexible-dose study, Simon et al. (2004) treated 20 patients with generalized social anxiety disorder for 8 weeks. Comorbid depressive and other anxiety disorders were permitted as long as they were considered secondary disorders for that patient. Participants had high levels of symptoms at baseline, with a mean CGI-S score of 6 and a mean LSAS score of 90.8. The mean endpoint dosage of levetiracetam was 2,013±948 mg/day (range 500–3,000 mg/day). The study found a 20-point decrease in LSAS scores. There were also decreases in CGI-S and Hamilton Anxiety Scale scores. Levetiracetam was generally well tolerated, with mild and transient side effects such as fatigue, sedation, and headache.

Subsequently, a small placebo-controlled pilot study randomly assigned 18 subjects to receive either placebo (n=7) or levetiracetam (n=11) at flexible dosages ranging from 500 to 3,000 mg/day for 7 weeks (Zhang et al. 2005). After the first visit, two subjects from the levetiracetam group dropped out because of early side effects (muscle spasms/pain and severe headache). An additional two subjects in this group had a relatively poor tolerance to the drug. The study found no differences on the measures of social anxiety (BSPS, LSAS, and SPIN). The mean dosage at study endpoint was 2,279 mg/day.

Gabapentin. Gabapentin has been approved since 1993 for use as an adjunctive treatment for refractory partial epilepsy; it is thought to work through voltage-gated calcium channels and to have GABAergic effects. Pande et al. (1999) conducted a randomized, double-blind trial in which 69 patients with social anxiety disorder were assigned to receive gabapentin (n=34) (dosage range 900–3,600 mg/day in three divided doses) or placebo (n=35) for 14 weeks. Patients had a low level of comorbidity. More patients taking gabapentin (62%) completed the study than those in the placebo group (51%). Twice as many of the patients taking gabapentin (n=11; 32%) as those taking placebo (n=5; 14%) were categorized as responders according to the defined criteria on the LSAS (≥50% improvement from baseline) in the intent-to-treat sample (P=0.08). Older patients (>35 years) exhibited a greater degree of effect than younger patients. Dizziness and dry mouth were among the most common side effects.

Pregabalin. The anticonvulsant pregabalin has been studied for various indications. It has been shown to have analgesic, anxiolytic, and anticonvulsant properties, thought to be mediated by a reduction of calcium influx in nerve terminals. In a 10-week double-blind trial, 135 patients with social anxiety disorder were randomly assigned to treatment with pregabalin 600 mg/day (n=47), pregabalin 150 mg/day (n=42), or placebo (n=46) (Pande et al. 2004). Patients were required to have a total score of 50 or more on the LSAS. Patients could have a secondary diagnosis of major depressive disorder, but patients with a score of 3 or more at screening on the 17-item Hamilton Rating Scale for Depression, item 1 (depressed mood), were excluded. The primary efficacy parameter was change in the LSAS total score. Ninety-four patients (70%) completed the study. The mean LSAS total score decreased significantly more with pregabalin 600 mg/day than with placebo. Pregabalin 600 mg/day was also superior to placebo as rated on the BSPS fear subscale. Pregabalin 150 mg/day was not significantly better than placebo on any outcome measure. Most of the reported adverse events were of moderate or mild intensity.

Nineteen patients withdrew from the study due to adverse events, 23.4% (n=11) in the pregabalin 600 mg/day group, 9.5% (n=4) in the pregabalin 150 mg/day group, and 8.7% (n=4) in the placebo group. In the pregabalin 600 mg/day group, seven patients (14.9%) reported sexual adverse events. No serious adverse event was considered related to use of the study medication. Headache occurred with similar frequency in all treatment groups. Further studies are needed to define the optimal dosage, magnitude of the effects, and long-term effects.

Tiagabine. Tiagabine, a selective GABA reuptake inhibitor, has received one open-label trial for patients with social anxiety disorder. Dunlop et al. (2007) treated 54 patients for 12 weeks with tiagabine at dosages ranging from 4 to 16 mg/day. The mean dosage for patients completing the trial was 12.2±4.0 mg/day. Twenty-two of the 54 subjects (40.7%) were considered responders (defined as a CGI-I score of ≤2), and this percentage was higher (63%) when considering only patients who completed the trial (17/27). Tiagabine has also been studied for the treatment of generalized anxiety disorder.

Valproic acid. The anticonvulsant valproic acid is well established as an efficacious agent for a variety of seizure and mood disorders. It has also been thought to have anxiolytic properties mediated by its enhancement of GABAergic activity in the central nervous system. Kinrys et al. (2003) conducted a 12-week flexible-dose, open-label trial of valproic acid (500–2,500 mg/day) in 17 patients with social anxiety disorder. The mean dosage was 1,985±454 mg/day. The mean reduction in LSAS scores was 19.1 points for all participants. Results showed that 41% of the participants were responders according to the CGI-I scores. Adverse effects were mild, and no severe adverse events were reported during the trial.

Atypical Antipsychotics

Olanzapine. Based on preliminary observations suggesting that this medication has anxiolytic effects, Barnett et al. (2002) randomly assigned 12 patients to receive olanzapine (n=7) or placebo (n=5). There were no differences between the groups in mean CGI-I scores at endpoint. However, patients receiving olanzapine showed a significantly greater improvement than placebo recipients on the BSPS and SPIN. Drowsiness and dry mouth were among the most common side effects. Larger studies are needed in order to clarify its effects.

Risperidone. Simon and colleagues (2006) conducted an 8-week open-label trial of risperidone as augmentation therapy in 30 patients with a primary diagnosis of generalized anxiety disorder, social anxiety disorder, or panic disorder who had undergone a trial with adequate (or maximally tolerated) doses of an SSRI or benzodiazepine for at least 8 weeks. Seven (23.3%) of the patients included in the study had a diagnosis of social anxiety disorder. The mean dosage of risperidone at study endpoint for all 30 patients in the study was 1.1 mg/day (SD=0.7 mg/day). The study found a significant decrease in the Hamilton Anxiety Scale and CGI-S scores across all patients in the trial. Patients with social anxiety disorder had their mean LSAS score decrease from 81.3 (SD=19.7) to 38.4 (SD=24.0).

Quetiapine. A small open-label trial included 13 patients with generalized social anxiety disorder treated with quetiapine at flexible dosages (150–300 mg/day) for 12 weeks (Schutters et al. 2005). Nine patients were considered responders (CGI scores <2), and mean total LSAS scores decreased by 37%. Three patients discontinued the trial due to adverse effects, consisting mainly of sedation.

Suggested Guidelines for Pharmacotherapy

Generalized Social Anxiety Disorder

The high frequency and unpredictability of anxiety-provoking situations that occur in the lives of patients with the generalized subtype of social anxiety disorder warrant standing daily doses of medication in these patients, because as-needed use becomes impractical. We believe that at the moment, SSRIs constitute the first-line medication treatment for generalized social anxiety disorder. They have been most extensively tested, are generally well tolerated, and treat comorbid depression. Results of double-blind studies support the efficacy of drugs like escitalopram, fluvoxamine, paroxetine, and sertraline. Studies of fluoxetine, however, have had inconsistent results. The SNRI venlafaxine has also emerged as first-line therapy due to response characteristics similar to those of the SSRIs (see Table 27–1).

Benzodiazepines remain a reasonable alternative. These are commonly used in patients who are unable to tolerate or are inadequately responsive to SSRIs or venlafaxine. The relatively long-acting agent clonazepam appears to be highly efficacious as shown in several studies. The role of alprazolam remains inconclusive. Benzodiazepines are not efficacious in the treatment of some of the comorbidities commonly associated with this disorder (e.g., major depressive disorder), and they should generally be avoided in most patients with a history of substance use disorders, which are moderately comorbid with social anxiety disorder.

Phenelzine has been the most studied MAOI for the treatment of generalized social anxiety disorder. It has proven to be efficacious, but the need to follow dietary restrictions has put it as an alternative at the present. It is generally well tolerated as demonstrated by several studies, and its use can be reserved for patients with refractory disease. Gabapentin and pregabalin have each been studied in only a single controlled trial. Preliminary results have shown their efficacy, but these must be followed by larger trials. Mirtazapine has also shown some efficacy (see Figure 27–1).

Nongeneralized Social Anxiety Disorder

Cases of nongeneralized social anxiety disorder, in which feared performance situations arise only occasionally and predictably (as with musicians or people making professional presentations), can be treated initially with beta-blockers used on an as-needed basis. If beta-blockers are ineffective or are contraindicated, an alternative is the use of a benzodiazepine. However, the benzodiazepine doses needed to control anxiety may interfere with functioning when the demands of the performance are high and may sometimes cause sedation. When performance situations arise frequently, treatments used for generalized social anxiety disorder might be preferable for most patients (see Table 27–2).

Outcome Predictors

A number of predictors have been examined to identify patients who may be most likely to respond to pharmacotherapy. To date, only later age of onset (in adulthood) of social anxiety disorder (Van Ameringen 2004b) and duration of treatment (D.J. Stein et al. 2002b) seem to predict treatment response. Other variables such as sex, age, duration of illness, and comorbidity have not been shown to be significant predictors of outcome (D.J. Stein et al. 2002b). Further work is needed to confirm these findings.

Long-Term Treatment Outcome

Although research has provided useful information on the acute treatment of social anxiety disorder, many questions remain to be answered regarding the appropriate length of pharmacological treatment in order to maintain achieved2 results. In an early study (M.B. Stein et al. 1996), patients treated with open-label paroxetine for

TABLE 27–1. Pharmacotherapy for generalized social anxiety disorder

Drug and class	Initial dosage (mg/day)	Target dosage (mg/day)	Main side effects
SSRIs			Sexual dysfunction, headache, nausea, sedation, insomnia, sweating, withdrawal syndrome
Escitalopram	5	5–20	
Fluvoxamine	50	50–300	
Paroxetine[a]	10	10–60	
Paroxetine CR[a]	12.5	12.5–75	
Sertraline[a]	50	50–200	
SNRIs			Same as SSRIs; also hypertension
Venlafaxine ER[a]	75	75–375	
MAOIs			Sedation, sleep disturbances, insomnia, hypotension, weight gain. *Note:* Low-tyramine diet is required to prevent hypertensive reaction. MAOIs are contraindicated in combination with an SSRI or SNRI (risk of serotonergic syndrome).
Phenelzine	15	30–90	
Other antidepressants			Sedation, weight gain, dry mouth
Mirtazapine	15–30	30–60	
Benzodiazepines			Sedation, cognitive impairment, ataxia, withdrawal syndrome
Clonazepam	0.25	0.5–4.0	
Other anticonvulsants			Sedation, ataxia, dizziness, dry mouth, nausea, asthenia, flatulence, decreased libido
Gabapentin	600	900–3,600	
Pregabalin	300	600	

Note. CR=controlled-release formulation; ER=extended-release formulation; MAOIs=monoamine oxidase inhibitors; SNRIs=serotonin-norepinephrine reuptake inhibitors; SSRIs=selective serotonin reuptake inhibitors.

[a]U.S. Food and Drug Administration approved for social phobia (social anxiety disorder).

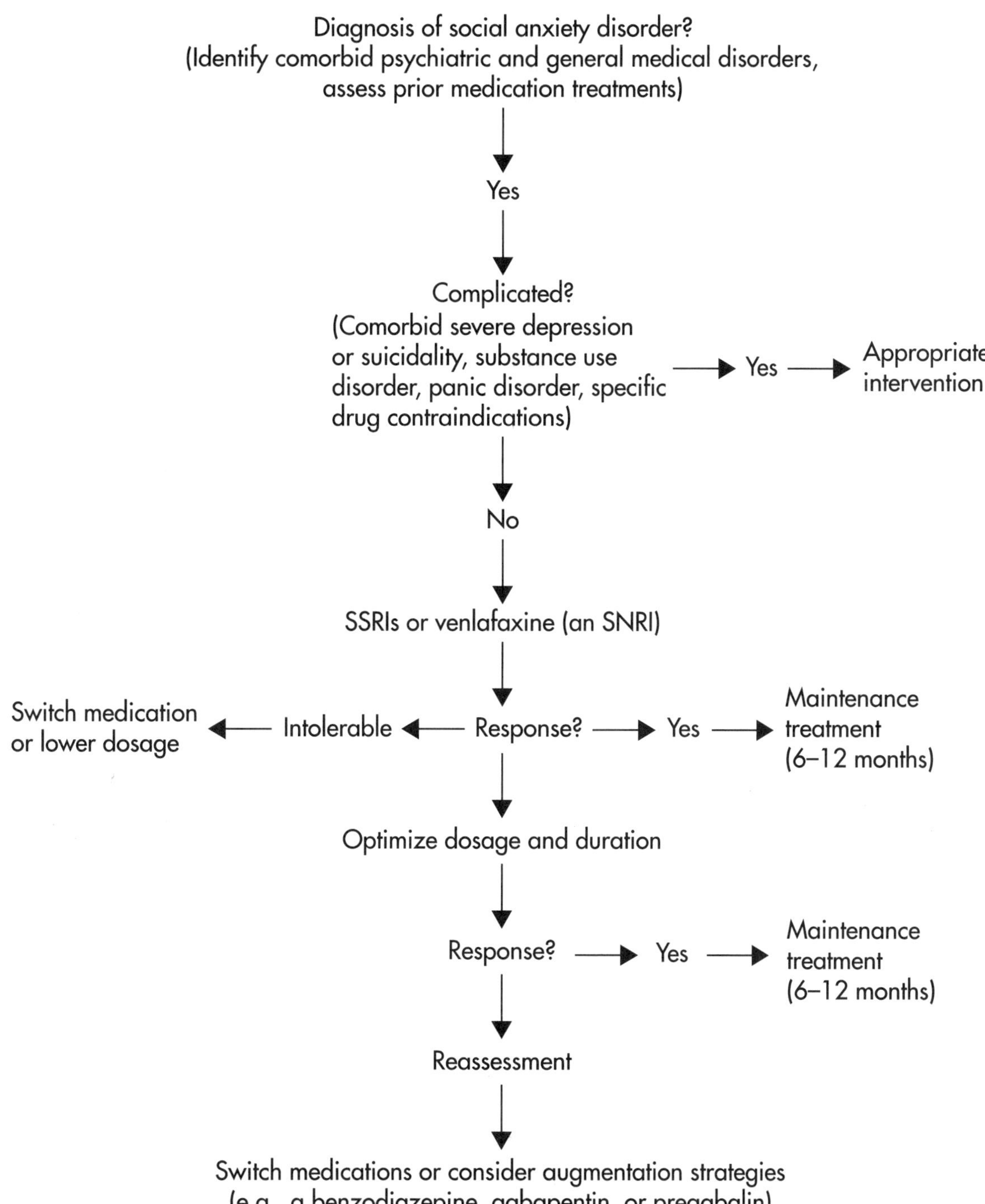

FIGURE 27–1. Algorithm for the pharmacological treatment of generalized social anxiety disorder.[a]
SNRI=serotonin-norepinephrine reuptake inhibitor; SSRIs=selective serotonin reuptake inhibitors.
[a]Consider cognitive-behavioral therapy at each point of the algorithm at which medication is not tolerated or efficacious.

11 weeks underwent a 12-week double-blind, placebo-controlled trial of paroxetine discontinuation. The trial showed a 13% relapse rate in the paroxetine continuation group versus a 63% relapse rate in the discontinuation (placebo) group. Similar results have been shown in other paroxetine trials (D.J. Stein et al. 2002b). In a study of sertraline discontinuation (described above in the "Sertraline" section) (Van Ameringen et al. 2001; Walker et al. 2000), individuals randomly selected to discontinue sertraline after 5 months of treatment had significantly

TABLE 27–2. Pharmacotherapy for nongeneralized social anxiety disorder

Drug and class	Initial dosage (mg/day)	Target dosage (mg/day)	Main side effects
Beta-blockers			Hypotension, bradycardia
Propranolol	10	10–40	
Benzodiazepines			Sedation, cognitive impairment, ataxia
Alprazolam[a]	0.25	0.25–1	
Lorazepam[a]	0.5	0.5–2	

[a]U.S. Food and Drug Administration approved for anxiety.

higher relapse rates than those who continued taking the medication for another 24 weeks. Other reports (Versiani et al. 1992) have shown up to 50% loss of treatment gains in the 2 months following discontinuation of phenelzine in responders after 16 weeks of treatment, measured as an increase in mean score on all parameters at week 24 relative to that at week 16. Similarly, other authors (Liebowitz et al. 1992) have reported that relapse occurred in up to one-third of patients in the 2 months following phenelzine discontinuation after 16 weeks of treatment. Other studies have shown that a sizeable percentage of patients maintain clinical improvements when continuing to take SSRIs (D.J. Stein et al. 2002c). Based on these data, it seems reasonable to treat patients for 6–12 months, with slow tapering and discontinuation, and follow up to monitor for relapse.

Few studies have made direct comparisons between CBT and pharmacotherapy for the treatment of social anxiety disorder. Although some studies suggest pharmacotherapy might have an earlier onset of effects, the major interest in studies seems to be the use of CBT in the assistance of tapering and discontinuation of medication. This is thought to provide patients with therapeutic tools that can help them deal with social anxiety symptoms once medication is discontinued. Limited data from trials comparing the outcomes of pharmacotherapy versus CBT at 6–12 months after discontinuation suggest that CBT may have a more durable effect (Liebowitz et al. 1999; Haug et al. 2003), although the sample sizes of those analyses suggest caution in interpreting the findings. Therefore, it has been suggested that the use of concomitant CBT may help maintain the gains following medication cessation, as seen in a trial by Gelernter et al. (1991), who reported no loss of phenelzine's efficacy after 2 months without treatment.

In summary, clinical improvement with pharmacotherapy seems to last at least 12 months with maintenance treatment, with relapse rates after discontinuation differing among pharmacological agents. Discontinuation of medication after 12–20 weeks of treatment seems to increase the risk for relapse compared with maintenance of medication after that time period. Close follow-up after discontinuation is warranted.

Special Populations

Treatment in Children

Onset of social anxiety disorder usually occurs in late childhood or early adolescence (Grant et al. 2005). Early treatment of social anxiety disorder would theoretically promise reduction of long-term morbidity. However, few studies to date have addressed this particular population, making the role of pharmacotherapy for treatment of this disorder uncertain in young patients. The degree to which most of the adult psychopharmacological data can be extended to this group remains to be clarified. Furthermore, there has been an increasing concern about studies reporting an increased risk of suicidal ideation among adolescents receiving therapy with SSRIs or SNRIs (Hammad et al. 2006). Even though these data come primarily from studies of depression, careful monitoring is warranted. Thus, there is a tension between the need to increase our empirical evidence about the treatment of social anxiety disorder in children and concern about the danger for children involved in the studies, both during treatment and in the surveillance periods.

Despite these concerns, several placebo-controlled trials have been conducted, providing substantial evidence of the efficacy of SSRIs and SNRIs in children ages 6–17 years. The first group of studies conducted in children included patients with a wide range of anxiety disorders, and some of the studies concentrated on children with selective mutism, a condition that has been shown to greatly overlap with social anxiety disorder.

Fairbanks et al. (1997) treated a group of children with mixed anxiety disorders who had not responded to psychotherapy. Treatment with fluoxetine was started at a dosage of 5 mg/day, which increased weekly by 5–10 mg/day for 6–9 weeks until improvement occurred or to a maximum of 40 mg/day (children <12 years) or 80 mg/day (adolescents). Of the 10 children with social anxiety disorder, 8 were much improved as assessed by the CGI scale. Simeon and Ferguson (1987) treated avoidant and overanxious disorders with open-label alprazolam in a group of children. Both child- and parent-rated anxiety symptoms decreased for both diagnostic groups, and cognitive functioning also improved with treatment. Subsequently, Simeon et al. (1992) compared alprazolam versus placebo treatment in 30 children with avoidant and overanxious disorders but found no significant differences between the treatment groups.

Reports of medication treatment of selective mutism include a study in which a 12-year-old girl who had not responded to two trials of psychotherapy was successfully treated with fluoxetine (20 mg/day) (Black et al. 1992). In another report, a 7-year-old girl who had failed to respond to previous trials of behavior therapy and amantadine (200 mg/day) responded to phenelzine (52.5 mg/day). Medication was tapered and withdrawn by week 24, with gains maintained at 5-month follow-up. Black and Uhde (1994) conducted a double-blind, placebo-controlled study of fluoxetine for the treatment of selective mutism. Six patients were assigned to the fluoxetine group and nine to the placebo group. Patients in the fluoxetine treatment group had significantly more improvement than placebo-treated patients on parents' ratings of mutism change and global change. Clinicians' and teachers' ratings did not show significant differences between treatment groups. Medication was well tolerated. Dummit et al. (1996) treated selective mutism in 21 children in a 9-week open-label trial of fluoxetine. The mean dose was 28.1 mg (range 10–60 mg/day). After fluoxetine treatment, the disorder improved in 76% of the children. Side effects were similar to those generally experienced by adults taking SSRIs.

In a trial conducted by the Research Unit on Pediatric Psychopharmacology Anxiety Study Group (2001), 153 children ages 6–17 years who met criteria for social anxiety disorder, separation anxiety disorder, or generalized anxiety disorder entered a 3-week psychoeducational program. Those who did not respond (n=128) were then randomly assigned to receive either placebo or fluvoxamine (50–300 mg/day). After 8 weeks of treatment, patients in the fluvoxamine group had improved significantly more than patients in the placebo group on the CGI-I scale and the Pediatric Anxiety Rating Scale.

Another trial, by Birmaher et al. (2003), studied subjects ages 7–17 years who met criteria for generalized anxiety disorder, separation anxiety disorder, and/or social anxiety disorder with significant impairment (Children's Global Assessment Scale [CGAS] score≤60). Seventy-four patients were randomly assigned to receive fluoxetine (n=37) or placebo (n=37). In this sample, 47% of individuals had separation anxiety disorder, 54% had social anxiety disorder, 63% had generalized anxiety disorder, 5% had selective mutism, 24% had simple phobia, and 1% had panic disorder. When specific diagnoses were analyzed, subjects with social anxiety disorder who received fluoxetine had a 76% response rate (CGI-I score ≤2), whereas those who received placebo had a 21% response rate. There was also a significant increase in functional improvement (CGAS score ≥70) in 45.5% of subjects with social anxiety disorder in the fluoxetine treatment group versus 10.5% in the placebo group.

Paroxetine was studied (Wagner et al. 2004) in a trial that included 322 children and adolescents with social anxiety disorder. Subjects were randomly assigned to paroxetine (10–50 mg/day) or placebo treatment. Seventy-seven percent of subjects in the paroxetine group and 38.3% of those in the placebo group were considered responders (CGI-I score ≤2). Significantly more patients taking paroxetine achieved remission, as defined by having a 70% reduction in the Liebowitz Social Anxiety Scale for Children and Adolescents (LSAS-CA; 47.2% vs. 13.3%) and by having a CGI-I score of 1 (47.8% vs. 14.9%).

In another large trial, March et al. (2007) randomly assigned 293 patients ages 8–17 years with generalized social anxiety disorder to receive venlafaxine ER (n=137) or placebo (n=148) for 16 weeks. The mean age was 13.6 years (SD=2.63) in the placebo group and 13.6 years (SD=2.46) in the venlafaxine ER group. Dosages ranged from 37.5 mg/day to a maximum of 225 mg/day. Primary efficacy outcomes were measured using LSAS-CA and CGI-I scores. Random regression analyses in the intent-to-treat groups showed venlafaxine ER treatment to be statistically significantly superior to placebo treatment (P=0.001) on the LSAS-CA. Following CGI-I criteria (a score of 1 or 2) for response, 56% (95% confidence interval [CI], 47%–64%) of venlafaxine ER–treated subjects responded, which was statistically superior to the 37% response rate (95% CI, 29%–45%) in placebo recipients. Adverse effects included nausea, anorexia, asthenia, pharyngitis, and mydriasis. Three subjects in the venlafaxine ER group developed suicidal ideation (two during the course of treatment and one during the tapering phase) versus none in the placebo group, but there were no suicide attempts.

Mrakotsky et al. (2008) conducted an 8-week open-label pilot study of mirtazapine in children with social anxiety disorder, ages 8–17 years. All participants began with a 15 mg/day baseline dosage. The mean final daily dosage of mirtazapine was 28.75 mg/day (SD=12.40) or 0.58 mg/kg/day (SD=0.19). Primary outcome measures were symptom improvement, based on clinician ratings and self-reports, and tolerability, based on rates of discontinuation due to adverse effects. Fifty-six percent (10/18) responded to treatment, and 17% (3/18) achieved full remission. Social anxiety disorder symptoms improved significantly during the first 2 weeks of treatment, as did symptoms of comorbid depression and anxiety. Eleven patients (61%) did not complete all 8 weeks of treatment; four (22%) discontinued due to adverse effects, including fatigue and irritability. The others discontinued due to study burden (28%) or insufficient response (6%) or to pursue herbal treatment (6%). Mirtazapine was associated with a mean weight gain of 3.27 kg (SD=2.57), a significant increase in weight.

Treatment-Refractory Social Anxiety Disorder

Significant gaps remain in our knowledge of how to treat social anxiety disorder. For example, although most acute medication trials result in 40%–60% of the subjects being rated as much or very much improved, most subjects do not achieve true remission. Other subjects appear to be more or less evenly divided between those who fail to respond to the drug and those who fail to complete the trial. Even among responders, typically defined by a CGI-I score of 1 or 2, considerable residual symptoms are still present in the majority of them, and these patients often continue to meet criteria that would have earned them study entry in the first place. Clinical experience suggests that patients who do not benefit from one medication may respond to another of the same or a different class or may respond to CBT. Partial responses to an SSRI or an SNRI may be augmented with CBT or with a benzodiazepine, gabapentin, or pregabalin (although the combination of an SSRI or an SNRI with an MAOI is absolutely contraindicated due to the risk of development of serotonergic syndrome). However, few empirical data are available to guide subsequent treatment of patients who show minimal or no improvement, or of patients who show much improvement but still exhibit meaningful symptoms and impairment. Clinically useful predictors of response to specific pharmacological treatments are also lacking.

In managing treatment-resistant patients, the first step is to identify possible reasons for treatment resistance. Therapeutic failure may be caused by nonadherence to treatment, resulting in suboptimal medication levels or treatment duration. Another reason for resistance is the presence of a comorbid psychiatric disorder. These are very common in patients with social anxiety disorder and are often exclusion criteria in clinical trials. The lack of information about the influence of comorbidity on treatment response can also be due to the fact that trials that allow comorbid disorders do not usually report treatment response stratified by the presence or absence of those conditions. Besides comorbid medical conditions, individual pharmacokinetic characteristics (drug interactions, rapid metabolizers) and perpetuating factors may be factors contributing to resistance.

Medications that are effective in partially reducing symptoms acutely may yield only limited further benefit during longer periods of treatment (Walker et al. 2000), suggesting the need for augmentation strategies. Although buspirone has not proven to be superior to placebo as monotherapy, a small trial conducted by Van Ameringen et al. (1996) studied buspirone as an augmenting agent with an SSRI for 8 weeks in 10 patients with generalized social anxiety disorder who had had a partial response to an adequate trial of the SSRI. The mean dosage at endpoint was 45 mg/day, with dosages ranging from 30 to 60 mg/day. Seven patients (70%) were considered responders according to CGI criteria. This approach has not been further studied. M.B. Stein et al. (2001) compared pindolol potentiation of paroxetine versus paroxetine plus placebo in a study that included 14 subjects with generalized social phobia who were rated as less than very much improved on the CGI scale after at least 10 weeks of treatment with a maximally tolerated dosage of paroxetine. Patients were given 15 mg of pindolol per day (in three divided doses) for 4 weeks or placebo in addition to a steady paroxetine dosage. Pindolol was not found to be superior to placebo as an augmenting agent.

Other approaches include the concurrent administration of paroxetine and clonazepam. Seedat and Stein (2004) randomly assigned 28 patients with generalized social anxiety disorder to receive paroxetine plus clonazepam or paroxetine plus placebo. More clonazepam recipients (79%) than placebo recipients (43%) were classified as CGI responders, but the effect was not statistically significant at $P=0.06$, due to the small sample size. The clonazepam group also showed greater changes on dimensional measures, including the LSAS, but these differences also failed to reach significance due to the limited power of the study. The study raised a question about the dosing strategy for clonazepam. The maximum dosage in this study was 2.0 mg/day, compared with 3.0 mg/day in other trials (e.g., Davidson et al. 1993). Clonazepam deserves further study as an augmentation or alternative treatment for patients whose illness does not respond completely to an initial SSRI trial.

One open-label trial (Altamura et al. 1999) demonstrated the efficacy of switching to venlafaxine in a group of 12 social anxiety disorder patients who had not responded to SSRI treatment (10 had received fluoxetine, 2 had received paroxetine). Another trial, previously referenced in this chapter (Pallanti and Quercioli 2006 ; see "Citalopram and Escitalopram"), found some efficacy with escitalopram in patients in whom paroxetine had not shown efficacy. Similar results have been found with citalopram (Simon et al. 2002) and risperidone (Simon et al. 2006).

Novel and Experimental Approaches

St. John's wort has been studied in a small pilot study for generalized social anxiety disorder (Kobak et al. 2005). This 12-week randomized trial included 40 subjects who received a flexible dose of St. John's wort (600–1,800 mg/day; $n=20$) or placebo ($n=20$). Results showed no significant difference in the mean change in the LSAS score with St. John's wort (11.4) versus placebo (13.2). Therefore, at the moment, available study results fail to provide evidence for the efficacy of St. John's wort in treating social anxiety disorder.

An exciting new development is the use of medication to augment the effect of CBT. Hofmann et al. (2006) studied the effect of D-cycloserine, an analog of D-alanine and a partial agonist at the *N*-methyl-D-aspartate (NMDA) receptor, in an attempt to boost treatment response in patients undergoing exposure therapy for social anxiety disorder. The rationale for this approach is the knowledge that fear learning and extinction are both blocked by antagonists at the glutamatergic NMDA receptor (which is involved in learning and memory) and the suggestion that D-cycloserine appears to augment learning in animal studies and in some human trials. Preliminary results showed that patients who received D-cycloserine (short-term treatment with 50 mg of D-cycloserine) in addition to attenuated exposure therapy reported significantly less social anxiety than patients who received placebo plus attenuated exposure therapy.

In addition to the pharmacological agents described in this chapter, other drugs currently under investigation include omega-3 fatty acids, ziprasidone, quetiapine, atomoxetine, and memantine for use as monotherapies or augmentation therapies in either generalized or nongeneralized social anxiety disorder. Further work is needed before preliminary evidence for their efficacy can be established.

Topical aluminum chloride preparations have been reported to be useful in treating some of the associated symptoms of social anxiety disorder (e.g., sweaty hands) (Bohn and Sternbach 1996). Other somatic treatments such as endoscopic sympathetic block (Pohjavaara et al. 2001, 2003; Telaranta 1998) have been suggested to be beneficial in generalized social anxiety disorder patients who had no therapeutic response to adequate medication trials or psychotherapy.

Treatment Recommendations

Case Vignette

A 32-year-old single man reports feeling anxious and self-conscious around people at school, at work, and in social interactions since his childhood. He appears shy and quiet. On questioning, he describes moderate to severe anxiety in social situations and a constant worry about becoming the center of attention when he finds himself with strangers. He fears everybody will look at him and notice what he is doing. He feels anxious when eating or drinking in a public place, as he fears people will notice his tremor and sweating hands. At work, he avoids meetings and group discussions, and he even turned down a promotion that required him to interact more with his colleagues. He frequently avoids meeting new people and dating. He wants to become more socially active but fears he will look ridiculous.

For most cases, as in the one described above, the first treatment options are usually an SSRI or venlafaxine. These are particularly useful in patients who prefer medication, have prominent depressive symptoms, or lack access to a trained therapist. The first recommendation is to start with a low dosage for 1 week in order to decrease the likelihood of side effects and then increase the dose to the usual effective dose for several weeks. If the response is incomplete, the dose should be gradually increased to the maximal dose, as tolerated. It is recommended that treatment be continued for 6–12 months, followed by tapering and discontinuation. However, the risk of relapse must be recognized. In patients with recurrent symptoms, treatment may be reinstituted for longer periods.

Conclusion

It seems reasonable to offer treatment, including pharmacotherapy, to any individual with social anxiety disorder when significant distress or impairment is present. Some patients may be surprised by the idea of taking medication for a problem that they see as a long-standing personality trait. Several complementary lines of reasoning support the use of pharmacotherapy in the treatment of social anxiety disorder (Liebowitz and Marshall 1995):

1. The research literature has clearly confirmed the efficacy of several drug classes in the treatment of social anxiety disorder.
2. Physical and cognitive symptoms of anxiety can interfere with optimal performance and ultimately encourage avoidance of feared situations; thus, medications that can directly decrease anxiety may help improve performance in social or professional situations.
3. Concerns about social comparisons and shyness are likely to be strongly biologically based, given the evolution of humans as a group-living species and evidence from twin and family studies that there is a significant genetic contribution to the disorder.

It is helpful to set reasonable expectations for response. In the short term, we expect to see symptomatic relief and improvements in social relatedness and performance. Over the long term, we hope to see increased vocational or educational functioning and improved capacity for more intimate relationships of all kinds. Although some patients have a complete remission of symptoms, more commonly seen is a substantial reduction of symptoms without alteration in the typical patient's self-perception as someone who tends to be shy. The choice of a pharmacological agent for use in a specific patient depends on the diagnostic subtype of social anxiety disorder, presence of comorbidity, and preference of the patient.

Key Clinical Points

- At present, SSRIs and venlafaxine (an SNRI) are considered the first-line pharmacological treatments for the generalized subtype of social anxiety disorder, with a proposed length of treatment of 6–12 months.
- In patients with generalized social anxiety disorder who cannot tolerate either an SSRI or venlafaxine, suggested pharmacotherapy includes long-acting benzodiazepines (e.g., clonazepam). However, these agents are not recommended in patients with comorbid major depressive disorder or in those with a history of substance abuse.
- MAOIs have been proven efficacious but at the moment are generally reserved for treating refractory disease, because patients must undergo dietary restrictions.
- Other agents that have been shown to improve symptoms of generalized social anxiety disorder include gabapentin, pregabalin, risperidone, and mirtazapine. Larger studies are needed to support their widespread use.
- For the nongeneralized subtype of social anxiety disorder, medication may be useful on an as-needed basis because feared situations occur predictably and with less than daily frequency. These medications include beta-blockers, such as propranolol, or benzodiazepines.
- Children and adolescents seem to benefit from SSRIs and SNRIs, but they must be closely monitored until further investigation assesses the agents' safety profile in this population, due to the reported increased risk of suicidal ideation among adolescents taking these agents.
- CBT and augmentation strategies seem to play an important role in both increasing response rates and maintaining improvement over time.

References

Aberg-Wistedt A, Agren H, Ekselius L, et al: Sertraline versus paroxetine in major depression: clinical outcome after six months of continuous therapy. J Clin Psychopharmacol 20:645–652, 2000

Allgulander C: Paroxetine in social anxiety disorder: a randomized placebo-controlled study. Acta Psychiatr Scand 100:193–198, 1999

Allgulander C, Mangano R, Zhang J, et al: Efficacy of Venlafaxine ER in patients with social anxiety disorder: a double-blind, placebo-controlled, parallel-group comparison with paroxetine. Hum Psychopharmacol 19:387–396, 2004

Altamura AC, Pioli R, Vitto M, et al: Venlafaxine in social phobia: a study in selective serotonin reuptake inhibitor non-responders. Int Clin Psychopharmacol 14:239–245, 1999

American Psychiatric Association: Diagnostic and Statistical Manual of Mental Disorders, 3rd Edition. Washington, DC, American Psychiatric Association, 1980

Atmaca M, Tezcan E, Kuloglu M: An open clinical trial of reboxetine in the treatment of social phobia. J Clin Psychopharmacol 23:417–419, 2003

Baldwin D, Bobes J, Stein DJ, et al: Paroxetine in social phobia/social anxiety disorder: randomised, double-blind, placebo-controlled study. Br J Psychiatry 175:120–126, 1999

Barnett SD, Kramer ML, Casat CD, et al: Efficacy of olanzapine in social anxiety disorder: a pilot study. J Psychopharmacol 16:365–368, 2002

Beaumont G: A large open multicenter trial of clomipramine in the management of phobic disorders. J Int Med Res 5 (suppl 5):116–129, 1977

Benca R, Matuzas W, Al-Sadir J: Social phobia, MVP, and response to imipramine. J Clin Psychopharmacol 6:50–51, 1986

Birmaher B, Axelson DA, Monk K, et al: Fluoxetine for the treatment of childhood anxiety disorders. J Am Acad Child Adolesc Psychiatry 42:415–423, 2003

Black B, Uhde TW: Treatment of elective mutism with fluoxetine: a double-blind, placebo-controlled study. J Am Acad Child Adolesc Psychiatry 33:1000–1006, 1994

Black B, Uhde TW, Tancer ME: Fluoxetine for the treatment of social phobia. J Clin Psychopharmacol 12:293–295, 1992

Blanco C, Schneier FR, Schmidt A, et al: Pharmacological treatment of social anxiety disorder: a meta-analysis. Depress Anxiety 18:29–40, 2003

Blomhoff S, Haug TT, Hellstrom K, et al: Randomised controlled general practice trial of sertraline, exposure therapy and combined treatment in generalised social phobia. Br J Psychiatry 179:23–30, 2001

Bohn P, Sternbach H: Topical aluminum chloride for social phobia-related hyperhidrosis (letter). Am J Psychiatry 153:1368, 1996

Clark DB, Agras WS: The assessment and treatment of performance anxiety in musicians. Am J Psychiatry 148:598–605, 1991

Clark DM, Ehlers A, McManus F, et al: Cognitive therapy versus fluoxetine in generalized social phobia: a randomized placebo-controlled trial. J Consult Clin Psychol 71:1058–1067, 2003

Crippa JA, Filho AS, Freitas MC, et al: Duloxetine in the treatment of social anxiety disorder (letter). J Clin Psychopharmacol 27:310, 2007

Davidson JR, Potts N, Richichi E, et al: Treatment of social phobia with clonazepam and placebo. J Clin Psychopharmacol 13:423–428, 1993

Davidson JR, Foa EB, Huppert JD, et al: Fluoxetine, comprehensive cognitive behavioral therapy, and placebo in generalized social phobia. Arch Gen Psychiatry 61:1005–1013, 2004a

Davidson J, Yaryura-Tobias J, DuPont R, et al: Fluvoxamine-controlled release formulation for the treatment of generalized social anxiety disorder. J Clin Psychopharmacol 24:118–125, 2004b

Deltito JA, Stam M: Psychopharmacological treatment of avoidant personality disorder. Compr Psychiatry 30:498–504, 1989

Dummit ES 3rd, Klein RG, Tancer NK: Fluoxetine treatment of children with selective mutism: an open trial. J Am Acad Child Adolesc Psychiatry 35:615–621, 1996

Dunlop BW, Papp L, Garlow SJ, et al: Tiagabine for social anxiety disorder. Hum Psychopharmacol 22:241–244, 2007

Dursun SM, Devarajan S: Accelerated weight loss after treating refractory depression with fluoxetine plus topiramate: possible mechanisms of action? Can J Psychiatry 46:287–288, 2001

Emmanuel NP, Lydiard RB, Ballenger JC: Treatment of social phobia with bupropion. J Clin Psychopharmacol 11:276–277, 1991

Emmanuel NP, Czepowicz VD, Villareal G, et al: Venlafaxine in social phobia: a case series. New Research Poster 113, presented at the 148th annual meeting of the American Psychiatric Association, Miami, FL, May 1995

Emmanuel NP, Brawman-Mintzer O, Morton WA, et al: Bupropion-SR in treatment of social phobia. Depress Anxiety 12:111–113, 2000

Fahlén T, Nilsson HL, Borg K, et al: Social phobia: the clinical efficacy and tolerability of the monoamine oxidase-A and serotonin uptake inhibitor brofaromine: a double-blind placebo-controlled study. Acta Psychiatr Scand 92:351–358, 1995

Fairbanks J, Pine DS, Tancer NK, et al: Open fluoxetine treatment of mixed anxiety disorders in children and adolescents. J Child Adolesc Psychopharmacol 7:17–29, 1997

Falloon IR, Lloyd GG, Harpin RE: The treatment of social phobia: real-life rehearsal with nonprofessional therapists. J Nerv Ment Dis 169:180–184, 1981

Fedoroff IC, Taylor S: Psychological and pharmacological treatments of social phobia: a meta-analysis. J Clin Psychopharmacol 21:311–324, 2001

Gelernter CS, Uhde TW, Cimbolic P, et al: Cognitive-behavioral and pharmacological treatments of social phobia: a controlled study. Arch Gen Psychiatry 48:938–945, 1991

Gorman JM, Liebowitz MR, Fyer AJ, et al: Treatment of social phobia with atenolol. J Clin Psychopharmacol 5:298–301, 1985

Gould RA, Buckminster S, Pollack MH, et al: Cognitive-behavioral and pharmacological treatment for social phobia: a meta-analysis. Clin Psychol (New York) 4:291–306, 1997

Grant BF, Hasin DS, Blanco C, et al: The epidemiology of social anxiety disorder in the United States: results from the National Epidemiologic Survey on Alcohol and Related Conditions. J Clin Psychiatry 66:1351–1361, 2005

Hedges DW, Brown BL, Shwalb DA, et al: The efficacy of selective serotonin reuptake inhibitors in adult social anxiety disorder: a meta-analysis of double-blind, placebo-controlled trials. J Psychopharmacol 21:102–111, 2007

Heimberg RG, Liebowitz MR, Hope DA, et al: Cognitive-behavioral group therapy versus phenelzine in social phobia: 12-week outcome. Arch Gen Psychiatry 55:1133–1141, 1998

Hofmann SG, Meuret AE, Smits JA, et al: Augmentation of exposure therapy with D-cycloserine for social anxiety disorder. Arch Gen Psychiatry 63:298–304, 2006

International Multicenter Clinical Trial Group on Moclobemide in Social Phobia: Moclobemide in social phobia: a double-blind, placebo-controlled clinical study. Eur Arch Psychiatry Clin Neurosci 247:71–80, 1997

Johnson BA: Recent advances in the development of treatments for alcohol and cocaine dependence: focus on topiramate and other modulators of GABA or glutamate function. CNS Drugs 19:873–896, 2005

Kasper S, Stein DJ, Loft H, et al: Escitalopram in the treatment of social anxiety disorder: randomised, placebo-controlled, flexible-dosage study. Br J Psychiatry 186:222–226, 2005

Katzelnick DJ, Kobak KA, Greist JH, et al: Sertraline for social phobia: a double-blind, placebo-controlled crossover study. Am J Psychiatry 152:1368–1371, 1995

Kinrys G, Pollack MH, Simon NM, et al: Valproic acid for the treatment of social anxiety disorder. Int Clin Psychopharmacol 18:169–172, 2003

Kobak KA, Griest JH, Jefferson JW, et al: Fluoxetine in social phobia: a double-blind placebo controlled pilot study. J Clin Psychopharmacol 22:257–262, 2002

Kobak KA, Taylor LV, Warner G, et al: St. John's wort versus placebo in social phobia: results from a placebo-controlled pilot study. J Clin Psychopharmacol 25:51–58, 2005

Lader M, Stender K, Bürger V, et al: Efficacy and tolerability of escitalopram in 12- and 24-week treatment of social anxiety disorder: randomised, double-blind, placebo-controlled, fixed-dose study. Depress Anxiety 19:241–248, 2004

Liebowitz MR: Social phobia. Mod Probl Pharmacopsychiatry 22:141–173, 1987

Liebowitz MR, Marshall RD: Pharmacological treatments: clinical applications, in Social Phobia: Diagnosis, Assessment, and Treatment. Edited by Heimberg RG, Liebowitz MR, Hope DA, et al. New York, Guilford, 1995, pp 366–383

Liebowitz MR, Schneier FR, Campeas R, et al: Phenelzine versus atenolol in social phobia: a placebo controlled comparison. Arch Gen Psychiatry 49:290–300, 1992

Liebowitz MR, Stein MB, Tancer M, et al: A randomized, double-blind, fixed-dose comparison of paroxetine and placebo in the treatment of generalized social anxiety disorder. J Clin Psychiatry 63:66–74, 2002

Liebowitz MR, DeMartinis NA, Weihs K, et al: Efficacy of sertraline in severe generalized social anxiety disorder: results of a double-blind, placebo-controlled study. J Clin Psychiatry 64:785–792, 2003

Liebowitz MR, Gelenberg AJ, Munjack D: Venlafaxine extended release vs placebo and paroxetine in social anxiety disorder. Arch Gen Psychiatry 62:190–198, 2005a

Liebowitz MR, Mangano RM, Bradwejn J, et al: SAD Study Group: A randomized controlled trial of venlafaxine extended release in generalized social anxiety disorder. J Clin Psychiatry 66:238–247, 2005b

Lott M, Greist JH, Jefferson JW, et al: Brofaromine for social phobia: a multicenter, placebo-controlled, double-blind study. J Clin Psychopharmacol 17:255–260, 1997

Lydiard RB, Laraia MT, Howell EF, et al: Alprazolam in the treatment of social phobia. J Clin Psychiatry 49:17–19, 1988

March JS, Entusah AR, Rynn M, et al: A randomized controlled trial of venlafaxine ER versus placebo in pediatric social anxiety disorder. Biol Psychiatry 62:1149–1154, 2007

Marks IM, Mathews AM: Brief standard self-rating for phobic patients. Behav Res Ther 17:263–267, 1979

Montgomery SA, Nil R, Durr-Pal N, et al: A 24-week randomized, double-blind, placebo-controlled study of escitalopram for the prevention of generalized social anxiety disorder. J Clin Psychiatry 66:1270–1278, 2005

Mrakotsky C, Masek B, Biederman J, et al: Prospective open-label pilot trial of mirtazapine in children and adolescents with social phobia. J Anxiety Disord 22:88–97, 2008

Muehlbacher M, Nickel MK, Nickel C, et al: Mirtazapine treatment of social phobia in women: a randomized, double-blind, placebo-controlled study. J Clin Psychopharmacol 25:580–583, 2005

Munjack DJ, Baltazar PL, Bohn PB, et al: Clonazepam in the treatment of social phobia: a pilot study. J Clin Psychiatry 51 (suppl 5):35–40, 1990

Munjack DJ, Bruns J, Baltazar P, et al: A pilot study of buspirone in the treatment of social phobia. J Anxiety Disord 5:87–98, 1991

Noyes R Jr, Moroz G, Davidson JR, et al: Moclobemide in social phobia: a controlled dose-response trial. J Clin Psychopharmacol 17:247–254, 1997

Ontiveros A, Fontaine R: Social phobia and clonazepam. Can J Psychiatry 35:439–441, 1990

Pallanti S, Quercioli L: Resistant social anxiety disorder response to escitalopram. Clin Pract Epidemol Ment Health 2:35, 2006

Pande AC, Davidson JR, Jefferson JW, et al: Treatment of social phobia with gabapentin: a placebo-controlled study. J Clin Psychopharmacol 19:341–348, 1999

Pande AC, Feltner DE, Jefferson JW, et al: Efficacy of the novel anxiolytic pregabalin in social anxiety disorder: a placebo-controlled, multicenter study. J Clin Psychopharmacol 24:141–149, 2004

Pecknold JC, McClure DJ, Appeltauer L, et al: Does tryptophan potentiate clomipramine in the treatment of agoraphobic and social phobic patients? Br J Psychiatry 140:484–490, 1982

Pohjavaara P, Telaranta T, Väisänen E: Endoscopic sympathetic block—new treatment of choice for social phobia? Ann Chir Gynaecol 90:177–184, 2001

Pohjavaara P, Telaranta T, Väisänen E: The role of the sympathetic nervous system in anxiety: is it possible to relieve anxiety with endoscopic sympathetic block? Nord J Psychiatry 57:55–60, 2003

Potts NLS, Davidson JRT: Pharmacological treatments: literature review, in Social Phobia: Diagnosis, Assessment, and Treatment. Edited by Heimberg RG, Liebowitz MR, Hope DA, et al. New York, Guilford, 1995, pp 334–366

Reich JR, Yates W: A pilot study of treatment of social phobia with alprazolam. Am J Psychiatry 145:590–594, 1988

Reiter SR, Pollack MH, Rosenbaum JF, et al: Clonazepam for the treatment of social phobia. J Clin Psychiatry 51:470–472, 1990

Research Unit on Pediatric Psychopharmacology Anxiety Study Group: Fluvoxamine for the treatment of anxiety disorders in children and adolescents. N Engl J Med 344:1279–1285, 2001

Rickels K, Mangano R, Khan A: A double-blind, placebo-controlled study of a flexible dose of venlafaxine ER in adult outpatients with generalized social anxiety disorder. J Clin Psychopharmacol 24:488–496, 2004

Schneier FR: Clinical assessment strategies for social phobia. Psychiatr Ann 25:550–553, 1995

Schneier FR, Chin SJ, Hollander E, et al: Fluoxetine in social phobia [letter]. J Clin Psychopharmacol 12:62–63, 1992

Schneier FR, Saoud JB, Campeas R, et al: Buspirone in social phobia. J Clin Psychopharmacol 13:251–256, 1993

Schneier FR, Goetz D, Campeas R, et al: Placebo-controlled trial of moclobemide in social phobia. Br J Psychiatry 172:70–77, 1998

Schutters SI, van Megen HJ, Westenberg HG: Efficacy of quetiapine in generalized social anxiety disorder: results from an open-label study. J Clin Psychiatry 66:540–542, 2005

Seedat S, Stein MB: Double-blind, placebo-controlled assessment of combined clonazepam with paroxetine compared with paroxetine monotherapy for generalized social anxiety disorder. J Clin Psychiatry 65:244–248, 2004

Simeon JG, Ferguson HB: Alprazolam effects in children with anxiety disorders. Can J Psychiatry 32:570–574, 1987

Simeon JG, Ferguson HB, Knott V: Clinical, cognitive, and neurophysiological effects of alprazolam effects in children and adolescents with overanxious disorder and avoidant disorders. J Am Acad Child Adolesc Psychiatry 31:29–33, 1992

Simon NM, Korbly NB, Worthington JJ, et al: Citalopram for social anxiety disorder: an open-label pilot in refractory and nonrefractory patients. CNS Spectr 7:655–657, 2002

Simon NM, Worthington JJ, Doyle AC, et al: An open-label study of levetiracetam for the treatment of social anxiety disorder. J Clin Psychiatry 65:1219–1222, 2004

Simon NM, Hoge EA, Fischmann D, et al: An open-label trial of risperidone augmentation for refractory anxiety disorders. J Clin Psychiatry 67:381–385, 2006

Simpson HB, Schneier FR, Campeas RB, et al: Imipramine in the treatment of social phobia. J Clin Psychopharmacol 18:132–135, 1998a

Simpson HB, Schneier FR, Marshall RD, et al: Low dose selegiline (l-deprenyl) in social phobia. Depress Anxiety 7:126–129, 1998b

Spielberger CD: Manual for the State-Trait Anxiety Inventory (Form V). Palo Alto, CA, Consulting Psychologists Press, 1983

Stein DJ, Cameron A, Amrein R, et al: Moclobemide Social Phobia Clinical Study Group: Moclobemide is effective and well tolerated in the long-term pharmacotherapy of social anxiety disorder with or without comorbid anxiety disorder. Int Clin Psychopharmacol 17:161–170, 2002a

Stein DJ, Stein MB, Pitts CD, et al: Predictors of response to pharmacotherapy in social anxiety disorder: an analysis of 3 placebo-controlled paroxetine trials. J Clin Psychiatry 63:152–155, 2002b

Stein DJ, Versiani M, Hair T, et al: Efficacy of paroxetine for relapse prevention in social anxiety disorder: a 24-week study. Arch Gen Psychiatry 59:1111–1118, 2002c

Stein DJ, Ipser JC, Balkom AJ: Pharmacotherapy for social phobia. Cochrane Database Syst Rev 4:CD001206, 2004a

Stein DJ, Kasper S, Andersen EW, et al: Escitalopram in the treatment of social anxiety disorder: analysis of efficacy for different clinical subgroups and symptom dimensions. Depress Anxiety 20:175–181, 2004b

Stein DJ, Andersen EW, Lader M: Escitalopram versus paroxetine for social anxiety disorder: an analysis of efficacy for different symptom dimensions. Eur Neuropsychopharmacol 16:33–38, 2006

Stein MB, Chartier MJ, Hazen AL, et al: Paroxetine in the treatment of generalized social phobia: open-label treatment and double-blind placebo-controlled discontinuation. J Clin Psychopharmacol 16:218–222, 1996

Stein MB, Fyer AJ, Davidson JR, et al: Fluvoxamine treatment of social phobia (social anxiety disorder): a double-blind, placebo-controlled study. Am J Psychiatry 156:756–760, 1999

Stein MB, Sareen J, Hami S, et al: Pindolol potentiation of paroxetine for generalized social phobia: a double-blind, placebo-controlled, cross-over study. Am J Psychiatry 158:1725–1727, 2001

Stein MB, Pollack MH, Bystritsky A, et al: Efficacy of low and higher dose extended-release venlafaxine in generalized social anxiety disorder: a 6-month randomized controlled trial. Psychopharmacology 177:280–288, 2005

Sternbach H: Fluoxetine treatment of social phobia. J Clin Psychopharmacol 10:230–231, 1990

Tata AL, Kockler DR: Topiramate for binge-eating disorder associated with obesity. Ann Pharmacother 40:1993–1997, 2006

Telaranta T: Treatment of social phobia by endoscopic thoracic sympathicotomy. Eur J Surg Suppl 580: 27–32, 1998

Turner SM, Beidel DC, Jacob RG: Social phobia: a comparison of behavior therapy and atenolol. J Consult Clin Psychol 62:350–358, 1994

Van Ameringen M, Mancini C, Streitner DL: Fluoxetine efficacy in social phobia. J Clin Psychiatry 54:27–32, 1993

Van Ameringen M, Mancini C, Wilson C: Buspirone augmentation of selective serotonin reuptake inhibitors (SSRIs) in social phobia. J Affect Disord 39:115–121, 1996

Van Ameringen MA, Lane RM, Walker JR, et al: Sertraline treatment of generalized social phobia: a 20-week, double-blind, placebo-controlled study. Am J Psychiatry 158:275–281, 2001

Van Ameringen M, Mancini C, Pipe B, et al: An open trial of topiramate in the treatment of generalized social phobia. J Clin Psychiatry 65:1674–1678, 2004a

Van Ameringen M, Oakman J, Mancini C, et al: Predictors of response in generalized social phobia: effect of age of onset. J Clin Psychopharmacology 24:42–48, 2004b

Van Ameringen M, Mancini C, Oakman J, et al: Nefazodone in the treatment of generalized social phobia: a randomized, placebo-controlled trial. J Clin Psychiatry 68:288–295, 2007

van der Linden GJ, Stein DJ, van Balkom AJ: The efficacy of the selective serotonin reuptake inhibitors for social anxiety disorder (social phobia): a meta-analysis of randomized controlled trials. Int Clin Psychopharmacol 15 (suppl 2):S15–S23, 2000

Van Veen JF, Van Vliet IM, Westenberg HG: Mirtazapine in social anxiety disorder: a pilot study. Int Clin Psychopharmacol 17:315–317, 2002

van Vliet IM, den Boer JA, Westenberg HG: Psychopharmacological treatment of social phobia: clinical and biochemical effects of brofaromine, a selective MAO-A inhibitor. Eur Neuropsychopharmacol 2:21–29, 1992

van Vliet IM, den Boer JA, Westenberg HG: Psychopharmacological treatment of social phobia: a double-blind placebo controlled study with fluvoxamine. Psychopharmacology 115:128–134, 1994

van Vliet IM, den Boer JA, Westenberg HG, et al: Clinical effects of buspirone in social phobia: a double-blind placebo-controlled study. J Clin Psychiatry 58:164–168, 1997

Vasudev K, Macritchie K, Geddes J, et al: Topiramate for acute affective episodes in bipolar disorder. Cochrane Database Syst Rev 1:CD003384, 2006

Versiani M, Mundim FD, Nardi AE, et al: Tranylcypromine in social phobia. J Clin Psychopharmacol 8:279–283, 1988

Versiani M, Nardi AE, Mundim FD: Fobia social [in Portuguese]. J Bras Psiquiatr 38:251–263, 1989

Versiani M, Nardi AE, Mundim FD, et al: Pharmacotherapy of social phobia: a controlled study with moclobemide and phenelzine. Br J Psychiatry 161:353–360, 1992

Versiani M, Nardi[a] AE, Figueira I, et al: Double-blind placebo controlled trials with bromazepam. J Bras Psiquiatr 46:167–171, 1997

Villarreal G, Johnson MR, Rubey R: Treatment of social phobia with the dopamine agonist pergolide. Depress Anxiety 11:45–47, 2000

Wagner KD, Berard R, Stein MB, et al: A multicenter, randomized, double-blind, placebo-controlled trial of paroxetine in children and adolescents with social anxiety disorder. Arch Gen Psychiatry 61:1153–1162, 2004

Walker JR, Van Ameringen MA, Swinson R: Prevention of relapse in generalized social phobia: results of a 24-week study in responders to 20 weeks of sertraline treatment. J Clin Psychopharmacol 6:636–644, 2000

Watson D, Friend R: Measurement of social evaluative anxiety. J Consult Clin Psychol 33:448–457, 1969

Westenberg HG, Stein DJ, Yang H, et al: A double-blind placebo-controlled study of controlled release fluvoxamine for the treatment of generalized social anxiety disorder. J Clin Psychopharmacol 24:49–55, 2004

Willoughby RR: Some properties of the Thrustone Personality Schedule and a suggested revision. J Soc Psychol 3:401–424, 1932

Zhang W, Connor KM, Davidson JR: Levetiracetam in social phobia: a placebo controlled pilot study. J Psychopharmacol 19:551–553, 2005

Zitrin CM, Klein DF, Woerner MG, et al: Treatment of phobias, I: a comparison of imipramine hydrochloride and placebo. Arch Gen Psychiatry 40:125–138, 1983

Recommended Readings

Grant BF, Hasin DS, Blanco C, et al: The epidemiology of social anxiety disorder in the United States: results from the National Epidemiologic Survey on Alcohol and Related Conditions. J Clin Psychiatry 66:1351–1361, 2005

Heimberg RG, Liebowitz MR, Hope DA, et al: Cognitive-behavioral group therapy versus phenelzine in social phobia: 12-week outcome. Arch Gen Psychiatry 55:1133–1141, 1998

Hofmann SG, Meuret AE, Smits JA, et al: Augmentation of exposure therapy with D-cycloserine for social anxiety disorder. Arch Gen Psychiatry 63:298–304, 2006

Research Unit on Pediatric Psychopharmacology Anxiety Study Group: Fluvoxamine for the treatment of anxiety disorders in children and adolescents. N Engl J Med 344:1279–1285, 2001

Schneier FR: Clinical practice: social anxiety disorder. N Engl J Med 355:1029–1036, 2006

Schneier FR, Welkowitz LA: The Hidden Face of Shyness. New York, Avon Books, 1996

Stein DJ, Stein MB, Pitts CD, et al: Predictors of response to pharmacotherapy in social anxiety disorder: an analysis of 3 placebo-controlled paroxetine trials. J Clin Psychiatry 63:152–155, 2002

Stein DJ, Ipser JC, Balkom AJ: Pharmacotherapy for social phobia. Cochrane Database Syst Rev 4:CD001206, 2004

Web Sites of Interest

Anxiety Disorders Association of America. http://www.adaa.org/GettingHelp/AnxietyDisorders/SocialPhobia.asp

National Institute of Mental Health. http://www.nimh.nih.gov/healthinformation/socialphobiamenu.cfm

Social Anxiety Research Clinic. http://www.columbia-socialanxiety.org

Chapter 28

Psychotherapy for Social Anxiety Disorder

Kristin E. Pontoski, M.A.
Richard G. Heimberg, Ph.D.
Cynthia L. Turk, Ph.D.
Meredith E. Coles, Ph.D.

Since the publication of DSM-III (American Psychiatric Association 1980), the body of literature focusing on the efficacy of psychological treatments for social phobia (social anxiety disorder) has matured. Nearly three decades of research has resulted in the development of several empirically supported cognitive-behavioral treatments, which include variations of exposure and cognitive restructuring techniques for adults presented in both group and individual formats. In addition, research has increasingly demonstrated the efficacy of cognitive-behavioral, psychosocial, and family interventions for children and adolescents with social anxiety disorder. More recent investigations have focused on specific factors that contribute to successful treatment outcome and enhancements to standard treatments that may increase long-term gains for patients with social anxiety disorders that are difficult to treat.

Cognitive-Behavioral Therapy

Theoretical Model Underlying Cognitive-Behavioral Therapy for Social Anxiety Disorder

The central concern of persons with social anxiety disorder is that they fear they will be negatively evaluated by others. Individuals with social anxiety worry that they will do or say something to elicit negative evaluation from others or that they will demonstrate physical symptoms during a social situation that will make them appear excessively anxious to others (American Psychiatric Association 2000). Rapee and Heimberg (1997) and D.M. Clark and Wells (1995) presented two similar models that described the maintenance of social anxiety and demonstrated why socially anxious individuals do not benefit from everyday interactions with others. Space limitations prohibit thorough explication of these models, and the reader is referred to the original sources. However, both models submitted that individuals with social anxiety disorder perceive social situations as dangerous and that the perception of potential evaluation by others initiates a cognitive routine that furthers the experience of anxiety. For instance, Rapee and Heimberg (1997) suggested that the perception of an evaluative audience leads the individual to focus on a mental representation of how he or she appears to that audience. This mental representation, which is likely to be negatively distorted, is compared with an estimate of what the person believes may be expected of him or her by that audience. As this discrepancy increases in a negative direction, the perceived probability of negative evaluation from the audience is increased. The person becomes hypervigilant for negative external cues (e.g., signs of boredom or disinterest from the audience) and internal cues (e.g., unpleasant physiological sensations), and these cues further inform the person's mental representation as seen by the perceived audience. The cycle repeats itself, with anxiety increasing as the person continually anticipates negative outcomes, and the situation comes to an end or the person escapes. Thereafter, the person may engage in postevent processing (Brozovich and Heimberg, in press), repeatedly reviewing and reconstructing the memory of the situation in a negative and ultimately maladaptive fashion. He or she is thus posed to experience equal or greater anxiety at the next occurrence of a similar situation.

This conceptualization and that of D.M. Clark and Wells (1995) suggest that it is critical to provide experiences that will allow the patient to reevaluate his or her cognitive construction of the self and others. Consistent with these conceptualizations, exposure, cognitive restructuring, and the combination of exposure and cognitive restructuring have been most commonly examined as a means of modifying patients' schemas and reducing symptoms of social anxiety. Several other cognitive and behavioral techniques have been utilized as well, including applied relaxation and social skills training.

Exposure Techniques

Exposure therapy is designed to give socially anxious patients access to their feared social situations via imagery (imaginal exposure) or direct confrontation (in vivo exposure) and has been recognized as an essential component of most successful treatments for anxiety for many years (Barlow and Wolfe 1981). According to behavioral models of social anxiety, exposure provides the opportunity for the naturally occurring process of habituation to the feared stimulus and increases contact with reinforcers for nonphobic behavior (McNeil et al. 2001). Cognitive models assert that exposure presents the opportunity for contact with powerful corrective information, which facilitates the modification of dysfunctional beliefs and the alteration of information processing biases, thereby decreasing anxiety (D.M. Clark and Wells 1995; Rapee and Heimberg 1997). Exposure techniques are maximally effective when patients are fully engaged in the emotional and physiological arousal associated with the feared situations (Foa and Kozak 1986), as is most likely to occur when patients are instructed to focus their attention fully on the exposure experience (Wells and Papageorgiou 1998). Research conducted since 2000 (see Bouton 2002) suggests that exposure produces new learning that competes with the previously learned fear response. However, much of that new learning may be context-specific, and the likelihood of return of fear after exposure increases with the degree of similarity of the new situation to the originally feared situation. Nevertheless, exposure techniques effectively reduce social anxiety (e.g., Fava et al. 1989). In comparative studies, exposure has proven superior to progressive muscle relaxation training (Al-Kubaisy et al. 1992; Alström et al. 1984), pill placebo (Turner et al. 1994b), wait-list control conditions (Butler et al. 1984; Newman et al. 1994), and a control therapy consisting of education, self-exposure instructions, and unspecified anxiolytic medication (Alström et al. 1984). However, there is some question as to the durability of gains when exposure is administered alone (Heimberg and Juster 1995), and exposure has often been combined with cognitive techniques in the treatment of social anxiety disorder. The effectiveness of this approach is discussed in the next section.

Combined Cognitive Restructuring and Exposure

Contemporary cognitive models of social anxiety disorder propose that anxiety is largely maintained by dysfunctional beliefs and biased information processing strategies; therefore, successful treatment will be associated with modification of these cognitive problems (e.g., D.M. Clark and Wells 1995; Rapee and Heimberg 1997). Socially anxious individuals who engage in self-exposure may not experience anxiety reduction, because they do not receive adequate feedback from their environment regarding the accuracy of their fear of negative evaluation (Butler 1985).

Several historical cognitive therapies have influenced the development of contemporary cognitive and behavioral techniques. Rational-emotive therapy (Ellis 1962) posits that individuals develop irrational beliefs that cause and sustain negative emotional states. Individuals with social anxiety disorder can be conceptualized as clinging to the irrational belief that one should be completely competent, adequate, and achieving in order to be viewed as a worthwhile person. The goal of rational-emotive therapy is to confront and modify these irrational beliefs through discussion and persuasion to change the patient's fundamental ideology. Modified versions of rational-emotive therapy have been associated with significant treatment gains among individuals with social anxiety disorder in several studies (e.g., DiGiuseppe et al. 1990; Emmelkamp et al. 1985; Mattick and Peters 1988; Mattick et al. 1989; Mersch et al. 1989). Treatment gains are durable, with patients maintaining their improvements at 18-month follow-up (Scholing and Emmelkamp 1996).

Beck's theoretical approach asserts that negative emotions are produced by cognitive processing errors such that patients label, interpret, and evaluate their experiences in a biased, highly personalized, overly arbitrary, or extreme manner (Beck 1976). Beck's cognitive therapy attempts to correct these errors through logic, Socratic discussion, and empirical testing of negative cognitions. The goal of therapy is to remold the patient's rigid, maladaptive rules to be more accurate, realistic, and flexible. Beck's cognitive therapy was influential in the development of cognitive-behavioral group therapy (CBGT) for social anxiety disorder (reviewed below). For the treatment of social anxiety disorder, Beck's cognitive therapy has been shown to produce treatment gains similar to those produced by rational-emotive therapy and superior to those produced by a wait-list control condition (DiGiuseppe et al. 1990).

Self-instructional training is a modified version of Meichenbaum's (1985) stress-inoculation training. In self-instructional training, patients observe and record the negative thoughts and feelings they experience in problematic situations to facilitate the development of more adaptive appraisals. They then work collaboratively with their therapists to develop coping thoughts and skills relevant to anticipating the problematic situation, engaging the situation, and thinking about the situation after it has concluded. Patients practice these coping thoughts and skills in imaginal rehearsal, role-plays, and real-life situations. In three studies, self-instructional training produced significant improvements among individuals with social anxiety disorder (DiGiuseppe et al. 1990; Emmelkamp et al. 1985; Jerremalm et al. 1986).

With few exceptions, most cognitive therapies for social anxiety disorder include systematic exposure to feared social situations and behavioral experiments (Juster and Heimberg 1998). Thus, these treatments are not "purely" cognitive. A growing body of research supports the efficacy of treatments incorporating both cognitive techniques and exposure. In comparative studies, these treatments have been shown to be superior to wait-list control conditions (Butler et al. 1984; D.M. Clark et al. 2006; DiGiuseppe et al. 1990; Hope et al. 1995a), an educational-supportive control therapy (Heimberg et al. 1990, 1993, 1998; Lucas and Telch 1993), and pill placebo (D.M. Clark et al. 2003; Heimberg et al. 1998).

Cognitive-Behavioral Group Therapy

A diverse literature has accumulated on the efficacy of CBGT, resulting in a treatment protocol designed specifically for social anxiety disorder (Heimberg and Becker 2002). CBGT consists of 12 weekly 2½-hour group sessions, the first two of which are designed to introduce the rationale for treatment, enhance the development of group cohesion, and teach cognitive restructuring concepts. Subsequent sessions focus on integrating cognitive restructuring skills with exposure so that patients learn to recognize, examine, and challenge their negative and inaccurate thoughts before, during, and after participating in role-plays of feared social situations in the group context. Exposures in session allow patients to test the accuracy of the automatic thoughts that arise during difficult social situations. Treatment in session ultimately focuses on exploring the core beliefs that underlie and maintain each patient's social concerns and on the adoption of achievable and objective goals in social situations rather than more abstract and unattainable ones (e.g., lack of nervousness, flawless performance). Patients also engage in exposures between sessions and practice applying cognitive restructuring skills to real-world anxiety-provoking situations with the goal of learning to be their own cognitive therapists.

A series of investigations contributed to the development and efficacy of this treatment protocol. CBGT was compared with educational-supportive group therapy (ES), a psychosocial treatment consisting of lectures, discussions, and group support (Heimberg et al. 1990). ES was designed to control for therapist attention, treatment credibility, and patient expectancies. A total of 49 patients meeting criteria for DSM-III social anxiety disorder were treated. Patient ratings confirmed that treatment credibility and outcome expectations were similar for CBGT and ES. Following treatment, clinical assessors assigned 75% of CBGT patients, but only 40% of ES patients, severity ratings below the level defined as clinically impaired. After treatment, CBGT patients reported less anxiety before and during an individualized behavior test than ES patients. Both groups showed similar improvement on self-report measures, but at 6-month follow-up, CBGT patients maintained their gains on self-report measures and remained more improved than ES patients on both assessor and behavior test anxiety ratings.

Of these patients, 19 participated in a long-term follow-up study in which the follow-up interval ranged from 4.5 to 6.25 years (Heimberg et al. 1993). The subset of follow-up participants was less impaired before and after treatment than nonparticipants. However, no pretreatment differences were found between CBGT and ES follow-up participants. At long-term follow-up, 89% of CBGT patients were rated below the clinical threshold by independent assessors, compared with 44% of ES patients. Assessor ratings indicated that CBGT patients experienced a level of anxiety not much greater than that of the general population. CBGT patients were rated as less anxious and more socially skilled during a behavior test than ES patients.

Lucas and Telch (1993) compared the effectiveness of CBGT, ES, and an individual version of the CBGT protocol (ICBT) in the treatment of 66 patients with DSM-III-R (American Psychiatric Association 1987) social anxiety disorder. This study replicated Heimberg et al.'s (1990) finding that patients treated with CBGT were more improved than patients treated with ES. CBGT and ICBT resulted in similar gains—both superior to ES. However, the group protocol was more cost-effective.

CBGT has also been compared with several pharmacotherapies that show proven efficacy for the treatment of social anxiety disorder. Heimberg et al. (1998) completed a two-site study in which 133 patients were randomly assigned to receive CBGT, the monoamine oxidase inhibitor (MAOI) phenelzine, ES, or pill placebo. All treatments were delivered at each site, one known for cognitive-behavioral treatment and the other for pharmacological treatment of anxiety disorders. At the week 6 (midtreatment) assessment, independent assessors rated phenelzine patients as more improved and less anxious than patients in all other conditions. At the 12-week (posttreatment) assessment, the independent assessors rated 75% of CBGT patients, 77% of phenelzine patients, 35% of ES patients, and 41% of placebo patients as treatment responders (either moderately or markedly improved). Thus, after 12 weeks of treatment, CBGT and phenelzine produced similar proportions of treatment responders, and both active treatments had higher proportions of responders than placebo or ES conditions. After 12 weeks, however, phenelzine patients were significantly more improved than CBGT patients on some measures. Encouragingly, there was no significant site-by-treatment interaction, suggesting that these treatments can be efficacious at facilities with differing theoretical orientations.

After the 12 weeks of acute treatment described above (Heimberg et al. 1998), patients demonstrating a positive response to either CBGT or phenelzine received monthly maintenance treatment for 6 months, which was followed by a 6-month follow-up (Liebowitz et al. 1999). Over the course of maintenance and follow-up, patients treated with CBGT were less likely to relapse than patients treated with phenelzine, and this was especially the case among patients with generalized social anxiety disorder. Thus, phenelzine may provide somewhat more immediate relief, but CBGT may provide greater protection against relapse.

CBGT has also been demonstrated to be roughly equivalent to the benzodiazepine clonazepam in acute efficacy (Otto et al. 2000). To investigate the efficacy of combining CBT with phenelzine, the same multisite research group completed a randomized, controlled trial comparing the efficacy of CBGT, phenelzine, combined CBGT/phenelzine, and pill placebo in 128 patients with social anxiety disorder (Heimberg 2003). Preliminary analyses suggested that the combined treatment outperformed pill placebo, fared better than phenelzine on some measures of social anxiety, and always produced better results than CBGT alone. A variant of CBGT, comprehensive cognitive-behavioral group therapy (CCBT; Foa EB, Herbert JD, Franklin ME, Bellack AS: "Comprehensive Cognitive Behavior Therapy for Generalized Social Phobia," unpublished manuscript, 1995), was compared with fluoxetine, placebo, and their combinations in a large multisite sample of individuals with generalized social anxiety disorder (Davidson et al. 2004). CCBT includes exposure and cognitive restructuring and an additional emphasis on social skills training to address deficits in social skills that could impede progress. After 14 weeks of treatment, all active treatments were documented as superior to the placebo condition, and the combined treatments did not seem to offer any additional efficacy over the individual therapies.

Heimberg and colleagues have adapted CBGT to an individual format (Hope et al. 2000, 2006). This workbook-driven, individual CBT involves 16 one-hour weekly sessions, conducted over 16–20 weeks, and consists of the same components as CBGT: psychoeducation, cognitive restructuring, and in-session and in vivo exposure. Zaider et al. (2003) demonstrated that this individualized CBT provided superior outcomes to a wait-list control condition and produced effect sizes similar to those in the group package.

Clark's Individual Cognitive Therapy for Social Anxiety Disorder

Clark's cognitive therapy (CT) has been widely applied to the individual treatment of social anxiety disorder. Based on the cognitive model of social anxiety discussed above (D.M. Clark and Wells 1995), this treatment focuses on the identification of specific safety behaviors that maintain socially anxious symptoms by fostering avoidance. The treatment consists of 16 weekly individual sessions during which the therapist and patient formulate a specified version of Clark's CT model with personalized thoughts, images, safety behaviors, and attentional strategies. An experiment is then conducted in which patients role-play a situation first using internal focus and safety behaviors and next attempting to focus outward and drop safety behaviors. Throughout the course of therapy, CT techniques are used to encourage patients to shift focus externally to gain a more accurate understanding of the way in which others interpret their behavior. In addition, video feedback (described below) is used to help correct distortions of self-imagery, and behavioral experiments are conducted to confront feared social situations while dropping safety behaviors and focusing attention externally, both in session and for homework.

Clark's CT has demonstrated efficacy in two randomized, controlled trials. D.M. Clark et al. (2003) compared CT to fluoxetine plus self-exposure and placebo plus self-exposure in 60 patients with social anxiety disorder. After 16 weeks, there were significant improvements from all three treatments, but CT was shown to be superior to both medication and placebo at midtreatment, posttreatment, and 12-month follow-up. It is unclear whether differences in session length or the inclusion of self-exposure instructions in the administration of medication and placebo confounded the interpretation of these results, although the difference between CT and the other conditions was substantial.

Clark's CT was next compared to exposure plus applied relaxation and a wait-list condition in a randomized, controlled trial of 60 individuals with social anxiety disorder (D.M. Clark et al. 2006). After 12 weeks of treatment, participants in both active treatment groups showed superior performance to those in the wait-list condition on most measures of distress and psychopathology, and the CT treatment was shown to be superior to exposure plus applied relaxation on the measures of social anxiety. These gains were maintained at 1-year follow-up. In particular, twice as many patients receiving CT were characterized as treatment responders, compared with those receiving exposure plus applied relaxation.

Group Cognitive-Behavioral Therapy Versus Individual Cognitive Therapy for Social Anxiety Disorder

Efforts have been made to compare the efficacy of individual CT (ICT) versus group CBT for social anxiety disorder. Stangier et al. (2003) compared Clark's CT with a group CBT based on Clark's model in a sample of individuals with social anxiety disorder. Both the individual and the group treatments resulted in improvements on general functioning and social anxiety, but gains on measures of social anxiety were larger among those receiving individual CBT. Mörtberg et al. (2007) compared ICT with a variant of group therapy called intensive group cognitive treatment (IGCT) and treatment as usual (pharmacotherapy with a selective serotonin reuptake inhibitor) in a sample of 100 patients with social anxiety disorder. After 14 weeks of treatment, all therapies showed some efficacy, and ICT demonstrated superiority to IGCT and treatment as usual. However, these results are difficult to interpret given that the IGCT was delivered in longer sessions over a 3-week period, whereas ICT and treatment as usual were delivered in weekly sessions over a 16-week period. Recall that Lucas and Telch (1993) found no differences between individual and group formats based on Heimberg's model. The results of meta-analyses (reported below) also failed to reveal differences in efficacy between group and individual CBT, leaving the question without a satisfactory answer.

Relaxation Techniques

Relaxation techniques are designed to help patients control the physiological component of their social anxiety, the rationale being that excessive arousal impedes performance in social situations. Several variations of relaxation have historically been used to treat social anxiety, either alone or paired with exposure to fear-evoking imagery. Progressive muscle relaxation training as a sole treatment has shown little efficacy for social anxiety disorder (Al-Kubaisy et al. 1992; Alström et al. 1984). Self-control desensitization, in which patients use progressive muscle relaxation in response to anxiety experienced while visualizing increasingly more anxiety-evoking scenes, and systematic desensitization, a technique that combines progressive muscle relaxation and the visualization of scenes of gradually increasing anxiety-evoking potential, both resulted in improvement on many measures, but this improvement was not found to be consistently superior to wait-list conditions (Kanter and Goldfried 1979; Marzillier et al. 1976).

Approaches in which individuals are specifically trained to apply relaxation skills in feared social situations have had more promising results (Jerremalm et al. 1986; Ost et al. 1981). In applied relaxation, patients learn to increase their awareness of the earliest signs of anxiety, to practice relaxation techniques until they are able to achieve a moderately relaxed state quickly, and then to apply their relaxation skills during anxiety provoking situations (Ost 1987). Thus, applied relaxation combines relaxation and exposure techniques, with relaxation skills being used as a means of coping with anxiety. As described in the earlier section "Clark's Individual Cognitive Therapy for Social Anxiety Disorder," D.M. Clark et al. (2006) compared cognitive therapy, exposure plus applied relaxation treatment, and a wait-list control condition for individuals with social anxiety disorder. Both active treatments showed significant treatment efficacy compared with the control group condition, but the cognitive therapy was more effective than the exposure plus relaxation treatment. Future studies should compare applied relaxation with exposure alone to determine whether the inclusion of relaxation enhances treatment efficacy; research should also focus on the combined efficacy of cognitive therapy, relaxation, and exposure.

Social Skills Training

Social skills training (SST) is another behavioral intervention designed to teach the skills necessary to achieve good social outcomes. SST is based on the assumption that socially anxious patients exhibit behavioral deficiencies (e.g., poor eye contact, difficulty maintaining a conversation) that elicit negative reactions from others and lead to perception of poor interpersonal outcomes (Lucock and Salkovskis 1988). Research examining the social skills of socially anxious individuals has produced mixed results, with some studies suggesting behavioral deficiencies (Halford and Foddy 1982; Stopa and Clark 1993) and others not (J.V. Clark and Arkowitz 1975; Glasgow and Arkowitz 1975; Rapee and Lim 1992). Even when behavioral deficits are observed, it is unclear whether they are a function of a lack of social knowledge or skill, behavioral inhibition produced by anxiety, or a combination of these and other factors. Socially anxious individuals often report a lack of skills to interact in various situations; however, observation of their performance during exposures often reveals their behavior to be within acceptable limits. This observation is consistent with research suggesting that individuals with social anxiety disorder often underestimate the adequacy of their social performance (e.g., Rapee and Lim 1992).

Techniques commonly used in social skills training include therapist modeling, behavioral rehearsal, corrective feedback, social reinforcement, and homework assignments. However, benefits attributed to social skills training could also be explained by training aspects (e.g., repeated practice of feared social behaviors), the exposure aspects (e.g., confrontation of feared situations), or the cognitive elements (e.g., corrective feedback about the adequacy of one's social behavior) inherent in the procedures (Heimberg 2003; Turk et al. 1999).

In the only controlled study of social skills training, 15 weeks of training failed to produce improvements in social anxiety, social skills, and overall clinical adjustment superior to those demonstrated by a wait-list control group (Marzillier et al. 1976). In several other studies, SST resulted in significant improvements in various aspects of social anxiety disorder such as reductions in self-reported anxiety, depression, and difficulty in social situations (Falloon et al. 1981; Lucock and Salkovskis 1988; Stravynski et al. 1982; Trower et al. 1978; Wlazlo et al. 1990). However, none of these studies included adequate control conditions. Turner et al. (1994a) reported in an uncontrolled study that social effectiveness therapy, a treatment that combines SST with psychoeducation and exposure, resulted in significant gains for patients with generalized social anxiety disorder and that these gains were maintained at 2-year follow-up (Turner et al. 1995). It is not possible to state with confidence from these uncontrolled studies that these treatments were responsible for successful outcomes or that SST is sufficient as a stand-alone treatment, and there is little evidence to support the latter conclusion (Ponniah and Hollon 2007). However, a 2005 study incorporated an SST module into standard CBGT and compared this treatment with CBGT alone for patients with generalized social anxiety disorder. Both treatments were efficacious, but the combination group demonstrated significantly greater gains (Herbert et al. 2005).

Meta-Analytic Findings

Several meta-analytic reviews of the efficacy of various cognitive-behavioral techniques for the treatment of social anxiety disorder have been conducted, resulting in the overall finding that cognitive-behavioral treatments tend to be superior to control conditions (Chambless and Hope 1996; Fedoroff and Taylor 2001; Feske and Chambless 1995; Gould et al. 1997; Taylor 1996).

Taylor (1996) examined individual trials for social anxiety disorder comparing several cognitive-behavioral treatments, including cognitive restructuring, SST, exposure, and exposure plus cognitive restructuring with wait-list and placebo control conditions. All active treatments were found to be superior to the wait-list condition, but only exposure combined with cognitive restructuring was shown to be superior to placebo. The active treatments demonstrated reductions in self-reported symptoms of social anxiety; these reductions were maintained, and often further improvements were made several months after treatment was discontinued. There were no differences among the active treatments in effect size at follow-up and no differences between group and individual treatment.

Gould et al. (1997) found no differences in outcome or attrition in their meta-analysis of CBT, pharmacotherapy, and combined treatment for social anxiety disorder. Gains resulting from CBT were maintained during follow-up. Exposure alone, cognitive restructuring plus exposure, and treatment with selective serotonin reuptake inhibitors had large effect sizes, whereas cognitive restructuring alone, SST, MAOIs, and benzodiazepines had moderate effect sizes. Like Taylor (1996), Gould et al. (1997) found no differences between group and individual treatment.

In the meta-analysis by Fedoroff and Taylor (2001), benzodiazepines and selective serotonin reuptake inhibitors were superior to wait-list, pill placebo, and attention placebo control conditions and applied relaxation. Benzodiazepines were superior to MAOIs, cognitive restructuring, cognitive restructuring plus exposure, and SST. Cognitive restructuring plus exposure was superior to applied relaxation and to attention placebo and wait-list controls. There were no other differences among the psychological treatments.

Factors Affecting Treatment Outcome in CBT for Social Anxiety Disorder

Subtype of Social Anxiety Disorder and Avoidant Personality Disorder

Individuals with generalized social anxiety disorder begin treatment with greater severity of symptoms and greater impairment than those with nongeneralized social anxiety disorder and are therefore less likely to achieve high end-state functioning after cognitive-behavioral treatment. In addition, the presence of avoidant personality disorder (APD), which is diagnosed in about 60% of individuals with social anxiety disorder, may also affect treatment outcome, but results are mixed. Some studies have found treatment to be less effective for individuals with social anxiety disorder and comorbid APD (Chambless et al. 1997; Feske et al. 1996), whereas others have found that APD does not significantly complicate treatment outcome (Brown et al. 1995; Hope et al. 1995b). Some researchers consider APD to be a more severe variant of social anxiety disorder (Heimberg 1996) and have noted that it remits with standard treatment for social anxiety disorder. For example, Brown et al. (1995) found that 47% of patients with social anxiety disorder and comorbid APD no longer met criteria for APD after CBT for social anxiety disorder.

Comorbid Anxiety and Mood Disorders

The effects of comorbid anxiety and mood disorders on the efficacy of CBT for social anxiety disorder have been investigated. Chambless et al. (1997) found that in a sample of individuals receiving CBGT for social anxiety disorder, a higher level of self-reported depression at pretreatment was related to a decreased posttreatment reduction in the level of anxious anticipation prior to a behavioral test; this pattern, however, was not found for clinician ratings of depression. Erwin et al. (2002) compared individuals with uncomplicated social anxiety disorder, comorbid anxiety disorder, and comorbid mood disorder. Those with comorbid mood disorder tended to have greater severity of symptoms both before and following 12 weeks of CBGT. Those with comorbid anxiety disorders fared as well as those with uncomplicated social anxiety disorder. Davidson et al. (2004) reported that higher levels of depressive symptoms were related to more severe social anxiety, less change in social anxiety, and greater attrition in a placebo-controlled study.

Moscovitch et al. (2005) found that in a sample of individuals receiving CBGT for social anxiety disorder, changes in depression were fully mediated by changes in social anxiety (accounting for 91% of the variance in depression scores), whereas changes in social anxiety were only partially mediated by changes in depression (accounting for only 6% of the variance in social anxiety scores), which suggests that improvements in the symptoms of depression tend to track improvements in the symptoms of social anxiety in this group of patients.

Comorbid Social Anxiety Disorder and Alcohol Abuse

Social anxiety disorder tends to co-occur at particularly high rates with alcohol use disorders. According to the National Epidemiological Survey on Alcohol and Related Conditions, nearly half of individuals with a lifetime diagnosis of social anxiety disorder also had a lifetime diagnosis of an alcohol use disorder (Grant et al. 2005). In addition, adolescent social anxiety disorder predicts later development of alcohol dependence by age 30 years, even when controlling for depression or other anxiety disorders (Buckner et al. 2008). Individuals with social anxiety disorder often report the use of alcohol as self-medication to reduce their anxiety in stressful situations (Buckner et al. 2006). Therefore, when the severity of alcohol use warrants a diagnosis of alcohol use disorder, patients might lack motivation to decrease their alcohol use. Motivational enhancement therapy (W.R. Miller et al. 1992) is a promising intervention for alcohol use disorder. The goal of motivational enhancement therapy is to resolve ambivalence around the desire to change problematic drinking behaviors. A case study demonstrated the successful treatment of a 33-year-old male with comorbid generalized social anxiety disorder and alcohol use disorder in which treatment consisted of a combined motivational enhancement therapy–CBT approach. After 19 sessions, the patient remitted from both disorders and continued to do well at 6-month follow-up (Buckner et al., in press). Controlled trials investigating the combination of these two treatments in this special population are necessary to better understand their efficacy.

Motivation, Expectancy, Homework Compliance, and Other Aspects of Treatment Process

Patients often have mixed reactions to treatment and may express ambivalence about their ability to make lasting changes. Several studies have examined the effects of treatment expectancy and homework compliance on treatment outcome in social anxiety disorder. In two studies, patients who found treatment to be credible and who expected treatment gains did better than those who held more negative expectations regarding treatment (Chambless et al. 1997; Safren et al. 1997). Homework compliance has also been related to treatment gains. Individuals who were more compliant made greater gains than less compliant individuals, both immediately following treatment (Leung and Heimberg 1996) and at a 6-month follow-up (Edelman and Chambless 1995). However, Woody and Adessky (2002) did not find support for this relationship.

Patients can also differ in their degree of motivation for therapy. A pilot study with a mixed group of patients with panic disorder, social anxiety disorder, and generalized anxiety disorder examined the benefit of adding three sessions of motivational interviewing prior to group CBT (Westra and Dozois 2006). Individuals who received motivational interviewing, as compared to those who received no pretreatment intervention, showed an increase in positive expectancy for anxiety change before treatment, were more compliant with assigned homework during CBT, and were more likely to be responders to CBT.

Other processes of treatment may influence outcome, and one of these may be group cohesion. Taube-Schiff et al. (2007) examined cohesion among persons receiving CBGT, finding that it increased over the life of the group. Importantly, controlling for baseline values, group cohesion predicted outcomes on measures of social anxiety, depression, and impairment. The nature of the alliance between therapist and patient may also be important in CBT for social anxiety disorder. S.A. Hayes et al. (2007) demonstrated that a strong alliance was associated with patients engaging in the session and finding the session helpful. However, a moderate alliance was most productive when the measure was the amount of anxiety reduction experienced during in-session exposures to feared situations. Speculatively, an alliance that is too weak may not provide a sufficient sense of safety for some patients, whereas a very strong alliance may suppress patients' anxiety experience and indirectly interfere with their ability to overcome it. Finally, in a study comparing group CBT, exposure group therapy, and wait-list control conditions, Hofmann (2004) examined whether changes in estimated social cost, or negative cognitive appraisal, mediated pretreatment to posttreatment changes in both active treatment groups. Only the group receiving group CBT showed continued improvement from posttreatment to the 6-month follow-up. Continued benefit was associated with an overall reduction in estimated social cost, suggesting that the cognitive-behavioral intervention was associated with greater treatment gains that are mediated through changes in estimated social cost.

Anger

We have also examined how patient anger affects treatment outcome. Individuals who experienced anger more frequently, were more quick-tempered, and were more likely to perceive unfair treatment by others were less likely to stay in treatment for the full 12-session course of CBGT (Erwin et al. 2003). Among those who completed treatment, patients who experienced more extreme anger and who were more likely to inhibit their anger made smaller treatment gains than less angry patients. One might speculate that anger interferes with the person's ability to engage fully in exposure to feared situations or to form a viable working alliance with the therapist or other group members.

The studies reviewed here have identified numerous variables that predict treatment outcome. Attempts to manipulate these predictors may serve to improve already effective treatments. For example, techniques for modifying negative expectancies, increasing homework compliance, or reducing anger may lead to better outcomes. These studies have also provided us with information about patients who may require additional or more intensive treatment, such as patients with generalized social disorder and/or comorbid depression.

Other Psychosocial Treatments for Social Anxiety Disorder

Cognitive-behavioral treatments are by far the most extensively researched psychosocial approaches for social anxiety disorder. However, in clinical practice, other approaches are often utilized. There is a small but growing body of literature on the efficacy of these approaches.

Psychodynamic Perspectives

Gabbard (1992) proposed three models for understanding the symptoms of social anxiety disorder: 1) shame experiences regarding unconscious wishes to be the center of attention, 2) guilt concerning wishes to eliminate competitors while doubting one's ability to actually do so, and 3) separation anxiety involving attempts for autonomy leading to long-term loss of a caregiver's love. An individual case of social anxiety disorder conceptualized from a psychodynamic perspective was presented by Zerbe (1997). Like Gabbard, Zerbe (1997) proposed that shame is an important underlying dynamic in social anxiety disorder. Zerbe presented the case of a woman with fears of performance situations (e.g., public speaking) and interaction situations (e.g., dating) based on the belief that she could never "measure up" to the demands of other people. Zerbe attributed the development of social anxiety disorder in this patient to a lack of nurturance and support from her parents during childhood. Zerbe (1997) asserted that "one can safely assume that the early traumatogenic environment of this patient played a substantial role in the etiology of her social phobia" (p. 10).

A short-term treatment manual has been developed for social anxiety disorder that is based on Luborsky's supportive-expressive therapy (Leichsenring et al. 2007). The treatment includes several elements, such as a focus on the core conflictual relationship theme that influences the patient's primary symptoms, goal setting, enhancing insight, and understanding the role of shame and unrealistic demands. In addition, there is a component similar to exposure in which patients are encouraged to confront feared social situations. This treatment manual is currently being used in a large-scale investigation comparing psychodynamic therapy to CBT for social anxiety disorder.

Interpersonal Psychotherapy

Interpersonal psychotherapy (IPT) is based on the assumption that psychiatric disorders occur and are maintained within a psychosocial and interpersonal context. The main goal of IPT is to improve the patient's interpersonal functioning as a means of achieving symptomatic recovery. IPT is a time-limited (12–16 week) therapy that is efficacious in the treatment of acute depression (for a review, see DeMello et al. 2005), dysthymic disorder (Markowitz 1994), and other disorders with an interpersonal component such as bulimia nervosa (Wilfley et al. 2002). Lipsitz et al. (1999) modified IPT for social anxiety disorder. In this treatment, core interpersonal problem areas are identified and then examined through multiple techniques (e.g., exploration of feelings and thoughts related to the problem area, encouragement of affective expression, clarification of feelings, communication and decisions analysis, and role-playing).

An initial uncontrolled study of IPT with nine individuals with social anxiety disorder yielded promising results (Lipsitz et al. 1999). Following treatment, 78% of patients were classified as responders by independent evaluators. Ratings of improvement were also significant on a clinician-administered measure of social anxiety, and self-ratings of global symptom severity and social distress also decreased following treatment. However, a randomized trial that compared IPT to a supportive therapy control for social anxiety disorder failed to replicate these initial findings (Lipsitz et al., in press). This study included 70 patients who received 14 weekly sessions of individual IPT or supportive therapy. Both groups demonstrated improvement on several measures of social anxiety, but the two treatment conditions were not significantly different on the majority of outcome measures or the proportion of treatment responders.

Another study did, however, provide some support for the efficacy of IPT for social anxiety disorder (Borge et al., in press). Conducted in an inpatient setting, this study compared 10 weeks of residential IPT to residential cognitive therapy in a sample of 80 individuals with social anxiety disorder. Treatments were modified to include individual and group components to best fit an inpatient setting. Both groups demonstrated improvements on measures of social anxiety, and these gains were maintained at 1-year follow-up. The efficacy of residential IPT was similar to that of IPT delivered in an outpatient setting. However, definitive conclusions about the efficacy of IPT for social anxiety disorder cannot be made, because there were few differences between the effects of residential IPT and CBT in this study (CBT was superior on a single secondary measure), and no control condition was included.

Morita Therapy

Morita therapy is a Japanese therapy for anxious patients that emphasizes behavior change and personal growth (Reynolds 1980). It encourages patients to relinquish control of emotions and redirect their attention toward more active and constructive pursuits. The experience of ego transcendence (i.e., forgetting oneself and one's symptoms) through immersion in activities is believed to play an integral role in patients' reformulation of themselves and their behavioral capacities. Although Morita therapy does contain some unique aspects (e.g., not explicitly attempting to reduce or eliminate anxious symptoms), it shares other components with Western therapies (e.g., use of reattribution, attentional refocusing, modifying of dysfunctional beliefs, positive reinterpretation). Morita therapy emphasizes that anxiety is not an abnormal experience or trait, that anxiety can be accepted as it is, and that attempts to manipulate or explicitly reduce anxiety often paradoxically result in increased preoccupation with symptoms. In feared situations, patients are instructed to persevere through anxious moments, focusing on the task at hand, to recognize they have a choice of action and not emotion, and to consider that the intensity of emotion is a reflection of the importance of the task.

A small body of literature has addressed the application of Morita therapy to shyness and social anxiety (Alden 1988; Ishiyama 1987). Ishiyama (1987) posited three fundamental philosophical premises in Morita therapy regarding social anxiety: 1) social anxiety is a normal human emotion, 2) social anxiety has a self-actualizing meaning, and 3) social anxiety can be used as a motivator-facilitator of constructive action. Case studies have shown Morita therapy to be successful in helping patients to accept their anxiety and redirect their attention away from it (Alfonso 1992; Ishiyama 1986). In a study of five socially anxious college students, Ishiyama (1991) found Morita therapy reduced patients' target complaints, increased coping effectiveness, and reduced social anxiety and avoidance.

Acceptance and Commitment Therapy

Acceptance and commitment therapy has been recently applied to the treatment of social anxiety disorder with promising results. Dalrymple and Herbert (2007) investigated the efficacy of a 12-week program integrating exposure therapy and acceptance and commitment therapy. Several measures were administered to assess social anxiety symptoms, experiential avoidance (the attempt to alter the form, frequency, or situational sensitivity of private events even when doing so causes behavioral harm; S.C. Hayes et al. 1996), and general quality of life. Nineteen participants received 12 weekly 1-hour sessions that included presentation of the four main components of acceptance and commitment therapy. The first stage (sessions 1 and 2) involved "creative helplessness," in which participants came to understand the futility of their past efforts to control anxiety. The next phase (starting with session 3) presented the concept of "willingness" to have unwanted or distressing thoughts while being exposed to difficult social situations. Mindfulness techniques were presented in the third stage (beginning in session 4) to help teach nonjudgmental experience and appraisal of anxious thoughts and to move toward cognitive defusion, the exercise of separating the self from internal experiences. The final stage (beginning in session 7) facilitated participation in experiences that reflected one's valued choices. These acceptance and commitment therapy concepts were demonstrated using metaphors and experiential exercises. The treatment also incorporated traditional behavior therapy techniques such as in-session role-plays, in vivo exposure, and social skills training.

Participants were assessed at posttreatment and at 3-month follow-up. They displayed a significant decrease in social anxiety, fear of negative evaluation, and experiential avoidance and a significant increase in quality of life. A midtreatment decrease in experiential avoidance predicted posttreatment decrease in anxiety. Similar results were reported in a small uncontrolled trial of acceptance and commitment therapy–based group therapy for social anxiety disorder (Ossman et al. 2006).

Meditation-Based Stress Reduction

A randomized trial compared CBGT and a meditation-based stress reduction program (MBSR; Koszycki et al. 2007). The authors suggested that MBSR might be beneficial for social anxiety disorder because it may help patients shift from a focus on threat-related social cues to an external focus on the social world. Mindfulness techniques may also help decrease physiological symptoms such as increased heart rate, blushing, trembling, and sweating, thus making social interactions more manageable (J.J. Miller et al. 1995). A total of 53 participants were randomly assigned to receive either group MBSR or CBGT. The CBGT group received 12 weekly 2-hour group sessions according to the Heimberg and Becker (2002) treatment manual delivered by therapists experienced in CBT for anxiety. The MBSR treatment included 8 weekly 2-hour sessions and 1 all-day meditation retreat delivered by a meditation instructor. The program included psychoeducation about meditation and yoga techniques and instruction to perform daily audiotape-guided meditation.

Both the MBSR and the CGBT conditions demonstrated clinically meaningful changes on measures of social anxiety, depression, and quality of life; however, patients receiving CBGT demonstrated greater reductions in self-reported fear of negative evaluation and clinician-rated behavioral avoidance. Although it was somewhat less efficacious than CBGT, MBSR appeared to produce meaningful improvements in socially anxious patients. MBSR could be disseminated to a variety of settings by lay people expert in meditation but not necessarily in mental health practice, perhaps helping to reach those socially anxious persons reluctant to pursue more traditional treatment options. Further research should be conducted investigating the efficacy of incorporating meditation/mindfulness techniques into standard CBT practices to see whether they enhance treatment outcome.

Long-Term Treatment

There is little research on long-term treatment of social anxiety disorder, and this is an important future research agenda. Follow-up data for short-term treatments suggest maintenance of gains for CBT for intervals up to 5 years (Heimberg et al. 1993; Taylor 1996) and modest relapse (Liebowitz et al. 1999). Nevertheless, there is a need for study of longer-term treatment, especially for patients who do not show complete response to acute treatments.

Special Populations

Cognitive-Behavioral Therapy for Children and Adolescents With Social Anxiety Disorder

As the field of psychology has moved to emphasize prevention of psychopathology, an important area of research focuses on the treatment of childhood and adolescent social anxiety disorder, and much more work is needed in this area. However, in most studies children with social anxiety disorder and children with other anxiety disorders were combined without considering possible diagnosis effects. Kendall (1994) and Kendall et al. (1997) investigated the efficacy of a 16-session cognitive-behavioral treatment program for anxiety disorders in two separate groups of children (ages 9–13 years). Both studies included samples of adolescents with overanxious disorder, separation anxiety disorder, and avoidant disorder (social anxiety disorder). Kendall (1994) showed cognitive-behavioral treatment to be superior to a wait-list condition, and improvements in the cognitive-behavioral group were maintained at 1-year follow-up. Kendall et al. (1997) replicated these findings, and more than 50% of treated children no longer met criteria for their primary anxiety disorder. At follow-up an average of 7.4 years after treatment, participants demonstrated continued improvements in anxiety, based on interviews of adolescents and their parents, and positive responders showed a reduced amount of substance abuse compared with responders who had shown less improvement in anxiety (Kendall et al. 2004).

To address the potential importance of family factors in the maintenance of anxiety, *family anxiety management* (Sanders and Dadds 1993) was designed as an adjunct to individual CBT for anxious children. Family anxiety management involves the training of parents to reward courageous behavior, extinguish anxious behavior, cope with their own anxiety, and help with communication and problem-solving skills. Barrett et al. (1996) compared CBT alone, CBT plus family anxiety management, and a wait-list condition in 79 children with overanxious disorder, separation anxiety disorder, or social anxiety disorder. Both treatment conditions were shown to be superior to the wait-list control condition, and family anxiety management augmented the efficacy of CBT. Rates of response did not differ by diagnosis.

Spence et al. (2000) also investigated the efficacy of child-focused CBT compared with CBT plus parent involvement and a wait-list control condition for 12 weekly group sessions. The CBT participants were to receive social skills training, relaxation training, gradual exposure to feared social situations, and cognitive restructuring; a total of 50 children with social anxiety disorder were randomly assigned to one of the three conditions. The parent involvement component was investigated to determine whether parents can learn how to model and reinforce social skills, discourage situational avoidance, and reinforce homework compliance. At posttreatment, children in both CBT conditions showed a greater decrease in social anxiety symptoms and greater parent-rated social skills than the wait-list group; these gains were maintained at 1-year follow-up. There was a trend toward greater improvement in the CBT plus parent involvement group, but differences were not statistically significant.

Other studies have examined interventions specifically designed for children and adolescents with a primary diagnosis of social anxiety disorder. A group treatment program based on Heimberg et al.'s (1990) CBGT was adapted for adolescents with social anxiety (Albano et al. 1995). The program included psychoeducation, problem-solving techniques, assertiveness training, cognitive restructuring, and graduated exposure to distressing social situations. Albano et al. demonstrated efficacy of CBGT adapted for adolescents with five patients, four of whom displayed subclinical levels of social anxiety disorder at posttreatment and at 1-year follow-up. Hayward et al. (2000) randomly assigned 35 female adolescents with social anxiety disorder to receive either CBGT for adolescents or no treatment. The treatment group displayed significant gains after 16 weeks compared with the no-treatment group; however, these gains were not maintained at 1-year follow-up.

Another CBT intervention was designed to target a younger group of children with social anxiety disorder (Gallagher et al. 2004). The investigation included 23 preadolescent children (ages 8–11 years) who were randomly assigned to either a 3-week cognitive-behavioral group intervention or a wait-list control group. Treatment was delivered over 3 weeks in 3 intensive group sessions that focused on psychoeducation, cognitive exercises, and behavioral exposure. Improvements in anxiety and depression at posttreatment in the active group were significantly greater than in the wait-list group, according to parent and child reports.

Beidel et al. (2000) compared social effectiveness therapy for children (SET-C) with an active nonspecific comparison treatment in children ages 8–12 years with social anxiety disorder. SET-C includes group SST, peer generalization sessions, and individually tailored in vivo exposure. Children in the SET-C group demonstrated increased social skills and social interaction and decreased social anxiety symptoms at posttreatment; 67% of the SET-C group, compared with 5% of the control condition, did not meet criteria for social anxiety disorder at posttreatment, and gains were maintained at 6-month follow-up. Furthermore, at a 3-year follow-up, 72% of the children in the SET-C group continued to be free of the diagnosis of social anxiety disorder (Beidel et al. 2005), and at 5-year follow-up the majority of improvements made during treatment continued to be maintained (Beidel et al. 2006). This finding is particularly compelling given that most participants had reached mid-adolescence—the period considered to be the peak age of onset for social anxiety disorder—by this time, yet treatment effects were maintained across measures of general psychopathology and social anxiety. These follow-up data suggest that individuals treated with the SET-C program acquire skills that they can continue to implement for several years after completing treatment and at 5-year follow-up.

Masia-Warner et al. (2005) completed a randomized, controlled trial investigating the efficacy of a school-based group treatment program, skills for social and academic success (SASS), compared with a wait-list control condition in a sample of 35 adolescents with social anxiety disorder. The program was designed to conform flexibly to the scheduling conflicts of a high school calendar and consisted of 12 weekly group school sessions (approximately 40 minutes each), two 15-minute individual meetings, and two group booster sessions. Additionally, four 90-minute weekend social events that included prosocial peers, called "peer assistants," provided real-world exposures and opportunities for skills generalization and feelings of mastery. Parents and teachers each attended two group meetings to help integrate the skills learned into both home and school settings. Adolescents in the SASS group demonstrated significantly greater reductions in social anxiety and avoidance and improved functioning compared with the wait-list group, as indicated by parent, adolescent, and assessor reports. Furthermore, 67% of treated subjects, compared with 6% of wait-list participants, no longer met criteria for social anxiety disorder following treatment. Importantly, this study demonstrates the effectiveness of disseminating CBT techniques to a school setting. In summary, several interventions have demonstrated efficacy for decreasing social anxiety and improving general quality of life in children and adolescents. Future studies should continue to investigate the potential advantage of parent and teacher involvement, the contextual factors that best foster long-term treatment gains (school, home, neighborhood, or clinic), and factors that affect treatment efficacy.

Minority Populations

Fink et al.'s (1996) treatment of a 39-year-old African American woman illustrates the importance of cultural factors in the treatment of social anxiety disorder. The patient presented in this case study initially reported fear of interacting with colleagues in the medical field. When her fears were further examined, it became evident that she was particularly fearful of interactions with Caucasian individuals, including settings in which she interacted with male Caucasian physicians and classroom settings in which she was the only African American student among many Caucasian students. Inclusion of these culturally relevant factors in the patient's imaginal exposure scenes and in vivo homework assignments (e.g., imagining or interacting with Caucasian doctors or students) enhanced the social-evaluative fear-provoking nature of the scene/event and enhanced the efficacy of the exposure exercise. Fink et al. (1996) argued that it is unlikely that the long-term success realized by their patient would have been observed if her core concerns regarding cultural factors had not been addressed.

Little empirical research has examined the effects of ethnicity or cultural factors on the outcome of treatment for social anxiety disorder. In a study by Treadwell et al. (1995), cognitive-behavioral treatment was equally effective among anxious children of different ethnic groups. However, this study did not specifically address social anxiety disorder.

Patients With Treatment-Refractory Social Anxiety Disorder

To date, CBT—delivered either in individual or group format—is the most efficacious psychological treatment for social anxiety disorder. Although these treatments tend to help the majority of patients, more work is needed on strategies to enhance treatment for patients with social anxiety that is more difficult to treat. One of the most logical options to pursue when CBT fails to produce significant treatment gains is augmentation with (or switch to) pharmacotherapy. However, little research has been devoted to the topic of treating patients with CBT-refractory social anxiety disorder, and options for patients who do not respond well to medication treatments or who prefer not to pursue pharmacotherapy are not well defined. Research that examines randomization to secondary treatments after an initial course of CBT has been insufficiently illuminating, and identifying patient or clinical variables that might moderate effects of the secondary treatments is an important agenda for future research.

One important aspect of treatment to revisit in patients with refractory disorders is an accurate and thorough case conceptualization. The information gathered in the beginning of therapy forms the foundation of a well-conceptualized case, but in cases that are difficult to treat, this information should be continually updated. As the therapist learns more about the patient, his or her complex difficulties could extend beyond the realm of a fundamental fear of negative evaluation and could, therefore, require additional techniques to address comorbid problems, such as depression, anger, or substance abuse (Wright et al. 2006). It is also helpful for therapists to speak directly with patients about how they understand the rationale of CBT and the ability for CBT techniques to adequately address their problems. A comparison of dropouts and completers of treatment for social anxiety found that completers rated the treatment to be more logical than dropouts (Hofmann and Suvak 2006). Other research reviewed in this chapter suggests that patients who do not believe in the credibility of their treatments are less likely to respond positively.

Practical Techniques and Experimental Approaches

In addition to the more traditional cognitive-behavioral techniques to treat social anxiety disorder, including exposure, cognitive restructuring, relaxation, and social skills training, some experimental techniques show promise for the future treatment of social anxiety disorder.

One very useful technique that deserves much further study is video feedback, employed in the individual therapies of both Clark and Heimberg. The data consistently demonstrate that patients with social anxiety disorder underestimate the quality of their behavioral performance, and this distortion begs for correction (Rapee and Lim 1992; Stopa and Clark 1993). In video feedback, after an in-session exposure, the patient and therapist view the tape, but they do so in a very specific manner, referred to in the literature as cognitive preparation. The patient is first asked to imagine what his or her performance may have been like and to specifically evaluate several behaviors of concern. He or she is then instructed to view the video from a stance of neutrality, as if watching the performance of a stranger. Several studies suggest that this strategy produces improvements in self-perception of behavior and that it may be most useful among those whose self-perceptions are most discrepant from the ratings of their behavior by others (Harvey et al. 2000; Kim et al. 2002; Rodebaugh and Chambless 2002; Rodebaugh and Rapee 2005). However, few studies have examined the efficacy of video feedback in clinical samples or as an integrated portion of an overall cognitive-behavioral approach, and not all investigators report positive results (e.g., see Smits et al. 2006).

A preliminary study has examined a technique to directly address memories of unpleasant social experiences among social anxiety patients (Wild et al. 2008). In one session lasting approximately 1.5 hours, patients were instructed in cognitive restructuring and a process called *memory rescripting*. During memory rescripting, patients imagine the event taking place at the age they were when it occurred, then imagine it at their current age watching their younger self and intervening if they wish, and finally imagine it as their younger self with the adult self in the room, intervening as before. In the control condition, a therapist encourages the patient to talk about the early memory and the image associated with it, providing supportive listening and reflection without challenging the patient. Individuals who received the rescripting session were less likely to fully believe the encapsulated belief represented in the memory, were less distressed by the memory, and gave lower anxiety ratings when visualizing feared social situations than control subjects. The utility of integrating this approach with other cognitive restructuring techniques should be evaluated in future research. Furthermore, techniques of this nature are consistent with the finding that some patients with social anxiety disorder react to memories of stressful social experiences as do patients with posttraumatic stress disorder after a traumatic event (Erwin et al. 2006); this suggests the potential utility of prolonged imaginal exposure to these "traumatic" memories as a potentially useful treatment intervention.

Virtual reality exposure offers an advantage over traditional exposure because it allows for the simulation of feared situations in session that may otherwise be difficult to coordinate (e.g., public speaking situations in which a sizable audience is required) or that the patient might be reluctant to approach in vivo. A preliminary open trial of individual CBT for public speaking anxiety using virtual reality exposure was recently conducted (Andersen et al. 2005). Ten participants received four sessions of anxiety management training and four sessions of virtual reality exposure. Decreases in self-reported public speaking anxiety were demonstrated at posttreatment and 3-month follow-up. In addition, an investigation of 36 socially anxious individuals compared virtual reality therapy to CBGT (Klinger et al. 2005). Participants in the virtual reality therapy group were exposed for 20-minute intervals to simulations of public speaking, assertiveness, scrutiny, and intimacy situations. Both treatments resulted in clinically significant reductions in social anxiety. The magnitude of effect of the two treatments was similar, suggesting that virtual reality therapy may be a viable alternative to more studied methods of treatment for social anxiety disorder. Additional study is clearly warranted.

Another area of great potential promise is augmentation of the efficacy of exposure or other forms of CBT with chemical aids. D-Cycloserine (DCS), a partial agonist of the *N*-methyl-D-aspartate receptor, has been shown to augment learning and memory, and doses of DCS received shortly after exposure facilitate extinction to feared stimuli in animals. The use of DCS in animal trials and in the treatment of human anxiety is summarized in Chapter 24, "Psychotherapy for Panic Disorder," in this volume. Hofmann et al. (2006) present very compelling pilot data of the utility of DCS in the cognitive-behavioral treatment of social anxiety disorder, and these findings were replicated by Guastella et al (2008).

An important future direction for the treatment of generalized social anxiety disorder is the development of treatments that are more accessible to those individuals reluctant to seek treatment because of fear or embarrassment associated with doing so (Newman et al. 2003). Individuals with social anxiety disorder who have not sought treatment list fear of negative evaluation by the treatment provider as a significant barrier to treatment seeking (Olfson et al. 2000). And there is a population of persons who use the Internet as a resource; the social anxiety symptoms of these individuals are more severe than those of persons who seek treatment (Erwin et al. 2004), making the dissemination of treatment via the Web an important priority. A trial of 64 individuals with generalized social anxiety disorder compared a type of therapy consisting of a 9-week Internet-based self-help CBT manual with a wait-list control condition (Andersson et al. 2006). In addition to receiving the manual, participants in the active treatment condition completed two in-person group exposure sessions and had e-mail contact with a therapist. The Internet-based therapy was associated with significant improvements in social anxiety, fear, avoidance, depression, and generalized anxiety compared with the wait-list control group, and these gains were maintained at 1-year follow-up. Future studies should compare the efficacy of such treatments (as well as fully self-administered, Web-based treatments) with empirically supported therapies such as CBGT.

Conclusion

At this point, there is considerable evidence supporting the efficacy of CBT for social anxiety disorder, and this appears to be the case whether treatment is delivered in group or individual therapy. (Note, however, that there is little research about ways in which these modalities might be usefully combined.) Exposure is certainly a key ingredient in the efficacy of CBT, and it is likely (although less definitively demonstrated) that the combination of exposure and cognitive restructuring yields the most clinically significant outcomes. Applied relaxation appears to have clinical utility. The support for social skills training is much more mixed, with the data suggesting it is not a sufficient stand-alone treatment, but it might have a role as an adjunct to other cognitive-behavioral techniques. Little is known about long-term treatment or the utility of booster sessions for social anxiety disorder. CBT compares well with pharmacotherapy in terms of acute efficacy, but so far as it has been evaluated, successful CBT appears to confer protection against relapse that is less likely with common pharmacotherapies. The data on the combination of CBT and pharmacotherapy do not provide us with clear direction; combined treatment is not clearly superior, and the role of either treatment in augmenting the efficacy of the other is largely unknown.

In adults, CBT outcome is predicted to a degree by the presence of generalized fear, avoidant personality disorder, and depression, although results for each of these variables are mixed, and all may be proxies for the severity of social anxiety disorder. The presence of other anxiety disorders does not seem to adversely affect outcome. Anger and substance abuse are certain to complicate the course of treatment, but solutions for these problems have not been studied. Expectancy for a positive treatment outcome, compliance with between-session therapy assignments, and group cohesion do appear to predict positive outcomes, and changes in cognition appear to mediate change in CBT.

Beyond CBT, the literature on treatment approaches to social anxiety disorder becomes sparse. Interpersonal therapy has been the most extensively studied, but with decidedly mixed results. Psychodynamic treatments lack empirical data, although a trial is currently under way. Acceptance and mindfulness strategies have yielded promising preliminary data but require much further research. Regardless of therapy approach, the use of the World Wide Web as a tool for reaching out to persons who might not otherwise access treatment is an important consideration for the future.

Much less is known about the treatment of children and adolescents with social anxiety disorder, partly because that literature does not tend to examine outcomes for separate anxiety disorders as a matter of course; however, much headway has been made in that direction, and CBT appears to be associated with significant positive change. Involvement of family members, especially for younger children, may be an important aspect of treatment, and involvement of peers is likely to be helpful for adolescents.

Key Clinical Points

The literature thus far on CBT for social anxiety disorder does not allow a consensus statement regarding an algorithm for optimal treatment outcome. It does appear that the following components of treatment are important:

- Psychoeducation about social anxiety disorder, including a cognitive-behavioral conceptualization of the patient's specific difficulties
- Training in the skills necessary to view and evaluate one's thinking and behavior from a distanced and objective perspective
- Exposure to feared social and/or performance situations in a graduated manner
- Behavioral experiments testing specific negative beliefs or predictions held by the patient
- Generalization of new learning across a number of environments
- Methods to help the patient develop an attitude of approach toward anxiety-evoking situations so that desired outcomes can be accomplished, with or without anxiety

References

Albano AM, Marten PA, Holt CS, et al: Cognitive-behavioral group treatment for social phobia in adolescents: a preliminary study. J Nerv Ment Dis 183:649–656, 1995

Alden LE: Morita therapy with socially avoidant clients. International Bulletin of Morita Therapy 1:43–51, 1988

Alfonso V: Brief Morita intervention with a socially anxious client: a case study. International Bulletin of Morita Therapy 5:26–34, 1992

Al-Kubaisy T, Marks IM, Logsdail S, et al: Role of exposure homework in phobia reduction: a controlled study. Behav Ther 23:599–621, 1992

Alström JE, Nordlund CL, Persson G, et al: Effects of four treatment methods on social phobic patients not suitable for insight-oriented psychotherapy. Acta Psychiatr Scand 70:97–110, 1984

American Psychiatric Association: Diagnostic and Statistical Manual of Mental Disorders, 3rd Edition. Washington, DC, American Psychiatric Association, 1980

American Psychiatric Association: Diagnostic and Statistical Manual of Mental Disorders, 3rd Edition, Revised. Washington, DC, American Psychiatric Association, 1987

American Psychiatric Association: Diagnostic and Statistical Manual of Mental Disorders, 4th Edition, Text Revision. Washington, DC, American Psychiatric Association, 2000

Anderson PL, Zimand E, Hodges LF, et al: Cognitive behavioral therapy for public-speaking anxiety using virtual reality for exposure. Depress Anxiety 22:156–158, 2005

Andersson G, Carlbring P, Holmström A, et al: Internet-based self-help with therapist feedback in vivo group exposure for social phobia: a randomized controlled trial. J Consult Clin Psychol 74:677–686, 2006

Barlow DH, Wolfe BE: Behavioral approaches to anxiety disorders: a report on the NIMH-SUNY, Albany, research conference. J Consult Clin Psychol 49:448–454, 1981

Barrett PM, Dadds MR, Rapee RM: Family treatment of childhood anxiety: a controlled trial. J Consult Clin Psychol 64:333–342, 1996

Beck AT: Cognitive Therapy and the Emotional Disorders. Oxford, UK, International Universities Press, 1976

Beidel DC, Turner SM, Morris TL: Behavioral treatment of childhood social phobia. J Consult Clin Psychol 68:1072–1080, 2000

Beidel DC, Turner SM, Young BJ, et al: Social effectiveness therapy for children: three-year follow up. J Consult Clinical Psychol 73:721–725, 2005

Beidel DC, Turner SM, Young BJ: Social effectiveness therapy for children: five years later. Behav Ther 37:416–425, 2006

Borge FM, Hoffart A, Sexton H, et al: Residential cognitive therapy versus residential interpersonal therapy for social phobia: a randomized clinical trial. J Anxiety Disord 22:991–1010, 2008

Bouton ME: Context, ambiguity, and unlearning: sources of relapse after behavioral extinction. Biol Psychiatry 52:976–986, 2002

Brown EB, Heimberg RG, Juster HR: Social phobia subtype and avoidant personality disorder: effect on severity of social phobia, impairment, and outcome of cognitive-behavioral treatment. Behav Ther 26:467–486, 1995

Brozovich F, Heimberg RG: An analysis of post-event processing in social anxiety disorder. Clin Psychol Rev 28:891–903, 2008

Buckner JD, Eggleston AM, Schmidt NB: Social anxiety and problematic alcohol consumption: the mediating role of drinking motives and situations. Behav Ther 37:381–391, 2006

Buckner JD, Schmidt NB, Lang AR, et al: Specificity of social anxiety disorder as a risk factor for alcohol and cannabis dependence. J Psychiatr Res 42:230–239, 2008

Buckner JD, Ledley DR, Heimberg RG, et al: Treating comorbid social anxiety and alcohol use disorders: combining motivation enhancement therapy with cognitive-behavioral therapy. Clinical Case Studies 7:208–223, 2008

Butler G: Exposure as a treatment for social phobia: some instructive difficulties. Behav Res Ther 23:651–657, 1985

Butler G, Cullington A, Munby M, et al: Exposure and anxiety management in the treatment of social phobia. J Consult Clin Psychol 52:642–650, 1984

Chambless DL, Hope DA: Cognitive approaches to the psychopathology and treatment of social phobia, in Frontiers of Cognitive Therapy. Edited by Salkovskis PM. New York, Guilford, 1996, pp 345–382

Chambless DL, Tran GQ, Glass CR: Predictors of response to cognitive-behavioral group therapy for social phobia. J Anxiety Disord 11:221–240, 1997

Clark DM, Wells A: A cognitive model of social phobia, in Social Phobia: Diagnosis, Assessment and Treatment. Edited by Heimberg RG, Liebowitz MR, Hope DA, et al. New York, Guilford, 1995, pp 69–93

Clark DM, Ehlers A, McManus F, et al: Cognitive therapy versus fluoxetine in generalized social phobia: a randomized placebo-controlled trial. J Consult Clin Psychol 71:1058–1067, 2003

Clark DM, Ehlers A, Hackmann A, et al: Cognitive therapy versus exposure and applied relaxation in social phobia: a randomized controlled trial. J Consult Clin Psychol 74:568–578, 2006

Clark JV, Arkowitz H: Social anxiety and self-evaluation of interpersonal performance. Psychol Rep 36:211–221, 1975

Dalrymple KL, Herbert JD: Acceptance and commitment therapy for generalized social anxiety disorder. Behav Modif 31:543–568, 2007

Davidson JRT, Foa EB, Huppert J, et al: Fluoxetine, comprehensive cognitive behavioral therapy, and placebo in generalized social phobia. Arch Gen Psychiatry 61:1005–1013, 2004

DeMello MF, de Jesus Mari J, Bacaltchuk J, et al: A systematic review of research findings on the efficacy of interpersonal therapy for depressive disorders. Eur Arch Psychiatry 255:75–82, 2005

DiGiuseppe R, McGowan L, Sutton-Simon K, et al: A comparative outcome study of four cognitive therapies in the treatment of social anxiety. Journal of Rational-Emotive and Cognitive-Behavior Therapy 8:129–146, 1990

Edelman RE, Chambless DL: Adherence during sessions and homework in cognitive-behavioral group treatment of social phobia. Behav Res Ther 33:573–577, 1995

Ellis A: Reason and Emotion in Psychotherapy. New York, Lyle Stuart, 1962

Emmelkamp PM, Mersch PP, Vissia E, et al: Social phobia: a comparative evaluation of cognitive and behavioral interventions. Behav Res Ther 23:365–369, 1985

Erwin BA, Heimberg RG, Juster H, et al: Comorbid anxiety and mood disorders among persons with social anxiety disorder. Behav Res Ther 40:19–35, 2002

Erwin BA, Heimberg RG, Schneier FR, et al: Anger experience and expression in social anxiety disorder: pretreatment profile and predictors of attrition and response to cognitive-behavioral treatment. Behav Ther 34:331–350, 2003

Erwin BA, Turk CL, Heimberg RG, et al: The Internet: home to a severe population of individuals with social anxiety disorder? J Anxiety Disord 18:629–646, 2004

Erwin BA, Heimberg RG, Marx BP, et al: Traumatic and socially stressful life events among persons with social anxiety disorder. J Anxiety Disord 20:896–914, 2006

Falloon IRH, Lloyd GG, Harpin RE: The treatment of social phobia: real-life rehearsal with nonprofessional therapists. J Nerv Ment Dis 169:180–184, 1981

Fava GA, Grandi S, Canestrari R: Treatment of social phobia by homework exposure. Psychother Psychosom 52:209–213, 1989

Fedoroff IC, Taylor S: Psychological and pharmacological treatments for social anxiety disorder: a meta-analysis. J Clin Psychopharmacol 21:311–324, 2001

Feske U, Chambless DL: Cognitive behavioral versus exposure only treatment for social phobia: a meta-analysis. Behav Ther 26:695–720, 1995

Feske U, Perry KJ, Chambless DL, et al: Avoidant personality disorder as a predictor for treatment outcome among generalized social phobics. J Pers Disord 10:174–184, 1996

Fink CM, Turner SM, Beidel DC: Culturally relevant factors in the behavioral treatment of social phobia: a case study. J Anxiety Disord 10:201–209, 1996

Foa EB, Kozak MJ: Emotional processing of fear: exposure to corrective information. Psychol Bull 99:20–35, 1986

Gabbard GO: Psychodynamics of panic disorder and social phobia. Bull Menninger Clin 56:A3–13, 1992

Gallagher HM, Rabian BA, McCloskey MS: A brief cognitive-behavioral intervention for social phobia in childhood. J Anxiety Disord 18:459–479, 2004

Glasgow RE, Arkowitz H: The behavioral assessment of male and female social competence in dyadic interactions. Behav Ther 6:488–498, 1975

Gould RA, Buckminster S, Pollack MH, et al: Cognitive-behavioral and pharmacological treatment for social phobia: a meta-analysis. Clin Psychol Sci Pract 4:291–306, 1997

Grant BF, Hasin DS, Blanco C, et al: The epidemiology of social anxiety disorder in the United States: results from the National Epidemiological Survey on Alcohol and Related Conditions. J Clin Psychiatry 66:1351–1361, 2005

Guastella AJ, Richardson R, Lovibond PF, et al: A randomized controlled trial of D-cycloserine enhancement of exposure therapy for social anxiety disorder. Biol Psychiatry 63:544–549, 2008

Halford K, Foddy M: Cognitive and social skills correlates of social anxiety. Br J Clin Psychol 21:17–28, 1982

Harvey AG, Clark DA, Ehlers A, et al: Social anxiety and self-impression: cognitive preparation enhances the beneficial effects of video feedback following a stressful social task. Behav Res Ther 38:1183–1192, 2000

Hayes SA, Hope DA, VanDyke M, et al: Working alliance for clients with social anxiety disorder: relationship with session helpfulness and within-session habituation. Cogn Behav Ther 36:34–42, 2007

Hayes SC, Wilson KG, Gifford EV, et al: Experiential avoidance and behavioral disorders: a functional dimensional approach to diagnosis and treatment. J Consult Clin Psychol 64:1152–1168, 1996

Hayward C, Varady S, Albana AM, et al: Cognitive-behavioral group therapy for social phobia in female adolescents: results of a pilot study. J Am Acad Child Adolesc Psychiatry 39:721–726, 2000

Heimberg RG: Social phobia, avoidant personality disorder, and the multiaxial conceptualization of interpersonal anxiety, in Trends in Cognitive and Behavioural Therapies. Edited by Salkovskis P. Sussex, UK, Wiley, 1996, pp 43–62

Heimberg RG: Cognitive-behavioral and psychotherapeutic strategies for social anxiety disorder. Paper presented at the annual meeting of the Anxiety Disorders Association of America, Toronto, Ontario, Canada, March 2003

Heimberg RG, Becker RE: Cognitive-Behavioral Group Therapy for Social Phobia: Basic Mechanisms and Clinical Strategies. New York, Guilford, 2002

Heimberg RG, Juster HR: Cognitive-behavioral treatments: literature review, in Social Phobia: Diagnosis, Assessment and Treatment. Edited by Heimberg RG, Liebowitz MR, Hope DA, et al. New York, Guilford, 1995, pp 261–309

Heimberg RG, Dodge CS, Hope DA, et al: Cognitive-behavioral group treatment of social phobia: comparison to a credible placebo control. Cognit Ther Res 14:1–23, 1990

Heimberg RG, Salzman DG, Holt CS, et al: Cognitive-behavioral group treatment for social phobia: effectiveness at five-year follow-up. Cogn Ther Res 17:325–339, 1993

Heimberg RG, Liebowitz MR, Hope DA, et al: Cognitive-behavioral group therapy versus phenelzine in social phobia: 12-week outcome. Arch Gen Psychiatry 55:1133–1141, 1998

Herbert JD, Gaudiano BA, Rheingold AA, et al: Social skills training augments the effectiveness of cognitive behavioral group therapy for social anxiety disorder. Behav Ther 36:125–138, 2005

Hofmann SG: Cognitive mediation of treatment change in social phobia. J Consult Clin Psychol 72:392–399, 2004

Hofmann SG, Suvak M: Treatment attrition during group therapy for social phobia. J Anxiety Disord 20:961–972, 2006

Hofmann SG, Meuret AE, Smits JA, et al: Augmentation of exposure therapy with D-cycloserine for social anxiety disorder. Arch Gen Psychiatry 63:298–304, 2006

Hope DA, Heimberg RG, Bruch MA: Dismantling cognitive-behavioral group therapy for social phobia. Behav Res Ther 33:637–650, 1995a

Hope DA, Herbert JD, White C: Diagnostic subtype, avoidant personality disorder, and efficacy of cognitive behavioral group therapy for social phobia. Cogn Ther Res 19:285–303, 1995b

Hope DA, Heimberg RG, Juster H, et al: Managing Social Anxiety: A Cognitive-Behavioral Therapy Approach (Client Workbook). New York, Oxford University Press, 2000

Hope DA, Heimberg RG, Turk CL: Managing Social Anxiety: A Cognitive-Behavioral Therapy Approach (Therapist Guide). New York, Oxford University Press, 2006

Ishiyama FI: Brief Morita therapy on social anxiety: a single case study of therapeutic changes. Canadian Journal of Counseling 20:56–65, 1986

Ishiyama FI: Use of Morita therapy in shyness counseling in the west: promoting clients' self-acceptance and action taking. J Couns Dev 65:547–551, 1987

Ishiyama FI: A Japanese reframing technique for brief social anxiety treatment: an exploratory study of cognitive and therapeutic effects of Morita therapy. Journal of Cognitive Psychotherapy 5:55–70, 1991

Jerremalm A, Jansson L, Ost LG: Cognitive and physiological reactivity and the effects of different behavioral methods in the treatment of social phobia. Behav Res Ther 24:171–180, 1986

Juster HR, Heimberg RG: Social phobia, in Comprehensive Clinical Psychology (Hersen M, Bellack AS, series eds), Vol 6: Adults: Clinical Formulation and Treatment. Edited by Salkovskis P. New York, Elsevier, 1998, pp 475–498

Kanter NJ, Goldfried MR: Relative effectiveness of rational restructuring and self-control desensitization in the reduction of interpersonal anxiety. Behav Ther 10:472–490, 1979

Kendall PC: Treating anxiety disorders in children: results of a randomized clinical trial. J Consult Clin Psychol 62:100–110, 1994

Kendall PC, Flannery-Schroeder E, Panichelli-Mindel SM, et al: Therapy for youths with anxiety disorders: a second randomized clinical trial. J Consult Clin Psychol 65:366–380, 1997

Kendall PC, Safford S, Flannery-Schroeder E: Child anxiety treatment: outcomes and impact on substance use and depression at 7.4-year follow-up. J Consult Clin Psychol 72:276–287, 2004

Kim H-Y, Lundh L-G, Harvey A: The enhancement of video feedback by cognitive preparation in the treatment of social anxiety: a single session experiment. J Behav Ther Exp Psychiatry 33:19–37, 2002

Klinger E, Bouchard S, Légeron P, et al: Virtual reality therapy versus cognitive therapy for social phobia: a preliminary controlled study. Cyberpsychol Behav 8:76–88, 2005

Koszycki D, Benger M, Shlik J, et al: Randomized trial of a meditation-based stress reduction program and cognitive behavior therapy in generalized social anxiety disorder. Behav Res Ther 45:2518–2526, 2007

Leichsenring F, Beutel M, Leibing E: Psychodynamic psychotherapy for social phobia: a treatment based on supportive-expressive therapy. Bull Menninger Clin 71:56–83, 2007

Leung AW, Heimberg RG: Homework compliance, perceptions of control, and outcome of cognitive-behavioral treatment of social phobia. Behav Res Ther 34:423–432, 1996

Liebowitz MR, Heimberg RG, Schneier FR, et al: Cognitive-behavioral group therapy versus phenelzine in social phobia: long-term outcome. Depress Anxiety 10:89–98, 1999

Lipsitz JD, Markowitz JC, Cherry S, et al: Open trial of interpersonal psychotherapy for the treatment of social phobia. Am J Psychiatry 156:1814–1816, 1999

Lipsitz JD, Gur M, Vermes D, et al: A randomized trial of interpersonal therapy versus supportive therapy for social anxiety disorder. Depress Anxiety 25:542–553, 2008

Lucas RA, Telch MJ: Group versus individual treatment of social phobia. Paper presented at the annual meeting of the Association for Advancement of Behavior Therapy, Atlanta, GA, November 1993

Lucock MP, Salkovskis PM: Cognitive factors in social anxiety and its treatment. Behav Res Ther 26:297–302, 1988

Markowitz JC: Psychotherapy of dysthymia. Am J Psychiatry 151:1114–1121, 1994

Marzillier JS, Lambert C, Kellet J: A controlled evaluation of systematic desensitization and social skills training for socially inadequate psychiatric patients. Behav Res Ther 14:225–238, 1976

Masia-Warner C, Klein RG, Dent HC, et al: School-based intervention for adolescents with social anxiety disorder: results of a controlled study. J Abnorm Child Psychol 33:707–722, 2005

Mattick RP, Peters L: Treatment of severe social phobia: effects of guided exposure with and without cognitive restructuring. J Consult Clin Psychol 56:251–260, 1988

Mattick RP, Peters L, Clarke JC: Exposure and cognitive restructuring for social phobia: a controlled study. Behav Ther 20:3–23, 1989

McNeil DW, Lejuez CW, Sorrell JT: Behavioral theories of social phobia: contributions of basic behavioral principles, in From Social Anxiety to Social Phobia: Multiple Perspectives. Edited by Hofmann SG, DiBartolo PM. Needham Heights, MA, Allyn & Bacon, 2001

Meichenbaum D: Stress Inoculation Training. New York, Pergamon, 1985

Mersch PPA, Emmelkamp PMG, Bögels SM, et al: Social phobia: individual response patterns and the effects of behavioral and cognitive interventions. Behav Res Ther 27:421–434, 1989

Miller JJ, Fletcher K, Kabat-Zinn J: Three-year follow-up and clinical implications of a mindfulness meditation-based stress reduction intervention in the treatment of anxiety disorders. Gen Hosp Psychiatry 17:192–200, 1995

Miller WR, Zweben A, DiClemente CC, et al: Motivational Enhancement Therapy Manual: A Clinical Research Guide for Therapists Treating Individuals With Alcohol Abuse and Dependence. Rockville, MD, National Institute on Alcohol Abuse and Alcoholism, 1992

Mörtberg E, Clark DM, Sundin O, et al: Intensive group cognitive treatment and individual cognitive therapy vs. treatment as usual in social phobia: a randomized controlled trial. Acta Psychiatr Scand 115:142–154, 2007

Moscovitch DA, Hofmann SG, Suvak MK, et al: Mediation of changes in anxiety and depression during treatment of social phobia. J Consult Clin Psychol 73:945–952, 2005

Newman MG, Hofmann SG, Trabert W, et al: Does behavioral treatment of social phobia lead to cognitive changes? Behav Ther 25:503–517, 1994

Newman MG, Erickson T, Przeworski A, et al: Self-help and minimal-contact therapies for anxiety disorders: is human contact necessary for therapeutic efficacy? J Consult Clin Psychol 69:251–274, 2003

Olfson M, Guardino M, Struening E, et al: Barriers to treatment of social anxiety. Am J Psychiatry 157:521–527, 2000

Ossman WA, Wilson KG, Storaasli RD, et al: A preliminary investigation of the use of acceptance and commitment therapy in a group treatment for social phobia. International Journal of Psychology and Psychological Therapy 6:397–416, 2006

Ost LG: Applied relaxation: description of a coping technique and review of controlled studies. Behav Res Ther 25:397–409, 1987

Ost LG, Jerremalm A, Johansson J: Individual response patterns and the effects of different behavioral methods in the treatment of social phobia. Behav Res Ther 19:1–16, 1981

Otto MW, Pollck MH, Gould, RA, et al: A comparison of the efficacy of clonazepam and cognitive-behavioral

group therapy for the treatment of social phobia. J Anxiety Disord 14:345–358, 2000
Ponniah K, Hollon SD: Empirically supported psychological interventions for social phobia in adults: a qualitative review of randomized controlled trials. Psychol Med 38:3–14, 2007
Rapee RM, Heimberg RG: A cognitive-behavioral model of anxiety in social phobia. Behav Res Ther 35:741–756, 1997
Rapee RM, Lim L: Discrepancy between self- and observer ratings of performance in social phobics. J Abnorm Psychol 101:728–731, 1992
Reynolds DK: The Quiet Therapies. Honolulu, HI, University Press of Hawaii, 1980
Rodebaugh TL, Chambless DL: The effects of video feedback on self-perception of performance: a replication and extension. Cognit Ther Res 26:629–644, 2002
Rodebaugh TL, Rapee RM: Those who think they look worst respond best: self-observer discrepancy predicts response to video feedback following a speech task. Cognit Ther Res 29:705–715, 2005
Safren SA, Heimberg RG, Juster HR: Client expectancies and their relationship to pretreatment symptomatology and outcome of cognitive behavioral group treatment for social phobia. J Consult Clin Psychol 65:694–698, 1997
Sanders MR, Dadds MR: Behavioral Family Intervention. New York, Pergamon, 1993
Scholing A, Emmelkamp PMG: Treatment of generalized social phobia: results at long-term follow-up. Behav Res Ther 34:447–452, 1996
Smits JA, Powers MB, Buxkamper R, et al: The efficacy of videotape feedback for enhancing the effects of exposure-based treatment for social anxiety disorder: a controlled investigation. Behav Res Ther 44:1773–1785, 2006
Spence SH, Donovan C, Brechman-Toussaint M: The treatment of childhood social phobia: the effectiveness of a social skills training-based, cognitive-behavioural intervention, with and without parental involvement. J Child Psychol Psychiatry 41:713–726, 2000
Stangier U, Heidenreich T, Peitz M, et al: Cognitive therapy for social phobia: individual versus group treatment. Behav Res Ther 41:991–1007, 2003
Stopa L, Clark DM: Cognitive processes in social phobia. Behav Res Ther 31:255–267, 1993
Stravynski A, Marks I, Yule W: Social skills problems in neurotic outpatients: social skills training with and without cognitive modification. Arch Gen Psychiatry 39:1378–1385, 1982
Taube-Schiff M, Suvak MK, Antony MM, et al: Group cohesion in cognitive-behavioral group therapy for social phobia. Behav Res Ther 45:687–698, 2007
Taylor S: Meta-analysis of cognitive-behavioral treatments for social phobia. J Behav Ther Exp Psychiatry 27:1–9, 1996
Treadwell KRH, Flannery-Schroeder, EC, Kendall PC: Ethnicity and gender in relation to adaptive functioning, diagnostic status, and treatment outcome in children from an anxiety clinic. J Anxiety Disord 9:373–383, 1995
Trower P, Yardley K, Bryant B, et al: The treatment of social failure: a comparison of anxiety-reduction and skills acquisition procedures on two social problems. Behav Modif 2:41–60, 1978
Turk CL, Fresco DM, Heimberg RG: Social phobia: cognitive behavior therapy, in Handbook of Comparative Treatments of Adult Disorders, 2nd Edition. Edited by Hersen M, Bellack AS. New York, Wiley, 1999, pp 287–316
Turner SM, Beidel DC, Cooley MR, et al: A multi-component behavioral treatment for social phobia: social effectiveness therapy. Behav Res Ther 32:381–390, 1994a
Turner SM, Beidel DC, Jacob RG: Social phobia: a comparison of behavior therapy and atenolol. J Consult Clin Psychol 62:350–358, 1994b
Turner SM, Beidel DC, Cooley-Quille MR: Two-year follow-up of social phobics treated with social effectiveness therapy. Behav Res Ther 33:553–555, 1995
Wells A, Papageorgiou C: Social phobia: effects of external attention in anxiety, negative beliefs, and perspective taking. Behav Ther 29:357–370, 1998
Westra HA, Dozois DJA: Preparing clients for cognitive behavioral therapy: a randomized pilot study of motivational interviewing for anxiety. Cognit Ther Res 30:481–498, 2006
Wild J, Hackmann A, Clark DM: Rescripting early memories linked to negative images in social phobia: a pilot study. Behav Ther 39:47–56, 2008
Wilfley DE, Welch RR, Stein RI, et al: A randomized comparison of group cognitive behavior therapy and group interpersonal therapy for the treatment of overweight individuals with binge-eating disorder. Arch Gen Psychiatry 59:713–721, 2002
Wlazlo Z, Schroeder-Hartwig K, Hand I, et al: Exposure in vivo vs. social skills training for social phobia: long-term outcome and differential effects. Behav Res Ther 28:181–193, 1990
Woody SR, Adessky RS: Therapeutic alliance, group cohesion, and homework compliance during cognitive-behavioral group treatment of social phobia. Behav Ther 33:5–27, 2002
Wright JH, Basco MR, Thase ME: Learning Cognitive-Behavior Therapy: An Illustrated Guide. Washington, DC, American Psychiatric Publishing, 2006
Zaider T, Heimberg RG, Roth DA, et al: Individual CBT for social anxiety disorder: preliminary findings. Paper presented at the annual meeting of the Association for Advancement of Behavior Therapy, Boston, MA, November 2003

Zerbe KJ: Uncharted waters: psychodynamic considerations in the diagnosis and treatment of social phobia, in Fear of Humiliation: Integrated Treatment of Social Phobia and Comorbid Conditions. Edited by Menninger WW. Northvale, NJ, Jason Aronson, 1997

Recommended Readings

Bandelow B, Stein DJ (eds): Social Anxiety Disorder. New York, Marcel Dekker, 2004

Crozier WR, Alden LE (eds): The Essential Handbook of Social Anxiety for Clinicians. Chichester, UK, Wiley, 2005

Heimberg RG, Becker RE: Cognitive-Behavioral Group Therapy for Social Phobia: Basic Mechanisms and Clinical Strategies. New York, Guilford, 2002

Hope DA, Heimberg RG, Juster H, et al: Managing Social Anxiety: A Cognitive-Behavioral Therapy Approach (Client Workbook). New York, Oxford University Press, 2000

Hope DA, Heimberg RG, Turk CL: Managing Social Anxiety: A Cognitive-Behavioral Therapy Approach (Therapist Guide). New York, Oxford University Press, 2006

Ledley DR, Heimberg RG: Social anxiety disorder, in Improving Outcomes and Preventing Relapse in Cognitive Behavioral Therapy. Edited by Antony MM, Ledley DR, Heimberg RG. New York, Guilford, 2005, pp 38–76

Turk CL, Heimberg RG, Magee L: Social anxiety disorder, in Clinical Handbook of Psychological Disorders, 4th Edition. Edited by Barlow DH. New York, Guilford, 2008, pp 123–163

Web Sites of Interest

Academy of Cognitive Therapy. http://www.academyofct.org

Adult Anxiety Clinic of Temple University. http://www.temple.edu/phobia

Anxiety Disorders Association of America. http://www.adaa.org/GettingHelp/AnxietyDisorders/SocialPhobia.asp

Association for Behavioral and Cognitive Therapies. http://www.abct.org

International Paruresis Association. http://www.paruresis.org

National Institute of Mental Health. http://www.nimh.nih.gov/health/topics/social-phobia-social-anxiety-disorder/index.shtml

National Mental Health Association. http://www.nmha.org/go/information/get-info/anxiety-disorders/social-phobias

Social Anxiety/Social Phobia Association. http://www.social-phobia.org

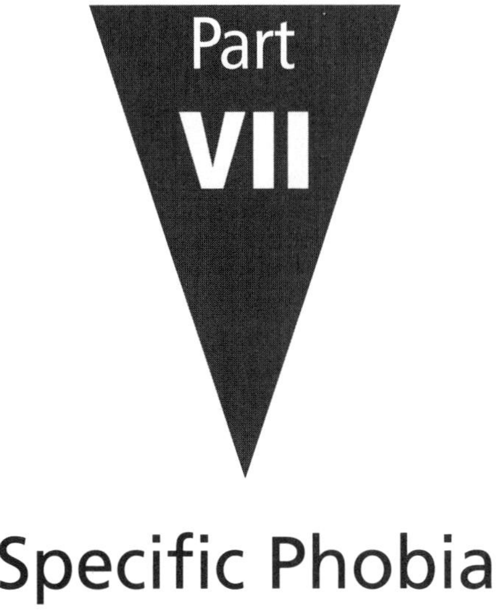

Specific Phobia

Chapter 29

Specific Phobia

Amanda L. Gamble , Ph.D.
Allison G. Harvey, Ph.D.
Ronald M. Rapee, Ph.D.

Specific phobia is a relatively common psychiatric disorder across the population. As suggested by its name, it is characterized by a marked fear of and a desire to avoid a specific situation or object. Typically, the objects that become the target of a phobia are those that cause distress and distaste in the general population. However, people with specific phobia overestimate the consequences of enduring exposure to the feared stimulus (Beck et al. 1985).

Relatively few individuals with specific phobia actually seek treatment (Essau et al. 2000; Stinson et al. 2007). This is perhaps because many people with specific phobia view the fear as a "normal" part of their personality. In addition, many phobic stimuli can be avoided in daily life with relatively little difficulty. For example, it usually causes little interference in life for a person with dog phobia to select routes where there are no dogs. When not confronted with the phobic stimulus, people with specific phobia are generally symptom free (Butler 1989). Indeed, epidemiological studies have found that specific phobia tends to include a larger number of mild cases than do other anxiety disorders (Kessler et al. 2005b; Wells et al. 2006). Nonetheless, for many individuals, a phobia can be a problem that interferes with life and requires treatment. Avoidant behavior in individuals with dental phobia and blood-injection-injury phobia can lead to serious medical complications (Milgrom et al. 1995), and in at least one case reported in the literature, specific phobia was implicated in suicide (Pegeron and Thyer 1986). Consequently, clinicians and researchers must be aware of the current issues relating to the nature, theory, and treatment of specific phobia. In addition, specific phobia represents a diagnosis that was of interest to the very earliest cognitive-behavioral therapists and researchers. A review of specific phobia thus also represents an interesting historical foray into the development of psychological theory and treatments.

In this chapter, we outline the symptomatology, differential diagnosis and most frequently encountered comorbidities, epidemiology, pathogenesis, and treatment of specific phobia.

Classification and Symptomatology

The early classification of phobias used a great many Greek words to describe the feared objects. More recent classification systems have distinguished between types of phobias based on statistical analysis of data collected from a large cohort of phobic individuals. For example, Beck and colleagues (1985) distinguished three classes of phobias: 1) those that are related to social rejection, 2) those that are agoraphobic in nature, and 3) those that are related to blood and injury. A factor analysis reported by Fredrikson et al. (1996) supported the classification of phobias into three slightly different categories: 1) situational phobias, 2) animal phobias, and 3) mutilation phobias. In a third attempt to organize phobic types, DSM-IV-TR (American Psychiatric Association 2000) distinguished four subtypes of phobia: 1) animal, 2) natural environment (e.g., storms, water), 3) blood-injection-injury, and 4) situational (e.g., flying, enclosed spaces). A fifth category ("other") is reserved for phobias (e.g., fear of vomiting) that do not fit into one of the four main categories.

Several studies have questioned the validity of subtyping phobias. "Specific" phobias tend not to be particularly specific, with most patients reporting multiple specific phobias (Curtis et al. 1998; Hofmann et al. 1997) and subclinical fears of other phobic stimuli (Goisman et al. 1998; Lipsitz et al. 2002). In a large epidemiological study, Stinson et al. (2007) found that only 28% of individuals with a specific phobia reported just a single specific fear, suggesting considerable overlap between subtypes from a clinical perspective. It is also difficult to differentiate phobia subtypes on physiological grounds. Antony et al. (1997) found that individuals with phobias of animals, of heights, of blood injections, and of driving report similar frequency of panic attacks, similar intensity of physical and cognitive symptoms, and similar awareness of, and anxiety about, physical sensations.

Others (e.g., Ware et al. 1994) have suggested that types of phobias can be distinguished in terms of the principal emotion they elicit—disgust or fear. Although the majority of phobias are motivated primarily by fear, disgust appears to play a particularly important role in small animal and blood-injection-injury phobias (Davey 1993; Kleinknecht et al. 1996). Individuals with small animal phobia and those with blood-injection-injury phobia report heightened disgust on exposure to fear-relevant stimuli (Tolin et al. 1997) and respond to phobic-related stimuli with a disgust-specific facial expression (de Jong et al. 2002). Individuals with blood-injection-injury phobia and small animal phobia also tend to show greater sensitivity to disgust, as measured by disgust sensitivity scales (Sawchuk et al. 2000; Tolin et al. 1997). This hypersensitivity may be an important factor in maintaining behavioral avoidance. For example, Mulkens et al. (1996) demonstrated that 75% of subjects with spider phobia would not eat a cookie after a spider had briefly touched it, compared with 30% of control subjects. Disgust sensitivity may also underpin the tendency for phobic individuals to preferentially allocate attention to disgust-relevant stimuli. For example, Charash and McKay (2002) found that disgust-sensitive individuals were more likely to allocate attention to words that elicit disgust, relative to neutral words, when primed with a disgustful story. Importantly, disgust sensitivity appears to be independent of any link with neuroticism (Mulkens et al. 1996). It is currently unclear whether disgust is a cause or a result of phobia; however, initial research suggests that disgust sensitivity may be a potential risk factor in the etiology of small animal and blood-injection-injury phobias (de Jong and Merckelbach 1998).

In terms of blood-injection-injury phobia, Page (1994) differentiated two subtypes of patients: those who manifest the sympathetic nervous system activation characteristic of most other specific phobias and those who are characterized by fainting, a response specific to blood-injection-injury phobias. The fainting is caused by the steep drop in blood pressure following an initial rise when the individual is initially exposed to blood- injection, or injury-related stimuli.

Apart from the patients with blood-injection-injury phobia who faint, all phobic individuals show two broad sets of symptoms (Mavissakalian and Barlow 1981):

1. The anxiety or sympathetic nervous system activation that occurs on anticipation of, or confrontation with, the phobic stimulus. The anxiety reaction typically includes any combination of the following symptoms: unsteadiness, feelings of unreality, perception of impending doom, dryness of the mouth, pounding heart, nausea, fear of dying, fear of going crazy, sweating, shortness of breath, feelings of choking or being smothered, chest pain, chest discomfort, faintness, and trembling (American Psychiatric Association 1980).
2. The desired or attempted avoidance that individuals with specific phobias engage in. Phobic individuals show a behavioral preference to minimize contact with the feared event. When the event cannot be avoided, it will be endured with a high level of anxiety, and the phobic individual will escape as soon as possible. Often, this tendency toward avoidance renders the individual quite restricted in his or her activities. However, the level of impairment experienced depends on the extent to which the target of the phobia can be readily avoided (Sturgis and Scott 1984).

A third characteristic of specific phobia added by Beck and colleagues (1985) is the insight that the individual usually has into the overly exaggerated nature of the phobia.

Turning now to formal diagnostic systems, the three aspects of specific phobia highlighted above form the basis of the DSM-IV-TR diagnostic criteria. Specifically, DSM-IV-TR stipulates that the fear must be "marked and persistent" (criterion A) and that, on exposure, the phobic individual must have an immediate increase in anxiety, which may take the form of a panic attack (criterion B). The individual must recognize this response as excessive (criterion C), and the symptoms must cause significant interference with the person's social or occupational functioning (criterion E). Criterion D reflects the avoidance aspect of the diagnosis (see Table 29–1 for the full criteria).

Differential Diagnosis and Comorbidity

As can be seen in Table 29–1, DSM-IV-TR states that the avoidance and anxiety manifested by a phobic individual should not be better accounted for by another mental disorder. To accurately diagnose specific phobia, a key differentiating factor is that the individual with specific phobia does not present as generally anxious. Instead, the anxiety typically is limited to the anticipation of exposure to or actual confrontation with the phobic stimulus.

In terms of differentiating specific phobia from other anxiety disorders, several points should be considered. First, like specific phobia, the fear in posttraumatic stress disorder (PTSD) is mostly specific, but the fear has been triggered by an external traumatic event; furthermore, PTSD is characterized by intrusions and nightmares that are not typical of specific phobia. Similarly, the hallmark symptoms of obsessive-compulsive disorder are obsessions and compulsions, which are not a feature of specific phobia. The feature that distinguishes social phobia from specific phobia is the focus on fear of negative evaluation in social situations.

The key factor in the differential diagnosis of psychosis and specific phobia is the insight that the individual with specific phobia has into the irrationality of the phobia and the resistance—delusional in its intensity—that the psychotic individual has to the alteration of the fear (Andrews et al. 1994).

Perhaps the more difficult differential diagnosis is between individuals with specific phobia who experi-

TABLE 29–1. DSM-IV-TR diagnostic criteria for specific phobia

A. Marked and persistent fear that is excessive or unreasonable, cued by the presence or anticipation of a specific object or situation (e.g., flying, heights, animals, receiving an injection, seeing blood).

B. Exposure to the phobic stimulus almost invariably provokes an immediate anxiety response, which may take the form of a situationally bound or situationally predisposed panic attack. **Note:** In children, the anxiety may be expressed by crying, tantrums, freezing, or clinging.

C. The person recognizes that the fear is excessive or unreasonable. **Note:** In children, this feature may be absent.

D. The phobic situation(s) is avoided or else is endured with intense anxiety or distress.

E. The avoidance, anxious anticipation, or distress in the feared situation(s) interferes significantly with the person's normal routine, occupational (or academic) functioning, or social activities or relationships, or there is marked distress about having the phobia.

F. In individuals under age 18 years, the duration is at least 6 months.

G. The anxiety, panic attacks, or phobic avoidance associated with the specific object or situation are not better accounted for by another mental disorder, such as obsessive-compulsive disorder (e.g., fear of dirt in someone with an obsession about contamination), posttraumatic stress disorder (e.g., avoidance of stimuli associated with a severe stressor), separation anxiety disorder (e.g., avoidance of school), social phobia (e.g., avoidance of social situations because of fear of embarrassment), panic disorder with agoraphobia, or agoraphobia without history of panic disorder.

Specify type:

Animal Type

Natural Environment Type (e.g., heights, storms, water)

Blood-Injection-Injury Type

Situational Type (e.g., airplanes, elevators, enclosed places)

Other Type (e.g., fear of choking, vomiting, or contracting an illness; in children, fear of loud sounds or costumed characters)

ence panic attacks and individuals who meet the diagnostic criteria for panic disorder. The key factor differentiating specific phobia from panic disorder is that in the latter, the fear is specifically focused on having a panic attack. A study illustrating this point was reported by McNally and Louro (1992). These authors compared a group of individuals who reported a fear of flying. Half were given diagnoses of panic disorder with agoraphobia, and half met the criteria for specific phobia. The comparison showed that individuals in the specific phobia group avoided flying because they feared crashing, whereas those in the agoraphobic group feared experiencing a panic attack. Given that the distinction can be difficult (Ehlers et al. 1994), requiring some clinical judgment, DSM-IV-TR recommends that information about the following be gathered and considered when making the diagnostic decision:

1. The situations that elicit the fear
2. The type and number of panic attacks
3. The range of situations that the individual avoids
4. The level of anxiety between episodes of fear on exposure to the situation

In terms of comorbidity, an individual with one anxiety disorder commonly also has one or more other anxiety disorders. This tendency for comorbidity among the anxiety disorders applies less to specific phobia than to the other anxiety disorders (Kendler et al. 1992; Sanderson et al. 1990). Nevertheless, in a national comorbidity survey (Magee et al. 1996), most individuals with specific phobia reported at least one additional lifetime disorder. A more recent comorbidity survey that examined 12-month prevalence (Kessler et al. 2005b) found that specific phobias are strongly comorbid with other phobias (agoraphobia and social phobia), other anxiety disorders, and the affective disorders. In particular, specific phobia is associated with increased risk of depression, even after adjusting for sociodemographic differences and other psychiatric comorbidity (Choy et al. 2007; Goodwin 2002). Specific phobias with onset in childhood may also predict the later development of substance use disorders in adolescence and adulthood (Essau et al. 2000).

Epidemiology

Age at Onset

The mean age at onset for specific phobia is reported to be around 7 years (Kessler et al. 2005a). However, collapsing across different specific phobias may mask interesting differences. Several studies have analyzed the age at onset of phobia subtypes and found that they are quite variable (Becker et al. 2007; Sturgis and Scott 1984). Overall, studies tend to indicate that animal and blood-injection-injury phobias begin in childhood, whereas situational phobias have a later age of onset (Becker et al. 2007; Himle et al. 1989; Lipsitz et al. 2002; Öst 1987). In one interesting longitudinal study, Agras and colleagues (1972) found that 100% of the patients with specific phobia who were younger than 20 years had improved at follow-up, but only 43% of the adults with specific phobia had improved. Similarly, 40% of the participants younger than age 20 were asymptomatic at follow-up, but no adults were asymptomatic. Based on these data, it could be suggested that many specific fears in youth are relatively transient, but those that extend into adulthood are more severe and persistent. Consistent with this idea, epidemiological studies of adults indicate that the mean duration of specific phobia is between 20.1 years and 24.5 years (Meyer et al. 2004; Stinson et al. 2007), far greater than the duration of other anxiety disorders and depressive illnesses (Meyer et al. 2004). This chronicity may be due to the relatively mild impact on day-to-day functioning and the tendency not to seek treatment.

Prevalence and Sex Ratio

Specific phobia is the most common anxiety disorder in the general population over a 12-month period (Kessler et al. 2005a, 2005b; Wells et al. 2006). Overall, the lifetime prevalence of specific phobia has been found to be between 8.8% and 12.5% (Kessler et al. 2005a; Magee et al. 1996; Reiger et al. 1988; Stinson et al. 2007). The variation in diagnostic rates may at least partly be attributable to the different thresholds used to judge the level of impairment.

Fredrikson et al. (1996) dissected the prevalence rates according to sex ratio and reported that women (21.2%) were more likely than men (10.9%) to meet the criteria for any single specific phobia. Women also reported higher rates of multiple phobias than did men (women, 5.4%; men, 1.5%). Similar rates were reported by Kessler et al. (1994), who found a lifetime prevalence rate for males of 6.7% and for females of 15.7%. Most of the different types of specific phobias occur in a considerably higher proportion of females; the exception is blood-injection-injury phobia. Several researchers have found relatively equal proportions of males and females with blood-injection-injury fears (Agras et al. 1969; Fredrikson et al. 1996; Himle et al. 1989). Prevalence may also be sensitive to racial background; an epidemiological survey of American adults found specific phobia to be significantly less common in Asian and Hispanic adults than in white adults (Stinson et al. 2007).

Pathogenesis

Conditioning

Several early researchers conceptualized the etiology of phobias within a classical conditioning framework. In the famous "Little Albert" study, Watson and Raynor (1920) reported that the pairing of a white rat (considered to be the neutral stimulus) with a loud noise (considered to be the aversive stimulus) produced a conditioned fear response when the participant was exposed to the rat on future occasions. Mowrer (1960) extended this classical conditioning model by proposing that conditioning is mediated by motivations such as the desire to reduce fear. Thus, the model was extended to account for avoidance behavior, a strategy that is reinforced by reduction in the fear response. Although the conditioning model is still influential in the field of phobias, it is now recognized to have some shortcomings (for review, see Rachman 1976, 1977, 1978, 1991). The most salient difficulties with the conditioning model are the following:

1. The distinct categories of fears noted in epidemiological studies, contrary to the proposal made by conditioning theorists that all stimuli can become feared stimuli (the *equipotentiality premise*)
2. The observation that many people experience aversive conditioning but do not develop a phobia (Ehlers et al. 1994; Hofmann et al. 1995)
3. The fact that a traumatic etiology is not reported by all, or even most, phobic individuals (Menzies and Clarke 1995c; Öst 1987)
4. The limited success of studies that have endeavored to condition stable fears in humans in an experimental setting (Bancroft 1969; Marks and Gelder 1967)
5. The evidence attesting to the indirect and vicarious modes of onset of fears (Rachman 1978)

Preparedness

To attempt to account for some of the limitations of the traditional Pavlovian account of phobias, Seligman (1971) developed the preparedness theory of fear acquisition. Seligman noted that the common feature of stimuli that become the target of a phobic reaction is that they are biologically threatening. He postulated that as a consequence of natural selection, human beings are biologically prepared to develop fears of stimuli that threaten personal safety; that is, phobias were conceptualized to be a result of prepared learning. Seligman defined four features of *prepared phobias*:

1. They are often acquired through one-trial conditioning (note that Seligman's account is still an associative theory in which phobias are acquired via conditioning, albeit in a single trial).
2. They are noncognitive in that they persist despite insight into the irrationality of the fear.
3. The object involves a threat relevant to humankind of the past and remains as a result of natural selection.
4. They are not easily extinguished.

Taking the findings relating to ease of acquisition first, McNally (1987) reviewed 17 studies that measured the acquisition stage of conditioning of fear-relevant and fear-irrelevant stimuli and found little evidence for the first prediction. Specifically, several studies have shown that in the laboratory, nonprepared stimuli can acquire aversive associations just as quickly as prepared stimuli (McNally 1987). The second hypothesis of the preparedness theory, that fears are not cognitive and thus will be held despite the knowledge that the phobic object will not cause harm, has received mixed support. For example, Öhman et al. (1975) showed subjects pictures of phobic stimuli and pictures of neutral stimuli and administered shock to half of the subjects when the phobic stimuli (pictures of snakes) were presented and to the other half when the neutral stimuli were presented. Both groups acquired the conditioned fear, as measured by skin conductance responses. However, instructing subjects that no more shocks would be administered was not effective in extinguishing the fear to the snake pictures. However, McNally (1981) found the opposite result with a different methodology. Taken together, no clear conclusion about the second assumption of preparedness theory can be drawn (McNally 1987). The third and perhaps most basic assumption of preparedness theory, that there is differential associativity for stimuli that are biologically prepared, has also failed to gather clear support. However, methodological problems have rendered this hypothesis difficult to test unequivocally (McNally 1987).

The final hypothesis, that phobias are difficult to extinguish, has received the most empirical support of the four predictions (e.g., Öhman and Dimberg 1978).

However, some studies were not able to replicate these findings (McNally 1986; McNally and Foa 1986). Furthermore, McNally (1987) outlined several alternative explanations for the studies that supported the notion of resistance to extinction, in an attempt to reconcile the contradictory findings. Taken together, the evidence suggests that three of the predictions of preparedness theory have not been supported empirically, and although some evidence has been gathered for the fourth prediction, alternative explanations are possible (McNally 1987). There is little doubt that the central premise of Seligman's theory—that certain stimuli are "evolutionarily prepared" to cause phobic responding—is well supported. However, the details of the theory, especially that phobic responding is acquired in a single associative experience, have not met with a great deal of support.

Multiple Pathways

In accord with the mixed support that has accumulated for the preparedness theory and the difficulties observed in using direct conditioning accounts to explain vicarious conditioning, Rachman (1991) suggested that there may be several alternative pathways to the acquisition of phobic fears. Specifically, he proposed that phobias could be acquired through modes such as direct conditioning, vicarious conditioning, and verbal acquisition.

Vicarious conditioning is difficult to test adequately, but evidence for this mode of acquisition has come from numerous sources. First, laboratory experiments with humans have found that learning can occur by way of observation. For example, Bandura and Rosenthal (1966) arranged for participants to view a person feigning a pain reaction to an electric shock. After a few trials, the buzzer that preceded the shock resulted in an increase in physiological responses, even though the participants had not had contact with the electric shock apparatus. Second, a similar pattern of results has been found with animals. Cook and Mineka (1989) reported two experiments in which rhesus monkeys watched videotapes of monkeys behaving fearfully to stimuli that were either fear relevant (snakes, crocodiles) or fear irrelevant (flowers, rabbits). Monkeys who observed the videotapes acquired a fear of the fear-relevant stimuli but not of the fear-irrelevant stimuli. This demonstration of a preparedness aspect to vicarious learning has been replicated across several studies (e.g., Cook et al. 1985; Mineka et al. 1984). Third, several studies that asked individuals to self-report on the perceived mode of onset of their phobia have consistently identified a small subgroup of subjects who nominate vicarious pathways (Fazio 1972; McNally and Steketee 1985; Menzies and Clarke 1993a, 1993b; Öst 1987; Rimm et al. 1977).

Evidence for the acquisition of phobias via verbal information can be seen in the epidemics of koro reported in Singapore and Thailand. Individuals with koro perceive that their genitals are shrinking, and they report an intense fear of dying. The epidemics were thought to have been caused by verbal transmission via the media (Rachman 1991; Tseng et al. 1988). Furthermore, many studies have reported increases in skin conductance in response to a target stimulus after participants were informed that the stimulus would be followed by a shock (Cook and Harris 1937).

Nonassociative Theory

The potential methods of fear acquisition described above are based on an associative theory of phobias. That is, the central mechanism in the development of phobias is believed to be the formation of an association between the feared stimulus (which was previously neutral) and a potentially threatening outcome. Some authors, however, have questioned such associative accounts of phobia acquisition. The nonassociative theory arose when evidence from various sources converged on the proposal that phobias may be acquired without previous direct or indirect associative learning (Menzies and Clarke 1995c).

The first source of evidence is that many phobic individuals report no direct or indirect contact with a conditioning event. For example, Menzies and Clarke (1993a) interviewed the parents of children with a water phobia. They found that only 1 parent out of 50 could recall a classical conditioning episode, and 58% of the parents reported that the fear had always been present. Retrospective reports from phobic adults have also indicated a lack of direct conditioning experience in height phobia (Menzies and Clarke 1995b) and spider phobia (Jones and Menzies 1995; Kleinknecht 1982). Importantly, prospective longitudinal studies have also supported the nonassociative account of phobia acquisition. Poulton et al. (1998) examined the relationship between serious falls that occurred before age 9 and fear of heights at ages 11 and 18 years. No individual with height phobia at age 18 reported having had a serious fall. Instead, individuals with a previous serious fall reported less fear than those who had never fallen. Similar results were also obtained in a prospective study examining the development of water phobia (Poulton et al. 1999).

The second source of evidence is Walk and Gibson's (1960) demonstration of the response of human infants to the "visual cliff" apparatus (Menzies and Clarke 1995c). Specifically, in the original study by Walk and Gibson, all 27 infants (100%) called by their mother crawled onto the shallow, visually safe side at least once, and only 3 infants (11%) crawled onto the deep, visually unsafe side on occasion. Importantly, this effect appears to be innate and is manifested at the time an infant is able to move independently (Bertenthal et al. 1984). Therefore, it is argued that natural selection has prepared humans with the ability to avoid, without prior experience, situations that could lead to significant harm. In this context, it has been proposed that fear is innate or is acquired in accord with a particular stage of development (Menzies and Clarke 1995c).

Further support for this position can be drawn from the research finding fear of strangers in both humans (Dennis 1940) and rhesus monkeys (Sackett 1966). These findings are particularly compelling in the latter study, in which the monkeys were reared alone; the fear manifested in response to pictures of threatening monkeys thus had obviously developed in the absence of a direct or an indirect conditioning episode. Finally, separation anxiety in human infants (Smith 1979) and several other mammals (Mineka 1982) has been found to be unrelated to past aversive experiences of separation (Bowlby 1973; Clarke and Jackson 1983; Poulton et al. 2001).

On the basis of these data, Menzies and Clarke (1995c) argued that learning experiences (either verbal, vicarious, or direct) are not necessary for the development of phobias. Instead, these normal childhood concerns are hypothesized to continue and to become phobias in adult life in some individuals by two means. First, some adults may have learned as children to successfully avoid an object in the domain of physical harm because their parents used avoidant coping styles or verbally reinforced the fears. In this way, the fear is maintained and in adulthood takes on phobic proportions (Menzies and Clarke 1995c). Second, a dishabituation of previous childhood fears may occur during particularly stressful periods (Clarke and Jackson 1983). For example, 16% of the students who feared heights reported that their fear developed during a stressful period (Menzies and Clarke 1993b).

When these studies are taken together, there is convincing evidence for nonassociative factors in the onset of specific phobia.

Biological Factors

Some evidence has also suggested that genetic variation may play a role in the etiology of phobias. For example, Fyer and colleagues (1990) reported a significantly higher risk for specific phobia among first-degree relatives of probands with specific phobia compared with the first-degree relatives of control subjects who had never received a diagnosis of a psychiatric disorder. Although these results suggest that specific phobia is a highly familial disorder, such data do not distinguish between genetic and shared environmental factors. Studies that have attempted to delineate genetic versus environmental contributions to specific phobia have produced mixed results depending on the age of those surveyed. In one study of 6-year-old twins, the heritability estimate for specific phobia was high (60%), with relatively little variance attributed to the nonshared environment and none attributed to the shared environment (Bolton et al. 2006). In contrast, studies of large cohorts of phobic adults have found lower heritability estimates and greater environmental contribution (e.g., Kendler et al. 1999, 2001). Genetic contribution may also vary according to phobia subtype; at least two studies have found a more specific genetic contribution for blood phobia (Fyer et al. 1990; Marks 1988). In summary, the evidence suggests that the mode of onset for specific phobia may be at least partially mediated by genetic transmission, and for children and individuals with blood-injection-injury phobia, heritability appears to be elevated.

Despite the prevalence of specific phobia, its neuropathophysiology remains poorly understood (Fyer 1998). Although hyperactivation of the amygdala is well documented in other anxiety disorders (e.g., Breiter and Rauch 1996; Rauch et al. 2000; Stein et al. 2002; Straube et al. 2004), results of functional magnetic resonance imaging studies have been less conclusive for specific phobia, with some studies showing hyperactivation in individuals with specific phobia (Goossens et al. 2007; Straube et al. 2006b) and others finding no differences (Paquette et al. 2003; Wik et al. 1996). A number of studies have found normalization of neural hyperactivity after cognitive-behavioral therapy (Paquette et al. 2003; Straube et al. 2006a). Several studies using positron emission tomography in phobic individuals (e.g., Fredrikson et al. 1995; Rauch et al. 1995) have found changes in regional cerebral blood flow within sensory areas involved in the detection of environmental stimuli, as well as paralimbic structures. The latter are thought to integrate sensory information with stored information about meaning and context, to assign priority to incoming information as the basis for action. Increased cortical thickness in these areas has also been documented

(Rauch et al. 2004), suggesting that greater functional involvement may be accompanied by structural change. However, at least one study failed to show increased cerebral blood flow in these areas (Mountz et al. 1989), indicating that results are far from ubiquitous. Accordingly, further work is required to delineate the role of the brain both functionally and structurally in specific phobia.

Cognitive Factors

Unlike behavioral and biological approaches, cognitive accounts of specific phobia focus on the role of dysfunctional thoughts and beliefs involving the feared object or situation. Although some theorists suggest that acquisition of phobias may be mediated by cognitive appraisal (Rachman 1991), most attention has focused on the role of cognitions in the maintenance of phobias (Thorpe and Salkovskis 1995). Specifically, it is proposed (Last 1987) that the focus of attention for an individual with social phobia is on 1) interpretation of the physiological changes that accompany the anxiety, 2) anticipatory plans to avoid the feared stimulus, and 3) thoughts relating to escape from the stimulus.

The cognitive approach argues that such cognitions increase arousal and anxiety and increase the likelihood that the phobic individual will attempt to avoid or escape the feared situation, an option that precludes habituation to the feared object (Last 1987). Empirically, several studies have supported this view.

Last and Blanchard (1982) found that when an individual with a specific phobia diagnosis is exposed to a feared situation, negative self-statements are triggered, which then heighten physiological activity. Similarly, Thorpe and Salkovskis (1995) found that most people with specific phobia reported at least one unrealistic belief about the harm that could befall them if they were exposed to the feared object or situation. Furthermore, a review of studies with phobic individuals (May 1977a, 1977b; Rimm et al. 1977; Wade et al. 1977) led Last (1987) to conclude that "maladaptive cognitions may be an important phenomenon in the genesis and maintenance of fear in clinically significant phobias" (p. 179).

Biases in information processing have also been implicated in the maintenance of phobias (Davey 1995). Specifically, the findings from several methodologies converge on the conclusion that phobic subjects have an attentional bias toward phobia-related threats. For example, Burgess et al. (1981) asked phobic and control subjects to complete a dichotic listening task. Participants were asked to speak out loud the information presented in one ear and indicate when either neutral or phobia-related words were presented in the other ear. Phobic subjects readily detected phobia-related words presented in the unattended ear, but control subjects did not.

The Stroop paradigm (for review, see J.M.G. Williams et al. 1996) is another methodology used to investigate the influence of cognitive processes in the maintenance of specific phobia. The Stroop test requires participants to rapidly name the color in which words are presented while ignoring the word content. Longer response latencies are assumed to reflect emotional interference in the processing of the color of the word. Several studies have found that phobic individuals are slower to name the color of threat-related words (Constantine et al. 2001; Kindt and Brosschot 1997; Thorpe and Salkovskis 1997) and pictures (Constantine et al. 2001; Lavy and van den Hout 1993). Vigilance for phobic stimuli has also been demonstrated using dot probe tasks in which pairs of phobic and neutral stimuli are presented for 500 milliseconds and replaced by a probe. An attentional bias for threat is indicated by faster detection of probes replacing phobic stimuli than of probes replacing neutral stimuli. Using this task, phobic individuals have demonstrated vigilance for pictures of phobic stimuli (Mogg et al. 2004). However, results with the dot probe task have been less consistent than results of the Stroop test, with several dot probe studies failing to replicate an attentional bias for phobic stimuli (e.g., Elsesser et al. 2006; Wenzel and Holt 1999). Importantly, attentional bias has also been demonstrated in phobic children (Martin and Jones 1995; Martin et al. 1992) and appears to be sensitive to diagnostic status, with several studies finding that attentional bias is reduced following treatment (van den Hout et al. 1997; Watts et al. 1986).

Researchers have also attempted to determine whether attentional bias occurs at an early (preconscious) level of processing or whether it relies on strategic (conscious) processing. Öhman and Soares (1994) included masked trials to assess whether the lower threshold for the detection of threat occurs below the level of conscious awareness. These authors found that masked phobia-related objects (in which subjects could not intentionally name the object) can elicit a physiological reaction in individuals with a phobia but not in control participants. Van den Hout et al. (1997) added to the strength of these findings by reporting that the intensity of phobic symptomatology was associated with a processing bias in both conscious (unmasked) and preconscious (masked) trials in individuals with a specific phobia. Öhman (1995) accounted for the preattentive bias toward threat by postulating that automatic preattentive attentional systems operate to maintain and detect threat in the environment. When threat is detected by these efficient involuntary systems, controlled or effortful attentional processes switch into operation to further ascertain the level and nature of the threat. If the stimuli are deemed to be threatening, the arousal system is activated.

Although the overall research consensus appears to be that phobic individuals are vigilant for threat in the early stages of attentional processing, little is known about what happens to attentional bias with extended exposure to a threatening stimulus. This is largely due to the fact that the Stroop and dot probe tasks depend on speeded responses to briefly presented stimuli (usually 500 milliseconds), thus providing only a static snapshot of attention. In real-life situations, however, phobic individuals generally encounter phobic events for longer than 500 milliseconds; it therefore seems important to examine changes in attention under more realistic viewing conditions. An alternative approach to assessing attentional bias has been to study the eye movements of anxious individuals while they are viewing pictures of phobic stimuli. Eye movement provides a dynamic "on-line" registration of attention, enabling researchers to examine the time course of selective attention over much longer stimulus durations than in the Stroop test or dot probe task. Using this methodology, Hermans et al. (1999) tracked the eye movements of spider-anxious individuals and control subjects while viewing slides containing a picture of a spider and a flower for 3 seconds. Spider-anxious individuals spent more time looking at spiders at the beginning of each presentation but more time viewing flowers toward the end, suggesting a tendency to focus on threat initially and then look away. Two further studies have replicated this vigilance-avoidance pattern of viewing behavior using similar designs (Pflugshaupt et al. 2007; Rinck and Becker 2006). Free-viewing paradigms in which phobic individuals self-determine viewing time for phobic pictures have also shown less viewing time for phobic pictures than for neutral pictures (Tolin et al. 1999). Findings such as these have led researchers to propose that anxiety is characterized by a vigilance-avoidance pattern of attentional allocation (Mogg et al. 1987, 1997). According to this two-stage model, individuals who are initially vigilant for threatening information avoid subsequent processing of the threat in an effort to alleviate their anxious mood.

Some authors have attempted to examine cognitive biases associated with specific phobias. A controversy in the literature on cognitive mediation in specific phobias has focused on two factors of potential importance. On one hand, S.L. Williams and colleagues (Williams and Watson 1985; Williams et al. 1985) argued that phobic avoidance and fear are principally mediated by low perceptions of self-efficacy. In contrast, Menzies and Clark (1995a) argued that phobic reactions are primarily mediated by exaggerated perceptions of danger and not by perceptions of self-efficacy. A study by Rapee (1997), however, implicated both self-efficacy and exaggerated perception of danger as additional cognitive factors that are likely to mediate phobic reactions.

Summary

This section has shown the possible utility of considering various theoretical approaches to understanding the causation of specific phobia. Consistent with this conclusion, Wilhelm and Roth (1997b) summarized five pathways to the development of phobias:

1. Direct conditioning
2. Vicarious conditioning
3. Verbal acquisition (Rachman 1991)
4. Nonassociative means (Menzies and Clarke 1995c)
5. Mediation by cognitive factors (Butler 1989; Last 1987; Wilhelm and Roth 1997b)

Whether each of these pathways in fact provides an alternative possible means to the acquisition of phobic avoidance or whether some will prove to be empirically unsupported awaits further investigation.

Treatment

Exposure Therapy

The earliest treatments for specific phobia were developed based on conditioning theory and thus were exposure based (Wolpe 1958). Consistent with the predictions of conditioning theory, systematic desensitization was found to be more effective than insight-oriented group or individual psychotherapy for specific phobia (Gelder et al. 1967). Today, the most compelling evidence for successful treatment remains with exposure-based treatments. The basic principle of exposure is that the prevention of escape or avoidance will result in learning that the feared outcome will not occur (Butler 1989). Specifically, flooding (Sherry and Levine 1980), in vivo exposure (Hecker 1990), modeling (Denney et al. 1977), and systematic desensitization (Curtis et al. 1976; Wolpe 1958) all have been found to provide successful treatment for specific phobia:

- *Flooding* involves the patient being exposed to the phobic stimulus in its most threatening form, with exposure continuing until the anxiety has dissipated. The extreme discomfort implicit in this method tends to discourage its wide use given the success of alternative methods of exposure.
- *In vivo exposure* involves live exposure to the phobic object and usually is conducted in a graded fashion, beginning with situations that elicit a small amount of anxiety and moving up the hierarchy of fears as the anxiety habituates and confidence increases.
- *Modeling* involves the therapist encouraging the patient to have contact with the phobic stimulus by providing demonstrations of approaching and contacting the phobic stimulus.
- *Systematic desensitization* (Wolpe 1958) relies on progressive muscle relaxation to manage the anxiety elicited during imaginal exposure to the phobic stimulus. That is, the patient is first trained in relaxation and is then asked to imagine a series of anxiety-provoking images while maintaining the incongruent relaxed state.

Although exposure techniques have proven efficacy in the treatment of specific phobia, research has delineated some considerations that should guide the specific treatment procedures. First, several studies (Barlow et al. 1969; Crowe et al. 1972; Emmelkamp and Wessels 1975; Gelder et al. 1973) have indicated that in vivo exposure is superior to imaginal exposure (Barlow 1988; Marks 1978). Furthermore, more recent research has indicated that in vivo exposure combined with modeling yields significantly better results in the treatment of spider phobia than direct observation (watching another patient being treated) and indirect observation (watching a videotape of a treatment session) (Öst et al. 1997). These recommendations make intuitive sense because the transfer of learning from imaginal or vicarious experiences of the feared object to real-life situations in which it is present could be difficult.

Second, longer exposure to the phobic stimulus has been recommended. It is theorized that moving away from the feared object prior to anxiety reduction will result in fear sensitization because it will cause escape and anxiety reduction to be paired (Öst 1989). Interestingly, however, empirical support for this intuitively appealing suggestion has been mixed (Rachman et al. 1986).

Finally, it has been proposed that exposure should be based on a graded hierarchy of fears (Barlow 1988). That is, the phobic patient should be asked to identify all the stimuli he or she is avoiding and place them in order, from those that elicit the least fear to those that elicit the most fear (see Butler 1989 for guidelines). After constructing the hierarchy, patients should be assisted in establishing experiments that involve exposure to each feared object or situation. Working to move up the hierarchy as the patient's anxiety habituates to each feared stimulus will increase the patient's comfort and compliance with treatment and between-session exposure tasks. In terms of the duration of treatment, a body of work has shown some exciting findings. Specifically, evidence has accumulated to suggest that one single intensive session of exposure-based treatment (2–3 hours) produces results comparable to those obtained over several sessions (Arntz and Lavy 1993; Hellström and Öst 1995; Öst 1989, 1996; Öst et al. 1991b).

As described by Öst (1989), the session for an individual with spider phobia begins with a detailed rationale for exposure that emphasizes the importance of staying in the exposure situation until the anxiety decreases. The individual is then exposed to four or five spiders of increasing sizes in turn. Each step is modeled by the therapist; then the patient attempts the same task. The first step involves teaching the patient to catch the spider with a glass and a piece of paper and to simulate throwing it out of the house. As the anxiety habituates, the amount of contact with the spider increases in the tasks. During the session, the patient is exposed to having a spider walking on his or her hand and even to having the spider on the patient's back or hair. This latter task exposes the patient to a situation in which he or she has no control over the spider. The end goal of the session is that the individual will be able to handle contact with a spider in everyday situations with little anxiety. Further evidence has indicated that the intensive single session is as successful with a group of patients as when individualized therapy is conducted (Öst et al. 1997).

Interestingly, the efficacy of exposure-based treatments may differ when disgust is an important underlying emotion. Several studies have found that disgust is slower to extinguish than fear in response to repeated exposure to a feared stimulus (Olatunji et al. 2007; Smits et al. 2002). Smits et al. (2002) repeatedly measured disgust and fear ratings of spider-phobic adults while undergoing 30 minutes of self-directed in vivo exposure to a tarantula. Although both fear and disgust ratings decreased significantly following the exposure session, disgust was significantly slower to attenuate than fear. Moreover, only spider-specific disgust ratings were reduced following treatment, whereas global disgust sensitivity (i.e., disgust for stimuli such as rotting food) remained unchanged. Given emerging evidence about the importance of disgust in maintaining phobia, it will be important for future research to examine how traditional exposure-based treatments can be used effectively to overcome disgust as well as fear.

Technological advances such as the advent of virtual reality have also had an impact on the theory of and research into exposure therapy. The use of virtual environments to provide phobic individuals with exposure opportunities to artificially created phobic events has been widespread. The efficacy of these treatments rests on the assumption that a virtual environment can elicit thoughts, feelings, and behaviors similar to those elicited by a real-life phobic situation, thereby providing opportunity for therapeutic change without some of the practical complications. To date, virtual reality has been used successfully in exposure-based treatments for various phobias. Randomized, controlled trials have shown that virtual exposure is as effective as in vivo exposure in the treatment of flying phobia (Rothbaum et al. 2000) and height phobia (Emmelkamp et al. 2002). Virtual reality has also proven superior to wait-list control conditions in individuals with spider phobia (Dewis et al. 2001; Garcia-Palacios et al. 2002) and height phobia (Hodges et al. 1995; Krijn et al. 2004). At least one study has also examined the efficacy of virtual reality as an adjunct to cognitive therapy (Mühlberger et al. 2003). This study compared cognitive therapy alone, cognitive therapy plus virtual reality, and a wait-list control group. The group that received adjunctive virtual reality fared better after treatment than the cognitive group or the wait-list control group.

Importantly, the effectiveness of virtual reality treatments appears to be maintained in the long term, with several studies demonstrating that the long-term effectiveness of virtual exposure is similar to the long-term efficacy of in vivo exposure (Emmelkamp et al. 2002; Rothbaum et al. 2002). From a practical perspective, virtual reality has a range of benefits compared with in vivo exposure. It is particularly useful when exposure to phobic stimuli is impractical because the stimulus itself is either not readily available (e.g., storms) or expensive, or when the phobic situation can be difficult to emulate in a graded way (e.g., flight phobia). Virtual environments also have the advantage of being tightly controlled: the therapist can manipulate specific situational determinants and program the occurrence of specific events, which cannot be guaranteed in real-life situations. Viewing such benefits in conjunction with mounting evidence for its efficacy, virtual reality remains an important and exciting avenue for future research.

Eye Movement Desensitization and Reprocessing

The efficacy of eye movement desensitization and reprocessing (EMDR) in the treatment of spider phobia in children has been tested (Muris et al. 1997). Shapiro (1995) described EMDR as a revolutionary treatment for psychological disorders that involve phobias and avoidance. The procedure involves many of the components of imaginal exposure therapy already outlined, except that during the desensitization a set of horizontal eye movements is elicited from the patient via hand movements by the therapist. The study by Muris et al. (1997) compared one session of EMDR with one session of in vivo exposure. Both treatments resulted in better performance on the self-report measures, but in vivo exposure was superior in reducing avoidance. It was concluded that there is no basis for suspecting that EMDR should replace in vivo exposure in the treatment of specific phobia.

Hypnotherapy

Several case studies have reported on the success of hypnosis in the treatment of specific phobia (Bird 1997; Ginsberg 1993; Morgan 2001). In terms of group studies, some either have not included a comparison group (Peretz et al. 1996) or have had many dropouts from treatment, markedly reducing statistical power (Hammarstrand et al. 1995). Two further studies, which found comparable effects for hypnotherapy and systematic desensitization (Moore et al. 1996, 2002), did not randomly assign participants to groups. Randomized, controlled trials of the efficacy of hypnosis in the treatment of specific phobia are therefore still required. Particular attention to the differentiation of hypnosis from imaginal exposure in terms of methodology (perhaps they are identical procedures) and in terms of outcomes is necessary.

Psychopharmacology

Few studies have tested the efficacy of psychopharmacology in the treatment of specific phobia. Bernadt et al. (1980) found positive initial results with diazepam and beta-blockers in decreasing avoidance behaviors and heart rate, respectively; however, subjective ratings of fear and avoidance were unchanged. Moreover, several studies using benzodiazepines have shown no evidence of long-term reductions in anxiety or avoidance (Campos et al. 1984; Whitehead et al. 1978; Wilhelm and Roth 1997a). For example, Wilhelm and Roth (1997a) found that individuals with a flying phobia who were given alprazolam reported less anxiety prior to taking a flight than did individuals who were given a placebo. However, these gains were short-lived. On a repeat flight 1 week later, the alprazolam group reported greater anxiety, more panic attacks, and greater physiological response than the placebo group. More recently, Johren et al. (2000) tested individuals with dental phobia who received either a single dose of midazolam, one session of applied relaxation, or no intervention prior to dental treatment. Although midazolam lowered anxiety prior to dental treatment, this effect was lost at 3 months, whereas individuals in the applied relaxation group continued to benefit from treatment. There has been some interesting work on the use of selective serotonin reuptake inhibitors (Benjamin et al. 2000), but larger studies are needed.

Based on these preliminary studies, it has been concluded that psychopharmacology is not the treatment of choice for specific phobia (Andrews et al. 1994; Barlow 1988; Fyer 1987; Roy-Byrne and Cowley 2007). However, there is some debate about whether pharmacotherapy may be a useful adjunct to behavior therapy. Researchers have theorized that reducing anxiety in the presence of the feared stimulus should lead to faster extinction of anxiety due to decreased avoidance (Whitehead et al. 1978), while others have argued that drug administration during exposure therapy will decrease the effectiveness of exposure and/or increase the likelihood of relapse (Wilhelm and Roth 1997a). This may occur because benzodiazepines at high doses can interfere with learning and their use may undermine a patient's ability to cope with the phobic situation without the drug. To test whether benzodiazepines facilitate or interfere with behavioral treatment, Coldwell et al. (2007) gave subjects with dental phobia one of two doses of alprazolam (0.5 mg or 0.75 mg) or a placebo. There was no advantage in combining alprazolam with systematic desensitization. Subjects in the alprazolam and placebo groups progressed through systematic desensitization treatment at the same rate, and dental fear was reduced similarly in all groups 1 year after study completion. On the basis of these results, Coldwell and colleagues concluded that there is no benefit in combining benzodiazepines with behavioral treatment of dental phobia.

There has been growing interest in the use of D-cycloserine, an *N*-methyl-D-aspartate receptor agonist, to potentiate the effects of exposure through enhanced learning. Ressler et al. (2004) gave subjects with height phobia either D-cycloserine or a pill placebo prior to virtual reality exposure. Those who took medication fared better than those in the placebo group, reporting lower anxiety and increasing their graded exposure practice to real height situations at 1-week and 3-month follow-ups. Despite these advances in pharmacotherapy, the utility of learning-enhancing drugs and the possibility of combining pharmacological and psychological treatments need further investigation.

Treatment of Blood-Injection-Injury Phobia

Treatment of blood-injection-injury phobia often becomes a priority when life-threatening illnesses can be averted by use of medical procedures that involve the feared object (e.g., injections, regular blood transfusions). As in the other types of phobias, exposure has been found to be a central component in the successful treatment of blood-injection-injury phobia (Curtis and Thyer 1983; Lloyd and Deakin 1975). Furthermore, initial evidence based on a single case report indicates that cognitive therapy may provide added assistance in the treatment of blood-injection-injury phobia (Wardle and Jarvis 1981).

Note that the treatment of this phobia can be complicated by fainting. Two treatment interventions have been highlighted by Page (1994) to protect the patient from fainting. The first technique, termed *applied tension*, involves instructing the patient to rapidly and frequently tense various muscle groups in his or her body during exposure, an activity that creates a physiological state that is incompatible with fainting. Indeed, Kozak and Montgomery (1981) successfully used exposure therapy in a group of individuals with blood-injection-injury phobia, with applied tension used an adjunct. In a more recent study, Öst and associates (1991a) compared three groups of patients with blood-injection-injury phobia: 1) those who were treated with exposure alone, 2) those who were treated with applied tension alone, and 3) those who were treated with applied tension plus exposure. The two applied-tension groups had better outcomes than the exposure-only group. This study raised the possibility that for blood-injection-injury phobia, the skill of applied tension is more important than the exposure component of treatment. In a case study, a second strategy was a successful adjunct to the treatment of blood-injection-injury phobia. This strategy involved eliciting the emotional state of anger from a patient during exposure in order to elicit a physiological change that is incompatible with fainting (Cohn et al. 1976). The patient was instructed to identify and to re-create in his or her mind, during exposure, four personal situations in which he or she felt particularly angry. If the patient does faint during exposure, the fainting response will probably subside over a few sessions if exposure continues as consciousness returns (Marks 1988).

Conclusion

The empirical evidence supports the proposal that there are multiple pathways to the onset of specific phobia. The most recent theoretical development has been in the domain of the nonassociative accounts of specific phobia, which argue that phobias may occur outside of direct or indirect contact with the feared object. Although such theoretical models focus on fear as the primary emotion elicited by the phobic stimulus or situation, disgust is receiving increasing attention as an important determinant of the phobic response. Future research into the treatment of disgust may provide important advances in treatment outcomes, particularly for those with animal or blood-injection-injury phobias where disgust is most clearly implicated. Furthermore, the consensus in the literature is that exposure therapy is the basis of a successful intervention for specific phobia. An exciting recent development in the treatment of specific phobia has been the one-session group treatment developed by the Swedish research group led by Öst. The use of virtual reality to provide tightly controlled, convenient opportunities for graded exposure represents an important development in the treatment of specific phobia, especially in cases where repeated exposure to the feared event is impractical or costly. Interventions such as these represent a cost-effective alternative to the four to six sessions of face-to-face therapy traditionally required for the treatment of specific phobia. Finally, the use of fear extinction–enhancing drugs such as D-cycloserine represents a potentially exciting innovation for the future of phobia treatments; however, considerable research is still required before the clinical efficacy of these agents can be established.

◀ Key Clinical Points ▶

- Specific phobia is characterized by a marked fear of, and a desire to avoid, a specific situation or object.
- Specific phobia is one of the most common psychiatric disorders across the population; however, many people do not seek treatment, especially when feared stimuli and situations can be avoided with relative ease.
- There are five different phobia subtypes: 1) animal, 2) natural environment (e.g., storms, water), 3) blood-injection-injury, and 4) situational type (e.g., flying, enclosed spaces). A fifth category (other) is reserved for phobias (e.g., fear of vomiting) that do not fit into one of the four main categories. Despite the tendency to subtype, there are more commonalities than differences among the phobias.
- Although most phobias are motivated primarily by fear, disgust appears to play an important role in small-animal and blood-injection-injury phobias.
- Behavioral, biological, and cognitive processes are all thought to be important in the etiology and maintenance of specific phobia.
- Behavioral accounts of specific phobia have developed over time and with some controversy. Conditioning models stressed the importance of learned associations between a feared stimulus (previously neutral) and a potentially threatening outcome. Associations can be made via direct experience, indirect experience (e.g., observational learning) and transmission of information. In contrast, nonassociative accounts have held that phobias may be acquired without previous direct or indirect associative learning. Today, it is generally accepted that one or all of these modes of onset may be involved in the etiology of phobia.
- Cognitive accounts of specific phobia have emphasized the importance of distorted negative thinking patterns and dysfunctional beliefs and attitudes, not simply as a result of the fear response, but as a critical factor in the etiology and maintenance of the disorder.

- There is evidence of genetic and neurological involvement in specific phobia; however, precise contributions and mechanisms await further research.
- Research has generally pointed toward cognitive and behavioral interventions as the treatment of choice for specific phobia, rather than pharmacotherapy.
- Traditional exposure-based treatments can be difficult to apply in persons with blood-injury-injection phobia because of these individuals' tendency to faint on exposure to the phobic stimulus. In such cases, applied tension (Page 1994) may be an effective addition to exposure treatment. It involves instructing the patient to rapidly and frequently tense various muscle groups during exposure, an activity that creates a physiological state incompatible with fainting.
- There is emerging evidence that learning-enhancing drugs, such as D-cycloserine, may potentiate the effects of exposure during CBT and ultimately enhance treatment outcome. This research is in its infancy, however, and the possibility of combining such pharmacological and psychological treatments needs further investigation.

References

Agras WS, Sylvester D, Oliveau D: The epidemiology of common fears and phobia. Compr Psychiatry 10:151–156, 1969

Agras WS, Chapin HM, Oliveau DC: The natural history of phobias: course and prognosis. Arch Gen Psychiatry 26:315–317, 1972

American Psychiatric Association: Diagnostic and Statistical Manual of Mental Disorders, 3rd Edition. Washington, DC, American Psychiatric Association, 1980

American Psychiatric Association: Diagnostic and Statistical Manual of Mental Disorders, 4th Edition, Text Revision. Washington, DC, American Psychiatric Association, 2000

Andrews G, Crino R, Lampe L, et al: The Treatment of Anxiety Disorders. New York, Cambridge University Press, 1994

Antony MM, Brown TA, Barlow DH: Heterogeneity among specific phobia types in DSM-IV. Behav Res Ther 35:1089–1100, 1997

Arntz A, Lavy E: Does stimulus elaboration potentiate exposure in-vivo treatment?: two forms of one-session treatment of spider phobia. Behavioural Psychotherapy 21:1–12, 1993

Bancroft J: Aversion therapy of homosexuality. Br J Psychiatry 115:1417–1431, 1969

Bandura A, Rosenthal TL: Vicarious classical conditioning as a function of arousal level. J Pers Soc Psychol 3:54–62, 1966

Barlow DH: Anxiety and Its Disorders: The Nature and Treatment of Anxiety and Panic. New York, Guilford, 1988

Barlow DH, Leitenberg H, Agras WS, et al: The transfer gap in systematic desensitization: an analogue study. Behav Res Ther 7:191–196, 1969

Beck AT, Emery G, Greenberg RL: Anxiety Disorders and Phobias: A Cognitive Perspective. New York, Basic Books, 1985

Becker ES, Rinck M, Turke V, et al: Epidemiology of specific phobia subtypes: findings from the Dresden Mental Health Study. Eur Psychiatry 22:69–74, 2007

Benjamin J, Ben-Zion IZ, Karbofsky E, et al: Double-blind placebo-controlled pilot study of paroxetine for specific phobia. Psychopharmacology 149:194–196, 2000

Bernadt MW, Silverstone T, Singleton W: Behavioural and subjective effects of beta-adrenergic blockade in phobic subjects. Br J Psychiatry 137:452–457, 1980

Bertenthal BI, Campos JJ, Barrett KC: Self-produced locomotion: an organizer of emotional, cognitive, and social development in infancy, in Continuities and Discontinuities in Development. Edited by Emde RN, Harmon RJ. New York, Plenum, 1984, pp 175–210

Bird N: Treatment of childhood dental phobia using a modified television visualization technique. Contemporary Hypnosis 14:80–83, 1997

Bolton D, Eley TC, O'Connor TG, et al: Prevalence and genetic and environmental influences on anxiety disorders in 6-year-old twins. Psychol Med 36:335–344, 2006

Bowlby J: Attachment and Loss, Vol 2: Separation: Anxiety and Anger. New York, Basic Books, 1973

Breiter HC, Rauch SL: Functional MRI and the study of OCD: from symptom provocation to cognitive-behavioral probes of cortico-striatal systems and the amygdala. Neuroimage 4:127–138, 1996

Burgess IS, Jones LM, Roberts SA, et al: The degree of control exerted by phobic and non-phobic verbal stimuli over the recognition behaviour of phobic and non-phobic subjects. Behav Res Ther 19:233–243, 1981

Butler G: Phobic disorders, in Cognitive Behaviour Therapy for Psychiatric Problems: A Practical Guide. Edited by

Hawton K, Salkovskis PM, Kirk J, et al. Oxford, UK, Oxford University Press, 1989, pp 95–128

Campos PE, Solyom L, Koelink A: The effects of timolol maleate on subjective and physiological component of air travel phobia. Can J Psychiatry 29:570–574, 1984

Charash M, McKay D: Attentional bias for disgust. J Anxiety Disord 16:529–541, 2002

Choy Y, Fyer AJ, Goodwin RD: Specific phobia and comorbid depression: a closer look at the National Comorbidity Survey data. Compr Psychiatry 48:132–136, 2007

Clarke JC, Jackson JA: Hypnosis and Behavior Therapy: The Treatment of Anxiety and Phobias. New York, Springer, 1983

Cohn CK, Kron RE, Brady JP: A case of blood-illness-injury phobia treated behaviorally. J Nerv Ment Dis 162:65–68, 1976

Coldwell SE, Wilhelm FH, Milgrom P, et al: Combining alprazolam with systematic desensitization therapy for dental injection phobia. J Anxiety Disord 21:871–887, 2007

Constantine R, McNally RJ, Hornig CD: Snake fear and the pictorial emotional Stroop paradigm. Cognit Ther Res 25:757–764, 2001

Cook M, Harris RE: The verbal conditioning of the galvanic skin reflex. J Exp Psychol 21:202–210, 1937

Cook M, Mineka S: Observational conditioning of fear to fear-relevant versus fear-irrelevant stimuli in rhesus monkeys. J Abnorm Psychol 98:448–459, 1989

Cook M, Mineka S, Wolkenstein B, et al: Observational conditioning of snake fear in unrelated rhesus monkeys. J Abnorm Psychol 94:591–610, 1985

Crowe MJ, Marks IM, Agras WS, et al: Time limited desensitization, implosion, and shaping for phobic patients: a crossover study. Behav Res Ther 10:319–328, 1972

Curtis GC, Thyer BA: Fainting on exposure to phobic stimuli. Am J Psychiatry 140:771–774, 1983

Curtis G, Nesse R, Buxton M, et al: Flooding in vivo as a research tool and treatment method for phobias: a preliminary report. Compr Psychiatry 17:153–160, 1976

Curtis GC, Magee WJ, Eaton WW, et al: Specific fears and phobias: epidemiology and classification. Br J Psychiatry 173:212–217, 1998

Davey GC: Factors influencing self-rated fear to a novel animal. Cogn Emot 7:461–471, 1993

Davey GC: Preparedness and phobias: specific evolved associations or a generalized expectancy bias? Behav Brain Sci 18:289–325, 1995

de Jong PJ, Merckelbach H: Blood-injection-injury phobia and fear of spiders: domain specific individual differences in disgust sensitivity. Pers Individ Dif 24:153–158, 1998

de Jong PJ, Peters M, Vanderhallen I: Disgust and disgust sensitivity in spider phobia: facial EMG in response to spider and oral disgust imagery. J Anxiety Disord 16:477–493, 2002

Denney DR, Sullivan BJ, Thiry MR: Participant modelling and self-verbalization training in the reduction of spider fears. J Behav Ther Exp Psychiatry 8:247–253, 1977

Dennis W: Does culture appreciably affect patterns of infant behavior? J Soc Psychol 12:305–317, 1940

Dewis LM, Kirkby KC, Martin F, et al: Computer-aided vicarious exposure versus live graded exposure for spider phobia in children. J Behav Ther Exp Psychiatry 32:17–27, 2001

Ehlers A, Hofmann SG, Herda CA, et al: Clinical characteristics of driving phobia. J Anxiety Disord 8:323–339, 1994

Elsesser K, Heuschen I, Pundt I, et al: Attentional bias and evoked heart-rate response in specific phobia. Cogn Emot 20:1092–1107, 2006

Emmelkamp PM, Wessels H: Flooding in imagination versus in vivo: a comparison with agoraphobics. Behav Res Ther 13:7–15, 1975

Emmelkamp PM, Krijn M, Hulsbosch AM, et al: Virtual reality treatment versus exposure in vivo: a comparative evaluation in acrophobia. Behav Res Ther 40:509–516, 2002

Essau CA, Conradt J, Petermann F: Frequency, comorbidity and psychosocial impairment of specific phobia in adolescents. J Clin Child Psychol 29:221–231, 2000

Fazio AF: Implosive therapy with semiclinical phobias. J Abnorm Psychol 80:183–188, 1972

Fredrikson M, Wik G, Annas P, et al: Functional neuroanatomy of visually elicited simple phobic fear: additional data and theoretical analysis. Psychophysiology 32:43–48, 1995

Fredrikson M, Annas P, Fischer H, et al: Gender and age differences in the prevalence of specific fears and phobias. Behav Res Ther 34:33–39, 1996

Fyer AJ: Simple phobia. Mod Probl Pharmacopsychiatry 22: 174–192, 1987

Fyer AJ: Current approaches to etiology and pathophysiology of specific phobia. Biol Psychiatry 44:1295–1304, 1998

Fyer AJ, Mannuzza S, Gallops MS, et al: Familial transmission of simple phobia and fears: a preliminary report. Arch Gen Psychiatry 47:252–256, 1990

Garcia-Palacios A, Hoffman H, Carlin A, et al: Virtual reality in the treatment of spider phobia: a controlled study. Behav Res Ther 40:983–993, 2002

Gelder MG, Marks IM, Wolff HE, et al: Desensitization and psychotherapy in the treatment of phobic states: a controlled inquiry. Br J Psychiatry 113:53–73, 1967

Gelder MG, Bancroft JH, Gath DH, et al: Specific and nonspecific factors in behaviour therapy. Br J Psychiatry 123:445–462, 1973

Ginsberg SH: Hypnosis as an adjunct to broad spectrum psychotherapy in the treatment of simple phobia. Australian Journal of Clinical and Experimental Hypnosis 21:39–59, 1993

Goisman RM, Allworth BA, Rogers MP, et al: Simple phobia as a comorbid anxiety disorder. Depress Anxiety 7:105–112, 1998

Goodwin RD: Anxiety disorders and the onset of depression among adults in the community. Psychol Med 32:1121–1124, 2002

Goossens L, Sunaert S, Peeters R, et al: Amygdala hyperfunction in phobic fear normalizes after exposure. Biol Psychiatry 62:1119–1125, 2007

Hammarstrand G, Berggren U, Hakeberg M: Psychophysiological therapy vs hypnotherapy in the treatment of patients with dental phobia. Eur J Oral Sci 103:399–404, 1995

Hecker JE: Emotional processing in the treatment of simple phobia: a comparison of imaginal and in vivo exposure. Behavioural Psychotherapy 18:21–34, 1990

Hellström K, Öst LG: One-session therapist directed exposure vs two forms of manual directed self-exposure in the treatment of spider phobia. Behav Res Ther 33:959–965, 1995

Hermans D, Vansteenwegen D, Eelen P: Eye movement registration as a continuous index of attention deployment: data from a group of spider anxious students. Cogn Emot 13:419–434, 1999

Himle JA, McPhee K, Cameron OG, et al: Simple phobia: evidence for heterogeneity. Psychiatry Res 28:25–30, 1989

Hodges LF, Kooper R, Meyer TC, et al: Virtual environments for treating the fear of heights. Computer 28:27–34, 1995

Hofmann SG, Ehlers A, Roth WT: Conditioning theory: a model for the etiology of public speaking anxiety? Behav Res Ther 33:567–571, 1995

Hofmann SG, Lehman CL, Barlow DH: How specific are specific phobias? J Behav Ther Exp Psychiatry 28:233–240, 1997

Johren P, Jackowski J, Gangler P, et al: Fear reduction in patients with dental treatment phobia. Br J Oral Maxillofac Surg 38:612–616, 2000

Jones MK, Menzies RG: The etiology of spider phobia. Anxiety Stress Coping 8:227–234, 1995

Kendler KS, Neale MC, Kessler RC, et al: The genetic epidemiology of phobias in women: the interrelationship of agoraphobia, social phobia, situational phobia, and simple phobia. Arch Gen Psychiatry 49:273–281, 1992

Kendler KS, Karkowski LM, Prescott CA: Fears and phobias: reliability and heritability. Psychol Med 29:539–553, 1999

Kendler KS, Myers J, Prescott CA, et al: The genetic epidemiology of irrational fears and phobias in men. Arch Gen Psychiatry 58:257–265, 2001

Kessler RC, McGonagle KA, Zhao S, et al: Lifetime and 12-month prevalence of DSM-III-R psychiatric disorders in the United States: results from the National Comorbidity Survey. Arch Gen Psychiatry 51:8–19, 1994

Kessler RC, Berglund PA, Demler O, et al: Lifetime prevalence and age-of-onset distributions of DSM-IV disorders in the National Comorbidity Survey Replication. Arch Gen Psychiatry 62:593–602, 2005a

Kessler RC, Chiu WT, Demler O, et al: Prevalence, severity, and comorbidity of 12-month DSM-IV disorders in the National Comorbidity Survey Replication. Arch Gen Psychiatry 62:617–627, 2005b

Kindt M, Brosschot JF: Phobia-related cognitive bias for pictorial and linguistic stimuli. J Abnorm Psychol 106:644–648, 1997

Kleinknecht RA: The origins and remission of fear in a group of tarantula enthusiasts. Behav Res Ther 20:437–443, 1982

Kleinknecht RA, Thorndike RM, Walls MM: Factorial dimensions and correlates of blood, injury, injection and related medical fears: cross validation of the medical fear survey. Behav Res Ther 34:323–331, 1996

Kozak MJ, Montgomery GK: Multimodal behavioral treatment of recurrent injury-scene-elicited fainting (vasodepressor syncope). Behavioural Psychotherapy 9:316–321, 1981

Krijn M, Emmelkamp PM, Biemond R, et al: Treatment of acrophobia in virtual reality: the role of immersion and presence. Behav Res Ther 42:229–239, 2004

Last CG: Simple phobias, in Anxiety and Stress Disorders: Cognitive-Behavioral Assessment and Treatment. Edited by Michelson L, Ascher LM. New York, Guilford, 1987, pp 176–190

Last CG, Blanchard EB: Classification of phobics versus fearful nonphobics: procedural and theoretical issues. Behav Assess 4:195–210, 1982

Lavy E, van den Hout M: Selective attention evidenced by pictorial and linguistic Stroop tasks. Behav Ther 24:645–657, 1993

Lipsitz JD, Barlow DH, Mannuzza S, et al: Clinical features of four DSM-IV specific phobic subtypes. J Nerv Ment Dis 170:471–478, 2002

Lloyd G, Deakin HG: Phobias complicating treatment of uterine carcinoma (case report). BMJ 4:440, 1975

Magee WJ, Eaton WW, Wittchen H-U, et al: Agoraphobia, simple phobia, and social phobia in the National Comorbidity Survey. Arch Gen Psychiatry 53:159–168, 1996

Marks I: Exposure treatments: clinical applications, in Behaviour Modification: Principles and Clinical Applications, 2nd Edition. Edited by Agras WS. Boston, MA, Little, Brown, 1978, pp 110–134

Marks I: Blood-injury phobia: a review. Am J Psychiatry 145:1207–1213, 1988

Marks IM, Gelder M: Transvestism and fetishism: clinical and psychological changes during faradic aversion. Br J Psychiatry 117:173–185, 1967

Martin M, Jones GV: Integral bias in the cognitive processing of emotionally linked pictures. Br J Psychol 86:419–435, 1995

Martin M, Horder P, Jones GV: Integral bias in naming of phobia-related words. Cogn Emot 6:479–486, 1992

Mavissakalian M, Barlow DH: Phobia: Psychological and Pharmacological Treatment. New York, Guilford, 1981

May JR: A psychophysiological study of self and externally regulated phobic thoughts. Behav Ther 8:849–861, 1977a

May JR: Psychophysiology of self-regulated phobic thoughts. Behav Ther 8:150–159, 1977b

McNally RJ: Phobias and preparedness: instructional reversal of electrodermal conditioning to fear-relevant stimuli. Psychol Rep 48:175–180, 1981

McNally RJ: Pavlovian conditioning and preparedness: effects of initial fear level. Behav Res Ther 24:27–33, 1986

McNally RJ: Preparedness and phobias: a review. Psychol Bull 101:283–303, 1987

McNally RJ, Foa EB: Preparedness and resistance to extinction to fear-relevant stimuli: a failure to replicate. Behav Res Ther 24:529–535, 1986

McNally RJ, Louro CE: Fear of flying in agoraphobia and simple phobia: distinguishing features. J Anxiety Disord 6:319–324, 1992

McNally RJ, Steketee GS: The etiology and maintenance of severe animal phobias. Behav Res Ther 23:431–435, 1985

Menzies RG, Clarke JC: The etiology of childhood water phobia. Behav Res Ther 31:499–501, 1993a

Menzies RG, Clarke JC: The etiology of fear of heights and its relationship to severity and individual response patterns. Behav Res Ther 31:355–365, 1993b

Menzies RG, Clarke JC: Danger expectancies and insight in acrophobia. Behav Res Ther 33:215–221, 1995a

Menzies RG, Clarke JC: The etiology of acrophobia and its relationship to severity and individual response patterns. Behav Res Ther 33:795–803, 1995b

Menzies RG, Clarke JC: The etiology of phobias: a nonassociative account. Clin Psychol Rev 15:23–48, 1995c

Meyer C, Rumpf H, Hapke U, et al: Impact of psychiatric disorders in the general population: satisfaction with life and the influence of comorbidity and disorder duration. Soc Psychiatry Psychiatr Epidemiol 39:435–441, 2004

Milgrom P, Weinstein P, Getz T: Treating Fearful Dental Patients: A Patient Management Handbook, 2nd Edition. Seattle, University of Washington, 1995

Mineka S: Depression and helplessness in primates, in Child Nurturance, Vol 3. Edited by Fitzgerald HE, Mullins JA, Gaze P. New York, Plenum, 1982, pp 197–242

Mineka S, Davidson M, Cook M, et al: Observational conditioning of snake fear in rhesus monkeys. J Abnorm Psychol 93:355–372, 1984

Mogg K, Mathews A, Weinman J: Memory bias in clinical anxiety. J Abnorm Psychol 96:94–98, 1987

Mogg K, Bradley BP, de Bono J, et al: Time course of attentional bias for threat information in non-clinical anxiety. Behav Res Ther 35:297–303, 1997

Mogg K, Bradley BP, Miles F, et al: Time course of attentional bias for threat scenes: testing the vigilance-avoidance hypothesis. Cogn Emot 18:689–700, 2004

Moore R, Abrahamsen R, Brødsgaard I: Hypnosis compared with group therapy and individual desensitization for dental anxiety. Eur J Oral Sci 104:612–618, 1996

Moore R, Brødsgaard I, Abrahamsen R: A 3-year comparison of dental anxiety treatment outcomes: hypnosis, group therapy and individual desensitization vs no specialist treatment. Eur J Oral Sci 110:287–295, 2002

Morgan S: Hypnosis and simple phobia. Australian Journal of Clinical and Experimental Hypnosis 29:17–25, 2001

Mountz JM, Modell JG, Wilson MW, et al: Positron emission tomographic evaluation of cerebral blood flow during state anxiety in simple phobia. Arch Gen Psychiatry 46: 501–504, 1989

Mowrer OH: Learning Theory and Behaviour. New York, Wiley, 1960

Mühlberger A, Wiedemann GC, Pauli P: Efficacy of a one-session virtual reality exposure treatment for fear of flying. Psychother Res 13:323–336, 2003

Mulkens S, de Jong PJ, Merckelbach H: Disgust and spider phobia. J Abnorm Psychol 105:464–468, 1996

Muris P, Merckelbach H, van Haaften H, et al: Eye movement desensitization and reprocessing versus exposure in vivo. Br J Psychiatry 17:82–86, 1997

Öhman A: Preferential preattentive processing of threat in anxiety: preparedness and attentional biases, in Current Controversies in the Anxiety Disorders. Edited by Rapee RM. New York, Guilford, 1995, pp 253–296

Öhman A, Dimberg U: Facial expressions as conditioned stimuli for electrodermal responses: a case of "preparedness"? J Pers Soc Psychol 36:1251–1258, 1978

Öhman A, Soares JJ: "Unconscious anxiety": phobic responses to masked stimuli. J Abnorm Psychol 103:231–240, 1994

Öhman A, Erixon G, Löfberg I: Phobias and preparedness: phobic versus neutral pictures as conditioned stimuli for human autonomic responses. J Abnorm Psychol 84:41–45, 1975

Olatunji BO, Forsyth JP, Cherian A: Evaluative differential conditioning of disgust: a sticky form of relational learning that is resistant to extinction. J Anxiety Disord 21:820–834, 2007

Öst LG: Age of onset in different phobias. J Abnorm Psychol 96:223–229, 1987

Öst LG: One-session treatment for specific phobias. Behav Res Ther 27:1–7, 1989

Öst LG: One session group treatment of spider phobia. Behav Res Ther 34:707–715, 1996

Öst LG, Fellenius J, Sterner U: Applied tension, exposure in vivo, and tension-only in the treatment of blood injury phobia. Behav Res Ther 29:561–574, 1991a

Öst LG, Salkovskis PM, Hellström K: One-session therapist directed exposure vs self-exposure in the treatment of spider phobia. Behav Ther 22:407–422, 1991b

Öst LG, Ferebee I, Furmark T: One-session group therapy of spider phobia: direct versus indirect treatments. Behav Res Ther 35:721–732, 1997

Page AC: Blood-injury phobia. Clin Psychol Rev 14:443–461, 1994

Paquette V, Lévesque J, Mensour B, et al: "Change the mind and you change the brain": effects of cognitive-behavioral therapy on the neural correlates of spider phobia. Neuroimage 18:401–409, 2003

Pegeron JP, Thyer BA: Simple phobia leading to suicide: a case report. The Behavior Therapist 9:134–135, 1986

Peretz B, Katz J, Zilburg I, et al: Treating dental phobic patients in the Israeli Defense Force. Int Dent J 46:108–112, 1996

Pflugshaupt T, Mosimann UP, Schmitt WJ, et al: To look or not to look at threat? Scanpath differences within a group of spider phobics. J Anxiety Disord 21:353–366, 2007

Poulton R, Davies S, Menzies RG, et al: Evidence for a non-associative model of the acquisition of a fear of heights. Behav Res Ther 36:537–544, 1998

Poulton R, Menzies RG, Craske MG, et al: Water trauma and swimming experiences up to age 9 and fear of water at age 18: a longitudinal study. Behav Res Ther 37:39–48, 1999

Poulton R, Milne B, Craske MG, et al: A longitudinal study of the etiology of separation anxiety. Behav Res Ther 39:1395–1410, 2001

Rachman S: The passing of the two-stage theory of fear and avoidance: fresh possibilities. Behav Res Ther 14:125–131, 1976

Rachman S: The conditioning theory of fear-acquisition: a critical examination. Behav Res Ther 15:375–387, 1977

Rachman S: Fear and Courage. San Francisco, CA, WH Freeman, 1978

Rachman S: Neo-conditioning and the classical theory of fear acquisition. Clin Psychol Rev 11:155–173, 1991

Rachman S, Craske M, Tallman K, et al: Does escape behavior strengthen agoraphobic avoidance? a replication. Behav Ther 17:366–384, 1986

Rapee RM: Perceived threat and perceived control as predictors of the degree of fear in physical and social situations. J Anxiety Disord 11:455–461, 1997

Rauch SL, Savage CR, Alpert NM, et al: A positron emission tomographic study of simple phobic symptom provocation. Arch Gen Psychiatry 52:20–28, 1995

Rauch SL, Whalen PJ, Shin LM, et al: Exaggerated amygdala response to masked facial stimuli in posttraumatic stress disorder: a functional MRI study. Biol Psychiatry 47:769–776, 2000

Rauch SL, Wright BM, Busa E, et al: A magnetic resonance imaging study of cortical thickness in animal phobia. Biol Psychiatry 55:946–952, 2004

Reiger DA, Boyd JH, Burke JD, et al: One-month prevalence of mental disorders in the United States. Arch Gen Psychiatry 45:977–986, 1988

Ressler KJ, Rothbaum BO, Tannenbaum L, et al: Cognitive enhancers as adjuncts to psychotherapy: use of D-cycloserine in phobic individuals to facilitate extinction of fear. Arch Gen Psychiatry 61:1136–1144, 2004

Rimm DC, Janda LH, Lancaster DW, et al: An exploratory investigation of the origin and maintenance of phobias. Behav Res Ther 15:231–238, 1977

Rinck M, Becker ES: Spider fearful individuals attend to threat, then quickly avoid it: evidence from eye movements. J Abnorm Psychol 115:231–238, 2006

Rothbaum BO, Hodges L, Smith S, et al: A controlled study of virtual reality exposure therapy for the fear of flying. J Consult Clin Psychol 68:1020–1026, 2000

Rothbaum BO, Hodges L, Anderson PL, et al: Twelve-month follow-up of virtual reality and standard exposure therapies for the fear of flying. J Consult Clin Psychol 70:428–432, 2002

Roy-Byrne P, Cowley D: Pharmacological treatments for panic disorder, generalized anxiety disorder, specific phobia, and social anxiety disorder, in A Guide to Treatments That Work. Edited by Nathan P, Gorman J. New York, Oxford University Press, 2007, pp 395–430

Sackett GP: Monkeys reared in isolation with pictures as visual input. Science 154:1468–1472, 1966

Sanderson WC, DiNardo PA, Rapee RM, et al: Syndrome comorbidity in patients diagnosed with a DSM-III-R anxiety disorder. J Abnorm Psychol 99:308–312, 1990

Sawchuk CN, Lohr JM, Tolin DF, et al: Disgust sensitivity and contamination fears in spider and blood-injury-injection phobias. Behav Res Ther 38:753–762, 2000

Seligman M: Phobias and preparedness. Behav Ther 2:307–320, 1971

Shapiro F: Eye Movement Desensitization and Reprocessing: Basic Principles, Protocols, and Procedures. New York, Guilford, 1995

Sherry GS, Levine BA: An examination of procedural variables in flooding therapy. Behav Ther 11:148–155, 1980

Smith PK: The ontogeny of fear in children, in Fear in Animals and Man. Edited by Slukin W. London, Van Nostrand Reinhold, 1979, pp 164–168

Smits JAJ, Telch MJ, Randall PK: An examination of the decline in fear and disgust during exposure-based treatment. Behav Res Ther 40:1243–1253, 2002

Stein MB, Goldin PR, Sareen J, et al: Increased amygdala activation to angry and contemptuous faces in generalized social phobia. Arch Gen Psychiatry 59:1027–1034, 2002

Stinson FS, Dawson DA, Chou PS, et al: The epidemiology of DSM-IV specific phobia in the USA: results from the National Epidemiologic Survey on Alcohol and Related Conditions. Psychol Med 37:1047–1059, 2007

Straube T, Kolassa IT, Glauer M, et al: Effect of task conditions on brain responses to threatening faces in social phobics: an event-related functional magnetic resonance imaging study. Biol Psychiatry 56:921–930, 2004

Straube T, Glauer M, Dilger S, et al: Effects of cognitive-behavioral therapy brain activation in specific phobia. Neuroimage 29:125–135, 2006a

Straube T, Mentzel H, Miltner W: Neural mechanisms of automatic and direct processing of phobogenic stimuli in specific phobia. Biol Psychiatry 59:162–170, 2006b

Sturgis ET, Scott R: Simple phobia, in Behavioral Theories and Treatment of Anxiety. Edited by Turner SM. New York, Plenum, 1984, pp 91–141

Thorpe SJ, Salkovskis PM: Phobic beliefs: do cognitive factors play a role in specific phobias. Behav Res Ther 33:805–816, 1995

Thorpe SJ, Salkovskis PM: Information processing in spider phobics: the Stroop colour naming task may indicate strategic but not automatic attentional bias. Behav Res Ther 35:131–144, 1997

Tolin DF, Lohr JM, Sawchuk CN, et al: Disgust and disgust sensitivity in blood-injection-injury and spider phobia. Behav Res Ther 35:949–953, 1997

Tolin DF, Lohr JM, Lee TC, et al: Visual avoidance in specific phobia. Behav Res Ther 37:63–70, 1999

Tseng W, Kan-Ming M, Hsu J, et al: A sociocultural study of koro epidemics in Guandong, China. Am J Psychiatry 145:1538–1543, 1988

van den Hout M, Tenney N, Huygens K, et al: Preconscious processing bias in specific phobia. Behav Res Ther 35:29–34, 1997

Wade TCW, Malloy TE, Proctor S: Imaginal correlates of self-reported fear and avoidance behavior. Behav Res Ther 15:17–22, 1977

Walk R, Gibson EJ: A comparative and analytic study of visual depth perception. Psychol Monogr 75:1–44, 1960

Wardle J, Jarvis M: The paradoxical fear response to blood, injury and illness: a treatment report. Behavioural Psychotherapy 9:13–24, 1981

Ware J, Jain K, Burgess I, et al: Disease-avoidance model: factor analysis of common animal fears. Behav Res Ther 32:57–63, 1994

Watson JB, Raynor R: Conditioned emotional reactions. J Exp Psychol 3:1–14, 1920

Watts FN, McKenna FP, Sharrock R, et al: Colour naming of phobia-related words. Br J Psychol 77:97–108, 1986

Wells EJ, Browne MA, Scott K, et al: Prevalence, interference with life and severity of 12-month DSM-IV disorders in Te Rau Hinengaro: The New Zealand Mental Health Survey. Aust N Z J Psychiatry 40:845–854, 2006

Wenzel A, Holt CS: Dot probe performance in two specific phobias. Br J Clin Psychol 38:407–410, 1999

Whitehead WE, Blackwell B, Robinson A: Effects of diazepam on phobic avoidance behavioral and phobic anxiety. Biol Psychiatry 13:59–64, 1978

Wik G, Fredrikson M, Fischer H: Cerebral correlates of anticipated fear: a PET study of specific phobia. Int J Neurosci 87:267–276, 1996

Wilhelm FH, Roth WT: Acute and delayed effects of alprazolam on flight phobics during exposure. Behav Res Ther 35:831–841, 1997a

Wilhelm FH, Roth WT: Clinical characteristics of flight phobia. J Anxiety Disord 11:241–261, 1997b

Williams JMG, Mathews A, MacLeod C: The emotional Stroop task and psychopathology. Psychol Bull 120:3–24, 1996

Williams SL, Watson N: Perceived danger and perceived self-efficacy as cognitive determinants of acrophobic behavior. Behav Ther 16:136–146, 1985

Williams SL, Turner SM, Peer DF: Guided mastery and performance desensitization treatments for severe acrophobia. J Consult Clin Psychol 53:237–247, 1985

Wolpe J: Psychotherapy by Reciprocal Inhibition. Stanford, CA, Stanford University Press, 1958

Recommended Readings

Choy Y, Fyer AJ, Lipsitz JD: Treatment of specific phobia in adults. Clin Psychol Rev 27:266–286, 2007

Fyer AJ: Current approaches to etiology and pathophysiology of specific phobia. Biol Psychiatry 44:1295–1304, 1998

Page AC: Blood-injury phobia. Clin Psychol Rev 14:443–461, 1994

Poulton R, Menzies RG: Non-associative fear acquisition: a review of the evidence from retrospective and longitudinal research. Behav Res Ther 40:127–149, 2002

Stinson FS, Dawson DA, Chou PS, et al: The epidemiology of DSM-IV specific phobia in the USA: results from the National Epidemiologic Survey on Alcohol and Related Conditions. Psychol Med 37:1047–1059, 2007

Posttraumatic Stress Disorder/ Acute Stress Disorder

Chapter 30

Phenomenology of Posttraumatic Stress Disorder

Alexander C. McFarlane, M.D.

The last two and a half decades have been a period of intense interest in psychological trauma, leading to a very fruitful period of research and changes in clinical practice that have had a significant effect on psychiatry in general. This interest is reflected in an exponential growth in the number of published articles in the field (Yehuda 2006). This interest has been triggered partly because, unlike most other psychiatric disorders, posttraumatic stress disorder (PTSD) is a disorder for which it is easy to date the onset (or at least the onset of the risk of its development) by the date of the exposure to some major or catastrophic event in an individual's life. Increasingly, this body of work has emphasized that development of PTSD is the exception rather than the rule following exposure to such events and that the stress response that underpins the condition is atypical in those individuals who go on to develop PTSD (Yehuda and McFarlane 1995).

PTSD was not included in the *Diagnostic and Statistical Manual of Mental Disorders* until DSM-III (American Psychiatric Association 1980), although *traumatic neurosis* had been a widely accepted term since the nineteenth century (Horowitz 1986). The lack of consistent conventions about diagnosis and nomenclature meant that several different diagnostic labels were used to describe traumatic reactions, such as *shell shock*, *war neurosis*, and *neurasthenia* (Glass 1974). The phenomenology had been well described prior to the publication of DSM-III, but there was a dispute about whether traumatic neurosis was a disorder distinct from the anxiety and depressive neuroses. This debate continues (Spitzer et al. 2007), with some questioning the uniqueness and specificity of PTSD as the main consequence of traumatic events. However, these controversies about the conceptualization of diagnostic entities are not unique to PTSD, and similar debates occur about depression and psychosis.

The Nature of Trauma

Traumatic events inflict both an external and an internal reality that attacks ideals and beliefs about safety, control, and freedom from pain. The external reality is of danger because these events have the capacity to kill, maim, brutalize, and destroy. Examples of such events are disasters, wars, rape, assault, motor vehicle accidents, and predatory violence. These events bring an internal reality of fear, horror, and lack of control because

This chapter was prepared with support of the Australian National Health and Medical Research Council project grant 201813 and program grant 300403.

the victim is confronted with potentially overwhelming threat. Often, the individual's sense of powerlessness is compounded in the aftermath of the event by the recurring and involuntary memory of his or her perceptions and emotions. This state is magnified by the memories of the trauma, which are triggered by often subtle and unrecognized reminders of the event. Previous life knowledge does little to equip people for these events.

Traumatic events have a range of practical effects. For some, these experiences leave only the scars of shattered assumptions of safety and personal invulnerability. However, they also may inflict personal injuries that disable, which means that the experience is colored with physical pain and suffering. If a relative is killed or a house destroyed, grief will further complicate the experience because although the victim tries to avoid disturbing memories of the experience, he or she also may wish to retain memories of the lost person or home. With certain traumas such as domestic violence and rape, the intentional cruelty of the perpetrator can radically disturb the victim's sense of trust. Relationships become a constant reminder of the danger and risk. The loss of personal autonomy in war, both in military service and during the experience of occupation, can reframe an individual's sense of self-effectiveness. Societies have a range of traditions and institutions to attempt to protect against these events or create philosophies to deal with the aftermath. The reaction to these experiences is a social issue as well as one of individual psychology.

Definition of the Stressor Criterion

One of the central issues for this field has been defining and observing a traumatic event. DSM-III adopted the definition of a traumatic event as "a stressor that would be markedly distressing to almost anyone" (American Psychiatric Association 1980, p. 247). The qualifier states that "the essential feature…is the development of characteristic symptoms following a psychologically distressing event that is outside the range of usual human experience" (American Psychiatric Association 1980, p. 247). The stressors described include combat, natural disasters, accidental man-made disasters, or deliberate man-made disasters. Also, some stressors may frequently produce the disorder (e.g., torture), whereas others produce it only occasionally (e.g., car accidents).

This definition was further clarified in DSM-III-R: "The most common traumata involve either a serious threat to one's life or physical integrity; a serious threat or harm to one's children, spouse, or other close relatives and friends; sudden destruction of one's home or community; or seeing another person who has recently been or is being seriously injured or killed as the result of an accident or physical violence" (American Psychiatric Association 1987, pp. 247–248).

The *International Statistical Classification of Diseases and Related Health Problems* (ICD-10) (World Health Organization 1992a) further elaborates with the current definition:

> PTSD arises from a delayed and/or protracted response to a stressful event or situation (either short lived or long lasting) of an exceptionally threatening or catastrophic nature which is likely to cause pervasive distress in almost everybody (e.g., natural or man-made disasters, combat, serious accidents, witnessing the violent death of others or being a victim or torture, terrorist, rape or other crime). Predisposing factors such as personality traits (e.g., compulsive asthenic) or previous history of neurotic illness may lower the threshold for the development of the syndrome or aggravate its course but is neither necessary nor sufficient to explain its occurrence. (p. 147)

DSM-IV (American Psychiatric Association 1994) introduced a further dimension in defining the stressor criterion:

> (1) the person experienced, witnessed, or was confronted with an event or events that involved actual or threatened death or serious injury, or a threat to the physical integrity of self or others
> (2) the person's response involved intense fear, helplessness, or horror. **Note:** in children, this may be expressed instead by disorganized or agitated behavior
> (DSM-IV-TR [American Psychiatric Association 2000], p. 467)

This definition acknowledges the possibility of a personal subjective response to a significantly greater degree. This dimension was included in an attempt to account for the role of subjective affective reactions to the trauma, which are presumed to be one determinant of the outcome. A significant disparity frequently exists between the perceived threat in a situation and the actual threat to the individual, posing a clinical dilemma. This is perhaps most apparent in considering cases of PTSD following rear-end motor vehicle collisions. The lack of opportunity for an individual to anticipate or prepare for the accident in this situation may be one of the reasons that such events are so readily perceived as being threatening.

Epidemiology

Traumatic Stress

Careful definition of the stressor criterion has provided a benchmark for conducting epidemiological research. Population-based research has identified a surprising frequency of the type of events qualifying as traumatic. The National Comorbidity Survey in the United States (Kessler et al. 1995) and the Australian Bureau of Statistics Epidemiology Study in Australia (Creamer et al. 2001) reported that more than half of the adult community has been exposed to traumatic experiences (Kessler et al. 1995; Norris 1992). This finding challenges the original notion that these are events outside the range of usual human experience. For example, in a U.S. study, 25% of the male population and 14% of the female population reported having been exposed to life-threatening accidents (Kessler et al. 1995). Hence, any discussion about an epidemic of PTSD is not justified by the empirical data. PTSD was found to be the most common anxiety disorder among females (Kessler et al. 1995). More recent, detailed examination of the prevalence of exposure to traumatic events suggests that with more in-depth questioning, lifetime rates of traumatic exposure may be as high as 90% (Breslau and Kessler 2001).

There is little doubt that many people experience the threat and distress of these events without being disabled or developing long-term psychological symptoms. Kessler et al. (1995) found that the most common causes of PTSD in men are engaging in combat and witnessing death or severe injury, whereas the most common causes of PTSD in women are being raped and sexually molested. Among the men in this representative sample of 5,877 persons ages 15–54 years, 61% had experienced a qualifying trauma, and a further 17% had been exposed to a trauma that produced intrusive recollections but was not covered by the stressor criterion. In contrast, 51% of the women had experienced a traumatic stressor. Significant differences by sex were found in the types of events experienced. For example, 25% of the men had had an accident, in contrast to 14% of the women, whereas 9% of the women had been raped, in contrast to 1% of the men. The capacity of these events to produce PTSD varied significantly, ranging from 48% of the female rape victims to 11% of the men witnessing death or serious injury.

In a study of 1,000 adults in the southern United States, Norris (1992) found that 69% of the sample had experienced a traumatic stressor in their lives, including 21% in the past year alone. The most common trauma was tragic death, with sexual assault leading to the highest rates of PTSD and motor vehicle accidents presenting the most adverse combination of frequency and effect. Both Norris (1992) and Kessler et al. (1995) found that a person's age, race, and sex have important effects on exposure to trauma and the likelihood of developing PTSD, although Norris did not recruit a strictly random sample. For example, Norris (1992) observed that black men were most vulnerable to the effect of trauma and that young people had the highest rates of PTSD. Kessler et al. (1995) found that women had twice the risk of developing PTSD following a trauma compared with men and that no age effect was seen in women because PTSD at an early age has increased in recent cohorts of women.

The majority of traumatized people are reluctant to seek treatment for their distress (Wang et al. 2005). The issues that individual victims face in declaring their predicament are complex, and many victims are highly ambivalent about describing their experience, for good reasons. For example, the female rape victim has to face not being believed, hurting her parents and partner, and confronting the pain and shame of self-disclosure. Women often have denied the existence of domestic violence because of the importance of the social illusion of harmony and the desire to avoid acknowledging their powerlessness. There are also circumstances in which a woman will initially admit domestic violence but later withdraw the allegation under pressure of the violent spouse, saying that she made the initial accusation "for revenge."

Posttraumatic Stress Disorder

A variety of different settings and methodologies are available for investigating the prevalence of PTSD. The studies that have had the greatest effect have examined large representative population samples. One of the striking findings is that generally only a minority of trauma-exposed individuals develop PTSD, emphasizing the importance of resilience as an issue for further consideration (Southwick et al. 2005). A discussion of that emerging field is beyond the scope of this chapter.

General Population

Seven studies have assessed the prevalence of PTSD in the general population, independent of exposure to specific stressful events. The most important of these was the National Comorbidity Survey mentioned earlier in this chapter (Kessler et al. 1995); this study was later replicated in Australia (Creamer et al. 2001). The latter study examined some of the effects of the use of ICD-

10 criteria versus DSM-IV criteria. In general, the two systems appeared to be reasonably similar, although there was a significantly lower threshold in ICD-10 than in DSM-IV.

Andrews et al. (1999) compared the equivalence of the two sets of criteria in a set of epidemiological data in Australia. A significant disparity in PTSD was found in this pilot data set for the Australian Bureau of Statistics (1998) study, in which there was only 35% concordance between the two diagnostic systems. Similar discordance existed for substance abuse. The 12-month prevalence of PTSD based on ICD-10 criteria was 7%, compared with 3% based on DSM-IV criteria. The discordance appears to emerge because of the avoidance and numbing symptoms required for a diagnosis of PTSD according to DSM-IV (DSM-IV criterion C). Although numbing is noted as a general feature in the *Clinical Descriptions and Diagnostic Guidelines* version of ICD-10 (World Health Organization 1992), it was not given the same prominence in the *Diagnostic Criteria for Research* version (World Health Organization 1993). Andrews et al. (1999) also noted some other important differences, such as a reference in ICD-10 to the timing of the onset as being important, whereas DSM-IV criterion E refers to the duration of the disturbance as being of great importance. Furthermore, ICD-10 does not refer to the patient's impairment in the diagnosis, whereas DSM-IV does. Peters et al. (1999) reported that the differences in qualifying for criterion C accounted for those in the Australian data set who met DSM-IV but not ICD-10 criteria. When subjects with a positive diagnosis based on ICD-10 but not DSM-IV criteria were examined similarly, it again appeared to be criteria D and F, which focus on the degree of distress and impairment, that accounted for the differences in diagnosis. In patients who had a negative diagnosis based on DSM-IV but a positive one based on ICD-10, the major difference emerged as the qualifying degree of distress and impairment.

Three studies have been carried out in the framework of the Epidemiologic Catchment Area (ECA) study (Robins and Regier 1991). These studies, summarized below, provide information about the total number of patients in different communities, which reflects both the prevalence of various traumas that may have affected the members of the community in question and the potency of the individual traumatic events to trigger PTSD.

1. In the first study, carried out in a sample of 2,493 people living in St. Louis, Missouri, lifetime PTSD rates of 0.5% among men and 1.3% among women (an overall rate of 1.4%) were found; however, the percentage of people who experienced some symptoms after a trauma was substantially higher (15% among men and 16% among women), with an average of 2.4 symptoms per person among those affected (Helzer et al. 1987). The rates found in subgroups such as veterans were less than would be expected from previous studies, such as the National Vietnam Veterans' Readjustment Study (Kulka et al. 1990), that specifically examined at-risk populations. This raises questions about the sensitivity of case detection in this and other general population samples.
2. At the St. Louis site, additional data were collected as part of the second wave of the same survey (Cottler et al. 1992). The overall rate of PTSD (1.35%) was very similar to that found in the first wave (1.4%). One of the main aims of this study was to assess the association between PTSD and substance use: cocaine or opiate users were more than three times more likely than control subjects to report a traumatic event.
3. At the North Carolina site of the ECA study, the lifetime and 6-month prevalence rates of PTSD in 2,985 subjects were 1.3% and 0.4%, respectively (Davidson et al. 1991). In comparison with subjects without any history of PTSD, those with PTSD reported significantly more job instability, family history of psychiatric illness, parental poverty, experiences of child abuse, and separation or divorce of parents before age 10.

A further survey was carried out in a random sample of 1,007 young adults (ages 21–30 years) from a large health maintenance organization in Detroit, Michigan (Breslau et al. 1991; Chilcoat and Breslau 1998). The lifetime exposure to traumatic events was 39.1% among the sample surveyed. The rate of PTSD in those who had been exposed to trauma was 23.6%, yielding an overall lifetime prevalence rate in the total sample of 9.2% and placing this diagnosis among the most common psychiatric disorders for this age-specific population group, preceded only by phobia, major depression, and alcohol and drug dependence. Among those who had been exposed to a traumatic event, a significant sex difference in the rate of the disorder was seen: 30.7% of the women met PTSD criteria as compared with 14.0% of the exposed men. Risk factors for PTSD following exposure included early separation from parents, neuroticism, preexisting anxiety or depression, and a family history of anxiety. It is unclear why the rates in this study were higher than those in the ECA study (Robins and Regier 1991), given that the population was not markedly atypical of the general population of individuals of similar age.

A number of studies have looked at different national samples (Breslau 2002), including one in Iceland (Lindal and Stefansson 1993) that reported very low lifetime prevalence rates of anxiety disorders, including PTSD, as assessed through the administration of an Icelandic translation of the U.S. National Institute of Mental Health Diagnostic Interview Schedule. The study cohort (N=862) consisted of half of those living in Iceland who were born in 1931. The overall prevalence of anxiety disorders was 44.2%, and the lifetime prevalence of PTSD was 0.6% of the whole sample. However, PTSD was found only in females (1.2% prevalence), and the mean age at onset was 39 years. Women with a diagnosis of PTSD had, on average, 3.2 additional diagnoses. The replication of the U.S. National Comorbidity Survey found a lifetime prevalence of 6.8% and a 12-month prevalence of 3.5%, with 36.6% of these disorders being classified as serious (Kessler et al. 2005a, 2005b).

War Veterans

The first Gulf War and the more recent wars in Iraq and Afghanistan have built on the earlier body of work with Vietnam War veterans. Sample sizes and compositions, study settings, assessment methods, prevalence periods (point, period, or lifetime), and inclusion of a comparison group differ remarkably among various studies. These differences are reflected in a marked variation in prevalence rates, ranging from a low of 2% (current prevalence) in the Centers for Disease Control Vietnam Experience Study (1988) to more than 70% found in five other studies (McFarlane 1990).

The National Vietnam Veterans' Readjustment Study was probably the most in-depth investigation of the overall psychological and psychosocial consequences of the Vietnam War among veterans (Kulka et al. 1990). It included an overall sample of 3,016 subjects whose symptoms were assessed with a variety of standardized instruments. This study reported that 15% of all male veterans who were involved in active war operations currently had PTSD, and an additional 11% had subsyndromal PTSD. These rates must be compared with a PTSD rate of 3% among Vietnam War era veterans who did not serve in Southeast Asia and a rate of 1% among civilian control subjects who were matched for age, sex, race/ethnicity, and occupation. Among the females who served in Vietnam, the estimated prevalence of PTSD was 9% (Jordan et al. 1991). The same study found few differences in the rate of other psychiatric disorders among the Vietnam veterans, other veterans from the Vietnam era, and civilian control subjects.

Another study evaluated the influence of military service during the Vietnam War era on the occurrence of PTSD among a sample of more than 2,000 pairs of male-male monozygotic veteran twins (Goldberg et al. 1990). A PTSD prevalence rate of almost 17% was found in twins who served in Southeast Asia compared with 5% in co-twins who did not. A ninefold increase in the rate of PTSD was seen among twins who experienced high levels of combat compared with those who did not serve in Vietnam.

Most studies found an association between severity and duration of combat exposure on the one hand and prevalence and persistence of PTSD on the other (Solomon et al. 1987). Having been wounded or involved in certain highly traumatic experiences (e.g., handling dead bodies, witnessing mutilation or atrocities) was generally strongly associated with PTSD. High comorbidity rates also have been found, showing that PTSD is only one of the possible psychopathological outcomes following exposure to combat and highly stressful situations.

Studies of veterans from the first Gulf War have highlighted the tendency for symptoms to increase with time and the importance of depression and PTSD (Ikin et al. 2004; Wolfe et al. 1999). Studies of veterans of the current conflicts in Afghanistan and Iraq have demonstrated similar patterns, with PTSD and depression being most marked in those with high levels of combat exposure and prolonged deployments (Hoge et al. 2006; Milliken et al. 2007). There have been some important differences in PTSD prevalence between U.K. forces and their reserves, but these are likely to be accounted for by the intensity of combat (Browne et al. 2007; Hotopf et al. 2006) and have highlighted that reserve personnel are a group at particular risk.

Other Populations

The number of studies that have assessed the prevalence of PTSD among victims of natural and technological disasters continues to grow. In a recent review of 225 studies, Norris (2006) highlighted that the quality of more recent studies is, if anything, declining, due to small samples and short follow-up periods. The published studies show that symptoms are similar after a variety of disastrous events but that rates are influenced by the levels of exposure and the postdisaster environment (Norris et al. 2002a; 2002b). Former prisoners of war and other types of prisoners, generally imprisoned for political reasons (e.g., Basoglu et al. 1994; Bauer et al. 1993), also have been extensively examined. In all of these studies, the PTSD rate was quite substantial: the prevalence rate in six studies was 50% or higher, and three studies showed prevalence rates of 70% or more. This prevalence probably indicates the severity of the effects of torture on many of the victims. In almost all of these studies, some patients had PTSD symptoms for the first time decades after the end of their imprisonment, and many others were still experiencing symptoms decades after the end of detention and the first appearance of the disorder.

The main form of political violence that has been investigated is terrorist attacks (Abenhaim et al. 1992; Bell et al. 1988; Curran et al. 1990; Murthy 2007; Perrin et al. 2007; Rubin et al. 2007; Shalev 1992; Weisaeth 1993). The rate of PTSD has been found to be substantial in the highly exposed. Following the September 11, 2001, terrorist attacks, investigation of the gradient of exposure showed that PTSD rates varied significantly according to the distance that an individual was from the site of the World Trade Center (Galea et al. 2004; Laugharne et al. 2007).

The PTSD rate also has been determined in samples of resettled refugees, mostly Southeast Asians (e.g., Carlson and Rosser-Hogan 1991; Hauff and Vaglum 1993). Six of these studies found a PTSD rate of 50% or higher. Refugees who have faced very difficult circumstances (including torture, starvation, and witnessing killings) represent a highly traumatized population and have a substantial rate of PTSD and other psychiatric disorders.

Many studies have assessed the prevalence of PTSD among victims of different types of violence (Welch and Mason 2007), including victims of crime, subjects exposed to multiple homicides, police officers involved in shooting experiences, children and adults exposed to sniper attacks, battered women, and victims of rape or other sexual violence. The latter topic has been investigated in various studies (Bownes et al. 1991; Burge 1988; Dahl 1989; Lopez et al. 1992; Riggs et al. 1992; Rothbaum et al. 1992). The rate of PTSD has been reported between 25% and 70%, suggesting the major impact of violence on mental health (Okasha 2007).

A variety of other populations have been examined to assess PTSD rates, including medical patients hospitalized or treated for different reasons (e.g., patients hospitalized because of major burns or accidental injuries, including injuries from motor vehicle accidents, or patients receiving treatment for pain) (Aghabeigi et al. 1992; Benedikt and Kolb 1986), psychiatric patients with other baseline diagnoses (Davidson and Smith 1990; Hryvniak and Rosse 1989; McGorry et al. 1991), and rescuers of disaster victims (Durham et al. 1985; Ersland et al. 1989; Perrin et al. 2007). Across these studies, the rates of PTSD vary depending on factors related to the type, severity, length, and consequences of the stressor and on the psychiatric status of the subjects before the traumatic event occurred. In particular, a substantial rate of PTSD has been found among psychiatric patients specifically evaluated on measures of PTSD symptomatology and among burn patients.

Clinical Features

Course

Blank (1993) highlighted the fact that the longitudinal course of PTSD has multiple variations and suggested that there needs to be a discrimination between the acute, delayed, chronic, intermittent, residual, and reactivated patterns. Also, he suggested that the available data indicate a need for the establishment of a posttraumatic stress *syndrome* when full diagnostic criteria for PTSD are not met (see discussion above about the need for considering the definition of *subsyndromal PTSD*). However, determining the longitudinal course of PTSD is a major problem because there are a number of challenges in following populations over time (Peleg and Shalev 2006).

The series of alterations of the DSM diagnostic criteria across editions reflects the way in which the perceived symptoms of the disorder have changed over time. The original criteria were substantially based on the observations made by Kardiner (1941) about World War I veterans with chronic morbidity. These suggested that the disorder had much in common with schizophrenia, particularly the constriction of affect and withdrawal.

The changes between DSM-III-R (1987) and DSM-IV (1994) were made largely to accommodate the findings of studies conducted in the interim. As a consequence, these criteria place greater emphasis on the role of acute traumatic emotional reactions. The utility of the criteria therefore may vary significantly with the duration of the disorder. The National Comorbidity Survey data (Kessler et al. 1995) suggested that

PTSD will resolve in the first 6 years in 60% of those who develop the disorder. For the remainder, the disorder has a chronic course, which poses a serious public health problem. Longitudinal studies have provided valuable information about how the sensitivity and specificity of symptoms change with time. For example, Solomon et al. (1987) found that the prominence of intrusive symptoms in Israeli servicemen decreased over a 2-year period, whereas symptoms of avoidance increased (Blank 1993). A more recent follow-up of this population indicated that symptoms rose again 17 years later (Solomon and Mikulincer 2006).

The relation between the acute symptoms of traumatic stress and the emergence of PTSD is also an issue of considerable theoretical and clinical importance. It appears that the timing of the point of maximal intensity and the progressive reinforcement of the traumatic response are critical to the emergence of chronicity (Weisaeth 1989). Foa (1997) noted that a poor response to treatment is predicted by delayed timing of the maximal traumatic response. She concluded that engagement with the traumatic memory is a critical dimension to the processing of the experience. A lack of engagement or delayed engagement means that the affect and intensity of the memory have been distanced. Anger and dissociation are two mechanisms that interfere with this process.

A number of studies of motor vehicle accident victims showed very few differences within the first 24 hours of the trauma between individuals who develop PTSD or major depressive disorder and the majority who have no long-term psychological sequelae (e.g., Atchison and McFarlane 1997; Carty et al. 2006). Those who develop PTSD have a progressive kindling of their reactions, which can be detected by the tenth day after the accident, but the severity of intrusions further increases over the next 6 months. This suggests that a progressive dysregulation occurs in the immediate posttraumatic period. Avoidance emerges as a secondary attempt at downregulating this distress. Investigation of the progression of PTSD has considerable relevance to the development of interventions targeted at acutely distressed populations.

Social and Cultural Issues

There has been some debate about the applicability of PTSD in Third World cultures and nations disrupted by war (Summerfield 2001, 2002; see also Chapter 39, "Cultural and Social Aspects of Anxiety Disorders," in this volume). Some view the application of concepts of traumatization in these settings as stigmatizing and object that recovery has been medicalized. Summerfield has argued that diagnosing the distress from traumatic events is an unnecessary intrusion of psychiatry into the complex social dynamics that allow societies to cope and rebuild from the fractures and suffering of war. However, a number of systematic studies of PTSD in non-European cultures have observed and documented the same constellation of symptoms and associated social disadvantages as in Western cultures (Rasmussen et al. 2007). Also, PTSD in the absence of comorbid depression appears to be the disorder that is a particular marker of continued risk of increasing symptomatic distress across time in Bosnian refugees (Mollica et al. 2007). A consistent observation is the greater degree to which symptoms of PTSD manifest as somatic distress in Asian cultures (Silove et al. 2007). Furthermore, PTSD has been well documented in children following events such as the 2004 Indian Ocean tsunami, suggesting the utility of the construct across age groups in non-European cultures (John et al. 2007).

Identifying the symptoms of distress in refugee and war-torn populations, it has been argued, allows advocacy for the recognition of the suffering of these populations rather than stigmatizes their distress (Silove et al. 1998). Ultimately there are a limited number of ways in which the human psyche, independent of one's culture, can react to extreme events because of the nature of the brain's biology. To argue that PTSD applies in one culture but not another is to ignore this basic commonality.

Impairment

The epidemiological data indicate that PTSD is not only highly prevalent but also associated with substantial morbidity. Also, a growing amount of literature details the negative effect of PTSD in terms of distress and dysfunction. For example, a comparison of PTSD patients and patients with other anxiety disorders showed that the PTSD patients had a worse outcome on a range of dimensions of functioning (Warshaw et al. 1993). In this longitudinal study in a clinical setting, PTSD had severe effects on quality of life in virtually all domains, including high levels of depression, suicide attempts and gestures, and alcohol abuse. These kinds of data reinforce the important role of psychological trauma in psychopathology and its sequelae.

The National Comorbidity Survey (Kessler and Frank 1997; Kessler et al. 1995) indicated that PTSD is often a chronic and disabling condition. These observations have led to the conclusion that there is an enduring pattern of chronic morbidity within this disorder that is long lasting and sometimes treatment resistant. In the Australian epidemiological study (Creamer et al. 2001), the work impairment in terms of days cut back per month was 2.8 days. This was significantly greater than the work impairment in people without PTSD. The odds ratio for current unemployment was 3.2 and the odds ratio for the increased use of outpatient health care was 28.2. Such findings led Kessler and colleagues to conclude that PTSD and major depression represent the most substantial causes of disease burden by psychological disorder (Kessler et al. 1995).

A number of studies have suggested that the psychoeconomic status of veterans is compromised (Kulka et al. 1990). The most carefully controlled examination of the socioeconomic effects of PTSD (McCarren et al. 1995) was a twin study in which one twin had PTSD and the other did not. The investigators found that employment was the one factor that was different in the PTSD twin. No difference was found in the combat-discordant twins that could account for this finding, indicating that the disadvantage in employment capacity was an effect of PTSD. An examination of the impact of PTSD in veterans suggested that significant gains could be made from moderate degrees of symptom improvement (Schnurr et al. 2005). A similar study of veterans found that the impairments extended into broad areas of social dysfunction and quality of life (Zatzick et al. 1997). A further recent community study by Jeon et al. (2006) found that severity of PTSD symptoms did not have a major impact on the associated dysfunction. Partial PTSD and the full-blown syndrome had similar patterns of morbidity. Treatment has been shown to have a beneficial impact on work performance (Duffy et al. 2007).

Clinical Features of the Traumatic Stress Response

DSM-IV-TR (American Psychiatric Association 2000) describes three main criteria (Table 30–1) for PTSD:

1. Reexperiencing of the traumatic event via intrusive remembrances, dreams, and flashbacks
2. Physical or emotional avoidance of stimuli associated with the trauma or a numbing of responsiveness (including symptoms such as restricted range of affect, feeling of detachment from others, and inability to recall important aspects of the trauma)
3. Persistence of symptoms of increased arousal, such as poor sleep, difficulty concentrating, and exaggerated startle response

Evidence has shown that the same pattern of symptoms emerges following a variety of traumatic events, such as natural disasters (McFarlane 1988), accidents (Schottenfeld and Cullen 1986), and wartime experiences (Foy et al. 1987; Keane and Fairbank 1983). This suggests that the underlying process of symptom formation is determined more by a shared response diathesis than by a trauma-specific pattern of distress. The critical dimension of PTSD that separates it from other psychiatric disorders is the recognition that extremely traumatic events can produce a disorder with a specific pattern of symptomatology in which the exposure plays a central organizing etiological role.

Two differing diagnostic systems—DSM-IV-TR and ICD-10 (World Health Organization 1992a)—are currently in use. Although many criticisms have been made of the diagnostic criteria of DSM-III, DSM-III-R, DSM-IV, and ICD-10, the provision of precise definitions has allowed a great deal of research to be conducted. Epidemiological and phenomenological research has made a central contribution and has allowed these definitions and their boundaries to be tested. By providing a benchmark, the definition of PTSD was an important step forward, particularly because it has allowed exploration of the nature of the reactions to these types of events.

The uniqueness of PTSD lies within DSM-IV-TR criterion B. Essentially, as van der Kolk and van der Hart (1991) emphasized, PTSD is a disorder of memory, in which the traumatic experience is not normally integrated. This is evident in the memory's dominance of the patient's consciousness. Thus, the reexperiencing of symptoms reflects the primary characteristic of the disorder. The definition in ICD-10 emphasizes this feature and does not require avoidance to be present all the time. The existence of the ICD-10 and DSM-IV-TR definitions with their differences in the stressor criterion definition and the extent of avoidance creates the possibility of these systems being used alternatively, with the clear potential for conflict in medicolegal settings. Similarly, important differences exist in the ICD-10 and DSM-IV-TR definitions of *acute stress reaction*, with the ICD-10 definition focusing on the polymorphic nature of acute reactions and the DSM-IV definition highlighting the dissociative aspect of the disorder. A brief description of the symptoms of PTSD follows.

Intrusive memories. Repeated involuntary memories may recur spontaneously or can be triggered by a variety of real and symbolic stimuli. These may involve intense sensory and visual memories of the event, which

TABLE 30–1. DSM-IV-TR diagnostic criteria for posttraumatic stress disorder

A. The person has been exposed to a traumatic event in which both of the following were present:

(1) the person experienced, witnessed, or was confronted with an event or events that involved actual or threatened death or serious injury, or a threat to the physical integrity of self or others

(2) the person's response involved intense fear, helplessness, or horror. **Note:** In children, this may be expressed instead by disorganized or agitated behavior

B. The traumatic event is persistently reexperienced in one (or more) of the following ways:

(1) recurrent and intrusive distressing recollections of the event, including images, thoughts, or perceptions. **Note:** In young children, repetitive play may occur in which themes or aspects of the trauma are expressed.

(2) recurrent distressing dreams of the event. **Note:** In children, there may be frightening dreams without recognizable content.

(3) acting or feeling as if the traumatic event were recurring (includes a sense of reliving the experience, illusions, hallucinations, and dissociative flashback episodes, including those that occur on awakening or when intoxicated). **Note:** In young children, trauma-specific reenactment may occur.

(4) intense psychological distress at exposure to internal or external cues that symbolize or resemble an aspect of the traumatic event

(5) physiological reactivity on exposure to internal or external cues that symbolize or resemble an aspect of the traumatic event

C. Persistent avoidance of stimuli associated with the trauma and numbing of general responsiveness (not present before the trauma), as indicated by three (or more) of the following:

(1) efforts to avoid thoughts, feelings, or conversations associated with the trauma

(2) efforts to avoid activities, places, or people that arouse recollections of the trauma

(3) inability to recall an important aspect of the trauma

(4) markedly diminished interest or participation in significant activities

(5) feeling of detachment or estrangement from others

(6) restricted range of affect (e.g., unable to have loving feelings)

(7) sense of a foreshortened future (e.g., does not expect to have a career, marriage, children, or a normal life span)

D. Persistent symptoms of increased arousal (not present before the trauma), as indicated by two (or more) of the following:

(1) difficulty falling or staying asleep

(2) irritability or outbursts of anger

(3) difficulty concentrating

(4) hypervigilance

(5) exaggerated startle response

E. Duration of the disturbance (symptoms in criteria B, C, and D) is more than 1 month.

F. The disturbance causes clinically significant distress or impairment in social, occupational, or other important areas of functioning.

Specify if:

Acute: if duration of symptoms is less than 3 months

Chronic: if duration of symptoms is 3 months or more

Specify if:

With Delayed Onset: if onset of symptoms is at least 6 months after the stressor may or may not be accompanied by extreme physiological and psychological distress. They may occur with a dissociative quality characteristic of flashbacks, and they may also occur in dreams.

Avoidance of stimuli and numbing. A second pattern of response that sometimes dominates the clinical picture is characterized by avoidance and numbing. Here, the individual enters a state of detachment, emotional blunting, and relative unresponsiveness to his or her surroundings. This is associated with an inability to gain the usual sense of pleasure from activities and an avoidance of situations that are reminiscent of the trauma.

Symptoms of increased arousal. Finally, the individual shows a pattern of increased arousal, which is indicated by sleep disturbance, difficulties with memory and concentration, hypervigilance, irritability, and an exaggerated startle response. In the more chronic forms of the disorder, hyperarousal and avoidance tend to be the predominant clinical features.

The manifestations of PTSD can best be understood as being driven by several simultaneous processes. The repetition of traumatic memories is a well-demonstrated consequence of traumatic experiences. This probably occurs in part because of the way in which these memories are laid down and the continued difficulties the individual has in processing them and forming a complete representation. The triggering of these memories is also a consequence of fear conditioning mechanisms (Wessa and Flor 2007), which are critical to many aspects of human learning. These serve to sustain and kindle the increased arousal (Post et al. 1997). Avoidance and numbing represent homeostatic mechanisms, whereby the individual attempts to modulate and shut down his or her hyperresponsiveness. The disorder arises because some individuals are unable to progressively quench or shut off the acute stress response, which is ubiquitous at times of exposure to such events. From a learning theory perspective, this process is seen as a failure of extinction or new learning in the aftermath of the fear conditioning that occurs at the time of the trauma.

Individuals with PTSD remain trapped by intense past experience to an unusual degree. This significantly interferes with their capacity to maintain involvement in current life activities and relationships. This disruption happens for two primary reasons. First, their pattern of numbing and decreased general responsiveness makes it difficult for them to gain the normal rewards from ongoing interactions with their environment. Second, their hyperarousal means that they readily become distressed by unexpected stimuli, which further encourages their withdrawal. Apart from their detachment, their propensity to experience triggered memories of the past highlights how their internal perceptual organization becomes attuned to detecting the subtle similarities between the present and the traumatic past. As a consequence, many neutral experiences become reinterpreted as having traumatic associations (McFarlane et al. 2002).

Another possible mechanism by which individuals may remain trapped by traumatic experience is dissociation. For an individual to integrate an experience, a coherent internal representation must be developed. Traumatic experiences have the capacity to disrupt this information-processing capacity of the brain. One view is that traumatic memories tend to be laid down as primary sensory memories with only partial linguistic transformation. The distress associated with the symptomatology tends to further encourage this pattern of dissociation. One consequence of dissociation is that it significantly decreases the individual's pattern of hyperarousal (Bryant 2007). However, as this psychological process becomes progressively more involuntary, it can lead to a significant disorganization of the individual's behavior because of his or her inability to deal with the present in an organized and integrated fashion. A complementary perspective focuses on the way that the individual's cognitive schemas are progressively modified by the sense of lack of control and perceived dangerousness about the world. These "meaning maps" drive the individual's behavior and reactivity to the demands of day-to-day life in the aftermath of the trauma.

A series of more recent examinations of the factor structure of the symptoms of PTSD has suggested that rather than being organized into the subgroups of intrusions, avoidance, and hyperarousal, a range of different aggregations of symptoms can been described (e.g., Elklit and Shevlin 2007) and will be need to be considered in any revision of the symptoms in DSM-V.

Somatic Symptoms

The question arises as to whether a specific pattern of associated physical symptoms occurs as part of the traumatic stress response. Historically, PTSD was described by a series of names that focused on the physical accompaniments of the response, such as "soldiers' heart" in the American Civil War (Trimble 1985). The controversy about the effects of herbicides on the physical health of Vietnam War veterans similarly highlights how even in more recent times, the physical symptoms associated with PTSD can be the primary concern of traumatized populations and their search for compensation (Hall 1986). The Gulf War syndrome has again incited this controversy (Kang et al. 2009). This is an important issue in traumatized individuals, who may or may not have been injured. In the injured patient, the significance of somatic distress is particularly likely to be missed or incorrectly attributed to ongoing sequelae of the physical injury.

Several studies have noted an increased reporting of physical symptoms in individuals with PTSD (Lipton and Schaffer 1988; Litz et al. 1992; Shalev et al. 1990; Solomon and Mikulincer 1987; van Kamp et al. 2006; White and Faustman 1989). Most of the studies that have examined the relationship between physical symptoms and trauma have been studies of war veterans. For example, Shalev and colleagues (1990) compared Lebanese war veterans who had chronic PTSD with matched combat veterans who did not have PTSD. Veterans in the PTSD group self-reported statistically significantly higher rates of cardiovascular, neurological, gastrointestinal, audiological, and pain symptoms than those in the non-PTSD group. A detailed medical examination, including chest X ray, electrocardiogram, spirometric tests, blood counts, and urinalysis, however, detected few differences between the two groups. Thus, either the physical symptoms are related to a psychological process or patients with PTSD generally report symptoms in a different way than do patients without PTSD. These same phenomena are being observed among combat veterans who served in the current Iraq war (Hoge et al. 2007). Somatic presentations are also common in refugee populations (Van Ommeren et al. 2002).

The nature of somatic symptoms as integral to the phenomenology of PTSD may be accounted for by the existence of several psychological mechanisms. Some authors (Spiegel 1988) see dissociation as a central part of the psychological mechanisms influencing symptom formation in PTSD that may therefore predispose the expression of distress in somatic forms. Growing evidence indicates that information processing is disordered in PTSD, and this may contribute to the presentation of somatic symptoms in PTSD (Galletly et al. 2001; McFarlane 2007). An impaired ability to process information and differentiate relevant from irrelevant information may be at the root of the disturbed concentration and memory found in PTSD patients. This problem with defining the salience of information may contribute to a focus on and misinterpretation of somatic sensations.

Evaluation

Rating Scales

Several rating scales have been developed for use in the trauma field. These include measures for assessing the number of traumatic events an individual has been exposed to, the symptoms of PTSD using self-report measures, and structured diagnostic instruments. The most commonly reported prevalence estimates of the number of traumatic exposures arise from use of the Composite International Diagnostic Interview (CIDI; World Health Organization 1990); this has been used in most of the large national epidemiology studies. Hence, it is an instrument that allows comparisons between populations. Of the available instruments, none is generally accepted within the field (see the review by Norris and Hamblen 2004).

Various instruments also have been developed for measuring exposure to specific traumatic events such as disasters or combat. Again, these tend to be highly specific and need to be carefully designed to address the full range of possibilities within the circumstances of a particular event. There are a number of issues about the psychometric structure and reliability of these instruments (McFarlane 1995).

Self-report scales have been developed that are widely used in both research and clinical settings. These include the following:

- The Posttraumatic Stress Diagnostic Scale (PDS) developed by Foa and her colleagues (1997), which follows DSM-IV closely. This instrument also has a 12-item checklist of traumatic events that then leads into the specific issue of the person identifying the most traumatic event before addressing the 17 symptoms of PTSD.
- The PTSD checklist (PCL; Weathers et al. 1999), which has been extensively used and is in the public domain. It was developed at the National Center for PTSD and has been shown to correlate highly with clinician-administered measures.
- The Davidson Trauma Scale (DTS; Davidson et al. 1997), which is reliable, valid, and sensitive in the measurement of treatment effects.
- The Impact of Events Scale (Revised) (Weiss 2004) is a further instrument that warrants consideration. This instrument was built on an earlier version, the IES, which only tapped into the elements of intrusion and avoidance. The latter edition's inclusion of hyperarousal symptoms means that the full range of

PTSD symptoms is covered. This measure has been used diagnostically but is also valuable in terms of assessing a dimensional response in trauma victims.

Structured clinical interviews play an important role in the assessment of PTSD in clinical and research settings. Instruments have been developed for use in both children and adults. A commonly used instrument is the Structured Clinical Interview for DSM-IV Axis I Disorders (SCID-I; First et al. 1997). The value of this instrument is that it can be incorporated into a broader assessment of psychopathology, including other Axis I disorders.

Perhaps the most widely accepted instrument is the Clinician-Administered PTSD Scale (CAPS) (Blake et al. 1990), which provides both a current and a lifetime diagnosis of PTSD according to DSM-IV criteria. Other instruments include the Structured Interview for PTSD (SI-PTSD). Originally introduced by Davidson and colleagues in 1989, this instrument has been updated to meet DSM-IV criteria (Davidson et al. 1998). Ultimately, clinicians and researchers should become skilled and proficient in the use of one instrument while being aware of its strengths and weaknesses.

Psychophysiological Assessment

PTSD, as reflected in DSM-IV-TR criterion B (5), has a particular pattern of psychophysiological reactivity that is thought to characterize the condition. Extensive research has been conducted into the specificity and sensitivity of changes in heart rate, electrodermal skin response, and blood pressure in response to exposure to traumatic triggers (Orr et al. 2002). Further research has objectively examined the exaggerated startle response and the disorders of memory and concentration in PTSD patients using event-related potentials. These domains of assessment have the potential to offer more objective methods of assessing PTSD in the not too distant future.

Differential Diagnosis

From a clinical perspective, the major differential diagnostic challenge is to determine which is the primary disorder when two or more disorders exist. If the disorders have emerged following exposure to trauma and PTSD is the first condition to emerge, this can be presumed to be the primary diagnosis. The challenge exists when subsyndromal PTSD was present and a disorder, such as major depressive disorder, emerges, leading to a worsening of the PTSD such that it then meets full diagnostic criteria. Given that the traumatic memory is central to the etiology of posttraumatic reactions, it is reasonable to presume that PTSD is the primary disorder. Another differential diagnostic challenge is to ascertain whether panic attacks are indicative of a trigger pattern of psychological and physiological distress (symptoms B4 and B5) or whether they are more typical of the spontaneous attacks consistent with a diagnosis of panic disorder. Also, triggered distress can present as simple phobia when the person does not consciously link the avoidance to the traumatic event.

Comorbidity and PTSD

The existence of any psychiatric disorder without the co-occurrence of other disorders in a clinical setting is the exception rather than the rule. Large epidemiological studies indicate that a range of other disorders, particularly affective disorders, panic disorder, and alcohol and substance abuse, frequently emerge in conjunction with PTSD in the significant majority of patients and that this is not isolated to treatment-seeking populations (McFarlane 2004). Patients with comorbid disorders are likely to have a worse long-term outcome than those without comorbidities and may require chronic maintenance therapy. Studies also have broadened attention as to the range of psychiatric disorders that may arise as a consequence of traumatic exposure.

The complexity of people's responses to trauma, and the comparative simplicity of the PTSD conceptualization, is illustrated by the intimate association between trauma, dissociation, and somatization (van der Kolk et al. 1996). Trauma can affect individuals on every level of functioning: biological, psychological, social, and spiritual. Merely focusing on the existence of PTSD symptoms does little justice to presenting an adequate description of the complexity of what is experienced and the extent of a victim's suffering. Excessive attention to the intrusion, numbing, and arousal phenomena in PTSD may severely limit accurate observations of how people react to trauma and may interfere with appropriate treatment. Recognition of the profound personality changes that can follow childhood trauma or prolonged exposure to trauma in adults is an important development because those changes are major sources of distress and disability. This issue is beginning to be recognized, as demonstrated by the inclusion of complex adaptations to trauma (in the form of disturbed affect regulation, aggression against the self and others, attention and dissociative problems, somatization, and altered relationships with oneself and others) among the "Associated Features and Disorders" in the "Posttraumatic Stress Disorder" section of DSM-IV-TR.

Complex PTSD: Dissociation and Personality Functioning

The contribution of trauma to the development of borderline personality disorder and multiple personality disorder is generally accepted (Herman 1992). Childhood trauma, particularly sexual and physical abuse, can lead to a range of changes in an individual's ability to modulate and tolerate affect, propensity toward dissociative behavior, and capacity for relationships (Saxe et al. 1993). ICD-10 has recognized that enduring personality change can occur after catastrophic experiences, such as being in a concentration camp or being tortured. These changes are characterized by a hostile or mistrustful attitude toward the world, social withdrawal, feelings of emptiness, a sense of constant threat, and estrangement. The relationship between such personality changes and PTSD has been investigated; findings suggest that it is uncommon for the personality changes to exist in the absence of PTSD (Herman 1992). Similarly, such changes are much more likely to occur as a response to childhood trauma than as a response to traumatic experiences in late adolescence or adulthood. Thus, the developmental stage of an individual can be an important determinant of the nature and duration of the consequences of a traumatic experience. DSM-IV-TR also incorporates several other specific diagnostic issues related to PTSD, as discussed below.

Acute stress reactions are specifically differentiated from PTSD because current diagnostic definitions imply that PTSD is established only after the symptoms have been present for a month. Although the concept of acute stress reaction was embodied relatively recently in DSM-IV and ICD-10, in military settings combat stress reactions have long been recognized as a specific pattern of reaction that requires particular treatment. This raises the question as to whether PTSD arises from the normal distress response or whether the immediate response of someone who develops PTSD is different from that of the individual who does not appear to have any specific adverse consequences of the trauma. The definition of acute stress reaction and the change in the DSM-IV stressor criterion reflect the presumed role of feelings of intense fear, horror, helplessness, or dissociation in close proximity to the traumatic event as playing an important role in any adverse outcome (Spiegel and Cardena 1991).

The issue has been raised, particularly regarding children, of whether a separate diagnosis should be developed to describe the developmental deviation associated with PTSD. The question of whether a separate diagnosis is required to best describe this condition is ongoing (Briere and Spinazzola 2005), but there is an empirical case to support this construct (van der Kolk et al. 2005). One argument is that the treatment strategy for such patients is considerably different from the strategy for patients with PTSD uncomplicated by developmental deviation, and that complex PTSD is a diagnosis that creates a more informed approach to treatment (Ford et al. 2005).

Subsyndromal PTSD

Clinicians at times have to contend with the challenge of how to diagnose and manage patients who do not satisfy the full diagnostic criteria for PTSD but are seeking treatment. The term *subsyndromal PTSD* has been coined to describe individuals who have some PTSD symptoms but do not satisfy the full DSM-IV-TR criteria. A number of studies have highlighted that the avoidance symptoms generally are the criteria that form the barrier to the diagnosis of PTSD (Peters et al. 1999). Interestingly, the ICD-10 criteria for PTSD do not require the presence of actual avoidance, referring instead to "preferred avoidance of reminders." This difference reflects the lack of objective consensus about the optimal threshold for these phenomena. The impact of subsyndromal PTSD has been examined systematically in several population studies, which suggest that the degree of disability it causes is similar to that of PTSD. Furthermore, subsyndromal PTSD has been associated with an increased risk of binge drinking of alcohol, potentially impeding recovery (Adams et al. 2006). Also, the pattern of health care utilization in individuals with subsyndromal PTSD has been found to more closely resemble the pattern seen with full PTSD than the pattern in individuals without symptoms (Gillock et al. 2005). It has been argued that the associated disability warrants subsyndromal PTSD being accepted as a subcategory in any revision of the diagnostic criteria (Mylle and Maes 2004). Another important issue is that patients with PTSD often have fluctuating symptoms and may therefore satisfy the full diagnostic criteria at one point in time but not at another. The utility of a diagnosis of subsyndromal PTSD is that it would capture such a longitudinal course of PTSD and would assist understanding of the nature of delayed-onset PTSD for clinical and research purposes (Bryant and Harvey 2002).

Conclusion

The major body of knowledge about the etiology and phenomenology of PTSD developed following the inclusion of PTSD in the DSM system of classification in 1980. PTSD, which was previously known by a variety of names such as traumatic neurosis, remains a diagnosis that requires further refinement. However, this diagnosis has had considerable utility in focusing attention on the impact of traumatic events as a significant cause of psychiatric morbidity. While it has emerged that disorders such as major depressive disorder not uncommonly arise after these events, PTSD has highlighted the role of traumatic memories as driving the adjustment after exposure to trauma. The diagnostic criteria for PTSD serve to focus a clinician's assessment on the way in which the event remains embedded in the person's awareness and drives behaviors such as avoidance of reminders. These phenomena often are not spontaneously reported, and hence the diagnosis contributes to a better understanding of what drives an individual's reactivity to a range of environmental triggers and the behaviors that arise in an attempt to modulate the consequent distress. Although the use of PTSD as a diagnosis has been criticized, particularly in refugee and Third World postconflict environments, there is a substantial body of work describing PTSD in a range of cultures. As a disorder, the construct has apparent face validity, underpinned by the universality of this dimension of human distress.

The subtyping of PTSD is an issue that has provoked particularly intense interest. The observational base for PTSD has established the validity of delayed-onset PTSD as a distinct subtype. However, it is recognized that many individuals diagnosed with delayed-onset PTSD have had subsyndromal symptoms prior to developing the full-blown disorder. One of the controversies that will need to be addressed in DSM-V is whether subsyndromal PTSD should be included as a distinct subtype. Although acute stress disorder has significant clinical utility, the role of dissociative symptoms (Bryant 2007) in the diagnostic criteria has been questioned. Acute stress disorder has particular utility as a construct because of the importance of defining individuals in the immediate aftermath of a trauma who have significant risk of developing PTSD in the long term. It is important to realize that the majority of people who develop chronic PTSD do not have clinically remarkable acute patterns of symptoms but that these emerge in the weeks following the traumatic exposure.

PTSD is a disorder that leads to substantial disadvantages in an individual's quality of life and work capacity. Accurate diagnosis plays a central role in instigating treatment, highlighting the importance of systematically assessing individuals who have experienced traumatic events for the symptoms of PTSD. Although the diagnostic criteria will continue to undergo further revision as more information about the patterns of adaptation to traumatic events continues to emerge, there is little doubt that this diagnosis has done much to create a focus on and interest in the effects of psychological trauma. Previously this interest was haphazard and sporadic, generally provoked by war.

Key Clinical Points

- The prevalence of the exposure to traumatic events is frequently underestimated and requires systematic direct enquiry when assessing patients.
- The core phenomenon of posttraumatic stress disorder is the presence of traumatic memories, which drive the hyperarousal, numbing, and avoidance. Traumatic memories are targeted in cognitive and behavioral treatments.
- Patients may not spontaneously volunteer the existence of traumatic memories due to the use of avoidance, and therefore specific exploration of their history is necessary. Assessment can be enhanced by the use of structured diagnostic interviews.
- PTSD is not the only psychopathological outcome of trauma. The presence of comorbid disorders, particularly depression and substance abuse, requires careful exploration and needs to be taken into account in developing a treatment plan. Major depressive disorder in the absence of PTSD is also a prevalent diagnosis following traumatic exposure.
- Somatic symptoms are frequently an important aspect of the clinical presentation and need specific consideration in treatment planning because they can be important triggers for the ongoing memories of the traumatic events.
- Through the processes of kindling and sensitization, symptoms increase in the months following trauma exposure in a significant group of individuals. As a consequence, the severity of acute symptoms is not necessarily a good predictor of the clinical course of an individual's distress, and there is often a delay in presenting for treatment.

References

Abenhaim L, Dab W, Salmi LR: Study of civilian victims of terrorist attacks (France 1982–1987). J Clin Epidemiol 45:103–109, 1992

Adams RE, Boscarino JA, Galea S: Alcohol use, mental health status and psychological well-being 2 years after the World Trade Center attacks in New York City. Am J Drug Alcohol Abuse 32:203–224, 2006

Aghabeigi B, Feinmann C, Harris M: Prevalence of post-traumatic stress disorder in patients with chronic idiopathic facial pain. Br J Oral Maxillofac Surg 30:360–364, 1992

American Psychiatric Association: Diagnostic and Statistical Manual of Mental Disorders, 3rd Edition. Washington, DC, American Psychiatric Association, 1980

American Psychiatric Association: Diagnostic and Statistical Manual of Mental Disorders, 3rd Edition, Revised. Washington, DC, American Psychiatric Association, 1987

American Psychiatric Association: Diagnostic and Statistical Manual of Mental Disorders, 4th Edition. Washington, DC, American Psychiatric Association, 1994

American Psychiatric Association: Diagnostic and Statistical Manual of Mental Disorders, 4th Edition, Text Revision. Washington, DC, American Psychiatric Association, 2000

Andrews G, Slade T, Peters L: Classification in psychiatry: ICD-10 versus DSM-IV. Br J Psychiatry 174:3–5, 1999

Atchison M, McFarlane A: Clinical patterns of acute psychological response to trauma, in The Aftermath of Road Accidents: Psychological, Social and Legal Consequences of an Everyday Trauma. Edited by Mitchell M. London, Routledge, 1997, pp 49–57

Australian Bureau of Statistics: Mental Health and Wellbeing: Profile of Adults, Australia 1997. Canberra, Australian Bureau of Statistics, 1998

Basoglu M, Paker M, Paker O, et al: Psychological effects of torture: a comparison of tortured with nontortured political activists in Turkey. Am J Psychiatry 151:76–81, 1994

Bauer M, Priebe S, Haring B, et al: Long-term mental sequelae of political imprisonment in East Germany. J Nerv Ment Dis 181:257–262, 1993

Bell P, Kee M, Loughrey GC, et al: Post-traumatic stress in Northern Ireland. Acta Psychiatr Scand 77:166–169, 1988

Benedikt RA, Kolb LC: Preliminary findings on chronic pain and posttraumatic stress disorder. Am J Psychiatry 143:908–910, 1986

Blake DD, Weathers FW, Nagy LM, et al: A clinician rating scale for assessing current and lifetime PTSD: the CAPS-1. Behav Ther 13:187–188, 1990

Blank A: The longitudinal course of posttraumatic stress disorder, in Posttraumatic Stress Disorder: DSM-IV and Beyond. Edited by Davidson JRT, Foa EB. Washington, DC, American Psychiatric Press, 1993, pp 3–22

Bownes IT, O'Gorman EC, Sayers A: Assault characteristics and posttraumatic stress disorder in rape victims. Acta Psychiatr Scand 83:27–30, 1991

Breslau N: Epidemiologic studies of trauma, posttraumatic stress disorder, and other psychiatric disorders. Can J Psychiatry 47:923–929, 2002

Breslau N, Davis GC, Andreski P, et al: Traumatic events and posttraumatic stress disorder in an urban population of young adults. Arch Gen Psychiatry 48:216–222, 1991

Briere J, Spinazzola J: Phenomenology and psychological assessment of complex posttraumatic states. J Trauma Stress 18:401–412, 2005

Browne T, Hull L, Horn O, et al: Explanations for the increase in mental health problems in UK reserve forces who have served in Iraq. Br J Psychiatry 190:484–489, 2007

Bryant RA: Does dissociation further our understanding of PTSD? J Anxiety Disord 21:183–191, 2007

Bryant RA, Harvey AG: Delayed onset posttraumatic stress disorder: a prospective evaluation. Aust N Z J Psychiatry 36:205–209, 2002

Burge SK: Post-traumatic stress disorder in victims of rape. J Trauma Stress 1:193–209, 1988

Carlson EB, Rosser-Hogan R: Trauma experiences, posttraumatic stress, dissociation, and depression in Cambodian refugees. Am J Psychiatry 148:1548–1551, 1991

Carty J, O'Donnell ML, Creamer M: Delayed-onset PTSD: a prospective study of injury survivors. J Affect Disord 90:257–261, 2006

Centers for Disease Control Vietnam Experience Study: Health status of Vietnam veterans, I: psychosocial characteristics. JAMA 259:2701–2707, 1988

Chilcoat HD, Breslau N: Investigations of causal pathways between PTSD and drug use disorders. Addict Behav 23:827–840, 1998

Cottler LB, Compton WM, Mager D, et al: Post-traumatic stress disorder among substance users from the general population. Am J Psychiatry 149:664–670, 1992

Creamer M, Burgess PM, McFarlane AC: Post-traumatic stress disorder: findings from the Australian National Survey of Mental Health and Wellbeing. Psychol Med 31:1237–1247, 2001

Curran PS, Bell P, Murray A, et al: Psychological consequences of the Enniskillen bombing. Br J Psychiatry 156:479–482, 1990

Dahl S: Acute response to rape: a PTSD variant. Acta Psychiatr Scand Suppl 80:56–62, 1989

Davidson J, Smith R: Traumatic experiences in psychiatric outpatients. J Trauma Stress 3:459–475, 1990

Davidson J, Smith R, Kudler H: Validity and reliability of the DSM-III criteria for posttraumatic stress disorder: experience with a structured interview. J Nerv Ment Dis 177:336–341, 1989

Davidson JR, Hughes D, Blazer DG, et al: Posttraumatic stress disorder in the community: an epidemiological study. Psychol Med 21:713–721, 1991

Davidson JR, Malik MA, Travers J: Structured interview for PTSD (SIP): psychometric validation for DSM-IV criteria. Depress Anxiety 5:127–129, 1997

Duffy M, Gillespie K, Clark DM: Post-traumatic stress disorder in the context of terrorism and other civil conflict in Northern Ireland: randomised controlled trial. BMJ 334:1147–1150, 2007

Durham TW, McCammon SL, Allison EJ: The psychological impact of disaster on rescue personnel. Ann Emerg Med 14:664–668, 1985

Elklit A, Shevlin M: The structure of PTSD symptoms: a test of alternative models using confirmatory factor analysis. Br J Clin Psychol 46:299–313, 2007

Ersland S, Weisaeth L, Sund A: The stress upon rescuers involved in an oil rig disaster: "Alexander L. Kielland" 1980. Acta Psychiatr Scand 80:38–49, 1989

First MB, Spitzer RL, Gibbon M, et al: Structured Clinical Interview for DSM-IV Axis I Disorders, Clinician Version (SCID-CV). Washington, DC, American Psychiatric Association, 1997

Foa EB: Psychological processes related to recovery from a trauma and an effective treatment for PTSD. Ann NY Acad Sci 821:410–424, 1997

Foa EB, Cashman L, Jaycox L, et al: The validation of a self-report measure of posttraumatic stress disorder: the Posttraumatic Diagnostic Scale. Psychol Assess 9:445–451, 1997

Ford JD, Courtois CA, Steele K, et al: Treatment of complex posttraumatic self-dysregulation. J Trauma Stress 18:437–447, 2005

Foy DW, Carrol EM, Donahoe CO: Etiological factors in the development of PTSD in clinical samples of Vietnam combat veterans. J Clin Psychol 43:17–27, 1987

Galea S, Vlahov D, Tracy M, et al: Hispanic ethnicity and post-traumatic stress disorder after a disaster: evidence from a general population survey after September 11, 2001. Ann Epidemiol 14:520–531, 2004

Galletly C, Clark CR, McFarlane AC, et al: Working memory in posttraumatic stress disorder—an event-related potential study. J Trauma Stress 14:295–309, 2001

Gillock KL, Zayfert CT, Mark T, et al: Posttraumatic stress disorder in primary care: prevalence and relationships with physical symptoms and medical utilization. Gen Hosp Psychiatry 27:392–399, 2005

Glass AJ: Mental health programs in the armed forces, in American Handbook of Psychiatry, 2nd Edition. Edited by Arieti S. New York, Basic Books, 1974

Goldberg J, True W, Eisen SA, et al: A twin study of the effects of the Vietnam War on posttraumatic stress disorder. JAMA 263:1227–1232, 1990

Hall W: The Agent Orange controversy after the Evatt Royal Commission. Med J Aust 145:219–225, 1986

Hauff E, Vaglum P: Vietnamese boat refugees: the influence of war and flight traumatization on mental health on arrival in the country of resettlement. Acta Psychiatr Scand 88:162–168, 1993

Helzer JE, Robins LN, McEvoy L: Posttraumatic stress disorder in the general population: findings of the Epidemiological Catchment Area survey. N Engl J Med 317: 1630–1634, 1987

Herman JL: Trauma and Recovery. New York, Basic Books, 1992

Hoge CW, Auchterlonie JL, Milliken CS: Mental health problems, use of mental health services, and attrition from military service after returning from deployment to Iraq or Afghanistan. JAMA 295:1023–1032, 2006

Hoge CW, Terhakopian A, Castro CA, et al: Association of posttraumatic stress disorder with somatic symptoms, health care visits, and absenteeism among Iraq war veterans. Am J Psychiatry 164:150–153, 2007

Horowitz MJ: Stress Response Syndromes, 2nd Edition. New York, Plenum, 1986

Hotopf M, Hull L, Fear NT, et al: The health of UK military personnel who deployed to the 2003 Iraq war: a cohort study. Lancet 367:1731–1734, 2006

Hryvniak MR, Rosse RB: Concurrent psychiatric illness in inpatients with post-traumatic stress disorder. Mil Med 154:399–401, 1989

Ikin JF, Sim MR, Creamer MC, et al: War-related psychological stressors and risk of psychological disorders in Australian veterans of the 1991 Gulf War. Br J Psychiatry 185:116–126, 2004

Jeon HJ, Suh T, Lee HJ, et al: Partial versus full PTSD in the Korean community: prevalence, duration, correlates, comorbidity, and dysfunctions. Depress Anxiety 24:577–585, 2006

John PB, Russell S, Russell PS: The prevalence of posttraumatic stress disorder among children and adolescents affected by tsunami disaster in Tamil Nadu. Disaster Manage Response 5:3–7, 2007

Jordan BK, Schlenger WE, Hough RL, et al: Lifetime and current prevalence of specific psychiatric disorders among Vietnam veterans and controls. Arch Gen Psychiatry 48:207–215, 1991

Kang HK, Li B, Mahan CM, et al: Health of US veterans of 1991 Gulf War: a follow-up survey in 10 years. J Occup Environ Med 51:401–410, 2009

Kardiner A: The Traumatic Neuroses of War. Menasha, WI, George Banta Publishing, 1941

Keane TM, Fairbank TA: Survey analysis of combat-related stress disorders in Vietnam veterans. Am J Psychiatry 140:348–350, 1983

Kessler RC, Frank RG: The impact of psychiatric disorders on work loss days. Psychol Med 27:861–873, 1997

Kessler RC, Sonnega A, Bromet E, et al: Posttraumatic stress disorder in the National Comorbidity Survey. Arch Gen Psychiatry 52:1048–1060, 1995

Kessler RC, Berglund P, Demler O, et al: Lifetime prevalence and age-of-onset distributions of DSM-IV disorders in the National Comorbidity Survey Replication. Arch Gen Psychiatry 62:593–602, 2005a

Kessler RC, Chiu WT, Demler O, et al: Prevalence, severity, and comorbidity of 12-month DSM-IV disorders in the National Comorbidity Survey Replication. Arch Gen Psychiatry 62:617–627, 2005b

Kulka R, Schlenger WE, Fairbank JA, et al: Trauma and the Vietnam War Generation: Report of the Findings From the National Vietnam Veterans' Readjustment Study. New York, Brunner/Mazel, 1990

Laugharne J, Janca A, Widiger T: Posttraumatic stress disorder and terrorism: 5 years after 9/11. Curr Opin Psychiatry 20:36–41, 2007

Lindal E, Stefansson JG: The lifetime prevalence of anxiety disorder in Iceland as estimated by the US National Institute of Mental Health Diagnostic Interview Schedule. Acta Psychiatr Scand 88:29–34, 1993

Lipton MI, Schaffer WR: Physical symptoms related to posttraumatic stress disorder in an aging population. Mil Med 153:316–318, 1988

Litz BT, Keane TM, Fisher L, et al: Physical health complaints in combat-related post-traumatic stress disorder: a preliminary report. J Trauma Stress 5:131–141, 1992

Lopez G, Piffaut G, Seguin A: Prise en charge psychologique des victimes d'agressions sexuelles: à propos d'une enquête des UMJ, Paris (436 questionnaires). Psychol Med (Paris) 24:286–288, 1992

McCarren M, Janes GR, Goldberg J, et al: A twin study of the association of post-traumatic stress disorder and combat exposure with long-term socioeconomic status in Vietnam veterans. J Trauma Stress 8:111–124, 1995

McFarlane AC: The phenomenology of posttraumatic stress disorders following a natural disaster. J Nerv Ment Dis 176:22–29, 1988

McFarlane AC: Vulnerability to posttraumatic stress disorder, in Posttraumatic Stress Disorder: Etiology, Phenomenology, and Treatment. Edited by Wolf ME, Mosnaim AD. Washington, DC, American Psychiatric Press, 1990, pp 3–20

McFarlane AC: The severity of the trauma: issues about its role in post-traumatic stress disorder, in Beyond Trauma: Cultural and Societal Dynamics. Edited by Kleber RJ, Figley CR, Gersons BPR. New York, Plenum, 1995, pp 31–54

McFarlane A: The contribution of epidemiology to the study of traumatic stress. Soc Psychiatry Psychiatr Epidemiol 39:874–882, 2004

McFarlane AC: Stress-related musculoskeletal pain. Best Pract Res Clin Rheumatol 21:549–565, 2007

McFarlane AC, Yehuda R, Clark CR: Biologic models of traumatic memories and post-traumatic stress disorder: the role of neural networks. Psychiatr Clin North Am 25:253–270, 2002

McGorry PD, Chanen A, McCarthy E, et al: Posttraumatic stress disorder following recent-onset psychosis: an unrecognized postpsychotic syndrome. J Nerv Ment Dis 179:253–258, 1991

Milliken CS, Auchterlonie JL, Hoge CW: Longitudinal assessment of mental health problems among active and reserve component soldiers returning from the Iraq war. JAMA 298:2141–2148, 2007

Mollica RF, Caridad KR, Massagli MP: Longitudinal study of posttraumatic stress disorder, depression, and changes in traumatic memories over time in Bosnian refugees. J Nerv Ment Dis 195:572–579, 2007

Murthy RS: Mass violence and mental health—recent epidemiological findings. Int Rev Psychiatry 19:183–192, 2007

Mylle J, Maes M: Partial posttraumatic stress disorder revisited. J Affect Disord 78:37–48, 2004

Norris FH: Epidemiology of trauma: frequency and impact of different potentially traumatic events on different demographic groups. J Consult Clin Psychol 60:409–418, 1992

Norris FH: Disaster research methods: past progress and future directions. J Trauma Stress 19:173–184, 2006

Norris FH, Hamblen JL: Standardised self-report measures of civilian trauma and PTSD, in Assessing Psychological Trauma and PTSD, 2nd Edition. Edited by Wilson JP, Keane TM. New York, Guilford, 2004, pp 63–102

Norris FH, Friedman MJ, Watson PJ, et al: 60,000 disaster victims speak: part I: an empirical review of the empirical literature, 1981–2001. Psychiatry 65:207–239, 2002a

Norris FH, Friedman MJ, Watson PJ: 60,000 disaster victims speak: part II: summary and implications of the disaster mental health research. Psychiatry 65:240–260, 2002b

Okasha A: Mental health and violence: WPA Cairo declaration—international perspectives for intervention. Int Rev Psychiatry 19:193–200, 2007

Orr SP, Metzger LJ, Pitman RK: Psychophysiology of post-traumatic stress disorder. Psychiatr Clin North Am 25:271–293, 2002

Perrin MA, DiGrande L, Wheeler K, et al: Differences in PTSD prevalence and associated risk factors among World Trade Center disaster rescue and recovery workers. Am J Psychiatry 164:1385–1394, 2007

Peters L, Slade T, Andrews G: A comparison of ICD-10 and DSM-IV criteria for post-traumatic stress disorder. J Trauma Stress 12:335–343, 1999

Peleg T, Shalev AY: Longitudinal studies of PTSD: overview of findings and methods. CNS Spectr 11:589–602, 2006

Post RM, Weiss SR, Smith M, et al: Kindling versus quenching: implications for the evolution and treatment of post-traumatic stress disorder. Ann N Y Acad Sci 821:285–295, 1997

Riggs DS, Dancu CV, Gershuny BS, et al: Anger and post-traumatic stress disorder in female crime victims. J Trauma Stress 5:613–624, 1992

Robins LN, Regier SA: Psychiatric Disorders in America. New York, Free Press, 1991

Rothbaum BO, Foa EB, Riggs DS, et al: A prospective examination of post-traumatic stress disorder in rape victims. J Trauma Stress 5:455–476, 1992

Rubin GJ, Brewin CR, Greenberg N, et al: Enduring consequences of terrorism: 7-month follow-up survey of reactions to the bombings in London on 7 July 2005. Br J Psychiatry 190:350–356, 2007

Saxe GN, van der Kolk BA, Berkowitz R, et al: Dissociative disorders in psychiatric inpatients. Am J Psychiatry 150:1037–1042, 1993

Schnurr PP, Lunney CA, Sengupta A, et al: A longitudinal study of retirement in older male veterans. J Consult Clin Psychol 73:561–566, 2005

Schottenfeld RS, Cullen MR: Recognition of occupational-induced PTSD. J Occup Med 28:365–369, 1986

Shalev AY: Posttraumatic stress disorder among injured survivors of a terrorist attack: predictive value of early intrusion and avoidance symptoms. J Nerv Ment Dis 180:505–509, 1992

Shalev A, Bleich A, Ursano RJ: Posttraumatic stress disorder: somatic comorbidity and effort tolerance. Psychosomatics 31:197–203, 1990

Silove D, Steel Z, McGorry P, et al: Trauma exposure, post-migration stressors, and symptoms of anxiety, depression and post-traumatic stress in Tamil asylum-seekers: comparison with refugees and immigrants. Acta Psychiatr Scand 97:175–181, 1998

Silove D, Steel Z, Bauman A, et al: Trauma, PTSD and the longer-term mental health burden amongst Vietnamese refugees: a comparison with the Australian-born population. Soc Psychiatry Psychiatr Epidemiol 42:467–476, 2007

Solomon Z, Mikulincer M: Combat stress reaction, posttraumatic stress disorder and somatic complaints among Israeli soldiers. J Psychosom Res 31:131–137, 1987

Solomon Z, Mikulincer M: Trajectories of PTSD: a 20-year longitudinal study. Am J Psychiatry 163:659–666, 2006

Solomon Z, Weisenberg M, Schwarzwald J, et al: Posttraumatic stress disorder amongst front line soldiers with combat stress reactions: the 1982 Israeli experience. Am J Psychiatry 144:448–454, 1987

Southwick SM, Vythilingam M, Charney DS: The psychobiology of depression and resilience to stress: implications for prevention and treatment. Annu Rev Clin Psychol 1:255–291, 2005

Spiegel D: Dissociation and hypnosis in post traumatic stress disorders. J Trauma Stress 1:17–33, 1988

Spiegel D, Cardena E: Disintegrated experience: the dissociative disorders revisited. J Abnorm Psychol 100:366–378, 1991

Spitzer RL, First MB, Wakefield JC: Saving PTSD from itself in DSM-V. J Anxiety Disord 21:233–241, 2007

Summerfield D: The invention of post-traumatic stress disorder and the social usefulness of a psychiatric category. BMJ 322:95–98, 2001

Summerfield D: Effects of war: moral knowledge, revenge, reconciliation, and medicalised concepts of "recovery." BMJ 325:1105–1107, 2002

Trimble MR: Posttraumatic stress disorder: history of a concept, in Trauma and Its Wake, Vol 5. Edited by Figley CR. New York, Brunner/Mazel, 1985, pp 5–14

van der Kolk BA, van der Hart O: The intrusive past: the flexibility of memory and the engraving of trauma. Am Imago 48:425–454, 1991

van der Kolk BA, Pelcovitz D, Roth S, et al: Dissociation, somatization and affect dysregulation: the complexity of adaptation to trauma. Am J Psychiatry 153 (7 suppl):83–93, 1996

van der Kolk BA, Roth S, Pelcovitz D, et al: Disorders of extreme stress: the empirical foundation of a complex adaptation to trauma. J Trauma Stress 18:389–399, 2005

van Kamp I, van der Velden PG, Stellato RK, et al: Physical and mental health shortly after a disaster: first results from the Enschede firework disaster study. Eur J Public Health 16:253–259, 2006

Van Ommeren M, Sharma B, Sharma GK, et al: The relationship between somatic and PTSD symptoms among Bhutanese refugee torture survivors: examination of comorbidity with anxiety and depression. J Trauma Stress 15:415–421, 2002

Wang PS, Berglund P, Olfson M, et al: Failure and delay in initial treatment contact after first onset of mental disorders in the National Comorbidity Survey Replication. Arch Gen Psychiatry 62:603–613, 2005

Warshaw MG, Fierman E, Pratt L, et al: Quality of life and dissociation in anxiety disorder patients with histories of trauma or PTSD. Am J Psychiatry 150:1512–1516, 1993

Weathers FW, Ruscio AM, Keane TM: Psychometric properties of nine scoring rules for the Clinician-Administered Posttraumatic Stress Disorder Scale. Psychol Assess 11:124–133, 1999

Weisaeth L: The stressors and the posttraumatic syndrome after an industrial disaster. Acta Psychiatr Scand Suppl 355:25–37, 1989

Weisaeth L: Torture of a Norwegian ship's crew: stress reactions, coping and psychiatric aftereffects, in International Handbook of Traumatic Stress Syndromes. Edited by Wilson JP, Raphael B. New York, Plenum, 1993, pp 743–750

Weiss DS: The Impact of Events Scale Revised in Assessing Psychological Trauma in PTSD, 2nd Edition. New York, Guilford, 2004

Welch J, Mason F: Rape and sexual assault. BMJ 334:1154–1158, 2007

Wessa M, Flor H: Failure of extinction of fear responses in posttraumatic stress disorder: evidence from second-order conditioning. Am J Psychiatry 164:1684–1692, 2007

White P, Faustman WO: Coexisting physical conditions among inpatients with post-traumatic stress disorder. Mil Med 154:66–71, 1989

Wolfe J, Erickson DJ, Sharkansky EJ, et al: Course and predictors of posttraumatic stress disorder among Gulf War veterans: a prospective analysis. J Consult Clin Psychol 67:520–528, 1999

World Health Organization: The Composite International Diagnostic Interview (CIDI). Geneva, Switzerland, World Health Organization, 1990

World Health Organization: The ICD-10 Classification of Mental and Behavioural Disorders: Clinical Descriptions and Diagnostic Guidelines. Geneva, Switzerland, World Health Organization, 1992

World Health Organization: The ICD-10 Classification of Mental and Behavioural Disorders: Diagnostic Criteria for Research. Geneva, Switzerland, World Health Organization, 1993

Yehuda R: Preface. Ann N Y Acad Sci 1071:xv–xxi, 2006

Yehuda R, McFarlane AC: Conflict between current knowledge about PTSD and its original conceptual basis. Am J Psychiatry 152:1705–1713, 1995

Zatzick DF, Marmar CR, Weiss DS, et al: Posttraumatic stress disorder and functioning and quality of life outcomes in a nationally representative sample of male Vietnam veterans. Am J Psychiatry 154:1690–1695, 1997

Recommended Readings

Reyes G, Elhai JD, Ford JD (eds): Encyclopedia of Psychological Trauma. Hoboken, NJ, Wiley, 2008

van der Kolk BA, McFarlane AC, Weisaeth L (eds): Traumatic Stress: The Effects of Overwhelming Experience on Mind, Body and Society. New York, Guilford, 2006

Wilson JP, Keane TM (eds): Assessing Psychological Trauma and PTSD, 2nd Edition. New York, Guilford, 2004

Chapter 31

Pathogenesis of Posttraumatic Stress Disorder and Acute Stress Disorder

Rachel Yehuda, Ph.D.
Casey Sarapas, B.S.

When the diagnosis of posttraumatic stress disorder (PTSD) was first established, the intent was to describe symptoms associated with a prolonged response to a traumatic event. Thus, chronic PTSD was not considered qualitatively different from the more acute response, but rather was considered to reflect a chronicity of the stress response. Research in the past two decades has now questioned the idea that PTSD is simply an extension of a more acute and short-term response to trauma. Rather, PTSD is only one of several types of responses to traumatic exposure (McFarlane 1988; Rothbaum and Foa 1993; Shalev et al. 1998), and a relatively rare one at that (Breslau et al. 1991; Kessler et al. 1995). Furthermore, and especially relevant to the acute stress disorder (ASD) diagnosis, its development cannot always be predicted from the short-term response to trauma (Kessler et al. 1995). PTSD symptoms can dramatically decline over time (Galea et al. 2003; Orcutt et al. 2002), or may, conversely, only develop later in life, sometimes appearing for the first time decades after trauma exposure (Adams and Boscarino 2006; Bryant and Harvey 2002; Carty et al. 2006; Gray et al. 2004). It is unknown whether this so-called *delayed PTSD* shares a mechanism with the more typical onset of PTSD, which begins immediately after trauma exposure. However, the phenomenon seems consistent with the observation that many who recover from PTSD experience a recrudescence (generally triggered by an adverse life event or traumatic reminder).

Clearly, PTSD is a clinical syndrome that can vary in its chronological presentation and in its longitudinal course. It is therefore interesting to evaluate the relationship between PTSD and ASD in this context, including the question of whether PTSD simply involves a continuation of an acute response to trauma. At the time the diagnosis was first established, this was widely assumed to be the case (Yehuda and McFarlane 1995), despite the fact that there were not, at that point, any longitudinal data—either retrospective or prospective—formally establishing the relation between acute and chronic posttraumatic symptoms.

This work was supported by National Institute of Mental Health grant R02 MH49555 (R.Y.), Merit Review, and U.S. Department of Defense Funding (R.Y.).

Although some studies have found that a majority of people with ASD do develop PTSD (reviewed in Yehuda et al. 2005a), ASD is not always predictive of PTSD and is, in particular, not associated with more chronic forms of PTSD. As a result, some have suggested extending the time frame for ASD to several months or years, with chronic PTSD being reserved for those who either fail to return to pretraumatic function or who have relapses. An alternative conclusion is simply that ASD is not an especially useful diagnosis, at least so long as its purpose is to predict chronic PTSD. Here, the acute response to trauma may not constitute evidence of a "disorder" (i.e., an abnormal, pathological process) so much as evidence of trauma exposure. To the extent that ASD represents a normative response to trauma that may resolve even without treatment, rather than developing into PTSD, the category of adjustment disorder may be more appropriate. If, alternatively, ASD is a good predictor of PTSD, it may be that this syndrome captures elements of a maladaptive response. What might justify the existence of ASD as a condition separate from an adjustment disorder would be a delineation of biological alterations that represent a disordered or failed acute stress response. The opportunity for studies of such alterations to be informative has dramatically increased, given that psychological and biological investigations of PTSD have suggested differences between what is observed, both acutely and chronically, in those who develop PTSD, compared with those who do not.

In this chapter, we suggest that the discussions that originally linked PTSD and ASD were based on conceptions of PTSD that are now outdated. To support this view, we review the biological and psychological underpinnings of what is currently known about PTSD and its relationship with ASD.

Risk Factors

The relative rareness of PTSD in trauma-exposed people supports the idea that risk factors unrelated to trauma exposure increase risk for PTSD (Andrews et al. 2000; Bromet et al. 1998; Heinrichs et al. 2005; Koenen et al. 2002, 2007; Macklin et al. 1998; McFarlane 2000; Perkonigg et al. 2000; Schumm et al. 2006; Yehuda 1999b, 2004). In theory, such factors could separately include features of the traumatic event or characteristics of the person (including preexisting traits and/or aspects of their individual response during or after the experience), each making distinct contributions to one's trauma response. In practice, such factors may be linked. The greater prevalence of PTSD following exposure to interpersonal violence rather than following accidents suggests that the former are more potent stressors and, accordingly, increase one's risk by providing an increased "dosage" of trauma. Yet, because exposure to interpersonal violence occurs less randomly among populations than accidents, the link between such exposures and PTSD may reflect demographic, socioeconomic, or even genetic predictors of event exposure (Breslau et al. 1991, 1998, 1999; Koenen et al. 2002; Stein et al. 2002a). One study demonstrated a higher concordance between monozygotic than dizygotic twins with respect to interpersonal violence and PTSD, implying shared genetic risk factors both for exposure to violence and for the development of PTSD (Stein et al. 2002b).

Knowledge has been hampered by the fact that information about risk factors has generally been collected retrospectively. For example, the subjective assessment of how distressing an event was in the past may be determined by how distressed one was, and continued to be, in the months and years that followed. However, data collected in the immediate aftermath of an event offer their own interpretative challenges. The immediate reactions of panic or dissociation that predict PTSD may reflect the intensity or severity of the current experience exclusively, or they may represent an exaggerated response, which itself results from earlier risk factors, such as prior trauma exposure (reviewed in McNally 2003). In particular, exposure to childhood physical or sexual abuse increases risk for PTSD to subsequent traumatization (Andrews et al. 2000; Bremner et al. 1993; Breslau et al. 1999; Donovan et al. 1996; Koenen et al. 2007; Yehuda et al. 2001b, 2001c). However, such experiences may also be associated with elevated risk for PTSD, because they increase the probability of subsequent exposure to traumatic events (Nishith et al. 2000; Storr et al. 2007). An augmented response to a subsequent traumatic event may therefore reflect either an accumulating "dose" of the stressor or changes in biological response characteristics resulting from earlier experiences.

Other risk factors for PTSD include a family history of psychopathology, and especially parental PTSD; cognitive factors, such as low IQ; female gender; preexisting avoidant, antisocial, or neurotic personality or behavioral problems; other traits, such as proneness to experiencing negative emotions; and poor social support (Bromet et al. 1998; Davidson et al. 1998; Macklin et al. 1998; Marmar et al. 2006; McNally 2003; Silva et al. 2000; Storr et al. 2007; Yehuda 1999a; Yehuda et al. 1998a, 2001a). These traits may reflect either genetic diatheses or early life experiences. Early abuse might lead to changes in personality and cognitive abilities, but may also be a consequence of these factors. Similarly, factors associated with heritable parental characteristics (e.g., psychopathology) may also increase risk for PTSD by increasing exposure to neglect or abuse. Such factors constitute important sources of individual variation in stress responses. The relevant question is, by what means do risk factors disrupt the fear response? That is, to what extent do they interfere with cognitive processing involved in fear acquisition, impede containment of the biological response to fear, and delay extinction? If risk factors are primarily involved in failure of recovery, then the risk factors associated with PTSD may be distinct from those observed in normal acute stress responses and even in ASD.

To date, risk factors for the development of ASD include female gender; high scores on the Beck Depression Inventory; avoidant coping style; and acute stress severity (Harvey and Bryant 1998). Bromet et al. (1998) examined risk factors for trauma exposure, regardless of whether the individual developed PTSD, and controlling for type of trauma. They found that history of affective or anxiety disorder and parental mental disorder both carried increased risk. The apparently higher number of risk factors for PTSD compared with ASD may be related to the relative newness of the latter diagnosis and the consequent lack of studies rather than to a lack of risk factors per se. Additional studies that assess vulnerability to both PTSD and ASD are needed to further clarify the distinct and overlapping risk factors for these entities.

Biological Factors

Neurochemistry

The classic work of Cannon (1914), followed by observations by Selye (1936), identified a range of physiological changes associated with acute exposure to a stressor, including increases in sympathetic and decreases in parasympathetic tone, and the release of adrenocorticotropic hormone (ACTH), cortisol and catecholamines from the pituitary, adrenal cortex, and adrenal medulla, respectively. These and related physiological adjustments of the autonomic nervous system (ANS) and certain organs (e.g., changes in heart rate, blood pressure, respiration, and skin conductance) were viewed as adaptive responses to stress in the short run, which could nonetheless have pathological consequences with prolonged exposure to stress. An important feature of this stress response was the return to baseline soon after the termination of the stressor. However, initial descriptions of combat veterans suggested a chronic and sustained physiological hyperarousal (Kardiner 1941). As early as 1918, World War I veterans with "irritable heart of soldiers" were reported as having increased heart rates in response to experimentally induced sounds of gunfire and exaggerated behavioral responses to epinephrine injections (Fraser and Wilson 1918; Meakins and Wilson 1918).

The first neurochemical and psychophysiological studies in PTSD were also performed in combat veterans. As hypothesized, these investigations generally reported alterations consistent with the classic picture of stress just described. Thus, in earlier studies, patients with chronic PTSD showed increases in peripheral catecholamine levels, increased sympathetic tone, and decreased parasympathetic tone. They also showed changes in heart rate, respiration, skin conductance, and other autonomic measures compared with control subjects; however, there is some question about whether these changes are observable under resting conditions or only under provocation (Bryant 2006; Buckley and Kaloupek 2001; Kosten et al. 1987; Mellman et al. 2004; O'Donnell et al. 2004; Southwick et al. 1997; Yehuda et al. 1992, 1998b).

Compared with control samples, then, catecholamine levels have generally been higher in PTSD (Table 31–1). Furthermore, there is a clear relationship between increased urinary norepinephrine (NE) and epinephrine and symptom exacerbation in PTSD, as evidenced by the substantially higher levels of these urinary measures observed in hospitalized Vietnam combat veterans with PTSD compared with other psychiatric groups (Kosten et al. 1987). These observations were confirmed and extended in a subsequent study that demonstrated increased urinary NE, epinephrine, and dopamine excretion in Vietnam combat veterans, particularly in those who were inpatients, compared with normal controls (Yehuda et al. 1992). It should be noted, however, that Mellman et al. (1995) did not observe significant elevations in urinary NE or 3-methoxy-4-hydroxyphenylglycol (MHPG) in Vietnam veterans. Moreover, Murburg et al. (1995) demonstrated that arterialized NE levels were actually lower in veterans with PTSD compared with healthy control subjects.

When plasma NE levels were examined every 30 minutes over a 24-hour period under controlled laboratory conditions, significantly higher levels of plasma NE were found in PTSD study participants without

TABLE 31–1. Catecholamine alterations in posttraumatic stress disorder

Study	Population	Findings
Meakins and Wilson 1918	Combat veterans	↑ BP with EPI
Kardiner 1941	Combat veterans	↑ BP with EPI
Kosten et al. 1987	Combat veterans	↑ Baseline catecholamines
Perry et al. 1987	Combat veterans	↓ α_2R
McFall et al. 1990	Combat veterans	No difference in baseline catecholamines; ↑ EPI to challenge
Perry et al. 1990	Combat veterans	No difference in baseline catecholamines
Blanchard et al. 1991	Combat veterans	No difference in baseline catecholamines; ↑ HR and NE to challenge
Yehuda et al. 1992	Combat veterans	↑ Baseline catecholamines
Southwick et al. 1993	Combat veterans	↑ Catecholamines after challenge
Mellman et al. 1995	Combat veterans	No difference in baseline catecholamines
Murburg et al. 1995	Combat veterans	↓ Baseline catecholamines
Yehuda et al. 1998b	Combat veterans	↑ Baseline catecholamines
Geracioti et al. 2001	Combat veterans	↑ Baseline catecholamines
Lemieux and Coe 1995	Sexual abuse victims	↑ Baseline catecholamines
Orr 1997	Sexual abuse victims	↑ Physiological response to challenge
Friedman et al. 2007	Sexual abuse victims	↑ Baseline catecholamines in those with adult sexual abuse
Goenjian et al. 1996	Earthquake survivors	↑ Baseline catecholamines
Perry 1994	Noncombat trauma victims	↓ α_2R
Maes et al. 1999	Noncombat trauma victims	↓ α_2R; ↑NE precursor availability
Marshall et al. 2002	Noncombat trauma victims	No difference in baseline catecholamines
Young and Breslau 2004	Noncombat trauma victims	↑ Baseline catecholamines

Note. BP=blood pressure; EPI=epinephrine; α_2R=α_2 adrenergic receptor; HR=heart rate; NE=norepinephrine.

comorbid depressive symptoms, compared with psychiatrically healthy and depressed participants (Yehuda et al. 1998b). After controlling for severity of depressive symptoms in this sample, a significant positive correlation (r=0.65) was apparent between the NE mesor and self-rated severity of PTSD symptoms. Curiously, inverse correlations were apparent between urinary levels of MHPG and intrusive symptoms (r=–0.67) and flashbacks (r=–0.63). Using a protocol in which salivary samples were obtained at three time points throughout the day, Goenjian et al. (1996) noted increased salivary MHPG levels in Armenian children with PTSD following an earthquake five years earlier, compared with children who lived much further away from the earthquake epicenter and had substantially fewer PTSD symptoms. The authors also noted changes in the circadian rhythm of salivary MHPG that were related to severity of PTSD symptoms.

The most important evidence of a neurochemical disturbance in PTSD comes from experiments in which the catecholamine system is provoked directly—these studies clearly link PTSD symptoms and catecholamines. Thus, Vietnam veterans with PTSD showed higher plasma NE and MHPG levels following neuroendocrine provocation (Southwick et al. 1993) and stress testing (McFall et al. 1990) compared with nonpsychiatric control subjects. Of particular interest is the finding that infusion of the selective α_2-antagonist yohimbine not only produced augmented MHPG responses in Vietnam combat veterans with PTSD, but also induced PTSD-related symptoms such as flashbacks and panic attacks (Southwick et al. 1993). Yohimbine blocks α_2 adrenergic autoreceptors, which causes an increase in the release of NE from noradrenergic terminals. Therefore, the exacerbation of symptoms in response to this intervention implies not only heightened sensitivity to the effects of catecholamines, but also a role for catecholamines in directly mediating the anxiety-related symptoms of PTSD. Elevated plasma catecholamine levels have been found in individuals during trauma-related imagery as part of an assessment of PTSD or trauma-related cues (Blanchard et al. 1991; McFall et al. 1990).

Neuropeptide Y (NPY) has more recently become of interest as a possible factor involved in PTSD resilience and recovery. NPY is a peptide that has neuroprotective effects in the hippocampus, and is thought to function as an anxiolytic (Heilig 2004; Smialowska et al. 2003). There are important functional interactions between NPY and corticotropin-releasing factor (CRF), such that NPY counteracts the anxiogenic effects of CRF (Heilig 2004; Sheriff et al. 2001). NPY also has counter-regulatory effects on NE in many brain areas associated with anxiety, fear, and depression (Guidi et al. 1999; Hastings et al. 2001; Pich et al. 1993; Thorsell et al. 1999). Preliminary studies have demonstrated that persons under extreme stress with high NPY levels show better performance than those with low levels of NPY (Morgan et al. 2000a, 2000b). Similarly, patients with PTSD have reduced baseline plasma NPY levels and a blunted yohimbine-induced NPY increase (Morgan et al. 2003; Rasmusson et al. 2000). Plasma NPY levels seem to be directly associated with recovery from PTSD, because they were significantly higher in combat veterans with past but not current PTSD, compared with veterans with current PTSD or veterans who never developed PTSD (Yehuda et al. 2006). Further research may establish whether and to what extent baseline NPY levels are associated with treatment response and with spontaneous symptom improvement or recovery.

Endocrine

Inconsistent with the classic conceptualization of stress, cortisol levels were not elevated in chronic PTSD (reviewed in Yehuda 2002a, 2005, 2006). In fact, the first published neuroendocrine study demonstrated significantly lower 24-hour mean urinary cortisol excretion in combat veterans with PTSD compared with veterans with other psychiatric disorders (Mason et al. 1986). Particularly interesting is that norepinephrine and epinephrine levels assayed from the same sample revealed sustained increases in these hormones in PTSD, thus emphasizing a dissociation between the two major endocrine makers of stress, catecholamines and cortisol (Mason et al. 1988). Although not all studies have reported similar observations, those in which cortisol levels were assessed via samples collected regularly over a 24-hour period under carefully controlled conditions did find evidence of reduced cortisol levels as well as alterations in the circadian rhythmicity of cortisol (Bremner et al. 2003a; Yehuda et al. 1996b).

At first, the apparent disconnection of cortisol levels and other markers of stress proved difficult to interpret. However, in the mid-1980s it became clear that in addition to its role in facilitating energy delivery to the body's vital organs, stress-activated cortisol release helps contain sympathetic activation and other stress-induced neural defensive reactions (Munck et al. 1984). Furthermore, just as cortisol suppresses stress-activated biological reactions, elevated cortisol levels also suppress the further release of cortisol itself, through negative feedback inhibition. Occupation of glucocorticoid receptors in the paraventricular nucleus of the hypothalamus and at the pituitary suppresses release of CRF and ACTH, respectively, which in turn results in a reduction in cortisol release and a restoration of basal hormone levels (E.R. de Kloet et al. 1986; McEwen 1979). It therefore followed that if the cortisol response to a stressor is muted, an increased or prolonged activation of the sympathetic nervous system could result (E.R. de Kloet et al. 2005; Yehuda 2002a).

Lower cortisol levels in PTSD may manifest at the time of acute traumatization. Studies examining cortisol levels within hours or days following trauma exposure demonstrate either an inverse relationship between cortisol levels and PTSD severity in the acute aftermath of trauma or a significantly attenuated rise in cortisol levels in people who subsequently developed PTSD (Anisman et al. 2001; Delahanty et al. 2000, 2003; McFarlane et al. 1997).

The paradox surrounding observations of low cortisol deepened as it became clear that CRF levels were elevated relative to control conditions (Baker et al. 1999; Bremner et al. 1997; Yehuda et al. 1996a), despite the fact that CRF is responsible for the release of ACTH and ACTH is responsible for the release of cortisol. People with PTSD were also significantly more likely to show enhanced cortisol negative feedback inhibition (C.S. de Kloet et al. 2006; Goenjian et al. 1996; Newport et al. 2004; Stein et al. 1997b; Yehuda et al. 1993, 2004a, 2004b), apparently resulting from increased responsiveness of glucocorticoid receptors (Bachmann et al. 2005; Rohleder et al. 2004; Yehuda et al. 1995, 2004c). It appeared, then, that CRF hypersecretion does not culminate in cortisol hypersecretion due to increased cortisol negative feedback inhibition (reviewed in Yehuda 2002a). This profile was clearly different from that observed in animal models of stress. It also differed from observations in humans with depression, in which elevated CRF resulted in increased cortisol levels and weaker cortisol negative feedback inhibition (Holsober 2003; Nemeroff 1998).

As these findings were emerging in the mid- to late 1990s, there were no precedents in the animal or human literature for understanding them as consequences of either an acute or chronic response to a single-event exposure. Rather, accumulating evidence began to suggest that cortisol-related alterations in PTSD reflected preexisting vulnerability factors that increase the probability of developing PTSD following trauma exposure. This was supported by observations that lower cortisol levels in the acute aftermath of trauma were correlated with two well-established risk factors: prior trauma exposure and parental PTSD. With respect to the former, a number of reports demonstrated an association between cortisol and, more importantly, measures reflecting enhanced glucocorticoid receptor responsiveness, and early trauma exposure (Delahanty et al. 2003; King et al. 2001; Resnick et al. 1995; Yehuda et al. 2004a). With respect to parental PTSD, adult offspring of Holocaust survivors with PTSD showed significantly lower urinary and plasma cortisol levels across the diurnal cycle (Yehuda et al. 2001b, 2007c) and demonstrated an enhanced cortisol negative feedback inhibition (Yehuda et al. 2007a), compared with offspring of Holocaust survivors without PTSD and control subjects with no Holocaust exposure. In these studies, offsprings' cortisol levels at baseline and in response to dexamethasone were negatively correlated with severity of parental PTSD symptoms, even after controlling for PTSD symptoms in the offspring. The association between low cortisol and parental PTSD was replicated in infants of mothers who developed PTSD following exposure to the World Trade Center attacks while pregnant. Infants of such mothers had significantly lower salivary cortisol levels than infants born to similarly exposed mothers who did not develop PTSD, particularly if the mothers were in their third trimester at the time of exposure (Yehuda et al. 2005b).

The data suggested that hypothalamic-pituitary-adrenal (HPA) axis alterations in PTSD might reflect a source of individual variation in stress responses that may be present prior to an event exposure. Such alterations might affect the stress response trajectory in a manner that impedes recovery. It was hypothesized that reduced cortisol signaling at the time of a trauma compromised the inhibition of stress-induced biological responses (e.g., during and following a traumatic event), resulting in prolonged physiological or emotional distress, which would then facilitate the development of PTSD (Yehuda 2002b). Low cortisol signaling might also explain the observation of a greater heart rate in those who develop PTSD. That measures reflecting glucocorticoid levels and responsiveness were demonstrated to be associated with pre-exposure vulnerability to PTSD provides a plausible explanation for the variability in detection of cortisol levels in PTSD. That is, lower cortisol levels may only be present in those trauma survivors showing specific risk factors associated with this marker, whereas cortisol levels may not be low in those who develop PTSD in the absence of certain pre-exposure risk factors.

Although many of the observations from discrete studies may show disagreement with one another, as observed previously in this chapter with respect to catecholamine alterations, most of the findings that have been observed in PTSD are compatible with enhanced negative feedback inhibition of the HPA axis in PTSD. In such a circumstance, there may be transient elevations in cortisol. However, if there is a greater responsiveness of glucocorticoid receptors at the pituitary, these increases would be shorter-lived due to a more efficient containment of ACTH release. This model posits that chronic or transient elevations in CRF stimulate the pituitary release of ACTH, which in turn stimulates the adrenal release of cortisol. However, an increased negative feedback inhibition would result in reduced cortisol levels under ambient conditions (Yehuda et al. 1996b). In contrast to other models of endocrinopathy, which identify specific and usually singular primary alterations in endocrine organs or regulation, the model of enhanced negative feedback inhibition in PTSD is, in large part, descriptive. The model currently offers little explanation for why some individuals show such alterations of the HPA axis following exposure to traumatic experiences and others do not, but represents an important development in the field of neuroendocrinology of PTSD by accounting for a substantial proportion of the findings observed, and can be put to further hypothesis testing. Table 31–2 demonstrates that almost all findings in PTSD are consistent with an enhanced negative feedback inhibition. Other potential explanatory models included reduced adrenal capacity, altered glucocorticoid metabolism, and differences in heterologous or homologous regulation of the HPA axis at multiple sites.

TABLE 31–2. Compatibility of findings in posttraumatic stress disorder with enhanced negative feedback inhibition

Finding in PTSD	Enhanced negative feedback
Lower ambient cortisol levels	Yes
Normal or variable cortisol levels	Yes
Higher cortisol levels	Yes[a]
Increased circadian rhythm of cortisol	Yes
Decreased circadian rhythm of cortisol	No
Normal ACTH levels	Yes
Low β-endorphin levels	Yes[b]
Increased CRF levels in cerebrospinal fluid	Yes
Increased glucocorticoid receptor number	Yes
Increased glucocorticoid receptor responsiveness	Yes
Normal cortisol levels following 1 mg DEX	Yes
Decreased cortisol levels following 0.5 mg DEX	Yes
Increased cortisol levels following 1 mg DEX	No
Decreased number of cytosolic glucocorticoid receptors following DEX compared with baseline receptors	Yes
Increased ACTH following DEX administration	Yes
Increased ACTH levels to high dose metyrapone	Yes
Decreased ACTH levels to low dose metyrapone	No
Decreased ACTH levels following CRF	Yes
Increased ACTH levels following CRF	No
Decreased ACTH levels following CCK-4	Yes
Increased ACTH levels following naloxone	No
Increased ACTH levels following stress	Yes
Increased cortisol response to ACTH	No
Decreased cortisol response to ACTH	Yes

Note. This table demonstrates that the model of enhanced negative feedback is compatible with 18 of these 24 observations of HPA alterations in PTSD. ACTH=adrenocorticotropic hormone; CCK=cholecystokinin; CRF=corticotropin-releasing factor; DEX=dexamethasone.

[a]Higher cortisol levels are only consistent with enhanced negative feedback to the extent that they represent transient elevations.

[b]To the extent that β-endorphin is co-released with ACTH and reflects ACTH, this finding is compatible.

Neuroimaging

Concurrent with the studies previously mentioned that examined peripheral markers of stress, developments in neuroimaging methods presented an opportunity to examine indices of brain structure and function. Early theories proposed that the hippocampus might be a region of central importance in PTSD because of its prominent role in both the neuroendocrine stress response and memory alterations that characterize PTSD (Landfield and Eldridge 1994; McEwen and Sapolsky 1995; Sapolsky 1994). Many, but not all, studies have now demonstrated smaller hippocampal volumes in PTSD (Bremner et al. 1995, 2003b; Gurvits et al. 1996; Hedges et al. 2003; Stein et al. 1997a). However, as with the neuroendocrine observations, debate continues regarding the etiology and significance of these findings.

Initial reports emphasized that smaller hippocampal volumes in PTSD most likely resulted from consequences of excess glucocorticoid release associated with trauma exposure (e.g., Bremner et al. 1995, 1997; Gurvits et al. 1996; Stein et al. 1997a). This hypothesis was based on evidence that repeated stress or glucocorticoid exposure results in decreased hippocampal volume and decreased dendritic branching in animals (McEwen et al. 1992; Sapolsky 1994, 2000). However, the finding that cortisol levels are not elevated in either the acute or chronic aftermath of trauma in those who develop PTSD challenged this view (reviewed in Yehuda and LeDoux 2007). In addition, parameters reflecting increased glucocorticoid levels or activity have not been generally shown to relate to hippocampal alterations in PTSD (Neylan et al. 2003; Yehuda et al. 2007b).

The idea that trauma exposure might result in smaller hippocampal volumes in PTSD, even without a direct effect of cortisol, has also been difficult to support. Only one study demonstrated a very clear negative correlation between severity of combat exposure and hippocampal volume in combat veterans with and without PTSD (Gurvits et al. 1996). Furthermore, Holocaust survivors, who were certainly exposed to severe and chronic trauma, were not found to have smaller hippocampal volumes relative to nonexposed subjects (Golier et al. 2005). Finally, prospective longitudinal studies also failed to show change in hippocampal volume over time in persons followed in the acute aftermath of trauma, and longitudinally (Bonne et al. 2001).

Instead, like cortisol, smaller hippocampal volume in PTSD appears to be associated with a preexisting trait risk factor, as was most evidenced by the finding that smaller volumes were found not only in combat-exposed Vietnam veterans with PTSD, but also in their nonexposed identical twins (Gilbertson et al. 2002; Pitman et al. 2006). That smaller hippocampal volumes are associated with preexisting risk was also supported by the demonstration of smaller hippocampal volume in veterans who developed PTSD following their first traumatic exposure; these subjects were compared with veterans who recovered from their first traumatic experiences but then developed PTSD in response to a subsequent event (Yehuda et al. 2007b). Researchers investigating trauma survivors at 1 and 6 months posttrauma failed to identify differences in hippocampal volume in those who developed PTSD (Bonne et al. 2001). Because smaller hippocampal volume is correlated with other constitutional factors that have been independently associated with increasing risk for the development of PTSD (Macklin et al. 1998), such as low IQ (Gurvits et al. 1996), this measure may represent a correlate of a constitutional trait or traits that predict difficulty in coping with adversity.

The preceding discussion of cortisol and hippocampal volume demonstrates that rather than reflecting normal consequences of stress exposure, many observed alterations in PTSD are likely to represent preexisting risk factors. Given that changes in these two parameters (cortisol and hippocampal volume) have been linked both conceptually and, in animal models of stress, empirically, a question arises regarding whether or not these two risk factors represent distinct measures with separate etiologies that confer risk through different mechanisms.

Reduced hippocampal volume may confer risk through an association with decreased cognitive capacity for necessary reinterpretation and adaptation of traumatic experiences. Cognitive deficits could impair functioning following a traumatic experience, regardless of whether there has been a sensitizing prior experience. Risk factors associated with reduced cortisol signaling, on the other hand, might confer risk by interfering with the neurochemical response to environmental stress and impeding reinstatement of physiological homeostasis.

There is likely to be a final common pathophysiology of PTSD that is independent of the contribution of individual risk factors. Nonetheless, it is important to identify biological correlates of specific risk factors, because they might explain clinically meaningful individual or cohort differences in areas such as treatment response, phenomenology, and pathophysiology. For example, smaller hippocampal volumes seem to be a more salient biological measure in combat veterans than in Holocaust survivors, even though these two groups demonstrated similar cognitive deficits associated with PTSD symptom severity when they were directly compared with one another (Yehuda et al. 2005c). In trying to conceptualize what might be appropriate targets for interventions, both individual differences and uniform processes are legitimate candidates.

Psychological Factors

Cognitive-Behavioral

The biological correlates of PTSD and PTSD risk described earlier could provide a biological basis for psychological theories pertaining to the development of PTSD, in which PTSD is conceived as a failure to mobilize psychological processes that underlie natural recovery (Foa 1997). In this view, traumatic events activate and/or promote distress and negative cognitions, such as that the world is dangerous and the victim is incompetent. Natural recovery occurs via repeated confrontations with trauma-related situations and emotional engagement with trauma-related thoughts and feelings (e.g., sharing the memories with others). In the absence of repeated traumatization, these natural exposures help disconfirm the common posttrauma cognition that the world is a dangerous place, and also lead to a reduction of distress because they provide opportunities for challenging dysfunctional cognitions (e.g., "I will never be safe again").

Chronic PTSD results from behavioral and cognitive avoidance of trauma reminders. Certain pretrauma schemata may render some individuals especially vulnerable to developing strong dysfunctional cognitions and associated distress. This excessive emotional reaction fosters severe avoidance that, in turn, reinforces dysfunctional cognitions by preventing exposure to disconfirming information. The reinforcement of these cognitions, such as that the world is indiscriminately dangerous and the victim is totally incompetent, further perpetuates the victim's distress.

The hypothesized psychological mechanism underlying the efficacy of cognitive-behavioral interventions is that encouraging confrontation with trauma-related situations and memories offsets patients' tendency to avoid trauma reminders. This provides survivors with the opportunity to obtain information that will correct the dysfunctional cognitions.

An Integrated Model

As previously mentioned, it seems that low cortisol levels at the time of the traumatic event contribute to a failure to adequately contain the sympathetic stress response. Accordingly, one model for the relationship between biological and psychological variables begins with the notion that individuals with lower cortisol going into a trauma may experience the event as more distressing, and will remain in a state of heightened arousal for a longer period of time, than those with higher ambient cortisol. This experience of an extreme, prolonged response to a stressor would foster the development and maintenance of cognitions that the world is extremely dangerous (e.g., continuously racing heart rate means "high threat" or "I'm very scared; therefore, I must be in danger") and that the self is incompetent (e.g., continuously racing heart rate signifies helplessness, or "I can't calm down; therefore, I can't cope"). Survivors' subjective distress would make it difficult for them to disconfirm these hypotheses, since these cognitions would be compatible with inner physiological states. Because a continuous, elevated stress response is highly aversive (and might be associated, in particular, with elevated NE levels), individuals would be more motivated to avoid reminders of the trauma, thereby reinforcing cognitions that anxiety will persist unless escape/avoidance occurs.

Political and Cultural Factors

The PTSD (and, later, ASD) diagnoses were established in part to validate symptoms of those who had been victimized and, as such, had been, unsurprisingly, politicized. Concerns about malingering and compensation neurosis have historically been and continue to be raised. As recently as 2005, for instance, the U.S. Veterans Affairs system proposed a review of PTSD diagnostic criteria and screening procedures in the face of rising costs of PTSD compensation claims (Vedantam 2005). Although neither PTSD nor any other medical syndrome exists in a cultural vacuum, it should be noted that politics and culture can only instigate the movement toward acknowledging that there are mental or physical consequences of exposure; they cannot, in essence, create these consequences where there are none. Although the diagnosis of PTSD was established in the absence of empirical data about the longitudinal course, phenomenology, and biology of PTSD, it could not have withstood the test of time in the absence of data ultimately supporting this idea. According to its original philosophical conception, biomarkers for PTSD should have been consistent with a normative biological fear response, compatible with models of chronic stress. Although little support was found for this model in particular, evidence of a strong biological basis for PTSD and PTSD risk, alongside a clear phenomenology that is consistent across individuals and cohorts exposed to various types of trauma, can now be used in lieu of political or cultural arguments about victimization. It is now time to similarly evaluate ASD to determine its true place in psychiatric nosology.

Conclusion

Although early ideas about the etiology of PTSD—that it represented or resulted from an extended but essentially normative stress response—seemed intuitive, they have not in all cases been supported by the prevalence of the disorder among persons exposed to a trauma or by research into its endocrine and neural correlates. Instead, this research has demonstrated that PTSD is one among several possible long-term responses to trauma, and that a specific individual's likelihood of responding in this way is tied to certain risk factors. One idea is that preexisting biological alterations increase the probability that the stress response will not be contained. This in turn might result in augmented hyperarousal.

The diagnostic category of ASD may have been established (several years after the emergence of PTSD) because of the heterogeneity in both short-term and long-term responses to trauma; particularly salient was the observation that some individuals were symptomatic for only a comparatively short time after trauma exposure. To date, it has been useful to conceptualize ASD and PTSD as two distinct but closely related conditions. Nonetheless, the nature of the diagnosis should be better characterized. In particular, it would be helpful to understand whether ASD represents a common, normative, short-term response to trauma, or, instead, a constellation of symptoms likely to persist and become PTSD.

This issue will be best resolved through further investigation of ASD and its relationship with PTSD. At present, it does seem that the disorders share similar symptoms, prevalence, risk factors, and neurobiological bases. ASD often, but not always, leads to the development of PTSD, although it is unclear whether it predicts more chronic, treatment-refractory PTSD. It will be interesting to know whether and to what extent the two conditions respond to similar treatments. Further research will likely be aimed at identifying subgroups of patients with ASD who are most likely to develop PTSD or recover from trauma.

Key Clinical Points

- Posttraumatic stress disorder is not a default or normative response to trauma exposure, but occurs only in a minority of trauma survivors and seems to represent the expression of a specific phenotype.
- The PTSD risk phenotype seems to carry certain biological markers. Among the most strongly supported of these are low cortisol, enhanced negative feedback inhibition of cortisol, and reduced hippocampal volumes.
- Environmental factors, such as childhood physical or sexual abuse or poor social support, also contribute to PTSD risk; these factors often offer interpretative challenges, given that many of them increase risk for trauma exposure itself as well as for PTSD.
- Although acute stress disorder shares some risk factors, biomarkers, and other characteristics with PTSD, it is currently unknown whether the disorder represents a general response to trauma, consistent with a normal physiological stress response, or a unique syndrome that represents, in essence, a prodromal phase of PTSD.

References

Adams RE, Boscarino JA: Predictors of PTSD and delayed PTSD after disaster: the impact of exposure and psychosocial resources. J Nerv Ment Dis 194:485–493, 2006

Andrews B, Brewin CR, Rose S, et al: Predicting PTSD symptoms in victims of violent crime: the role of shame, anger, and childhood abuse. J Abnorm Psychol 109:69–73, 2000

Anisman H, Griffiths J, Matheson K, et al: Posttraumatic stress symptoms and salivary cortisol levels. Am J Psychiatry 158:1509–1511, 2001

Bachmann AW, Sedgley TL, Jackson RV, et al: Glucocorticoid receptor polymorphisms and post-traumatic stress disorder. Psychoneuroendocrinology 30:297–306, 2005

Baker DG, West SA, Nicholson WE, et al: Serial CSF corticotropin-releasing hormone levels and adrenocortical activity in combat veterans with posttraumatic stress disorder. Am J Psychiatry 156:585–588, 1999 [erratum published in: Am J Psychiatry 156:986, 1999]

Blanchard EB, Kolb LC, Prins A, et al: Changes in plasma norepinephrine to combat-related stimuli among Vietnam veterans with posttraumatic stress disorder. J Nerv Ment Dis 179:371–373, 1991

Bonne O, Brandes D, Gilboa A, et al: Longitudinal MRI study of hippocampal volume in trauma survivors with PTSD. Am J Psychiatry 158:1248–1251, 2001

Bremner JD, Southwick SM, Johnson DR, et al: Childhood physical abuse and combat-related posttraumatic stress disorder in Vietnam veterans. Am J Psychiatry 150:235–239, 1993

Bremner JD, Randall P, Scott TM, et al: MRI-based measurement of hippocampal volume in patients with combat-related PTSD. Am J Psychiatry 152:973–981, 1995

Bremner JD, Licinio J, Darnell A, et al: Elevated CSF corticotropin releasing factor concentrations in posttraumatic stress disorder. Am J Psychiatry 154:624–629, 1997

Bremner JD, Vythilingam M, Anderson G, et al: Assessment of the hypothalamic-pituitary-adrenal axis over a 24-hour diurnal period and in response to neuroendocrine challenges in women with and without childhood sexual abuse and posttraumatic stress disorder. Biol Psychiatry 54:710–718, 2003a

Bremner JD, Vythilingam M, Vermetten E, et al: MRI and PET study of deficits in hippocampal structure and function in women with childhood sexual abuse and posttraumatic stress disorder. Am J Psychiatry 160:924–932, 2003b

Breslau N, Davis GC, Andreski P, et al: Traumatic events and posttraumatic stress disorder in an urban population of young adults. Arch Gen Psychiatry 48:216–222, 1991

Breslau N, Kessler RC, Chilcoat HD, et al: Trauma and posttraumatic stress disorder: the 1996 Detroit area survey of trauma. Arch Gen Psychiatry 55:626–632, 1998

Breslau N, Chilcoat HD, Kessler RC, et al: Previous exposure to trauma and PTSD effects of subsequent trauma: results from the Detroit Area Survey of Trauma. Am J Psychiatry 156:902–907, 1999

Bromet E, Sonnega A, Kessler RC: Risk factors for DSM-III-R posttraumatic stress disorder: findings from the National Comorbidity Survey. Am J Epidemiol 147:353–361, 1998

Bryant RA: Longitudinal psychophysiological studies of heart rate: mediating effects and implications for treatment. Ann NY Acad Sci 1071:19–26, 2006

Bryant RA, Harvey AG: Delayed-onset posttraumatic stress disorder: a prospective study. Aust N Z J Psychiatry 36:205–209, 2002

Buckley TC, Kaloupek DG: A meta-analytic examination of basal cardiovascular activity in posttraumatic stress disorder. Psychosom Med 63:585–594, 2001

Cannon WB: The emergency function of the adrenal medulla in pain and the major emotions. Am J Physiol 33:356–372, 1914

Carty J, O'Donnell ML, Creamer M: Delayed-onset PTSD: a prospective study of injury survivors. J Affect Disord 90:257–261, 2006

Davidson JR, Tupler LA, Wilson WH, et al: A family study of chronic post-traumatic stress disorder following rape trauma. J Psychiatr Res 32:301–309, 1998

de Kloet CS, Vermetten E, Geuze E, et al: Assessment of HPA-axis function in posttraumatic stress disorder: pharmacological and non-pharmacological challenge tests, a review. J Psychiatr Res 40:550–567, 2006

de Kloet ER, Reul JM, de Ronde FS, et al: Function and plasticity of brain corticosteroid receptor systems: action of neuropeptides. J Steroid Biochem 25:723–731, 1986

de Kloet ER, Joels M, Holsboer F: Stress and the brain: from adaptation to disease. Nat Rev Neurosci 6:463–475, 2005

Delahanty DL, Raimonde AJ, Spoonster E: Initial posttraumatic urinary cortisol levels predict subsequent PTSD symptoms in motor vehicle accident victims. Biol Psychiatry 48:940–947, 2000

Delahanty DL, Raimonde AJ, Spoonster E, et al: Injury severity, prior trauma history, urinary cortisol levels, and acute PTSD in motor vehicle accident victims. J Anxiety Disord 17:149–164, 2003

Donovan BS, Padin-Rivera E, Dowd T, et al: Childhood factors and war zone stress in chronic PTSD. J Trauma Stress 9:361–368, 1996

Foa EB: Psychological processes related to recovery from a trauma and an effective treatment for PTSD. Ann NY Acad Sci 821:410–424, 1997

Fraser F, Wilson RM: The sympathetic nervous system and the "irritable heart of soldiers." Br Med J 2:27–29, 1918

Friedman MJ, Jalowiec J, McHugo G, et al: Adult sexual abuse is associated with elevated neurohormone levels among women with PTSD due to childhood sexual abuse. J Trauma Stress 20:611–617, 2007

Galea S, Boscarino J, Resnik H, et al: Trends of probable post-traumatic stress disorder in New York City after the September 11 terrorist attacks. Am J Epidemiol 158:514–524, 2003

Geracioti TD Jr, Baker DG, Ekhator NN, et al: CSF norepinephrine concentrations in posttraumatic stress disorder. Am J Psychiatry 158:1227–1230, 2001

Gilbertson MW, Shenton ME, Ciszewski A, et al: Smaller hippocampal volume predicts pathologic vulnerability to psychological trauma. Nat Neurosci 5:1242–1247, 2002

Goenjian AK, Yehuda R, Pynoos RS, et al: Basal cortisol, dexamethasone suppression of cortisol, and MHPG in adolescents after the 1988 earthquake in Armenia. Am J Psychiatry 153:929–934, 1996

Golier JA, Yehuda R, De Santi S, et al: Absence of hippocampal volume differences in survivors of the Nazi Holocaust with and without PTSD. Psychiatry Res 139:53–64, 2005

Gray MJ, Bolton EE, Litz BT: A longitudinal analysis of PTSD symptom course: delayed-onset PTSD in Somalia peacekeepers. J Consult Clin Psychol 72:909–913, 2004

Guidi L, Tricerri A, Vangeli M, et al: Neuropeptide Y plasma levels and immunological changes during academic stress. Neuropsychobiology 4:188–195, 1999

Gurvits TV, Shenton ME, Hokama H, et al: Magnetic resonance imaging study of hippocampal volume in chronic, combat-related posttraumatic stress disorder. Biol Psychiatry 40:1091–1099, 1996

Harvey AG, Bryant RA: Acute stress disorder after mild traumatic brain injury. J Nerv Ment Dis 186:333–337, 1998

Hastings JA, McClure-Sharp JM, Morris MJ: NPY Y1 receptors exert opposite effects on corticotropin releasing factor and noradrenaline overflow from the rat hypothalamus in vitro. Brain Res 890:32–37, 2001

Hedges DW, Allen S, Tate DF, et al: Reduced hippocampal volume in alcohol and substance naïve Vietnam combat veterans with posttraumatic stress disorder. Cogn Behav Neurol 16:219–224, 2003

Heilig M: The NPY system in stress, anxiety and depression. Neuropeptides 38:213–224, 2004

Heinrichs M, Wagner D, Schoch W, et al: Predicting posttraumatic stress symptoms from pretraumatic risk factors: a 2-year prospective follow-up study in firefighters. Am J Psychiatry 162:2276–2286, 2005

Holsboer F: Corticotropin-releasing hormone modulators and depression. Curr Opin Investig Drugs 4:46–50, 2003

Kardiner A: The Traumatic Neuroses of War. New York, Hoeber, 1941

Kessler RC, Sonnega A, Bromet E, et al: Posttraumatic stress disorder in the National Comorbidity Survey. Arch Gen Psychiatry 52:1048–1060, 1995

King JA, Mandansky D, King S, et al: Early sexual abuse and low cortisol. Psychiatry Clin Neurosci 55:71–74, 2001

Koenen KC, Harley R, Lyons MJ, et al: A twin registry study of familial and individual risk factors for trauma exposure and posttraumatic stress disorder. J Nerv Ment Dis 190:209–218, 2002

Koenen KC, Moffitt TE, Poulton R, et al: Early childhood factors associated with the development of post-traumatic stress disorder: results from a longitudinal birth cohort. Psychol Med 37:181–192, 2007

Kosten TR, Mason JW, Giller EL, et al: Sustained urinary norepinephrine and epinephrine levels in post-traumatic stress disorder. Psychoneuroendocrinology 12:13–20, 1987

Landfield PW, Eldridge JC: The glucocorticoid hypothesis of age-related hippocampal neurodegeneration: role of dysregulated intraneuronal calcium. Ann NY Acad Sci 746:308–326, 1994

Lemieux AM, Coe CL: Abuse-related posttraumatic stress disorder: evidence for chronic neuroendocrine activation in women. Psychosom Med 57:105–115, 1995

Macklin ML, Metzger LJ, Litz BT, et al: Lower precombat intelligence is a risk factor for posttraumatic stress disorder. J Consult Clin Psychol 66:323–326, 1998

Maes M, Lin AH, Verkerk R, et al: Serotonergic and noradrenergic markers of post-traumatic stress disorder with and without major depression. Neuropsychopharmacology 20:188–197, 1999

Marmar CR, McCaslin SE, Metzler TJ, et al: Predictors of posttraumatic stress in police and other first responders. Ann NY Acad Sci 1071:1–18, 2006

Marshall RD, Blanco C, Printz D, et al: A pilot study of noradrenergic and HPA axis functioning in PTSD vs. panic disorder. Psychiatry Res 110:219–230, 2002

Mason JW, Giller EL, Kosten TR, et al: Urinary-free cortisol in posttraumatic stress disorder. J Nerv Ment Dis 174:145–149, 1986

Mason JW, Giller EL, Kosten TR, et al: Elevation of urinary norepinephrine/cortisol ratio in posttraumatic stress disorder. J Nerv Ment Dis 176:498–502, 1988

McEwen BS: Influences of adrenocortical hormones on pituitary and brain function. Monogr Endocrinol 12:467–492, 1979

McEwen BS, Sapolsky RM: Stress and cognitive function. Curr Opin Neurobiol 5:205-216, 1995

McEwen BS, Gould EA, Sakai RR: The vulnerability of the hippocampus to protective and destructive effects of glucocorticoids in relation to stress. Br J Psychiatry Suppl 15:18–23, 1992

McFall ME, Murburg MM, Ko GN, et al: Autonomic responses to stress in Vietnam combat veterans with posttraumatic stress disorder. Biol Psychiatry 27:1165–1175, 1990

McFarlane AC: The longitudinal course of posttraumatic morbidity: the range of outcomes and their predictors. J Nerv Ment Dis 176:30–39, 1988

McFarlane AC: Posttraumatic stress disorder: a model of the longitudinal course and the role of risk factors. J Clin Psychiatry 61 (suppl 5):15–20; discussion 21–23, 2000

McFarlane AC, Atchison M, Yehuda R: The acute stress response following motor vehicle accidents and its relation to PTSD. Ann NY Acad Sci 821:437–441, 1997

McNally RJ: Psychological mechanisms in acute response to trauma. Biol Psychiatry 53:779–788, 2003

Meakins JC, Wilson RM: The effect of certain sensory stimulation on the respiratory rate in cases of so-called "irritable heart." Heart 7:17–22, 1918

Mellman TA, Kumar A, Kulick-Bell R, et al: Nocturnal/ daytime urine noradrenergic measures and sleep in combat-related PTSD. Biol Psychiatry 38:174–179, 1995

Mellman TA, Knorr BR, Pigeon WR, et al: Heart rate variability during sleep and the early development of posttraumatic stress disorder. Biol Psychiatry 55:953–956, 2004

Morgan CA 3rd, Wang S, Mason J, et al: Hormone profiles in humans experiencing military survival training. Biol Psychiatry 47:891–901, 2000a

Morgan CA 3rd, Wang S, Southwick SM, et al: Plasma neuropeptide-Y concentrations in humans exposed to military survival training. Biol Psychiatry 47:902–909, 2000b

Morgan CA 3rd, Rasmusson AM, Winters B, et al: Trauma exposure rather than posttraumatic stress disorder is associated with reduced baseline plasma neuropeptide-Y levels. Biol Psychiatry 54:1087–1091, 2003

Munck A, Guyre PM, Holbrook NJ: Physiological functions of glucocorticoids in stress and their relation to pharmacological actions. Endocr Rev 5:25–44, 1984

Murburg MM, McFall ME, Lewis N, et al: Plasma norepinephrine kinetics in patients with posttraumatic stress disorder. Biol Psychiatry 38:819–825, 1995

Nemeroff CB: Psychopharmacology of affective disorders in the 21st century. Biol Psychiatry 4:517–525, 1998

Newport DJ, Heim C, Bonsall R, et al: Pituitary-adrenal responses to standard and low-dose dexamethasone suppression tests in adult survivors of child abuse. Biol Psychiatry 55:10–20, 2004

Neylan TC, Schuff N, Lenoci M, et al: Cortisol levels are positively correlated with hippocampal N-acetylaspartate. Biol Psychiatry 54:1118–1121, 2003

Nishith P, Mechanic MB, Resick PA: Prior interpersonal trauma: the contribution to current PTSD symptoms in female rape victims. J Abnorm Psychol 109:20–25, 2000

O'Donnell T, Hegadoren KM, Coupland NC: Noradrenergic mechanisms in the pathophysiology of post-traumatic stress disorder. Neuropsychobiology 50:273–283, 2004

Orcutt HK, Erickson DJ, Wolfe, J: A prospective analysis of trauma exposure: the mediating role of PTSD symptomatology. J Trauma Stress 15:259–266, 2002

Orr SP: Psychophysiologic reactivity to trauma-related imagery in PTSD: diagnostic and theoretical implications of recent findings. Ann NY Acad Sci 821:114–124, 1997

Perkonigg A, Kessler RC, Storz S, et al: Traumatic events and post traumatic stress disorder in the community: prevalence, risk factors and comorbidity. Acta Psychiatr Scand 101:46–59, 2000

Perry BD: Neurobiological sequelae of childhood trauma: PTSD in children, in Catecholamine Function in Posttraumatic Stress Disorder: Emerging Concepts. Edited by Murburg MM. Washington, DC, American Psychiatric Press, 1994, pp 233–255

Perry BD, Giller EL, Southwick SM: Altered platelet alpha2-adrenergic binding sites in post-traumatic stress disorder. Am J Psychiatry 144:1511–1512, 1987

Perry BD, Southwick SM, Yehuda R, et al: Adrenergic receptor regulation in post-traumatic stress disorder, in Biological Assessment and Treatment of Posttraumatic Stress Disorder. Edited by Giller EL Jr. Washington, DC, American Psychiatric Press, 1990, pp 87–114

Pich EM, Agnati LF, Zini I, et al: Neuropeptide Y produces anxiolytic effects in spontaneously hypertensive rats. Peptides 14:909–912, 1993

Pitman RK, Gilbertson MW, Gurvits TV, et al: Clarifying the origin of biological abnormalities in PTSD through the study of identical twins discordant for combat exposure. Ann NY Acad Sci 1071:242–254, 2006

Rasmusson AM, Hauger RL, Morgan CA, et al: Low baseline and yohimbine-stimulated plasma neuropeptide Y (NPY) levels in combat-related PTSD. Biol Psychiatry 47:526–539, 2000

Resnick HS, Yehuda R, Pitman RK, et al: Effect of previous trauma on acute plasma cortisol level following rape. Am J Psychiatry 152:1675–1677, 1995

Rohleder N, Joksimovic L, Wolf JM, et al: Hypocortisolism and increased glucocorticoid sensitivity of pro-inflammatory cytokine production in Bosnian war refugees with posttraumatic stress disorder. Biol Psychiatry 55:745–751, 2004

Rothbaum BO, Foa EB: Subtypes of posttraumatic stress disorder and duration of symptoms, in Posttraumatic Stress Disorder: DSM-IV and Beyond. Edited by Davidson JRT, Foa EB. Washington, DC, American Psychiatric Press, 1993, pp 23–35

Sapolsky RM: The physiological relevance of glucocorticoid endangerment of the hippocampus. Ann NY Acad Sci 746:294–304; discussion 304–307, 1994

Sapolsky RM: Glucocorticoids and hippocampal atrophy in neuropsychiatric disorders. Arch Gen Psychiatry 57:925–935, 2000

Schumm JA, Briggs-Phillips M, Hobfoll SE: Cumulative interpersonal traumas and social support as risk and resiliency factors in predicting PTSD and depression among inner-city women. J Trauma Stress 19:825–836, 2006

Selye H: A syndrome produced by various nocuous agents. Nature 138:32–34, 1936

Shalev AY, Freedman S, Brandes D, et al: PTSD and depression following trauma. Am J Psychiatry 155:630–637, 1998

Sheriff S, Dautzenberg FM, Mulchahey JJ, et al: Interaction of neuropeptide Y and corticotropin-releasing factor signaling pathways in AR-5 amygdalar cells. Peptides 22:2083–2089, 2001

Silva RR, Alpert M, Munoz DM, et al: Stress and vulnerability to posttraumatic stress disorder in children and adolescents. Am J Psychiatry 157:1229–1235, 2000

Smialowska M, Wieronska JM, Szewczyk B: Neuroprotective effect of NPY on kainate neurotoxicity in the hippocampus. Pol J Pharmacol 55:979–986, 2003

Southwick SM, Krystal JH, Morgan CA, et al: Abnormal noradrenergic function in posttraumatic stress disorder. Arch Gen Psychiatry 50:266–274, 1993

Southwick SM, Krystal JH, Bremner JD, et al: Noradrenergic and serotonergic function in posttraumatic stress disorder. Arch Gen Psychiatry 54:749–758, 1997

Stein MB, Koverola C, Hanna C, et al: Hippocampal volume in women victimized by childhood sexual abuse. Psychol Med 27:951–959, 1997a

Stein MB, Yehuda R, Koverola C, et al: Enhanced dexamethasone suppression of plasma cortisol in adult women traumatized by childhood sexual abuse. Biol Psychiatry 42:680–686, 1997b

Stein MB, Hofler M, Perkonigg A, et al: Patterns of incidence and psychiatric risk factors for traumatic events. Int J Methods Psychiatr Res 11:143–153, 2002a

Stein MB, Jang KL, Taylor S, et al: Genetic and environmental influences on trauma exposure and posttraumatic stress disorder symptoms: a twin study. Am J Psychiatry 159:1675–1681, 2002b

Storr CL, Ialongo NS, Anthony JC, et al: Childhood antecedents of exposure to traumatic events and posttraumatic stress disorder. Am J Psychiatry 164:119–125, 2007

Thorsell A, Carlsson K, Ekman R, et al: Behavioral and endocrine adaptation, and up-regulation of NPY expression in rat amygdala following repeated restraint stress. Neuroreport 10:3003–3007, 1999

Vedantam V: A political debate on stress disorder: as claims rise, VA takes stock. The Washington Post, December 27, 2005, p A1

Yehuda R: Biological factors associated with susceptibility to posttraumatic stress disorder. Can J Psychiatry 44:34–39, 1999a

Yehuda R (ed): Risk Factors for Posttraumatic Stress Disorder. Washington, DC, American Psychiatric Press, 1999b

Yehuda R: Current status of cortisol findings in post-traumatic stress disorder. Psychiatr Clin North Am 25:341–368, vii, 2002a

Yehuda R: Post-traumatic stress disorder. N Engl J Med 346:108–114, 2002b

Yehuda R: Risk and resilience in posttraumatic stress disorder. J Clin Psychiatry 65(suppl):29–36, 2004

Yehuda R: Neuroendocrine aspects of PTSD. Handb Exp Pharmacol (169):371–403, 2005

Yehuda R: Advances in understanding neuroendocrine alterations in PTSD and their therapeutic implications. Ann NY Acad Sci 1071:137–166, 2006

Yehuda R, LeDoux J: Response variation following trauma: a translational neuroscience approach to understanding PTSD. Neuron 56:19–32, 2007

Yehuda R, McFarlane AC: Conflict between current knowledge about posttraumatic stress disorder and its original conceptual basis. Am J Psychiatry 152:1705–1713, 1995

Yehuda R, Southwick S, Giller EL, et al: Urinary catecholamine excretion and severity of PTSD symptoms in Vietnam combat veterans. J Nerv Ment Dis 180:321–325, 1992

Yehuda R, Southwick SM, Krystal JH, et al: Enhanced suppression of cortisol following dexamethasone administration in posttraumatic stress disorder. Am J Psychiatry 150:83–86, 1993

Yehuda R, Boisoneau D, Lowy MT, et al: Dose-response changes in plasma cortisol and lymphocyte glucocorticoid receptors following dexamethasone administration in combat veterans with and without posttraumatic stress disorder. Arch Gen Psychiatry 52:583–593, 1995

Yehuda R, Levengood RA, Schmeidler J, et al: Increased pituitary activation following metyrapone administration in post-traumatic stress disorder. Psychoneuroendocrinology 21:1–16, 1996a

Yehuda R, Teicher MH, Trestman RL, et al: Cortisol regulation in post-traumatic stress disorder and major depression: a chronobiological analysis. Biol Psychiatry 40:79–88, 1996b

Yehuda R, Schmeidler J, Wainberg M, et al: Vulnerability to posttraumatic stress disorder in adult offspring of Holocaust survivors. Am J Psychiatry 155:1163–1171, 1998a

Yehuda R, Siever LJ, Teicher MH, et al: Plasma norepinephrine and 3-methoxy-4-hydroxyphenylglycol concentrations and severity of depression in combat posttraumatic stress disorder and major depressive disorder. Biol Psychiatry 44:56–63, 1998b

Yehuda R, Halligan SL, Bierer LM: Relationship of parental trauma exposure and PTSD to PTSD, depressive and anxiety disorders in offspring. J Psychiatr Res 35:261–270, 2001a

Yehuda R, Halligan SL, Grossman R: Childhood trauma and risk for PTSD: relationship to intergenerational effects of trauma, parental PTSD, and cortisol excretion. Dev Psychopathol 13:733–753, 2001b

Yehuda R, Spertus IL, Golier JA: Relationship between childhood traumatic experiences and PTSD in adults. Annu Rev Psychiatry 20:117–158, 2001c

Yehuda R, Golier JA, Halligan SL, et al: The ACTH response to dexamethasone in PTSD. Am J Psychiatry 161:1397–1403, 2004a

Yehuda R, Golier JA, Yang RK, et al: Enhanced sensitivity to glucocorticoids in peripheral mononuclear leukocytes in posttraumatic stress disorder. Biol Psychiatry 55:1110–1116, 2004b

Yehuda R, Halligan SL, Golier JA, et al: Effects of trauma exposure on the cortisol response to dexamethasone administration in PTSD and major depressive disorder. Psychoneuroendocrinology 29:389–404, 2004c

Yehuda R, Bryant R, Marmar C, et al: Pathological responses to terrorism. Neuropsychopharmacology 30:1793–1805, 2005a

Yehuda R, Engel SM, Brand SR, et al: Transgenerational effects of PTSD in babies of mothers exposed to the WTC attacks during pregnancy. J Clin Endocrinol Metab 90:4115–4118, 2005b

Yehuda R, Stavitsky K, Tischler L, et al: Learning and memory in aging trauma survivors with PTSD, in Neuropsychology of PTSD: Biological, Cognitive, and Clinical Perspectives. Edited by Vasterling JJ, Brewin CR. New York, Guilford, 2005c, pp 208–229

Yehuda R, Brand S, Yang RK: Plasma neuropeptide Y concentrations in combat exposed veterans: relationship to trauma exposure, recovery from PTSD, and coping. Biol Psychiatry 59:660–663, 2006

Yehuda R, Blair W, Labinsky E, et al: Effects of parental PTSD on the cortisol response to dexamethasone administration in their adult offspring. Am J Psychiatry 164:163–166, 2007a

Yehuda R, Golier JA, Tischler L: Hippocampal volume in aging combat veterans with and without post-traumatic stress disorder: relation to risk and resilience factors. 41:435–445, 2007b

Yehuda R, Teicher MH, Seckl JR, et al: Parental posttraumatic stress disorder as a vulnerability factor for low cortisol trait in offspring of holocaust survivors. Arch Gen Psychiatry 64:1040–1048, 2007c

Young EA, Breslau N: Cortisol and catecholamines in posttraumatic stress disorder: an epidemiologic community study. Arch Gen Psychiatry 61:394–401, 2004

Recommended Readings

Andrews B, Brewin CR, Philpott R, et al: Delayed-onset posttraumatic stress disorder: a systematic review of the evidence. Am J Psychiatry 164:1319–1326, 2007

Bisson JI: Post-traumatic stress disorder. BMJ 334:789–793, 2007

Bisson J, Andrew M: Psychological treatment of post-traumatic stress disorder (PTSD). Cochrane Database Syst Rev 18:CD003388, 2007

Bremner JD: Neuroimaging in posttraumatic stress disorder and other stress-related disorders. Neuroimaging Clin North Am 17:523–538, ix, 2007

Koenen KC: Genetics of posttraumatic stress disorder: Review and recommendations for future studies. J Trauma Stress 20:737–750, 2007

Yehuda R, Bierer LM: Transgenerational transmission of cortisol and PTSD risk. Prog Brain Res 167:121–135, 2008

Yehuda R, LeDoux J: Response variation following trauma: a translational neuroscience approach to understanding PTSD. Neuron 56:19–32, 2007

Yehuda R, Bryant R, Marmar C, et al: Pathological responses to terrorism. Neuropsychopharmacology 30:1793–1805, 2005

Zatzick DF, Galea S: An epidemiologic approach to the development of early trauma focused intervention. J Trauma Stress 20:401–412, 2007

Web Sites of Interest

National Center for PTSD. 2007. http://www.ncptsd.va.gov

National Institutes of Mental Health: Posttraumatic Stress Disorder. 2009. http://www.nimh.nih.gov/health/topics/post-traumatic-stress-disorder-ptsd/index.shtml

Chapter 32

Pharmacotherapy for Posttraumatic Stress Disorder

Wei Zhang, M.D., Ph.D.
Jonathan R.T. Davidson, M.D.

Posttraumatic stress disorder (PTSD) is a heterogeneous and complex disorder that may require a multifaceted treatment approach. Clinical studies have provided sufficient evidence for the efficacy and safety of both pharmacological and psychosocial interventions. Furthermore, increasing evidence now indicates that severe trauma can produce neurobiological changes (Garakani et al. 2006; Hageman et al. 2001), providing a framework for a rational psychopharmacological treatment of PTSD.

Historically, various agents have been used to treat traumatic stress. Casualties from the American Civil War were observed more than 100 years ago by Weir Mitchell, who commented on the use of bromides, opium, chloral, and brandy (Davidson and van der Kolk 1996). The issue of self-medication arose even then, and it continues to the present with the abuse of narcotics, alcohol, and illicit drugs. Wagner-Jauregg tried electrical stimulation for PTSD in Austrian soldiers in the early twentieth century. World War II brought more consideration of treatments for acute and chronic PTSD. These included barbiturates, insulin, stimulants, and ether. Sargant and Slater (1972) administered carbon dioxide in the 1960s for chronic PTSD and later suggested that antidepressant drugs might be applicable to chronic PTSD. Following combat stress reported after the Vietnam War, phenelzine was evaluated for efficacy in PTSD (Hogben and Cornfield 1981). Phenelzine, a monoamine oxidase inhibitor (MAOI), could enhance psychotherapy by promoting an abreaction. Thus, pharmacotherapy emerged as having either a primary therapeutic effect or an enhancing effect on psychotherapy. More recently, antidepressants, and especially the selective serotonin reuptake inhibitors (SSRIs), which are now the first-line pharmacotherapy for PTSD, have been used widely to treat PTSD and its comorbid conditions such as depression and other anxiety disorders. Other agents such as atypical antipsychotics, adrenergic suppressors, and anticonvulsants have also emerged as effective augmentation strategies.

Clinical guidelines for PTSD treatment include (but are not limited to) those published by 1) the American Psychiatric Association (2004); 2) the U.S. Department of Veterans Health Administration/Department of Defense (2003); 3) the International Psychopharmacology Algorithm Project (IPAP) (2005), of which the flowchart is presented in Figure 32–1; 4) the British Association for Psychopharmacology (Baldwin et al. 2005); and 5) the National Institute of Clinical Excellence (http://www.nice.org.uk/nicemedia/pdf/CG026fullguideline.pdf)

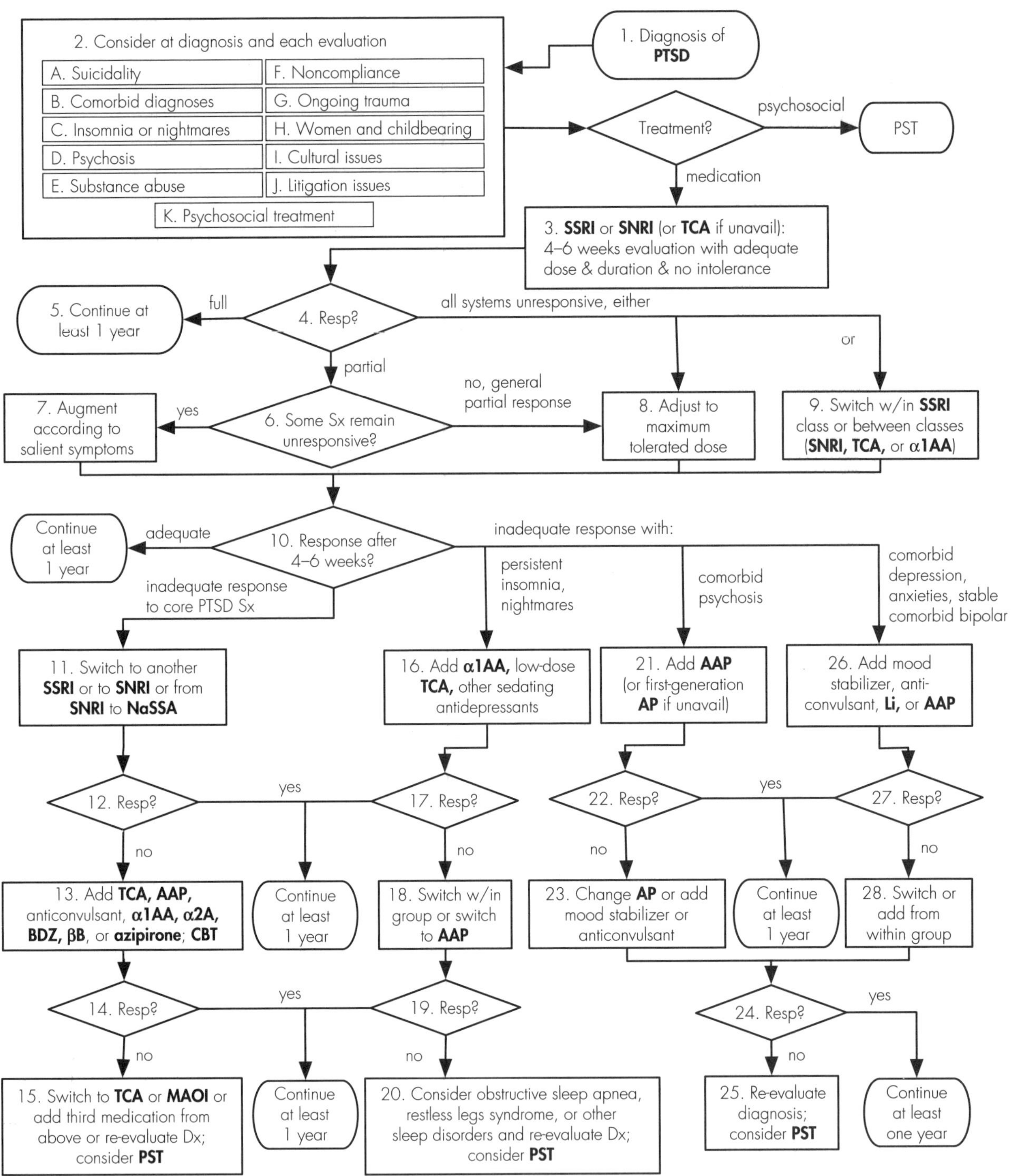

FIGURE 32–1. IPAP posttraumatic stress disorder (PTSD) algorithm version 1.0 (June 2005).

α1AA=α_1-adrenergic antagonist; α2A=α_2-agonist; AAP=atypical antipsychotic; AP=antipsychotic; βB=beta-blocker; BDZ=benzodiazepine; CBT=cognitive-behavioral therapy; Dx=diagnosis; MAOI=monoamine oxidase inhibitor; NaSSA=noradrenergic and selective serotonergic antidepressant; PST=psychosocial treatment; SNRI=serotonin-norepinephrine reuptake inhibitor; SSRI=selective serotonin reuptake inhibitor; Sx=symptoms; TCA=tricyclic antidepressant.

Source. Copyright ©2005 International Psychopharmacology Algorithm Project, http://www.ipap.org. Permission granted by IPAP for reprint in this edition for descriptive, not prescriptive, purposes.

Medication Treatments

Goals of Pharmacological Therapy for PTSD

The symptoms of PTSD represent both psychological and biological responses to a definable stressor, an environmental event. Two main categories of PTSD symptoms respond to medication: core symptoms and secondary symptoms (Davidson 1997). The core symptoms include the basic symptom cluster, as defined by DSM-IV-TR (American Psychiatric Association 2000): 1) intrusive reexperiencing of the original trauma (e.g., nightmares and flashbacks); 2) avoidance of stimuli associated with the trauma; 3) numbing, estrangement, and anhedonia; and 4) hyperarousal. The secondary symptoms include impaired function, poor resilience to stress, and comorbid conditions.

Medication theoretically may have different roles in treatment of PTSD: one is to seal over the distress and allow resumption of normal life activities, and another is to be part of a treatment plan designed to uncover the distress and allow for resolution of the traumatic experience. In the latter role, medication could serve as an adjunct to psychotherapy in working through the distress and trauma. Medication used with the intent of sealing over the pain was an early concept of treatment in the work of Sargant and Slater (1972). They found that when fears were repressed, patients improved; they also found that MAOIs and tricyclic antidepressants (TCAs) were more valuable than abreaction. In later years, the concept of medications that enhanced psychotherapy and abreaction gained recognition. Hogben and Cornfield (1981) noted that phenelzine enhanced psychotherapy in five combat veterans.

The goals of pharmacological therapy for PTSD are the same regardless of the conceptual model:

1. To reduce core PTSD symptoms in all clusters
2. To restore function
3. To improve life quality
4. To enhance resilience to stress or trauma
5. To minimize comorbidity such as depression, other anxiety disorders, and substance abuse
6. To prevent relapse
7. To prevent the development of PTSD in candidates at high risk of nonrecovery after a trauma

Review of Pharmacotherapy Literature in PTSD

The diverse presentation of symptoms in PTSD and the number of neurobiological systems that may be affected present a challenge in the search for effective pharmacological agents in treatment. However, a growing number of placebo-controlled clinical studies have provided evidence of efficacy for various pharmacological agents in PTSD (Table 32–1).

Selective Serotonin Reuptake Inhibitors

The SSRIs are now widely used in anxiety disorders, including PTSD. There are underlying reasons for the relevance of serotonin to PTSD. In some animal models, evidence suggests that serotonin receptor pathways are mediators of conditioned avoidance and learned helplessness as well as resilience to stress (Graeff et al. 1996). Clinically, certain symptoms such as poor impulse control, sleep disturbances, and repetitive responses to intrusive recollections seem compatible with postulated abnormalities in 5-hydroxytryptophan. Challenge studies with *m*-chlorophenylpiperazine (m-CPP) can produce aggravation of PTSD symptoms in a portion of subjects. The most preponderant evidence for the effectiveness of pharmacotherapy in treating PTSD is for the SSRIs, which are the first-line medications for PTSD recommended by most guidelines, including practice guidelines from the American Psychiatric Association (Ursano et al. 2004), International Consensus Group on Depression and Anxiety (Ballenger et al. 2004), and International Psychopharmacology Algorithm Project (2005). Sertraline and paroxetine are the two U.S. Food and Drug Administration (FDA)–approved agents for PTSD.

Citalopram. There has been only one placebo-controlled study of citalopram, in which the drug was compared against sertraline and placebo in a sample (N=58) of civilian PTSD patients and failed to show benefit of either drug for PTSD on the Clinician-Administered PTSD Scale (CAPS; Blake et al. 1995) total score and subscales of reexperiencing and physiological arousal relative to placebo (Tucker et al. 2003).

Fluoxetine. Eight placebo-controlled studies (six acute, two relapse prevention) of fluoxetine for PTSD have been published.

Van der Kolk et al. (1994) conducted a 5-week randomized, double-blind trial comparing fluoxetine and placebo in a diverse population of 22 women and 42 men, of whom 31 were veterans and 33 were nonveterans. Dropout rates for patients receiving fluoxetine were higher than those for patients receiving placebo; no intent-to-treat analysis was performed. Results indicated that by week 5 the active drug significantly reduced the

TABLE 32–1. Placebo-controlled drug studies in posttraumatic stress disorder

Study	*N*	Active drug, daily dosage (mg)[a]	Treatment length (weeks)[a]	Results
SSRIs				
Citalopram				
Tucker et al. 2003	58	Citalopram, 20–50 Sertraline, 50–200	10	No superiority of citalopram or sertraline over placebo
Fluoxetine				
van der Kolk et al. 1994	64	Fluoxetine, 20–60	5	Fluoxetine superior to placebo
Connor et al. 1999	53	Fluoxetine, 20–60	12	Fluoxetine superior to placebo
Martenyi et al. 2002b	301	Fluoxetine, 20–80	12	Fluoxetine superior to placebo
Martenyi et al. 2002a	131	Fluoxetine, 20–80	24 randomization	Fluoxetine superior to placebo in relapse prevention
Davidson et al. 2005	62	Fluoxetine, 10–60	24 randomization	Fluoxetine superior to placebo in relapse prevention
Hertzberg et al. 2000	12	Fluoxetine, 10–60	12	No superiority of fluoxetine over placebo
Martenyi et al. 2007	411	Fluoxetine, 20, 40	12	No superiority of fluoxetine over placebo
van der Kolk et al. 2007	88	Fluoxetine, 10–60 Eye movement desensitization and reprocessing (EMDR)	8	No superiority of fluoxetine over placebo
Paroxetine				
Marshall et al. 2001	551	Paroxetine, 20, 40	12	Paroxetine superior to placebo
Tucker et al. 2001	307	Paroxetine, 20–50	12	Paroxetine superior to placebo
Stein et al. 2003	322	Paroxetine, 20–50	12	Paroxetine superior to placebo
Marshall et al. 2007	70	Paroxetine, 20–60	10	Paroxetine superior to placebo, including dissociative symptoms
Unpublished data[b]	127	Paroxetine, 20–50	24 randomization	No superiority of paroxetine over placebo in relapse prevention
Sertraline				
Brady et al. 2000	187	Sertraline, 50–200	12	Sertraline superior to placebo
Davidson et al. 2001b	208	Sertraline, 50–200	12	Sertraline superior to placebo
Davidson et al. 2001a	96	Sertraline, 50–200	28	Sertraline superior to placebo in relapse prevention
Zohar et al. 2002	42	Sertraline, 50–200	10	Numeric but no statistical superiority of sertraline over placebo

TABLE 32–1. Placebo-controlled drug studies in posttraumatic stress disorder *(continued)*

Study	*N*	Active drug, daily dosage (mg)[a]	Treatment length (weeks)[a]	Results
Tucker et al. 2003	58	Sertraline, 50–200 Citalopram, 20–50	10	No superiority of citalopram or sertraline over placebo
Brady et al. 2005	94	Sertraline, 150	12	No superiority of sertraline over placebo in PTSD or depressive symptoms
Davidson et al. 2006a	538	Sertraline, 25–200 Venlafaxine ER 37.5–300	12	Sertraline superior to placebo on secondary measures
Friedman et al. 2007	129	Sertraline, 25–200	12	No superiority of sertraline over placebo
SNRIs				
Davidson et al. 2003	29	Mirtazapine up to 45	8	Mirtazapine superior to placebo
Davidson et al. 2006a	538	Venlafaxine ER 37.5–300 Sertraline, 25–200	12	Venlafaxine ER superior to placebo, not superior to sertraline
Davidson et al. 2006b	329	Venlafaxine XR 37.5–300	24	Venlafaxine XR superior to placebo
TCAs				
Reist et al. 1989	18	Desipramine, 100–200	4	Desipramine superior to placebo on depression but not PTSD measures
Davidson et al. 1990, 1993	62	Amitriptyline, 50–300	8	Amitriptyline superior to placebo on anxiety, depression, and IES scores
Kosten et al. 1991	60	Imipramine, 50–300 Phenelzine, 15–75	8	Both active drugs superior to placebo
MAOIs/RIMAs				
Shestatzky et al. 1988	13	Phenelzine, 45–75	5 crossover	No difference
Kosten et al. 1991	60	Imipramine, 50–300 Phenelzine, 15–75	8	Both active drugs superior to placebo
Katz et al. 1994	68	Brofaromine, 50–150	14	No statistical superiority of brofaromine over placebo
Baker et al. 1995	114	Brofaromine, titrated to 150	12	No difference in CAPS, but brofaromine superior on CGI
Other antidepressants				
Davis et al. 2004	41	Nefazodone 100–600	12	Nefazodone superior to placebo

TABLE 32–1. Placebo-controlled drug studies in posttraumatic stress disorder *(continued)*

Study	*N*	Active drug, daily dosage (mg)[a]	Treatment length (weeks)[a]	Results
Hertzberg et al. 2001	15	Adjunctive bupropion SR, 150–300	12	Bupropion SR superior to placebo in smoking cessation (primary outcome), but not PTSD
Becker et al. 2007	30	Adjunctive bupropion SR, 100–300	8	No superiority of bupropion SR over placebo
Antipsychotics				
Olanzapine				
Butterfield et al. 2001	15	Olanzapine, 5–20	10	No difference
Stein et al. 2002	19	Adjunctive olanzapine, 10–20	8	Significant decrease in CAPS total, CES-D and PSQI
Risperidone				
Hamner et al. 2003	40	Adjunctive risperidone, 1–6	5	Significant decrease in PANSS and CAPS reexperiencing
Monnelly et al. 2003	15	Adjunctive risperidone, 0.5–2	6	Significant decrease in OAS-M irritability, and PCL-M intrusive thoughts
Reich et al. 2004	21	Risperidone, 0.5–8	8	Significant decrease in CAPS-2 total, intrusive, hyperarousal
Bartzokis et al. 2005	73	Adjunctive risperidone, 1–3	16	Significant decrease in CAPS total, hyperarousal, Ham-A, PANSS positive
Padala et al. 2006	20	Risperidone, 4–6	10	Risperidone superior to placebo
Adrenergic suppressors				
Raskind et al. 2003	10	Adjunctive prazosin, 1–10	20 crossover	Prazosin superior to placebo in sleep and overall PTSD (CGI-I) symptoms
Raskind et al. 2007	40	Adjunctive prazosin, 1–15	8	Prazosin superior to placebo in sleep and overall PTSD (CGI-I) symptoms
Taylor et al. 2007	13	Adjunctive prazosin, 2–6	7 crossover	Prazosin superior to placebo in sleep and PTSD symptoms
Neylan et al. 2006	63	Adjunctive guanfacine, 1–3	8	No effect of guanfacine on sleep or PTSD symptoms
Anticonvulsants				
Hertzberg et al. 1999	15	Lamotrigine, 25–500	12	No significant superiority of lamotrigine
Davidson et al. 2007	232	Tiagabine, 2–16	12	No superiority of tiagabine over placebo
Tucker et al. 2007	38	Topiramate, 25–400	12	Topiramate superior to placebo on secondary measures

TABLE 32–1. Placebo-controlled drug studies in posttraumatic stress disorder *(continued)*

Study	*N*	Active drug, daily dosage (mg)[a]	Treatment length (weeks)[a]	Results
Benzodiazepines				
Braun et al. 1990	10	Alprazolam, 2.5–4.25	5	No change in PTSD
Cates et al. 2004	6	Adjunctive clonazepam, 2	2-week single-blind crossover	No change in PTSD
Other				
Kaplan et al. 1996	13	Inositol, 12 g	4	No effect of inositol on PTSD
Heresco-Levy et al. 2002	11	D-Cycloserine, 50	12 crossover	No effect of D-cycloserine on PTSD
Aerni et al. 2004	3	Cortisol, 10	1-month crossover	Cortisol superior to placebo in PTSD symptoms

Note. CAPS=Clinician Administered PTSD Scale; CES-D=Center for Epidemiologic Studies Depression Scale; CGI=Clinical Global Impression; CGI-I=CGI-Improvement; ER=extended release; Ham-A=Hamilton Rating Scale for Anxiety; Ham-D=Hamilton Rating Scale for Depression; IES=Impact of Event Scale; MAOIs/RIMAs=monoamine oxidase inhibitors/reversible inhibitors of monoamine oxidase–A; OAS-M=Overt Aggression Scale–Modified for Outpatients; PANSS=Positive and Negative Syndrome Scale for Schizophrenia; PCL-M=Patient Checklist for PTSD–Military Version; PSQI=Pittsburgh Sleep Quality Inventory; PTSD=posttraumatic stress disorder; SNRIs=serotonin-norepinephrine reuptake inhibitors; SR=sustained release; SSRIs=selective serotonin reuptake inhibitors; TCAs=tricyclic antidepressants.

[a]Except where indicated otherwise.
[b]http://www.nice.org.uk/pdf/CG026fullguideline.pdf.

overall PTSD symptoms (as assessed by the CAPS score), most notably in arousal and numbing. Nonveteran patients did better than the veteran patients, who had a higher level of symptomatology at week 5; depression improved more in the veterans taking fluoxetine than in those taking placebo. Connor and colleagues (1999) compared fluoxetine (up to 60 mg/day) and placebo in 53 civilians with PTSD in a 12-week double-blind study. Fluoxetine was more effective than placebo on most measures of PTSD severity at 12 weeks. The efficacy of fluoxetine in PTSD was also confirmed in the 12-week studies by Martenyi et al. (2002b), in which strong efficacy was found for fluoxetine over placebo in male combat veterans, communicating that SSRI therapy can be of benefit in this population and that combat-related PTSD itself does not automatically denote treatment resistance.

Other trials of fluoxetine have not been as encouraging. In a double-blind evaluation of fluoxetine and placebo in 12 male veterans (Hertzberg et al. 2000), fluoxetine failed to show efficacy. In a 12-week multicenter U.S. trial of two fixed doses of fluoxetine versus placebo, Martenyi et al. (2007) failed to demonstrate any significant differences between the groups; however, their findings might have been influenced by sampling (predominantly female), study design (fixed-dose, with a lower mean daily dose than their previous positive study) (Martenyi et al. 2002b), and other issues (higher placebo response of 38%). In an 8-week trial of fixed-flexible dose fluoxetine, eye movement desensitization and reprocessing (EMDR) and placebo (van der Kolk et al. 2007), between-group treatment difference was detected only between EMDR and placebo among completers on the CAPS total score, with no differences between fluoxetine and placebo on all measures, including those for PTSD and depressive symptoms. In the more important intent-to-treat comparison, no between-group differences were found.

Paroxetine. Paroxetine was approved in December 2001 by the FDA as a treatment of PTSD. Five placebo-controlled studies (four acute, one relapse prevention) have been published for PTSD. Two 12-week randomized, double-blind, placebo-controlled fixed-dose (20 and 40 mg/day) and flexible-dose (20–50 mg/day) trials of paroxetine, conducted by Marshall et al. (2001) and Tucker et al. (2001), respectively, showed benefits of paroxetine in PTSD across all trauma types and in both genders. Improvement appeared to be significant for all three symptom clusters (reexperiencing, avoidance/numbing, hyperarousal) and was associated with significant reduction in disability and comorbid depression. In addition, a pooled analysis of the above trials and a third 12-week placebo-controlled trial, which was partially positive on secondary outcomes, confirmed that paroxetine treatment resulted in significant improvement in all symptom clusters of PTSD, in sleep disturbance, and in response and remission rates (Stein et al. 2003). Additional data obtained in an urban, predominantly ethnic-minority sample, with Hispanic subjects being the majority (65%), supported efficacy for 10-week treatment of paroxetine versus placebo on core PTSD symptoms and associated symptoms (such as dissociation), with suggestions of benefit in areas of interpersonal difficulty (such as those involving affiliation and power) (Marshall et al. 2007).

Sertraline. Sertraline was approved by the FDA in December 1999 as a treatment for PTSD. Eight placebo-controlled studies (seven acute, one relapse prevention) have been published for PTSD.

Brady et al. (2000) studied 187 patients with PTSD in a 12-week double-blind, placebo-controlled multicenter trial with sertraline (50–200 mg). Sertraline was more effective than placebo across a spectrum of outcome measures. Similarly, Davidson et al. (2001b) reported significantly greater benefits with sertraline on most outcome measures, including CAPS total score and patient-rated Impact of Event Scale (IES). Interestingly, Davidson et al. (2002) also noticed in their mixed-model analysis of the two early studies that anger was more sensitive to sertraline treatment than other symptoms of PTSD, with substantial improvement as early as 1 week and persisting throughout the remainder of the treatment period.

In a 10-week pilot placebo-controlled study by Zohar et al. (2002), sertraline only showed only numeric but not statistical improvements over placebo on the primary outcome measure (CAPS-2) among subjects with predominantly combat-related PTSD. Other placebo-controlled trials of sertraline also have failed to show greater effect for drug over placebo, including the one mentioned earlier of sertraline and citalopram (Tucker et al. 2003), the one by Brady et al. (2005) in patients with PTSD and co-occurring alcohol dependence, and the report by Friedman et al. (2007). In addition, the efficacy of sertraline in the short-term treatment of PTSD was only partly confirmed by a three-arm (venlafaxine extended release [XR], sertraline, and placebo) study by Davidson et al. (2006b).

Two studies have examined the effects of combining sertraline with cognitive-behavioral therapy (CBT) in PTSD. A small 10-patient study of Cambodian refugees demonstrated greater benefit for the combination over sertraline alone in refractory patients (Otto et al. 2003), whereas a later and larger trial by Rothbaum et al. (2006) showed no overall advantage for combining treatments as augmentation to sertraline alone, although the investigators did find additional gains for the combination in those with a partial initial response to drug alone.

Serotonergic-Noradrenergic Antidepressants

Mirtazapine. Mirtazapine, a dual-acting antidepressant with antagonism at the serotonin types 2 and 3 (5-HT_2, 5-HT_3) and central presynaptic α_2 receptors, was found to be superior to placebo in PTSD response rate on the Short Posttraumatic Stress Disorder Rating Interview (SPRINT; Connor and Davidson 2001) in an 8-week pilot study (Davidson et al. 2003).

Venlafaxine. The serotonin-norepinephrine reuptake inhibitor (SNRI) venlafaxine XR has demonstrated efficacy in PTSD in both short-term as well as long-term studies of PTSD. Venlafaxine XR was effective and well tolerated in a 12-week three-arm (venlafaxine XR, sertraline, and placebo) treatment of PTSD (Davidson et al. 2006b).

Tricyclic Antidepressants

The three agents that have been studied in published placebo-controlled trials of TCAs in chronic PTSD are desipramine, amitriptyline, and imipramine. The outcomes may reflect, in part, differences among these drugs and other factors such as length of trials, dosages, or symptom profiles.

Desipramine was studied in 18 war veterans in a 4-week crossover trial (Reist et al. 1989). The results indicated no efficacy for the active drug. One limitation of the study was the brief trial period. Subsequent trials with TCAs did not find placebo differences until after the fourth week of treatment. An additional limitation was the dosage, which was relatively low (i.e., in the 100–200 mg/day range).

Amitriptyline (in dosages ranging from 50 to 300 mg/day) was studied in 46 subjects for 8 weeks and compared with placebo (Davidson et al. 1990). Results indicated a significant benefit (50% vs. 17%) compared with placebo on overall PTSD symptoms and also depressive and anxiety symptoms. Residual symptoms remained in many subjects, some of whom continued to meet criteria for PTSD at treatment end (45% of the subjects taking active drug compared with 74% taking placebo). In a subsequent study of the same sample, extended with 16 additional subjects, predictors of drug response were studied. Predictor analysis showed a greater response with amitriptyline in the less severely symptomatic veterans. The poorer responses were related to higher baseline levels of combat intensity, depression, neuroticism, anxious mood, impaired concentration, somatic symptoms, and feelings of guilt (Davidson et al. 1993).

In a study by Kosten et al. (1991), 60 veterans were studied over 8 weeks with a comparison of imipramine, phenelzine, and placebo. This study is discussed in the section below, "Monoamine Oxidase Inhibitors."

In summary, only three double-blind trials of TCAs for chronic PTSD are available. All of these studies involved veteran populations. Common to all studies was a lack of placebo response in war veterans with chronic PTSD. Two studies showed some improvement in PTSD; amitriptyline may have a preferential effect on avoidant symptoms, and imipramine may affect intrusive symptoms.

Monoamine Oxidase Inhibitors

Phenelzine. Two double-blind, placebo-controlled studies of phenelzine have been done in patients with PTSD.

In a study by Shestatzky et al. (1988) of 13 patients with PTSD and mixed trauma histories, subjects received phenelzine or placebo over 5 weeks; phenelzine was given in the range of 45–75 mg/day. No difference between medication and placebo was seen; the overall improvement could not be attributed to the active drug. The limitations of this study were the brief trial and the small sample size. The dropout rate was high (3 of the 10 patients receiving active drug), and the crossover design itself had some shortcomings.

The largest study was an 8-week randomized trial comparing two active pharmacotherapies—imipramine and phenelzine—with placebo in 60 veterans with PTSD (Kosten et al. 1991). Both phenelzine and imipramine were superior to placebo and preferentially beneficial for intrusive symptoms over avoidant symptoms. The response rate was 68% for phenelzine and 65% for imipramine, compared with 28% for placebo, on the IES. A unique strength of the study was the presumed therapeutic drug levels obtained by measuring platelet MAOI or imipramine plasma levels.

Brofaromine. Two double-blind, placebo-controlled studies of brofaromine have been done in patients with PTSD.

A controlled multicenter trial of brofaromine, a combined monoamine oxidase type A (MAO-A) and serotonin transport inhibitor, was conducted in 68 patients with primarily noncombat PTSD (Katz et al. 1994). Subjects received up to 150 mg/day of brofaromine. No difference between active drug and placebo was seen. In a subgroup with more chronic PTSD with symptom duration of at least 1 year, active drug significantly reduced PTSD symptoms.

In a second study in the United States, brofaromine was administered to 114 patients with PTSD, in whom the disorder arose mostly from combat trauma (Baker et al. 1995). This study was a 12-week randomized, double-blind, flexible-dose comparative design with two parallel groups. The primary outcome measure was change in the CAPS score. Both brofaromine and placebo groups showed significant reductions in the CAPS scores, but no difference between drug and placebo was found. Although brofaromine was somewhat promising in civilians with PTSD, the difference was modest, and the role of reversible inhibitors of MAO-A in PTSD is still very unclear. In addition, brofaromine has never been commercially available.

Other Antidepressants

The SSRI nefazodone was superior to placebo on overall symptoms of PTSD, as measured by CAPS total score, in a double-blind, placebo-controlled study conducted by Davis et al. (2004) among predominantly male combat veterans. However, nefazodone is associated with an increased risk of hepatotoxicity (28.96 cases per 100,000 patient-years) (Lucena et al. 2003) and even liver failure, and should not be used in people with liver disease. Trazodone is widely used to treat PTSD-related or drug-induced sleep problems, but its efficacy in PTSD has not been examined in well-designed or controlled studies. Bupropion sustained release (SR) has been evaluated in two double-blind, randomized, placebo-controlled trials of mainly combat veterans with PTSD. In the first of these studies (Hertzberg et al. 2001), the drug was associated with greater benefit on the primary outcome measure (i.e., smoking cessation) than was placebo, but no advantage accrued on PTSD measures. In the second trial, Becker et al. (2007) found no greater benefit for the drug over placebo on PTSD symptoms. In both studies, the majority of subjects were taking other psychotropic drugs.

Antipsychotics

The newer atypical antipsychotics show promise in their effects on mood and anxiety, as well as on psychosis. Psychotic features may be related to the core PTSD symptoms as part of the reexperiencing phenomenon or may be secondary to comorbid disorders such as major depression or substance abuse (Hamner 1997).

A growing number of studies have evaluated the use of atypical antipsychotic agents as adjunctive therapy for PTSD. It is particularly worth mentioning that all except one (Rothbaum et al. 2008) of the double-blind, placebo-controlled augmentation trials of antipsychotics in SSRI partial responders have yielded positive results on one or more measures in combat veterans.

In a small 10-week pilot study with a predominantly female veteran cohort, olanzapine monotherapy failed to outperform the placebo control, perhaps determined partly by a response rate of 60% in the placebo group (Butterfield et al. 2001). However, olanzapine was superior to placebo as adjunctive therapy for SSRI-resistant combat-related PTSD on PTSD-specific measures as well as comorbid depressive and sleep disorder symptoms (Stein et al. 2002).

Risperidone has been examined in four double-blind, randomized, placebo-controlled studies as adjunctive therapy for combat-related PTSD. A 5-week study by Hamner et al. (2003) demonstrated a superiority of adjunctive risperidone over placebo in improving reexperiencing symptoms of PTSD and comorbid psychotic symptoms. A small study by Monnelly et al. (2003) suggested that a low dose of add-on risperidone (0.5–2.0 mg/day) reduced PTSD-related irritability and intrusive thoughts. A third study, by Reich et al. (2004), evaluated the effectiveness of risperidone with or without the concomitant use of a antidepressant or a benzodiazepine in adult women with history of childhood abuses and found that risperidone was more helpful than placebo in reducing overall (measured by the CAPS total score) as well as intrusive and hyperarousal symptoms of PTSD. Additionally, Bartzokis et al. (2005) showed in a 4-month study that adjunctive risperidone improved a broad range of symptoms among patients with chronic combat-related PTSD, including core PTSD symptoms as measured by CAPS-2 total score and hyperarousal symptoms as well as overall anxiety and psychotic symptoms.

In one small pilot study (Padala et al. 2006), risperidone monotherapy also was found to be superior to placebo in reducing core PTSD symptoms as measured by

Treatment Outcomes Posttraumatic Stress Disorder Scale-8 (TOPS-8; Davidson and Colket 1997).

Adrenergic Suppressors

Autonomic arousal symptoms such as anxiety, restlessness, insomnia, hypervigilance, exaggerated startle response, and irritability are the core symptoms of PTSD. The locus coeruleus, a norepinephrine-rich area of the brain, is integrally involved in the moderation of adaptive and maladaptive responses to stress, as well as sleep, suggesting that noradrenergic suppression may have a possible benefit.

Raskind et al. (2003) conducted a double-blind, placebo-controlled crossover study and found add-on prazosin given at bedtime was superior to placebo in reducing trauma-related nightmares, sleep disturbance, and overall PTSD symptoms in patients already taking SSRI drugs. A more recent parallel placebo-controlled study with a larger sample size by the same group (Raskind et al. 2007) also confirmed findings in the initial study. Another placebo-controlled study, by Taylor et al. (2007), found that prazosin reduced nighttime PTSD symptoms in civilian PTSD subjects and that the effects were accompanied by increased total sleep time, rapid eye movement (REM) sleep time, and mean REM period duration without sedative-like effect on sleep onset latency. The pharmacological mechanisms of prazosin as possibly a "problem-specific" agent for improving sleep quality and nightmares are still under debate, but they may involve α_1-receptor-mediated modulation of REM (Krystal and Davidson 2007; Raskind et al. 2007).

Clonidine and guanfacine have been tested in open-label monotherapies or combination therapies and showed promise in treating PTSD-related sleep problems in children and adults (Harmon and Riggs 1996; Horrigan 1996; Horrigan and Barnhill 1996; Kinzie and Leung 1989; Kinzie et al. 1994). Standing in contrast is a negative placebo-controlled study of guanfacine (Neylan et al. 2006) in patients who, unlike those in the previous studies, were not preselected for having troublesome nightmares. In this study, guanfacine failed to show effect on PTSD symptoms, depression, general psychological distress, subjective sleep quality, or quality of life and was associated with significantly more side effects than placebo.

Propranolol has been studied mostly for the prevention of PTSD and is discussed in the section "Treatment of Acute Stress Disorder and Early Prevention of PTSD" later in this chapter.

Anticonvulsants

The rationale for the use of anticonvulsants/mood stabilizers is based on two premises: 1) patients with PTSD have affective instability, and 2) the mechanism of kindling may contribute to exaggerated reaction to stressors or to less stress being needed to induce a major pathological response. The kindling model suggests that antikindling drugs might be efficacious in PTSD (Friedman 1991).

Most preliminary evidence of the benefit of mood stabilizers or anticonvulsants in PTSD comes from open-label studies of lithium, carbamazepine, valproic acid, topiramate, and gabapentin. One of the few controlled studies, a 12-week, double-blind, placebo-controlled pilot trial of lamotrigine (Hertzberg et al. 1999), suggested superiority of lamotrigine over placebo for reexperiencing and avoidance/numbing symptoms of PTSD. However, the small sample size may have precluded these differences from being statistically significant. Tiagabine, a selective γ-aminobutyric acid (GABA) reuptake inhibitor (SGRI) was effective in reducing PTSD symptoms, including nightmares, in an open-label study (Connor et al. 2006), but a large placebo-controlled multicenter trial failed to show any advantage for drug over placebo (Davidson et al. 2007). Tucker et al. (2007) have reported mixed findings for topiramate versus placebo in a single-site study. No other replicative data have been presented in other controlled trials, so the role of this compound remains poorly understood in PTSD.

Benzodiazepines

Although anxiolytics such as benzodiazepines appear to be used widely in PTSD (Mellman et al. 2003), existing evidence does not yet support such use. In addition, withdrawal symptoms can be problematic, and adverse effects of benzodiazepines on mood, including severe rage reactions, have been noted (Risse et al. 1990).

The only randomized, double-blind study with benzodiazepines was a 5-week crossover trial with a 2-week interim phase, which compared alprazolam with placebo in a group of 10 Israeli patients with both combat- and civilian-related stress. Minimal efficacy was reported with maximum daily dosages of 4.25 mg/day of alprazolam (Braun et al. 1990). Although anxiety was slightly reduced, no effect on the core symptoms of PTSD was seen.

In a 2-week single-blind crossover study in which clonazepam 2 mg or placebo was added to preexisting treatment of PTSD, no difference was found between clonazepam and placebo in controlling nightmares (Cates et al. 2004).

An open-label study of alprazolam and clonazepam in 13 outpatients with PTSD found reduced hyperarousal symptoms but no change in intrusion or avoidance/numbing (Gelpin et al. 1996). Lowenstein et al. (1988) conducted an open-label study of clonazepam in subjects with PTSD and multiple personality disorder. In the five subjects described, dosages ranging from 1 to 6 mg/day over 6–21 months resulted in improvement in nightmares, insomnia, intrusive recollections, flashbacks, and panic. A shortcoming of this report was that many other subjects had received clonazepam but failed to respond, yet only those who responded were described in detail.

Brief Review of Comparator Trials and Predictors of Outcome

There have been four head-to-head comparator trials to our knowledge; each has been reviewed earlier under the specific medication category. They are citalopram versus sertraline (Tucker et al. 2003), fluoxetine versus EMDR (van der Kolk et al. 2007), sertraline versus venlafaxine ER (Davidson et al. 2006b), and imipramine versus phenelzine (Kosten et al. 1991). It would be premature to draw any specific conclusion based on these results as to whether one specific medication is superior to the others. Studies of PTSD similar in design to the Clinical Antipsychotic Trials of Intervention Effectiveness (CATIE) study for schizophrenia (Gorwood 2006) and the Sequenced Treatment Alternatives to Relieve Depression (STAR*D) for major depressive disorder (Fava et al. 2003) would provide important information regarding the comparative effectiveness of medications on key outcome measures of treatment efficacy, continuation, prolonged recovery, and health outcomes in PTSD.

Limited studies of predictors of treatment suggest that lower baseline levels of PTSD, depression, and anxiety symptoms, as well as intensity of trauma, were more predictive of favorable treatment outcome (Connor et al. 2001; Davidson et al. 1993). In one study with fluoxetine treatment (Davidson 2000), how well patients had done in the short term at month 3 was predictive of treatment response at month 15; with each 10-point increase on the self-rating Davidson Trauma Scale (Davidson et al. 1997) at month 3, there was a 29% lower chance of being a responder at month 15.

Treatment of Acute Stress Disorder and Early Prevention of PTSD

Although there has been widespread interest in the pharmacological prevention of acute stress disorder (ASD) or early PTSD, research in this area is limited and for the most part has been conceptually driven.

Two controlled studies—a randomized study by Pitman et al. (2002) and a nonrandomized study by Vaiva et al. (2003)—suggested that posttrauma propranolol may be preventive of some symptoms of PTSD, especially the physiological responses to subsequent trauma reminders. However, the methodological problems of both studies (e.g., small sample sizes, lack of control for comorbidity including substance abuse, concurrent medication use, and degree of β-receptor blockade) reduce the confidence that can be placed in their results.

Another randomized, double-blind prospective pilot study by Robert et al. (1999) in children with severe burn and ASD found that treatment with a low dose of imipramine for 1 week was more effective than chloral hydrate in relieving ASD symptoms, suggesting that antidepressants might work quickly and effectively in ASD.

Schelling and colleagues also have conducted three randomized, controlled studies on the effect of hydrocortisone in preventing PTSD following traumatic medical events, with one placebo (Weis et al. 2006) and one standard treatment (for perioperative period of cardiac surgery) (Schelling et al. 2004) controlled trial among patients undergoing cardiac surgery, and one placebo-controlled trial among septic shock patients (Schelling et al. 2001). Overall, they reported a lower intensity of PTSD symptoms related or unrelated to traumatic memories from the cardiovascular intensive care unit at 6–31 months follow-up and some benefits in shortening of medical treatment. However, the study population appeared be a medically heterogeneous group, and cardiac procedures and medications that could potentially affect PTSD symptoms were not well controlled. In addition, no baseline PTSD measures were collected.

Benzodiazepines are useful in controlling anxiety and agitation and in assisting sleep; however, they have not been proven to be particularly beneficial in ASD or early PTSD. In one controlled study by Gelpin et al. (1996), more subjects in the early treatment group with benzodiazepine (clonazepam or alprazolam) met criteria for PTSD at 6 months after the trauma (69%) than in the pair-matched control group (23%). Similar results at 6 weeks were also found in the study by Mellman et al.

(2002) comparing temazepam versus placebo among trauma survivors exhibiting early PTSD symptoms.

Long-Term Treatment and Relapse Prevention

Long-term and/or relapse prevention studies for PTSD are available for fluoxetine, paroxetine, and venlafaxine. The double-blind, placebo-controlled relapse prevention study of positive responders to the 12-week studies by Martenyi et al. (2002b), in which strong efficacy was found for fluoxetine over placebo in male combat veterans, also showed that subjects were less likely to relapse with a further 6 months of fluoxetine therapy (6%) than those with placebo therapy (16%) (Martenyi et al. 2002a). Further, in a 6-month open-label study with fluoxetine that was followed by 6-month double-blind, randomized treatment with fluoxetine or placebo, Davidson et al. (2005) reported that 22% of the subjects treated with fluoxetine versus 50% with placebo had a major relapse.

One relapse prevention study of paroxetine suggests that when the drug is discontinued after 12 weeks with a double-blind switch to placebo, and patients are followed for 6 months, there is no greater likelihood of relapse than in those who remain on the drug—the likelihood of relapse being low in both groups (http://www.nice.org.uk/nicemedia/pdf/CG026fullguideline.pdf).

In a relapse prevention study with sertraline, Davidson et al. (2001a) found the risk of relapse to be significantly less with drug (16%) than with placebo (48%) after 9 months of treatment, and the mean CAPS-2 score continued to improve from 45 (mild PTSD) at 3 months to 20 (minimal or no PTSD symptoms) at 9 months.

One large-scale study by Davidson et al. (2006a) of long-term (24-week) treatment with venlafaxine XR and placebo showed improvement in stress vulnerability and resilience, along with other primary and secondary measures of PTSD with treatment, and the highest effect size for venlafaxine XR over placebo was observed on the Connor-Davidson Resilience Scale (CD-RISC; Connor and Davidson 2003), relative to all other outcome measures. Remission rates were 51% for venlafaxine XR and 38% for placebo at 6 months, suggesting that with the passage of time beyond 3 months, additional new cases of remission accrue from continued treatment.

Special Populations

Comorbidity

According to the National Comorbidity Survey (Kessler et al. 1995), 79%–88% of the individuals with PTSD met criteria for at least one other disorder. It is important to factor this into our understanding of treatment response. In one study (Davidson and March 1995), the effect of amitriptyline was somewhat less in the face of multiple comorbidities, but we do not yet know if this is a general finding in PTSD. Certain individuals with comorbid alcohol dependence may respond favorably to an SSRI treatment, as indicated in an earlier study (Brady et al. 1995). In a double-blind trial to further substantiate the authors' promising open-label findings, no differences were found between sertraline and placebo (Brady et al. 2005).

Gender Issues and Treatment in Women of Childbearing Age

Most published studies of pharmacotherapy for PTSD involved male combat subjects and were negative or only weakly positive, yet evidence is increasing that women are more likely to develop PTSD than men (Breslau et al. 1997). On the other hand, for antipsychotic augmentation, most of the studies, which have been positive, took place in males. Do men and women with PTSD respond in similar ways to specific drugs? Are the sex differences in central serotonin synthesis of importance? The question of treatment and safety of medication in childbearing women is also an important issue. A guide for the pharmacological treatment of women of childbearing potential with PTSD and perinatal treatment of PTSD can be found on the IPAP PTSD Algorithm Web site (International Psychopharmacology Algorithm Project 2005). In severe or decompensating PTSD during pregnancy, the question of whether psychosocial treatment is adequate as a nonpharmacological alternative must be addressed.

Treatment in Children and the Elderly

There is a lack of studies assessing the efficacy and safety of pharmacotherapy of children with PTSD. SSRIs have been shown to be effective in other anxiety disorders, such as obsessive-compulsive disorder, social anxiety disorder, and generalized anxiety disorder, in children. Although these data might support indirectly the use for PTSD among children in clinical practice, PTSD-specific trials are needed. In addition, concerns for safety, such as suicidal ideation, seem to be a particularly important issue to monitor and address in this age population.

In elderly patients who present with PTSD symptoms, it is important to consider comorbid psychiatric and medical conditions as well as drug-drug interactions. Elderly PTSD patients appeared to have significantly higher rates of other psychiatric conditions, especially depression and anxiety disorders, than their non-PTSD control subjects (Spitzer et al. 2008). Appropriate medical workup may be necessary when there is an exacerbation of symptoms without apparent psychological triggers. Also, pharmacokinetic and pharmacodynamic considerations should be kept in mind, in particular the greater likelihood of accumulation of those drugs that are metabolized by oxidation and that have longer half-lives. The general rule of "start low and go slow" should be followed when treating an elderly patient with a pharmacological agent.

Cultural and Ethnic Issues

There is a paucity of data on the effect of cultural factors on either the diagnosis or the treatment of PTSD. Generally, studies have been conducted in a limited number of countries, and it has not yet been possible to compare a given treatment across cultures or across ethnic groups within a country. There may be important differences in dosage, metabolism (Lin 2001), and diet, as well as a lack of validation with respect to rating scales, in a particular culture. Limited evidence suggests that CBT emphasizing information, exposure, and cognitive restructuring might be successfully modified for subjects with different culture backgrounds to achieve additional gain when added to pharmacotherapy for PTSD, as indicated in a pilot study of Khmer-speaking Cambodian refugees (Otto et al. 2003). In addition, in a group of severely traumatized Cambodian refugee patients, both chronic PTSD and major depression symptoms improved significantly when patients were treated with a combination of clonidine and imipramine (Kinzie and Leung 1989).

Treatment Resistance

Response rates to current treatment strategies are approximately 60%–80%, with even lower remission rates (30% or less) after short-term treatment (Masand 2003). Many patients fail to adhere to treatment because of troublesome side effects such as gastrointestinal symptoms, sleep impairment, sedation, agitation, sexual dysfunction, or weight gain. Thus, strategies should be implemented to improve adherence, such as a thorough discussion of risks versus benefits, shared decision making with the patients, and close monitoring, especially during the initiation and titration of the medications.

When initial therapy with sufficient dose and duration fails, switching drugs within the same class or to a difference class, or augmentation with a sedating antidepressant, an atypical antipsychotic, a mood stabilizer, an anticonvulsant, or psychosocial treatment may be warranted. Of the existing psychosocial treatments, cognitive-behavioral therapies, including exposure therapy (particularly prolonged exposure therapy), anxiety management or stress inoculation, and cognitive therapy, have the strongest evidence of efficacy and produce significant improvement (Foa 2006). Although data are limited on the combination of drug therapy with CBT, preliminary results for the augmentation of existing drug therapy with CBT are modestly encouraging, especially among those who had a partial initial response to drug alone (Otto et al. 2003; Rothbaum et al. 2006). The only study to evaluate augmentation of ongoing CBT with drug therapy failed to find any advantage over augmentation with placebo (Simon et al. 2008). Psychosocial management, when effective, also appears to persist over time after completion of treatment.

Evidence supporting the above approaches is discussed earlier in the chapter under each medication category. In addition, references can be obtained from the IPAP algorithm for PTSD (International Psychopharmacology Algorithm Project 2005), where a stepwise approach to the pharmacotherapy of PTSD is outlined, taking into account salient symptomatology, comorbidity, and extent of response. Special issues, including suicidality, comorbidity, insomnia, psychosis, substance abuse, treatment adherence, ongoing trauma, women and childbearing, and cross-cultural and litigations issues, are discussed as well.

Novel and Experimental Approaches

Other interventions that have been studied include negative placebo-controlled trials of inositol (Kaplan et al. 1996) and D-cycloserine (Heresco-Levy et al. 2002) and a positive trial of low-dose cortisol (10 mg) in a placebo-controlled crossover study in three patients (Aerni et al. 2004).

There has also been one pilot study (Hollifield et al. 2007) suggesting that acupuncture, similarly to group CBT, yielded significantly better treatment response than a wait-list control group, as measured by self-reported PTSD symptoms. Symptom reductions at end of treatment were maintained at 3-month follow-up for both acupuncture and group CBT interventions. To our knowledge, no other trials have been reported on other alternative or herbal treatments of PTSD.

EMDR was superior to placebo on CAPS total score, but only among completers, not in the intent-to-treat population, in an 8-week trial of fixed and flexible-dose fluoxetine versus EMDR and placebo, as discussed earlier in the chapter.

Clinical Vignette

Mr. A is a 45-year-old Caucasian male who was involved in a motor vehicle collision on his way to work about 1 year ago. He was only mildly injured, with superficial skin lacerations, and recovered well physically without any complications. However, since the motor vehicle accident he had been feeling very anxious about driving and had only been able to manage driving to work on a different route so he can avoid the intersection where the accident occurred, and the new route took him 20 minutes longer to get to work. He had frequent nightmares about being trapped and not being able to escape and often woke up in the middle of the night in a cold sweat. He found it hard to concentrate on his work as an accountant and was startled easily whenever a car sped by or if he heard the siren of an ambulance. Three months after the accident, he finally went to his family physician, Dr. B, for his symptoms and distress. Dr. B prescribed a low dose of lorazepam at night and sertraline, which was titrated to 200 mg/day. Although Mr. A's overall anxiety about driving lessened after about 2 months on these medications, his nightmares persisted and even became more vivid on sertraline. He was able to fall asleep on lorazepam but woke up tired. He was then referred to a psychiatrist, Dr. C, who tapered him off lorazepam but added trazodone, which significantly improved his quality of sleep. Three months after being on the combination of sertraline and trazodone, he felt significantly better, with only two remaining problems: he still had significant fear about driving through that particular intersection where his car was hit, and from time to time he still struggled with nightmares. Prazosin was then added and titrated to 6 mg at bedtime, which controlled his nightmares. He was also referred to a nearby medical center, where he worked with a therapist on prolonged exposure therapy for driving through the intersection. Recently he has been doing very well. In his own words, "I feel like my old self again." Mr. A has been able to sleep well, without significant nightmares, and wakes up fresh with adequate energy. Work has become enjoyable again, and most of all he has been able to drive through that intersection without feeling panicky and has not been late for work since.

Conclusion

The field of pharmacological treatment of PTSD has observed a rapid growth in literature in recent years, and a wide range of medications have proven benefits in treating symptoms of PTSD, with the strongest evidence of efficacy for antidepressants (SSRIs, TCAs, MAOIs, SNRIs). Among the antidepressants, fluoxetine, sertraline, paroxetine, and venlafaxine XR are the most extensively studied in double-blind, placebo-controlled trials. Efficacy of SSRIs/SNRIs for reducing core symptoms of PTSD has been demonstrated in both short-term (4–12 weeks) and long-term (12 weeks and beyond) studies. These agents also appear to prevent relapse, strengthen resilience, and benefit some comorbid psychiatric disorders, although substance use disorders with PTSD continue to remain a major treatment challenge. Older antidepressants such as TCAs and MAOIs are of demonstrated efficacy in PTSD, especially among combat veterans with chronic PTSD. However, there have been few controlled trials in civilian populations, and issues of toxicity such as cardiovascular and anticholinergic side effects, seizure risks with TCAs, and dietary restrictions and risk of hypertensive crisis with MAOIs have precluded them from more frequent use.

Encouraging evidence also exists for atypical antipsychotic agents (as adjunctive therapies), adrenergic-inhibiting agents, and glucocorticoid agents (in the case of early prevention and perhaps even for treatment of chronic PTSD). However, most of these studies are open-label in design or limited in their sample sizes and are usually limited to short-term duration. The effects of anticonvulsants are ill defined, and efficacy data have not been particularly encouraging. It is unclear whether this reflects sampling characteristics, dosing problems, or intrinsic lack of efficacy of the drugs so far studied.

Despite existing effective pharmacotherapies for PTSD, many questions remain unanswered. Areas for future pharmacological research include management of the immediate aftermath of trauma to prevent the development of PTSD; improvement in drug tolerability, response, and remission rate; development of effective combination therapies; utilization of biological or genetic markers to direct population-specific treatment strategies; and naturalistic longitudinal studies to explore the disease course and treatment outcome of PTSD.

◀ Key Clinical Points ▶

- Effective treatments exist for posttraumatic stress disorder, including both pharmacological and psychosocial management.
- SSRIs and SNRIs are considered first-line pharmacological choices for the treatment of PTSD.
- An adequate medication trial requires treatment with an adequate dose for a sufficient duration (of at least 4–6 weeks when tolerated).
- Switching or augmentation strategies are recommended when an initial adequate trial of monotherapy fails. Approaches such as adding an atypical antipsychotic, an adrenergic agent, or cognitive-behavioral therapy have been proven beneficial as well.
- Treatment should aim not only to reduce symptoms for those with PTSD and other comorbid disorders but also to enhance psychological resilience to stress or trauma, prevent relapse, and restore function and quality of life.

References

Aerni A, Traber R, Hock C, et al: Low-dose cortisol for symptoms of posttraumatic stress disorder. Am J Psychiatry 161:1488–1490, 2004

American Psychiatric Association: Diagnostic and Statistical Manual of Mental Disorders, 4th Edition. Washington, DC, American Psychiatric Association, 2000

American Psychiatric Association: Treatment of patients with acute stress disorder and posttraumatic stress disorder. 2004. Available at http://www.psychiatryonline.com/pracGuide/pracGuideChapToc_11.aspx. Accessed January 2, 2009.

Baker DG, Diamond BI, Gillette G, et al: A double-blind, randomized, placebo-controlled, multi-center study of brofaromine in the treatment of post-traumatic stress disorder. Psychopharmacology (Berl) 122:386–389, 1995

Baldwin DS, Anderson IM, Nutt DJ, et al: Evidence-based guidelines for the pharmacological treatment of anxiety disorders: recommendations from the British Association for Psychopharmacology. J Psychopharmacol (Oxf) 19:567–596, 2005

Ballenger JC, Davidson JR, Lecrubier Y, et al: Consensus statement update on posttraumatic stress disorder from the International Consensus Group on Depression and Anxiety. J Clin Psychiatry 1:55–62, 2004

Bartzokis G, Lu PH, Turner J, et al: Adjunctive risperidone in the treatment of chronic combat-related posttraumatic stress disorder. Biol Psychiatry 57:474–479, 2005

Becker ME, Hertzberg MA, Moore SD, et al: A placebo-controlled trial of bupropion SR in the treatment of chronic posttraumatic stress disorder. J Clin Psychopharmacol 27:193–197, 2007

Blake DD, Weathers FW, Nagy LM, et al: The development of a Clinician-Administered PTSD Scale. J Trauma Stress 8:75–90, 1995

Brady KT, Sonne SC, Roberts JM: Sertraline treatment of comorbid posttraumatic stress disorder and alcohol dependence. J Clin Psychiatry 56:502–505, 1995

Brady K, Pearlstein T, Asnis GM, et al: Efficacy and safety of sertraline treatment of posttraumatic stress disorder: a randomized controlled trial. JAMA 283:1837–1844, 2000

Brady KT, Sonne S, Anton RF, et al: Sertraline in the treatment of co-occurring alcohol dependence and posttraumatic stress disorder. Alcohol Clin Exp Res 29:395–401, 2005

Braun P, Greenberg D, Dasberg H, et al: Core symptoms of posttraumatic stress disorder unimproved by alprazolam treatment. J Clin Psychiatry 51:236–238, 1990

Breslau N, Davis GC, Andreski P, et al: Sex differences in posttraumatic stress disorder. Arch Gen Psychiatry 54:1044–1048, 1997

Butterfield MI, Becker ME, Connor KM, et al: Olanzapine in the treatment of post-traumatic stress disorder: a pilot study. Int Clin Psychopharmacol 16:197–203, 2001

Cates ME, Bishop MH, Davis LL, et al: Clonazepam for treatment of sleep disturbances associated with combat-related posttraumatic stress disorder. Ann Pharmacother 38:1395–1399, 2004

Connor KM, Davidson JR: SPRINT: a brief global assessment of post-traumatic stress disorder. Int Clin Psychopharmacol 16:279–284, 2001

Connor KM, Davidson JRT: Development of a new resilience scale: The Connor-Davidson Resilience Scale (CD-RISC). Depress Anxiety 18:76–82, 2003

Connor KM, Sutherland SM, Tupler LA, et al: Fluoxetine in post-traumatic stress disorder. Randomised, double-blind study. Br J Psychiatry 175:17–22, 1999

Connor KM, Hidalgo RB, Crockett B, et al: Predictors of treatment response in patients with posttraumatic stress disorder. Prog Neuropsychopharmacol Biol Psychiatry 25:337–345, 2001

Connor KM, Davidson JR, Weisler RH, et al: Tiagabine for posttraumatic stress disorder: effects of open-label and double-blind discontinuation treatment. Psychopharmacology (Berl) 184:21–25, 2006

Davidson JR: Biological therapies for posttraumatic stress disorder: an overview. J Clin Psychiatry 58 (suppl 9):29–32, 1997

Davidson JR: Pharmacotherapy of posttraumatic stress disorder: treatment options, long-term follow-up, and predictors of outcome. J Clin Psychiatry 61:52–59, 2000

Davidson JRT, March JS: Traumatic stress disorders, in Psychiatry. Edited by Tasman A, Kay J, Lieberman J. Philadelphia, PA, WB Saunders, 1995, pp 1085–1099

Davidson JR, Colket JT: The eight-item treatment-outcome post-traumatic stress disorder scale: a brief measure to assess treatment outcome in post-traumatic stress disorder. Int Clin Psychopharmacol 12:41–45, 1997

Davidson JRT, van der Kolk BA: The psychopharmacologic treatment of posttraumatic stress disorder, in Traumatic Stress: The Effects of Overwhelming Experience on Mind, Body, and Society. Edited by van der Kolk BA, McFarlane AC, Weisaeth L. New York, Guilford, 1996, pp 510–524

Davidson J, Kudler H, Smith R, et al: Treatment of posttraumatic stress disorder with amitriptyline and placebo. Arch Gen Psychiatry 47:259–266, 1990

Davidson JR, Kudler HS, Saunders WB, et al: Predicting response to amitriptyline in posttraumatic stress disorder. Am J Psychiatry 150:1024–1029, 1993

Davidson JR, Book SW, Colket JT, et al: Assessment of a new self-rating scale for post-traumatic stress disorder. Psychol Med 27:153–160, 1997

Davidson J, Pearlstein T, Londborg P, et al: Efficacy of sertraline in preventing relapse of posttraumatic stress disorder: results of a 28-week double-blind, placebo-controlled study. Am J Psychiatry 158:1974–1981, 2001a

Davidson JR, Rothbaum BO, van der Kolk BA, et al: Multicenter, double-blind comparison of sertraline and placebo in the treatment of posttraumatic stress disorder. Arch Gen Psychiatry 58:485–492, 2001b

Davidson JR, Landerman LR, Farfel GM, et al: Characterizing the effects of sertraline in post-traumatic stress disorder. Psychol Med 32:661–670, 2002

Davidson JR, Weisler RH, Butterfield MI, et al: Mirtazapine vs placebo in posttraumatic stress disorder: a pilot trial. Biol Psychiatry 53:188–191, 2003

Davidson JR, Connor KM, Hertzberg MA, et al: Maintenance therapy with fluoxetine in posttraumatic stress disorder: a placebo-controlled discontinuation study. J Clin Psychopharmacol 25:166–169, 2005

Davidson J, Baldwin D, Stein DJ, et al: Treatment of posttraumatic stress disorder with venlafaxine extended release: a 6-month randomized controlled trial. Arch Gen Psychiatry 63:1158–1165, 2006a

Davidson J, Rothbaum BO, Tucker P, et al: Venlafaxine extended release in posttraumatic stress disorder: a sertraline- and placebo-controlled study. J Clin Psychopharmacol 26:259–267, 2006b

Davidson JR, Brady K, Mellman TA, et al: The efficacy and tolerability of tiagabine in adult patients with posttraumatic stress disorder. J Clin Psychopharmacol 27:85–88, 2007

Davis LL, Jewell ME, Ambrose S, et al: A placebo-controlled study of nefazodone for the treatment of chronic posttraumatic stress disorder: a preliminary study. J Clin Psychopharmacol 24:291–297, 2004

Fava M, Rush AJ, Trivedi MH, et al: Background and rationale for the Sequenced Treatment Alternatives to Relieve Depression (STAR*D) study. Psychiatr Clin North Am 26:457–494, 2003

Foa EB: Psychosocial therapy for posttraumatic stress disorder. J Clin Psychiatry 67 (suppl 2):40–45, 2006

Friedman MJ: Biological approaches to the diagnosis and treatment of post-traumatic stress disorder. J Trauma Stress 4:67–91, 1991

Friedman MJ, Marmar CR, Baker DG, et al: Randomized, double-blind comparison of sertraline and placebo for posttraumatic stress disorder in a department of veterans affairs setting. J Clin Psychiatry 68:711–720, 2007

Garakani A, Mathew SJ, Charney DS, et al: Neurobiology of anxiety disorders and implications for treatment. Mt Sinai J Med 73:941–949, 2006

Gelpin E, Bonne O, Peri T, et al: Treatment of recent trauma survivors with benzodiazepines: a prospective study. J Clin Psychiatry 57:390–394, 1996

Gorwood P: Meeting everyday challenges: antipsychotic therapy in the real world. Eur Neuropsychopharmacol 16 (suppl 3):S156–S162, 2006

Graeff FG, Guimaraes FS, De Andrade TG, et al: Role of 5-HT in stress, anxiety, and depression. Pharmacol Biochem Behav 54:129–141, 1996

Hageman I, Andersen HS, Jorgensen MB: Post-traumatic stress disorder: a review of psychobiology and pharmacotherapy. Acta Psychiatr Scand 104:411–422, 2001

Hamner MB: Psychotic features and combat-associated PTSD. Depress Anxiety 5:34–38, 1997

Hamner MB, Faldowski RA, Ulmer HG, et al: Adjunctive risperidone treatment in post-traumatic stress disorder: a preliminary controlled trial of effects on comorbid psychotic symptoms. Int Clin Psychopharmacol 18:1–8, 2003

Harmon RJ, Riggs PD: Clonidine for posttraumatic stress disorder in preschool children. J Am Acad Child Adolesc Psychiatry 35:1247–1249, 1996

Heresco-Levy U, Kremer I, Javitt DC, et al: Pilot-controlled trial of D-cycloserine for the treatment of post-traumatic stress disorder. Int J Neuropsychopharmacol 5:301–307, 2002

Hertzberg MA, Butterfield MI, Feldman ME, et al: A preliminary study of lamotrigine for the treatment of posttraumatic stress disorder. Biol Psychiatry 45:1226–1229, 1999

Hertzberg MA, Feldman ME, Beckham JC, et al: Lack of efficacy for fluoxetine in PTSD: a placebo controlled trial in combat veterans. Ann Clin Psychiatry 12:101–105, 2000

Hertzberg MA, Moore SD, Feldman ME, et al: A preliminary study of bupropion sustained-release for smoking cessation in patients with chronic posttraumatic stress disorder. J Clin Psychopharmacol 21:94–98, 2001

Hogben GL, Cornfield RB: Treatment of traumatic war neurosis with phenelzine. Arch Gen Psychiatry 38:440–445, 1981

Hollifield M, Sinclair-Lian N, Warner TD, et al: Acupuncture for posttraumatic stress disorder: a randomized controlled pilot trial. J Nerv Ment Dis 195:504–513, 2007

Horrigan JP: Guanfacine for PTSD nightmares. J Am Acad Child Adolesc Psychiatry 35:975–976, 1996

Horrigan JP, Barnhill LJ: The suppression of nightmares with guanfacine. J Clin Psychiatry 57:371, 1996

International Psychopharmacology Algorithm Project. 2005. Available at http://www.ipap.org/ptsd. Accessed April 24, 2009.

Kaplan Z, Amir M, Swartz M, et al: Inositol treatment of post-traumatic stress disorder. Anxiety 2:51–52, 1996

Katz RJ, Lott MH, Arbus P, et al: Pharmacotherapy of posttraumatic stress disorder with a novel psychotropic. Anxiety 1:169–174, 1994

Kessler RC, Sonnega A, Bromet E, et al: Posttraumatic stress disorder in the National Comorbidity Survey. Arch Gen Psychiatry 52:1048–1060, 1995

Kinzie JD, Leung P: Clonidine in Cambodian patients with posttraumatic stress disorder. J Nerv Ment Dis 177:546–550, 1989

Kinzie JD, Sack RL, Riley CM: The polysomnographic effects of clonidine on sleep disorders in posttraumatic stress disorder: a pilot study with Cambodian patients. J Nerv Ment Dis 182:585–587, 1994

Kosten TR, Frank JB, Dan E, et al: Pharmacotherapy for posttraumatic stress disorder using phenelzine or imipramine. J Nerv Ment Dis 179:366–370, 1991

Krystal AD, Davidson JR: The use of prazosin for the treatment of trauma nightmares and sleep disturbance in combat veterans with post-traumatic stress disorder. Biol Psychiatry 61:925–927, 2007

Lin KM: Biological differences in depression and anxiety across races and ethnic groups. J Clin Psychiatry 62 (suppl 13):13–19, 2001

Lowenstein RJ, Hornstein N, Farber B: Open trial of clonazepam in the treatment of posttraumatic stress symptoms in MPD. Dissociation 1:3–12, 1988

Lucena MI, Carvajal A, Andrade RJ, et al: Antidepressant-induced hepatotoxicity. Expert Opin Drug Saf 2:249–262, 2003

Marshall RD, Beebe KL, Oldham M, et al: Efficacy and safety of paroxetine treatment for chronic PTSD: a fixed-dose, placebo-controlled study. Am J Psychiatry 158:1982–1988, 2001

Marshall RD, Lewis-Fernandez R, Blanco C, et al: A controlled trial of paroxetine for chronic PTSD, dissociation, and interpersonal problems in mostly minority adults. Depress Anxiety 24:77–84, 2007

Martenyi F, Brown EB, Zhang H, et al: Fluoxetine vs placebo in prevention of relapse in post-traumatic stress disorder. Br J Psychiatry 181:315–320, 2002a

Martenyi F, Brown EB, Zhang H, et al: Fluoxetine versus placebo in posttraumatic stress disorder. J Clin Psychiatry 63:199–206, 2002b

Martenyi F, Brown EB, Caldwell CD: Failed efficacy of fluoxetine in the treatment of posttraumatic stress disorder: results of a fixed-dose, placebo-controlled study. J Clin Psychopharmacol 27:166–170, 2007

Masand PS: Tolerability and adherence issues in antidepressant therapy. Clin Ther 25:2289–2304, 2003

Mellman TA, Bustamante V, David D, et al: Hypnotic medication in the aftermath of trauma. J Clin Psychiatry 63:1183–1184, 2002

Mellman TA, Clark RE, Peacock WJ: Prescribing patterns for patients with posttraumatic stress disorder. Psychiatr Serv 54:1618–1621, 2003

Monnelly EP, Ciraulo DA, Knapp C, et al: Low-dose risperidone as adjunctive therapy for irritable aggression in posttraumatic stress disorder. J Clin Psychopharmacol 23:193–196, 2003

Neylan TC, Lenoci M, Samuelson KW, et al: No improvement of posttraumatic stress disorder symptoms with guanfacine treatment. Am J Psychiatry 163:2186–2188, 2006

Otto MW, Hinton D, Korbly NB, et al: Treatment of pharmacotherapy-refractory posttraumatic stress disorder among Cambodian refugees: a pilot study of combination treatment with cognitive-behavior therapy vs sertraline alone. Behav Res Ther 41:1271–1276, 2003

Padala PR, Madison J, Monnahan M, et al: Risperidone monotherapy for post-traumatic stress disorder related to sexual assault and domestic abuse in women. Int Clin Psychopharmacol 21:275–280, 2006

Pitman RK, Sanders KM, Zusman RM, et al: Pilot study of secondary prevention of posttraumatic stress disorder with propranolol. Biol Psychiatry 51:189–192, 2002

Raskind MA, Peskind ER, Kanter ED, et al: Reduction of nightmares and other PTSD symptoms in combat veterans by prazosin: a placebo-controlled study. Am J Psychiatry 160:371–373, 2003

Raskind MA, Peskind ER, Hoff DJ, et al: A parallel group placebo controlled study of prazosin for trauma nightmares and sleep disturbance in combat veterans with post-traumatic stress disorder. Biol Psychiatry 61:928–934, 2007

Reich DB, Winternitz S, Hennen J, et al: A preliminary study of risperidone in the treatment of posttraumatic stress disorder related to childhood abuse in women. J Clin Psychiatry 65:1601–1606, 2004

Reist C, Kauffmann CD, Haier RJ, et al: A controlled trial of desipramine in 18 men with posttraumatic stress disorder. Am J Psychiatry 146:513–516, 1989

Risse SC, Whitters A, Burke J, et al: Severe withdrawal symptoms after discontinuation of alprazolam in eight patients with combat-induced posttraumatic stress disorder. J Clin Psychiatry 51:206–209, 1990

Robert R, Blakeney PE, Villarreal C, et al: Imipramine treatment in pediatric burn patients with symptoms of acute stress disorder: a pilot study. J Am Acad Child Adolesc Psychiatry 38:873–882, 1999

Rothbaum BO, Cahill SP, Foa EB, et al: Augmentation of sertraline with prolonged exposure in the treatment of posttraumatic stress disorder. J Trauma Stress 19:625–638, 2006

Rothbaum BO, Brady KT, Davidson JR, et al: Placebo-controlled trial of risperidone augmentation for selective serotonin reuptake inhibitor-resistant civilian posttraumatic stress disorder. J Clin Psychiatry 69:520–525, 2008

Sargant WW, Slater E: The use of drugs in psychotherapy, in An Introduction to Physical Methods of Treatment in Psychiatry. Edited by Sargant WW, Slater E, Kelly D. New York, Science House, 1972, pp 142–162

Schelling G, Briegel J, Roozendaal B, et al: The effect of stress doses of hydrocortisone during septic shock on posttraumatic stress disorder in survivors. Biol Psychiatry 50:978–985, 2001

Schelling G, Kilger E, Roozendaal B, et al: Stress doses of hydrocortisone, traumatic memories, and symptoms of posttraumatic stress disorder in patients after cardiac surgery: a randomized study. Biol Psychiatry 55:627–633, 2004

Shestatzky M, Greenberg D, Lerer B: A controlled trial of phenelzine in posttraumatic stress disorder. Psychiatry Res 24:149–155, 1988

Simon NM, Connor KM, Lang AJ, et al: Paroxetine CR augmentation for posttraumatic stress disorder refractory to prolonged exposure therapy. J Clin Psychiatry 69:400–405, 2008

Spitzer C, Barnow S, Volzke H, et al: Trauma and Posttraumatic Stress Disorder in the Elderly: Findings From a German Community Study. J Clin Psychiatry 69:693–700, 2008

Stein MB, Kline NA, Matloff JL: Adjunctive olanzapine for SSRI-resistant combat-related PTSD: a double-blind, placebo-controlled study. Am J Psychiatry 159:1777–1779, 2002

Stein DJ, Davidson J, Seedat S, et al: Paroxetine in the treatment of post-traumatic stress disorder: pooled analysis of placebo-controlled studies. Expert Opin Pharmacother 4:1829–1838, 2003

Taylor FB, Martin P, Thompson C, et al: Prazosin effects on objective sleep measures and clinical symptoms in civilian trauma posttraumatic stress disorder: a placebo-controlled study. Biol Psychiatry 63:629–632, 2007

Tucker P, Zaninelli R, Yehuda R, et al: Paroxetine in the treatment of chronic posttraumatic stress disorder: results of a placebo-controlled, flexible-dosage trial. J Clin Psychiatry 62:860–868, 2001

Tucker P, Potter-Kimball R, Wyatt DB, et al: Can physiologic assessment and side effects tease out differences in PTSD trials? A double-blind comparison of citalopram, sertraline, and placebo. Psychopharmacol Bull 37:135–149, 2003

Tucker P, Trautman RP, Wyatt DB, et al: Efficacy and safety of topiramate monotherapy in civilian posttraumatic stress disorder: a randomized, double-blind, placebo-controlled study. J Clin Psychiatry 68:201–206, 2007

U.S. Department of Veterans Health Administration/Department of Defense: Clinical Practice Guideline for Posttraumatic Stress Disorder. 2003. Available at http://www.oqp.med.va.gov/cpg/ptsd/ptsd_gol.htm. Accessed January 2, 2009.

Ursano RJ, Bell C, Eth S, et al: Practice guideline for the treatment of patients with acute stress disorder and posttraumatic stress disorder. Am J Psychiatry 161:3–31, 2004

Vaiva G, Ducrocq F, Jezequel K, et al: Immediate treatment with propranolol decreases posttraumatic stress disorder two months after trauma. Biol Psychiatry 54:947–949, 2003

van der Kolk BA, Dreyfuss D, Michaels M, et al: Fluoxetine in posttraumatic stress disorder. J Clin Psychiatry 55:517–522, 1994

van der Kolk BA, Spinazzola J, Blaustein ME, et al: A randomized clinical trial of eye movement desensitization and reprocessing (EMDR), fluoxetine, and pill placebo in the treatment of posttraumatic stress disorder: treatment effects and long-term maintenance. J Clin Psychiatry 68:37–46, 2007

Weis F, Kilger E, Roozendaal B, et al: Stress doses of hydrocortisone reduce chronic stress symptoms and improve health-related quality of life in high-risk patients after cardiac surgery: a randomized study. J Thorac Cardiovasc Surg 131:277–282, 2006

Zohar J, Amital D, Miodownik C, et al: Double-blind placebo-controlled pilot study of sertraline in military veterans with posttraumatic stress disorder. J Clin Psychopharmacol 22:190–195, 2002

Recommended Readings

American Psychiatric Association: Diagnostic and Statistical Manual of Mental Disorders, 4th Edition. Washington, DC, American Psychiatric Association, 2000

Ballenger JC, Davidson JR, Lecrubier Y, et al: Consensus statement update on posttraumatic stress disorder from the International Consensus Group on Depression and Anxiety. J Clin Psychiatry 1:55–62, 2004

Connor KM, Zhang W: Recent advances in the understanding and treatment of anxiety disorders. Resilience: determinants, measurement, and treatment responsiveness. CNS Spectr 11 (10, suppl 12):5–12, 2006

Connor KM, Hidalgo RB, Crockett B, et al: Predictors of treatment response in patients with posttraumatic stress disorder. Prog Neuropsychopharmacol Biol Psychiatry 25:337–345, 2001

Davidson JR: Pharmacotherapy of posttraumatic stress disorder: treatment options, long-term follow-up, and predictors of outcome. J Clin Psychiatry 61:52–59, 2000

Davidson JR, Kudler HS, Saunders WB, et al: Predicting response to amitriptyline in posttraumatic stress disorder. Am J Psychiatry 150:1024–1029, 1993

Davidson JRT, van der Kolk BA: The psychopharmacologic treatment of posttraumatic stress disorder, in Traumatic Stress: The Effects of Overwhelming Experience on Mind, Body, and Society. Edited by van der Kolk BA, McFarlane AC, Weisaeth L. New York, Guilford, 1996, pp 510–524

Davidson JRT, Book SW, Colket JT, et al: Assessment of a new self-rating scale for post-traumatic stress disorder. Psychol Med 27:153–160, 1997

Fava M, Rush AJ, Trivedi MH, et al: Background and rationale for the sequenced treatment alternatives to relieve depression (STAR*D) study. Psychiatr Clin North Am 26:457–494, 2003

Foa EB: Psychosocial therapy for posttraumatic stress disorder. J Clin Psychiatry 67 (suppl 2):40–45, 2006

Gorwood P: Meeting everyday challenges: antipsychotic therapy in the real world. Eur Neuropsychopharmacol 16 (suppl 3):S156–S162, 2006

Hageman I, Andersen HS, Jorgensen MB: Post-traumatic stress disorder: a review of psychobiology and pharmacotherapy. Acta Psychiatr Scand 104:411–422, 2001

Masand PS: Tolerability and adherence issues in antidepressant therapy. Clin Ther 25:2289–2304, 2003

Rothbaum BO, Brady KT, Davidson JR, et al: Placebo-controlled trial of risperidone augmentation for selective serotonin reuptake inhibitor-resistant civilian posttraumatic stress disorder. J Clin Psychiatry 69:520–525, 2008

Simon NM, Connor KM, Lang AJ, et al: Paroxetine CR augmentation for posttraumatic stress disorder refractory to prolonged exposure therapy. J Clin Psychiatry 69:400–405, 2008

Web Sites of Interest

American Psychiatric Association. http://www.psych.org

Anxiety Disorders Association of America. http://www.adaa.org

British Association for Psychopharmacology. http://www.bap.org.uk

International Psychopharmacology Algorithm Project. http://www.ipap.org

National Institute for Health and Clinical Excellence. http://www.nice.org.uk

Chapter 33

Psychotherapy for Posttraumatic Stress Disorder

Monnica T. Williams, Ph.D.
Shawn P. Cahill, Ph.D.
Edna B. Foa, Ph.D.

Historical Background

Throughout the history of psychiatry and psychology, much has been written about the treatment of traumatized individuals, with special attention to combat-related experiences (e.g., Grinker and Spiegel 1944; Hurst 1919). This reflects the wide recognition that chronic psychological disturbances after traumatic experiences are a common occurrence, frequently requiring therapeutic intervention.

Learning theory provides a rich body of knowledge that has influenced current conceptualizations and treatments of traumatic reactions. In this tradition, chronic posttraumatic symptoms were viewed as severe fear reactions acquired through Pavlovian conditioning. Indeed, that conceptualization of traumatic reactions as the prototype of pathological fear is exemplified in the work of Dollard and Miller (1950). To illustrate how phobias are learned, the authors describe the case of a fighter pilot who developed extreme fear and avoidance of airplanes after being exposed to intensely fear-provoking stimuli during one of his missions. Rachman's work (1978) on fear and courage also exemplified the conception of traumatic reactions as rooted in fear and anxiety. To study basic mechanisms of fear and courage, Rachman chose military personnel as subjects for his experiments (as Dollard and Miller had). Correspondingly, Rachman (1980) conceptualized natural processes of recovery from a traumatic event in terms of reductions in anxiety reactions.

The official placement of posttraumatic stress disorder (PTSD) among the anxiety disorders in DSM-III (American Psychiatric Association 1980) acknowledges that anxiety is a common and potentially chronic reaction to trauma. The symptoms of PTSD overlap considerably with those of other anxiety disorders. For example, arousal symptoms such as hypervigilance, sleep disturbances, irritability, and difficulty concentrating are common to both PTSD and generalized anxiety disorder (GAD). Fear and avoidance are common to PTSD, specific phobia, social phobia, and panic disorder with agoraphobia. Furthermore, escape/avoidance behaviors in PTSD sufferers, like many avoidance behaviors in individuals with other anxiety disorders, are driven by the strong desire of anxious individuals to prevent states of high anxiety as well as a tendency toward exaggerating the probability of threat and the cost associated with the threat (Foa and Kozak 1986; Foa et al. 1989b, 1996). Hence, with the codification of PTSD, cognitive-behavioral theories of PTSD have conceptualized the disorder as a phobia with an especially extensive generalization (e.g., Foa et al. 1989b; Keane et al. 1985).

The conceptualization of the acquisition and extinction of pathological fear within learning theory prompted extensive research on the measurement and treatment of fear and anxiety with cognitive-behavioral therapy (CBT) techniques beginning in the 1960s. The first CBT techniques that were successfully applied to treating morbid anxiety were variants of exposure therapy (Foa et al. 1989a). Techniques involving imaginal and in vivo exposure to feared objects, situations, and memories had already been shown to be effective in the treatment of specific phobias (e.g., Bandura et al. 1969; Wolpe 1958), agoraphobia (e.g., Emmelkamp and Wessels 1975; Mathews et al. 1977), public speaking phobia (Paul 1996), and obsessive-compulsive disorder (e.g., Foa and Goldstein 1978; Meyer 1966).

Interestingly, the discovery that people who suffer trauma-related disturbances can be helped by exposure to trauma reminders, including traumatic memories, comes in part from the wide recognition that traumatic reactions are predominately anxiety related. The exposure principle is clearly imbedded in the early literature on treatment of trauma-related disturbances. For example, in 1893 Freud and Breuer described the phenomenology and treatment of hysteria, a condition that would likely be called PTSD in current diagnostic systems; hysterical symptoms disappeared when the therapist succeeded in bringing to light the memory of the traumatic event and the patient then described the event in the greatest possible detail and put the accompanying affect into words (see Freud 1973). A similar formulation was offered by emotional processing theory (Foa and Kozak 1986) and the treatment of PTSD that has ensued from that theory, which is focused on systematic, repeated recounting (i.e., imaginal exposure) of the traumatic memory.

The 1970s witnessed a new development in the treatment of anxiety disorders that parallels the development of exposure therapy described above. This approach is called *anxiety management training* (e.g., Suinn and Richardson 1971) and *stress inoculation training* (SIT; e.g., Meichenbaum 2007). The basic tenet of this treatment is that anxiety symptoms can be ameliorated by educating patients about anxiety symptoms, teaching them how to manage the symptoms, and providing skills to cope with future stresses and anxiety-evoking situations. SIT has been successfully applied to phobic patients (Meichenbaum 1974).

To understand the continuity between treatment of anxiety disorders developed prior to 1980 and treatments developed specifically for PTSD after 1980, it is important to recognize that researchers studying CBT interventions did not view themselves as developing specific treatments for specific disorders per se. Rather, they viewed themselves as studying processes related to fear reduction in general, with the assumption that knowledge gained from investigating methods of fear reduction with one group of individuals (e.g., those with agoraphobia) would be relevant to fear reduction among other anxious individuals (e.g., those with obsessive-compulsive disorder).

Recognition that the basis of PTSD lies in pathological anxiety and that CBT is effective for anxiety disorders led to the application of these procedures to the treatment of trauma victims with PTSD. Initial reports took the form of case studies of treatment for combat veterans (e.g., Black and Keane 1982; Fairbank and Keane 1982), rape victims (e.g., Rothbaum and Foa 1991; Wolff 1977), and motor vehicle accident victims (Kraft and Al-Issa 1965; Kushner 1965). These early case reports demonstrated trauma experts' recognition that the treatment for anxiety could naturally be applied to trauma-related psychological difficulties.

At first, exposure therapy programs were generally employed with veterans (e.g., Cooper and Clum 1989; Keane et al. 1989), and anxiety management programs such as SIT were generally employed with female assault victims (Veronen and Kilpatrick 1983). Foa et al. (1991) were the first to examine the efficacy of both exposure therapy and SIT with female victims of rape. More recent CBT studies have examined the efficacy of exposure therapy in combination with SIT, cognitive therapy, or other emotion regulation skills and included patients with traumatic experiences other than combat and assault; they included victims of childhood sexual abuse (e.g., Cloitre et al. 2002), refugees (Paunovic and Ost 2001), female assault victims (Foa et al. 1999, 2005), and mixed trauma samples (e.g., Marks et al. 1998). These studies suggested that the addition of SIT or cognitive restructuring did not add to the efficacy of exposure therapy alone (Foa et al. 2003).

In summary, from early on it was widely recognized that trauma-related psychological problems were rooted in fear and anxiety. In the 1960s and 1970s, there was already a great deal of knowledge concerning the effectiveness of CBT, in particular exposure therapy, in reducing anxiety symptoms in a variety of anxiety disorders. The traditional descriptions of successful treatments for posttraumatic disturbances converge with modern developments in the area of PTSD, both advocating exposure to the traumatic memory and reminders of the trauma. There was also evidence for the effectiveness of stress inoculation programs for anxiety disorders. In anxiety clinics, where behavioral and cognitive therapies were conducted, trauma victims were viewed as suffering from pathological anxiety and were treated in the same manner as other anxiety patients. These techniques were later validated in larger, randomized studies on trauma-related disturbances and PTSD (e.g., Foa et al. 1991, 1999, 2005; Keane et al. 1989; Marks et al. 1998; Resick et al. 2002).

Cognitive-Behavioral Therapy

Cognitive-Behavioral Interventions for PTSD: An Overview

CBT is not a single technique but rather a broad approach that includes a range of techniques, the goals of which are to reduce the intensity and frequency of distressing negative emotional reactions, to modify erroneous cognitions, and to promote functioning. In the field of PTSD the most-studied and best-supported treatments are all forms of CBT and include exposure therapy, SIT, and variations of cognitive therapy. Each of these interventions has been administered as a primary intervention or combined with other interventions to form a more comprehensive treatment package. A fourth treatment for PTSD that has received empirical support is eye movement desensitization and reprocessing (EMDR; Shapiro 2001), a treatment that utilizes elements of exposure and cognitive restructuring but also includes therapist-directed rapid eye movements or other laterally alternating activities. Two recent innovations in the treatment of PTSD are the application of imagery rehearsal therapy to PTSD-related nightmares and the use of technology to assist in the implementation of CBT, such as the use of virtual reality technology to implement exposure therapy and the administration of therapy via the Internet.

Exposure Therapy

PTSD is characterized by the reexperiencing of the traumatic event through intrusive and distressing memories, nightmares, and flashbacks and by strong emotional and physiological reactions triggered by trauma-related reminders. In addition, most individuals with PTSD attempt to ward off the intrusive symptoms and avoid the trauma reminders, even when such trigger stimuli are not inherently dangerous. Given these two broad categories of feared stimuli (the traumatic memories and triggers that are reminders of the trauma), the core components of exposure programs for the disorder are:

1. *Imaginal exposure*, revisiting the traumatic memory, repeatedly recounting it aloud, and processing the revisiting experience
2. *In vivo exposure*, the repeated confrontation with trauma-related situations and objects that evoke excessive anxiety but are not inherently dangerous

The goal of this treatment is to promote processing of the traumatic memory (Foa et al. 2006a) and to reduce distress and avoidance elicited by the trauma reminders. Additionally, individuals with pronounced symptoms of emotional numbing and depression are encouraged to engage in pleasurable activities even if these activities have dropped out of their repertoire due to loss of interest rather than because they elicit fear or anxiety (Foa et al. 2007). The rationale for this is similar to the use of behavioral activation strategies in the treatment of depression (Martell et al. 2001).

Exposure therapy programs that have been evaluated in randomized, controlled studies differ in which exposure techniques are implemented and how they are implemented, along with what other nonexposure techniques are utilized. For example, some researchers have relied exclusively on imaginal exposure (e.g., Bryant et al. 2003a; Cooper and Clum 1989; Keane et al. 1989; Tarrier et al. 1999), whereas Basoglu and colleagues (2005) have relied exclusively on in vivo exposure. By contrast, the prolonged exposure program developed by Foa and colleagues (1991, 1999, 2005, 2007; see also Resick et al. 2002; Rothbaum et al. 2005, 2006; Schnurr et al. 2007) and a similar program developed by Marks and colleagues (1998; see also Richards et al. 1994; Taylor et al. 2003) utilize both imaginal and in vivo techniques. Exposure therapy programs also differ in the extent to which exposure techniques are the primary focus in therapy (they are the primary focus in the programs developed by Foa and colleagues and Marks and colleagues) or are substantially supplemented with other CBT techniques such as stress inoculation and cognitive therapy procedures, as they are in the CBT program developed by Blanchard, Hickling, and colleagues (2003a; Hickling and Blanchard 1997; see also Maercker et al. 2006). In some programs, such as Resick's cognitive processing therapy (CPT) program (a CBT treatment with a smaller imaginal component) and the Blanchard and Hickling program just mentioned, exposure to the traumatic memory is implemented through narrative writing exercises.

Stress Inoculation Training

Veronen and Kilpatrick (1983) adopted Meichenbaum's (2007) SIT approach for the treatment of PTSD symptoms in female rape victims. As applied to PTSD, the SIT program includes education about trauma-related symptoms as well as anxiety management techniques such as controlled breathing and relaxation training, cognitive restructuring, guided (task-enhancing) self-dialogue, assertiveness training, role playing, covert modeling, and thought stopping. Once the various techniques have been introduced, the therapist and patient work together to select and implement the techniques in a flexible manner to address patients' current concerns or specific symptoms. As with exposure therapy, SIT programs vary from one another, the most notable difference being that some programs include an exposure component (e.g., Veronen and Kilpatrick 1983) whereas others do not (e.g., Foa et al. 1991, 1999). Although interest in the study of SIT for PTSD has diminished, one innovative use of SIT has been to target anger among veterans with chronic PTSD and significant anger problems (Chemtob et al. 1997).

Cognitive Therapy

Cognitive therapy for PTSD is derived from Beck's model of treatment for depression (A.T. Beck et al. 1979) and its extension to anxiety (A.T. Beck et al. 1985), wherein the goal of therapy is to help patients identify trauma-related dysfunctional beliefs that influence emotional and behavioral responses to a situation (Marks et al. 1998; Tarrier et al. 1999). Once these are identified, patients are taught to evaluate the thoughts in a logical, evidence-based manner. Information that supports or refutes the belief is examined, as are alternative ways of interpreting the problematic situation. The therapist helps patients weigh the evidence and consider alternative interpretations before deciding whether the belief accurately reflects reality, and, if it does not, to replace or modify it. As with other treatment programs already discussed, cognitive therapy programs differ in the length and number of sessions. Moreover, some cognitive therapy programs include an exposure component—such as Resick's CPT program (Resick and Schnicke 1992; Resick et al. 2002) and the cognitive therapy program based on Ehlers' and Clark's cognitive theory of PTSD (Ehlers and Clark 2000; Ehlers et al. 2003, 2005)—whereas other cognitive therapy programs do not (e.g., Marks et al. 1998; Tarrier et al. 1999).

Eye Movement Desensitization and Reprocessing

In EMDR (Shapiro 1989, 1991, 2001), the therapist asks the patient to generate images, thoughts, and feelings about the trauma; evaluate their aversive qualities; and make alternative cognitive appraisals of the trauma or their behavior during it. As the patient initially focuses on the distressing images and thoughts, and later focuses on the alternative cognition, the therapist elicits rapid, laterally alternating eye movements by instructing the patient to visually track the therapist's finger as it moves back and forth across the patient's visual field. Originally, Shapiro (1991) regarded these eye movements as essential to the processing of the traumatic memory, but the importance of the eye movements has not gained empirical support (for a review, see Spates et al. 2008). Some EMDR programs have replaced the eye movement component with other procedures (e.g., having the patient alternate finger tapping from the right to the left hand; Shapiro 2001), indicating that equivalent mechanisms underlie the various procedures. However, dismantling studies have not demonstrated that these movements affect symptom reduction (Cahill et al. 1999), and well-designed research studies assessing treatment outcomes have found no advantage of using EMDR versus exposure therapy alone (Rothbaum et al. 2005; Taylor et al. 2003).

Outcome of Clinical Trials for Chronic PTSD

The efficacy of CBT in the treatment of PTSD among adults has been the focus of considerable research in the past 20 years that has been summarized in several narrative and meta-analytic reviews. For example, in the second edition of the International Society for Traumatic Stress Studies (ISTSS) treatment guidelines (Foa et al. 2008), Cahill et al. (2008) identified 64 studies in which participants were randomly assigned to some form of CBT or at least one other study group. The single most common comparison was a wait-list control condition (39 studies), though several (19) studies used some form of nonspecific control treatment, such as relaxation, supportive counseling, psychoeducation, or treatment as usual. In addition, 12 studies directly compared two or more CBT programs (excluding EMDR). These included studies of some form of exposure therapy compared with SIT (Foa et al., 1991, 1999) or cognitive therapy (Marks et al. 1998; Resick et al. 2002;

Tarrier et al. 1999), as well as comparisons of individual CBT programs versus combined programs, including exposure therapy plus either SIT or cognitive therapy versus: exposure therapy alone (Foa et al. 1999, 2005; Marks et al. 1998; Paunovic and Ost 2001), SIT alone (Foa et al. 1999), or cognitive therapy alone (Bryant et al. 2003a; Marks et al. 1998; Resick et al. 2008).

Another seven studies directly compared EMDR to some other CBT program (Devilly and Spence 1999; Ironson et al. 2002; Lee et al. 2002; Power et al. 2002; Rothbaum et al. 2005; Taylor et al. 2003; Vaughan et al. 1994), although concerns have been raised about the randomization procedures used in the Devilly and Spence study (1999). Separate chapters on EMDR in the earlier (Chemtob et al. 2000) and revised (Spates et al. 2008) editions of the ISTSS guidelines together identify a total of 18 studies—including the already-mentioned seven studies comparing EMDR to other types of CBT—that either assessed the efficacy of EMDR or attempted to dismantle the components of EMDR, such as eye movements and other laterally alternating stimuli (e.g., finger tapping; Pitman et al. 1996a), and its cognitive restructuring component (Cusack and Spates 1999).

In broad summary of the 75 studies reviewed in the ISTSS guideline chapters (Foa et al. 2008), the vast majority found that treatment with CBT was associated with significant improvement on measures of PTSD symptoms and, frequently, other associated emotional reactions such as depression and anxiety. Moreover, CBT is routinely found to be significantly more efficacious than wait-list control conditions and to be as efficacious as or more efficacious than nonspecific control treatments. However, studies directly comparing different CBT treatments have found only small differences between treatment conditions, differences that generally fail to achieve statistical significance, possibly due in part to sample sizes that are not large enough to detect small differences. In addition, the direction of the differences between conditions does not reliably replicate. For example, the first study to directly compare exposure therapy versus SIT (Foa et al. 1991) found some evidence of a slight advantage for SIT, particularly immediately posttreatment, whereas a subsequent study (Foa et al. 1999) found some evidence for a slight advantage for exposure therapy. Similarly, among the seven studies comparing EMDR with some other CBT program, three provided some evidence of a slight advantage for CBT (Devilly and Spence 1999; Rothbaum et al. 2005; Taylor et al. 2003) and three found some evidence of a slight advantage for EMDR (Lee et al. 2002; Power et al. 2002; Vaughan et al. 1994). In the seventh study (Ironson et al. 2002), there was not even a hint of superiority for one treatment over the other. In general, then, the differences between CBT and wait-list conditions are substantially larger than the differences among the various CBT programs, and when differences do occur among active treatments, the direction of the difference is not consistent across studies—suggesting that different CBT programs yield similar degrees of improvement. It is important to note that exposure therapy has gained much more empirical evidence for its efficacy than other forms of CBT, including EMDR.

Just as different CBT programs appear to yield similar improvement, studies that have compared combined CBT programs and the constituent components (e.g., exposure therapy plus SIT vs. exposure therapy alone vs. SIT alone) have generally failed to find significant benefit for the combined treatment compared to the individual treatment. Again, this may in part be attributed to low statistical power to detect small differences due to low sample size, although two relevant studies utilized samples comprising 50 or more participants in each condition. Foa and colleagues (2005) compared exposure therapy alone ($n=79$) versus exposure therapy plus cognitive restructuring ($n=74$). Both treatments were clearly superior to a wait-list control condition, and the degree of improvement from pretreatment to posttreatment, expressed in terms of standard deviation units (i.e., within-group effect sizes), was similar for the two treatments but was numerically larger for the exposure therapy group (Cohen's $d=1.45$) than for the combined condition ($d=1.30$).

Resick and colleagues (2008) compared standard CPT ($n=53$), which includes some exposure through writing and reading a traumatic narrative, with a version of CPT in which writing and reading the traumatic narrative are removed ($n=51$). A third comparison group in this study was one in which participants engaged in repeated writing about the trauma and reading the narrative without any formal cognitive therapy ($n=50$). All three treatments were associated with significant improvement. However, group comparisons conducted posttreatment indicated the CPT treatment without writing was superior to the writing treatment, whereas results with standard CPT were not different from results with either the writing treatment or the CPT variation without the writing component. It should be noted, however, that the writing-only treatment included six sessions conducted every 2 weeks whereas the other two treatments included 12 sessions, each conducted weekly. This procedural difference might have reduced the efficacy of the writing-only treatment. Thus, Foa et al. (2005) found that adding cognitive therapy did not enhance the combination of imaginal plus in vivo exposure, and Resick et al. (2008) found that omitting exposure via writing and reading the trauma narrative did not reduce the efficacy of CPT.

Dismantling studies of EMDR, in which participants were individuals with PTSD or trauma-related symptoms, indicate that variations of EMDR in which eye movements are replaced by other laterally alternating stimuli (e.g., Pitman et al. 1996a) or simply removed (e.g., Boudewyns and Hyer 1996; Renfrey and Spates 1994)—and in which the formal cognitive restructuring (i.e., "reprocessing") procedures are replaced with more desensitization trials (Cusack and Spates 1999)—produce similar improvement. As with most studies comparing different CBT programs, the EMDR dismantling studies are limited by small samples with adequate power to detect only large differences between treatment conditions, although the pattern of means in these studies suggests that if there are differences between EMDR and the dismantled variations, the differences are quite small.

Similar conclusions about the general efficacy of different CBT programs were drawn from a meta-analysis of psychotherapy for PTSD by Bradley et al. (2005). These authors reviewed 26 studies that used a total of 44 active treatment conditions, 15 wait-list control conditions, and 8 nonspecific control treatment conditions (e.g., supportive counseling). The mean within-group effect size for active treatments was 1.43 (95% confidence interval [CI], 1.23–1.64), which was superior to that of a wait-list control condition (d=0.35; 95% CI, 0.19–0.51) and nonspecific control condition (d=0.59; 95% CI, 0.30–0.88). The various specific CBT approaches yielded similar effect sizes with overlapping confidence intervals:

- Exposure therapy: d=1.57; 95% CI, 1.11–2.04
- SIT or cognitive therapy: d=1.65; 95% CI, 0.96–2.35
- Exposure therapy plus SIT or cognitive therapy: d=1.66; 95% CI, 1.18–2.14
- EMDR: d=1.43; 95% CI, 1.02–1.83)

Somewhat more-guarded conclusions were drawn from a recent meta-analysis conducted under the auspices of the Institute of Medicine (2008). This meta-analysis focused only on the highest quality studies and included in their evaluation consideration of data that were lost due to dropouts and the statistical methods used to deal with such missing data. Based on the study selection criteria used by the Institute of Medicine, the review committee considered 24 randomized, controlled studies of some form of exposure therapy (alone, or in combination with SIT or cognitive therapy; notably, CPT was designated as an exposure therapy for the purposes of this review); 10 studies of EMDR; three studies of cognitive therapy; and four studies of coping skills training, which included SIT treatment and relaxation control conditions. Consistent with the previous reviews, the Institute of Medicine concluded that regarding exposure therapy, "the evidence is sufficient to conclude the efficacy of exposure therapies in the treatment of PTSD" (p. 8). By contrast, regarding EMDR, cognitive therapy, and coping skills training, the Institute of Medicine concluded that the evidence is "inadequate to determine the efficacy" (p. 9) of these other treatments.

Innovations

Among the 64 randomized studies of CBT for PTSD included in the Cahill et al. (2008) review previously discussed are a small number of studies of recent treatment innovations. One such innovation is the specific targeting of nightmares and other sleep disturbances, two common symptoms of PTSD. Little is currently known about the efficacy of the various CBT programs discussed thus far for the resolution of such symptoms (Maher et al. 2006), and at least one study found that nearly half (48%) of patients who no longer met criteria for PTSD following CBT experienced at least some insomnia posttreatment, and 30% of patients reported severe insomnia (Zayfert and DeViva 2004). Imagery rehearsal therapy is a CBT program that combines sleep hygiene and cognitive restructuring with imaginal exposure to the content of a nightmare. However, during the exposure practice, the content of the nightmare is intentionally altered in some way.

Research into this treatment program is just beginning, but the results of two randomized studies are promising. In the first of these, Krakow and colleagues (2001) found that three group-administered sessions resulted in a significant reduction in the number of nightmares, improvement in sleep quality, and a decrease in other symptoms of PTSD. In a second study, Davis and Wright (2007) modified imagery rehearsal therapy to include relaxation training, additional exposure through writing and talking about the nightmares, and education about common trauma-related themes included in CPT. As in the Krakow et al. (2001) study, the modified imagery rehearsal therapy was superior to wait-list conditions on measures of nightmare frequency, sleep quality, and PTSD. At present, however, there are no studies directly comparing imagery rehearsal therapy with other treatments for PTSD to determine the relative merits of targeting PTSD versus the more narrow focus on sleep and combating nightmares specifically in terms of patient outcome.

Two additional innovations enlist the use of computer technology to administer therapy: virtual reality technology and the use of the Internet to deliver therapy. Virtual reality technology has been developed as a method to implement exposure therapy in the treatment of anxiety disorders. A meta-analysis (Powers and Emmelkamp 2008) found 16 group studies in which virtual reality exposure therapy was compared with a wait-list or some other minimal control condition (11 studies) or in vivo exposure (five studies) in the treatment of phobias (11 studies), panic disorder (two studies), social phobia (two studies), and PTSD (one study). The overall effect size (Cohen's *d*) for treatments versus control conditions in these studies was 1.11, and the overall effect size for virtual reality exposure versus in vivo exposure was 0.35 in favor of virtual reality exposure (P=0.06). In the only controlled study of PTSD and virtual reality exposure therapy, Difede et al. (2007a) conducted a small investigation comparing this therapy to a wait-list control condition in the treatment of PTSD related to the September 11, 2001, terrorist attacks on the World Trade Center. Exposure was conducted according to a hierarchy beginning with images of a jet flying over the Twin Towers but not crashing into them, working gradually to witnessing a full sequence of events that included jets crashing into both towers, people screaming, people jumping from the buildings, and finally both towers collapsing. Completers received between 6 and 13 sessions (mean=7.5) and demonstrated a significant reduction in PTSD severity scores whereas patients in the wait-list control group had a slight increase in their scores. The posttreatment effect size for completers was large (d=1.54).

In a related use of technology, Basoglu et al. (2007) provided Turkish earthquake survivors with a single session of exposure to simulated tremors. The earthquake simulator consisted of a small house mounted on a shake plate that could simulate earth tremors of differing magnitude, under control of the patient. Length of time in the simulator was permitted to vary and ranged from 9 to 70 minutes. Results indicated significant reductions in PTSD severity measured 4 and 8 weeks after completion of treatment relative to severity in wait-list control subjects over the same time period.

The second innovative approach using computer technology is the use of the Internet to deliver therapy. Lange and his colleagues (2003) have developed a treatment program titled *Interapy* that is used to conduct all aspects of treatment over the Internet, including initial screening for eligibility, informed consent, baseline assessment, implementation of the treatment, and posttreatment assessment. The treatment involves patients writing 10 essays over a period of 5 weeks. Four essays involve exposure to the trauma, four essays encourage cognitive reappraisal by instructing patients to provide advice to a hypothetical friend who went through the same experience, and the final two essays involve writing a letter of closure addressed either to the self or to some significant other. Seven times throughout the treatment, patients receive written feedback on their essays from a therapist making suggestions as to how to proceed.

Two randomized studies of Interapy have been conducted thus far, the first using a population of undergraduate psychology students reporting traumatic symptoms who received research credit for their participation (Lange et al. 2001). In the second study the treatment was made more broadly available to the residents of Amsterdam (Lange et al. 2003). Both studies found significant reductions in trauma-related reexperiencing and avoidance among treatment completers compared to wait-list control subjects. In a third study, Hirai and Clum (2005) evaluated an 8-week Internet-administered treatment that included anxiety management training (relaxation and controlled breathing), cognitive restructuring, and exposure via writing. Except for a telephone screening to determine eligibility, all assessment measures were completed online or submitted through the mail. Patients were drawn from psychology students at Virginia Polytechnic Institute and State University who were seeking extra credit and from the larger Blacksburg, Virginia, community. Treatment completers showed greater reductions in PTSD symptoms, anxiety, and depression and increases in coping abilities and self-efficacy than patients assigned to a wait-list condition.

Using the Internet (or postal services) to conduct assessments and administer therapy has important potential advantages, as it makes treatment available to individuals who may not be otherwise willing to seek mental health services due to the perceived stigma, as well as to those who live in areas where mental health services are not otherwise available. However, this is balanced by concerns raised about providing mental health services to someone sight unseen, including concerns about patient safety, the practice of psychotherapy across state and even international borders, and the accuracy of the information obtained. This final concern is of particular relevance to research evaluating the efficacy of therapy administered via the Internet, as the structured clinical interview administered by a well-trained independent evaluator blinded to the treatment used is considered the industry standard for psychotherapy outcome research.

Litz et al. (2007; see Litz et al. 2004 for greater details of the intervention program) conducted a study that combined live therapy delivered through the Internet and in-person assessment. Patients in the study were active-duty Department of Defense personnel with PTSD resulting from exposure to the September 11, 2001, terrorist attacks on the U.S. Pentagon or from subsequent combat in Iraq or Afghanistan. The 8-week CBT program involved an initial in-person visit with a therapist to complete the pretreatment evaluation, provide psychoeducation in stress management and cognitive reframing techniques, begin the development of a hierarchy of stressful situations, and orient patients to the use of the De-Stress (Litz et al. 2007) Internet program. Thereafter, patients were instructed to log in at least once per day, and the program provided information and instruction about the use of stress management techniques, self-monitoring to identify stressful situations, and graduated in vivo exposure. After week 6 a telephone contact with the therapist was scheduled to assess the patient's readiness to confront the memory of the trauma through writing a trauma narrative and repeatedly reading it. Throughout the study, patients had ad lib access to the information on the Web site and were able to contact their therapist through e-mail and by telephone. Results revealed that treatment completers showed significantly greater reduction in PTSD severity than did those who received supportive counseling similarly administered through the Internet, although no differences were seen in the intent-to-treat analyses.

Treatment of Acute Stress Reactions/ Prevention of Chronic PTSD

Although studied less extensively, two approaches for preventing chronic posttraumatic psychopathology that have received empirical scrutiny are psychological debriefing and brief CBT (B-CBT) packages.

Following the original ISTSS practice guidelines (Foa et al. 2000), we use the term *psychological debriefing* in a general way to refer to very brief interventions (consisting of one or a few sessions), which are usually implemented shortly after the occurrence of a traumatic event (typically within 72 hours) and share a number of features. These shared features comprise discussion of the facts of the traumatic event and the trauma survivors' beliefs about what happened; an opportunity to express thoughts, impressions, and emotional reactions; provision of information to normalize the trauma survivors' reactions; and planning for coping with the trauma and its consequences (Bisson et al. 2000).

Proponents of psychological debriefing (e.g., Everly et al. 2001) have emphasized that psychological debriefing should not be viewed as a stand-alone treatment, but rather should be implemented in the larger context of the more comprehensive Critical Incident Stress Management (CISM) protocol and that psychological debriefing was intended to be implemented as a group intervention rather than an individual intervention. By contrast, the randomized, controlled studies of psychological debriefing have focused primarily on individually administered psychological debriefing implemented as a stand-alone intervention; some studies have utilized groups, but these were not randomized (e.g., Carlier et al. 1998, 2000; Deahl et al. 2000; Eid et al. 2001). To our knowledge, no randomized, controlled studies have been conducted evaluating group psychological debriefing in the context of CISM. With the preceding caveats in mind, the results of randomized, controlled studies of individual psychological debriefing are somewhat mixed, but a potentially important pattern appears to be emerging. Specifically, although participants receiving psychological debriefing in general report high levels of consumer satisfaction with the intervention and studies utilizing valid and reliable measures of PTSD symptoms find improvement over time, studies that included an untreated control condition have not found any benefit on specific PTSD measures (e.g., Conlon et al. 1999; Rose et al. 1999). Thus, symptom reduction following psychological debriefing in these studies is better attributed to natural recovery rather than an effect of treatment. Even more concerning, however, is the possibility of an iatrogenic effect of psychological debriefing, such that the intervention may impede natural recovery among some individuals, such as those with the most severe initial traumatic reactions (e.g., Bisson et al. 1997; Carlier et al. 1998, 2000; Mayou et al. 2000).

A more promising, but as yet still underresearched, approach is the application of brief (4–5 sessions) CBT utilizing the same anxiety management and exposure therapy techniques developed for the treatment of chronic PTSD. B-CBT is typically initiated 2–4 weeks posttrauma and appears to speed recovery from early PTSD symptoms (Foa et al. 1995a, 2006b) and acute stress disorder, and may reduce the incidence of PTSD 6 months later (Bryant et al. 1998, 1999, 2003b), although long-term (≥1 year) follow-up studies of intent-to-treat samples have found similar rates of PTSD for B-CBT and supportive counseling (Bryant et al. 2003b). Mirroring the research on treatment for chronic PTSD, the only study to directly compare the combination of exposure therapy plus anxiety management training versus exposure therapy alone (Bryant et al. 1999) found no significant differences between the two treatments. In a recent study (Bryant et al. 2008), participants who received exposure therapy improved much more than those receiving cognitive restructuring, whose improvement did not differ from that of wait-list control subjects. It seems that the specific active component in B-CBT is exposure.

One of the major factors limiting progress in the development of highly efficacious prevention programs is the phenomenon of natural recovery. As longitudinal studies of trauma survivors have shown, most individuals exposed to a traumatic event will show a decline in PTSD symptoms in the weeks and months immediately following the traumatic event (e.g., Blanchard et al. 1996; Riggs et al. 1995; Rothbaum et al. 1992). Thus, either efficacious preventative programs must promote more rapid or complete recovery than would occur naturally, or researchers need to be able to reliably identify subpopulations least likely to recover in the absence of intervention, as has been generally true of the diagnostic criteria for acute stress disorder (e.g., Harvey and Bryant 2002). Despite this limitation, the extant research suggests that brief versions (i.e., 4–5 sessions compared to 9 or more sessions) of the same CBT programs that are effective in the treatment of chronic PTSD, when administered starting within a few weeks of the trauma, can speed recovery for some individuals displaying PTSD symptoms.

Discussion of Factors Affecting Outcome

In contrast to the large body of literature on the efficacy of various treatments for PTSD, studies examining predictors of treatment outcome are few. The factors that have been investigated as predictors of treatment outcome for CBT may be classified into three types: 1) pretreatment variables, which include trauma-related variables (e.g., type of trauma, prior history of trauma) and personal characteristics (e.g., anger reactions); 2) general treatment-related factors, such as treatment attendance; and 3) specific treatment-related factors, such as fear activation during exposure therapy exercises followed by subsequent fear reduction. The potential utility of identifying pretreatment predictors of treatment outcome is to provide individuals with accurate expectations about the efficacy of treatment and, in cases where different treatments are found more or less effective for certain kinds of individuals, to match patients with the most effective treatments. By contrast, the potential utility of identifying treatment-related predictors of outcome is to provide therapists with guidance as to which factors to focus on in sessions in order to optimize treatment outcome.

Among the pretreatment predictors of treatment outcome, some studies found that initial PTSD severity was associated with poor outcome (Blanchard et al. 2003b; van Minnen et al. 2002). However, as noted below, Foa and Cahill (2002) found PTSD severity to predict poor outcome with SIT but not with prolonged exposure. To the extent that high severity impedes improvement with some treatments, this may reflect in part an artifact that is related to the practice in most randomized, controlled studies of providing a single dose of treatment regardless of patient response to treatment. Specifically, even when there are no differences in the *rate* of improvement between individuals with different initial PTSD severity levels, those with higher PTSD levels pretreatment will also have higher levels posttreatment unless the dose of treatment selected is enough for optimal outcome among those with the highest pretreatment levels. For this reason, what is important is to identify predictors of change from pre- to posttreatment or predictors of posttreatment PTSD severity after controlling for pretreatment severity. Trauma-related characteristics that have been associated with poorer outcome include the following:

- A history of childhood trauma prior to the index event (Hembree et al. 2004a; van Minnen et al. 2002)
- Multiple traumas or a personal trauma (e.g., interpersonal assault), as opposed to impersonal trauma (e.g., natural disaster) (van Minnen et al. 2002)
- Time since the trauma (van Minnen et al. 2002)
- The receipt of injury during the trauma (Hembree et al. 2004a)

Pretreatment patient characteristics that have been associated with poorer response to treatment include the following:

- Male gender (Tarrier et al. 2000)
- Suicide risk (as judged by the therapist) (Tarrier et al. 2000)
- Living alone (Tarrier et al. 2000)
- Comborbid GAD (Tarrier et al. 2000) and depression (Taylor et al. 2001)
- Pain severity and interference due to the trauma (Taylor et al. 2001) as well as days of work missed (Blanchard et al. 2003b)
- Pretreatment anger problems (Foa et al. 1995c; Taylor et al. 2001; van Minnen et al. 2002)
- The use or increased use of psychiatric medication during the treatment period (Taylor et al. 2001), particularly benzodiazepine use (van Minnen et al. 2002)

Interestingly, several of the factors that have been associated with poorer treatment outcome (e.g., multiple traumas or trauma prior to the index trauma) have also been found to be associated with development of chronic PTSD (for meta-analytic reviews of factors related to the development of chronic PTSD, see Brewin et al. 2000 and Ozer et al. 2003).

Although several trauma and patient characteristics have been identified as predictors of treatment outcome, few have been studied across a range of samples to evaluate their reliability. Indeed, some factors that have been studied in multiple samples fail to replicate as predictors of outcome. For example, whereas Hembree et al. (2004a) and van Minnen et al. (2002) found that prior history of childhood trauma was associated with poorer treatment outcome, Resick and colleagues (2003) did not find any difference in treatment response between rape victims with and those without a prior history of childhood sexual abuse. Pretreatment anger variables have been associated with poorer outcome in several studies (Foa et al. 1995c; Taylor et al. 2001; van Minnen et al. 2002); however, Cahill et al. (2003) found not only that pretreatment anger was associated with poor outcome but also that CBT for PTSD significantly reduced anger, even among patients with clinically elevated anger levels at pretreatment. Similarly, although comorbidity with depression (Taylor et al. 2001) and GAD (Tarrier et al. 2000) has been associated with poorer response to treatment in some studies, CBT for PTSD has been found to reduce the prevalence of these conditions (Blanchard et al. 2003a).

In an attempt to answer the question of matching treatments to patients, Foa and Cahill (2002) examined differential predictors for outcome of prolonged exposure and SIT. They found that a greater level of general anxiety prior to treatment was associated with more severe PTSD symptoms posttreatment. However, high pretreatment severity of PTSD, depression, and poor social functioning were not related to treatment outcome of prolonged exposure. In contrast, poorer general social functioning at pretreatment predicted poorer social functioning and greater depression after treatment with SIT. Also, greater levels of pretreatment PTSD and depression predicted greater PTSD severity following treatment with SIT. These findings suggest that prolonged exposure may be more suitable for patients who initially present with poor social functioning, severe PTSD, or severe depression.

General treatment-related variables that were found to be associated with poorer outcome were the following:

- Patient ratings of low credibility of treatment, therapist ratings of low patient motivation for treatment, a great number of missed sessions (Tarrier et al. 1999), or patients requiring a longer period of time to complete treatment (Tarrier et al. 2000)
- Low patient engagement or high avoidance in therapy (Taylor et al. 2001)
- Less completed homework (Marks et al. 1998)
- A poor working alliance during the early portion of therapy (Cloitre et al. 2004)

Interestingly, Cloitre et al. (2004) found that the effect of the working alliance on outcome was mediated through its effect on increased negative mood regulation. Specifically, a strong working alliance early in therapy was associated with greater regulation of negative mood during subsequent sessions, which in turn was associated with greater symptom improvement. Consistent with mediation, the direct relationship between the working alliance and treatment outcome was no longer significant after taking into consideration the effect of negative mood regulation on treatment outcome (Baron and Kenny 1986).

Lastly, several studies have investigated specific treatment-related factors that according to Foa and Kozak's (1986) emotional processing theory are expected to be associated with better outcome in the treatment of PTSD. According to emotional processing theory, anxiety, such as is seen in PTSD, reflects the activation of a fear structure encoded in memory that contains information about fear-relevant stimuli and responses, as well as the meanings attributed to these stimuli and responses. Fear is pathological when the fear structure contains erroneous associations such that harmless stimuli are associated with the meaning of "danger" and trigger intense fear and avoidance reactions. Fear reduction requires modification of the fear structure through activation of the fear structure and the incorporation of corrective information. Foa and Kozak (1986) suggested three indicators for emotional processing (i.e., modification of the fear memory in ways to promote fear reduction): 1) fear activation, indicating the fear network has been accessed, 2) within-session fear reduction, and 3) between-session fear reduction (i.e., *habituation*), which may serve as part of the corrective information (e.g., evidence that arousal does not last indefinitely) as well as be indicative of change in the underlying fear structure. Consistent with emotional processing theory, studies have found evidence that outcome of exposure therapy is associated with the following:

- Activation of fear during exposure (Foa et al. 1995c; Jaycox et al. 1998; Pitman et al. 1996b)
- Habituation of fear within exposure sessions (Pitman et al. 1996b)
- Habituation across sessions (Jaycox et al. 1998; Pitman et al. 1996b)

Also consistent with the tenets of emotional processing theory, and consistent with other cognitive theories of PTSD (e.g., Ehlers and Clark 2000), is evidence of cognitive change following treatment for PTSD (e.g., Foa and Rauch 2004) and evidence that improvement following treatment is associated with changes in the trauma narrative such that reduced fragmentation in the narrative is associated with reduced anxiety and increased organization is associated with reduced depression (Foa et al. 1995b).

As noted earlier, most randomized, controlled treatment outcome studies select a single arbitrary dose of treatment. Yet it is possible that some individuals may require more treatment than others to obtain a good outcome. Thus, one strategy for improving outcomes is to provide the same treatment for longer duration, as is commonly done in clinical practice: when a patient is showing improvement but has not yet fully responded to treatment, sometimes the most sensible approach is to continue with more of the same. Foa et al. (2005) incorporated such flexible dosing. Patients whose PTSD symptoms decreased by at least 70% at session 8 terminated treatment at session 9. The remaining patients were offered additional sessions, to a maximum of 12. Fifty-eight percent of patients received extension sessions; these patients had showed an average reduction of PTSD severity of 31% by session 8. Further improvement was achieved during the extension period, such that after the extension sessions the average reduction in PTSD severity from pretreatment was 60%. Thus, research is beginning to address the need to develop and evaluate strategies for enhancing treatment outcome for those who show partial response to existing treatment programs, but further research is needed.

Other Psychosocial Approaches

Psychodynamic Therapy

Psychodynamic treatment attempts to reengage normal mechanisms for adaptive behavior by bringing unconscious conflicts into the conscious mind. This is done by investigating the psychological meaning of the traumatic event with the patient. It may include the exploration of wishes, fears, and defense mechanisms evoked by the event, and the relationship between the patient and therapist is considered a key element in the treatment (Kudler et al. 2000). In a study of prototypical community treatments for PTSD, Schottenbauer et al. (2006) identified several key factors that define psychodynamic treatment:

1. One factor consists of items that would be classified as *expressive therapy*. Expressive therapy aims to increase insight and self-knowledge, using the techniques of questioning, confrontation, clarification, and interpretation (Wallerstein and Dewitt 1997). The therapist takes a neutral position toward the patient, and the therapeutic relationship itself is a mechanism for treatment, as well as the interpretation of transference. Expressive techniques deemed most important by therapists included the patient feeling anxiety and having a discomforting affect, the therapist conveying a sense of nonjudgmental acceptance, and the therapist asking for more information.
2. Another psychodynamic factor corresponds to what has been termed *supportive therapy* in the psychodynamic tradition, an approach that reduces mental anguish and attempts to strengthen defenses to increase the adaptation of the ego in daily life (Wallerstein and Dewitt 1997). Supportive psychotherapy also aims to help the patient develop more

effective defense mechanisms. Not unlike CBT clinicians, psychodynamic therapists administering supportive therapy may intervene with regard to the patient's daily life. The therapist may suggest specific activities to do between sessions, giving explicit advice and providing guidance as needed, although this was considered a less important aspect of treatment in the Schottenbauer et al. (2006) study.

3. A third factor, termed *psychodynamic-integrative*, includes components such as challenging the patient's views, encouraging action, focusing on feelings of guilt, and emphasizing emotional experiences.

Although individual psychodynamic treatment is offered widely by professionals for PTSD (Becker et al. 2004), only one randomized, controlled trial has included a psychodynamic component for PTSD (Brom et al. 1989), so this modality has not yet been established as an empirically supported treatment for trauma.

Group Therapies

Group therapy has been frequently prescribed for both acutely and chronically traumatized individuals. It has been used to treat trauma following assault (Mitchell 1983), natural disaster (Lystad 1988; Raphael 1986), childhood sexual abuse (Ganzarian and Buchele 1993; Herman and Schatzow 1987), rape (Yassen and Glass 1984), domestic violence (Rounsaville et al. 1979), concentration camp internment (Laub and Auerhahn 1993), and war (Parson 1985). The task of group therapy is to help victims regain a sense of safety, connection, and competence. Sharing one's experience with other victims may be considered an effective intervention because the shared history of trauma can form the basis of reestablishing a sense of community in individuals who may feel cut off from others. For chronically traumatized individuals, group psychotherapy may provide a sense of mutuality and a forum to explore concerns about safety and trust that have been affected by the trauma (van der Kolk et al. 2002).

There are three primary types of group therapies, which can be broadly classified as supportive, psychodynamic, and cognitive-behavioral, although some treatments may use a blend of approaches. Although the approaches may differ in their underlying formulations of symptom etiology and maintenance, they share many similar features including the following:

- Membership in the group by survivors of the same type of trauma (e.g., combat veterans, rape victims)
- Validation of the traumatic exposure
- Normalization of traumatic responses
- Adoption of a nonjudgmental stance toward the patient's response to the trauma

Incorporating these principles facilitates the development of a safe therapeutic environment.

Since the establishment of PTSD as a separate diagnosis in DSM, relatively little research has focused on the evaluation of group therapy techniques. Only a handful of group psychotherapy outcome studies have been published since the late 1990s, eight of which were studies of CBT (J.G. Beck et al. 2009; Falsetti et al. 2001, 2005; Hollifield et al. 2007; Krakow et al. 2000, 2001; Schnurr et al. 2003; Zlotnick et al. 1997), two on psychodynamic therapy (Classen et al. 2001; Spiegel et al. 2004), and one using an insight-oriented feminist model (Stalker and Fry 1999). Other studies have been nonrandomized or lacked a control condition, which limits the conclusions that can be drawn. Importantly, most randomized, controlled studies failed to account for clustering observations within groups, which limits the power of these studies to draw clear conclusions about the efficacy of treatment.

Other than the fact that most group studies demonstrate some positive benefit for participants, little is known about the factors that moderate or mediate outcome for a PTSD therapy group of any type. Neither of the two studies that compared group CBT to an active comparison condition found any advantage for one treatment over the other. In a study of 325 male veterans, Schnurr et al. (2003) did not find any advantage for the trauma-focused CBT condition compared to present-focused supportive group therapy (Schnurr et al. 2003). In a much smaller study of 84 men and women with PTSD resulting from a variety of civilian traumas, Hollifield et al. (2007) found that both group CBT and individually administered acupuncture were superior to a wait-list control condition but that there were no differences between the two treatments. There is also evidence that the presence of a borderline member in a group hampers recovery among all members (Cloitre and Koenen 2001). Research on group therapy as a means of delivering PTSD treatment is still in the early stages, and more research is needed before it can be considered an empirically validated modality. In particular, there is a need to compare the same treatment delivered in group versus individual sessions to determine whether changing the format changes the efficacy of treatment.

Special Populations

CBT has been used successfully in controlled studies to relieve the symptoms of PTSD in the following groups:

- Adult female survivors of rape (e.g., Echeburua et al. 1997; Foa et al. 1991, 1999, 2005; Resick et al. 2002, 2008; Rothbaum et al. 2005), physical assault (e.g., Foa et al. 1999, 2005; Resick et al. 2008), domestic violence (Kubany et al. 2003, 2004), and childhood abuse (e.g., Chard 2005; Cloitre et al. 2002; Foa et al. 2005; Resick et al. 2008)
- Male and female veterans (e.g., Cooper and Clum 1989; Glynn et al. 1999; Keane et al. 1989; Monson et al. 2006; Schnurr et al. 2007)
- Motor vehicle accident victims (e.g., Blanchard et al. 2003a; Ehlers et al. 2003; Fecteau and Nicki 1999)
- Refugees (e.g., Neuner et al. 2004; Otto et al. 2003; Paunovic and Ost 2001)
- Earthquake victims (Basoglu et al. 2005, 2007)
- Emergency responders (e.g., Difede et al. 2007b)
- Victims of terrorism (Difede et al. 2007a; Duffy et al. 2007)
- Mixed accident and assault victims (e.g., Bryant et al. 2003a; Ehlers et al. 2005; Marks et al. 1998)

Additional groups have been studied in open trials and in some randomized trials of CBT, with promising results. These samples included men and women receiving treatment for PTSD comorbid with the following conditions:

- Cocaine dependence (Back et al. 2001; Brady et al. 2001)
- Other substance use disorders (Najavits et al. 2005, 2006)
- Traumatic grief (K. Shear et al. 2005; M.K. Shear et al. 2001)
- Severe mental illness, such as bipolar disorder (Mueser et al. 2007, 2008)

Patients with PTSD and other comorbid disorders may also benefit from CBT, as treatments that reduce PTSD symptoms also reduce symptoms of general anxiety and depression. Studies have found that CBT treatment for PTSD decreases anger (e.g., Cahill et al. 2003), trauma-related guilt (Kubany et al. 2003; Resick et al. 2002), and shame (Kubany et al. 2003). Simultaneously, it increases self-esteem (Kubany et al. 2003) and reduces maladaptive trauma-related cognitions (Foa and Rauch 2004; Paunovic and Ost 2001). Cloitre et al. (2002) implemented a treatment for PTSD from childhood abuse that combined skills training in affect regulation and interpersonal relationships followed by imaginal exposure. Although improvement at posttreatment was associated with the strength of the therapeutic alliance developed during the skills training phase of treatment, within-group effect sizes for the exposure therapy phase of treatment were as large as or larger than the corresponding effect sizes for the skills training phase on measures of dissociation, alexithymia, and depression (Cahill et al. 2004b).

Certain comorbid conditions may reduce the effectiveness of CBT for PTSD. As noted previously, Tarrier et al. (2000) and Taylor et al. (2001) found that the presence of comorbid GAD predicted poorer outcomes, although Blanchard et al. (2003a) found that CBT for PTSD resulted in significant reductions in comorbid and major depression compared to either supportive counseling or a wait-list condition. Feeny et al. (2002) reanalyzed data from the Foa et al. (1999) study of prolonged exposure, SIT, and prolonged exposure/SIT to investigate whether treatment for PTSD would be less efficacious in patients with borderline personality characteristics. Results revealed no significant differences among treatment completers in their response to measures of PTSD severity, depression, or state- or trait-anxiety. In an analysis of data from the Foa et al. (2005) study of prolonged exposure alone and in combination with cognitive restructuring, Hembree et al. (2004a) found no difference in the percentage of patients who no longer met diagnostic criteria following treatment between participants with and without personality disorders.

Falsetti et al. (2001, 2005) evaluated the efficacy of a treatment called multichannel exposure therapy (M-CET) that combined Resick and Schnicke's (1992) CPT program with parts of Barlow and colleagues' (1994) panic control treatment for the treatment of women with PTSD and comorbid panic attacks. Compared to a wait-list control condition, treatment with M-CET resulted in a significant decrease in both PTSD severity and panic frequency. Hinton and colleagues (2005b, 2006a) have studied a combination CBT treatment that also incorporates elements of panic control treatment for use in the treatment of Cambodian and Vietnamese refugees with PTSD, who also frequently reported physical symptoms similar to those of panic. Results of three small randomized, controlled studies (Hinton et al. 2004, 2005a, 2006b) have found the treatment to be associated with superior outcome compared with wait-list control conditions on measures of both PTSD severity and anxiety sensitivity, the latter being a cognitive vulnerability factor associated with panic disorder (Taylor 1999).

In summary, CBT for PTSD has been found to be efficacious across a range of study populations, including populations with a range of specific traumas and individuals with a range of comorbid conditions. Successful treatment of PTSD is frequently associated with improvement using many different types of outcome measures and with a reduction in some common comorbid conditions. In addition, CBT for PTSD has been successfully integrated with CBT treatments for other specific comorbid conditions, although no dismantling or comparative outcome studies have been published to determine whether the addition of other CBT elements targeting the comorbid condition is necessary to achieve optimal outcome.

Practical Techniques

Treatment of PTSD

At the Center for the Treatment and Study of Anxiety, we have been studying interventions for the prevention (Foa et al. 1995a, 2006b) and treatment of PTSD since the mid-1980s (Foa et al. 1991, 1999, 2005; Rothbaum et al. 2006). Although there are many effective treatment options for people with PTSD, at present we believe the evidence favors prolonged exposure—the combination of imaginal and in vivo exposure therapy—as the treatment of choice, for four primary reasons (Cahill and Foa 2004):

1. The efficacy of exposure therapy has been repeatedly demonstrated in randomized, controlled trials across a wide range of trauma populations by researchers in the United States and internationally.
2. Prolonged exposure is the only treatment that has been directly compared with each of the other major treatments (i.e., SIT, variations of cognitive therapy, and EMDR); these studies have generally found that prolonged exposure produces outcomes that are as good as or somewhat better than outcomes with the comparison treatments.
3. Attempts to enhance the efficacy of prolonged exposure by adding elements of other CBT programs, such as SIT or cognitive therapy, have not resulted in a demonstrably better outcome than prolonged exposure alone.
4. The results of our initial work evaluating the efficacy of prolonged exposure when administered by community therapists have been quite successful (Foa et al. 2005; Schnur et al. 2007).

No other treatment program has yet established as complete and successful a track record as prolonged exposure. Therefore, this section is devoted to the treatment of PTSD with prolonged exposure.

Prolonged exposure is typically administered in 9–12 ninety-minute sessions delivered once or twice weekly. The two primary techniques employed in the administration of prolonged exposure are imaginal exposure to the traumatic memory, where the patient is helped to mentally visualize the feared traumatic memory and recount it aloud, and in vivo exposure to traumatic reminders and safe stimuli (people, places, things, or activities) that trigger trauma-related distress in daily life. Typically, the techniques are used in combination.

In the first therapy session, following a thorough intake evaluation to determine that PTSD symptoms are the patient's primary psychological difficulties, the therapist obtains further information about the patient's trauma history and begins the process of psychoeducation. The first two sessions consist of education about the nature of trauma, which includes common reactions to trauma, factors that maintain PTSD symptoms, and the rationale for treatment by prolonged exposure. Together, the therapist and patient agree on the details of the treatment plan (e.g., creating a hierarchy of feared objects and situations for in vivo practice), and the patient receives training in controlled breathing. Importantly, controlled breathing is presented as a method to manage stress in the course of daily life, not as a method to control anxiety during exposure exercises. In vivo exposure is discussed in depth in the second session, and the first in vivo exposure homework assignment is assigned for the patient to implement between the second and third sessions. To monitor progress, the patient is taught to quantify the level of distress or anxiety at the beginning, peak, and end of each in vivo exercise using the common Subjective Units of Distress Scale (described in Foa et al. 2007) that ranges from 0 (no anxiety/distress) to 100 (most anxiety/distress ever).

During sessions 3 through 5, imaginal exposures are conducted with the therapist, and the patient describes the entire traumatic memory from beginning to end. Patients are instructed to close their eyes, imagine the traumatic event as vividly as possible, and describe it out loud in detail, including a description of the thoughts and emotions they experienced during trauma. The patient is instructed to describe the traumatic event in the present tense and is encouraged to become emotionally engaged with the memory. The therapist asks the patient to report his or her Subjective Units of Distress levels approximately every 5 minutes during the imaginal exposure. The exposure is conducted for 30–60 minutes and is audiorecorded each time for the patient to listen to as part of daily homework. At the end of each imaginal exposure session, the therapist and patient spend about 20 minutes discussing the patient's experience during the imaginal revisiting of the trauma. Often the patient will report new details and insights about the trauma during the discussion. This phase of the session, called *processing*, helps patients to integrate the new information and insights into their understanding of the event. In this way, prolonged exposure reduces the distress associated with the unpleasant memories and ultimately results in a more realistic perspective about the experience.

By the fifth or sixth session, the focus of the imaginal exposure is shifted to specific segments within the traumatic narrative. By this point in therapy, patients are generally able to recount the trauma more easily, but there are usually a few specific parts of the story that are more upsetting than the rest, which we refer to as *hot spots*. Imaginal exposure is then focused on repeating the parts of the story that constitute these hot spots, one at a time, until anxiety to the hot spot diminishes. In the final session, the patient puts the whole story back together again and narrates the trauma from beginning to end. A more detailed description of the treatment can be found in Foa et al. (2007).

Clinical Issues

Use of Exposure in Clinical Practice

Effective treatments for PTSD, such as prolonged exposure and other forms of CBT, cannot benefit traumatized patients unless mental health care providers make use of the treatments. Evidence suggests that given an informed choice, consumers would select exposure or another form of CBT as their most preferred treatment for PTSD (Becker et al. 2007; Zoellner et al. 2003). However, many consumers of mental health services are unaware that different types of therapy exist and that some treatments have greater evidence of efficacy than others. They may rely on their therapists to determine what treatment is appropriate for their needs. Unfortunately, most clinicians who treat PTSD rarely use exposure therapy (Cahill et al. 2006).

Becker et al. (2004) surveyed a large sample of psychologists who treat PTSD. Among the therapists in the study, the most common theoretical orientations were eclectic (37%), psychodynamic/analytic (28%), behavioral/cognitive-behavioral (21%), and cognitive (9%). The therapists were asked whether they used imaginal exposure with their PTSD patients and if not, their reasons. Only 27% reported that they had been trained in the use of imaginal exposure for PTSD, and only 9% reported using imaginal exposure with the majority of their PTSD patients. Thus, not only were the majority of PTSD therapists untrained in the use of exposure therapy, even fewer regularly used exposure to treat PTSD. Becker et al. (2004) further found that the three most frequently cited reasons for not using exposure therapy with PTSD patients were lack of training (60%), resistance to the use of manualized treatments (25%), and fears that patients would decompensate (22%). Therefore, to increase the number of therapists using exposure therapy for PTSD, clinicians' concerns must be adequately addressed.

Tolerability and Safety of Exposure Therapy

Concern about the tolerability and safety of exposure therapy has existed since its initial development. Wolpe (1958), a pioneer of systematic desensitization, was concerned that evoking too much anxiety during treatment could actually sensitize the patient, resulting in greater distress to reminders of the trauma. Although there was mounting evidence that more intense exposure therapy techniques, such as imaginal and in vivo flooding, safely and effectively reduced anxiety symptoms for obsessive-compulsive disorder and agoraphobia, concerns over the sensitization of PTSD patients remained (Barlow 2002).

Safety concerns about exposure therapy have generally been dispelled for most anxiety disorders, yet many clinicians continue to regard PTSD patients as too fragile for exposure-based treatment. One concern is that distressed patients may retreat from exposure therapy before they can benefit from it. To address this concern, Hembree et al. (2003) conducted a meta-analysis of dropout rates from 25 studies of various CBT programs for PTSD. Patients were significantly less likely to drop out when assigned to a control condition (11.4%, combining wait-list, supportive counseling, and relaxation) than when receiving active treatment of any type. Among the active treatments compared, most did not differ significantly from each other in dropout rates: 20.5% with exposure therapy alone, 22.1% with SIT or cognitive therapy alone, and 26.9% with exposure therapy plus SIT or cognitive therapy alone. The only exception was EMDR, with a dropout rate of 18.9%, which did not differ significantly from the dropout rates in either control groups or active treatment groups. Thus, although dropout rates were higher in active treatment groups than in control groups, dropout rates with exposure therapy alone were no different than those with other active treatments.

A second concern is that exposure therapy may actually worsen symptoms of PTSD. Two reports that have advanced this idea are a case series by Pitman et al. (1991) and a randomized study by Tarrier et al. (1999). Pitman et al. (1991) described six cases taken from a larger study (*N*=20; Pitman et al. 1996b) of imaginal exposure therapy with veterans. Although each of the cases described some form of worsening of symptoms (e.g., increased trauma or depressive symptoms, or relapse of a preexisting condition such as alcohol abuse), the study from which the cases came did not include a comparison condition. Thus, it is not known how patients would have fared with no treatment at all.

Tarrier et al. (1999) examined the relative rates of numerical symptom worsening following treatment with either imaginal exposure or cognitive therapy (*N*=72). Numerical symptom worsening was defined as an increase from pre- to posttreatment of at least one point on the Clinician-Administered PTSD Scale (CAPS; Blake et al. 1995). Despite comparable overall improvement in the two conditions across several outcome measures, 9% of patients receiving cognitive therapy reported numerical worsening compared with 31% of those receiving exposure therapy. The interpretation of this finding, however, is limited by three considerations. First, an increase of one point on the CAPS is within the measurement error of the instrument (Devilly and Foa 2001); therefore it is not clear whether these patients' symptoms actually got worse or simply did not improve. Second, as in the Pitman et al. (1991) study, Tarrier et al. (1999) did not include a no-treatment control condition. Thus, it is not clear how their finding compares with the natural course of the disorder. Third, the high rate of relative numerical worsening seen in Tarrier et al.'s (1999) exposure therapy condition has not been replicated.

Taylor et al. (2003) evaluated rates of numerical symptom worsening following exposure therapy, EMDR, and relaxation therapy. Of 45 participants who completed treatment, only one patient showed numerical symptom worsening on the CAPS, and that patient received relaxation therapy. Unpublished analyses of numerical symptom worsening among completers from studies by Foa et al. (1999, 2005), Resick et al. (2002), and Rothbaum et al. (2005) also found low rates of PTSD numerical symptom worsening following prolonged exposure (<10%), which were not different from rates seen with other CBT treatments and were significantly lower than rates of symptom worsening with no-treatment control conditions (Cahill et al. 2004a). Cloitre et al. (2002) investigated the efficacy of a PTSD treatment for childhood abuse (*N*=58) that combined imaginal exposure with skills training in interpersonal relationships and affect regulation, based on principles of dialectical behavior therapy (Linehan 1993). Approximately 5% of patients receiving the treatment showed numerical symptom worsening compared with approximately 25% of patients assigned to a wait-list condition. Thus, the evidence suggests that treatment reduces the likelihood of symptom worsening and that rates of numerical symptom worsening are not higher following exposure therapy than following other treatments.

Foa et al. (2002) evaluated whether *reliable symptom worsening*, an increase larger than the standard error of the difference between two measurement occasions (Devilly and Foa 2001), was associated with the initiation of imaginal exposure, increased dropout from treatment, or poorer treatment outcome. Utilizing data from the Foa et al. (2005) study comparing prolonged exposure versus prolonged exposure plus cognitive restructuring (prolonged exposure/CR), Foa et al. (2002) examined reliable symptom increases in self-reported PTSD severity occurring between sessions 2 and 4. Patients assigned to the prolonged exposure condition began imaginal exposure in session 3, whereas patients assigned to prolonged exposure/CR learned cognitive restructuring in session 3, with imaginal exposure starting at session 4. This design allowed comparison of those patients showing symptom increases between sessions 2 and 4 with patients randomly assigned to either begin imaginal exposure or begin cognitive restructuring. A minority of patients (7 of 73; 9.6%) displayed reliable PTSD symptom worsening between sessions 2 and 4, although a greater percentage of such cases occurred after initiation of imaginal exposure (6 of 7; 85.7%) than cognitive restructuring (1 of 7; 14.3%). This phenomenon, if observed in clinical practice, might lead a concerned clinician to abandon imaginal exposure in favor of another technique. However, the prudent approach would be to continue treatment in the same manner, as the increase in PTSD symptoms is only temporary. Foa et al.'s study (2002) showed that this short-lived symptom worsening was associated with neither poorer treatment outcome nor increased dropout rates.

Conclusion

It has been widely recognized that traumatic events can lead to psychological disturbances and chronic distress. Popular therapeutic approaches, such as psychodynamic therapy and group therapy, are not yet considered empirically supported treatments due to the lack of randomized, controlled trials documenting their efficacy. There are at least four treatment approaches that have empirical support for PTSD, all forms of CBT; these include exposure therapy, cognitive therapy, SIT, and EMDR. CBT has been shown to significantly reduce symptoms of PTSD from a wide variety of traumas, including combat, natural disasters, sexual assault, nonsexual physical assault, childhood abuse, and a combination of traumas. Prolonged exposure, a specific CBT exposure therapy program, is currently the best-supported approach to treatment. Concerns about this approach linger, despite evidence of safety and tolerability comparable to that of other forms of CBT. Prolonged exposure is a relatively short-term treatment that can be administered effectively by clinicians who have limited experience with CBT. An important challenge at the present time is disseminating information about effective treatment programs to therapists, patients, and the general public.

◄ Key Clinical Points ►

- Chronic psychological disturbances following traumatic experiences are a common occurrence that frequently requires therapeutic intervention.
- Psychological debriefing, a frequently proposed early intervention, has not been demonstrated to be more effective than natural recovery or compassionate assessment.
- Cognitive-behavioral techniques have been demonstrated to significantly reduce symptoms of chronic posttraumatic stress disorder and may promote more rapid recovery following trauma.
- Prolonged exposure is a highly effective CBT-based method of reducing PTSD symptoms.
- Most clinicians do not use imaginal exposure with their PTSD patients.
- Exposure therapy is not associated with a worsening of symptoms or early dropout from treatment.
- Psychodynamic and group therapies are common treatments for PTSD but are not yet empirically validated.

References

American Psychiatric Association: Diagnostic and Statistical Manual of Mental Disorders, 3rd Edition. Washington, DC, American Psychiatric Association, 1980

Back SE, Dansky BS, Carroll KM, et al: Exposure therapy in the treatment of PTSD among cocaine-dependent individuals: description of procedures. J Subst Abuse Treat 21:35–45, 2001

Bandura A, Blanchard EB, Ritter B: The relative efficacy of desensitization and modeling approaches for inducing behavioral, affective, and cognitive changes. J Pers Soc Psychol 13:173–199, 1969

Barlow DH: Anxiety and Its Disorders: The Nature and Treatment of Anxiety and Panic, 2nd Edition. New York, Guilford, 2002

Barlow DH, Brown TA, Craske MG: Definitions of panic attacks and panic disorder in the DSM–IV: implications for research. J Abnorm Psychol 103:553–564, 1994

Baron RM, Kenny DA: The moderator-mediator variable distinction in social psychological research. J Pers Soc Psychol 51:1173–1182, 1986

Basoglu M, Salcioglu E, Livanou M, et al: Single-session behavioral treatment of earthquake-related posttraumatic stress disorder: a randomized waiting list controlled trial. J Trauma Stress 18:1–11, 2005

Basoglu M, Salcioglu E, Livanou M: A randomized controlled study of single-session behavioral treatment of earthquake-related post-traumatic stress disorder using an earthquake simulator. Psychol Med 37:203–213, 2007

Beck AT, Rush AJ, Shaw BF, et al: Cognitive Therapy of Depression. New York, Guilford, 1979

Beck AT, Emery G, Greenberg RL: Anxiety Disorders and Phobias: A Cognitive Perspective. New York, Basic Books, 1985

Beck JG, Coffey SF, Foy DW, et al: Group cognitive behavior therapy for chronic posttraumatic stress disorder: an initial randomized pilot study. Behav Ther 40:82–92, 2009

Becker CB, Zayfert C, Anderson E: A survey of psychologists' attitudes towards and utilization of exposure therapy for PTSD. Behav Res Ther 42:277–292, 2004

Becker CB, Darius E, Schaumberg K: An analog study of patient preferences for exposure versus alternative treatments for posttraumatic stress disorder. Behav Res Ther 45:2861–2873, 2007

Bisson J, Jenkins P, Alexander J, et al: A randomised controlled trial of psychological debriefing for victims of acute burn trauma. Br J Psychiatry 171:78–81, 1997

Bisson JI, McFarlane AC, Rose S: Psychological debriefing, in Effective Treatments for PTSD: Practice Guidelines From the International Society for Traumatic Stress Studies. Edited by Foa EB, Keane TM, Friedman MJ. New York, Guilford, 2000, pp 39–59

Black JL, Keane TM: Implosive therapy in the treatment of combat related fears in a World War II veteran. J Behav Ther Exp Psychiatry 13:163–165, 1982

Blake DD, Weathers FW, Nagy LM, et al: The development of a Clinician-Administered PTSD Scale. J Trauma Stress 8:75–90, 1995

Blanchard EB, Hickling EJ, Barton KA, et al: One-year prospective follow-up of motor vehicle accident victims. Behav Res Ther 34:775–786, 1996

Blanchard EB, Hickling EJ, Devineni T, et al: A controlled evaluation of cognitive behavioral therapy for posttraumatic stress in motor vehicle accident survivors. Behav Res Ther 41:79–96, 2003a

Blanchard EB, Hickling EJ, Malta LS, et al: Prediction of response to psychological treatment among motor vehicle accident survivors with PTSD. Behav Ther 34:351–363, 2003b

Boudewyns PA, Hyer L: Eye movement desensitization and reprocessing (EMDR) as treatment for post-traumatic stress disorder (PTSD). Clin Psychol Psychother 3:185–195, 1996

Bradley R, Greene J, Russ E, et al: A multidimensional meta-analysis of psychotherapy for PTSD. Am J Psychiatry 162:214–227, 2005

Brady KT, Dansky BS, Back SE, et al: Exposure therapy in the treatment of PTSD among cocaine-dependent individuals: preliminary findings. J Subst Abuse Treat 21:47–54, 2001

Brewin CR, Andrews B, Valentine JD: Meta-analysis of risk factors for posttraumatic stress disorder in trauma-exposed adults. J Consult Clin Psychology 68:748–766, 2000

Brom D, Kleber RJ, Defares PB: Brief psychotherapy for post-traumatic stress disorder. J Consult Clin Psychology 57:607–612, 1989

Bryant RA, Harvey AG, Sackville T, et al: Treatment of acute stress disorder: a comparison between cognitive-behavioral therapy and supportive counseling. J Consult Clin Psychology 66:862–866, 1998

Bryant RA, Sackville T, Dangh ST, et al: Treating acute stress disorder: an evaluation of cognitive behavior therapy and supportive counseling techniques. Am J Psychiatry 156:1780–1786, 1999

Bryant RA, Moulds ML, Guthrie RM, et al: Imaginal exposure alone and imaginal exposure with cognitive restructuring in treatment of posttraumatic stress disorder. J Consult Clin Psychology 71:706–712, 2003a

Bryant RA, Moulds ML, Nixon RDV: Cognitive behaviour therapy of acute stress disorder: a four-year follow-up. Behav Res Ther 41:489–494, 2003b

Bryant RA, Mastrodomenico J, Felmingham KL, et al: Treatment of acute stress disorder: a randomized controlled trial. Arch Gen Psychiatry 65:659–667, 2008

Cahill SP, Foa EB: A glass half empty or half full? Where we are and directions for future research in the treatment of PTSD, in Advances in the Treatment of Posttraumatic Stress Disorder: Cognitive-Behavioral Perspectives. Edited by Taylor S. New York, Springer, 2004, pp 267–313

Cahill SP, Carrigan MH, Frueh BC: Does EMDR work? And if so, why? A critical review of controlled outcome and dismantling research. J Anxiety Disord 13:5–33, 1999

Cahill SP, Rauch SAM, Hembree EA, et al: Effect of cognitive-behavioral treatments for PTSD on anger. Journal of Cognitive Psychotherapy 17:113–131, 2003

Cahill SP, Foa EB, Rothbaum BO, et al: First do no harm: worsening or improvement after prolonged exposure. Poster presented at the annual meeting of the International Society for Traumatic Stress Studies, New Orleans, LA, November 2004a

Cahill SP, Zoellner LA, Feeny NC, et al: Sequential treatment for child abuse-related posttraumatic stress disorder: methodological comment on Cloitre, Koenen, Cohen, and Han (2002). J Consult Clin Psychol 72:543–548, 2004b

Cahill SP, Foa EB, Hembree EA, et al: Dissemination of exposure therapy in the treatment of PTSD. J Trauma Stress 19:597–610, 2006

Cahill SP, Rothbaum BO, Resick PA, et al: Cognitive-behavior therapy for adults, in Effective Treatments for PTSD: Practice Guidelines From the International Society for Traumatic Stress Studies, 2nd Edition. Edited by Foa EB, Keane TM, Friedman MJ, et al. New York, Guilford, 2008

Carlier IV, Lamberts RD, Van Uchelen AJ, et al: Disaster related stress in police officers: a field study of the impact of debriefing. Stress Med 14:143–148, 1998

Carlier IV, Voerman AE, Gersons BP: The influence of occupational debriefing on post-traumatic stress symptomatology in traumatized police officers. Br J Med Psychol 73:87–98, 2000

Chard KM: An evaluation of cognitive processing therapy for the treatment of posttraumatic stress disorder related to childhood sexual abuse. J Consult Clin Psychol 73:965–971, 2005

Chemtob CM, Novaco RW, Hamada RS, et al: Cognitive-behavioral treatment of severe anger in posttraumatic stress disorder. J Consult Clin Psychol 65:184–189, 1997

Chemtob CM, Tolin DF, van der Kolk BA, et al: Eye movement desensitization and reprocessing, in Effective Treatments for PTSD: Practice Guidelines From the International Society for Traumatic Stress Studies. Edited by Foa EB, Keane TM, Friedman MJ. New York, Guilford, 2000, pp 139–154

Classen C, Koopman C, Nevill-Manning K: A preliminary report comparing trauma-focused and present-focused group therapy against a wait-listed condition among childhood sexual abuse survivors. Journal of Aggression, Maltreatment and Trauma 4:265–288, 2001

Cloitre M, Koenen KC: The impact of borderline personality disorder on process group outcome among women with posttraumatic stress disorder related to childhood abuse. Int J Group Psychother 51:379–398, 2001

Cloitre M, Koenen K, Cohen LR, et al: Skills training in affective and interpersonal regulation followed by exposure: a phase-based treatment for PTSD related to childhood abuse. J Consult Clin Psychol 70:1067–1074, 2002

Cloitre M, Stovall-McClough K, Miranda R, et al: Therapeutic alliance, negative mood regulation, and treatment outcome in child abuse-related posttraumatic stress disorder. J Consult Clin Psychol 72:411–416, 2004

Conlon L, Fahy TJ, Conroy R: PTSD in ambulant RTA victims: a randomized controlled trial of debriefing. J Psychosom Res 46:37–44, 1999

Cooper NA, Clum GA: Imaginal flooding as a supplementary treatment for PTSD in combat veterans: a controlled study. Behav Ther 20:381–391, 1989

Cusack K, Spates CR: The cognitive dismantling of Eye Movement Desensitization and Reprocessing (EMD/R) treatment of posttraumatic stress disorder (PTSD). J Anxiety Disord 13:87–99, 1999

Davis JL, Wright DC: Randomized clinical trial for treatment of chronic nightmares in trauma-exposed adults. J Trauma Stress 20:123–133, 2007

Deahl MP, Srinivasan M, Jones N, et al: Preventing psychological trauma in soldiers: the role of operational stress training and psychological debriefing. Br J Med Psychol 73:77–85, 2000

Devilly GJ, Foa EB: Comments on Tarrier et al.'s study and the investigation of exposure and cognitive therapy. J Consult Clin Psychol 69:114–116, 2001

Devilly GJ, Spence SH: The relative efficacy and treatment distress of EMDR and a cognitive-behavior trauma treat protocol in the amelioration of posttraumatic stress disorder. J Anxiety Disord 13:131–157, 1999

Difede J, Cukor J, Jayasinghe N, et al: Virtual reality exposure therapy for the treatment of posttraumatic stress disorder following September 11, 2001. J Clin Psychiatry 68:1639–1647, 2007a

Difede J, Malta LS, Best S, et al: A randomized controlled clinical treatment trial for World Trade Center attack-related PTSD in disaster workers. J Nerv Ment Dis 195:861–865, 2007b

Dollard J, Miller NE: Personality and Psychotherapy. New York, McGraw-Hill, 1950

Duffy M, Gillespie K, Clark DM: Post-traumatic stress disorder in the context of terrorism and other civil conflict in Northern Ireland: randomised controlled trial. BMJ 334:1147–1150, 2007

Echeburua E, Corral PD, Zubizarreta I, et al: Psychological treatment of chronic posttraumatic stress disorder in victims of sexual aggression. Behav Modif 21:433–456, 1997

Ehlers A, Clark DM: A cognitive model of posttraumatic stress disorder. Behav Res Ther 38:319–345, 2000

Ehlers A, Clark DM, Hackmann A, et al: A randomized controlled trial of cognitive therapy, self-help booklet, and repeated assessment as early interventions for PTSD. Arch Gen Psychiatry 60:1024–1032, 2003

Ehlers A, Clark DM, Hackmann A, et al: Cognitive therapy for post-traumatic stress disorder: development and evaluation. Behav Res Ther 43:413–431, 2005

Eid J, Johnsen BH, Weisaeth L: The effects of group psychological debriefing on acute stress reactions following a traffic accident: a quasi-experimental approach. Int J Emerg Ment Health 3:145–154, 2001

Emmelkamp PMG, Wessels H: Flooding in imagination vs flooding in vivo: a comparison with agoraphobics. Behav Res Ther 13:7–16, 1975

Everly GS Jr, Flannery RB Jr, Eyler V, et al: Sufficiency analysis of an integrated multicomponent approach to crisis intervention: Critical Incident Stress Management. Adv Mind Body Med 17:174–183, 2001

Fairbank JA, Keane TM: Flooding for combat-related stress disorders: assessment of anxiety reduction across traumatic memories. Behav Ther 13:499–510, 1982

Falsetti SA, Resnick HS, Davis J, et al: Treatment of posttraumatic stress disorder with comorbid panic attacks: combining cognitive processing therapy with panic control treatment techniques. Group Dyn 5:252–260, 2001

Falsetti SA, Resnick HS, Davis J: Multiple Channel Exposure Therapy: Combining cognitive-behavioral therapies for the treatment of posttraumatic stress disorder with panic attacks. Behav Modif 29:70–94, 2005

Fecteau G, Nicki R: Cognitive behavioural treatment of post traumatic stress disorder after motor vehicle accident. Behav Cogn Psychother 27:201–214, 1999

Feeny NC, Zoellner LA, Foa EB: Treatment outcome for chronic PTSD among female assault victims with borderline personality characteristics: a preliminary examination. J Personal Disord 16:30–40, 2002

Foa EB, Cahill SP: Specialized treatment for PTSD: matching survivors to the appropriate modality, in Treating Trauma Survivors With PTSD. Edited by Yehuda R. Washington, DC, American Psychiatric Publishing, 2002, pp 43–62

Foa EB, Goldstein A: Continuous exposure and complete response prevention in the treatment of obsessive-compulsive neurosis. Behav Ther 9:821–829, 1978

Foa EB, Kozak MJ: Emotional processing of fear: exposure to corrective information. Psychol Bull 99:20–35, 1986

Foa EB, Rauch SA: Cognitive changes during prolonged exposure versus prolonged exposure plus cognitive restructuring in female assault survivors with posttraumatic stress disorder. J Consult Clin Psychol 72:879–884, 2004

Foa EB, Rothbaum BO, Kozak MJ: Behavioural treatments of anxiety and depression, in Anxiety and Depression: Distinctive and Overlapping Features. Edited by Kendall P, Watson D. New York, Academic Press, 1989a

Foa EB, Steketee G, Rothbaum B: Behavioral/cognitive conceptualizations of post-traumatic stress disorder. Behav Ther 20:155–176, 1989b

Foa EB, Rothbaum BO, Riggs DS, et al: Treatment of posttraumatic stress disorder in rape victims: a comparison between cognitive-behavioral procedures and counseling. J Consult Clin Psychol 59:715–723, 1991

Foa EB, Hearst-Ikeda D, Perry KJ: Evaluation of a brief cognitive-behavioral program for the prevention of chronic PTSD in recent assault victims. J Consult Clin Psychol 63:948–955, 1995a

Foa EB, Molnar C, Cashman L: Change in rape narratives during exposure therapy for posttraumatic stress disorder. J Trauma Stress 8:675–690, 1995b

Foa EB, Riggs DS, Massie ED, et al: The impact of fear activation and anger on the efficacy of exposure treatment for posttraumatic stress disorder. Behav Ther 26:487–499, 1995c

Foa EB, Franklin ME, Perry KJ, et al: Cognitive biases in generalized social phobia. J Abnorm Psychol 105:433–439, 1996

Foa EB, Dancu CV, Hembree EA, et al: A comparison of exposure therapy, stress inoculation training, and their combination for reducing posttraumatic stress disorder in female assault victims. J Consult Clin Psychol 67:194–200, 1999

Foa EB, Zoellner LA, Feeny NC, et al: Does imaginal exposure exacerbate PTSD symptoms? J Consult Clin Psychol 70:1022–1028, 2002

Foa EB, Rothbaum BO, Furr JM: Augmenting exposure therapy with other CBT procedures. Psychiatr Ann 33:47–53, 2003

Foa EB, Hembree EA, Cahill SP, et al: Randomized trial of prolonged exposure for PTSD with and without cognitive restructuring: outcome at academic and community clinics. J Consult Clin Psychol 73:953–964, 2005

Foa EB, Huppert JD, Cahill SP: Emotional processing theory: an update, in Pathological Anxiety: Emotional Processing in Etiology and Treatment. Edited by Rothbaum BO. Guilford, New York, 2006a, pp 3–24

Foa EB, Zoellner LA, Feeny NC: An evaluation of three brief programs for facilitating recovery after assault. J Trauma Stress 19:29–43, 2006b

Foa EB, Hembree EA, Rothbaum BO: Prolonged Exposure Therapy for PTSD: Emotional Processing of Traumatic Experiences: Therapist Guide. New York, Oxford University Press, 2007

Foa EB, Keane TM, Friedman MJ, et al (eds): Effective Treatments for PTSD: Practice Guidelines From the International Society for Traumatic Stress Studies, 2nd Edition. New York, Guilford, 2008

Freud S: The New Introductory Lectures in Psychoanalysis. New York, Penguin, 1973

Ganzarian R, Buchele BJ: Group psychotherapy for adults with a history of incest, in Comprehensive Group Psychotherapy, 3rd Edition. Edited by Kaplan HI, Sadock BJ. Baltimore, MD, Williams & Wilkins, 1993, pp 515–525

Glynn SM, Eth S, Randolph ET, et al: A test of behavioral family therapy to augment exposure for combat-related posttraumatic stress disorder. J Consult Clin Psychol 67:243–251, 1999

Grinker RR, Spiegel JP: Brief psychotherapy in war neuroses. J Psychosom Med 6:123–131, 1944

Harvey AG, Bryant RA: Acute stress disorder: a synthesis and critique. Psychol Bull 128:886–902, 2002

Hembree EA, Rauch SAM, Foa EB: Beyond the manual: the insider's guide to prolonged exposure for PTSD. Cogn Behav Pract 10:22–30, 2003

Hembree EA, Cahill SP, Foa EB: Impact of personality disorders on treatment outcome for female assault survivors with chronic PTSD. J Personal Disord 18:117–127, 2004a

Hembree EA, Street GP, Riggs DS, et al: Do assault-related variables predict response to cognitive behavioral treatment for PTSD? J Consult Clin Psychol 72:531–534, 2004b

Herman JL, Schatzow E: Recovery and verification of memories of childhood sexual trauma. Psychoanalytic Psychology 4:1–14, 1987

Hickling EJ, Blanchard EB: The private practice psychologist and manual-based treatments: post-traumatic stress disorder secondary to motor vehicle accidents. Behav Res Ther 35:191–203, 1997

Hinton DE, Pham T, Tran M, et al: CBT for Vietnamese refugees with treatment-resistant PTSD and panic attacks: a pilot study. J Trauma Stress 17:429–433, 2004

Hinton DE, Chhean D, Pich V, et al: A randomized controlled trial of cognitive-behavior therapy for Cambodian refugees with treatment-resistant PTSD and panic attack: a cross-over design. J Trauma Stress 18:617–629, 2005a

Hinton DE, Pollack MH, Pich V, et al: Orthostatically induced panic attacks among Cambodian refugees: flashbacks, catastrophic cognitions, and associated psychopathology. Cogn Behav Pract 12:301–311, 2005b

Hinton DE, Chhean D, Pich V, et al: Neck-focused panic attacks among Cambodian refugees: a logistic and linear regression analysis. J Anxiety Disord 20:119–138, 2006a

Hinton DE, Pich V, Chhean D, et al: Somatic-focused therapy for traumatized refugees: treating posttraumatic stress disorder and comorbid neck-focused panic attacks among Cambodian refugees. Psychotherapy: Theory, Research, Practice, Training 43:491–505, 2006b

Hirai M, Clum GA: An Internet-based self-change program for traumatic event related fear, distress, and maladaptive coping. J Trauma Stress 18:631–636, 2005

Hollifield M, Sinclair-Lian N, Warner TD, et al: Acupuncture for posttraumatic stress disorder: a randomized controlled pilot trial. J Nerv Ment Dis 195:504–513, 2007

Hurst AF: Hysteria in the light of the experience of war. J Educ Res 20:771–774, 1919

Institute of Medicine: Treatment of Posttraumatic Stress Disorder: An Assessment of the Evidence. Washington, DC, National Academies Press, 2008

Ironson G, Freund B, Strauss JL, et al: Comparison of two treatments for traumatic stress: a community-based study of EMDR and prolonged exposure. J Clin Psychol 58:113–128, 2002

Jaycox LH, Foa EB, Morral AR: Influence of emotional engagement and habituation on exposure therapy for PTSD. J Consult Clin Psychol 66:185–192, 1998

Keane TM, Zimering RT, Caddell JM: A behavioral formulation of PTSD in Vietnam veterans. The Behavior Therapist 8:9–12, 1985

Keane TM, Fairbank JA, Caddell JM, et al: Implosive (flooding) therapy reduces symptoms of PTSD in Vietnam combat veterans. Behav Ther 20:245–260, 1989

Kraft T, Al-Issa I: The application of learning theory to the treatment of traffic phobia. Br J Psychiatry 111:277–279, 1965

Krakow B, Hollifield M, Scharader R, et al: A controlled study of imagery rehearsal for chronic nightmares with PTSD: a preliminary report. J Trauma Stress 13:589–609, 2000

Krakow B, Hollifield M, Johnston L, et al: Imagery rehearsal therapy for chronic nightmares in sexual assault survivors with posttraumatic stress disorder: a randomized controlled trial. JAMA 286:537–545, 2001

Kubany ES, Hill EE, Owens JA: Cognitive trauma therapy for battered women with PTSD: preliminary findings. J Trauma Stress 16:81–91, 2003

Kubany ES, Hill EE, Owens JA, et al: Cognitive trauma therapy for battered women with PTSD (CTT-BW). J Consult Clin Psychol 72:3–18, 2004

Kudler HS, Blank AS, Krupnick JL: Psychodynamic therapy, in Effective Treatments for PTSD: Practice Guidelines From the International Society for Traumatic Stress Studies. Edited by Foa EB, Keane TM, Friedman MJ. New York, Guilford, 2000, pp 176–198

Kushner M: Desensitization of a posttraumatic phobia, in Case Studies in Behavior Modification. Edited by Ullmann LP, Krasner L. New York, Holt, Rinehart, & Winston, 1965, pp 193–196

Lange A, van de Ven JP, Schrieken B, et al: Interapy, a treatment of posttraumatic stress through the Internet: a controlled trial. J Behav Ther Exp Psychiatry 32:73–90, 2001

Lange A, Rietdijk D, Hudcovicova M, et al: Interapy: a controlled randomized trial of the standardized treatment of posttraumatic stress through the Internet. J Consult Clin Psychol 71:901–909, 2003

Laub D, Auerhahn NC: Knowing and not knowing massive psychic trauma: forms of traumatic memory. Int J Psychoanal 74:287–301, 1993

Lee C, Gavriel H, Drummond P, et al: Treatment of PTSD: Stress inoculation training with prolonged exposure compared to EMDR. J Clin Psychol 58:1071–1089, 2002

Linehan MM: Cognitive-Behavioral Treatment of Borderline Personality Disorder. New York, Guilford, 1993

Litz BT, Williams L, Wang J, et al: A therapist-assisted Internet self-help program for traumatic stress. Prof Psychol Res Pr 35:628–634, 2004

Litz BT, Engel CC, Bryant RA, et al: A randomized, controlled proof-of-concept trial of an Internet-based, therapist-assisted self-management treatment for posttraumatic stress disorder. Am J Psychiatry 164:1676–1683, 2007

Lystad M: Mental Health Response to Mass Emergencies. New York, Brunner/Mazel, 1988

Maercker A, Zollner T, Menning H, et al: Dresden PTSD treatment study: randomized controlled trial of motor vehicle accident survivors. BMC Psychiatry 6:29, 2006

Maher MJ, Rego SA, Asnis GM: Sleep disturbances in patients with post-traumatic stress disorder: epidemiology, impact, and approaches to management. CNS Drugs 20:567–590, 2006

Marks I, Lovell K, Noshirvani H, et al: Treatment of posttraumatic stress disorder by exposure and/or cognitive restructuring. Arch Gen Psychiatry 55:317–325, 1998

Martell CR, Addis ME, Jacobson NS: Depression in Context: Strategies for Guided Action. New York, WW Norton, 2001

Mathews A, Teasdale J, Munby M, et al: A home-based treatment program for agoraphobia. Behav Ther 8:915–924, 1977

Mayou RA, Ehlers A, Hobbs M: Psychological debriefing for road traffic accident victims. Br J Psychiatry 176:589–593, 2000

Meichenbaum D: Cognitive Behavior Modification. Morristown, NJ, General Learning Press, 1974

Meichenbaum D: Stress inoculation training: a preventative and treatment approach, in Principles and Practice of Stress Management, 3rd Edition. Edited by Lehrer PM, Woolfolk RL, Sime WE, et al. New York, Guilford, 2007, pp 497–516

Meyer V: Modification of expectations in cases with obsessional rituals. Behav Res Ther 4:273–280, 1966

Mitchell J: When disaster strikes... the critical incident stress debriefing process. JEMS 8:36–39, 1983

Monson CM, Schnurr PP, Resick PA, et al: Cognitive processing therapy for veterans with military-related posttraumatic stress disorder. J Consult Clin Psychol 74:898–907, 2006

Mueser KT, Bolton E, Carty PC, et al: The trauma recovery group: a cognitive-behavioral program for post-traumatic stress disorder in persons with severe mental illness. Community Ment Health J 43:281–304, 2007

Mueser KT, Rosenberg SD, Xie H, et al: A randomized controlled trial of cognitive-behavioral treatment for posttraumatic stress disorder in severe mental illness. J Consult Clin Psychol 76:259–271, 2008

Najavits LM, Schmitz M, Gotthardt S, et al: Seeking safety plus exposure therapy: an outcome study on dual diagnosis men. J Psychoactive Drugs 37:425–435, 2005

Najavits LM, Gallop RJ, Weiss RD: Seeking Safety therapy for adolescent girls with PTSD and substance use disorder: a randomized controlled trial. J Behav Health Serv Res 33:453–463, 2006

Neuner F, Schauer M, Klaschik C, et al: A comparison of narrative exposure therapy, supportive counseling, and psychoeducation for treating posttraumatic stress disorder in an African refugee settlement. J Consult Clin Psychol 72:579–587, 2004

Otto MW, Hinton D, Korbly NB, et al: Treatment of pharmacotherapy-refractory posttraumatic stress disorder among Cambodian refugees: a pilot study of combination treatment with cognitive-behavior therapy vs sertraline alone. Behav Res Ther 41:1271–1276, 2003

Ozer EJ, Best SR, Lipsey TL, et al: Predictors of posttraumatic stress disorder and symptoms in adults: a meta-analysis. Psychol Bull 129:52–73, 2003

Parson ER: Post-traumatic accelerated cohesions: its recognition and management in group treatment of Vietnam veterans. Group 9:10–23, 1985

Paul GL: Insight vs Desensitization in Psychotherapy. Stanford, CA, Stanford University Press, 1996

Paunovic N, Ost LG: Cognitive-behavior therapy vs exposure therapy in the treatment of PTSD in refugees. Behav Res Ther 39:1183–1197, 2001

Pitman RK, Altman B, Greenwald E, et al: Psychiatric complications during flooding therapy for posttraumatic stress disorder. J Clin Psychiatry 52:17–20, 1991

Pitman RK, Orr SP, Altman B, et al: Emotional processing during eye movement desensitization and reprocessing therapy of Vietnam veterans with chronic posttraumatic stress disorder. Compr Psychiatry 37:419–429, 1996a

Pitman RK, Orr SP, Altman B, et al: Emotional processing and outcome of imaginal flooding therapy in Vietnam veterans with chronic posttraumatic stress disorder. Compr Psychiatry 37:409–418, 1996b

Power KG, McGoldrick T, Brown K, et al: A controlled comparison of eye movement desensitization and reprocessing versus exposure plus cognitive restructuring, versus waiting list in the treatment of posttraumatic stress disorder. J Clin Psychol Psychother 9:299–318, 2002

Powers MB, Emmelkamp PM: Virtual reality exposure therapy for anxiety disorders: a meta-analysis. J Anxiety Disord 22:561–569, 2008

Rachman SJ: Fear and Courage. San Francisco, CA, WH Freeman, 1978

Rachman S: Emotional processing. Behav Res Ther 18:51–60, 1980

Raphael B: When Disaster Strikes. New York, Basic Books, 1986

Renfrey G, Spates CR: Eye movement desensitization: a partial dismantling study. J Behav Ther Exp Psychiatry 25:231–239, 1994

Resick PA, Schnicke MK: Cognitive processing therapy for sexual assault victims. J Consult Clin Psychol 60:748–756, 1992

Resick PA, Nishith P, Weaver TL, et al: A comparison of cognitive processing therapy with prolonged exposure and a waiting condition for the treatment of chronic posttraumatic stress disorder in female rape victims. J Consult Clin Psychol 70:867–879, 2002

Resick PA, Nishith P, Griffin MG: How well does cognitive-behavioral therapy treat symptoms of complex PTSD? An examination of child sexual abuse survivors within a clinical trial. CNS Spectr 8:340–355, 2003

Resick PA, Galovski TE, Uhlmansiek MO, et al: A randomized clinical trial to dismantle components of cognitive processing therapy for posttraumatic stress disorder in female victims of interpersonal violence. J Consult Clin Psychol 76:243–258, 2008

Richards DA, Lovell K, Marks IM: Post-traumatic stress disorder: evaluation of a behavioral treatment program. J Trauma Stress 7:669–680, 1994

Riggs DS, Rothbaum BO, Foa EB: A prospective examination of symptoms of posttraumatic stress disorder in victims of nonsexual assault. J Interpers Violence 10:201–214, 1995

Rose S, Brewin CR, Andrews B, et al: A randomized controlled trial of individual psychological debriefing for victims of violent crime. Psychol Med 29:793–799, 1999

Rothbaum B, Foa EB: Exposure treatment of PTSD concomitant with conversion mutism: a case study. Behav Ther 22:449–456, 1991

Rothbaum BO, Foa EB, Riggs DS, et al: A prospective examination of post-traumatic stress disorder in rape victims. J Trauma Stress 5:455–475, 1992

Rothbaum BO, Astin MC, Marsteller F: Prolonged exposure versus eye movement desensitization and reprocessing (EMDR) for PTSD rape victims. J Trauma Stress 18:607–616, 2005

Rothbaum BO, Cahill SP, Foa EB, et al: Augmentation of sertraline with prolonged exposure in the treatment of PTSD. J Trauma Stress 19:625–638, 2006

Rounsaville BJ, Weissman MM, Prusoff BA, et al: Marital disputes and treatment outcome in depressed women. Compr Psychiatry 20:483–490, 1979

Schnurr PP, Friedman MJ, Foy DW, et al: Randomized trial of trauma-focused group therapy for posttraumatic stress disorder. Arch Gen Psychiatry 60:481–488, 2003

Schnurr PP, Friedman MJ, Engel CC, et al: Cognitive behavioral therapy for posttraumatic stress disorder in women: a randomized controlled trial. JAMA 297:820–830, 2007

Schottenbauer MA, Arnkoff DB, Glass CR, et al: Psychotherapy for posttraumatic stress disorder in the community: reported prototypical treatments. Clin Psychol Psychother 13:108–122, 2006

Shapiro F: Efficacy of eye movement desensitization procedure in the treatment of traumatic memories. J Trauma Stress 2:199–223, 1989

Shapiro F: Eye movement desensitization and reprocessing procedure: from EMD to EMDR: a new treatment model for anxiety and related traumata. The Behavior Therapist 14:133–135, 1991

Shapiro F: Eye Movement Desensitization and Reprocessing: Basic Principles, Protocols, and Procedures, 2nd Edition. New York, Guilford, 2001

Shear K, Frank E, Houck PR, et al: Treatment of complicated grief: a randomized controlled trial. JAMA 293:2601–2608, 2005

Shear MK, Frank E, Foa E, et al: Traumatic grief treatment: a pilot study. Am J Psychiatry 158:1506–1508, 2001

Spates CR, Koch E, Pagoto S, et al: Eye movement desensitization and reprocessing, in Effective Treatments for PTSD: Practice Guidelines From the International Society for Traumatic Stress Studies, 2nd Edition. Edited by Foa EB, Keane TM, Friedman MJ, et al. New York, Guilford 2008

Spiegel D, Classen C, Thurston E, et al: Trauma-focused versus present-focused models of group therapy for women sexually abused in childhood, in From Childhood Sexual Abuse to Adult Sexual Risk: Trauma, Revictimization, and Intervention. Edited by Koenig LJ, Doll LS, O'Leary A, et al. Washington, DC, American Psychological Association, 2004, pp 251–268

Stalker C, Fry R: A comparison of short-term group and individual therapy for sexually abused women. Can J Psychiatry 44:168–174, 1999

Suinn RM, Richardson F: Anxiety management training: a nonspecific behavior therapy program for anxiety control. Behav Ther 2:498–510, 1971

Tarrier N, Pilgrim H, Sommerfield C, et al: A randomized trial of cognitive therapy and imaginal exposure in the treatment of chronic posttraumatic stress disorder. J Consult Clin Psychol 67:13–18, 1999

Tarrier N, Sommerfield C, Pilgrim H, et al: Factors associated with outcome of cognitive-behavioural treatment of chronic post-traumatic stress disorder. Behav Res Ther 38:191–202, 2000

Taylor S: Anxiety Sensitivity: Theory, Research, and Treatment of the Fear of Anxiety. Mahwah, NJ, Erlbaum, 1999

Taylor S, Fedoroff IC, Koch WJ, et al: Posttraumatic Stress Disorder Arising After Road Traffic Collisions: Patterns of Response to Cognitive–Behavior Therapy. J Consult Clin Psychol 69:541–551, 2001

Taylor S, Thordarson DS, Maxfield L, et al: Efficacy, speed, and adverse effects of three PTSD treatments: exposure therapy, relaxation training, and EMDR. J Consult Clin Psychol 71:330–338, 2003

van der Kolk BA, McFarlane AC, van der Hart O: Psychotherapy for posttraumatic stress disorder and other trauma-related disorders, in The American Psychiatric Publishing Textbook of Anxiety Disorders [1st edition]. Edited by Stein DJ, Hollander E. Washington, DC, American Psychiatric Publishing, 2002, pp 403–411

van Minnen A, Arntz A, Keijsers GPJ: Prolonged exposure in patients with chronic PTSD: predictors of treatment outcome and dropout. Behav Res Ther 40:439–457, 2002

Vaughan K, Armstrong MS, Gold R, et al: A trial of eye movement desensitization compared to image habituation training and applied muscle relaxation in posttraumatic stress disorder. J Behav Ther Exp Psychiatry 25:283–291, 1994

Veronen LJ, Kilpatrick DG: Stress management for rape victims, in Stress Reduction and Prevention. Edited by Meichenbaum D, Jaremko ME. New York, Plenum, 1983, pp 341–374

Wallerstein RS, DeWitt KN: Intervention modes in psychoanalysis and psychoanalytic psychotherapies: a revised classification. Journal of Psychotherapy Integration 7:129–150, 1997

Wolff R: Systematic desensitization and negative practice to alter the aftereffects of a rape attempt. J Behav Ther Exp Psychiatry 8:423–425, 1977

Wolpe J: Psychotherapy by Reciprocal Inhibition. Stanford, CA, Stanford University Press, 1958

Yassen J, Glass L: Sexual assault survivor groups: a feminist practice perspective. Soc Work 29:252–257, 1984

Zayfert C, DeViva JC: Residual insomnia following cognitive behavioral therapy for PTSD. J Trauma Stress 17:69–73, 2004

Zlotnick C, Warshaw M, Shea MT, et al: Trauma and chronic depression among patients with anxiety disorders. J Consult Clin Psychol 65:333–336, 1997

Zoellner LA, Feeny NC, Cochran B, et al: Treatment choice for PTSD. Behav Res Ther 41:879–886, 2003

Recommended Readings

Foa EB, Chrestman KR, Gilboa-Schechtman E: Prolonged Exposure Therapy for PTSD: Emotional Process of Traumatic Experiences: Therapist Guide. Oxford, UK, Oxford University Press, 2009

Follette VM, Ruzek JI: Cognitive-Behavioral Therapies for Trauma, 2nd Edition. New York, Guilford, 2006

Taylor S: Clinician's Guide to PTSD: A Cognitive-Behavioral Approach. New York, Guilford, 2006

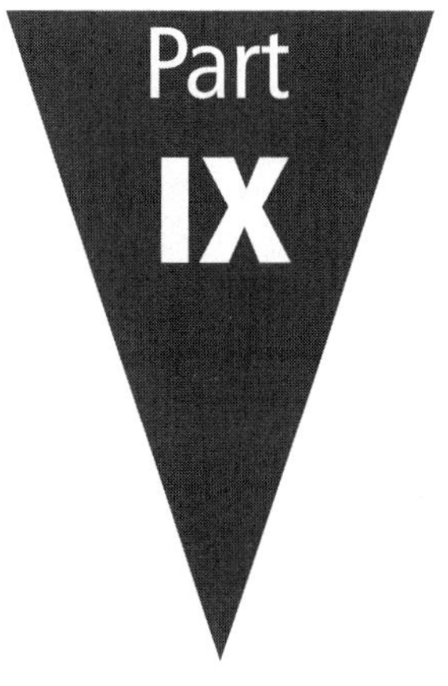

Anxiety Disorders in Special Populations

Chapter 34

Anxiety Disorders in Children and Adolescents

Phoebe S. Moore, Ph.D.
John S. March, M.D., M.P.H.
Anne Marie Albano, Ph.D., ABPP
Margo Thienemann, M.D.

Presumably because they are associated with significant suffering and disruption in normal psychosocial and academic development and family functioning, disorders characterized by excessive fear are among the more common causes of referral of children to mental health care (Morris and March 2004). Prevalence studies indicate that between 6% and 20% of children have at least one clinically diagnosable anxiety disorder (Costello et al. 2004); and this striking statistic does not include obsessive-compulsive disorder (OCD), which affects another 0.5%–1.0% of children (Flament et al. 1988). As many as 54% of affected young persons will experience a major depressive episode as part of their anxiety syndrome (Costello et al. 2004; Kessler et al. 1994), with consequent increases in morbidity and perhaps mortality (Curry et al. 2004).

Echoing many of the findings elsewhere in this book on adult anxiety disorders, in this chapter we provide an overview of the anxiety disorders that have a specific onset during childhood or adolescence: generalized anxiety disorder, separation anxiety disorder, social phobia, and specific phobia. For more detailed reviews on etiopathogenesis (Sweeney and Pine 2004), assessment (Fonseca and Perrin 2001; Greco and Morris 2004), epidemiology (Costello and Angold 1995b; Costello et al. 2004), psychosocial treatments (Flannery-Schroeder and Kendall 2000; Kendall et al. 2004), family treatment (Barmish and Kendall 2005; Barrett et al. 1996, 2001), medication management (Reinblatt and Riddle 2007; Reinblatt and Walkup 2005), and combined treatment (March and Ollendick 2004), please see the "Recommended Readings" at the end of the chapter.

This work was supported in part by National Institute of Mental Health grant 1 K24 MH01557 to Dr. March. Portions of this chapter were adapted from March JS: "Assessment of Pediatric Posttraumatic Stress Disorder," in *Posttraumatic Stress Disorder: A Comprehensive Text.* Edited by Saigh PA, Bremner JD. Boston, MA, Allyn & Bacon, 1999, Chapter 10, and from Kratochvil C, Kutcher S, Reiter S, et al: "Psychopharmacology of Pediatric Anxiety Disorders," in *Handbook of Psychotherapies With Children and Families* (Issues in Clinical Child Psychology). Edited by Russ SW, Ollendick TH. New York, Kluwer Academic/Plenum, 1999, Chapter 18.

Overview of Anxiety in Children and Adolescents

Most fears occurring during childhood and adolescence are developmentally appropriate to the context in which they occur. Anxiety is a normal and basic emotion, deeply rooted in the neurobiological system to promote protection and survival (Barlow 2002). *Anxiety, worry,* and *fear* are all terms describing the process of anticipating threat or harm. At certain levels and under certain conditions, anxiety, worry, and fear serve an adaptive function. For example, the experience of anxiety in anticipation of a musical performance will motivate an individual to rehearse; worry about the consequences of smoking may lead to ceasing smoking or not starting to smoke; and fear of being victimized may prevent an individual from walking alone through high-crime areas late at night.

In contrast to these normal processes, the clinical manifestation of anxiety usually refers to developmentally inappropriate fears or to developmentally appropriate fears that produce excessive distress or dysfunction (Silverman 1987). Excessive anxiety underlies each of the clinical manifestations of anxiety disorders, with the focus of that anxiety distinguishing between the conditions (Barlow 2002). Phobias are fears that are attached to specific objects or situations and that usually provoke avoidance, such as the fear of doctors, enclosed spaces, animals, or heights. Panic is the clinical manifestation of fear, whereby experience of the fight-or-flight reaction occurs in the absence of an objective threat (Barlow 2002). Worry, in generalized anxiety disorder, is typically a more diffuse anxiety state, is focused on many different situations and events, and is experienced as excessive and uncontrollable. The remaining anxiety disorders, such as separation anxiety disorder or social phobia, are also circumscribed to specific foci, such as being away from loved ones in the former or fear of negative evaluation in the latter.

Anxiety disorders in youths are composed of sets of clinically relevant fears that are among the common, but normative, fears present at one time or another in many children and adolescents. From a diagnostic point of view, such fears and worries are ubiquitous, so clinicians and researchers interested in childhood anxiety disorders face the daunting task of differentiating pathological anxiety from fears that occur as a part of normal developmental processes (Costello and Angold 1995b).

One approach to this taxonomic problem has been the development of rating scales that inventory common fears in children and adolescents (March and Albano 1996). The Multidimensional Anxiety Scale for Children (MASC; March 1998; March et al. 1997b) illustrates the general approach. The MASC was developed to sample key anxiety symptoms from the universe of anxiety symptoms that have concerned clinicians and researchers working with anxious children and adolescents. Only the most important symptoms and symptom clusters survived the scale development process, so that the MASC can be seen as representing the population factor structure of anxiety in both children and adolescents. As summarized in Table 34–1, the MASC contains four main factors, three of which can be divided into subfactors. To a large extent, the empirically derived factor structure of the MASC matches the DSM-IV-TR (American Psychiatric Association 2000) diagnostic clusters of social phobia, separation anxiety disorder, panic, and, averaged across all four factors, generalized anxiety disorder (Baldwin and Dadds 2007; Dierker et al. 2001; Grills-Taquechel et al. 2008). In addition, the hypothesized division of harm avoidance into perfectionism and anxious coping has also received empirical support (March 1998); this along with sex and age norms allows empirical quantification of distress and impairment, which is essential to establishing clinical severity, and thus diagnoses.

In contrast to scalar approaches, DSM-III-R (American Psychiatric Association 1987) took the tack of introducing a categorically defined subclass of anxiety disorders of childhood and adolescence; DSM-IV (American Psychiatric Association 1994) and its text revision in 2000 (DSM-IV-TR) both refined these con-

TABLE 34–1. Factor structure of anxiety from the Multidimensional Anxiety Scale for Children

Physical symptoms
Tense symptoms
Somatic symptoms
Harm avoidance
Perfectionism
Anxious coping
Social anxiety
Humiliation fears
Performance fears
Separation/panic anxiety

structs and established a greater degree of continuity—developmental and nosological—with the adult anxiety disorders. The DSM taxonomy in essence reflects an expert consensus regarding the actual clustering of anxiety in pediatric population samples (Shaffer et al. 1989), but empirical support in some cases is questionable (Beidel 1991). More specifically, several DSM-III-R anxiety disorders of childhood (overanxious and avoidant disorders, in particular) were collapsed in DSM-IV into the adult categories (generalized anxiety disorder and social phobia, respectively). However, the DSM-IV criteria sets themselves do not in general reflect a developmental perspective (Angold and Costello 1995; Cantwell and Baker 1988), so the clinician must translate the DSM-IV criteria into terms that are relevant for the age, sex, and cultural background of the child.

When considering how best to inventory anxiety symptoms, the severity and prevalence of fears must be considered, as well as their timing in the developmental trajectory (for a review, see Warren and Sroufe 2004). For example, certain specific phobias, such as nighttime fears, are age dependent in that they are much more common in children during the preschool and early elementary school years (King et al. 1992). In older children, however, the presence of such fears may more reliably be seen as indicating pathological anxiety. Similarly, separation anxiety seems more prominent in younger children, in whom it is developmentally appropriate, and becomes increasingly less appropriate as the child moves through middle childhood into adolescence (Black 1992). Other fears, such as fears about self-presentation and consequent social anxiety, become more common as children mature into adolescence (Costello and Angold 1995a).

In the DSM taxonomy, children with generalized anxiety disorder typically are characterized as perfectionistic "worriers" who are constantly asking for reassurance (Beidel and Turner 2005). The diagnostic category of generalized anxiety disorder in DSM-IV subsumes the childhood-only diagnosis of overanxious disorder from DSM-III-R. Children with social phobia show an exaggerated concern with self-presentation. They constantly fear saying or doing something foolish or embarrassing, are exquisitely sensitive to rejection and humiliation, and often feel socially scrutinized, which they usually handle by avoiding social interchange, particularly when it involves public speaking (Beidel et al. 2004). Social phobia now subsumes another childhood-only DSM-III-R disorder, avoidant disorder. Selective mutism can be conceptualized as an age-appropriate variant of specific (public speaking) or generalized social phobia, dependent on the extent of other areas of social inhibition, in which usually younger children will not talk (despite normal language development) to anyone other than "safe" friends and adults (Bergman et al. 2002; Freeman et al. 2004). Separation anxiety disorder is characterized by an intense fear of harm surrounding important attachment figures. Other anxiety disorders occurring in childhood include OCD, characterized by intrusive, unwanted, anxiety-provoking thoughts and anxiety-relieving rituals; panic disorder, with or without agoraphobia, which manifests in attacks of extreme fear and somatic symptoms, often leading to situational avoidance; and posttraumatic stress disorder (PTSD), which occurs after a trauma and manifests as intrusive reexperiencing of the trauma through memories, hypervigilance and hyperarousal, and avoidance of reminders of the trauma, accompanied by restricted affect or feelings of detachment or anhedonia.

Epidemiological surveys reveal that the anxiety disorders, particularly when assessed via symptoms rather than via functional impairment, are highly evident in children and adolescents. Costello et al. (2004), in their extensive review of the existing epidemiological evidence, note that lifetime estimates of any anxiety disorder in pediatric samples can range from approximately 14% or 15% (Warren et al. 1997; Wittchen et al. 1998) to as high as 25% (Brady et al. 2000; Kessler et al. 1994). Requiring a more stringent definition of anxiety disorder by including an impairment or disability criterion reduces rates by half or more; Costello et al. (2004) cite data from the Methods for Epidemiology of Child and Adolescent Mental Disorders (MECA) study (N=1,285), which showed that requiring at least moderate impairment for an anxiety diagnosis reduced the size of the "any anxiety diagnosis" group from 20.5% of the full sample to 7.2%. However, even when this more stringent criterion is applied, anxiety disorders seem to afflict a substantial minority of youths and must be considered a significant public health concern. In addition, it is notable that anxiety symptoms that do not reach a diagnostic threshold can often be associated with significant disability or impairment (Angold et al. 1999).

Overall, current or 3-month prevalence estimates in children and adolescents for any anxiety disorder tend to range from 2% to 4%, while 6-month to 12-month estimates show rates of 10%–20%, and lifetime estimates are only a bit higher (Costello et al. 2004). Generalized anxiety disorder and its now-defunct sister diagnosis, overanxious disorder, appear to be the most common, followed by separation anxiety, social phobia, and the specific phobias. Less common are PTSD, OCD, and panic disorder, which tend to reach less than 1% prevalence in population samples (Costello et al. 2004). Epidemiological data show that girls are affected more often than boys, with an overall ratio of 2:1 for anxiety diagnoses (with some variability by diagnosis), which holds steady throughout childhood and adolescence (Costello et al. 2004; Lewinsohn et al. 1998).

Finally, comorbidity among the anxiety disorders, and between the anxiety disorders and other internalizing and externalizing disorders, complicates both diagnosis and treatment (Costello et al. 2004; Curry et al. 2004). For example, a wide variety of specific phobias commonly accompany the anxiety disorders, including fear of the dark, monsters, kidnappers, bugs, small animals, heights, and open or enclosed spaces. Nighttime fears, resistance to going to bed, difficulty falling asleep alone or sleeping through the night alone, and nightmares involving separation themes are not uncommon. These specific phobic symptoms are common triggers for panic or separation anxiety and are responsible for many of the avoidance and ritualized anxiety-reducing behaviors (Black 1995). Anxious children also show high rates of comorbid depression (Costello et al. 2004; Curry et al. 2004). Children and adolescents with both anxiety and depression have a significantly worse long-term prognosis than those with anxiety alone (Pine et al. 1998), with a higher-than-expected risk for suicide (Lewinsohn et al. 1995). Youths with social anxiety and panic disorder may also be at risk for substance abuse disorders (Clark and Neighbors 1996).

Assessment

As noted earlier in this chapter, a wide variety of normal fears and worries are omnipresent among youths; pathological anxieties are less common but not rare (Costello et al. 2004; Ollendick et al. 1985); thus, both research requirements and clinical needs demand high quality, developmentally tailored instruments for the measurement of anxiety symptomatology and severity in youths. The past decade has seen a much-needed focus on the development and refinement of several promising assessment tools for pediatric anxiety (Silverman and Ollendick 2005). These newer instruments strive to take into account the unique aspects of anxiety as it manifests early in development, including the developmentally sanctioned progression in anxiety symptoms (Keller et al. 1992; Last et al. 1987) and the differences in day-to-day environments from those most typically experienced by adults, so that the presentation of anxiety also differs, as in *school phobia*. However, despite recent improvements in the availability of wide- and narrow-band self-report instruments, as well as the availability of structured clinical interviews for anxiety diagnosis, tools are lacking for parent and teacher reports of anxiety (Greco and Morris 2004). Likewise, measures of observed behavior, which may be particularly illuminating in the case of this set of psychiatric disorders, are seldom used and, as of yet, are neither normed nor standardized.

Silverman and Ollendick (2005) provide a critical and thoughtful, in-depth review of the field of evidence-based assessment of anxiety in youths, with specific recommendations for research and clinical applications. Additional information about assessment of pediatric anxiety disorders is available in Greco and Morris 2004; Langley et al. 2002; Schniering et al. 2000; and Wood et al. 2002.

Checklist Measures

Some anxiety symptoms, such as refusing to attend school in the patient with panic disorder and agoraphobia, are readily observable; other symptoms are open only to child introspection and thus to child self-reporting. For this and other reasons, self-report measures of anxiety, which provide an opportunity for the child to reveal his or her internal or "hidden" experience, have found wide application in both clinical and research settings (March and Albano 1996).

Typically, self-report measures use a Likert scale format in which a child is asked to rate each questionnaire item in an ordinal format anchored to frequency or distress/impairment or a combination of the two. For example, a child might be asked to rate "I feel tense" on a four-point frequency dimension that ranges from "almost never" to "often." Self-report measures are easy to administer, require a minimum of the clinician's time, and economically capture a wide range of important anxiety dimensions from the child's point of view. Taken together, these features make self-report measures ideally suited to gathering data before the initial evaluation because self-report measures used in this fashion increase clinician efficiency by facilitating accurate assessment of the prior probability that a particular child will or will not have symptoms within a specific symptom domain.

Earlier self-report measures of anxiety generally represented age-downward extensions of adult measures

(March and Albano 1996). These include the Revised Fear Survey Schedule for Children (Ollendick 1983), the Revised Children's Manifest Anxiety Scale (Reynolds and Paget 1981), and the State-Trait Anxiety Inventory for Children (Spielberger et al. 1976). The consensus regarding these measures currently is that although they may provide reliable and valid indices of global patient distress, they lack discriminant validity and thus confound anxiety with commonly comorbid conditions such as depression and attention-deficit/hyperactivity disorders (Greco and Morris 2004).

The identified need for more anxiety-specific scales that correspond more effectively to DSM-IV led to the development of three newer global anxiety measures: the MASC (described earlier), the Screen for Child Anxiety Related Emotional Disorders (SCARED; Birmaher et al. 1997, 1999), and the Spence Children's Anxiety Scale (Spence 1998) and its refinement by Chorpita and colleagues, the Revised Child Anxiety and Depression Scale (RCADS; Chorpita et al. 2000). These measures each present unique improvements on the above-reviewed instruments. The MASC, currently considered the gold standard of anxiety self-report assessment, is a normed instrument that produces both global and narrow-band scores reflecting developmentally tailored indices of severity. Its psychometric properties have been shown to be robust (Dierker et al. 2001; Grills-Taquechel et al. 2008; Wood et al. 2002). In addition to norms, the MASC has the unique strengths of having a validity index and a harm avoidance scale. The factor structure identified in the child-report version of the scale has been shown to hold for a parent-report version as well (Baldwin and Dadds 2007).

The SCARED instrument also shows strong psychometrics and validity data (Birmaher et al. 1997, 1999) and maps directly onto DSM-IV anxiety categories. It has parallel parent and child forms. This measure has been shown to be sensitive to treatment exposure (Muris et al. 2001). The revision of the Spence Children's Anxiety Scale, the RCADS, shares many of the strengths of the SCARED (Chorpita et al. 2000) but is newer and thus less tested in the research and clinical literature. As noted by Greco and Morris (2004), research is needed to delineate the relative strengths and unique contributions of each of these newer measures.

Parent-report versions of the SCARED and the MASC assessment tools are now available, allowing increased depth of knowledge to be attained via these checklist measures. However, few checklist measures of pediatric anxiety symptomatology or severity exist for teachers beyond such wide-band measures as the Teacher Report Form (Achenbach and Rescorla 2001).

Finally, some useful narrow-band measures for the assessment of specific anxiety disorders exist, including the Social Anxiety Scale for Children—Revised (La Greca and Stone 1993), the Children's Yale-Brown Obsessive Compulsive Scale (Goodman et al. 1991), and the Child PTSD Symptom Scale (Foa et al. 2001).

Diagnostic Interviews

Dimensional measures, such as the MASC, SCARED, and RCADS, can point clinicians toward clinically relevant symptoms and, precisely because of their dimensionality, are more able to gauge severity of symptoms. Conversely, establishing a DSM-IV-TR diagnosis generally requires an interview-based approach. Thus, it is not surprising that investigators have long called for an increased use of valid and standardized diagnostic procedures to compare data across settings (e.g., Albano et al. 1995). The clinical interview has become one such method of standardizing data collection while minimizing factors that confound the reliability and validity of the diagnostic process (Eisen and Kearney 1995). Structured and semistructured interviews allow the quantification of clinical data, reduce the potential for interviewer bias, and enhance diagnostic reliability (Silverman 1987). Virtually all such interviews used with clinically anxious children cover the same general age range (7–17 years), providing evaluation of both children and adolescents. Clinically, semistructured interviews have an advantage over structured interviews because they present diagnostic criteria and related clinical inquiries in a standardized format, while allowing the clinician a limited range of flexibility for elaboration and probing. Thus, a clinician may adapt the wording of a particular question to meet the cognitive developmental level of the child.

Most diagnostic interviews require that both parent and child be interviewed with complementary versions of the assessment instrument, which makes these instruments cumbersome for clinical practice. However, use of both parent and child interviews has the strength of allowing evaluators to assign diagnoses based on DSM-IV-TR criteria as seen from multiple perspectives. For example, the Anxiety Disorders Interview Schedule for DSM-IV (ADIS), child and parent versions (Silverman and Albano 1996), developed specifically to facilitate clinical research with anxious children and adolescents but now widely used in clinical settings as well, is a semistructured clinical interview that assesses the range of anxiety disorders, mood disorders, and related behavioral disturbances in children and adolescents. The ADIS is appropriate for administration to children ages 7–17, with developmentally appropriate wording and descriptors incorporated within the interview. The ADIS usually is administered by one evaluator and generally takes up to 3 hours to administer. Parents are interviewed separately from the child, with the general rule that data gained from one source not be used when interviewing the second source or divulged to the second source.

For each diagnosis, an initial inquiry section in the ADIS provides questions that probe for the presence of specific diagnostic criteria for each individual disorder, with skipouts strategically placed if threshold criteria are not met. An interference section provides an assessment of the child's and parent's subjective reporting of the degree of distress and impairment resulting from each diagnosis. If the clinician is interested in obtaining only diagnostic status, then just these two sections are required to assign a DSM-IV-TR diagnosis. Additional questions are provided to more fully examine the phenomenology of the disorders, to determine the degree of impairment in specific areas of functioning, and to explore relevant research questions pertaining to these disorders in youths. In addition, the ADIS provides an efficient mechanism for tracking overall treatment progress and patterns of symptom remission through follow-up assessments. In particular, the clinician is able to access information about the child's beliefs and interpretation of the problem; rate the child's physiological reactivity and assess for panic symptomatology; and gain an understanding of the behavioral mechanisms involved in escape, avoidance, or other methods of coping with the anxiety, each of which helps considerably with treatment planning and implementation.

Behavioral Observation

Although checklist and interview measures can provide useful information on symptomatology and the diagnostic profile, these measures can provide an incomplete or biased picture of patient functioning. Problems of agreement between raters (parents, teachers, and children; Epkins and Meyers 1994) can cloud the clinical picture, as can issues of various types of response bias, such as social desirability (Barrios and Hartmann 1997) and cognitive distortions characteristic of anxiety and internalizing symptomatology (Kendall and Flannery-Schroeder 1998). Thus, an assessment battery that utilizes samples of child behavior in anxiety-provoking situations has unique advantages for objective assessment. Currently there are no standardized behavioral measures of anxiety, but it is recommended that the thoughtful clinician attempt to obtain samples of anxious behaviors by the use of in-session unstructured observation, appropriate in-session behavioral avoidance tests (e.g., requesting that a socially anxious child go ask a question of the clinic's receptionist and observing the child's response), home observation, and/or school observation.

Clinical Application

To further anticipate the relevance of a careful diagnostic assessment to treatment, it cannot be overemphasized that the cornerstone of both pharmacological and psychosocial management of pediatric anxiety disorders is a careful functional analysis of problem behaviors. In terms of the disease management model, modern psychiatric treatment requires clear specification of the behavioral or emotional syndrome (e.g., anxiety); and within the syndrome, problems (e.g., avoidance of speaking in front of others); and within problems, symptoms (e.g., will not answer questions in class) targeted for intervention. Consequently, a thorough diagnostic assessment, including both a clinical interview with behavioral observation and a multimethod, multi-informant, multidomain scalar evaluation, is thought to be essential to generating a cognitive-behavioral treatment plan (March et al. 1995). The overall assessment goal is to move from the presenting complaint through a DSM-IV-TR diagnosis based on Axes I through V to a tailored treatment plan based on an idiographic portrayal of the problems besetting the child or adolescent. Such an evaluation might begin with a review of the patient's demographics and developmental, treatment, and psychiatric or medical history; a review of findings from normed rating scale data, school records, and previous mental health treatment records; a clinical interview of the child and his or her parents covering Axes I through V of DSM-IV-TR; a formal mental status examination; one or more behavioral observations; and, in some cases, a specialized neuropsychological evaluation. Ideally, a structured interview, such as the ADIS Child Version (Silverman and Albano 1996), also should be part of every diagnostic assessment.

Treatment

Overview

With the emergence of a rich psychopathology literature covering all the important domains of child and adolescent symptomatology, pediatric psychiatry and psychology have moved away from nonspecific interventions toward problem-focused treatments keyed to specific DSM diagnoses (Kazdin 1997; Kazdin and Weisz 2003; Kendall and Panichelli-Mindel 1995). In particular, the past 40 years have seen the emergence of diverse, sophisticated, empirically supported cognitive-behavioral therapy (CBT) methods for a range of childhood-onset mental disorders (Hibbs and Jensen 2005). Although psychodynamic psychotherapy (Keith 1995) is generally accepted as a treatment approach for anxious youths, largely because of uncontrolled case descriptions, individual (e.g., Kendall 1994) and family-centered (e.g., Barrett et al. 1996) CBT is the only treatment that has to date received solid empirical support. As a result of a significant body of research evidence, many now affirm that CBT administered within an evidence-based disease management model is the psychotherapeutic treatment of choice for pediatric anxiety disorders (see, for example, March et al. 1997a).

Cognitive-Behavioral Therapy

Historically, behavior therapy evolved within the theoretical framework of classical and operant conditioning, with cognitive interventions assuming a more prominent role with the increasing recognition that person-environment interactions are powerfully mediated by cognitive processes (Van Hasselt and Hersen 1993). Viewed in the context of situational and/or cognitive processes, behavior therapy is sometimes referred to as nonmediational (emphasizing the direct influence of situations on behavior) and cognitive therapy as mediational (emphasizing that thoughts and feelings underlie behavior). Behavioral psychotherapists work with patients to change behaviors and thereby reduce distressing thoughts and feelings. Cognitive therapists work to first change thoughts and feelings, with improvements in functional behavior following in turn. Despite their seeming differences, virtually all cognitive-behavioral interventions (including those for disruptive behaviors and depression) share four qualities:

1. An emphasis on psychoeducation
2. A detailed behavioral analysis of the problem and the factors that maintain or extinguish it
3. Problem-specific treatment interventions designed to ameliorate the symptoms of concern
4. Relapse prevention and generalization training at the end of treatment

CBT thus fits nicely into the current medical practice environment that appropriately values brief, empirically supported, problem-focused treatments. The major techniques used in CBT for pediatric anxiety disorders are summarized in Table 34–2.

Historically, the behavioral treatment of fear and anxiety in children dates back to the classic work of Jones (1924a, 1924b) and the elimination of the fear of rabbits in a small boy referred to as "Peter." Treatment consisted of progressive exposure of Peter to the rabbit while he was engaged in a pleasurable activity (eating) incompatible with fear. Following treatment, Peter's fear dissipated in response to both the rabbit and other, similar stimuli to which the fear had generalized. Building on Jones's early work, Wolpe (1958) developed a "graduated deconditioning" technique that he called *systematic desensitization*. The rationale for systematic desensitization is that anxiety is a set of classically conditioned responses that can be unlearned or counter-conditioned through associative pairing with anxiety-incompatible stimuli and responses. In systematic desensitization, anxiety-arousing stimuli are systematically and gradually paired (imaginally or in vivo) with competing stimuli such as food, praise, imagery, or cues generated from muscular relaxation. Systematic desensitization with children consists of three basic steps:

1. Training in progressive muscle relaxation
2. Rank ordering of fearful situations from lowest to highest
3. Hierarchically presenting fear stimuli via imagery while the child is in a relaxed state (Eisen and Kearney 1995)

Systematic desensitization appears to work well with older children and adolescents. Younger children, however, often have difficulty with both obtaining vivid imagery and acquiring the incompatible muscular relaxation. Strategies such as use of developmentally appropriate imagery and adjunctive use of workbooks may increase the effectiveness of these procedures with younger children.

Typically, anxious children and adolescents do not remain in the presence of anxiety-arousing stimuli for a sufficient length of time to allow extinction to occur in

TABLE 34–2. Techniques used in cognitive-behavioral therapy for pediatric anxiety disorders

Term	Definition	Examples
Cognitive restructuring	Active altering of maladaptive thought patterns; replacing these negative thoughts with more constructive adaptive cognitions and beliefs	Challenging aberrant risk appraisal in the patient with panic disorder
Contrived exposure	Exposure in which the patient seeks out and confronts anxiety-provoking situations or triggers	Intentionally going back to school (a child with separation anxiety)
Differential reinforcement of appropriate behavior	Attending to and positively rewarding appropriate behavior, especially when incompatible with inappropriate behavior	Praising (and maybe paying) the child with social phobia for answering the telephone in the therapist's office or at home when a responsible adult is not present
Exposure	Prolonged contact with the phobic stimulus in the absence of real threat to decrease anxiety; may be contrived (sought-out contact with feared stimuli) or not contrived (unavoidable contact with feared stimuli)	A patient with fear of heights goes up a ladder: the first time, it is scary; the tenth time, it is boring
Extinction	Conventionally defined as the elimination of problem behaviors through removal of parental positive reinforcement; technically defined as removing the negative reinforcement effect of the problem behavior so that it no longer persists	Refusal to reassure the anxious patient; refusal by the mother to cave in to the anxious oppositional child's tantrums by withdrawing a command
Generalization training	Moving the methods and success of problem-focused interventions to targets not specifically addressed in treatment	Exposure and response prevention in imagination for developmentally appropriate fears, even if not particularly bothersome or not specifically addressed in treatment
Negative reinforcement	Self-reinforcing purposeful removal of an aversive stimulus; stated differently, the termination of an aversive stimulus, which, when stopped, increases or stamps in the behavior that removed the aversive stimulus	Obtaining reassurance from a parent provides short-term relief of anxiety in a child. Eliminating reassurance, which at the same time blocks the negative reinforcement for answering by the parent when the child's distress and thus difficult behavior decreases, is a prime goal of treatment.
Positive reinforcement	Imposing a pleasurable stimulus to increase a desirable behavior	Praising the selectively mute youngster who talks to the teacher
Prompting, guiding, and shaping	External commands and suggestions that increasingly direct the child toward more adaptive behavior that is then reinforced; typically, shaping procedures rapidly fade in preference to generalization training	Gradually encouraging and helping the youngster with social phobia to talk in class and with other children
Punishment	Imposing an aversive stimulus to decrease an undesirable behavior	"Time-out" because of unacceptable behavior or overcorrection (as in extra chores to make restitution for aggressive behavior); typically, punishment worsens anxiety disorders

TABLE 34–2. Techniques used in cognitive-behavioral therapy for pediatric anxiety disorders *(continued)*

Term	Definition	Examples
Relapse prevention	Interventions designed to anticipate triggers for reemergence of symptoms; practicing skillful coping in advance	Imaginal exposure to a possible new fear followed by use of cognitive therapy and response prevention to successfully resist the incursion of anxiety-driven operant reinforcers
Response cost	Removal of positive reinforcer as a consequence of undesirable behavior	Loss of points in a token economy
Response prevention	Assisting patient to resist completion of an anxiety-maintaining behavior	Typically used to treat obsessive-compulsive disorder, in which response prevention means not performing rituals, the principle also applies in other situations, such as eliminating an avoidance or escape withdrawal behavior in the socially anxious or agoraphobic patient
Restructuring the environment	Changes in setting or stimuli that decrease problem behaviors and/or facilitate adaptive behavior	Intervening to protect the anxious child from punishment by the teacher or teasing by peers
Stimulus hierarchy	A list of phobic stimuli ranked from least to most difficult to resist, with fear thermometer rating scores	Unique list of exposure targets ranked by fear thermometer score; an individual patient may have one or more hierarchies, depending on the complexity of symptoms (e.g., a particular patient may have separate hierarchies for social fears and for separation anxiety)

the natural environment. Following the adult treatment literature (Barlow and Craske 1989), this avoidance led to the development of exposure-based interventions for a wide range of pediatric anxiety disorders (March 1995; Morris and March 2004). Because escape and avoidance behaviors are negatively reinforced by cessation of anxiety, exposure-based procedures require extended presentation of fear stimuli with concurrent prevention of escape and avoidance behaviors in order for the extinction of the conditioned responses to occur. Unlike systematic desensitization, stimulus presentation is not accompanied by progressive muscle relaxation. Rather, graduated imaginal or in vivo exposure to hierarchically presented fear stimuli is used to attenuate anxiety to phobic stimuli. Gradual exposure, with the consent of the child, is generally considered to produce less stress for the patient (and therapist) and thus is often preferred over the use of more prescriptive techniques, especially flooding.

Cognitive interventions, usually combined with exposure, also play a prominent role in CBT for anxious children and adolescents. For example, Kendall and colleagues (1992) developed a comprehensive cognitive-behavioral protocol for anxious youths that focused on transmitting coping skills to children in need. Based on the premise that anxious children view the world through a template of threat, automatic questioning (e.g., "What if ...?"), and behavioral avoidance, treatment focuses on providing educational experiences to build a new coping template for the child. Therapists help children to reconceptualize anxiety-provoking situations as problems to be solved, situations to be coped with. Various cognitive-behavioral components assist the therapist and child in building the coping template: relaxation training, imagery, correction of maladaptive self-talk, problem-solving skills, and management of reinforcers. Therapists use coping modeling, role-play rehearsals, in vivo exposure, and a collaborative therapeutic relationship with the child to facilitate treatment progress. Parents are actively involved in all facets of treatment as collaborators in the process of change. Moreover, this demonstrably effective treatment program (Kendall and Southam-Gerow 1996; Kendall et al. 1997, 2004) incorporates an innovative relapse prevention component, during which the child assumes the role of an expert and produces a video- or audiotaped "commercial" for the management of anxiety and fear.

Clinically, when parents or other significant others are trapped in the child's anxiety symptoms, it is crucial to help the child encourage them to stop participating in the avoidance strategies or rituals. To test the hypothesis that adding a family anxiety management component would boost treatment effectiveness, Barrett and colleagues (1996, 2001) developed a family program, parallel to Kendall's "Coping Cat" (Kendall and Southam-Gerow 1996), based on behavioral family intervention strategies found effective for the treatment of externalizing disorders in youths. Following the completion of each child session with the therapist, the child and parents participate in a family anxiety management session with the therapist. The point of the program is to empower parents and children by forming an "expert team" to overcome and master anxiety. Parents are trained in reinforcement strategies, with emphasis on differential reinforcement and systematic ignoring of excessive complaining and anxious behavior. Contingency management strategies are the main methods for reducing conflict and increasing cooperation and communication in the family. Moreover, parents receive training in communication and problem-solving skills so that they will be better able to function as a team in solving future problems. Results gathered over time suggest that combined treatment, although providing results comparable to the results of individual treatment at long-term follow-up (Barrett et al. 2001), may result in quicker and more dramatic improvement in the shorter term (Barrett et al. 1996).

In much the same vein, several investigators have confirmed the wisdom of tailored family involvement in the treatment of OCD in children and adolescents (Barrett et al. 2004, 2005; Freeman et al. 2003; Knox et al. 1996; Piacentini et al. 1994). March and Mulle (1998) have suggested that unilateral extinction strategies, such as when a parent returns a child with school phobia to school by force, have significant disadvantages:

1. Parents often have no workable strategy for managing the child's distress.
2. The treatment relationship is disrupted.
3. Symptoms that are not seen by parents and teachers cannot be targeted.
4. Most important, these approaches do not help the child internalize a more skillful strategy for coping with current and potential future anxiety symptomatology.

Thus, parents must be assisted by the skillful clinician to collaborate with the child-driven hierarchical exposure plan rather than pushing ritualizing children to "just stop" or intervening by force. Barrett and colleagues

(2004, 2005) determined that a potentially cost-effective way to administer family treatment for pediatric OCD is via group therapy.

Pharmacotherapy

With advances in the identification of child- and adolescent-onset anxiety (March and Albano 1998) came a concomitant increase in the application of pharmacological treatments borrowed in part from successful strategies applied in adults with similar disorders (Allen et al. 1995). Psychopharmacological interventions are increasingly recognized as an essential part of the treatment armamentarium for anxious youths (American Academy of Child and Adolescent Psychiatry 2007), with selective serotonin reuptake inhibitors (SSRIs) being the first-line medications.

Table 34–3 summarizes the general approach to prescribing medication for anxious youths, Table 34–4 inventories the drugs most commonly used for this purpose, including common side effects, and Table 34–5 provides brand name and dosing information.

Randomized clinical trials indicate that SSRI treatment is both beneficial and well tolerated in anxious children and adolescents (Birmaher et al. 2003; Black and Uhde 1994; The Research Unit on Pediatric Psychopharmacology Anxiety Study Group 2001; Rynn et al. 2001; Wagner et al. 2004). Although the U.S. Food and Drug Administration in 2004 required a black box warning for SSRI medications due to concerns about increased suicidality in youths taking these and other antidepressant medications, pooled analysis of controlled trials of these medications show no increase in the relative risk for suicidality in children and adolescents with anxiety disorders (as opposed to depression; Hammad 2004, as cited in Reinblatt and Walkup 2005). Bridge et al. (2007) pooled data from 27 trials of children or adolescents with major depressive disorder, OCD, or non-OCD anxiety, and found strong evidence for effectiveness of antidepressants, particularly for the non-OCD anxiety disorders. They noted that "[b]enefits of antidepressants appear to be much greater than risks from suicidal ideation/suicide attempt across indications, although comparison of benefit to risk varies as a function of indication, age, chronicity, and study conditions" (Bridge et al. 2007, p. 1683). Clearly, in clinical practice, careful monitoring of children and adolescents taking prescribed SSRIs is required. Specific questioning about suicidal ideation and intent is necessary to rule out this uncommon but severe adverse event.

TABLE 34–3. Approach to prescribing psychotropic medication for anxious youths

- Conduct a comprehensive baseline evaluation, including rating scales and, if indicated, laboratory measures
- Carefully consider the question of differential therapeutics to identify potential targets for medication treatment as distinct from psychosocial treatments when possible
- Establish risk-benefit ratios for each treatment, and obtain informed consent
- In general, begin with least-complicated and least-risky drug strategies
- Define indicators for each important outcome domain to better track potential benefits and side effects
- Insofar as possible, use only one medication at a time to minimize confusion in tracking outcome
- When adjusting medications, be sure to consider both dose-response (intensity) and time-response (temporal) characteristics of the chosen medication in relation to the patient's psychiatric disorder
- Use an evidence-based stages of treatment model, and establish a defined end point at which a decision can be made about whether the expected benefit has occurred and whether additional treatment(s) can or should be implemented

As this book was going to press, a large randomized, controlled study directly comparing CBT to an SSRI (sertraline), to placebo, and to the combination of CBT and sertraline was completed and the initial report became available (Walkup et al. 2008). This study, the Child-Adolescent Anxiety Multimodal Study (CAMS), has important implications for treatment planning by clinicians treating anxious youths. Both of the monotherapies (CBT alone and sertraline alone) were found to be efficacious, with 59.7% of youths responding to CBT alone and 54.9% to sertraline alone after 12 weeks of treatment. effect sizes were moderate for each monotherapy: 0.31 for CBT and 0.45 for sertraline, and the number needed to treat was 3.2 for sertraline and 2.8 for CBT. This suggests that either treatment course is effective; moreover, the low incidence of adverse events in the study may be encouraging to parents considering a medication-based approach for their child.

Interestingly, the combination of CBT and sertraline was found to be particularly powerful in this study, with 80.7% of children in the combination treatment group

TABLE 34–4. Commonly used medications for pediatric anxiety disorders

Psychotropic class	Drug	Therapeutic applications	Side effects	Comments
SSRIs	Citalopram Escitalopram Fluoxetine Fluvoxamine Paroxetine Sertraline	SSRIs may be useful in all anxiety disorders except specific phobia. Demonstrated efficacy in placebo-controlled trials for selective mutism, social phobia, separation anxiety disorder, generalized anxiety disorder No controlled studies for childhood-onset panic; open trials and chart reviews show benefit for adolescents with panic.	Generally well tolerated More common: gastrointestinal symptoms, headaches, increased motor activity, insomnia Less common: disinhibition, tremor Watch for restlessness, akathisia. An excessive dose for a particular patient may cause apathy and amotivation; this side effect may also occur with long-term use.	SSRIs are first-line compounds, with broad-spectrum activity in many mood and anxiety disorders and unique activity in OCD; well tolerated compared with TCAs Black box warning advises clinicians to monitor youths taking SSRIs for worsening symptoms of depression, agitation, and/or suicidal ideation or behavior Benefits and risks of long-term use have not been studied No empirical evidence that any particular SSRI is more effective than any other for pediatric anxiety; decision usually made based on side-effect profile, duration of action, and/or positive response to a particular SSRI in a first-degree relative with anxiety No specific dosing guidelines; literature suggests starting at low doses and monitoring side effects closely, then increasing slowly based on treatment response and tolerability. Some research indicates the need for an increase in SSRI dose if significant improvement is not achieved by week 4 of treatment. With paroxetine, interdose withdrawal symptoms, marked withdrawal symptoms on drug tapering, and sexual side effects limit usefulness
SNRIs	Venlafaxine Duloxetine	Generalized anxiety disorder Social phobia	Nausea, anorexia, asthenia, pharyngitis, mydriasis	Clinically, second line after SSRIs May be useful in patients with comorbid ADHD Extended-release form of venlafaxine is preferred Duloxetine has not been evaluated in children and adolescents
TCAs	Imipramine Nortriptyline Desipramine Clomipramine	All anxiety disorders except OCD and specific phobia Only TCA used for OCD	Anticholinergic side effects: Dry mouth, tremor, sweating, constipation, fatigue, dizziness, insomnia, postural hypotension Close cardiac monitoring is required for all TCA use.	Require ECG and laboratory monitoring Not effective in treating comorbid depression Controlled trials show mixed results. Use after two to three failed SSRI trials. Should be introduced at a low dose with patients closely monitored for anticholinergic and cardiac side effects

TABLE 34–4. Commonly used medications for pediatric anxiety disorders *(continued)*

Psychotropic class	Drug	Therapeutic applications	Side effects	Comments
Benzodiazepines	Alprazolam Clonazepam Lorazepam	Situation and anticipatory anxiety across all anxiety disorders Have not shown efficacy in controlled trials in child anxiety, despite established benefit in adult anxiety	Sedation, disinhibition, cognitive impairment, difficulty with discontinuation Impairs learning of new material while taking it Contraindicated in adolescents with substance abuse	Best for short-term control of anticipatory anxiety and panic while waiting for an SSRI to "kick in" Disinhibition and physiological dependence may be problematic. Abrupt discontinuation can provoke withdrawal seizures May permit exposure work in CBT in extremely phobic individuals
Other drugs	Buspirone Propranolol	Generalized anxiety disorder Specific social phobia	Light-headedness, headache, stomachache Generally well tolerated	Buspirone is broadly anxiolytic; it is not effective in panic disorder with agoraphobia or OCD. May be useful in place of a benzodiazepine when substance abuse is an issue. Propranolol and other beta-blockers are useful primarily in acute performance anxiety

Note. ADHD=attention-deficit/hyperactivity disorder; CBT=cognitive-behavioral therapy; ECG=electrocardiogram; OCD=obsessive-compulsive disorder; SNRIs=serotonin-norepinephrine reuptake inhibitors; SSRIs=selective serotonin reuptake inhibitors; TCAs=tricyclic antidepressants.

TABLE 34–5. Trade names and usual dosages of commonly prescribed medications

Drug and class	Trade name	Usual dosage for children and adolescents
SSRIs		
Citalopram	Celexa	10–60 mg/day
Escitalopram	Lexapro	5–30 mg/day
Fluoxetine	Prozac	2.5–60 mg/day
Fluvoxamine	Luvox	50–300 mg/day
Paroxetine	Paxil	10–60 mg/day
Sertraline	Zoloft	25–200 mg/day
SNRIs		
Duloxetine	Cymbalta	/[a]
Venlafaxine	Effexor	37.5–225 mg/day
TCAs		
Desipramine Imipramine Nortriptyline	Norpramin Tofranil Pamelor	Proper dosage is best established via monitoring blood levels
Clomipramine	Anafranil	100–250 mg
Benzodiazepines		
Alprazolam	Xanax	Maximum 4 mg/day
Clonazepam	Klonopin	Maximum 3 mg/day
Lorazepam	Ativan	Maximum 6 mg/day
Other drugs		
Buspirone	BuSpar	5–30 mg bid for adolescents; 5–7.5 mg bid for children
Propranolol	Inderal	Maximum 16 mg/kg/day

Note. SNRIs=serotonin-norepinephrine reuptake inhibitors; SSRIs=selective serotonin reuptake inhibitors; TCAs=tricyclic antidepressants.

[a]Inadequate research base precludes usual dosage recommendation at this time.

responding within 12 weeks (effect size, 0.86; number needed to treat, 1.7). This suggests that using both treatment modalities offers the best possible chance of speedy and effective treatment for anxious youths. The authors note that their findings suggest that all three treatment modalities (CBT, sertraline, combination) are efficacious and that patient-specific considerations may drive the selection of the particular treatment approach. These factors may include CBT availability in the patient's area, patient or parent preference, anxiety symptoms that cause moderate to severe difficulty in treatment participation, or severe or multiple comorbidity or suicidality. At this time, moderator and predictor analyses from the CAMS data set are not available. Once published, these findings may shed light on the most appropriate sequence of treatment for various anxiety presentations in youths.

Using psychotropic medication in pediatric patients entails other complexities not present with most adults. For example:

- Children less commonly seek treatment themselves. Alternatively, parents are sometimes "cornered into treatment" by pressure from school or social service agencies.
- Children commonly fear being labeled a "mental patient" by peers or extended family, so exploring the meaning of the medication to the child is important.

- Prescribing medication in a medical context, that is, for an illness that is bothering the child and from which he or she wants relief, increases compliance.
- The form and taste of medication, as well as route of administration, influence compliance, especially in younger children.
- If the cost of the drug is prohibitive, or it is not available locally, treatment may be interrupted.
- Although many methods are available to assess compliance, such as direct monitoring, questionnaires, pill counts, and measuring levels in body fluids, none is completely reliable.
- The factors most likely to result in a positive outcome are the following: a good therapeutic alliance, a careful explanation of benefits and risks coupled with written informed consent, a combination of medication with targeted psychosocial therapies, and thoughtful monitoring.
- Friendly and collegial communication with pediatricians, family doctors, and other professionals involved in the child's care also enhances compliance.
- Similarly, patients and their families must be informed that not all medicines help everybody and that a period of medication trial and error may be necessary to find the medication that is most helpful.
- Finally, the monitoring of side effects and adverse events related to medication use requires careful attention and direct questioning about known medication side effects that may not be spontaneously volunteered (e.g., sexual side effects for adolescents; suicidal ideation). Such information should result in tailoring of the dosing regimen, including reducing the dosage, changing the specified medication, and/or adding behavioral or pharmaceutical interventions to address side effects.

When patients' symptoms do not respond or only partially respond to initial pharmacotherapy, the clinician must reassess whether treatment targets have been appropriately identified and whether treatments have been appropriately implemented. Conversely, increasing the intensity of the treatment—for example, by adding behavioral family therapy, increasing the dose of the medication, or changing medications—may be necessary (March et al. 1997a). The efficacy of augmentation treatment (e.g., adding an antipsychotic medication to an SSRI for treatment-refractory OCD) is not well researched, although it is sometimes used clinically for partial responders. In many cases, partial improvement is all that can be expected; distinguishing between improvement and residual impairment in the context of the natural history of the disorder is an important part of differential therapeutics and of the psychoeducational process.

As noted in Table 34–4, other medications besides the SSRIs may be useful in the treatment of anxiety disorders in youths. Comorbid conditions may be an important guide in the selection of the appropriate medication. Some evidence suggests that venlafaxine (a serotonin-norepinephrine reuptake inhibitor) may be useful in treating generalized anxiety disorder (Rynn et al. 2007) and social phobia (March et al. 2007). Targeted propranolol (a beta-blocker) may be useful to treat performance anxiety in patients with nongeneralized social phobia (Faigel 1991).

Some medications may be less useful, precluded in certain comorbid presentations, or prescribed only with caution and ongoing monitoring. Despite research supporting the use of benzodiazepines in adults with anxiety disorder, these medications have not shown efficacy in clinical trials with anxious children and adolescents ages 7–18 (Bernstein et al. 1990; Graae et al. 1994; Simeon et al. 1992). They may have some limited utility as short-term agents to assist in the early phases of exposure treatment (e.g., in treating school phobia; see Kratochvil et al. 1999). Buspirone is a potentially useful agent in treating generalized anxiety disorder in children and adolescents (Salazar et al. 2001), but although side effects are generally considered benign with this medication, one study of its use in inpatient prepubertal children with anxiety plus aggression reported agitation and symptoms suggestive of mania in a significant portion of the sample (Pfeffer et al. 1997). Finally, tricyclic antidepressants and antipsychotics should be avoided when possible because of their lack of demonstrated efficacy and high potential for serious side effects.

Other agents have a smaller role, if any, to play, although combinations of various compounds may be useful in treatment-resistant patients. In every patient, careful attention to dose-response relationships (the intensity dimension) and time-action effects (the temporal dimension) is critical to maximize the benefit and minimize side effects.

Conclusion

Anxiety disorders are common in the pediatric population, and their treatment is a pressing public health need given that untreated anxiety in childhood or adolescence predicts significant morbidity later in life. There are limitations in the current research literature regarding long-term outcome of treated versus untreated youths; efficacious combination of cognitive-behavioral and pharmacological treatments; and treatment effectiveness across divergent patient characteristics such as culture, age, ethnicity, comorbidity profile, and symptom severity. However, the empirical literature is generally positive regarding the benefits of short-term cognitive-behavioral psychotherapy and pharmacotherapy for anxiety disorders in children and adolescents. Encouraging research also supports the durability of improvements achieved with CBT over time. At this stage of our understanding, it is reasonable to say that a combination of targeted psychosocial therapies, particularly CBT, alone or in combination with psychotropic medication, skillfully applied over time, affords the most plausible basis for sustained benefit in anxious children and adolescents.

Key Clinical Points

- Anxiety disorders are common in youth, and even subthreshold cases of anxiety may cause clinically significant impairment and require treatment.
- Anxieties and fears as they present in the child or adolescent must be considered in their developmental context. Severity and prevalence of fears, as well as functional impairment, should be evaluated to determine the need for treatment.
- Before beginning treatment, a thorough assessment utilizing dimensional (checklist) measures, interviews, and behavioral observation is recommended. Repeated assessment over the course of treatment is useful for determining progress.
- CBT is typically the first-line treatment for pediatric anxiety disorders, due to its demonstrated efficacy and benign side-effect profile.
- Family involvement is often helpful in psychotherapy for child/adolescent anxiety, and may lead to quicker and/or more substantial gains in treatment.
- The first-line psychopharmacological agents for the treatment of pediatric anxiety disorders are the SSRIs. Side effects, particularly emerging suicidal ideation or behavior, must be carefully monitored.
- Other classes of medications—such as serotonin-norepinephrine reuptake inhibitors, beta-blockers, benzodiazepines, buspirone, or tricyclic antidepressants—may be considered as alternative or augmentative medication strategies in cases of nonresponse to SSRIs.

References

Achenbach TM, Rescorla LA: Manual for the ASEBA School-Age Forms and Profiles. Burlington, University of Vermont Research Centre for Children, Youth and Families, 2001

Albano A, Kendall P: Cognitive behavioural therapy for children and adolescents with anxiety disorders: clinical research advances. Int Rev Psychiatry 14:129–134, 2002

Albano AM, DiBartolo PM, Heimberg RG, et al: Children and adolescents: assessment and treatment, in Social Phobia: Diagnosis, Assessment, and Treatment. Edited by Heimberg RG, Liebowitz MR, Hope DA, et al. New York, Guilford, 1995, pp 387–425

Allen AJ, Leonard H, Swedo SE: Current knowledge of medications for the treatment of childhood anxiety disorders. J Am Acad Child Adolesc Psychiatry 34:976–986, 1995

American Academy of Child and Adolescent Psychiatry: Practice parameters for the assessment and treatment of children and adolescents with anxiety disorders. J Am Acad Child Adolesc Psychiatry 46:267–283, 2007

American Psychiatric Association: Diagnostic and Statistical Manual of Mental Disorders, 3rd Edition, Revised. Washington, DC, American Psychiatric Association, 1987

American Psychiatric Association: Diagnostic and Statistical Manual of Mental Disorders, 4th Edition. Washington, DC, American Psychiatric Association, 1994

American Psychiatric Association: Diagnostic and Statistical Manual of Mental Disorders, 4th Edition, Text Revision.

Washington, DC, American Psychiatric Association, 2000

Angold A, Costello EJ: Developmental epidemiology. Epidemiol Rev 17:74–82, 1995

Angold A, Costello EJ, Farmer EM, et al: Impaired but undiagnosed. J Am Acad Child Adolesc Psychiatry 38:129–137, 1999

Baldwin JS, Dadds MR: Reliability and validity of parent and child versions of the Multidimensional Anxiety Scale for Children in community samples. J Am Acad Child Adolesc Psychiatry 46:252–260, 2007

Barlow DH: Anxiety and Its Disorders, 2nd Edition. New York, Guilford, 2002

Barlow DH, Craske MG: Mastery of Your Anxiety and Panic. Albany, NY, Graywind, 1989

Barrett PM, Dadds MR, Rapee RM: Family treatment of childhood anxiety: a controlled trial. J Consult Clin Psychol 64:333–342, 1996

Barrett PM, Duffy AL, Dadds MR, et al: Cognitive-behavioral treatment of anxiety disorders in children: long term (6-year) follow-up. J Consult Clin Psychol 69:135–141, 2001

Barrett PM, Healy Farrell L, March J: Cognitive-behavioral family treatment of childhood obsessive compulsive disorder: a controlled trial. J Am Acad Child Adolesc Psychiatry 43:46–62, 2004

Barrett PM, Farrell L, Dadds MR, et al: Cognitive-behavioral family treatment of childhood obsessive-compulsive disorder: long-term follow-up and predictors of outcome. J Am Acad Child Adolesc Psychiatry 44:1005–1014, 2005

Barrios BA, Hartmann DP: Fears and anxieties, in Assessment of Childhood Disorders, 3rd Edition. Edited by Mash EJ, Terdal LG. New York, Guilford, 1997, pp 230–327

Beidel DC: Social phobia and overanxious disorder in school-age children. J Am Acad Child Adolesc Psychiatry 30:545–552, 1991

Beidel DC, Turner SM: Childhood Anxiety Disorders: A Guide to Research and Treatment. New York, Routledge, 2005

Beidel DC, Morris TL, Turner MW: Social phobia, in Anxiety Disorders in Children and Adolescents, 2nd Edition. Edited by Morris TL, March JS. New York, Guilford, 2004, pp 141–163

Bergman RL, Piacentini J, McCracken JT: Prevalence and description of selective mutism in a school-based sample. J Am Acad Child Adolesc Psychiatry 41:938–946, 2002

Bernstein GA, Garfinkel BD, Borchardt CM: Comparative studies of pharmacotherapy for school refusal. J Am Acad Child Adolesc Psychiatry 29:773–781, 1990

Birmaher B, Khetarpal S, Brent D, et al: The Screen for Child Anxiety Related Emotional Disorders (SCARED): scale construction and psychometric characteristics. J Am Acad Child Adolesc Psychiatry 36:545–553, 1997

Birmaher B, Khetarpal S, Brent D, et al: The Screen for Child Anxiety Related Emotional Disorders (SCARED): a replication study. J Am Acad Child Adolesc Psychiatry 38:1230–1236, 1999

Birmaher B, Axelson DA, Monk K, et al: Fluoxetine for the treatment of childhood anxiety disorders. J Am Acad Child Adolesc Psychiatry 42:415–423, 2003

Black B: Anxiety disorders. New Dir Ment Health Serv 54(Summer):65–70, 1992

Black B: Separation anxiety disorder and panic disorder, in Anxiety Disorders in Children and Adolescents. Edited by March J. New York, Guilford, 1995, pp 212–234

Black B, Uhde TW: Treatment of elective mutism with fluoxetine: a double-blind, placebo-controlled study. J Am Acad Child Adolesc Psychiatry 33:1000–1006, 1994

Brady KT, Killeen TK, Bewerton T, et al: Comorbidity of psychiatric disorders and posttraumatic stress disorder. J Clin Psychiatry 61 (suppl 7):22–32, 2000

Bridge JA, Iyengar S, Salary CB, et al: Clinical response and risk for reported suicidal ideation and suicide attempts in pediatric antidepressant treatment: a meta-analysis of randomized controlled trials. JAMA 297:1683–1696, 2007

Cantwell DP, Baker L: Issues in the classification of child and adolescent psychopathology. J Am Acad Child Adolesc Psychiatry 27:521–533, 1988

Chorpita BF, Yim L, Moffitt C, et al: Assessment of symptoms of DSM-IV anxiety and depression in children: a revised child anxiety and depression scale. Behav Res Ther 35:835–855, 2000

Clark DB, Neighbors B: Adolescent substance abuse and internalizing disorders. Child Adolesc Psychiatr Clin N Am 5:45–55, 1996

Costello EJ, Angold A: Developmental Epidemiology. New York, Wiley, 1995a

Costello EJ, Angold A: Epidemiology, in Anxiety Disorders in Children and Adolescents. Edited by March J. New York, Guilford, 1995b, pp 109–124

Costello EJ, Egger HL, Angold A: Developmental epidemiology of anxiety disorders, in Phobic and Anxiety Disorders in Children and Adolescents: A Clinician's Guide to Effective Psychosocial and Pharmacological Interventions. Edited by Ollendick TH, March JS. New York, Oxford University Press, 2004, pp 61–91

Curry JF, March JS, Hervey AS: Comorbidity of childhood and adolescent anxiety disorders: prevalence and implications, in Phobic and Anxiety Disorders in Children and Adolescents: A Clinician's Guide to Effective Psychosocial and Pharmacological Interventions. Edited by Ollendick TH, March JS. New York, Oxford University Press, 2004, pp 116–140

Dierker LC, Albano AM, Clarke GN, et al: Screening for anxiety and depression in early adolescence. J Am Acad Child Adolesc Psychiatry 40:929–936, 2001

Eisen AR, Kearney CA: Practitioner's Guide to Treating Fear and Anxiety in Children and Adolescents : A Cognitive-Behavioral Approach. Northvale, NJ, Jason Aronson, 1995

Epkins CC, Meyers AW: Assessment of childhood depression, anxiety, and aggression: convergent and discriminant validity of self-, parent-, teacher-, and peer-report measures. J Pers Assess 62:364–381, 1994

Faigel HC: The effect of beta blockade on stress-induced cognitive dysfunction in adolescents. Clin Pediatr (Phila) 30:441–445, 1991

Flament MF, Whitaker A, Rapoport JL, et al: Obsessive compulsive disorder in adolescence: an epidemiological study. J Am Acad Child Adolesc Psychiatry 27:764–771, 1988

Foa EB, Johnson KM, Feeny NC, et al: The Child PTSD Symptom Scale: a preliminary examination of its psychometric properties. J Clin Child Adolesc Psychol 30:376–384, 2001

Freeman JB, Garcia AM, Fucci C, et al: Family based treatment of early onset obsessive compulsive disorder. J Child Adolesc Psychopharmacol 13 (suppl 1):S71–S80, 2003

Freeman JB, Garcia AM, Miller LM, et al: Selective mutism, in Anxiety Disorders in Children and Adolescents, 2nd Edition. Edited by Morris TL, March JS. New York, Guilford, 2004, pp 280–304

Goodman W, Price L, Rasmussen S, et al: Children's Yale-Brown Obsessive-Compulsive Scale (CY-BOCS). New Haven, CT, Yale University School of Medicine, 1991

Graae F, Milner J, Rizzotto L, et al: Clonazepam in childhood anxiety disorders. J Am Acad Child Adolesc Psychiatry 33:372–376, 1994

Greco LA, Morris TL: Assessment, in Anxiety Disorders in Children and Adolescents, 2nd Edition. Edited by Morris TL, March JS. New York, Guilford, 2004, pp 98–121

Grills-Taquechel AE, Ollendick TH, Fisak B: Reexamination of the MASC factor structure and discriminant ability in a mixed clinical outpatient sample. Depress Anxiety 25:942–950, 2008

Hammad TA: Review and evaluation of clinical data: relationship between psychotropic drugs and pediatric suicidality. 2004. Available at http://www.fda.gov/ohrms/dockets/ac/04/briefing/2004-4065b1-10-TAB08-Hammads-Review.pdf. Accessed October 21, 2007.

Hibbs E, Jensen PS: Psychosocial Treatments for Child and Adolescent Disorders: Empirically Based Strategies for Clinical Practice. Washington, DC, American Psychological Association, 2005

Jones MC: The elimination of children's fears. J Exp Psychol 7:383–390, 1924a

Jones MC: A laboratory study of fear: the case of Peter. Pedagogical Seminary 31:308–315, 1924b

Kazdin AE: A model for developing effective treatments: progression and interplay of theory, research, and practice. J Clin Child Psychol 26:114–129, 1997

Kazdin AE, Weisz JR (eds): Evidence-Based Psychotherapies for Children and Adolescents. New York, Guilford, 2003

Keith C: Psychodynamic psychotherapy, in Anxiety Disorders in Children and Adolescents. Edited by March J. New York, Guilford, 1995, pp 386–400

Keller MB, Lavori PW, Wunder J, et al: Chronic course of anxiety disorders in children and adolescents. J Am Acad Child Adolesc Psychiatry 31:595–599, 1992

Kendall PC: Treating anxiety disorders in children: results of a randomized clinical trial. J Consult Clin Psychol 62:100–110, 1994

Kendall PC, Flannery-Schroeder E: Methodological issues in treatment research for anxiety disorders in youth. J Ab norm Child Psychol 26:27–38, 1998

Kendall PC, Panichelli-Mindel SM: Cognitive-behavioral treatments. J Abnorm Child Psychol 23:107–124, 1995

Kendall PC, Southam-Gerow MA: Long-term follow-up of a cognitive-behavioral therapy for anxiety-disordered youth. J Consult Clin Psychol 64:724–730, 1996

Kendall P, Chansky T, Kane M, et al: Anxiety Disorders in Youth: Cognitive-Behavioral Interventions. Needham Heights, MA, Allyn & Bacon, 1992

Kendall PC, Flannery-Schroeder E, Panichelli-Mindel SM, et al: Therapy for youths with anxiety disorders: a second randomized clinical trial. J Consult Clin Psychol 65:366–380, 1997

Kendall PC, Safford S, Flannery-Schroeder E, et al: Child anxiety treatment: outcomes in adolescence and impact on substance use and depression at 7.4 year follow-up. J Consult Clin Psychol 72:276–287, 2004

Kessler RC, McGonagle KA, Zhao S, et al: Lifetime and 12-month prevalence of DSM-III-R psychiatric disorders in the United States: results from the National Comorbidity Study. Arch Gen Psychiatry 51:8–19, 1994

King NJ, Tonge BJ, Ollendick TH: Night-time fears in children. J Paediatr Child Health 28:347–350, 1992

Knox LS, Albano AM, Barlow DH: Parental involvement in the treatment of childhood compulsive disorder: a multiple-baseline examination incorporating parents. Behav Ther 27:93–114, 1996

Kratochvil C, Kutcher S, Reiter S, et al: Psychopharmacology of pediatric anxiety disorders, in Handbook of Psychotherapies With Children and Families (Issues in Clinical Child Psychology). Edited by Russ SW, Ollendick TH. New York, Kluwer Academic/Plenum, 1999, pp 345–366

La Greca AM, Stone WL: Social Anxiety Scale for Children–Revised: factor structure and concurrent validity. J Clin Child Psychol 22:17–27, 1993

Langley AK, Bergman RL, Piacentini JC: Assessment of childhood anxiety. Int Rev Psychiatry 14:102–113, 2002

Last CG, Strauss CC, Francis G: Comorbidity among childhood anxiety disorders. J Nerv Ment Dis 175:726–730, 1987

Lewinsohn PM, Rohde P, Seeley JR: Adolescent psychopathology, III: the clinical consequences of comorbidity. J Am Acad Child Adolesc Psychiatry 34:510–519, 1995

Lewinsohn PM, Lewinsohn M, Gotlib IH, et al: Gender differences in anxiety disorders and anxiety symptoms in adolescents. J Abnorm Psychol 107:109–117, 1998

March JS (ed): Anxiety Disorders in Children and Adolescents. New York, Guilford, 1995

March JS: Manual for the Multidimensional Anxiety Scale for Children (MASC). Toronto, Ontario, MultiHealth Systems, 1998

March JS: Assessment of pediatric posttraumatic stress disorder, in Posttraumatic Stress Disorder: A Comprehensive Text. Edited by Saigh PA, Bremner JD. Boston, MA, Allyn & Bacon, 1999, pp 199–218

March JS, Albano A: Assessment of anxiety in children and adolescents, in American Psychiatric Press Review of Psychiatry, Vol 15. Edited by Dickstein L, Riba MB, Oldham JM. Washington, DC, American Psychiatric Press, 1996, pp 405–427

March JS, Albano A: New developments in assessing pediatric anxiety disorders, in Advances in Child Psychology, Vol 20. Edited by Ollendick T, Prinz R. New York, Plenum, 1998, pp 213–242

March JS, Mulle K: OCD in Children and Adolescents: A Cognitive-Behavioral Treatment Manual. New York, Guilford, 1998

March JS, Ollendick TH: Integrated psychosocial and pharmacological treatment, in Phobic and Anxiety Disorders in Children and Adolescents: A Clinician's Guide to Effective Psychosocial and Pharmacological Interventions. Edited by Ollendick TH, March JS. New York, Oxford University Press, 2004, pp 141–172

March JS, Mulle K, Stallings P, et al: Organizing an anxiety disorders clinic, in Anxiety Disorders in Children and Adolescents. Edited by March J. New York, Guilford, 1995, pp 420–435

March J, Frances A, Kahn D, et al: Expert consensus guidelines: treatment of obsessive-compulsive disorder. J Clin Psychiatry 58 (suppl 4):1–72, 1997a

March JS, Parker JD, Sullivan K, et al: The Multidimensional Anxiety Scale for Children (MASC): factor structure, reliability, and validity. J Am Acad Child Adolesc Psychiatry 36:554–565, 1997b

March JS, Entusah AR, Rynn M, et al: A randomized controlled trial of venlafaxine ER versus placebo in pediatric social anxiety disorder. Biol Psychiatry 62:1149–1154, 2007

Morris TL, March JS (eds): Anxiety Disorders in Children and Adolescents, 2nd Edition. New York, Guilford, 2004

Muris P, Mayer B, Batelds E, et al: The revised version of the Screen for Child Anxiety Related Emotional Disorders (SCARED-R): treatment sensitivity in an early intervention trial for childhood anxiety disorders. Br J Clin Psychol 40:323–336, 2001

Ollendick TH: Reliability and validity of the Revised Fear Survey Schedule for Children (FSSC-R). Behav Res Ther 21:685–692, 1983

Ollendick TH, March JS (eds): Phobic and Anxiety Disorders in Children and Adolescents: A Clinician's Guide to Effective Psychosocial and Pharmacological Interventions. New York, Oxford University Press, 2004

Ollendick TH, Matson JL, Helsel WJ: Fears in children and adolescents: normative data. Behav Res Ther 23:465–467, 1985

Pfeffer CR, Jiang H, Domeshek LJ: Buspirone treatment of psychiatrically hospitalized prepubertal children with symptoms of anxiety and moderately severe aggression. J Child Adolesc Psychopharmacol 7:145–155, 1997

Piacentini J, Gitow A, Jaffer M, et al: Outpatient behavioral treatment of child and adolescent obsessive compulsive disorder. J Anxiety Disord 8:277–289, 1994

Pine DS, Cohen P, Gurley D, et al: The risk for early adulthood anxiety and depressive disorders in adolescents with anxiety and depressive disorders. Arch Gen Psychiatry 55:56–64, 1998

Reinblatt SP, Riddle MA: The pharmacological management of childhood anxiety disorders: a review. Psychopharmacology (Berl) 191:67–86, 2007

Reinblatt SP, Walkup JT: Psychopharmacologic treatment of pediatric anxiety disorders. Child Adolesc Psychiatr Clin N Am 14:877–908, 2005

The Research Unit on Pediatric Psychopharmacology Anxiety Study Group: Fluvoxamine for the treatment of anxiety disorders in children and adolescents. N Engl J Med 344:1279–1285, 2001

Reynolds CR, Paget KD: Factor analysis of the Revised Children's Manifest Anxiety Scale for blacks, whites, males and females with a national normative sample. J Consult Clin Psychol 49:352–359, 1981

Rynn MA, Siqueland L, Rickels K: Placebo-controlled trial of sertraline in the treatment of children with generalized anxiety disorder. Am J Psychiatry 158:2008–2014, 2001

Rynn MA, Riddle MA, Yeung PP, et al: Efficacy and safety of extended-release venlafaxine in the treatment of generalized anxiety disorder in children and adolescents: two placebo-controlled trials. Am J Psychiatry 164:290–300, 2007

Salazar DE, Frackiewicz EJ, Dockens R, et al: Pharmacokinetics and tolerability of buspirone during oral administration to children and adolescents with anxiety disorder and normal healthy adults. J Clin Pharmacol 41:1351–1358, 2001

Schniering CA, Hudson JL, Rapee RM: Issues in the diagnosis and assessment of anxiety disorders in children and adolescents. Clin Psychol Rev 20:453–478, 2000

Shaffer D, Campbell M, Cantwell D, et al: Child and adolescent psychiatric disorders in DSM-IV: issues facing the work group. J Am Acad Child Adolesc Psychiatry 28:830–835, 1989

Silverman WK: Childhood anxiety disorders: diagnostic issues, empirical support, and future research. Journal of Child and Adolescent Psychotherapy 4:121–126, 1987

Silverman WK, Albano A: The Anxiety Disorders Interview Schedule for DSM-IV, Child and Parent Versions. New York, Oxford University Press, 1996

Silverman WK, Ollendick TH: Evidence-based assessment of anxiety and its disorders in children and adolescents. J Clin Child Adolesc Psychol 34:380–411, 2005

Simeon JG, Ferguson HB, Knott V, et al: Clinical, cognitive, and neurophysiological effects of alprazolam in children and adolescents with overanxious and avoidant disorders. J Am Acad Child Adolesc Psychiatry 31:29–33, 1992

Spence SH: A measure of anxiety symptoms among children. Behav Res Ther 36:545–566, 1998

Spielberger CD, Gorsuch RL, Lushene RE: Manual for the State-Trait Anxiety Inventory. Palo Alto, CA, Consulting Psychologists Press, 1976

Van Hasselt V, Hersen M: Overview of behavior therapy, in Handbook of Behavior Therapy and Pharmacotherapy for Children. Edited by Van Hasselt V, Hersen M. Boston, MA, Longwood, 1993, pp 1–12

Wagner KD, Berard R, Stein MB, et al: A multicenter, randomized, double-blind, placebo-controlled trial of paroxetine in children and adolescents with social anxiety disorder. Arch Gen Psychiatry 61:1153–1163, 2004

Walkup JT, Albano AM, Piacentini J, et al: Cognitive behavioral therapy, sertraline, or a combination in childhood anxiety. New Engl J Med 359:2753–2766, 2008

Warren SL, Sroufe LA: Developmental issues, in Children and Adolescents: A Clinician's Guide to Effective Psychosocial and Pharmacological Interventions. Edited by Ollendick TH, March JS. New York, Oxford University Press, 2004, pp 92–115

Warren SL, Huston L, Egeland B, et al: Child and adolescent anxiety disorders and early attachment. J Am Acad Child Adolesc Psychiatry 36:627–633, 1997

Wittchen HU, Nelson CB, Lachner G: Prevalence of mental disorders and psychosocial impairments in adolescents and young adults. Psychol Med 28:109–126, 1998

Wolpe J: Psychotherapy by Reciprocal Inhibition. Stanford, CA, Stanford University Press, 1958

Wood JJ, Piacentini JC, Bergman RL, et al: Concurrent validity of the anxiety disorders section of the Anxiety Disorders Interview Schedule for DSM-IV: child and parent versions. J Clin Child Adolesc Psychol 31:335–342, 2002

Recommended Readings

Albano A, Kendall P: Cognitive behavioural therapy for children and adolescents with anxiety disorders: clinical research advances. Int Rev Psychiatry 14:129–134, 2002

American Academy of Child and Adolescent Psychiatry: Practice parameters for the assessment and treatment of children and adolescents with anxiety disorders. J Am Acad Child Adolesc Psychiatry 46:267–283, 2007

Barlow DH: Anxiety and Its Disorders, 2nd Edition. New York, Guilford, 2002

Barmish AJ, Kendall PC: Should parents be co-clients in cognitive-behavioral therapy for anxious youth? J Clin Child Adolesc Psychol 34:569–581, 2005

Barrett PM, Dadds MR, Rapee RM: Family treatment of childhood anxiety: a controlled trial. J Consult Clin Psychol 64:333–342, 1996

Barrett PM, Duffy AL, Dadds MR, et al: Cognitive-behavioral treatment of anxiety disorders in children: long term (6-year) follow-up. J Consult Clin Psychol 69:135–141, 2001

Compton SN, March JS, Brent D, et al: Cognitive-behavioural psychotherapy for anxiety and depressive disorders in children and adolescents: an evidence based medicine review. J Am Acad Child Adolesc Psychiatry 43:930–959, 2004

Costello EJ, Angold A: Epidemiology, in Anxiety Disorders in Children and Adolescents. Edited by March J. New York, Guilford, 1995b, pp 109–124

Costello EJ, Egger HL, Angold A: Developmental epidemiology of anxiety disorders, in Phobic and Anxiety Disorders in Children and Adolescents: A Clinician's Guide to Effective Psychosocial and Pharmacological Interventions. Edited by Ollendick TH, March JS. New York, Oxford University Press, 2004, pp 61–91

Flannery-Schroeder EC, Kendall PC: Group and individual cognitive behavioral treatments for youth with anxiety disorders: a randomized clinical trial. Cognit Ther Res 24:251–278, 2000

Fonseca AC, Perrin S: Clinical phenomenology, classification and assessment of anxiety in children and adolescents, in Anxiety Disorders in Children and Adolescents: Research, Assessment, and Intervention. Edited by Silverman WK, Treffers PDA. Cambridge, UK, Cambridge University Press, 2001, pp 126–158

Greco LA, Morris TL: Assessment, in Anxiety Disorders in Children and Adolescents, 2nd Edition. Edited by Morris TL, March JS. New York, Guilford, 2004, pp 98–121

Kendall PC, Safford S, Flannery-Schroeder E, et al: Child anxiety treatment: outcomes in adolescence and impact on substance use and depression at 7.4 year follow-up. J Consult Clin Psychol 72:276–287, 2004

March JS, Ollendick TH: Integrated psychosocial and pharmacological treatment, in Phobic and Anxiety Disorders in Children and Adolescents: A Clinician's Guide to Effective Psychosocial and Pharmacological Interventions. Edited by Ollendick TH, March JS. New York, Oxford University Press, 2004, pp 141–272

Langley AK, Bergman RL, Piacentini JC: Assessment of childhood anxiety. Int Rev Psychiatry 14:102–113, 2002

Moore PS, Mariaskin A, March JS, et al: Obsessive-compulsive disorder in children and adolescents: diagnosis, comorbidity, and developmental factors, in Handbook of Child and Adolescent Obsessive-Compulsive Disorder. Edited by Storch EA, Geffken G, Murphy TK. New York, Routledge, 2007, pp 17–46

Morris TL, March JS (eds): Anxiety Disorders in Children and Adolescents, 2nd Edition. New York, Guilford, 2004

Ollendick TH, March JS (eds): Phobic and Anxiety Disorders in Children and Adolescents: A Clinician's Guide to Effective Psychosocial and Pharmacological Interventions. New York, Oxford University Press, 2004

Reinblatt SP, Riddle MA: The pharmacological management of childhood anxiety disorders: a review. Psychopharmacology (Berl) 191:67–86, 2007

Reinblatt SP, Walkup JT: Psychopharmacologic treatment of pediatric anxiety disorders. Child Adolesc Psychiatr Clin N Am 14:877–908, 2005

Sweeney M, Pine D: Etiology of fear and anxiety, in Phobic and Anxiety Disorders in Children and Adolescents: A Clinician's Guide to Effective Psychosocial and Pharmacological Interventions. Edited by Ollendick TH, March JS. New York, Oxford University Press, 2004, pp 34–60

Vasey MW, Dadds MR: The Developmental Psychopathology of Anxiety. New York, Oxford University Press, 2001

Web Sites of Interest

American Academy of Child and Adolescent Psychiatry. http://aacap.org

Anxiety Disorders Association of America. http://www.adaa.org

Obsessive Compulsive Foundation. http://www.ocfoundation.org

Chapter 35

Anxiety Disorders in the Elderly

Eric J. Lenze, M.D.

Anxiety symptoms and DSM-IV-TR (American Psychiatric Association 2000) anxiety disorders are common in elderly persons, but study of this population has lagged behind that of other age groups. Such disorders can cause considerable distress or disability, yet are often undetected and untreated.

The overall goal in this chapter is to review the important aging-related issues in the anxiety disorders field. To this end, I survey the epidemiology, course, and presentation of anxiety in elderly persons; review the literature on treatment of late-life anxiety; highlight challenges in the detection and management of anxiety in this age group; and highlight gaps in the research literature.

Epidemiology and Presentation

Epidemiology

Epidemiological studies have produced fairly wide variation in the estimates of prevalence in elderly persons. For example, prevalence of generalized anxiety disorder (GAD) in this age group has varied from 0.7% to 7.3% (Beekman et al. 1998; Flint 1994). As a result, opinion on the prevalence of this disorder among the elderly varies from being viewed as "relatively uncommon" to highly prevalent and potentially more so than among young adults.

Table 35–1 shows the prevalence estimates from several large epidemiological studies that focus on elderly persons. As a whole, the studies suggest that GAD is at least as common in late life as in younger adults, whereas some other anxiety disorders (panic disorder, obsessive-compulsive disorder [OCD], and social phobia) are more rare. But it is worth noting that many researchers have raised the issue of whether epidemiological studies using methodology designed for younger adults can adequately capture the prevalence of mental disorders in older adults (O'Connor 2006). This issue is particularly relevant to anxiety disorders, in which disorders may present differently (Lawton et al. 1993), existing measures may not capture fear or anxiety as conceptualized by older adults (Kogan et al. 2004), and symptoms could be attributed to medical conditions. In other words, the prevalence of anxiety disorders among the elderly may be significantly higher than rates reflected in the studies cited Table 35–1.

Age of Onset

Risk factors for anxiety disorders in elderly persons include female gender, neurotic personality, early-life stress, chronic medical conditions, and chronic disability in self or spouse (Beekman et al. 2000; Vink et al. 2008).

In geriatric psychiatry, anxiety disorders have been dichotomized as either early- or late-onset, with late-onset illness often thought to have a different etiology (e.g., cerebrovascular or neurodegenerative). Less has been written about early- versus late-onset anxiety disorders, compared to depression or dementia.

Some reviews have suggested that late-onset anxiety disorders are rare (Flint 2005b), and that anxiety disor-

TABLE 35–1. Prevalence of anxiety disorders in elderly persons

	Studies in elderly					Adult comparator
	Longitudinal Aging Study Amsterdam (LASA)	Epidemiologic Catchment Area (ECA)	Amsterdam Study of the Elderly (AMSTEL)	Australian National Mental Health and Well-Being Study (NMHWS)	Canadian Community Health Survey (CCHS)	National Comorbidity Study Replication (NCS-R)
N	3,107	5,702	4,051	1,792	12,792	9,282
Age, years	55–85	≥65	65–84	≥65	≥55	≥18
Any anxiety disorder	10.2%	5.5%	N/A	4.4%	N/A	18.1%
GAD	7.3%	1.9%[a]	3.2%	2.4%	N/A	3.1%
Any phobic disorder	3.1%	4.8%	N/A	N/A	N/A	8.7%
Social phobia	N/A	N/A	N/A	0.6%	1.3%	6.8%
Agoraphobia	N/A	N/A	N/A	N/A	0.6%	0.8%
Panic disorder	1.0%	0.1%	N/A	0.8%[b]	0.8%	2.7%
OCD	0.6%	0.8%	N/A	0.1%	N/A	1.0%
PTSD	N/A	N/A	N/A	1.0%	N/A	3.5%

Note. GAD=generalized anxiety disorder; N/A=not applicable; OCD=obsessive-compulsive disorder; PTSD=posttraumatic stress disorder.

[a]This estimate is from one site of the ECA study; the overall study did not assess GAD.

[b]The NMHWS study combined panic disorder and agoraphobia for this prevalence rate.

ders usually have onset in childhood or early adulthood (Kessler et al. 2007). However, examinations of some clinical samples of elderly anxiety disorder patients (e.g., GAD, panic disorder, posttraumatic stress disorder [PTSD]) have found that many have late onset of illness, at least when measured retrospectively (Le Roux et al. 2005; Lenze et al. 2005a; Sheikh et al. 2004b; van Zelst et al. 2003).

Mechanisms in aging could be protective of anxiety, depending on the type of anxiety disorder. Negative affect, which is thought to underlie anxiety disorders, appears to decrease with aging in the population, at least until individuals reach their 70s (Charles et al. 2001; Teachman 2007). The low rates of panic and social phobia are consistent with the observation by some that elderly persons are inoculated over time against the anxiety-producing nature of stressors (Jarvik and Russell 1979). Finally, age-related changes in brain structure or function (e.g., due to neurodegeneration or normal aging) may reduce the propensity for panic or other highly autonomic responses (Flint 1994).

Aging could also be a risk factor for anxiety disorders. Several anxiogenic stressors are associated with aging: chronic illness and disability (in self or loved ones), bereavement, or worries related to fixed or intractable financial issues; these might interact with long-term vulnerability factors such as personality (de Beurs et al. 2000) or genetic factors. In a related manner, our group has frequently observed that aging brings many life changes—retirement, less involvement with children or social networks—which may have kept anxiety at bay as a coping mechanism. Thus, many late-onset GAD subjects have described themselves as "a worrier all my life," but also stated that their anxiety was controllable until retirement or other major life changes occurred.

Degeneration in brain regions associated with adaptive responses to anxiety (e.g., the dorsolateral prefrontal cortex) may reduce the ability to manage anxiogenic situations, essentially wiping out protective factors that otherwise kept an anxiety disorder from presenting earlier. Consistent with this assertion is evidence that stroke can cause GAD (Aström 1996) or OCD (Swoboda and Jenike 1995); however, there is less evidence that cognitive impairment itself (a marker for these brain changes) is a risk factor for anxiety in late life (Vink et al. 2008). In contrast, anxiety symptoms appear to predict cognitive decline in older adults (Wetherell et al. 2002).

Overall, very little research has been done on the pathophysiology of late-onset anxiety. Some studies have examined the hypothalamic-pituitary-adrenal (HPA) axis in late-life GAD, given that HPA axis dysfunction is common in young adults with anxiety disorders and that aging appears to confer increased risk of HPA axis disturbance, resulting in hypercortisolemia (Lupien et al. 2005). Late-life GAD is associated with up to 50% higher diurnal cortisol levels than in psychiatrically healthy elderly persons (Mantella et al. 2007). Other research has shown that cortisol levels in GAD decrease with pharmacologic treatment in older but not younger adults with GAD, suggesting some important age-related differences (Pomara et al. 2005). Interestingly, these findings in late-life GAD may differ from research results on PTSD, in which a study in a primarily older sample found lower cortisol among veterans with PTSD, as compared with subjects who did not have PTSD (Yehuda et al. 2007).

Assessing Late-Onset Anxiety Disorders

Late-onset anxiety disorders usually require a clinical search for their pathogenesis. Some prescription medications can induce anxiety, including frequently prescribed psychiatric medications such as psychostimulants or antidepressants; conversely, withdrawal from medications (such as sedative/hypnotics or antidepressants) can cause anxiety. Table 35–2 lists the medications believed to have anxiogenic potential either by their use or withdrawal. It is my experience that ambulatory elderly persons usually know (or, if anything, overinterpret) that a medication they are taking causes anxiety. However, hospitalized, institutionalized, or cognitively impaired elderly persons are much less likely to be aware of medication changes in a way that would give them insight into a medication cause. Clinicians should also note that elderly persons are likely to have polypharmacy, such that combinations of fairly benign medications might result in cumulative or interactive effects (for example, combination of several anticholinergics or one drug inhibiting the metabolism of another).

Anxiety disorders presenting in later life may have a different nature (Flint 2005a) and, as such, the DSM-IV-TR diagnoses, created for younger adults, may not adequately describe anxiety in older adults. Dementia is a common contributor to anxiety that presents as agitation (Mintzer et al. 1996), hoarding syndrome (Saxena 2007), or other atypical symptoms (Starkstein et al. 2007). Many common medical conditions are highly anxiogenic, including heart disease (Todaro et al. 2007), lung disease (Yohannes et al. 2006), or neurological diseases such as Parkinson's disease. Comorbid anxiety is also extremely common in late-life depression

TABLE 35–2. Commonly prescribed medications that can cause anxiety

Psychiatric medications
Anticholinergics (e.g., benztropine)
Antidepressants (e.g., bupropion, SSRIs/SNRIs)
Antipsychotics
Psychostimulants (e.g., methylphenidate)
Anticholinergics, nonpsychiatric
Diphenhydramine
Oxybutynin, tolterodine
Corticosteroids
Sympathomimetics (e.g., albuterol)
Over-the-counter medications or other substances
Alcohol (withdrawal from)
Caffeine
Nicotine
Stimulants, cold medicines
Withdrawal from:
Anticholinergics
Anticonvulsants (e.g., gabapentin)
Antidepressants
Narcotics (e.g., opiate pain medications)
Sedatives (e.g., benzodiazepines)

Note. SNRIs=serotonin-norepinephrine reuptake inhibitors; SSRIs= selective serotonin reuptake inhibitors.

(Beekman et al. 2000; Lenze et al. 2000). Finally, the decline of function that occurs with aging, creating frailty and gait instability, can result in fear of falling (Gagnon et al. 2005; Nagaratnam et al. 2005) or agoraphobic-like behavior, which may not be discerned by standard epidemiological assessments or methodology.

Thus, a consideration of the wide variation in prevalence estimates, combined with the atypical nature of many anxiety presentations, suggests that late-onset anxiety disorders are probably much more common than is appreciated in these studies. Further study is needed.

Generalized Anxiety Disorder in Older Adults

GAD is perhaps the most widely studied anxiety disorder in older adults. The central feature of GAD is excessive, difficult-to-control worry. In older adults, the areas of worry content in GAD typical for this age group include concerns about health or disability, family relationships, or finances (Diefenbach et al. 2001). Thus, many older adults with GAD will be harder to diagnose than younger individuals because they do not view their worry as "excessive." Clinicians should thus focus on the amount of time spent worrying, the effortful nature of trying to control it, and the degree of distress or impairment (e.g., due to avoidance), not whether the patient believes the worry is realistic.

Elderly persons with GAD are unlikely to present for mental health treatment (Ettner and Hermann 1997) unless there is coexisting depression or other comorbidity. Instead, their presentation in primary or other medical care typically involves the associated features of GAD: muscle tension, restlessness (feeling keyed up or on edge), sleep difficulties, concentration problems (often felt by older adults to be memory problems), fatigue, and irritability. As in young adults, GAD among the elderly population appears to have a chronic course: studies on elderly patients presenting for treatment in research clinics have found that the mean length of GAD symptoms was anywhere from 20 (Lenze et al. 2005a) to more than 30 years (Stanley et al. 2003a; Wetherell et al. 2003b). However, other investigators reported that GAD often develops with aging into a somatization condition (Rubio et al. 2007) or mixed GAD/major depressive disorder (MDD) (Schoevers et al. 2003). The high comorbidity of GAD with MDD is not surprising, given the overlap of symptoms such as impaired sleep, poor concentration (often described subjectively as memory complaints), low energy, and irritability. Yet some studies have found that "pure" GAD is more common than comorbid GAD/MDD (Beekman et al. 2000; Schoevers et al. 2003).

Some reports have focused on neuropsychological features in late-life GAD. One preliminary study found impaired short-term and delayed memory in GAD, but not the executive deficits that are seen in MDD (Mantella et al. 2007). These results are consistent with another study on late-life GAD, which found that increased anxiety severity was associated with memory impairments (Caudle et al. 2007). It has been suggested that memory impairment in late-life mental disorders could be due to hippocampal dysfunction, either causing or a result of the disorder; however, more research is needed. In particular, no longitudinal study of anxiety disorders has been carried out in which the pathophysiology of cognitive decline, or even dementia, were examined.

In summary, GAD is one of the most common mental disorders in elderly persons (Beekman et al. 1998), particularly in medical settings such as cardiovascular disease or primary care (Todaro et al. 2007; Tolin et al. 2005). GAD may be chronic, but may also change in quality or nature with aging (Flint 2005a).

Other Anxiety Disorders in Older Adults

PTSD can stem from traumatic experiences that are common in elderly persons, such as combat experience for veterans of WWII and other conflicts (Frueh et al. 2007), or as a result of medical events in which danger and horror are felt (Dew et al. 2001). Interestingly, an epidemiological report focused on older African Americans stated that PTSD (and not GAD or phobias) was the most common anxiety disorder found in this population. In this study, PTSD had the highest 12-month prevalence of any mental disorder (Ford et al. 2007), suggesting that this ethnic group has unique risks in aging. The research on late-life PTSD is lagging, however, and few conclusions can be made about its biology or presentation in this age group (van Zelst et al. 2003).

Panic disorder appears to have a low prevalence in community elderly, compared with young adults; in particular, late-onset panic disorder appears to be very rare. Elderly persons may be less able to mount an autonomic response to panicogenic stimuli (Flint et al. 2002), perhaps because of the reduction in locus coeruleus function associated with aging. On the other hand, the low prevalence seen in epidemiological studies may reflect a limitation in the existing diagnostic measures for panic disorder. Some research suggests that "fear," the core feature of panic and phobias, is conceptualized differently by older adults, compared with younger adults, suggesting that measures of panic would need to be adapted or created for this age group (Kogan et al. 2004). Late-onset panic should result in a search for medical or neurological causes. Elderly persons with panic disorder have less severe and less frequent panic attacks, compared with young adults, who frequently have daily attacks (Sheikh et al. 2004b). Nonetheless, panic attacks can lead to disabling agoraphobic avoidance in older adults and can also result in costly medical workups.

Phobias are unlikely to remit spontaneously, but they may appear less prevalent in elderly persons for the reasons described previously. Also, elderly persons may have had enough exposure with adequate coping throughout life to reduce the extent of phobia, or they may have accommodated their lifestyle to the phobia. These latter explanations seem to apply for public-speaking phobia, which often seems to diminish over decades and in any case may be difficult to diagnose in a person who has not had an indication to speak publicly for several decades. An epidemiological study of social phobia (Cairney et al. 2007) found that aging was associated with reduced prevalence of social phobia, although the condition still remained fairly common in old age. Another difficulty in diagnosing phobias lies in the possibility that the patient is more likely to realize that the fear is excessive or unreasonable, and some have suggested this diagnostic criterion be dropped for older adults (Flint 2005a).

Agoraphobia can present within the context of panic attacks, but in elderly persons it frequently arises without a clear diagnosis of panic disorder (McCabe et al. 2006). Agoraphobia can appear de novo in the context of a stroke or other medical event, in which it can be highly disabling, leading to inhibition of activities necessary for restoration after the event (Burvill et al. 1995). The largest study to examine agoraphobia in older adults reported it to be rare (0.6% prevalence) (McCabe et al. 2006), but the condition itself might lead to decreased detection in epidemiological studies. As with other anxiety disorders, agoraphobia may be difficult to detect clinically because elderly persons may not realize that their fear or activity restriction is excessive, or they may attribute it to a medical problem (e.g., stating that disability is due to the stroke rather than agoraphobia arising from the stroke).

Most epidemiological studies have concluded that OCD is rare in elderly persons and is rarely of late onset. The exception is a report from the Epidemiologic Catchment Area study that indicated a second peak of OCD incidence in women ages 65 years and older (Nestadt et al. 1998); these later-onset cases are less likely to be associated with a genetic predisposition (Nestadt et al. 2000). OCD has not been the topic of research in this age group (Velayudhan and Katz 2006), other than a few case reports and case series (e.g., Chacko et al. 2000; Weiss and Jenike 2000). Some of these reports have indicated the existence of cerebral lesions, often in the basal ganglia, in patients with late-onset OCD, supporting the assertion that neurodegenerative changes underlie many cases of late-onset anxiety disorders. The phenomenon of hoarding and other compulsive behavior in dementia (particularly when of cerebrovascular origin), together with greater neuropsychological impairment in late-onset OCD (Hwang et al. 2007), is more evidence of this connection between neurodegenerative illness and late-onset anxiety.

Comorbidity of Anxiety With Depression in the Elderly

Studies indicate that depressed elderly people with comorbid anxiety have greater somatic symptoms, greater likelihood of suicidal ideation (Jeste et al. 2006; Lenze et al. 2000), and a higher risk of suicide (Allgulander and Lavori 1993). These findings, along with observations that response to antidepressants is delayed or diminished in the context of comorbid anxiety symptoms or anxiety disorders, have garnered interest in the issue of anxiety comorbidity within the late-life depression field.

Longitudinally, anxiety symptoms appear to be more stable than depressive symptoms and more likely to lead to depressive symptoms than vice versa (Wetherell et al. 2001). Moreover, studies on young adults (Hettema et al. 2006) suggest that anxiety disorders could be a risk factor for late-life depression. Conversely, depression may precede anxiety symptoms (or the combination may appear simultaneously) (Lenze et al. 2005a); in this case, anxiety symptoms often persist after remission of depression and increase risk for depressive relapse (Dombrovski et al. 2007; Flint and Rifat 1997). Thus, it may be the greater persistence of anxiety symptoms over time that leads to poorer outcomes in late-life depression that is comorbid with anxiety.

Many studies have demonstrated a longer time to response in depression, and/or a reduced response rate, in association with anxiety symptoms (Alexopoulos et al. 2005; Andreescu et al. 2007; Dew et al. 1997) or an anxiety disorder (Flint and Rifat 1997; Steffens et al. 2005). Additionally, some (Andreescu et al. 2007), but not all (Flint and Rifat 1997), studies have indicated that even after elderly patients achieve full remission from late-life depression, the condition is more likely to recur if the patient initially experienced high levels of baseline anxiety symptoms. Finally, there is some preliminary research suggesting that comorbid anxiety predicts greater decline in memory during long-term follow-up of late-life depression (DeLuca et al. 2005).

A meta-analysis of placebo-controlled antidepressant trials in late-life depression concluded that comorbid anxiety symptoms did not predict poorer treatment outcomes (Nelson et al. 2009). However, it should be noted that this meta-analysis used a cutoff score on various Hamilton Rating Scale for Depression items as the definition of anxiety comorbidity, and this measure may not be adequately sensitive to this comorbidity. Other comprehensive reviews (e.g., Whyte et al. 2004) have concluded that comorbid anxiety is a predictor of poor treatment outcomes.

As a whole, these studies support the conceptualization of late-life "anxious depression" as a severe, treatment-relevant subtype. Missing from the literature, however, is an understanding of what exactly this comorbidity reflects. Further research is needed to elucidate whether anxious depression simply reflects substantial overlap of the diagnostic picture, dimensions of these syndromes, a common neurobiological underpinning (e.g., rumination/worry underlying depression/GAD, respectively), or some additional pathology—and whether anxious depression is a particularly relevant subtype in geriatrics (e.g., owing to more severe cognitive decline).

Treatment

Anxiety disorders in elderly persons are highly prevalent, tend to be chronic (Schuurmans et al. 2005), and may produce quality-of-life impairments and disability similar to what is seen in late-life depression (de Beurs et al. 1999; Wetherell et al. 2004). Despite these observations about the importance of anxiety disorders in the elderly, there has been surprisingly little research into their treatment in this age group.

Both psychotherapy and pharmacotherapy appear to be effective treatment options in this age group (Pinquart et al. 2007; Wetherell et al. 2005b), although there is no consensus about whether psychotherapy or medication should be first-line treatment.

Psychotherapy

Cognitive-behavioral therapy (CBT) is recommended for anxiety disorders in older adults who are able to learn new skills in CBT and use them effectively (Wetherell et al. 2005a). Several studies have demonstrated the effectiveness of CBT compared with waitlist control conditions, minimal-contact control conditions, or usual care (Stanley et al. 2003a, 2003b; Wetherell et al. 2003a). Most of these studies have been carried out in groups of elderly subjects with GAD, although some studies have also been carried out in mixed groups that included individuals with panic disorder (Barrowclough et al. 2001; Schuurmans et al. 2006).

More recently, a study in primary care demonstrated the effectiveness of CBT, compared to usual care, for older adults with GAD (Stanley et al. 2009).

A few studies have compared CBT with another active condition, either psychotherapy (Stanley et al.

1996; Wetherell et al. 2003a) or medication (Schuurmans et al. 2006). Results of these investigations have been more mixed, lacking a clear demonstration of the superiority of CBT. Thus, overall, data obtained from these studies suggest that CBT is efficacious for anxiety disorders in older adults. The results are preliminary, and additional studies are in progress.

In elderly persons, the most effective ingredient of CBT may be relaxation (Thorp et al. 2009). CBT packages for late-life anxiety typically involve education about anxiety, relaxation, cognitive therapy, problem-solving skills training, exposure exercises, and sleep hygiene instructions—all similar to treatment options offered to young adults (Stanley et al. 2004). Adaptations are recommended for using CBT in elderly persons. Consistent with the observation that recall diminishes with aging (particularly in anxiety), these adaptations include increased repetition and increased time spent on reviewing previous sessions (Mohlman et al. 2003). It is unclear whether these enhancements lead to additional efficacy of CBT in this age group. Another enhancement under consideration by several research groups involves combining or sequencing CBT with antidepressant medication. However, it is unclear whether this represents an effective approach, given long-held concerns about combining these two treatment modalities.

Pharmacotherapy

The evidence base for pharmacotherapy in older adults is limited and consists mainly of several small clinical trials, many quite old and in mixed populations.

Two studies have demonstrated the acute efficacy of benzodiazepines in reducing symptoms of late-life anxiety (Bresolin et al. 1988; Koepke et al. 1982). However, their use is already common in this age group (van Balkom et al. 2000). Benzodiazepines, like any sedatives, have a poorer risk-benefit ratio in elderly persons than in young adults. They are associated with an increased risk of falling in elderly persons (Landi et al. 2005; Paterniti et al. 2002), who are already in the age group in which falls and fall-related injuries are most relevant. Using medications with shorter half-life and less complicated elimination (e.g., lorazepam rather than diazepam) seems reasonable but has not been demonstrated to reduce the risk of falls or fall-related injuries. Furthermore, benzodiazepines appear to cause cognitive impairment in this age group, particularly in recall (Pomara et al. 1998). This cognitive problem is more likely with higher doses of benzodiazepines and in elderly persons who already have predisposition for cognitive impairment. Therefore, long-term use of benzodiazepines appears unfavorable in this age group. A common recommendation, then, is to use these medications at low dose as a short-term adjunct, in which case they may provide some early relief and improve adherence to the treatment regimen.

Serotonin-specific reuptake inhibitors (SSRIs) and serotonin-norepinephrine reuptake inhibitors (SNRIs) have been examined in some small or retrospective evaluations. A retrospective examination of phase 3 data for extended-release venlafaxine found the drug to be efficacious in adults ages 60 and older, with an effect size (drug-placebo difference) and side-effect profile similar to that found in younger adults. However, other research has demonstrated that venlafaxine, particularly at higher doses, can be associated with cardiac concerns such as orthostatic blood pressure changes. In an open-label trial of 62 elderly patients with major depressive disorder, venlafaxine at a mean final dose of 196 mg/day was generally well tolerated, but 24% of participants experienced an increase in blood pressure, 29% developed orthostatic hypotension, and 3% experienced an increase in QTc (Johnson et al. 2006). These side effects are consistent with venlafaxine's norepinephrine transporter inhibition at higher doses and suggest that lower doses should be used if possible, and that monitoring of electrocardiogram and vital signs is needed, particularly at higher doses.

Some small studies have demonstrated the efficacy of the SSRIs citalopram and sertraline for late-life anxiety disorders (Lenze et al. 2005b; Schuurmans et al. 2006). However, it is important to note that these were small preliminary studies. For example, in a sample of 34 subjects with various anxiety disorders (30 of 34 had GAD), Lenze et al. (2005b) found that response rate was 65% with citalopram versus 24% with placebo; however, the small sample size makes estimates of the efficacy (i.e., in terms of number needed to treat, or risk-benefit ratio) unclear. These studies found similar side effects in elderly persons and younger adults; however, the studies were not designed to determine some of the more recently reported potential risks of SSRIs in the elderly population, including gait impairment, which increases risk for falls (Herings et al. 1995; Landi et al. 2003), gastrointestinal bleeding (Yuan et al. 2006), bone loss (Diem et al. 2007), and hyponatremia induced by the syndrome of inappropriate secretion of antidiuretic hormone (Fabian et al. 2004). Such reports suggest that the risk-benefit ratio for acute and long-term SSRI use is not the same as in younger adults. I would not interpret these additional potential risks of SSRIs as evidence that such medications should be avoided as first-line treatment for late-life anxiety disorders; in contrast, clinically, they appear to be generally benign in acute and maintenance treatment. However, these added concerns will merit closer monitoring of geriatric patients, particularly those who are at least 70 years old, frail, or medically ill.

More recently, a 12-week placebo-controlled full-scale study demonstrated the efficacy of the SSRI escitalopram (Lenze et al. 2009). In that study, cumulative response rate was 69% for SSRI-treated subjects, compared to 51% for placebo. Escitalopram was efficacious for improvements in worry severity and role function, which is typically impaired in GAD. Also, in an exploratory analysis, subjects with high blood pressure at baseline showed a greater decrease with escitalopram than with placebo. Thus, this report confirms smaller preliminary studies in demonstrating the efficacy of SSRIs in older adults with GAD.

Thus, based on these preliminary studies, the use of SSRIs and SNRIs as first-line treatment in late-life anxiety disorders is recommended. The long-term or maintenance treatment of late-life anxiety with medication has not been studied.

The only augmentation study to be published to date was a small study with risperidone (Moríñigo et al. 2005). As with younger adults, the use of atypical antipsychotics in elderly patients is potentially problematic, given concerns about weight gain and metabolic effects (Newcomer and Haupt 2006). Additionally, results of a meta-analysis (Schneider et al. 2005) indicated a higher mortality with atypical agents compared with placebo in older patients with dementia, resulting in a black-box warning being isssued by the U.S. Food and Drug Administration for the entire class of atypical antipsychotics. It remains unclear what the increased mortality resulted from, although possibilities include the sedating properties of these agents (leading to falls or aspiration pneumonia), QT prolongation (leading to arrhythmias and sudden cardiac death), venous thromboembolism leading to pulmonary embolism, and other cardiovascular or cerebrovascular events (Gill et al. 2007; Schneider et al. 2005). It is unknown whether these risks apply to elders without dementia. A third type of adverse event involves extrapyramidal side effects and other (nonvascular) neurological problems. Age-associated reductions in dopamine and in D_2 receptors make elderly individuals more sensitive to antipsychotics. For all of these reasons, antipsychotics may have a poorer risk-benefit ratio in older adults. However, further research is needed to clarify the efficacy versus tolerability of these medications in late-life anxiety (as well as depression).

It should also be noted that the studies mentioned here have largely focused on GAD. Three studies have been carried out in mixed-age populations (mean age, 55–60 years, suggesting that most are elderly). One finding supported the use of citalopram (English et al. 2006), another supported superiority of mirtazapine over an SSRI (Chung et al. 2004), and a third found evidence that the α-adrenergic antagonist prazosin is efficacious, particularly for sleep-related concerns (Raskind et al. 2007). A small open-label study in late-life panic disorder found evidence of benefit from sertraline (Sheikh et al. 2004a). These studies are also preliminary. At the time of this writing, no large-scale prospective clinical trials of pharmacotherapy for late-life anxiety disorders have been published, although some studies are under way.

Given the high human and economic burden of anxiety disorders in older adults, it is surprising that little research has examined prevention strategies (Smit et al. 2006, 2007). A recent study found that stepped-care prevention of depression and anxiety disorders in older adults was effective (van't Veer-Tazelaar et al. 2009). This study used watchful waiting, bibliotherapy, and group CBT to reduce the onset of both anxiety disorders and depression by 50% in a high-risk population. These intervention components are likely to be extremely cost-effective, suggesting their consideration for more widespread implementation in at-risk older adults.

Clinical Challenges in the Detection and Management of Anxiety in Elderly Persons

This section describes the clinical challenges, and some solutions, facing clinicians who treat older adults.

Detection

Detecting the anxiety is a necessary step to managing it, yet it is often the most overlooked step in mental health assessments of the elderly. As noted, elderly persons may conceptualize anxiety differently from younger adults, and they may not find the same terms relevant (e.g., "panic" or "social anxiety" may be less relevant than "concerns" or "worries" about health or other issues). Elderly persons with anxiety are less likely to view themselves as having a mental disorder. This possibly explains the low rate of mental healthcare seeking by this population. With respect to generalized anxiety, or even fear responses (e.g., in a specific phobia or agoraphobia), elderly individuals may assert that anxiety or fear is a realistic response to their environment or current stressors. Thus, clinicians need to set a low bar for suspecting anxiety is present. Rather than introducing the topic with a question about anxiety or fear, it may be more helpful to ask about reactions to stress. Thus, "How do you feel in times of stress?" is a useful opener in detecting anxiety symptoms. Patients who report anxiety terms (e.g., "anxious," "concerned," "worried") can then be queried: for example, they may be asked, "How often does it occur?" and "What do you do to manage these feelings?" Inquiring whether anxiety is "excessive" or "uncontrollable" is unlikely to be fruitful. Rather, the clinician wants to know how much the anxiety symptoms bother the patient, what strategies they are trying in order to control or avoid the symptoms, and how much of their time is spent in the effort. Asking about somatic symptoms is helpful, because these may be a source of concern or distress. For example, patients with panic symptoms may not endorse "panic attacks" but may admit to brief periods with multiple physical symptoms (particularly autonomic symptoms, such as palpitations). Likewise, patients with GAD may downplay the effects of worrying on their lives, but may complain more readily about distress from sleep disturbance or difficulty concentrating (regarding the latter, patients often interpret difficulty with concentration as memory problems, and elderly anxious patients often express concerns about Alzheimer's disease).

Diagnosis and Differential

Uppermost in the minds of most clinicians will be differentiating anxiety from depression. However, it appears that if asked, elderly patients are able to clarify whether they view themselves as depressed or not. It is useful to determine whether depression or anxiety appears to be the principal diagnosis, given that this distinction will affect management considerations. Table 35-3 provides a differential of anxiety from other common problems in late life.

Pharmacological Management

Elderly persons will vary from young adults in terms of increased comorbid medical conditions, pharmacokinetic changes, frailty, drug interactions, and side effects. In particular, older and frailer or medically ill individuals need close monitoring (e.g., of gait, vital signs, or any incident medical issues that arise in the context of treatment, and the potential role of antianxiety medication in these).

It is also important to remember that the patient's anxiety will affect his or her views about treatment. This is particularly true in the case of medications, especially antidepressants, which can initially have a stimulating or mildly anxiogenic effect. As with young adults, older

TABLE 35–3. A brief differential of anxiety in elderly persons

Diagnosis	Clues	Questions
Primary anxiety disorder (most likely: GAD)	Anxiety presenting as chronic worry, often starting early in life and escalating in later years.	Are you a worrier? How long has this gone on? Have there been any changes in your life that have made the anxiety worse?
Anxiety secondary to dementia	Cognitive decline, often with anxiety as a prodrome. Late-onset. Agitation (yelling, pacing), and hoarding are frequent syndromes.	Has the family noticed any memory problems? Are there activities the person can no longer do as well, such as driving, paying bills, shopping, or balancing a checkbook? Does he repeat himself during conversations?
Anxiety secondary to depression	Marked anhedonia, guilt, thoughts of death.	Would you describe your problem more as anxiety or as depression?
Anxiety secondary to a medical condition	Usually abrupt onset; often atypical or autonomic symptoms.	Consider: thyroid disease, B_{12} deficiency, hypoxia, ischemia, hypoglycemia, delirium, pheochromocytoma, arrhythmia
Anxiety secondary to medications (or to medication withdrawal)	High index of suspicion for recent onset in hospitalized, institutionalized, or cognitively impaired elderly	Have you made any recent changes to your medications? Were there medications you were taking that you no longer are?

adults with anxiety disorders often report that they are sensitive or intolerant of antidepressant medications, which appears to stem from their anticipatory concern about side effects, their vigilance toward interoceptive stimuli, and their tendency to catastrophize about any interoceptive sensations they detect (even if unrelated to the antidepressant). In other words, the manifestations of the anxiety itself interfere in many ways with acceptance of, and adherence to, pharmacotherapy.

Older adults with anxiety disorders seem at particular risk for believing that medication side effects might somehow be toxic or incapacitating, despite the relatively benign nature of most medications used to treat these disorders. Explanation of the benign and usually short-lived nature of side effects is helpful at baseline, during close follow-up, and after dose titration. I have found that patients who do develop side effects are likely to be less distressed by the side effect itself than by worries that it will get worse. Additionally, clinicians should realize that reported side effects are often simply anxiety-related symptoms that preceded the start of the medicine and are now being attributed to the medicine. Arguing etiology of the side effects is unlikely to be helpful, but it can be explained that the medication should reduce these symptoms over time.

In spite of these management efforts, many patients will perceive that they cannot tolerate first-line SSRI treatment, or will refuse to initiate it. The early use of benzodiazepines may produce a fast anxiolytic action that could improve compliance; however, the long-term use of these medications is discouraged.

Gaps in the Research Literature

Despite their prevalence and morbidity, anxiety disorders in elderly persons have not received the same level of research attention that they have attracted in children or young adults; nor have they received as much attention as depression in the elderly (Lenze and Wetherell 2009).

Presentation and Neurobiology

As previously mentioned, the epidemiological studies of anxiety disorders in older adults tend to suffer from the use of measures and methodology that have been developed in young adults. As the anxiety disorders begin to shift to DSM-V nosology, study focused on examining the various categorizations underlying anxiety and depression (e.g., neuroticism vs. extraversion, fear vs. worry), and their distinct genetic diatheses, neurocircuitry, and neuroendocrine responses, is needed in all age groups. Along with this study is needed terminology that is adapted for, or specifically created for, older adults.

Longitudinal Course and Sequelae

Longitudinal studies can clarify the course of disorders and also the pathways from chronic anxiety to depression, cognitive impairment, or health outcomes. Yet, largely absent are longitudinal or mechanistic studies that would shed light on aging-related pathophysiology for the anxiety disorders, eventually leading to new treatments for anxiety or their consequences in this age group.

Treatment

At this time, several studies are ongoing that should clarify the effectiveness of SSRIs for late-life GAD, as well as CBT for late-life anxiety disorders. Yet augmentation or maintenance studies are largely absent. Anxiety disorders in elderly persons usually present in primary care or other medical settings, but not specialty mental health care. However, care models for detecting and effectively managing anxiety in this age group have not been developed or tested.

Conclusion

The detection and management of anxiety disorders in elderly persons are challenging, but the high prevalence and significant morbidity associated with these disorders highlight the importance of understanding them. It is expected that as our knowledge base (in diagnosis, etiology, and treatment) of these disorders improves, our ability to detect and effectively manage these disorders in elderly persons will improve as well, resulting in significant improvement in the function and quality of life of this population.

Key Clinical Points

- Anxiety disorders are common in elderly persons but may present differently in elderly persons, limiting efforts to adequately detect them in research or in clinical care.
- Effective treatment of anxiety disorders in this age group includes SSRIs and CBT, but further work is needed to clarify the acute and long-term effectiveness of these modalities.
- Anxiety research in elderly persons has lagged well behind that in other age groups, leading to gaps in our basic understanding of the presentation, course, and treatment of these disorders.

References

Alexopoulos GS, Katz IR, Bruce ML, et al: Remission in depressed geriatric primary care patients: a report from the PROSPECT study. Am J Psychiatry 162:718–724, 2005

Allgulander C, Lavori PW: Causes of death among 936 elderly patients with "pure" anxiety neurosis in Stockholm County, Sweden, and in patients with depressive neurosis or both diagnoses. Compr Psychiatry 34:299–302, 1993

American Psychiatric Association: Diagnostic and Statistical Manual of Mental Disorders, 4th Edition, Text Revision. Washington, DC, American Psychiatric Association, 2000

Andreescu C, Lenze EJ, Dew MA, et al: Comorbid anxiety in elderly patients with depression: impact on response and recurrence of major depressive disorder. Br J Psychiatry 190:344–349, 2007

Aström M: Generalized anxiety disorder in stroke patients: a 3-year longitudinal study. Stroke 27:270–275, 1996

Barrowclough C, King P, Colville J, et al: A randomized trial of the effectiveness of cognitive-behavioral therapy and supportive counseling for anxiety symptoms in older adults. J Consult Clin Psychol 69:756–762, 2001

Beekman AT, Bremmer MA, Deeg DJ, et al: Anxiety disorders in later life: a report from the Longitudinal Aging Study Amsterdam. Int J Geriatr Psychiatry 13:717–726, 1998

Beekman AT, de Beurs E, van Balkom AJLM, et al: Anxiety and depression in later life: co-occurrence and communality of risk factors. Am J Psychiatry 157:89–95, 2000

Bresolin N, Monza G, Scarpini E, et al: Treatment of anxiety with ketazolam in elderly patients. Clin Ther 10:536–546, 1988

Burvill PW, Johnson GA, Jamrozik KD, et al: Anxiety disorders after stroke: results from the Perth Community Stroke Study. Br J Psychiatry 166:328–332, 1995

Cairney J, McCabe L, Veldhuizen S, et al: Epidemiology of social phobia in later life. Am J Geriatr Psychiatry 15:224–233, 2007

Caudle DD, Senior AC, Wetherell JL, et al: Cognitive errors, symptom severity, and response to cognitive behavior therapy in older adults with generalized anxiety disorder. Am J Geriatr Psychiatry 15:680–689, 2007

Chacko RC, Corbin MA, Harper RG: Acquired obsessive compulsive disorder associated with basal ganglia lesions. J Neuropsychiatry Clin Neurosci 12:269–272, 2000

Charles ST, Reynolds CA, Gatz M: Age-related differences and change in positive and negative affect over 23 years. J Pers Soc Psychol 80:136–151, 2001

Chung MY, Min KH, Jun YJ, et al: Efficacy and tolerability of mirtazapine and sertraline in Korean veterans with posttraumatic stress disorder: a randomized open label trial. Hum Psychopharmacol 19:489–494, 2004

de Beurs E, Beekman ATF, van Balkom AJLM, et al: Consequences of anxiety in older persons: its effect on disability, well-being and use of health services. Psychol Med 29:583–593, 1999

de Beurs E, Beekman AT, Deeg DJ, et al: Predictors of change in anxiety symptoms of older persons: results from the Longitudinal Aging Study Amsterdam. Psychol Med 30:515–527, 2000

DeLuca AK, Lenze EJ, Mulsant BH, et al: Comorbid anxiety disorder in late-life depression: association with memory decline over four years. Int J Geriatr Psychiatry 20:848–854, 2005

Dew MA, Reynolds CF 3rd, Houck PR, et al: Temporal profiles of the course of depression during treatment: predictors of pathways toward recovery in the elderly. Arch Gen Psychiatry 54:1016–1024, 1997

Dew MA, Kormos RL, DiMartini AF, et al: Prevalence and risk of depression and anxiety-related disorders during the first three years after heart transplantation. Psychosomatics 42:300–313, 2001

Diefenach GJ, Stanley MA, Beck JG: Worry content reported by older adults with and without generalized anxiety disorder. Aging Mental Health 5:269–274, 2001

Diem SJ, Blackwell TL, Stone KL, et al: Use of antidepressants and rates of hip bone loss in older women: the study of osteoporotic fractures. Arch Intern Med 167:1240–1245, 2007

Dombrovski AY, Mulsant BH, Houck PR, et al: Residual symptoms and recurrence during maintenance treatment of late-life depression. J Affect Disord 103:77–82, 2007

English BA, Jewell M, Jewell G, et al: Treatment of chronic posttraumatic stress disorder in combat veterans with citalopram: an open trial. J Clin Psychopharmacol 26:84–88, 2006

Ettner SL, Hermann RC: Provider specialty choice among Medicare beneficiaries treated for psychiatric disorders. Health Care Financ Rev 18:43–59, 1997

Fabian TJ, Amico JA, Kroboth PD, et al: Paroxetine-induced hyponatremia in older adults: a twelve-week prospective study. Arch Int Med 164:327–332, 2004

Flint A: Epidemiology and comorbidity of anxiety disorders in the elderly. Am J Psychiatry 151:640–649, 1994

Flint A: Anxiety and its disorders in late life: moving the field forward. Am J Geriatr Psychiatry 13:3–6, 2005a

Flint A: Generalised anxiety disorder in elderly patients: epidemiology, diagnosis and treatment options. Drugs Aging 22:101–114, 2005b

Flint AJ, Rifat SL: Two-year outcome of elderly patients with anxious depression. Psychiatry Res 66:23–31, 1997

Flint A, Bradwejn J, Vaccarino F, et al: Aging and panicogenic response to cholecystokinin tetrapeptide: an examination of the cholecystokinin system. Neuropsychopharmacology 27:663–671, 2002

Ford BC, Bullard KM, Taylor RJ, et al: Lifetime and 12-month prevalence of DSM-IV disorders among older African Americans: findings from the National Survey of American Life (NSAL). Am J Geriatr Psychiatry 15:652–659, 2007

Frueh BC, Grubaugh AL, Acierno R, et al: Age differences on PTSD, psychiatric disorders, and healthcare service use among veterans in Veterans Affairs primary care clinics. Am J Geriatr Psychiatry 15:660–672, 2007

Gagnon N, Flint AJ, Naglie G, et al: Affective correlates of fear of falling in elderly persons. Am J Geriatr Psychiatry 13:7–14, 2005

Gill SS, Bronskill SE, Normand SL, et al: Antipsychotic drug use and mortality in older adults with dementia. Ann Intern Med 146:775–786, 2007

Herings RM, Stricker BH, de Boer A, et al: Benzodiazepines and the risk of falling leading to femur fractures: dosage more important than elimination half-life. Arch Intern Med 155:1801–1807, 1995

Hettema JM, Kuhn JW, Prescott CA, et al: The impact of generalized anxiety disorder and stressful life events on risk for major depressive episodes. Psychol Med 36:789–795, 2006

Hwang SH, Kwon JS, Shin YW, et al: Neuropsychological profiles of patients with obsessive-compulsive disorder: early onset versus late onset. J Int Neuropsychol Soc 13:30–37, 2007

Jarvik LJ, Russell D: Anxiety, aging, and the third emergency response. J Gerontol 37:197–200, 1979

Jeste ND, Hays JC, Steffens DC: Clinical correlates of anxious depression among elderly patients with depression. J Affect Disord 90:37–41, 2006

Johnson E, Whyte EM ,Mulsant BH, et al: Cardiovascular changes associated with venlafaxine in the treatment of late-life depression. Am J Geriatr Psychiatry 14:796–802, 2006

Kessler RC, Amminger GP, Aguilar-Gaxiola S, et al: Age of onset of mental disorders: a review of recent literature. Curr Opin Psychiatry 20:359–364, 2007

Koepke HH, Gold RL, Linden ME, et al: Multicenter controlled study of oxazepam in anxious elderly outpatients. Psychosomatics 23:641–645, 1982

Kogan JN, Edelstein BA: Modification and psychometric examination of a self-report measure of fear in older adults. J Anxiety Disord 18:397–409, 2004

Landi F, Onder G, Cesari M, et al: Psychotropic medications and risk for falls among community-dwelling frail older people: an observational study. J Gerontol A Biol Sci Med Sci 60:622–626, 2005

Lawton MP, Kleban MH, Dean J: Affect and age: cross-sectional comparisons of structure and prevalence. Psychol Aging 8:165–175, 1993

Le Roux H, Gatz M, Wetherell JL: Age at onset of generalized anxiety disorder in older adults. Am J Geriatr Psychiatry 13:23–30, 2005

Lenze EJ, Wetherell JL: Bringing the bedside to the bench, and then to the community: a prospectus for intervention research in late-life anxiety disorders. Int J Geriatr Psychiatry 24:1–14, 2009

Lenze EJ, Mulsant BH, Shear MK, et al: Anxiety disorders in depressed elderly patients. Am J Psychiatry 15:722–728, 2000

Lenze EJ, Mulsant BH, Mohlman J, et al: Generalized anxiety disorder in late life: lifetime course and comorbidity with major depressive disorder. Am J Geriatr Psychiatry 13:77–80, 2005a

Lenze EJ, Mulsant BH, Shear MK, et al: Efficacy and tolerability of citalopram in the treatment of late-life anxiety disorders: results from an 8-week randomized, placebo-controlled trial. Am J Psychiatry 162:146–150, 2005b

Lenze EJ, Rollman BL, Shear MK, et al: Escitalopram for older adults with generalized anxiety disorder: a placebo-controlled trial. JAMA 301:296–303, 2009

Lupien SJ, Fiocco A, Wan N, et al: Stress hormones and human memory function across the lifespan. Psychoneuroendocrinology 30:225–242, 2005

Mantella RC, Butters MA, Dew MA, et al: Cognitive impairment in late-life generalized anxiety disorder. Am J Geriatr Psychiatry 15:673–679, 2007

McCabe L, Cairney J, Veldhuizen S, et al: Prevalence and correlates of agoraphobia in older adults. Am J Geriatr Psychiatry 14:515–522, 2006

Mintzer JE, Brawman-Mintzer O: Agitation as a possible expression of generalized anxiety disorder in demented elderly patients: toward a treatment approach. J Clin Psychiatry 57(suppl):55–63, 1996

Mohlman J, Gorenstein EE, Kleber M, et al: Standard and enhanced cognitive-behavior therapy for late-life generalized anxiety disorder: two pilot investigations. Am J Geriatr Psychiatry 11:24–32, 2003

Moríñigo A, Blanco M, Labrador J, et al: Risperidone for resistant anxiety in elderly persons. Am J Geriatr Psychiatry 13:81–82, 2005

Nagaratnam N, Ip J, Bou-Haidar P: The vestibular dysfunction and anxiety disorder interface: a descriptive study with special reference to the elderly. Arch Gerontol Geriatr 40:253–264, 2005

Nelson JC, Delucchi K, Schneider LS: Anxiety does not predict response to antidepressant treatment in late life depression: results of a meta-analysis. Int J Geriatr Psychiatry 24:539–544, 2009

Nestadt G, Bienvenu OJ, Cai G, et al: Incidence of obsessive-compulsive disorder in adults. J Nerv Ment Dis 186:401–406, 1998

Nestadt G, Samuels J, Riddle M, et al: A family study of obsessive-compulsive disorder. Arch Gen Psychiatry 57:358–363, 2000

Newcomer JW, Haupt DW: The metabolic effects of antipsychotic medications. Can J Psychiatry 51:480–491, 2006

O'Connor DW: Do older Australians truly have low rates of anxiety and depression? A critique of the 1997 National Survey of Mental Health and Wellbeing. Aust N Z J Psychiatry 40:623–631, 2006

Paterniti S, DuFouil C, Alperovitch A: Long-term benzodiazepine use and cognitive decline in the elderly: the Epidemiology of Vascular Aging Study. J Clin Psychopharmacol 22:285–293, 2002

Pinquart M, Duberstein PR: Treatment of anxiety disorders in older adults: a meta-analytic comparison of behavioral and pharmacological interventions. Am J Geriatr Psychiatry 15:639–651, 2007

Pomara N, Tun H, DaSilva D, et al: The acute and chronic performance effects of alprazolam and lorazepam in the elderly: relationship to duration of treatment and self-rated sedation. Psychopharmacol Bull 34:139–153, 1998

Pomara N, Willoughby LM, Sidtis JJ, et al: Cortisol response to diazepam: its relationship to age, dose, duration of treatment, and presence of generalized anxiety disorder. Psychopharmacology (Berl) 178:1–8, 2005

Raskind MA, Peskind ER, Hoff DJ, et al: A parallel group placebo controlled study of prazosin for trauma nightmares and sleep disturbance in combat veterans with post-traumatic stress disorder. Biol Psychiatry 61:928–934, 2007

Rubio G, Lopez-Ibor JJ: Generalized anxiety disorder: a 40-year follow-up study. Acta Psychiatr Scand 115:372–379, 2007

Saxena S: Is compulsive hoarding a genetically and neurobiologically discrete syndrome? Implications for diagnostic classification. Am J Psychiatry 164:380–384, 2007

Schneider LS, Dagerman KS, Insel P: Risk of death with atypical antipsychotic drug treatment for dementia: meta-analysis of randomized placebo-controlled trials. JAMA 294:1934–1943, 2005

Schoevers RA, Beekman ATF, Deeg DJH, et al: Comorbidity and risk-patterns of depression, generalised anxiety disorder and mixed anxiety-depression in later life: results from the AMSTEL study. Int J Geriatr Psychiatry 18:994–1001, 2003

Schuurmans J, Comijs HC, Beekman ATF, et al: The outcome of anxiety disorders in older people at 6-year follow-up: results from the Longitudinal Aging Study Amsterdam. Acta Psychiatr Scand 111:420–428, 2005

Schuurmans J, Comijs H, Emmelkamp PM, et al: A randomized, controlled trial of the effectiveness of cognitive-behavioral therapy and sertraline versus a waitlist control group for anxiety disorders in older adults. Am J Geriatr Psychiatry 14:255–263, 2006

Sheikh JI, Lauderdale SA, Cassidy EL: Efficacy of sertraline for panic disorder in older adults: a preliminary open-label trial. Am J Geriatr Psychiatry 12:230, 2004a

Sheikh JI, Swales PJ, Carlson EB, et al: Aging and panic disorder: phenomenology, comorbidity, and risk factors. Am J Geriatr Psychiatry 12:102–109, 2004b

Smit F, Ederveen A, Cuijpers P, et al: Opportunities for cost-effective prevention of late-life depression: an epidemiological approach. Arch Gen Psychiatry 63:290–296, 2006

Smit F, Comijs H, Schoevers R, et al: Target groups for the prevention of late-life anxiety. Br J Psychiatry 190:428–434, 2007

Stanley MA, Beck JG, DeWitt Glassco J: Treatment of generalized anxiety in older adults: a preliminary comparison of cognitive-behavioral and supportive approaches. Behav Ther 27:565–582, 1996

Stanley MA, Beck JG, Novy DM, et al: Cognitive-behavioral treatment of late-life generalized anxiety disorder. J Consult Clin Psychol 71:309–319, 2003a

Stanley MA, Hopko DR, Diefenbach GJ, et al: Cognitive-behavior therapy for late-life generalized anxiety disorder in primary care: preliminary findings. Am J Geriatr Psychiatry 11:92–96, 2003b

Stanley MA, Diefenbach GJ, Hopko DR: Cognitive behavioral treatment for older adults with generalized anxiety disorder: a therapist manual for primary care settings. Behav Modif 28:73–117, 2004

Stanley MA, Wilson NL, Novy DM, et al: Cognitive behavior therapy for generalized anxiety disorder among older adults in primary care: a randomized clinical trial. JAMA 301:1460–1467, 2009

Starkstein SE, Jorge R, Petracca G, et al: The construct of generalized anxiety disorder in Alzheimer disease. Am J Geriatr Psychiatry 15:42–49, 2007

Steffens DC, McQuoid DR: Impact of symptoms of generalized anxiety disorder on the course of late-life depression. Am J Geriatr Psychiatry 13:40–47, 2005

Swoboda KJ, Jenike MA: Frontal abnormalities in a patient with obsessive-compulsive disorder: the role of structural lesions in obsessive-compulsive behavior. Neurology 45:2130–2134, 1995

Teachman BA: Aging and negative affect: the rise and fall and rise of anxiety and depression symptoms. Psychol Aging 21:201–207, 2007

Thorp SR, Ayers CR, Nuevo R, et al: Meta-analysis comparing different behavioral treatments for late-life anxiety. Am J Geriatr Psychiatry 17:105–115, 2009

Todaro JF, Shen BJ, Raffa SD, et al: Prevalence of anxiety disorders in men and women with established coronary heart disease. J Cardiopulm Rehabil Prev 27:86–91, 2007

Tolin DF, Robison JT, Gaztambide S, et al: Anxiety disorders in older Puerto Rican primary care patients. Am J Geriatr Psychiatry 13:150–156, 2005

van Balkom AJ, Beekman AT, de Beurs E, et al: Comorbidity of the anxiety disorders in a community-based older population in The Netherlands. Acta Psychiatr Scand 101:37–45, 2000

van't Veer-Tazelaar PJ, van Marwijk HW, van Oppen P, et al: Stepped-care prevention of anxiety and depression in late life: a randomized controlled trial. Arch Gen Psychiatry 66:297–304, 2009

van Zelst WH, de Beurs E, Beekman AT, et al: Prevalence and risk factors of posttraumatic stress disorder in older adults. Psychother Psychosom 72:333–342, 2003

Velayudhan L, Katz AW: Late-onset obsessive-compulsive disorder: the role of stressful life events. Int Psychogeriatr 18:341–344, 2006

Vink D, Aartsen MJ, Schoevers RA: Risk factors for anxiety and depression in the elderly: a review. J Affect Disord 106:29–44, 2008

Weiss AP, Jenike MA: Late-onset obsessive-compulsive disorder: a case series. J Neuropsychiatry Clin Neurosci 12:265–268, 2000

Wetherell JL, Gatz M, Pedersen NL: A longitudinal analysis of anxiety and depressive symptoms. Psychol Aging 16:187–195, 2001

Wetherell JL, Reynolds CA, Gatz M, et al: Anxiety, cognitive performance, and cognitive decline in normal aging. J Gerontol Psychol Sci 57B:P246–P255, 2002

Wetherell JL, Gatz M, Craske MG: Treatment of generalized anxiety disorder in older adults. J Consult Clin Psychol 71:31–40, 2003a

Wetherell JL, Le Roux H, Gatz M: DSM-IV criteria for generalized anxiety disorder in older adults: distinguishing the worried from the well. Psychol Aging 18:622–627, 2003b

Wetherell JL, Thorp SR, Patterson TL, et al: Quality of life in geriatric generalized anxiety disorder: a preliminary investigation. J Psychiatr Res 38:305–312, 2004

Wetherell JL, Hopko DR, Diefenbach GJ, et al: Cognitive-behavioral therapy for late-life generalized anxiety disorder: who gets better? Behav Ther 36:147–156, 2005a

Wetherell JL, Lenze EJ, Stanley MA: Evidence-based treatment of geriatric anxiety disorders. Psychiatr Clin North Am 28:871–896, 2005b

Whyte EM, Dew MA, Gildengers A, et al: Time course of response to antidepressants in late-life major depression: therapeutic implications. Drugs Aging 21:531–554, 2004

Yehuda R, Golier JA, Tischler L, et al: Hippocampal volume in aging combat veterans with and without post-traumatic stress disorder: relation to risk and resilience factors. J Psychiatr Res 41:435–445, 2007

Yohannes AM, Baldwin RC, Connolly MJ: Depression and anxiety in elderly patients with chronic obstructive pulmonary disease. Age Ageing 35:457–459, 2006

Yuan Y, Tsoi K, Hunt RH: Selective serotonin reuptake inhibitors and risk of upper GI bleeding: confusion or confounding? Am J Med 119:719–727, 2006

Recommended Readings

Lenze EJ, Wetherell JL: Bringing the bedside to the bench, and then to the community: a prospectus for intervention research in late-life anxiety disorders. Int J Geriatr Psychiatry 24:1–14, 2009

Lenze EJ, Rollman BL, Shear MK, et al: Escitalopram for older adults with generalized anxiety disorder: a placebo-controlled trial. JAMA 301:296–303, 2009

Stanley MA, Wilson NL, Novy DM, et al: Cognitive behavior therapy for generalized anxiety disorder among older adults in primary care: a randomized clinical trial. JAMA 301:1460–1467, 2009

van't Veer-Tazelaar PJ, van Marwijk HW, van Oppen P, et al: Stepped-care prevention of anxiety and depression in late life: a randomized controlled trial. Arch Gen Psychiatry 66:297–304, 2009

Chapter 36

Anxiety in the Context of Substance Abuse

Sudie E. Back, Ph.D.
Angela E. Waldrop, Ph.D.
Kathleen T. Brady, M.D., Ph.D.

The relationship between anxiety disorders and substance use disorders (SUDs) is complex and bidirectional. As described in this chapter, studies of treatment-seeking individuals as well as epidemiological surveys indicate that anxiety disorders, symptoms of anxiety, and SUDs commonly co-occur. The interaction between substance use and anxiety is multifaceted and variable. Anxiety disorders may be a risk factor for the development of substance abuse and dependence. Furthermore, anxiety disorders are likely to modify the presentation and outcome of treatment for SUDs, just as substance use and SUDs modify the presentation and outcome of treatment for anxiety disorders. In addition, anxiety symptoms may emerge during the course of chronic intoxication and withdrawal from alcohol or drugs. The interplay of these variables is likely to differ among individual cases and between different anxiety disorders. In this chapter, we review the epidemiology of co-occurring anxiety disorders and SUDs, etiological relationships, and diagnostic considerations, and we discuss in detail each of the primary anxiety disorders as they relate to SUDs.

Epidemiology

General Population

Several epidemiological studies conducted in the United States over the past 20 years have concluded that anxiety disorders and SUDs co-occur more commonly than would be expected by chance alone (Kessler et al. 1994, 1997; Regier et al. 1990). Table 36–1 presents prevalence rates for substance use and anxiety disorders. The National Epidemiological Survey on Alcohol and Related Conditions (NESARC) is the most recent and largest comorbidity study to date, with a sample of more than 43,000 adults. The study was designed to distinguish between independent mood and anxiety disorders (i.e., those that cannot be attributed to withdrawal or intoxication), and substance-induced mood and anxiety disorders. Results indicated that over 17% (17.7%) of respondents with an SUD in the prior 12 months met criteria for an independent anxiety disorder. Among respondents with any anxiety disorder in the prior 12 months, approximately 15% had at least one co-occurring SUD (Grant et al. 2004). The relationship between anxiety and drug use disorders (odds ratio [OR] = 2.8) was stronger than for anxiety and alcohol use disorders (OR = 1.7).

TABLE 36–1. Prevalence of substance use and anxiety disorders per 100 people in the United States

	ECA (lifetime prevalence)	NCS-R (lifetime prevalence)	NESARC (12-month prevalence)
Alcohol abuse	5.6	13.2	4.7
Alcohol dependence	7.9	5.4	3.8
Drug abuse	2.6	7.9	1.4
Drug dependence	3.5	3.0	0.6
Generalized anxiety disorder	—	5.7	2.1
Social phobia	2.8	12.1	2.8
Obsessive-compulsive disorder	2.5	1.6	—
Posttraumatic stress disorder	—	6.8	—
Panic disorder			
with agoraphobia	0.5	1.1	0.6
without agoraphobia	—	3.7	1.6

Note. ECA=Epidemiologic Catchment Area Study (Regier et al. 1990); NCS-R=National Comorbidity Survey–Replication (Kessler et al. 2006); NESARC=National Epidemiologic Survey on Alcohol and Related Conditions (Grant et al. 2004; Hasin et al. 2007).

Using data from NESARC, Hasin and colleagues explored 12-month and lifetime diagnoses (2007). The 12-month prevalence of an alcohol use disorder was 8.5%, and lifetime prevalence was 30.3%. The odds ratio of alcohol use disorders co-occurring with any anxiety disorder was 1.9 for 12-month diagnoses and 10.4 for lifetime diagnoses, when adjusted for several sociodemographic variables (Hasin et al. 2007).

A secondary analysis of six international epidemiological data sets, including the National Comorbidity Survey (NCS), examined co-occurring anxiety disorders and SUDs among 14- to 64-year-olds (Merikangas et al. 1998). Averaged across sites, 32% of individuals with lifetime alcohol dependence and 45% of individuals with lifetime drug dependence also met criteria for a lifetime anxiety disorder. Merikangas and colleagues note that although patterns of comorbidity tended to be similar for men and women, the magnitude of the relationships (indicated by odds ratios) was stronger for women.

Treatment-Seeking and Other Clinical Populations

Patients with anxiety disorders are more frequent users of all types of health services compared with individuals without anxiety disorders (Gurmankin Levy et al. 2007). In a large sample of primary care patients, among respondents with panic disorder with or without agoraphobia, 15% also had at least one SUD (Rodriguez et al. 2004).

A study of opioid abusers in a needle exchange program found that approximately 15% also had a lifetime anxiety disorder diagnosis: 12% in men and 21% in women (Kidorf et al. 2004). In a sample of substance use treatment clinics, 80% of patients had at least one co-occurring anxiety disorder, and comorbidity had a significant relationship to overall mental distress at initial interview and 6 years later (Bakken et al. 2007). The presence of agoraphobia predicted a higher risk for relapse in these patients (Landheim et al. 2006).

Order of Onset

The order of onset of co-occurring disorders can help in understanding etiological connections. Analysis of data from the National Comorbidity Survey Replication (NCS-R) indicated that the age at onset for different psychiatric disorders varies, with anxiety disorders tending to have an earlier age at onset than mood disorders (Kessler et al. 2005a). The epidemiological studies reviewed by Merikangas et al. (1998) allowed for the examination of the order of onset of SUDs versus anxiety disorders. In cases that included both alcohol dependence and an anxiety disorder, the anxiety disorder typically preceded alcohol dependence (56.7% to 79.4% across sites). In cases that included both drug dependence and an anxiety disorder, the proportion of cases in which the anxiety began first was even larger, ranging from 67.6% to 100% across sites (Merikangas et al. 1998).

A review by Kushner and colleagues (1990) indicated that order of onset differs by anxiety diagnoses. Social phobia, panic, and agoraphobia generally precede SUDs. The findings regarding generalized anxiety disorder (GAD) were less clear but suggested that GAD tends to develop near the same time as or after alcohol problems (Kushner et al. 1990). The same pattern of results was found in a later study of SUD patients in treatment (Compton et al. 2000).

Neurobiological Connections Between Anxiety Disorders and SUDs

Numerous studies have focused on etiological relationships between anxiety and addiction. A growing body of evidence implicates common neurobiological pathways and abnormalities involved in both disorders. One of the bridging constructs between several psychiatric disorders and SUDs involves the role of stress. Corticotropin releasing factor, one of the key hormones involved in the stress response, has been implicated in the pathophysiology of anxiety and affective and addictive disorders (Koob and Kreek 2007). Preclinical evidence suggested that corticotropin-releasing factor and noradrenergic pathways are involved in stress-induced reinstatement of drug-seeking behavior in drug-dependent laboratory animals (Piazza and Le Moal 1998). Similarly, human laboratory studies have shown that emotional stress and negative affect states increase drug craving in drug-dependent individuals (Cooney et al. 1997). In animal models, early-life stress and chronic stress resulted in long-term changes in stress responses, altering the sensitivity of the dopamine system to stress and increasing susceptibility to drug self-administration (Meaney et al. 2002). Other neurobiological systems also implicated in both anxiety disorders and SUDs include the endogenous opiate, noradrenergic, neuropeptide Y, nociceptin, orexin, and vasopressin systems.

Diagnostic Considerations

One concern in the area of comorbid anxiety disorders and SUDs is accurate diagnosis and differentiation between drug-induced states and primary anxiety diagnoses. The active use of some substances (e.g., marijuana, stimulants) is associated with anxiety symptoms, and withdrawal from other substances (e.g., opiates, benzodiazepines) is marked by anxiety states. It is also likely that chronic use of substances of abuse, which have powerful effects on neurotransmitter systems involved in the production of anxiety disorders, may unmask vulnerability or lead to neurobiological changes that manifest as anxiety disorders.

The best way to differentiate transient, substance-induced symptoms from true anxiety symptoms is through observation during a period of abstinence. A key issue is the duration of abstinence necessary for accurate diagnosis. The necessary abstinent time for diagnostic purposes will vary by diagnosis and by the substance being used. For long half-life drugs (e.g., some benzodiazepines, methadone), withdrawal symptoms may be quite protracted, and several weeks of abstinence may be essential for accurate diagnoses. For shorter-acting substances (e.g., cocaine, short-half-life benzodiazepines), both the acute intoxication and withdrawal duration are likely to be briefer, and it may be possible to make diagnoses after shorter periods of abstinence. In cases where the diagnosis remains unclear, the following factors weigh in favor of an anxiety disorder diagnosis: positive family history of anxiety disorders, onset of anxiety symptoms before the onset of SUD, and sustained anxiety symptoms during lengthy periods of abstinence.

Because anxiety is so commonly seen in association with substance use, any patient presenting for treatment of anxiety should be screened for alcohol and other drug use. Several brief screening tools for SUDs have demonstrated usefulness in psychiatric settings, including the Alcohol Use Disorders Identification Test (AUDIT; Bohn et al. 1995), Michigan Alcohol Screening Test (MAST; Teitelbaum and Carey 2000), Drug and Alcohol Screening Test (DAST; Maisto et al. 2000), and CAGE questions (Ewing 1984). It is important to bear in mind that caffeine and some over-the-counter medications (e.g., pseudoephedrine, diet pills) can cause substantial anxiety (Kendler et al. 2006), and although the use of these substances in an individual case might not constitute substance abuse, decreasing their use may be of enormous benefit in decreasing symptoms of anxiety.

The remainder of this chapter is divided into sections that address individual anxiety disorders. For each disorder, the prevalence of comorbidity as well as diagnostic and treatment considerations will be discussed. For many of the disorders discussed, few data exist. Relatively more studies have been conducted that explore the relationship between anxiety disorders and alcoholism. In areas where data are lacking, relevant studies concerning alcohol and anxiety disorders will be cited and general principles guiding appropriate clinical management of comorbid patients will be reviewed.

Anxiety Disorders

Generalized Anxiety Disorder

Epidemiology

Second to major depression, SUDs are the most common comorbid psychiatric disorder among individuals with generalized anxiety disorder (GAD) (Wittchen et al. 1994). An epidemiological study of 5,877 adults found that GAD was the anxiety disorder most often associated with using alcohol or drugs to self-medicate symptoms (Bolton and Sareen 2006). Similarly, data from the NESARC showed a strong association between 12-month prevalence rates of GAD and alcohol use disorders (odds ratio=2.0) and drug use disorders (odds ratio=4.5) (Grant et al. 2005). Comorbid GAD is associated with an accelerated progression from first use to the onset of dependence. For example, among 1,269 adolescents and young adults (mean age=20.1 years), Sartor and colleagues (2007) found that GAD was associated with a 3.5-fold increase in rate of progression from first drink to the onset of alcohol dependence. Furthermore, the presence of comorbid SUDs has been shown to significantly decrease the likelihood of recovery from GAD (Bruce et al. 2005).

Differential Diagnosis

GAD is particularly hard to diagnose in the face of SUDs because every symptom of GAD can be mimicked by substance use or withdrawal. To help ensure accurate diagnosis, the assessment of GAD should be delayed until intoxication or withdrawal has terminated. As mentioned earlier, for short-acting drugs (e.g., cocaine), it may be possible to assess GAD after 1 week of abstinence, but longer periods of time (e.g., 4–8 weeks) may be required for longer-acting drugs (e.g., methadone, valium) (McKeehan and Martin 2002; Schuckit and Monteiro 1988). DSM-IV-TR (American Psychiatric Association 2000) requires that a core number of anxiety symptoms be present for at least 6 months in order to meet diagnostic criteria for GAD. Substance use during those 6 months must be considered, and symptoms of GAD must have been present during times other than when the patient was using or recovering from alcohol or drugs. This can be challenging to assess because many SUD patients presenting for treatment and complaining of anxiety will not have had 6 months of abstinence.

A nosological issue concerning the diagnosis of GAD is whether the symptoms reflect a true anxiety disorder or are the result of other comorbid psychiatric conditions (Grant et al. 2005; Stein 2001). Because chronic use of alcohol and drugs can result in occupational, interpersonal, and physical health impairments, it can be difficult to discern whether the anxiety symptoms resulting from such impairments represent a true anxiety disorder. These are complicated and difficult issues to resolve. Consultation with colleagues on a case-by-case basis is recommended in order to design appropriate treatment plans. In addition, following the patient and reassessing the diagnosis of GAD is important. As the patient becomes abstinent and functioning improves, the course of anxiety symptoms will provide useful information regarding diagnosis.

Pharmacological Treatment

The treatment of GAD in the context of addiction can be challenging. Although benzodiazepines are effective in the treatment of GAD, their use in individuals with current or previous SUDs is controversial because of their abuse liability. Some authors (Kosten et al. 2000; Posternak and Mueller 2001) posit, however, that the empirical evidence regarding the dangers of treatment in individuals with SUDs is insufficient and that benzodiazepines may be safely used to treat anxiety disorders in some SUD patients. In some studies, buspirone, a partial 5-hydroxytryptamine 5-HT_{1A} agonist with low abuse potential, has been shown to be efficacious in alcoholics with anxiety (Kranzler et al. 1994; Malec et al. 1996; McKeehan and Martin 2002), but results are inconsistent. For example, Tollefson et al. (1992) found that patients treated with buspirone, as compared with placebo, evidenced significantly lower Hamilton Anxiety Scale test scores and self-reports of alcohol intake. In contrast, Malcolm et al. (1992) found no between-group differences in anxiety or alcohol use severity among patients treated with buspirone or placebo. Another randomized trial of buspirone among anxious opiate-dependent individuals found that buspirone was associated with trends toward improvements in depressive symptomatology and a slower return to substance use but no significant improvements in anxiety symptoms (McRae et al. 2004). Clearly, more research is needed to help clarify the spectrum of efficacy, but there is some evidence supporting the use of buspirone in SUD patients with GAD. Selective serotonin reuptake inhibitors (SSRIs) are efficacious in reducing GAD symptoms (Lydiard et al. 1988); however, no clinical trials of SSRIs in individuals with comorbid GAD and SUDs have been conducted.

Psychosocial Treatment

Among psychosocial treatments, cognitive-behavioral therapy (CBT) has been shown to decrease both anxiety symptoms and relapse in individuals with SUDs. Techniques such as relaxation, coping skills, behavioral activation, problem solving, and sleep hygiene can assist patients with both disorders (McKeehan and Martin 2002). Nutritional counseling and regular exercise may also be useful in helping individuals with GAD and comorbid SUDs to learn alternative strategies for coping with anxiety, but empirical trials are lacking.

Conclusions

SUDs and GAD commonly co-occur, so all patients with GAD should be screened for alcohol and drug use disorders, for subsyndromal use of substances to self-medicate anxiety symptoms, and for the use of over-the-counter substances that can induce anxiety (e.g., caffeine, diet pills). Identifying SUDs in GAD patients early in the course of illness is critical, because GAD is associated with significantly faster progression from initial use to addiction, and because once an SUD has developed, the likelihood of recovery from GAD is significantly compromised. Care should be taken in diagnosing GAD among individuals with SUDs, given that intoxication or withdrawal can mimic GAD symptoms. Findings regarding the use of buspirone treatment among patients with SUDs and GAD are mixed, but some support for its efficacy exists. The use of SSRIs, which are effective in treating GAD, has not been explored in patients with co-occurring SUDs and GAD. This would be a helpful area for future investigations. More research on the use of benzodiazepines and on development of psychosocial treatments is needed to advance the treatment of comorbid GAD and SUDs.

Social Phobia

Epidemiology

Individuals with social phobia are two to three times more likely than individuals without this phobia to develop an alcohol use disorder (Kushner et al. 1990), the most common substance of abuse among social phobia patients. Social phobia is also associated with illicit drug use, with odds ratios from community samples ranging from 1.6 to 2.3 (Sareen et al. 2006). In particular, generalized social phobia, as compared with fears of public speaking only, is associated with increased drug use (Sareen et al. 2006). Consistent with the self-medication model, SUDs generally follow the onset of social phobia symptoms (Carrigan and Randall 2003; Khantzian 1985; Myrick and Brady 1996; Sareen et al. 2001; Terra et al. 2006). Many socially anxious individuals report consuming alcohol or drugs to help reduce fear of criticism or embarrassment (Carrigan and Randall 2003; Thomas et al. 2003). In the NCS data, 16.4% of socially phobic individuals endorsed self-medicating with alcohol and drugs (Bolton et al. 2006).

Differential Diagnosis

Compared with other anxiety disorders, less abstinence may be needed to establish a diagnosis of social phobia for several reasons. Because the average onset of social phobia is before adolescence, symptoms of social anxiety are often present before the initiation of alcohol or drug use (Bakken et al. 2005; Sareen et al. 2001). Also, the cardinal symptom of social phobia, fear of public scrutiny, is fairly specific and not mimicked by substance use and withdrawal. Social anxiety symptoms that arise only in the context of acute intoxication or withdrawal are not sufficient to meet criteria for a diagnosis of social phobia.

Pharmacological Treatment

In a placebo-controlled trial, Randall et al. (2001a) examined the effectiveness of paroxetine, an SSRI, in 15 outpatients with alcohol dependence and social phobia. The paroxetine-treated group had significantly lower social phobia symptoms at the end of the 8-week trial, as compared with the placebo group. No significant group differences in measures of alcohol-use frequency or quantity were revealed, but significant improvement in the Clinical Global Index was found.

Gabapentin is an anticonvulsant agent with demonstrated efficacy in a placebo-controlled, double-blind trial for the treatment of social phobia (Pande et al. 1999). This is particularly noteworthy because gabapentin has also demonstrated efficacy in the treatment of alcohol withdrawal (Malcolm et al. 2001; Myrick et al. 1998; Voris et al. 2003), and unlike benzodiazepines, gabapentin has no abuse potential. There is one case report of a polysubstance-dependent individual with comorbid social phobia who demonstrated significant improvement in craving and substance use with gabapentin treatment (Verduin et al. 2007). However, there are no controlled trials examining the efficacy of gabapentin in co-occurring social phobia and SUDs. Future directions in the treatment of co-occurring social phobia and SUDs should include further exploration of anxiolytic anticonvulsant agents.

Psychosocial Treatment

There have been several controlled trials of psychosocial treatment for co-occurring social phobia and SUDs. In 93 outpatients with social phobia and alcohol dependence, Randall et al. (2001b) compared the efficacy of a 12-week manual-based CBT for alcohol dependence alone with an integrated manual-based CBT for both disorders. Contrary to their hypothesis, patients who received the alcohol-dependence-only treatment evidenced better outcomes than patients who received the integrated treatment. The authors hypothesized that exposure to feared social situations during early recovery may have led to increases in alcohol use to cope.

Schade et al. (2004) randomly assigned 96 individuals with alcohol dependence and comorbid social phobia and/or agoraphobia to receive either relapse prevention alone or relapse prevention plus CBT for the anxiety disorder. The majority (89 of 96) of the sample had social phobia. Both groups were offered concomitant SSRI pharmacotherapy (fluvoxamine), but more than half the total number of participants (53%) refused it. Individuals who received the combined psychosocial treatment (for alcohol dependence plus anxiety) had significantly greater improvement in anxiety symptoms than those who received treatment addressing alcohol dependence only. No significant between-group differences in alcohol use severity were observed, and the use of fluvoxamine did not predict improved outcome for anxiety or alcohol use severity.

Conclusions

Individuals with social phobia often use alcohol or drugs to self-medicate anxiety symptoms. In the majority of cases, social phobia precedes the development of SUDs—thus, preventive efforts are critical. SSRIs show promise in the treatment of co-occurring social phobia and alcohol dependence, but further study is needed. Gabapentin has also been shown in separate studies to decrease symptoms of social phobia and alcohol withdrawal. Examination of gabapentin among patients with this comorbidity would be a useful next step. Studies comparing psychosocial treatments of SUDs-only and combined treatments addressing both SUD and social phobia have shown mixed results, and it remains unclear whether and for whom integrated treatments are superior to single-diagnosis treatments.

Obsessive-Compulsive Disorder

Epidemiology

The association between obsessive-compulsive disorder (OCD) and SUDs is less robust when compared with associations with other anxiety disorders (Kessler et al. 2005b; Schuckit et al. 1997; Terra et al. 2006). In a clinical sample of 254 individuals, approximately 4% of OCD patients met criteria for a lifetime SUD (Sbrana et al. 2005). Schuckit et al. (1997) estimated lifetime rates of OCD among 3,632 individuals at 1.3% for alcohol-dependent individuals and 0.9% for control subjects, which was not significantly different. Individuals with OCD are not prone to impulsive or spontaneous behaviors, often have high levels of harm avoidance, and do not enjoy the sensations related to a loss of control, which drugs and alcohol often produce. When patients with OCD do use substances, they typically choose sedating substances (e.g., alcohol). The most commonly used illicit drug among individuals with OCD is marijuana (Sbrana et al. 2005).

Differential Diagnosis

SUDs contain elements of obsessions and compulsions (Modell et al. 1992). For example, individuals with SUDs have recurrent intrusive thoughts about using alcohol or drugs, often feel compelled to use alcohol or drugs, and may feel that if they use, the distressing thoughts or cravings will be quelled. For people with SUDs, however, the content of the cognitions and compulsions is restricted to alcohol or drug use. Furthermore, unlike compulsions, the substance use behaviors are not engaged in according to rigid rules that must be followed. Finally, the use of substances is connected in a realistic way with the cravings SUD patients experience.

Substances of abuse, such as alcohol or stimulants, and some medications such as benzodiazepines have been found to be associated with the occurrence of obsessive-compulsive behaviors (McKeehan and Martin 2002). Case reports have also described the emergence of obsessive-compulsive symptoms during acute intoxication of cocaine and other stimulants (Satel and McDougle 1991). However, the differential diagnosis of OCD in individuals with SUDs is not as difficult as that of some of the other anxiety disorders because there is less symptom overlap. Obsessions and compulsions focused on procuring and using drugs alone or that occur only during intoxication do not meet diagnostic criteria for OCD.

Pharmacological Treatment

There has been little research on the treatment of comorbid OCD and SUDs. In one case report (Chatterjee and Ringold 1999) on the use of gabapentin, an anticonvulsant, to augment paroxetine treatment in a 38-year-old man with OCD and alcohol dependence, a significant decrease was reported in craving and alcohol consumption after the man was given gabapentin, but the impact on OCD symptoms was mixed. SSRIs are efficacious in the treatment of OCD (Greist et al. 1995), but they have not been systematically tested in individuals with OCD and comorbid SUDs.

Psychosocial Treatment

There is also a dearth of literature regarding the psychosocial treatment of comorbid OCD and SUDs. Fals-Stewart and Schafer (1992) randomly assigned 60 patients dually diagnosed with OCD and an SUD to receive integrated psychotherapy for OCD and SUDs, therapy for SUDs only, or a progressive muscle relaxation–attention control group. The integrated-treatment group, as compared with the other two groups, evidenced significantly greater reductions in OCD symptoms, alcohol abstinence rates, and treatment retention.

Conclusions

SUDs are relatively rare among patients with OCD. Some substances of abuse and medications can produce obsessive-compulsive behaviors. This potential confound should be ruled out when diagnosing OCD among SUD patients. Little research on the treatment of co-occurring OCD and SUDs has been conducted to date, and there are no randomized, controlled trials examining the use of a pharmacological treatment for this patient population. SSRIs have been shown to be effective in treating OCD among non-substance-dependent patients and would likely be helpful among SUD patients, but this has not been systematically tested. One controlled clinical trial demonstrated promising results for an integrated psychotherapy addressing both OCD and SUD symptoms.

Posttraumatic Stress Disorder

Epidemiology

The comorbidity of posttraumatic stress disorder (PTSD) and SUDs is particularly striking. The NCS showed that adults with PTSD were two to four times more likely than those without PTSD to have a comorbid SUD (Kessler et al. 1995). Similarly, data from the Australian National Survey of Mental Health and Well-Being (N=10,000) found that 34.4% of respondents with PTSD had at least one SUD, with alcohol use disorders being the most common (Mills et al. 2006). Among treatment-seeking substance abusers, the prevalence of lifetime PTSD has been reported as high as 50% or greater (Dansky et al. 1994; Triffleman et al. 1995). In the majority of cases, the development of PTSD precedes the development of the SUD (Back et al. 2005, 2006b; Jacobsen et al. 2001; Stewart and Conrod 2003).

Differential Diagnosis

A characteristic unique to the diagnosis of PTSD, as compared with other anxiety disorders, is the fact that the diagnosis is dependent on exposure to a traumatic event. Thus, less abstinence is often needed to establish the diagnosis of PTSD among SUD patients. Intrusive symptoms (e.g., recurrent thoughts or images related to the trauma, psychological or physiological reactivity upon exposure to reminders of the trauma) are particularly characteristic of PTSD and are unlikely to be mimicked by substance use or withdrawal. Other symptoms (e.g., irritability, sleep impairment, difficulty concentrating, exaggerated startle response) could be exacerbated by the use of or withdrawal from alcohol and drugs and should be carefully assessed.

Pharmacological Treatment

Compared with investigation of SUDs in the context of other anxiety disorders, more empirical research is available on the treatment of comorbid PTSD and SUDs, although it is still in early stages. In a 12-week double-blind, placebo-controlled, trial, Brady and colleagues (2005) investigated the use of sertraline, which is approved by the U.S. Food and Drug Administration (FDA) for the treatment of PTSD, in 94 individuals with PTSD and alcohol dependence. Those who presented with less severe alcohol dependence and early-onset PTSD demonstrated greater improvement in alcohol use severity when treated with sertraline, as compared with placebo. In contrast, individuals with more severe alcohol dependence and later-onset PTSD demonstrated better alcohol use outcomes when treated with placebo as compared with sertraline. The sertraline-treated group also showed a trend toward greater PTSD improvement when compared with the placebo-treated group.

Among 254 outpatients with alcohol dependence and a variety of comorbid psychiatric disorders (42.9%

met DSM-IV-TR criteria for comorbid PTSD), Petrakis et al. (2005) investigated the efficacy of disulfiram and naltrexone or their combination in a 12-week randomized trial. Participants treated with naltrexone or disulfiram, as compared with placebo, had more consecutive weeks of abstinence and fewer drinking days per week. In comparison with naltrexone-treated participants, disulfiram-treated participants reported less craving from pre- to posttreatment. Although the authors did not investigate the effects of the medications by specific comorbid psychiatric disorder, participants treated with active medication evidenced greater symptom improvement (e.g., less anxiety) as measured by the Brief Symptom Inventory over the course of the trial. No clear advantage of combining disulfiram and naltrexone was observed.

Psychosocial Treatment

Numerous psychosocial studies for the treatment of co-occurring PTSD and SUDs have been conducted. These studies have shown promise and have demonstrated that the addition of trauma-focused interventions to SUD treatments typically result in significant decreases in both PTSD and SUD symptoms (Brady et al. 2001; Foa et al. 2006; Morrissey et al. 2005; Najavits et al. 1998, 2005; Triffleman 2000). Furthermore, a large percentage of PTSD/SUD patients indicate that they prefer to receive integrated treatments that address both disorders (Back et al. 2006a; Brown et al. 1998; Najavits et al. 2004).

The most widely studied integrated psychosocial treatment is Seeking Safety, a 25-session manualized treatment (Najavits 2002; Najavits et al. 1998) designed to bolster stabilization and safety by providing psychoeducation and by teaching coping skills. In one controlled study (Hien et al. 2004), 107 women were randomly assigned to Seeking Safety, relapse prevention, or treatment as usual. Patients who received treatment as usual failed to demonstrate significant improvement or, in the case of PTSD symptoms, worsened over time. Patients who received either Seeking Safety or relapse prevention demonstrated significant improvement in substance use, PTSD, and psychiatric symptom severity, but there was no significant difference between the Seeking Safety and relapse prevention treatment groups. More controlled studies in this area are needed.

Prolonged exposure therapy, a gold standard treatment for PTSD, may also be useful among SUD patients. Two studies have systematically examined treatments that integrate exposure-based techniques for PTSD with empirically validated treatments for SUD; however, neither study included a control group. Triffleman et al. (1999) developed a 20-week, manualized treatment that utilized relapse prevention, coping skills, psychoeducation, and in vivo exposure. In a small pilot trial (*N*= 19) using methadone-maintained, primary cocaine-abusing subjects, the integrated treatment was compared with Twelve-Step Facilitation therapy (Triffleman 2000). Both treatments were associated with improvements in PTSD and drug use, and no significant differences between treatment conditions were found. The small sample size, with less than 10 patients per treatment group, may have limited the statistical power to detect significant differences.

In a larger trial, Brady and colleagues (Back et al. 2001; Brady et al. 2001) developed a 16-session manualized treatment consisting of combined imaginal and in vivo exposure therapy for PTSD, and cognitive-behavioral relapse prevention techniques for cocaine dependence. Results of an uncontrolled preliminary study (*N*= 39) indicated that the treatment was associated with significant reductions in all three clusters of PTSD symptoms and cocaine use. Furthermore, these improvements were maintained over a 6-month follow-up period. Clearly, a controlled trial of prolonged exposure in co-occurring PTSD and SUDs is needed.

Several other studies have preliminarily explored the use of psychosocial treatments among PTSD/SUD patients with favorable results. For example, Donovan et al. (2001) developed a partial hospitalization program, called Transcend, for combat PTSD and comorbid SUDs. Transcend is eclectic in nature, employing therapeutic strategies from a variety of orientations such as psychodynamic, CBT, and Twelve-Step Facilitation therapy. The treatment is time-intensive and involves 10 hours of weekly group therapy for 12 weeks. Half the program is focused on trauma processing. An uncontrolled pilot study among 46 male veterans suggested Transcend may be helpful in improving PTSD symptoms (Donovan et al. 2001). Controlled studies and assessments of substance use severity and relapse are needed.

Finally, the Trauma Recovery and Empowerment Model (TREM) is a manualized group intervention designed for sexually and/or physically abused women (Harris 1998). TREM involves approximately 9 months of weekly 75-minute sessions emphasizing cognitive restructuring, survivor empowerment, peer support, and skill building. In addition, psychoeducation regarding the impact of violence, in particular PTSD, depression, and substance abuse, is provided. In a study of 170 women in residential substance abuse treatment, a modified version of TREM (reduced to 24 sessions and accompanied by a trauma workbook) showed promise in reducing trauma-related symptoms (Toussaint et al., in press). More systematic and controlled research on TREM is also needed.

Conclusions

SUDs are extremely common among patients with PTSD. All patients presenting with trauma and/or PTSD should be screened for SUDs and for subsyndromal use of substances to self-medicate PTSD symptoms. An impressive increase in research on the treatment of PTSD and comorbid SUDs has occurred over the past decade, particularly in the area of psychosocial treatments. A number of investigations have now shown that addressing trauma and PTSD among SUD patients is beneficial and typically leads to significant reductions in PTSD and SUD symptoms. More randomized, controlled trials are needed, however, to help elucidate whether integrated PTSD/SUD treatments are superior to SUD-only treatments. More research on the effectiveness of exposure-based techniques, the gold standard treatment of PTSD, among substance-dependent patients is also warranted. Pharmacological trials in this area are lacking. One study (Brady et al. 2005) suggests that there may be subtypes of PTSD/SUD patients that respond better to SSRIs. Given the FDA approval of SSRIs to treat PTSD, there are many opportunities for investigating their use among PTSD/SUD patients. Finally, the use of naltrexone or disulfiram among SUD patients has been shown to improve anxiety symptoms and alcohol use, but their effects on PTSD anxiety symptoms remains unknown.

Panic Attacks, Panic Disorder, and Agoraphobia

Epidemiology

In the NESARC study (Grant et al. 2004), panic disorder with agoraphobia was the anxiety disorder with the strongest association with SUDs. The 12-month odds of individuals experiencing panic disorder with agoraphobia were 1.4 with alcohol abuse, 3.6 with alcohol dependence, 3.5 with any drug abuse, and 10.5 with any drug dependence (Grant et al. 2004). The 12-month odds of having panic disorder without agoraphobia were 0.8 with alcohol abuse, 3.4 with alcohol dependence, 1.6 with any drug abuse, and 7.6 with any drug dependence (Grant et al. 2004). In one analysis of the NESARC data (Hasin et al. 2007), the 12-month odds ratio of alcohol use disorders comorbid with panic disorder with agoraphobia was 2.7, and panic disorder without agoraphobia was 2.1.

The NCS-R study also indicates that limited panic attacks, in addition to full-blown panic disorder, are significantly associated with SUDs (Kessler et al. 2006). Among respondents with panic disorder only, agoraphobia only, or their combination, 35.3% had an alcohol use disorder and 20.6% had an illicit drug use disorder. Among those with a history of panic attacks without the full disorder, 19.3% had an alcohol use disorder and 13.0% had an illicit drug use disorder, indicating significant risk associated even with subsyndromal panic symptoms.

The relationship between nicotine use and panic disorder is particularly interesting. Prospective data suggest that smoking enhances the risk for panic attacks and panic disorder, and panic, in turn, may increase the risk for nicotine dependence (Breslau et al. 2004; Isensee et al. 2003; Johnson et al. 2000). A review of longitudinal epidemiological data from the National Household Survey on Drug Abuse indicated that the risk for panic attacks is increased more than threefold in adults who have used cocaine (O'Brien et al. 2005). A recent review examined 20 studies to clarify any direct links between panic disorder and alcohol use disorders (Cosci et al. 2007). The authors concluded that panic and alcohol use disorders can precipitate one another. These findings were attributed to heritability of comorbidity, the pharmacological properties of alcohol that reduce subjective and physiological panic symptoms, and the tendency for heavy alcohol use to increase carbon dioxide sensitivity, perhaps increasing the likelihood for a panic attack (Cosci et al. 2007).

Differential Diagnosis

The ubiquitous nature of panic attacks in many other psychiatric disorders and the ability of some substances to evoke panic-like symptoms indicate the need for careful differential diagnosis when panic attacks are reported. As noted earlier, heavy alcohol use increases sensitivity to carbon dioxide, thereby increasing the possibility of a panic attack in heavy drinkers (Cosci et al. 2007). Because of noradrenergic stimulation, stimulant drugs can induce panic attacks that are not necessarily implicated in panic disorder but may develop into full-blown panic disorder over time (Louie et al. 1996). MDMA ("Ecstasy") has also been associated with the development of panic disorder in some clinical case studies (Pallanti and Mazzi 1992). One of the primary points to consider in differential diagnosis of panic disorder in the context of any other Axis I diagnosis is whether the panic attacks are ever untriggered or unexpected. The diagnosis also requires persistent worry about having an attack and symptoms that cause significant distress or impairment in at least one area of functioning (American Psychiatric Association 2000).

Pharmacological Treatment

Clinical trials for the treatment of anxiety disorders, including panic disorder, generally exclude participants with active SUDs. Thus, to date there are no pharmacotherapy trials for the treatment of co-occurring panic disorder and SUDs. SSRIs, however, are FDA approved for the treatment of panic disorder.

Psychosocial Treatment

Two treatment studies have investigated psychosocial treatments for panic disorder in individuals with a co-occurring SUD. Among alcohol-dependent inpatients with panic disorder (with or without agoraphobia), Bowen and colleagues (2000) compared treatment as usual for alcohol dependence with a CBT-oriented group treatment for panic disorder plus treatment as usual. The panic disorder–focused CBT component was based on a model of panic treatment that has significant empirical support (e.g., Craske et al. 1991). Although the combined treatment group received an additional 12 hours of treatment, no significant differences between groups were observed in anxiety symptoms or drinking measures (Bowen et al. 2000). Moreover, both groups showed improvement on measures of anxiety and alcohol abstinence up to 1 year after treatment completion. Among the hypothesized reasons for these findings were resistance from inpatient staff to the CBT intervention, limited cognitive skills and motivation for engagement among patients, and the severity of symptoms associated with inpatient populations (Bowen et al. 2000).

In a study conducted in a partial hospitalization program for addictions, a group cognitive-behavioral intervention for co-occurring panic and alcohol dependence was developed and tested (Kushner et al. 2006). The integrated treatment model was added to treatment as usual in an intensive program. The treatment was based on the Craske and Barlow model and contained three modules: psychoeducation, cognitive restructuring, and exposure. The treatment explicitly addressed links between patients' alcohol use, panic symptoms, and agoraphobia. Although the sample was small (N=48), participants who completed the additional panic treatment were significantly less likely to meet criteria for panic disorder at the 4-month follow-up. Relapse rates did not differ, but patients who participated in the integrated treatment had less severe relapses (i.e., fewer drinks and fewer drinking binges) (Kushner et al. 2006).

Conclusions

Panic disorder is strongly associated with SUDs. Patients with panic disorder and agoraphobia appear particularly vulnerable to increased substance use. Because acute intoxication or withdrawal from some substances of abuse can precipitate panic-like symptoms, careful assessment among SUD patients is required. To date, no pharmacological trials and only two psychosocial studies have examined the treatment of comorbid panic disorder and SUDs. Integrated CBT approaches have shown mixed results, and further study is necessary. Several medications, particularly SSRIs, have proven efficacious for the treatment of panic disorder and may be useful in patients with SUDs, but this needs to be systematically studied. The high rate of panic disorder and SUD comorbidity and the lack of tested treatments present a tremendous opportunity for growth in the development of treatments in this area.

Conclusion

Interest in the co-occurrence of anxiety disorders and SUDs has grown tremendously in recent years. It is clear that co-occurrence of these disorders is common and has a significant impact on prognosis and treatment. Furthermore, treatment of anxiety disorders may be associated with decreased substance use. Although there are promising developments in both pharmacotherapeutic and psychotherapeutic treatments that provide cause for considerable optimism, much work remains to be done.

◀ Key Clinical Points ▶

- Because substance intoxication and withdrawal are often associated with significant symptoms of anxiety, diagnostic clarity in the face of active use or during early abstinence is challenging. For generalized anxiety disorder in particular, symptom overlap with many withdrawal states is substantial, and the diagnosis must be carefully assessed and reassessed as individuals attain more time in recovery.
- The use of over-the-counter medications and excessive use of caffeine should be carefully assessed in anyone with significant anxiety.
- Advances in the pharmacotherapy of anxiety disorders have led to the development of newer agents with less toxicity, fewer side effects, and fewer interactions with substances of abuse. Although there are not many studies of pharmacotherapeutic treatment in individuals with co-occurring disorders, those that have been conducted indicate that similar pharmacotherapeutic agents work well for anxiety disorders with or without substance use disorders (SUDs).
- In the absence of specific data about the treatment of co-occurring disorders, the use of agents with known efficacy in the treatment of the anxiety disorder is recommended once the diagnosis has been clearly established. However, special considerations include potential toxic interactions with drugs and alcohol should relapse occur, medical conditions that are particularly common in individuals with SUDs, and the abuse potential of the agent being used.
- Poor medication adherence is a problem in individuals with SUDs as a result of complex and conflicting feelings and attitudes about the use of medications. It is therefore important to address the need for adherence to medications early in treatment, proactively and directly, and then engage in close follow-up to monitor adherence and clinical response.
- The use of agents that target substance use specifically, such as naltrexone or disulfiram, as add-on treatment for individuals with comorbid SUDs and anxiety disorders has not been systematically explored. The pharmacotherapy of SUDs is a rapidly developing area, and the use of adjunctive pharmacotherapeutic treatment is likely to become more relevant.
- It is important to maximize the use of nonpharmacological treatments. The ability to self-regulate subjective states and the confidence that can result from successful mastery through behavioral therapy can be extremely helpful to individuals in recovery. Learning strategies to self-regulate anxiety symptoms may help patients break out of the mindset of using external agents to combat intolerable subjective states and help them to acquire healthy alternative coping strategies.
- A number of studies demonstrate that cognitive-behavioral therapies are among the most effective treatments for both anxiety disorders and SUDs, and integrated approaches to the treatment of several anxiety disorders have shown promise. However, one study reported poorer outcomes among individuals with co-occurring alcohol dependence and social phobia who were treated with an integrated approach, so further investigation is needed.

References

American Psychiatric Association: Diagnostic and Statistical Manual of Mental Disorders, 4th Edition, Text Revision. Washington, DC, American Psychiatric Association, 2000

Back SE, Dansky BS, Carroll KM, et al: Exposure therapy in the treatment of PTSD among cocaine-dependent individuals: description of procedures. J Subst Abuse Treat 21:35–45, 2001

Back SE, Jackson JL, Sonne SC, et al: Alcohol dependence and posttraumatic stress disorder: differences in clinical presentation and response to cognitive-behavioral therapy by order of onset. J Subst Abuse Treat 29:29–37, 2005

Back SE, Brady KT, Jaanimägi U, et al: Cocaine dependence and PTSD: a pilot study of symptom interplay and treatment preferences. Addict Behav 31:351–354, 2006a

Back SE, Brady KT, Sonne SC, et al: Symptom improvement in co-occurring PTSD and alcohol dependence. J Nerv Ment Dis 194:690–696, 2006b

Bakken K, Landheim AS, Vaglum P: Substance-dependent patients with and without social anxiety disorder: occurrence and clinical differences—a study of a consecutive sample of alcohol-dependent and poly substance-dependent patients treated in two counties in Norway. Drug Alcohol Depend 80:321–328, 2005

Bakken K, Landheim AS, Vaglum P: Axis I and II disorders as long-term predictors of mental distress: a six-year prospective follow-up of substance-dependent patients. BMC Psychiatry 7:29, 2007

Bohn MJ, Babor TF, Kranzler HR: The Alcohol Use Disorders Identification Test (AUDIT): validation of a screening instrument for use in medical settings. J Stud Alcohol 56:423–432, 1995

Bolton J, Sareen J: Lifetime mood, anxiety, and drug use disorders are common in the United States population. Evid Based Ment Health 9:113, 2006

Bolton J, Cox B, Clara I, et al: Use of alcohol and drugs to self-medicate anxiety disorders in a nationally representative sample. J Nerv Ment Dis 194:818–825, 2006

Bowen R, D'Arcy C, Keegan D, et al: A controlled trial of cognitive behavioral treatment of panic in alcoholic inpatients with comorbid panic disorder. Addict Behav 25:593–597, 2000

Brady KT, Dansky BS, Back SE, et al: Exposure therapy in the treatment of PTSD among cocaine-dependent individuals: preliminary findings. J Subst Abuse Treat 21:47–54, 2001

Brady KT, Sonne S, Anton RF, et al: Sertraline in the treatment of co-occurring alcohol dependence and posttraumatic stress disorder. Alcohol Clin Exp Res 29:395–401, 2005

Breslau N, Novak SP, Kessler RC: Daily smoking and the subsequent onset of psychiatric disorders. Psychol Med 34:323–333, 2004

Brown PJ, Stout RL, Gannon-Rowley J: Substance use disorder-PTSD comorbidity: patients' perceptions of symptom interplay and treatment issues. J Subst Abuse Treat 15:445–448, 1998

Bruce SE, Yonkers KA, Otto MW, et al: Influence of psychiatric comorbidity on recovery and recurrence in generalized anxiety disorder, social phobia, and panic disorder: a 12-year prospective study. Am J Psychiatry 162:1179–1187, 2005

Carrigan MH, Randall CL: Self-medication in social phobia: a review of the alcohol literature. Addict Behav 28:269–284, 2003

Chatterjee CR, Ringold AL: A case report of reduction in alcohol craving and protection against alcohol withdrawal by gabapentin. J Clin Psychiatry 60:617, 1999

Compton WM 3rd, Cottler LB, Phelps DL, et al: Psychiatric disorders among drug dependent subjects: are they primary or secondary? Am J Addict 9:126–134, 2000

Cooney NL, Litt MD, Morse PA, et al: Alcohol cue reactivity, negative-mood reactivity, and relapse in treated alcoholic men. J Abnorm Psychol 106:243–250, 1997

Cosci F, Schruers KR, Abrams K, et al: Alcohol use disorders and panic disorder: a review of the evidence of a direct relationship. J Clin Psychiatry 68:874–880, 2007

Craske MG, Brown TA, Barlow DH: Behavioral treatment of panic disorder: a two-year follow-up. Behav Ther 22:289–304, 1991

Dansky BS, Brady KT, Roberts JT: Post-traumatic stress disorder and substance abuse: empirical findings and clinical issues. Subst Abus 15:247–257, 1994

Donovan B, Padin-Rivera E, Kowaliw S: "Transcend": initial outcomes from a posttraumatic stress disorder/substance abuse treatment program. J Trauma Stress 14:757–772, 2001

Ewing JA: Detecting alcoholism: the CAGE questionnaire. JAMA 252:1905–1907, 1984

Fals-Stewart W, Schafer J: The treatment of substance abusers diagnosed with obsessive-compulsive disorder: an outcome study. J Subst Abuse Treat 9:365–370, 1992

Foa E, Chrestman K, Riggs DS: Integrating prolonged exposure therapy and substance abuse treatment. Paper presented at the annual meeting of the International Society for Traumatic Stress Studies, Los Angeles, CA, November 2006

Grant BF, Stinson FS, Dawson DA, et al: Prevalence and co-occurrence of substance use disorders and independent mood and anxiety disorders: results from the National Epidemiologic Survey on Alcohol and Related Conditions. Arch Gen Psychiatry 61:807–816, 2004

Grant BF, Hasin DS, Stinson FS, et al: Co-occurrence of 12-month mood and anxiety disorders and personality disorders in the US: results from the national epidemiologic survey on alcohol and related conditions. J Psychiatr Res 39:1–9, 2005

Greist J, Chouinard G, DuBoff E, et al: Double-blind parallel comparison of three dosages of sertraline and placebo in outpatients with obsessive-compulsive disorder. Arch Gen Psychiatry 52:289–295, 1995

Gurmankin Levy A, Maselko J, Bauer M, et al: Why do people with an anxiety disorder utilize more nonmental health care than those without? Health Psychol 26:545–553, 2007

Harris M: Trauma Recovery and Empowerment: A Clinician's Guide for Working With Women in Groups. New York, Free Press, 1998

Hasin DS, Stinson FS, Ogburn E, et al: Prevalence, correlates, disability, and comorbidity of DSM-IV alcohol abuse and dependence in the United States: results from the National Epidemiologic Survey on Alcohol and Related Conditions. Arch Gen Psychiatry 64:830–842, 2007

Hien DA, Cohen LR, Miele GM, et al: Promising treatments for women with comorbid PTSD and substance use disorders. Am J Psychiatry 161:1426–1432, 2004

Isensee B, Wittchen HU, Stein MB, et al: Smoking increases the risk of panic: findings from a prospective community study. Arch Gen Psychiatry 60:692–700, 2003

Jacobsen LK, Southwick SM, Kosten TR: Substance use disorders in patients with posttraumatic stress disorder: a review of the literature. Am J Psychiatry 158:1184–1190, 2001

Johnson JG, Cohen P, Pine DS, et al: Association between cigarette smoking and anxiety disorders during adolescence and early adulthood. JAMA 284:2348–2351, 2000

Kendler KS, Myers J, Gardner CO: Caffeine intake, toxicity and dependence and lifetime risk for psychiatric and substance use disorders: an epidemiologic and co-twin control analysis. Psychol Med 36:1717–1725, 2006

Kessler RC, McGonagle KA, Zhao S, et al: Lifetime and 12-month prevalence of DSM-III-R psychiatric disorders in the United States: results from the National Comorbidity Study. Arch Gen Psychiatry 51:8–19, 1994

Kessler R, Sonnega A, Bromet E, et al: Posttraumatic stress disorder in the National Comorbidity Survey. Arch Gen Psychiatry 52:1048–1060, 1995

Kessler RC, Crum RM, Warner LA, et al: Lifetime co-occurrence of DSM-III-R alcohol abuse and dependence with other psychiatric disorders in the National Comorbidity Survey. Arch Gen Psychiatry 54:313–321, 1997

Kessler RC, Berglund P, Demler O, et al: Lifetime prevalence and age-of-onset distributions of DSM-IV disorders in the National Comorbidity Survey Replication. Arch Gen Psychiatry 62:593–602, 2005a

Kessler RC, Chiu WT, Demler O, et al: Prevalence, severity, and comorbidity of 12-month DSM-IV disorders in the National Comorbidity Survey Replication. Arch Gen Psychiatry 62:617–627, 2005b

Kessler RC, Chiu WT, Jin R, et al: The epidemiology of panic attacks, panic disorder, and agoraphobia in the National Comorbidity Survey Replication. Arch Gen Psychiatry 63:415–424, 2006

Khantzian E: The self-medication hypothesis of addictive disorders: focus on heroin and cocaine dependence. Am J Psychiatry 142:1259–1264, 1985

Kidorf M, Disney ER, King VL, et al: Prevalence of psychiatric and substance use disorders in opioid abusers in a community syringe exchange program. Drug Alcohol Depend 74:115–122, 2004

Koob G, Kreek MJ: Stress, dysregulation of drug reward pathways, and the transition to drug dependence. Am J Psychiatry 164:1149–1159, 2007

Kosten TR, Fontana A, Sernyak MJ, et al: Benzodiazepine use in posttraumatic stress disorder among veterans with substance abuse. J Nerv Ment Dis 188:454–459, 2000

Kranzler HR, Burleson JA, Del Boca FK, et al: Buspirone treatment of anxious alcoholics: a placebo-controlled trial. Arch Gen Psychiatry 51:720–731, 1994

Kushner MG, Sher KJ, Beitman BD: The relation between alcohol problems and the anxiety disorders. Am J Psychiatry 147:685–695, 1990

Kushner MG, Donahue C, Sletten S, et al: Cognitive behavioral treatment of comorbid anxiety disorder in alcoholism treatment patients: presentation of a prototype program and future directions. Journal of Mental Health 15:697–707, 2006

Landheim AS, Bakken K, Vaglum P: Impact of comorbid psychiatric disorders on the outcome of substance abusers: a six year prospective follow-up in two Norwegian counties. BMC Psychiatry 6:44, 2006

Louie AK, Lannon RA, Rutzick EA, et al: Clinical features of cocaine-induced panic. Biol Psychiatry 40:938–940, 1996

Lydiard RB, Roy-Byrne PP, Ballenger JC: Recent advances in the psychopharmacological treatment of anxiety disorders. Hosp Community Psychiatry 39:1157–1165, 1988

Maisto SA, Carey MP, Carey KB, et al: Use of the AUDIT and the DAST-10 to identify alcohol and drug use disorders among adults with a severe and persistent mental illness. Psychol Assess 12:186–192, 2000

Malcolm R, Anton RF, Randall CL, et al: A placebo-controlled trial of buspirone in anxious inpatient alcoholics. Alcohol Clin Exp Res 16:1007–1013, 1992

Malcolm R, Myrick H, Brady KT, et al: Update on anticonvulsants for the treatment of alcohol withdrawal. Am J Addict 10(suppl):16–23, 2001

Malec E, Malec T, Gagne MA, et al: Buspirone in the treatment of alcohol dependence: a placebo-controlled trial. Alcohol Clin Exp Res 20:307–312, 1996

McKeehan MB, Martin D: Assessment and treatment of anxiety disorders and co-morbid alcohol/other drug dependency. Alcohol Treat Q 20:45–59, 2002

McRae AL, Sonne SC, Brady KT, et al: A randomized, placebo-controlled trial of buspirone for the treatment of anxiety in opioid-dependent individuals. Am J Addict 13:53–63, 2004

Meaney M, Brake W, Gratton A: Environmental regulation of the development of mesolimbic dopamine systems: a neurobiological mechanism for vulnerability to drug abuse? Psychoneuroendocrinology 27:127–138, 2002

Merikangas KR, Mehta RL, Molnar BE, et al: Comorbidity of substance use disorders with mood and anxiety disorders: results of the International Consortium in Psychiatric Epidemiology. Addict Behav 23:893–907, 1998

Mills KL, Teesson M, Ross J, et al: Trauma, PTSD, and substance use disorders: findings from the Australian National Survey of Mental Health and Well-Being. Am J Psychiatry 163:652–658, 2006

Modell JG, Glaser FB, Cyr L, et al: Obsessive and compulsive characteristics of craving for alcohol in alcohol abuse and dependence. Alcohol Clin Exp Res 16:272–274, 1992

Morrissey JP, Jackson EW, Ellis AR, et al: Twelve-month outcomes of trauma-informed interventions for women with co-occurring disorders. Psychiatr Serv 56:1213–1222, 2005

Myrick DH, Brady KT: Social phobia in cocaine-dependent individuals. Am J Addict 6:99–104, 1996

Myrick DH, Malcolm R, Brady KT: Gabapentin treatment of alcohol withdrawal. Am J Psychiatry 155:1632, 1998

Najavits LM: Seeking Safety: A Treatment Manual for PTSD and Substance Abuse. New York, Guilford, 2002

Najavits LM, Weiss RD, Shaw SR, et al: "Seeking safety": outcome of a new cognitive-behavioral psychotherapy for women with posttraumatic stress disorder and substance dependence. J Trauma Stress 11:437–456, 1998

Najavits LM, Sullivan TP, Schmitz M, et al: Treatment utilization by women with PTSD and substance dependence. Am J Addict 13:215–224, 2004

Najavits LM, Schmitz M, Gotthardt S, et al: Seeking safety plus exposure therapy: an outcome study on dual diagnosis men. J Psychoactive Drugs 37:425–435, 2005

O'Brien MS, Wu LT, Anthony JC: Cocaine use and the occurrence of panic attacks in the community: a case-crossover approach. Subst Use Misuse 40:285–297, 2005

Pallanti S, Mazzi D: MDMA (ecstasy) precipitation of panic disorder. Biol Psychiatry 32:91–95, 1992

Pande AC, Davidson JR, Jefferson JW, et al: Treatment of social phobia with gabapentin: a placebo-controlled study. J Clin Psychopharmacol 19:341–348, 1999

Petrakis IL, Poling J, Levinson C, et al: Naltrexone and disulfiram in patients with alcohol dependence and comorbid psychiatric disorders. Biol Psychiatry 57:1128–1137, 2005

Piazza PV, Le Moal M: The role of stress in drug self-administration. Trends Pharmacol Sci 19:67–74, 1998

Posternak MA, Mueller TI: Assessing the risks and benefits of benzodiazepines for anxiety disorders in patients with a history of substance abuse or dependence. Am J Addict 10:48–68, 2001

Randall CL, Johnson MR, Thevos AK, et al: Paroxetine for social anxiety and alcohol use in dual-diagnosed patients. Depress Anxiety 14:255–262, 2001a

Randall CL, Thomas S, Thevos AK: Concurrent alcoholism and social anxiety disorder: a first step toward developing effective treatments. Alcohol Clin Exp Res 25:210–220, 2001b

Regier DA, Farmer ME, Rae DS, et al: Comorbidity of mental disorders with alcohol and other drug abuse: results from the Epidemiologic Catchment Area (ECA) Study. JAMA 264:2511–2518, 1990

Rodriguez BF, Weisberg RB, Pagano ME, et al: Frequency and patterns of psychiatric comorbidity in a sample of primary care patients with anxiety disorders. Compr Psychiatry 45:129–137, 2004

Sareen J, Chartier M, Kjernisted KD, et al: Comorbidity of phobic disorders with alcoholism in a Canadian community sample. Can J Psychiatry 46:733–740, 2001

Sareen J, Chartier M, Paulus MP, et al: Illicit drug use and anxiety disorders: findings from two community surveys. Psychiatry Res 142:11–17, 2006

Sartor CE, Lynskey MT, Heath AC, et al: The role of childhood risk factors in initiation of alcohol use and progression to alcohol dependence. Addiction 102:216–225, 2007

Satel SL, McDougle CJ: Obsessions and compulsions associated with cocaine abuse. Am J Psychiatry 148:947, 1991

Sbrana A, Bizzarri JV, Rucci P, et al: The spectrum of substance use in mood and anxiety disorders. Compr Psychiatry 46:6–13, 2005

Schade A, Marquenie LA, Van Balkom AJ, et al: Alcohol-dependent patients with comorbid phobic disorders: a comparison between comorbid patients, pure alcohol-dependent and pure phobic patients. Alcohol 39:241–246, 2004

Schuckit MA, Monteiro MG: Alcoholism, anxiety and depression. Br J Addict 83:1373–1380, 1988

Schuckit MA, Tipp JE, Bergman M, et al: Comparison of induced and independent major depressive disorders in 2,945 alcoholics. Am J Psychiatry 154:948–957, 1997

Stein DJ: Comorbidity in generalized anxiety disorder: impact and implications. J Clin Psychiatry 62(suppl):29–34, 2001

Stewart SH, Conrod PJ: Psychosocial models of functional associations between posttraumatic stress disorder and substance use disorder, in Trauma and Substance Abuse: Causes, Consequences, and Treatment of Comorbid Disorders. Edited by Ouimette P, Brown PJ. Washington, DC, American Psychological Association, 2003, pp 29–55

Teitelbaum LM, Carey KB: Temporal stability of alcohol screening measures in a psychiatric setting. Psychol Addict Behav 14:401–404, 2000

Terra MB, Barros HM, Stein AT, et al: Social anxiety disorder in 300 patients hospitalized for alcoholism in Brazil: high prevalence and undertreatment. Compr Psychiatry 47:463–467, 2006

Thomas SE, Randall CL, Carrigan MH: Drinking to cope in socially anxious individuals: a controlled study. Alcohol Clin Exp Res 27:1937–1943, 2003

Tollefson GD, Montague-Clouse J, Tollefson SL: Treatment of comorbid generalized anxiety in a recently detoxified alcoholic population with a selective serotonergic drug (buspirone). J Clin Psychopharmacol 12:19–26, 1992

Toussaint D, VanDeMark N, Bornemann A, et al: Modifications to the Trauma Recovery and Empowerment Model (TREM) for substance-abusing women with histories of violence: outcomes and lessons learned at a Colorado substance abuse treatment center. Journal of Community Psychology 7:879–894, 2007

Triffleman E: Gender differences in a controlled pilot study of psychosocial treatments in substance dependent patients with post-traumatic stress disorder: design considerations and outcomes. Alcohol Treat Q 18:113–126, 2000

Triffleman E, Marmar CR, Delucchi KL, et al: Childhood trauma and posttraumatic stress disorder in substance abuse inpatients. J Nerv Ment Dis 183:172–176, 1995

Triffleman E, Carroll K, Kellogg S: Substance dependence posttraumatic stress disorder therapy: an integrated cognitive-behavioral approach. J Subst Abuse Treat 17:3–14, 1999

Verduin ML, McKay S, Brady KT: Gabapentin in comorbid anxiety and substance use. Am J Addict 16:142–143, 2007

Voris J, Smith NL, Rao SM, et al: Gabapentin for the treatment of ethanol withdrawal. Subst Abus 24:129–132, 2003

Wittchen H-U, Zhao S, Kessler RC, et al: DSM-III-R generalized anxiety disorder in the National Comorbidity Survey. Arch Gen Psychiatry 51:355–364, 1994

Recommended Readings

Bolton J, Cox B, Clara I, et al: Use of alcohol and drugs to self-medicate anxiety disorders in a nationally representative sample. J Nerv Ment Dis 194:818–825, 2006

Compton WM, Cottler LB, Jacobs JL, et al: The role of psychiatric disorders in predicting drug dependence treatment outcome. Am J Psychiatry 160:890–895, 2003

Dunner DL: Management of anxiety disorders: the added challenge of comorbidity. Depress Anxiety 13:57–71, 2001

Merikangas KR, Mehta RL, Molnar BE, et al: Comorbidity of substance use disorders with mood and anxiety disorders: results of the International Consortium in Psychiatric Epidemiology. Addict Behav 23:893–907, 1998

Posternak MA, Mueller TI: Assessing the risks and benefits of benzodiazepines for anxiety disorders in patients with a history of substance abuse or dependence. Am J Addict 10:48–68, 2001

Tiet QQ, Mausbach B: Treatments for patients with dual diagnosis: a review. Alcohol Clin Exp Res 31:513–536, 2007

Web Sites of Interest

National Institute on Drug Abuse. http://www.nida.nih.gov

Substance Abuse and Mental Health Services Administration. http://www.samhsa.gov

Teen Drug Abuse. http://www.teendrugabuse.us

Chapter 37

Anxiety and Anxiety Disorders in Medical Settings

Thomas N. Wise, M.D.
Michael J. Marcangelo, M.D.
Danielle L. Anderson, M.D.

Health concerns rank with financial issues as the major sources of anxiety for individuals (Warr 1978; Wisocki 1988). Both disease states and medical settings foster such fears. Wells et al. (1988) noted that 6-month and lifetime prevalence rates of anxiety disorders in patients with chronic medical conditions were 15.3% and 21.3%, respectively. These rates were significantly higher than those found in the general population (6-month prevalence of 6.6% and lifetime prevalence of 12.9%). Therefore, before a particular patient is even admitted to the general hospital, the astute clinician should be prepared to consider in the initial differential diagnosis a primary anxiety disorder, regardless of what the medical illness may be. In outpatient medical settings, 4%–8% of patients have anxiety disorders, whereas in hospitalized patients, the prevalence can rise to 23% (Carroll et al. 1993; Levenson et al. 1986–1987). Although anxiety is often comorbid with depression, the two affects are different. Anxiety is a dysphoric affect, and dread of a future event is an essential feature. Depression is anguish over a loss that is directed toward the past and present.

A Framework of Perspectives

McHugh and Slavney (1998) argued that psychiatry should be viewed from multiple perspectives. Each perspective has a specific logic or internal grammar of its own, with both strengths and weaknesses (McHugh and Slavney 1998; M.A. Schwartz and Wiggins 1988). This approach is useful for the clinician working in the medical setting. The four perspectives are 1) the disease approach, 2) the life history perspective, 3) intersubject differences, and 4) motivated behavior.

Disease Approach

The disease approach is based on the medical model, in which a syndromic category is defined based on signs and symptoms that allow categorical designation to be developed and investigated for pathophysiological causes (McHugh and Slavney 1982). The validation process of a diagnosis involves designation of demographic and clinical factors, laboratory studies, syndromal demarcation from other disorders, follow-up studies to ascertain the course of the disorder, investigation of genetic and environmental factors, and documentation of response to various treatments. This is the essence of DSM-IV-TR and ICD-10 (American Psychiatric Association 2000; World Health Organization 1992). The strength of the disease model is the fact that rational treatment can be developed if organic etiologies are found. Its limitation is that it formally objectifies the entity by designating *what* the patient has but not *who* he or she is.

DSM-IV-TR catalogues a variety of syndromes in which anxiety is the main symptom. DSM iterations have partitioned anxiety into a variety of separate categories, such as panic disorder with or without agoraphobia, generalized anxiety disorder, social phobia, specific phobia, posttraumatic stress disorder, obsessive-compulsive disorder, adjustment disorder with anxiety, and acute stress disorder. Goldenberg et al. (1996) showed that "pure culture" of these diagnoses is rare because comorbidity among them is common and concurrent affective disorders or substance abuse frequently exists.

When considering anxiety states in the medically ill, clinicians often underdiagnose such syndromes because they rationalize that it is normal to be anxious about health issues (Jackson et al. 2007). The time limitations in a busy primary care practice may hinder accurate diagnosis. Somatic symptoms are often considered medically unexplained but not necessarily part of anxiety disorder. This underrecognition demands more effective screening instruments. The 7-item Generalized Anxiety Disorder Scale (GAD-7) has been demonstrated to be well accepted by primary care patients and easy to score. Two questions—"Have you felt nervous, anxious, or on edge for the past two weeks?" and "Are you unable to control the worrying?"—identify anxious patients quite well, with sensitivities ranging from 0.85 to 0.91 and specificities ranging from 0.62 to 0.70, if both questions are answered in the affirmative (Kroenke et al. 2007).

The disease perspective should remind the clinician that the role of organic anxiety must be considered, in that a variety of medical conditions, such as congestive heart failure, hyperthyroid disease, and metabolic disorders, may foster anxiety (Table 37–1) (Hall 1980). Thus, appropriate endocrine, laboratory, and imaging studies should be considered if they have not already been done. Laboratory data such as blood counts to consider anemia, thyroid screening to assess thyroid function, and CT or MRI scanning for complaints that could involve central nervous system disease are among commonly available studies to help rule out medical disorders, which anxiety can mimic. Furthermore, various drugs, such as caffeine or steroids, have the potential to cause anxiety in some patients. The clinician must assess both the nature and degree of anxiety in any categorical diagnosis to best manage the situation. Common categorical disorders in DSM-IV-TR that may apply to medical settings (Cassem 1990) are discussed in the remainder of this section.

Panic disorder denotes the acute onset of intense fear and physiological arousal with a variety of physiological symptoms, including palpitations, dyspnea, sweating, trembling, a sense of choking, chest pain, nausea or abdominal distress, and numbness and tingling sensations, which all may be interpreted as the onset of a serious illness. Thus, patients with panic disorder use an excess amount of medical care as a consequence of misinterpretation of their symptomatology (Katon 1996). The clinician must accurately diagnose this disorder and institute the proper psychopharmacological and psychotherapeutic treatment. A critical step is to educate the patient that his or her symptoms are part of a panic disorder rather than another serious illness (Colon et al. 1995). Patients with pulmonary disease and postpartum women have an increased incidence of panic disorder (Karajgi et al. 1990; Yellowlees et al. 1987).

Adjustment disorder with anxiety is one of the most common psychiatric entities in medically ill patients (Wilson-Barnett 1992). This diagnosis is complicated, because it is made in the context of a clearly defined stressor such as a physical illness, but the diagnosis requires that the individual have marked distress that is in excess of what would be expected from exposure to the stressor. Often, it is not clear what is an appropriate or an inappropriate response. The presence of occupational or social impairment experienced as a consequence of the patient's anxiety should allow the clinician to be more confident in making the diagnosis.

Acute stress disorder may also be seen in the medical setting and is characterized by a dissociation and detachment from painful affects. The presence of frightening images and dreams about the traumatic event and avoidance of stimuli differentiate this disorder from adjustment disorder. The exact incidence of acute stress disorder within medical settings is not known. That entity as well as posttraumatic stress disorder, however, may be found in both patients with serious illnesses and caregivers who have worked in disaster settings.

Finally, individuals with *generalized anxiety disorder* who have a chronic anxiety state with both psychological and physical symptomatology may also use medical care to a greater degree than do those without such disorders. Such individuals may demand both medical evaluations and pharmacological intervention.

Life History Perspective

In the life history perspective (Slavney and McHugh 1984), each patient's developmental vicissitudes will create a personal biography with a variety of specialized meanings (Engel 1997). The goal of understanding such meaningful connections is the essence of dynamic

TABLE 37–1. Common medical conditions that may cause anxiety

Cardiovascular	Metabolic	Neurological
Anemia	Acidosis	Cerebral anoxia
Arrhythmia	Hyperthermia	Cerebral vascular disease
Congestive heart failure	Hypocalcemia	Encephalopathy (i.e., delirium)
Coronary artery disease	Hypokalemia	Huntington's chorea
Hypovolemic states	Hypophosphatemia	Mass lesion of the brain[a]
Mitral valve prolapse	Acute intermittent porphyria	Multiple sclerosis
Respiratory	Vitamin B_{12} deficiency	Myasthenia gravis
Asthma and COPD	**Substance intoxication**	Pain
Hyperventilation	Alcohol	Parkinson's disease
Hypoxia	Amphetamines	Polyneuritis
Oat cell carcinoma	Caffeine	Postconcussion syndrome
Pneumonia	Cannabis	Postencephalitic disorders
Pneumothorax	Cocaine	Posterolateral sclerosis
Pulmonary embolism	Hallucinogens	Simple or complex partial seizure
Endocrinological	Inhalants	Vestibular dysfunction–related vertigo
Adrenal gland dysfunction	Phencyclidine	**Toxicological**
Hypoglycemia	**Substance withdrawal**	Carbon dioxide
Menopause and ovarian dysfunction	*Medications*	Carbon monoxide
Parathyroid disease	Anxiolytics	Gasoline
Pheochromocytoma	Clonidine	Heavy metals
Pituitary disorders	Hypnotics and sedatives	Insecticides and organophosphates
Premenstrual syndrome	SSRIs and TCAs	Paint
Thyroid dysfunction	*Other substances*	
	Alcohol	
	Cocaine	
	Nicotine	
	Opiates	

Note. COPD = chronic obstructive pulmonary disease; SSRIs = selective serotonin reuptake inhibitors; TCAs = tricyclic antidepressants.

[a]Especially third ventricle.

psychiatry. In individuals who are medically ill, it is essential to understand how they perceive their illness and what personalized meaning and expectations they attach to the situation in which they find themselves. Such data will begin to define "who" the patient is. This is best done by understanding the individual's life history. Health anxieties may be caused by the presence of illness in the patient's parents, family members, or friends. The life history perspective is also essential to understanding how a patient will react to a specific diagnosis. The patient's knowledge of a disease as well as fears and fantasies that he or she has gleaned from family or friends may distort his or her understanding about his or her condition. Such information may lead to catastrophic thinking when a diagnosis is given and foster both anxiety and depression. Unrealistic fears about medications are also common and may have their origins in the patient's experience with others. The clinician should use his or her own empathic abilities to better understand how the patient is reacting uniquely to his or her condition.

Intersubject Differences

In the *intersubject differences perspective,* individuals differ along a variety of dimensions such as height, weight, intelligence, and personality traits. In conceptualizing anxiety within medically ill populations, it may be useful to consider that beliefs about health exist along a dimension. Health worries that are normally found in populations include fears about health and development of illness as well as other common anxieties such as financial concerns and fears about the family. Health worries appear to increase as one gets older (Hocking and Koenig 1995). When fears about illness become paramount, such a condition may be labeled *health anxiety*. Health anxiety is considered pathological if it leads to sufficient distress to promote dysfunction in either caring for one's personal sense of well-being or completing daily tasks at work or home. Health anxiety could then clearly evolve into the disease perspective category of hypochondriasis, if such distress without a medical basis leads to frequent medical use and dysfunction. Individuals with panic disorder may well have sufficient autonomic arousal to precipitate hypochondriacal symptoms, which ultimately lead them to medical facilities. Such individuals often misinterpret these physiological events as the onset of a serious illness. Both psychiatric disorders could coexist, as demonstrated by Barsky et al. (1992) in a study that documented high levels of comorbidity with anxiety disorders in hypochondriacal patients. Finally, the diagnosis of obsessive-compulsive disorder should be considered in patients with obsessive hypochondriacal concerns that cause dysfunction and personal distress.

Like health anxiety, personality traits can also be viewed from a *dimensional* perspective. The tendency to worry, the need to be around others, agreeableness, conscientiousness, and openness to new or different ideas are all descriptions of personality traits that are measured along a dimension. Characteristic personality patterns predispose an individual to predictable reactions, given a provocation such as illness or the stress of a hospital setting. One method of describing such personality domains is that of the *five-factor model*, which divides personality into five basic domains: neuroticism, extraversion, openness, agreeableness, and conscientiousness (Costa and McCrae 1988). Neuroticism is the predisposition to experience anxiety, depression, self-consciousness, vulnerability, and hostility (Costa and McCrae 1990). It is not surprising that individuals with high neuroticism have augmented health worries. Russo et al. (1994, 1997) found that elevated neuroticism levels predicted excess medical use. Individuals who are introverted might find the public setting of hospitals with unfamiliar roommates extremely stressful. Individuals with high levels of conscientiousness, who like order, planning, and purpose, may find schedules not kept exactly within the hospital routine, such as waiting for tests or meals, exceedingly difficult. Those individuals who score low on the agreeableness dimension may express hostility to health care providers and provoke negative reactions among doctors, nurses, and other staff members. Understanding these basic personality traits can better allow the clinician to understand untoward responses.

Motivated Behavior

Motivated behavior is a goal-directed activity that lowers anxiety or craving. For example, a patient who is very anxious may constantly call a nurse for reassurance. Anxiety will certainly augment such "cravings" unless treated. It is useful to analyze the components of a behavior so that a rational intervention can be used. In the case of a patient frequently calling a nurse, behavioral assessment may show that whenever catastrophic thoughts about the symptom of pain occur, anxiety escalates, and the patient pushes the call button. The proper intervention would be cognitive reframing that the pain does not indicate a dire situation. Many goal-directed activities lead to a specific behavior that lowers anxiety. Thus, a patient who is quite disruptive within a medical setting because of repeated demands on the nursing staff may be initially evaluated by an examination of the various components that lead to this disruptive behavior.

Medical Environment

For individuals in hospital settings, anxiety may be caused by the nature of the environment. The hospital setting is often a strange and frightening place (Imboden and Wise 1984). Patients enter an unfamiliar world when they set foot in either the medical clinic or the hospital setting. One's unique self is depersonalized when the "ticket to admission" to any medical setting is proof that one has third-party insurance. The search and review by an unfamiliar clerk for insurance information sets up a journey through the medical system that can indeed provoke anxiety and enhance such cognitive fears. Separated from familiar surroundings and social supports, the hospitalized patient is often placed in a room with a complete stranger. Unfamiliar health care professionals ask a series of personal questions and perform physical examinations that include uncomfortable and embarrassing probing of orifices. Simple issues such as cold rooms can enhance anxiety.

The actual medical evaluation may well be a variety of tests. From needle phobia appearing when blood is drawn to a sense of confinement causing an anxiety reaction during imaging studies, phobic reactions and anxiety are quite common during a medical workup. Many patients are not, in fact, adequately prepared for imaging studies. The confined nature of such studies may provoke claustrophobia; the loud noises caused by the magnet during imaging will foster such fear. It is not surprising, in this setting, that as many as 20% of patients are unable to finish imaging studies because of such anxieties (Lukins et al. 1997; Murphy and Brunberg 1997).

After a medical evaluation is completed, a diagnosis is made that may or may not precipitate anxiety. If no serious disorder is found, the patient may often feel relieved. If he or she continues to experience discomfort, however, anxiety may persist. If a disease is identified, it is almost always perceived as a threat (Imboden and Wise 1984). The patient usually views serious illness as a potential loss. The most basic fear is loss of life, but the patient will also fear disability and dysfunction. Furthermore, disease states may deprive the patient of the characteristic behavior or lifestyle that has been important to preserving his or her self-esteem and happiness (Wise 1974). An individual with a myocardial infarction may find his or her career hopes dashed as a result of the stigma of disease. A young mother with breast cancer may fear that she will never live to see her children fully grown. Financial burdens of illness will also stress the individual and his or her family.

The coronary care unit (CCU) is a specific medical environment where anxiety can predominate and be a burden to patient recovery. Hackett et al. (1968) reported that at least one-half of the CCU patients in their sample were clinically anxious or depressed, whereas others have observed up to two-thirds of subjects with anxiety disorders (Cay et al. 1972). In a more formal study of CCU patients in which the Clinical Interview Schedule was used, at least 35 of 100 patients had either an anxiety or a depressive disorder (Lloyd and Cawley 1982).

Following a myocardial infarction, the typical pattern of reactions begins with initial fear and anxiety, which is replaced by a feeling that symptoms were a false alarm (denial); eventually, during days 3 through 7, the patient realizes what happened, which leads to demoralization and depression. For the clinician, not only the CCU setting and the phenomenology of anxiety but also the day of admission to the CCU offer helpful clues to identifying underlying anxiety (Cassem and Hackett 1971). The consequences of not being alert to the presence of such anxiety can be grave, if not life-threatening, for the cardiac patient. Moser and Dracup (1996) measured anxiety symptoms in 56 patients with confirmed myocardial infarctions in the 48-hour period following the infarctions and found more complications in patients with higher levels of anxiety than in patients with lower levels of anxiety (19.6% vs. 6%). These complications consisted of reinfarction, new-onset ischemia, ventricular fibrillation, sustained ventricular tachycardia, and in-hospital death. Even after controlling for clinical and sociodemographic factors that could influence these complications, Moser and Dracup discovered that anxiety level was independently predictive of these complications. Given these findings, it could be argued that anxiety early after myocardial infarction onset should be considered among the conventional risk factors for in-hospital acute myocardial infarction complications.

This relation of anxiety to medical complications is not just specific to the CCU setting. An earlier study conducted by Levenson et al. (1992) reported on the relation between general psychopathology and resource use in medical inpatients. They identified 22% of their sample of 1,020 inpatients as very anxious and found that this subcategory of patients had longer stays and higher costs during the index hospitalization. This association was determined to be independent of the severity of medical illness.

The surgical ward has also been reported to be associated with significant anxiety states. Strain (1985) estimated that up to 5% of general surgical patients have preoperative panic. Preexisting anxiety and new-onset anxiety in the context of serious medical illness were both thought to contribute to this frequency. Such preoperative anxiety was believed to predict postoperative states, but the literature has not been consistent on confirming this relation (Mathews and Ridgeway 1981).

Several studies clearly indicate that anxiety does occur in the postsurgical period and that this anxiety usually consists of posttraumatic stress disorder or its associated symptoms. Patients who remember the actual surgery because of inadequate anesthesia are at greater risk for developing posttraumatic stress disorder complications (Blacher 1975; Mcleod and Maycock 1992). Memory for events during any part of the anesthesia has been well-documented in controlled trials, and postoperative anxiety has been reported to predict such recall in a series of patients who underwent cardiopulmonary bypass surgery (Bennett et al. 1985; Goldmann et al. 1987).

Anxiety can predominate and be disabling in two patient populations besides CCU and surgical patients. In renal dialysis patients, anxiety is as common as depression, and the presence of any psychiatric disorder is associated with poor outcome (Farmer et al. 1979). Patients on ventilators have also been reported to be significantly anxious, and anxiety can affect the weaning process because it can transiently increase metabolic demands and cardiac work (Bergbom-Engberg and Haljamae 1989; Cassem and Hackett 1991; Parker et al. 1984).

Cardiac Disease and Anxiety

Anxiety and its relation to the heart deserve special consideration, given the extensive literature addressing the nature and extent of this relation. Osler's descriptions of early-onset angina may represent the first attempt at defining what we have come to know as type A behavior (Friedman and Rosenman 1974). Another early observer of the heart's connection to anxiety was Jacob Mendes DaCosta, who reported on cardiac symptoms of Civil War soldiers for which he could not identify objective cardiac findings. "DaCosta's syndrome" was further elaborated by Sir William Lewis (1918) during World War I, when he coined the term *effort syndrome.* These functional syndromes may represent the early efforts of medical practitioners to define panic attacks and the functional cardiac symptoms that accompanied them. Modern researchers have also observed that patients with cardiac symptoms such as chest pain who have no objective cardiac findings on angiography have a high prevalence (between 43% and 61%) of panic disorder (Beitman et al. 1987; Katon et al. 1988; Zinbarg et al. 1994).

Because of these early reports, modern research data have emerged that have been organized around the scientific delineation of anxiety and its psychobiological relation to cardiovascular disease. Researchers who used animal models showed that myriad cardiac abnormalities were produced when animals were exposed to some form of laboratory stress. Human studies have also generated compelling evidence for a psychophysiological relation between anxiety and the heart. In susceptible patients, cognitive stressors such as mental arithmetic can induce arrhythmias much more reliably than physical maneuvers designed to affect the cardiovascular system. Type A behaviors may correlate with coronary artery disease, although the research is inconsistent. Along with arrhythmias and coronary artery disease, human studies have found that myocardial necrosis and hypertension are attributable to stress. In animal and human research, the sympathoadrenal system is thought to be the final common pathway that explains the psychophysiological connection between stress and the heart (Henry and Stephens 1977). The activation of this system alters a variety of cardiovascular parameters (heart rate, platelet aggregation, myocardial contractility, arterial tone), which can be adaptive but can also potentially cause deleterious cardiac effects in susceptible individuals, such as those with cardiomyopathy (Kahn et al. 1987, 1990; Markovitz and Matthews 1991; Pauletto et al. 1991).

Psychiatric research designed to define and measure anxiety more rigorously has produced data that validate the data derived from the previously mentioned animal and human studies on the effects of stress on the heart. In a retrospective study, for example, Coryell et al. (1982) examined mortality rates of 113 inpatients with panic disorder to find that panic disorder in males was associated with significantly increased mortality from circulatory disease. In two prospective studies, Kawachi et al. (1994a, 1995) reported that anxiety symptoms in two male cohorts, as measured by the Crown-Crisp Index and the Cornell Medical Index, were also associated with an increased risk of mortality from sudden cardiac death.

Because patients with panic disorder and other anxiety symptoms have been found to have significantly decreased heart rate variability and because decreased heart rate variability has been associated with sudden cardiac death, it has been hypothesized that patients with pathological anxiety are vulnerable to developing cardiac arrhythmias that may be fatal (Kawachi et al. 1994b, 1995; Klein et al. 1995; Yeragani et al. 1993). Panic attacks have been demonstrated to impair myocardial perfusion in patients with cardiac disease, even when antiarrhythmic cardiac medication is administered (Fleet et al. 2005). Further research is required in this area, because other researchers have found no association between anxiety (panic disorder or social phobia) and decreased heart rate variability (Asmundson and Stein 1994). Fleet and colleagues reviewed the complex issues in investigating such associations (Fleet et al. 2000). Other psychophysiological theories have revolved around the issue of panic disorder and mitral valve prolapse. Originally, it was thought that because these two diseases share similar clinical symptoms, demographic features, and prevalence within the general population, the two may be subsumed within a single classification of mitral valve prolapse syndrome (Pariser et al. 1978; Savage et al. 1983a; Wooley 1976). And because mitral valve prolapse can be associated with potentially life-threatening cardiac illness (arrhythmias, sudden cardiac death, endocarditis, progressive mitral valve regurgitation), patients with panic disorder, mediated by mitral valve prolapse, were considered to be at possible increased risk for sudden cardiac death. These theoretical points, however, have not been borne out in the literature. Although patients with panic disorder may be at increased risk for mitral valve prolapse, these patients are thought to have the more benign form of this cardiac condition (Dager et al. 1986). Also, mitral valve prolapse within the general population has not been shown to be significantly correlated with increased cardiac abnormalities (Savage et al. 1983b). Alpert et al. (1991) offer a good review on this matter.

Some findings suggest that anxiety may be an independent risk factor for poor prognosis in patients with cardiovascular disease. Controlling for cardiac status, age, depression, and use of antidepressants, Strik et al. (2003) reported that anxiety was associated with future cardiac events in a cohort of men following a first myocardial infarction. Similar findings were found in a larger cohort of both men and women in a cardiac rehabilitation program, suggesting that anxiety was a stronger predictor of prognosis than depression (Rothenbacher et al. 2007). Finally, preoperative anxiety robustly predicted postoperative morbidity and mortality in patients undergoing cardiac surgery (Szekely et al. 2007).

Taking the findings as a whole, then, it is clear that the relation between anxiety and the heart has been carefully explored and delineated since the time of De-Costa and Osler. In fact, the literature generated from the question of this relationship may serve as a useful template to more broadly understand the complex interface between anxiety and a variety of other medical illnesses.

Management of Anxiety in Medical Settings

Physician-Patient Relationship

The physician must establish a working therapeutic alliance with any patient (Wise 1990). In the crisis of cancer, heart disease, or surgery, the physician is viewed as the individual who can literally save one's life and, thus, has a unique task. This role demands supportive and empathic care in both imparting information and offering hope, regardless of how serious the situation is. A study that found that placebo was as effective as alprazolam in reducing anxiety in cancer patients reinforced the role of the empathic supportive physician (Wald et al. 1993). In fact, it is often left to staff to convey critical information to patients, and to clarify medical opinions that may seem confusing or conflicting, so that patients can make informed treatment choices. Clearly it is inappropriate for staff members to make treatment choices for patients, but offering information and letting the patient know that it is his or her choice and that it will be an appropriate one, or that he or she can talk with various physicians and family members, can ease the patient's burden.

Supportive Psychotherapy

Listening to a patient's fears may be a uniquely supportive activity. Viederman and Perry (1980) outlined an assessment of the individual's life trajectory, in which the consultant attempts to understand where the patient is in his or her life and how the disease has modified hopes and dreams. Understanding the patient's marital relationship and how the spouse is coping with the crisis of a serious disease will further elucidate the social system in which the patient resides (Spiegel 1997). It is also essential for the psychiatric consultant to pay attention to the patient's wider support system, such as friends and employers. Group support has shown promise of benefit. Studies have shown that supportive group therapy is associated with longer survival in breast cancer patients (Spiegel and Kato 1996). Cognitive-behavioral and supportive therapies have improved the prognosis in melanoma patients (F.I. Fawzy 1995; N.W. Fawzy 1995).

Behavioral Medicine in Medically Ill Patients

The field of behavioral medicine has expanded beyond its original scope and has come to play an integral part in the understanding and treatment of anxiety in medically ill patients (G.E. Schwartz and Weiss 1978). Although fundamentally based on principles of classical and operant learning theories, behavioral medicine has broadened its concept of psychological life to include not only behaviors but also cognitions, emotions, and psychosocial environments. Along with this conceptual shift, many behavioral techniques have been developed, ranging from relaxation, hypnosis, and biofeedback training to environmental modification, cognitive-behavioral psychotherapy, and group education. These techniques have been applied to a variety of medically ill populations to successfully reduce anxiety and its effect on the outcome of disease processes. Several studies have documented the success of such behavioral treatments.

A significant amount of research in this area has been conducted with patients with cardiac illness. Anxiety states are one of the most common problems associated with this illness; most effective treatments have resulted in decreases in anxiety levels and changes in cardiac outcome. For example, stress reduction diminishes the risk of cardiac mortality and reinfarction (Frasure-Smith 1991). Indeed, for postmyocardial infarction patients, behavior therapies are superior to nearly all other methods of treatment in reducing risk of nonfatal myocardial infarction and cardiac death (the exceptions being the use of aspirin in patients with unstable angina and bypass surgery in patients classified as "high risk") (Ketterer 1993). Behavioral treatments have also been effective in treating the anxiety that accompanies other medical illnesses. For example, relaxation training helped to reduce preoperative anxiety in ambulatory surgery patients (Domar et al. 1987). Progressive relaxation and biofeedback have been particularly useful in chronic obstructive pulmonary disease and asthma, because these techniques do not have the respiratory depressant side effects of various anxiolytic medications (Davis et al. 1973; Hock et al. 1978).

Interestingly, though, not all patients respond to these behavior therapies. As in any other form of psychotherapeutic treatment, contraindications have been found (e.g., psychoanalysis with the schizophrenic patient). These include biofeedback for some extroverted patients and relaxation for patients with panic disorder and, possibly, patients with generalized anxiety disorder (Adler et al. 1987; Braith et al. 1988; Heide and Borkovec 1983; Leboeuf 1977; Ley 1988). In some studies, relaxation-induced anxiety correlated with measures indicating high internal locus of control and high fear of losing control.

Psychotropic Medications

For situations in which anxiety cannot be quickly relieved via psychotherapy or behavior therapies, the use of medication is indicated. Medications commonly used in physically healthy patients can be adopted with special considerations for the nature of the medical illness and concurrent medications being taken (Gorman 1987).

Benzodiazepines

Common issues that complicate benzodiazepine administration in medically ill patients are impaired pulmonary function, liver disease, pregnancy, and diminished cognitive capacity (Stoudemire et al. 1993). Central respiratory suppression should be closely monitored, especially in patients with compromised pulmonary function (Crawen and Sutherland 1991; Thompson and Thompson 1993). In patients with liver impairment, lorazepam and oxazepam should be considered because they do not undergo hepatic oxidation but are excreted via the kidney after glucuronidation (Epstein et al. 1993). In pregnancy, fetal congenital anomalies are associated with first-trimester benzodiazepine exposure. Studies have focused mostly on diazepam and alprazolam. In patients exposed to any benzodiazepines during the first trimester, the rate of oral cleft can be as high as 0.7%, which is 10 times higher than in the general population (Cohen and Rosenbaum 1998). Weinstock et al. (2001) studied 27 female subjects exposed to clonazepam, however, and found no evidence of congenital anomalies or fetal withdrawal syndromes and high Apgar scores in all the neonates. Nevertheless, clonazepam use may pose risks, given that there are early reports of both floppy baby syndrome and withdrawal syndromes in the infants whose mothers were taking this longer-acting benzodiazepine (Fisher et al. 1985).

The effects of benzodiazepines on the central nervous system are also important in the elderly or cognitively compromised patient. Impaired memory can affect recall, especially in elderly patients, or cause anterograde amnesia. In delirious patients or those with dementia, such drugs may foster confusion or disinhibition. Although benzodiazepines can cause amnesia, they can also be used to exploit this side effect. Intravenous use or oral intake of high-potency, short-half-life benzodiazepines such as lorazepam can be useful in the settings of painful and frightening procedures (Wolkowitz et al. 1987).

Benzodiazepines can also be useful in managing anticipatory anxiety. When patients are preparing for chemotherapy, benzodiazepines—either alone or with dexamethasone and ondansetron—decrease nausea and vomiting (Greenberg 1991). In medical settings, patients often have multiple-drug regimens, and thus drug interactions should be considered (Nemeroff et al. 1996; Preskorn 1996). Benzodiazepines may increase phenytoin and digoxin levels (Ochs et al. 1985).

Nonbenzodiazepine Anxiolytics

Antipsychotics. Low-dose antipsychotics can be useful in treating severe and persistent anxiety when benzodiazepine treatment fails (Colon et al. 1995). For steroid-induced anxiety and anxiety secondary to organic causes, especially delirium, low-dose antipsychotics are very effective (Hall 1980). This population has been reported to be more prone to neuropsychiatric side effects when given antipsychotics, so low doses should be initiated (Edelstein and Knight 1987). Extrapyramidal side effects and the possibility of neuroleptic malignant syndrome should be carefully monitored.

Beta-blockers. By directly blocking β-adrenergic stimulation, beta-blockers can be effective in treating anxiety symptoms secondary to hyperadrenergic states, such as hyperthyroidism. In such cases, they can improve both somatic and affective symptoms of anxiety (Granville-Grossman and Turner 1966; Kathol et al. 1980; Tyrer and Lader 1974). Nevertheless, depression and some parasomnias, such as hypnagogic hallucinations, have been reported (Fraser and Carr 1976; Gershon et al. 1979). Beta-blockers may decrease maximum exercise tolerance as a result of limitations of sympathomimetic response during exercise. Finally, patients with asthma, chronic obstructive pulmonary disease, diabetes, or bradycardia should avoid beta-blockers.

Antidepressants. The side effects of tricyclic antidepressants make them more difficult to use in medically ill patients. The newer generation of antidepressants, such as serotonin reuptake inhibitors and nefazodone, are safely used in the medically ill. At low doses, such as 50–100 mg, trazodone can ameliorate anxiety and sleep difficulties in anxious patients. As with benzodiazepines, drug-drug interactions must be considered when a patient is taking other medications in addition to the antidepressant (Nemeroff et al. 1996).

Buspirone. Buspirone is an effective agent for generalized anxiety disorder but not panic. It is well tolerated in the elderly and medically ill. Although buspirone has a lag time of 3–4 weeks before full effect becomes apparent, it has the advantage of not causing sedation or respiratory depression and might improve pulmonary ventilation (Garner et al. 1989; Rapaport and Mendelson 1989). It is thus useful for patients on mechanical ventilators or with poor respiratory drive (Crawen and Sutherland 1991; Mendelson et al. 1991).

Antihistamines. If respiratory function is a major concern or benzodiazepine abuse is present, antihistamines can be used to treat anxiety, because they have minimal pulmonary depression (Bluestine and Lesko 1994). Because of its mild anxiolytic, sedative, and analgesic effects, hydroxyzine is especially useful in treating terminally ill patients with pain (Breitbart and Jacobsen 1996). Antihistamines are not as potent as benzodiazepines and can potentially lower the seizure threshold as well as increase anticholinergic effects (Derogatis and Wise 1989).

Others. Intravenous anesthetics not only control pain but also help make the experience of pain be forgotten. In dying patients, methotrimeprazine has been recognized as a unique treatment for their anxiety as well as pain (Bruera et al. 1987). Child patients who need bone marrow biopsy and aspiration can benefit from fentanyl or ketamine. However, ketamine causes visual hallucinations in adult patients and therefore should be avoided (Bluestine and Lesko 1994).

Drug-Drug Interactions

Drug-drug interactions can be easily overlooked with dire consequences. In the patient with multiple medical illnesses, it becomes increasingly important to attempt to predict and prevent potential interactions. Given the complexity of pharmacologic treatment today, it is not possible to foresee all drug interactions before they occur. However, the possibility of a drug-drug interaction should always be kept in mind when there is a change in response to a drug or when new side effects arise when a new drug is added. Tracking the onset and course of adverse events in relation to medication changes is a useful technique for detecting the offending agents responsible for either a side effect or an interaction. This becomes more difficult to do if multiple medication changes are made at the same time.

The detection of interactions is often difficult, but a number of factors can suggest that an effect is due to such an interaction. Previous reports of interactions between two medications can assist with detecting drug-drug interactions. Other clues include whether or not there is resolution of the unwanted event with discontinuation of the suspected interacting drug and whether the adverse event worsened when the drug was increased. Drawing blood levels of medications to detect toxic or subtherapeutic serum concentrations of medications that were previously in the normal range can also help. Computer-based programs are now available to detect known interactions.

Drug-drug interactions are either due to pharmacodynamic or pharmacokinetic interactions. Pharmacodynamic drug-drug interactions are those in which there is a synergistic, additive, or antagonistic effect from administration of two medications. Pharmacokinetic interactions are the effects that one drug has on another drug's metabolism, absorption, excretion, or distribution. An example of this type of interaction involves two drugs that are both protein bound. Addition of the second drug results in the displacement of the first medication from its protein binding sites and an increase in its active serum form.

Many drugs are metabolized in the liver by cytochrome P450 (CYP) isoenzymes. (see Table 37–2) Most commonly, they are oxidized for easier elimination from the body. There are six main isoenzymes that are estimated to be responsible for 90% of drug oxidation in humans: CYP 1A2, 2C9, 2C19, 2D6, 2E1, and 3A4 (Tanaka and Hisawa 1999). Some medications can either inhibit or induce certain CYP isoenzymes. Competitive inhibition results when two medications compete for the same binding site on the isoenzyme. This reduces the isoenzyme's effectiveness and increases the level of the drugs oxidized by that protein.

Complementary and alternative medicines, though not regulated by the U.S. Food and Drug Administration, exert considerable influence on CYP isoenzymes. St. John's wort, commonly used to treat depression, has been linked in some reports to inhibition of CYP 3A4. This could lead to an increase in HIV protease inhibitors, antifungals, and macrolide antibiotics (Pal and Mitra 2006). Given the high number of over-the-counter medications that patients are using and the uncertain nature of many of the compounds, careful examination of the effects of complementary medications is in order. If an adverse drug reaction arises in the context of these substances, the alternative medication should be considered the cause until proven otherwise.

Benzodiazepines. There are multiple metabolism pathways for benzodiazepines. Alprazolam, triazolam, and midazolam are hydroxylated by CYP 3A4. Lorazepam, temazepam, and oxazepam are conjugated; thus, their metabolism is not altered by organ failure or drug-drug interactions (Crone and Gabriel 2004). In the context of liver failure, this may be advantageous. However, the glucuronidation of these drugs is stimulated by ritonavir and nelfinavir, antiretrovirals used in the treatment of HIV. This can lead to lower serum levels of these medications (Thompson et al. 2006).

Benzodiazepines alter gait and station and decrease respiratory drive. To avoid injury from falls, benzodiazepines should be used with caution in the elderly and alcohol dependent. A study found that 45.3% of patients who were taking benzodiazepines were also taking a medication listed as having a "major interaction" with them, per Micromedex (an online drug information database). The odds of an injury requiring medical care were more than doubled when a benzodiazepine and a medication with a "major interaction" were used concurrently (French et al. 2005). Major interactions with benzodiazepines may occur with antifungals, barbiturates, muscle relaxants, opioids, and chloral hydrate (French et al. 2005). Concurrent use with clozapine may result in respiratory depression (Brown et al. 1999). Midazolam, triazolam, estazolam, and alprazolam are CYP 3A4 substrates and have decreased clearance when used with any 3A4 inhibitors (Huyse et al. 2006; Thompson et al. 2006). These medication levels decrease with CYP 3A inducers such as carbamazepine, phenytoin, rifampin, and barbiturates. Benzodiazepines are considered to be inert with regard to interaction with oral anticoagulants (Van den Bemt et al. 2002). Note that midazolam is both a substrate of 3A4 and, due to some of its metabolites, an inhibitor.

Beta-blockers. Beta-blockers are primarily used to treat cardiac disease and hypertension but also have anxiolytic properties. Beta-blockers have additive effects on lowering blood pressure when used with other antihypertensives; there are also additive hypotensive effects via peripheral vasodilation when beta-blockers are combined with alpha-antagonists. Patients receiving this drug combination should be monitored for orthostasis. When clonidine is used with a beta-blocker, an exaggerated clonidine withdrawal response (acute hypertension) may occur. Concurrent use of amiodarone and beta-blockers may result in hypotension, bradycardia, or cardiac arrest. Propranolol and pindolol increase the plasma concentrations of thioridazine and increase the likelihood of pigmented retinopathy (Markowitz et al. 1995). This combination should be avoided.

Selective serotonin reuptake inhibitors and related compounds. The selective serotonin reuptake inhibitors (SSRIs) have become the most widely used antidepressants and anxiolytics and are felt to be safe in the context of many medical illnesses. Patients are often receiving other medications while taking SSRIs, and familiarity with metabolism of SSRIs has become an important part of their clinical use. Fluvoxamine has substantial inhibition of CYP 1A2 and 3A4 and a lesser degree of inhibition of CYP 2C9, 2C19, and 3A4 (Crone and Gabriel 2004). This leads to a number of clinically significant drug-drug interactions, perhaps the most important of which is the resultant increase in

TABLE 37–2. Drug-drug interactions

Antianxiety medication	Enzyme	Inhibition/Induction	Interactions
Benzodiazepines			
Lorazepam, temazepam, oxazepam	No liver metabolism-glucuronidation	None	Decreased by ritonavir, nelfinavir
Alprazolam, triazolam, estazolam	3A4	None	Increased by carbamazepine, phenytoin, rifampin, barbiturates, ritonavir, delavirdine, macrolides, calcium channel blockers, fluvoxamine, erythromycin, nefazodone, fluoxetine, sertraline, midazolam
Midazolam	3A4	Inhibits 3A4	Increased by the same medications as alprazolam, triazolam, estazolam
Beta-blockers			
Atenolol	Minimal metabolism		Additive effects with other hypertensive medications Exaggerated clonidine withdrawal Hypotension with trazodone, thioridazine, chlorpromazine, olanzapine, risperidone, quetiapine, tricyclics
Metoprolol	2D6		
Propranolol	2D6, 2C19		
SSRIs			
Fluvoxamine	Unknown	Inhibits 1A2, 3A4 Less inhibition of 2C19, 2C9, 3A4	Increases warfarin levels/INR, amiodarone, quinidine, simvastatin, calcium channel blockers
Fluoxetine, paroxetine	2D6	Inhibit 2D6	Increased by beta-blockers, ritonavir, protease inhibitors, many antiarrhythmics
Antipsychotics			
Haloperidol, perphenazine	2D6		Increased by fluoxetine, paroxetine, fluvoxamine Increase carbamazepine Decreased by carbamazepine
Clozapine	1A2 (primary) 2D6 (secondary)		Increased by fluoxetine, paroxetine, fluvoxamine, sertraline Decreased by carbamazepine
Risperidone	2D6		Altered by same medications as haloperidol and perphenazine
Olanzapine	1A2		Altered by same medications as clozapine
Quetiapine, ziprasidone	3A4		Altered by same medications as alprazolam, triazolam, and estazolam
Other			
Buspirone	3A4		Altered by the same medications as alprazolam, triazolam, and estazolam

Note. INR=international normalized ratio; SSRIs=selective serotonin reuptake inhibitors.

Source. Crone and Gabriel 2004; DeVane and Markowitz 2000; Dresser et al. 2000; Markowitz et al. 1995; Prior and Baker 2003; Tanaka and Hisawa 1999.

warfarin levels, prothrombin times, and international normalized rates. Due to fluvoxamine's inhibition of CYP 1A2, a significant interaction is expected with lidocaine, mexiletine, and propafenone (DeVane and Markowitz 2000). Fluvoxamine's inhibition of CYP 3A4 can lead to increased concentrations of amiodarone, quinidine, disopyramide, lovastatin, simvastatin (Crone and Gabriel 2004), and calcium channel blockers (DeVane and Markowitz 2000). It is also expected to affect angiotensin II blockers metabolized through CYP 2C9 (Crone and Gabriel 2004).

Fluoxetine and paroxetine are CYP 2D6 substrates and inhibitors. This has the effect of increasing the level of beta-blockers and potentiating their effects. Fluoxetine and paroxetine increase the level of ritonavir and protease inhibitors (Thompson et al. 2006) and should be used cautiously with antiarrhythmics, especially flecainide, mexiletine, and propafenone (Crone and Gabriel 2004; DeVane and Markowitz 2000). Fluoxetine may increase angiotensin II antagonists via inhibition of CYP 2C9 and calcium channel blockers via inhibition of CYP 3A4 (Crone and Gabriel 2004). Of the SSRIs, citalopram, escitalopram, and sertraline have the lowest liability to drug-drug interactions in general, whereas fluvoxamine and citalopram have the least potential to inhibit CYP 2D6. However, even medications with low liability to drug-drug interaction can cause important reactions. For example, a case has been reported in which citalopram and sertraline were found to have decreased efficacy in the face of concurrent rifampin treatment (Kukoyi et al. 2005). The use of SSRIs has been linked to upper gastrointestinal bleeding in some reports, but the risk is likely limited to individuals receiving nonsteroidal anti-inflammatory drugs (NSAIDs) or aspirin and those with other risk factors for bleeding (Yuan et al. 2006).

A serious danger when using SSRIs is serotonin syndrome. This syndrome is characterized by diarrhea, restlessness, agitation, hyperreflexia, myoclonus, autonomic instability, mental status changes, status epilepticus, coma, and death. This syndrome may occur with exposure to more than one serotonergic agent and when SSRIs are combined with monoamine oxidase inhibitors (MAOIs), meperidine, tryptophan, amphetamine derivatives, tramadol (Karunatilake and Buckley 2006), tricyclic antidepressants (TCAs), pethidine, pentazocine (Huyse et al. 2006), and, in at least one case report, oxycodone (Karunatilake and Buckley 2006). Lidocaine, midazolam, and fentanyl compete with protein-binding sites to increase SSRI levels and may potentially precipitate serotonin syndrome (Huyse et al. 2006). Some individuals with HIV have experienced serotonin syndrome while on the antiretroviral ritonavir, a strong inhibitor of CYP 2D6, and fluoxetine (DeSilva et al. 2001).

SSRIs and other antidepressants have been linked with alterations in the international normalized ratio (INR) in patients treated with warfarin. Warfarin is known to be metabolized by CYP 1A2, 2C9, 2C19, and 3A4 (Glueck et al. 2006), and reports of interactions with paroxetine, fluoxetine, and fluvoxamine have been published (Duncan et al. 1998). A large survey of patients receiving warfarin revealed that the drug most commonly linked to elevated INRs was trazodone (Wittkowsky et al. 2004). A report of increased INR in a patient treated with duloxetine and warfarin suggested that duloxetine may be exerting this effect through the 1A2 isoenzyme (Glueck et al. 2006). In patients being coadministered warfarin and antidepressants, careful monitoring of the INR is needed.

Tricyclic antidepressants. As mentioned previously, the side-effect profile of TCAs makes their use difficult in the medically ill. TCAs are eliminated by cytochrome P450 isoenzymes as well as by conjugation. In addition to the reaction with beta-blockers already cited, quinidine, a CYP 2D6 inhibitor, increases the clearance of imipramine and desipramine (DeVane and Markowitz 2000). Propafenone increases the concentration of desipramine, suggesting competitive inhibition of these two drugs, given that they are both substrates of 2D6 (Katz 1991). Reported interactions involving tricyclics include seizure activity when used with enflurane and potentiated effects of antimuscarinics. Tricyclics also interact with sympathomimetics, such that arrhythmia, hypertension, and tachycardia may result (Huyse et al. 2006).

Antipsychotics. Antipsychotics are playing an increasing role in the treatment of anxiety. This is particularly true on medical wards, where patients are likely to be receiving other medications and are at greater risk of drug-drug interactions. Many antipsychotics are predominantly metabolized through CYP 2D6, resulting in increased levels when used in conjunction with drugs that are known to inhibit CYP 2D6, such as paroxetine, quinidine, risperidone, and fluoxetine. Levels of haloperidol are increased when it is coadministered with fluoxetine or fluvoxamine (Tanaka and Hisawa 1999). Perphenazine plasma concentrations are increased with coadministration of paroxetine because of the latter's inhibition of CYP

2D6. As mentioned earlier in this chapter, propranolol and pindolol increase thioridazine levels. Angiotensin-converting enzyme inhibitors have additive hypotensive effects when combined with chlorpromazine. Clonidine has additive hypotensive effects when combined with chlorpromazine and fluphenazine (DeVane and Markowitz 2000). Haloperidol and carbamazepine, when coadministered, lead to increased carbamazepine levels and decreased haloperidol levels. Therapeutic phenobarbital or phenytoin levels lead to significant lowering of haloperidol and clozapine levels (Besag and Berry 2006).

Unlike other antipsychotics, clozapine is metabolized primarily by CYP 1A2 and secondarily through 2D6. Clozapine levels are increased by many SSRIs, including fluoxetine, fluvoxamine, paroxetine, and sertraline (Tanaka and Hisawa 1999). Clozapine's hypotensive effects are exacerbated by angiotensin-converting enzyme inhibitors. Clozapine levels are decreased by carbamazepine, secondary to enzyme induction (Tanaka and Hisawa 1999).

The atypical, or second-generation, antipsychotics have become the most widely used antipsychotic agents. Risperidone, like the first-generation antipsychotics, is metabolized by CYP 2D6. Olanzapine, like clozapine, is metabolized by CYP 1A2, whereas quetiapine and ziprasidone are metabolized by 3A4 (Prior and Baker 2003). It appears that among the atypical antipsychotics, risperidone has the greatest effects on the metabolism of other medications, but it is likely that more reports of interactions with all these agents will emerge.

Buspirone. Buspirone is an anxiolytic that preferentially binds to 5-HT_{1A} serotonin receptors. Since it does not bind to GABA receptors, it has lower liability to be abused and no cross-reaction with alcohol. It is metabolized primarily by CYP 3A4. The level of buspirone is increased by enzyme inhibitors including itraconazole, verapamil, diltiazem, nefazodone, and erythromycin (Dresser et al. 2000; Mahmood and Sahajwalla 1999). This increases its effective dose and the likelihood of side effects, including possible sedation and respiratory depression. Rifampin decreases the effects of buspirone (Lamberg et al. 1998), an effect that suggests that phenytoin and carbamazepine may do the same. Concurrent use with MAOIs may cause hypertensive crisis.

Conclusion

Anxiety is common in a wide variety of medical settings. Whether the environment is a physician's office, a medical laboratory, a radiology suite, or a hospital floor, the patient may be frightened because of the meaning of the illness that is being evaluated or treated and because of the realistic pain, disability, and potential mortality inherent in serious disease states. The clinician should approach the patient from a variety of perspectives. First, the clinician must ascertain *what* the patient has. The physician may use the disease model to differentiate psychiatric from medical and medication-related causes of anxiety or determine that both factors are present. Second, the clinician must understand *who* the patient is, based on past and present experiences, fears, and fantasies. Third, the clinician should understand the patient's general *beliefs* about health and his or her personality, in order to allow understanding of reactions to a provoking medical disorder or setting. Finally, the clinician should understand a patient's *behaviors* because they can reflect the patient's motivation to reduce anxiety. By systematically assessing each of these perspectives, the physician can offer the anxious medical patient a rational treatment that uses both biological and psychological interventions.

Key Clinical Points

- Anxiety is common in patients experiencing a medical illness and may occur in various forms, such as panic disorder or generalized anxiety disorder. Medical causes for anxiety, which can include endocrine, neurological, and cardiac diseases, must be identified before making the assumption that the patient's distress is solely due to psychiatric factors.
- It is important for the clinician to diagnose the form of the anxiety disorder and to understand the elements of the patient's fears that are realistic and those that are unrealistic. It is also essential to understand the patient's basic personality dimensions and whether they include a propensity for worry and fear.
- Treatment includes a supportive physician-patient relationship, utilization of supportive help to modify factors that foster anxiety, and use of rational psychopharmacology that is effective but also safe and tolerable.

References

Adler CM, Craske MG, Barlow DH: The use of modified relaxation in the experimental induction of anxiety and panic. Paper presented at the annual meeting of the Association for the Advancement of Behavior Therapy, Boston, MA, November 1987

Alpert MA, Mukerji V, Sabeti M, et al: Mitral valve prolapse, panic disorder, and chest pain. Med Clin North Am 75:1119–1133, 1991

American Psychiatric Association: Diagnostic and Statistical Manual of Mental Disorders, 4th Edition, Text Revision. Washington, DC, American Psychiatric Association, 2000

Asmundson GJ, Stein MB: Vagal attenuation in panic disorder: an assessment of parasympathetic nervous system function and subjective reactivity to respiratory manipulations. Psychosom Med 56:187–193, 1994

Barsky AJ, Wyshak G, Klerman G: Psychiatric comorbidity in DSM-III-R hypochondriasis. Arch Gen Psychiatry 49:101–108, 1992

Beitman BD, Basha I, Flaker G, et al: Atypical or nonanginal chest pain: panic disorder or coronary artery disease? Arch Intern Med 147:1548–1552, 1987

Bennett HL, Davis HS, Giannini JA: Non-verbal response to intraoperative conversion. Br J Anaesth 57:174–179, 1985

Bergbom-Engberg I, Haljamae H: Assessment of patients' experience of discomforts during respirator therapy. Crit Care Med 17:1068–1072, 1989

Besag FM, Berry D: Interactions between antiepileptic and antipsychotic drugs. Drug Saf 29:95–118, 2006

Blacher RS: On awakening paralyzed during surgery: a syndrome of traumatic neurosis. JAMA 234:67–68, 1975

Bluestine S, Lesko L: Psychotropic medications in oncology and in AIDS patients. Adv Psychosom Med 21:107–137, 1994

Braith JA, McCullough JP, Bush JP: Relaxation-induced anxiety in a subclinical sample of chronically anxious subjects. J Behav Ther Exp Psychiatry 19:193–198, 1988

Breitbart W, Jacobsen PB: Psychiatric symptom management in terminal care. Clin Geriatr Med 12:329–347, 1996

Brown CS, Markowitz JS, Moore, TR, et al: Atypical antipsychotics, part II: adverse effects, drug interactions, and costs. Ann Pharmacother 33:210–217, 1999

Bruera E, Chadwick S, Brennels C, et al: Methylphenidate associated with narcotics for the treatment of cancer pain. Cancer Treat Rep 71:67–70, 1987

Carroll BT, Kathol RG, Noyes R, et al: Screening for depression and anxiety in cancer patients using the hospital anxiety and depression scale. Gen Hosp Psychiatry 15:69–74, 1993

Cassem NH: Depression and anxiety secondary to medical illness. Psychiatr Clin North Am 13:597–612, 1990

Cassem NH, Hackett TP: Psychiatric consultation in a CCU. Ann Intern Med 75:9–14, 1971

Cassem NH, Hackett TP: The setting of intensive care, in Massachusetts General Hospital Handbook of General Hospital Psychiatry. Edited by Cassem NH. St. Louis, MO, Mosby, 1991, pp 373–399

Cay EL, Vetter N, Philip AE, et al: Psychological status during recovery from an acute heart attack. J Psychosom Res 16:425–435, 1972

Cohen LS, Rosenbaum JF: Psychotropic drug use during pregnancy: weighing the risks. J Clin Psychiatry 59(suppl):18–28, 1998

Colon EA, Popkin MK, Hocking LB, et al: Anxiety and panic anxiety in medically ill older patients: a review and update (review). Int J Psychiatry Med 25:221–238, 1995

Coryell W, Noyes R, Clancy J: Excess mortality in panic disorder. Arch Gen Psychiatry 39:701–703, 1982

Costa PT, McCrae RR: Personality in adulthood: a six-year longitudinal study of self-reports and spouse ratings on the NEO Personality Inventory. J Pers Soc Psychol 54:853–863, 1988

Costa PT, McCrae RR: Personality disorders and the five factor model of personality. J Personal Disord 4:362–371, 1990

Crawen J, Sutherland A: Buspirone for anxiety disorders in patients with severe lung disease (letter). Lancet 338:249, 1991

Crone CC, Gabriel GM: Treatment of anxiety and depression in transplant patients: pharmacokinetic considerations. Clin Pharmacokinet 43:361–394, 2004

Dager SR, Comess KA, Saal AK, et al: Mitral valve prolapse in a psychiatric setting: diagnostic assessment, research and clinical implications. Integr Psychiatry 4:211–223, 1986

Davis MH, Saunders DR, Creer TH, et al: Relaxation training facilitated by biofeedback apparatus as a supplemental treatment in bronchial asthma. J Psychosom Res 17:121–128, 1973

Derogatis LR, Wise TN: Anxiety and Depressive Disorders in the Medical Patient. Washington, DC, American Psychiatric Press, 1989

DeSilva KE, Le Flore DB, Marston BJ, et al: Serotonin syndrome in HIV-infected individuals receiving antiretroviral therapy and fluoxetine. AIDS 15:1281–1285, 2001

DeVane CL, Markowitz JS: Avoiding psychotropic drug interactions in the cardiovascular patient. Bull Menninger Clin 64:49–59, 2000

Domar AD, Noe JM, Benson H: The preoperative use of the relaxation response with ambulatory surgery patients. J Human Stress 13:101–107, 1987

Dresser GK, Spence JD, Bailey DG: Pharmacokinetic-pharmacodynamic consequences and clinical relevance of cytochrome P450 3A4 inhibition. Clin Pharmacokinet 38:41–57, 2000

Duncan D, Sayal K, McConnell H, et al: Antidepressant interactions with warfarin. Int Clin Psychopharmacol 13:87–94, 1998

Edelstein H, Knight RT: Severe parkinsonism in two AIDS patients taking prochlorperazine (letter). Lancet 2:341–342, 1987

Engel GL: From biomedical to biopsychosocial: being scientific in the human domain. Psychosomatics 38:521–528, 1997

Epstein SA, Wise TN, Goldberg RL: Gastroenterology, in Psychiatric Care of the Medical Patient. Edited by Stoudemire A, Fogel BS. New York, Oxford University Press, 1993, pp 611–626

Farmer CJ, Bewick M, Parsons V, et al: Survival on home haemodialysis: its relationship with physical symptomatology, psychosocial background and psychiatric morbidity. Psychol Med 9:515–523, 1979

Fawzy FI: A short-term psychoeducational intervention for patients newly diagnosed with cancer. Support Care Cancer 3:235–238, 1995

Fawzy NW: A psychoeducational nursing intervention to enhance coping and affective state in newly diagnosed malignant melanoma patients. Cancer Nurs 18:427–438, 1995

Fisher JB, Edgren BE, Mammel MD, et al: Neonatal apnea associated with maternal clonazepam therapy: a case report. Obstet Gynecol 66:345–355, 1985

Fleet R, Lavoie K, Beitman BD: Is panic disorder associated with coronary artery disease? A critical review of the literature. J Psychosom Res 48:347–356, 2000

Fleet R, Lesperance F, Arsenault A et al: Myocardial perfusion study of panic attacks in patients with coronary artery disease. Am J Cardiol 96:1064–1068, 2005

Fraser HS, Carr AC: Propranolol psychosis. Br J Psychiatry 129:508–509, 1976

Frasure-Smith N: In hospital symptoms of psychological stress as predictors of long term outcome after acute myocardial infarction in men. Am J Cardiol 67:121–127, 1991

French DD, Chirikos TN, Spehar A, et al: Effect of concomitant use of benzodiazepines and other drugs on the risk of injury in a veterans population. Drug Saf 28:1141–1150, 2005

Friedman M, Rosenman RH: Type A Behavior and Your Heart. New York, Knopf, 1974

Garner SJ, Eldridge FL, Wagner PG, et al: Buspirone, an anxiolytic drug that stimulates respiration. Am Rev Respir Dis 139:946–950, 1989

Gershon ES, Goldstein RE, Moss AJ, et al: Psychosis with ordinary doses of propranolol. Ann Intern Med 90:938–940, 1979

Glueck CJ, Khalil Q, Winiarska M, et al: Interaction of duloxetine and warfarin causing severe elevation of international normalized ratio (letter). JAMA 295:1517–1518, 2006

Goldenberg IM, White K, Yonkers K, et al: The infrequency of "pure culture" diagnoses among the anxiety disorders. J Clin Psychiatry 57:528–533, 1996

Goldmann L, Shah MV, Hebden MW: Memory of cardiac anaesthesia. Anaesthesia 42:596–603, 1987

Gorman J: Anxiety: is it a condition to be worried about? AAOHN J 35:90–91, 1987

Granville-Grossman KL, Turner P: The effect of propranolol on anxiety. Lancet 1:788–790, 1966

Greenberg DB: Strategic use of benzodiazepines in cancer patients. Oncology (Huntingt) 5:83–88, 1991

Hackett TP, Cassem NH, Wishnie HA: The coronary care unit: an appraisal of its psychological hazards. N Engl J Med 279:1365–1370, 1968

Hall RCW: Anxiety, in Psychiatric Presentations of Medical Illness: Somatopsychic Disorders. Edited by Hall RCW. New York, Spectrum, 1980, pp 180–210

Heide FJ, Borkovec TD: Relaxation-induced anxiety: paradoxical anxiety enhancement due to relaxation training. J Consult Clin Psychol 51:171–182, 1983

Henry JP, Stephens PM: Stress, Health, and the Social Environment: A Sociobiological Approach to Medicine. New York, Springer-Verlag New York, 1977

Hock RA, Rodgers CH, Redd C, et al: Medical-psychological interventions in male asthmatic children: an evaluation of psychological change. Psychosom Med 40:210–215, 1978

Hocking LB, Koenig HG: Anxiety in medically ill older patients: a review and update. Int J Psychiatry Med 25:221–238, 1995

Huyse FJ, Touw DJ, van Schijndel RS, et al: Psychotropic drugs and the preoperative period: a proposal for a guideline in elective surgery. Psychosomatics 47:8–22, 2006

Imboden JB, Wise TN: The stresses associated with physical illness, in The Principles and Practice of Medicine. Edited by Harvey AM, Johns RJ, McKusick VA, et al. Norwalk, CT, Appleton-Century-Crofts, 1984, pp 1354–1357

Jackson JL, Passamonti M, Kroenke K: Outcome and impact of mental disorders in primary care at 5 years. Psychosom Med 69:270–276, 2007

Kahn JP, Drusin RE, Klein DF: Idiopathic cardiomyopathy and panic disorder: clinical association in cardiac transplant candidates. Am J Psychiatry 144:1327–1330, 1987

Kahn JP, Gorman J, King D, et al: Cardiac left ventricular hypertrophy and chamber dilation in panic disorder patients: implications for idiopathic dilated cardiomyopathy. J Psychiatr Res 32:55–61, 1990

Karajgi B, Rifkin A, Doddi S, et al: The prevalence of anxiety disorders in patients with chronic obstructive pulmonary disease. Am J Psychiatry 147:200–201, 1990

Karunatilake H, Buckley NA: Serotonin syndrome induced by fluvoxamine and oxycodone. Ann Pharmacother 40:155–157, 2006

Kathol RG, Noyes R, Slymen DJ, et al: Propranolol in chronic anxiety disorders: a controlled study. Arch Gen Psychiatry 37:1361–1365, 1980

Katon W: Panic disorder: relationship to high medical utilization, unexplained physical symptoms, and medical costs. J Clin Psychiatry 57(suppl):11–18, 1996

Katon W, Hall ML, Russo J, et al: Chest pain: the relationship of psychiatric illness to coronary arteriography results. Am J Med 84:1–9, 1988

Katz MR: Raised serum levels of desipramine with the antiarrhythmic propafenone. J Clin Psychiatry 52:432–433, 1991

Kawachi I, Colditz GA, Ascherio A, et al: Prospective study of phobic anxiety and risk of coronary heart disease in men. Circulation 89:1992–1997, 1994a

Kawachi I, Sparrow D, Vokonas PS, et al: Symptoms of anxiety and risk of coronary heart disease: the Normative Aging Study. Circulation 90:2225–2229, 1994b

Kawachi I, Sparrow D, Vokonas PS, et al: Decreased heart rate variability in men with phobic anxiety (data from the Normative Aging Study). Am J Cardiol 75:882–885, 1995

Ketterer MW: Secondary prevention of ischemic heart disease: the case for aggressive behavioral monitoring and intervention. Psychosomatics 34:478–484, 1993

Klein E, Cnaani E, Harel T, et al: Altered heart rate variability in panic disorder patients. Biol Psychiatry 37:18–24, 1995

Kroenke K, Spitzer RL, Williams JB, et al: Anxiety disorders in primary care: prevalence, impairment, comorbidity, and detection. Ann Intern Med 146:317–325, 2007

Kukoyi O, Argo TR, Carnahan RM: Exacerbation of panic disorder with rifampin therapy in a patient receiving citalopram. Pharmacotherapy 25:435–437, 2005

Lamberg TS, Kivisto KT, Neuvonen PJ: Concentrations and effects of buspirone are considerably reduced by rifampicin. Br J Clin Pharmacol 45:381–385, 1998

Leboeuf A: The effects of EMG feedback training on state anxiety in introverts and extroverts. J Clin Psychol 33:251–253, 1977

Levenson JL, Hamer RM, Silverman JJ, et al: Psychopathology in medical inpatients and its relationship to length of hospital stay: a pilot study. Int J Psychiatry Med 16:231–236, 1986–1987

Levenson JL, Hamer RM, Rossiter C: Psychopathology and pain in medical inpatients: predict resource use during hospitalization but not rehospitalization. J Psychosom Res 36:585–592, 1992

Lewis W: The Soldiers Heart and the Effort Syndrome. London, England, Shaw and Sons, 1918

Ley R: Panic attacks during relaxation and relaxation-induced anxiety: a hyperventilation interpretation. J Behav Ther Exp Psychiatry 19:253–259, 1988

Lloyd GG, Cawley RH: Psychiatric morbidity after myocardial infarction. QJ Med 51:33–42, 1982

Lukins R, Davan IG, Drummond PD: A cognitive behavioural approach to preventing anxiety during magnetic resonance imaging. J Behav Ther Exp Psychiatry 28:97–104, 1997

Mahmood I, Sahajwalla C: Clinical pharmacokinetics and pharmacodynamics of buspirone, an anxiolytic drug. Clin Pharmacokinet 36:277–287, 1999

Markovitz JH, Matthews KA: Platelets and coronary heart disease: potential psychophysiologic mechanisms. Psychosom Med 53:643–668, 1991

Markowitz JS, Wells BG, Carson WH: Interactions between antipsychotic and antihypertensive drugs. Ann Pharmacother 29:603–609, 1995

Mathews A, Ridgeway V: Personality and surgical recovery: a review. Br J Clin Psychol 20:243–249, 1981

McHugh PR, Slavney PR: Methods of reasoning in psychopathology: conflict and resolution. Compr Psychiatry 23:197–215, 1982

McHugh PR, Slavney PR: The Perspectives of Psychiatry, 2nd Edition. Baltimore, MD, Johns Hopkins University Press, 1998

Mcleod AD, Maycock E: Awareness during anaesthesia and post-traumatic stress disorder. Anaesth Intensive Care 20:378–382, 1992

Mendelson WH, Maczaj M, Holt J: Buspirone administration to sleep apnea patients. J Clin Psychopharmacol 11:71–72, 1991

Moser DK, Dracup K: Is anxiety early after myocardial infarction associated with subsequent ischemic and arrhythmic events? Psychosom Med 58:395–401, 1996

Murphy KJ, Brunberg JA: Adult claustrophobia, anxiety and sedation in MRI. Magn Reson Imaging 15:51–54, 1997

Nemeroff CB, DeVane CL, Pollock BG: Newer antidepressants and the cytochrome P450 system. Am J Psychiatry 153:311–320, 1996

Ochs HR, Greenblatt DJ, Verburg-Ochs B: Effect of alprazolam on digoxin kinetics and creatinine clearance. Clin Pharmacol Ther 38:595–598, 1985

Pal D, Mitra AK: MDR- and CYP3A4-mediated drug-herbal interactions. Life Sci 78:2131–2145, 2006

Pariser SF, Pinta ER, Jones BA: Mitral valve prolapse syndrome and anxiety neurosis/panic disorder. Am J Psychiatry 135:246–247, 1978

Parker MM, Schubert W, Shelhamer JH, et al: Perceptions of a critically ill patient experiencing therapeutic paralysis in an ICU. Crit Care Med 12:69–71, 1984

Pauletto P, Scannaoieco G, Pessina AC: Sympathetic drive and vascular damage in hypertension and atherosclerosis. Hypertension 17:75–81, 1991

Preskorn SH: Clinical Pharmacology of Selective Serotonin Reuptake Inhibitors. Caddo, OK, Professional Communications, 1996

Prior TI, Baker GB: Interactions between the cytochrome P450 system and the second-generation antipsychotics. J Psychiatry Neurosci 28:99–112, 2003

Rapaport DM, Mendelson WH: Buspirone: a new respiratory stimulant (abstract). Am Rev Respir Dis 139:A625, 1989

Rothenbacher D, Hahmann H, Wusten B et al: Symptoms of anxiety and depression in patients with stable coronary heart disease: prognostic value and consideration of pathogenetic links. Eur J Cardiovasc Prev Rehabil 14:547–554, 2007

Russo J, Katon W, Sullivan M, et al: Severity of somatization and its relationship to psychiatric disorders and personality. Psychosomatics 35:546–556, 1994

Russo J, Katon W, Lin EHB, et al: Neuroticism and extraversion as predictors of health outcomes in depressed primary care patients. Psychosomatics 38:339–348, 1997

Savage DD, Garrison RJ, Devereux RB, et al: Mitral valve prolapse in the general population, I: epidemiological features. The Framingham study. Am Heart J 106:571–576, 1983a

Savage DD, Levy D, Garrison RJ, et al: Mitral valve prolapse in the general population, III: dysrhythmias. The Framingham study. Am Heart J 106:582–586, 1983b

Schwartz GE, Weiss SM: Behavioral medicine revisited: an amended definition. J Behav Med 1:249–251, 1978

Schwartz MA, Wiggins OP: Perspectivisim and the methods of psychiatry. Compr Psychiatry 29:237–251, 1988

Slavney PR, McHugh PR: Life stories and meaningful connections: reflections on a clinical method in psychiatry and medicine. Perspect Biol Med 27:279–288, 1984

Spiegel D: Psychosocial aspects of breast cancer treatment (review). Semin Oncol 24:S1-36–S1-47, 1997

Spiegel D, Kato PM: Psychosocial influences on cancer incidence and progression (review). Harv Rev Psychiatry 4:10–26, 1996

Stoudemire A, Fogel BS, Gulley LR, et al: Psychopharmacology in the medical patient, in Psychiatric Care of the Medical Patient. Edited by Stoudemire A, Fogel BS. New York, Oxford University Press, 1993, pp 155–206

Strain JJ: The surgical patient, in Psychiatry. Edited by Michels R, Cazenar JO. Philadelphia, PA, JB Lippincott, 1985, pp 1–11

Strik JM, Denollet J, Lousberg R, et al: Comparing symptoms of depression and anxiety as predictors of cardiac events and increased health care consumption after myocardial infarction. J Am Coll Cardiol 42:1801–1807, 2003

Szekely A, Balog P, Benki E, et al: Anxiety predicts mortality and morbidity after coronary artery and valve surgery: a 4-year follow up study. Psychosom Med 69:625–631, 2007

Tanaka E, Hisawa S: Clinically significant pharmacokinetic drug interactions with psychoactive drugs: antidepressants and antipsychotics and the cytochrome P450 system. J Clin Pharmacol Ther 24:7–16, 1999

Thompson A, Silverman B, Dzeng L, et al: Psychotropic medications and HIV. Clin Infect Dis 42:1305–1310, 2006

Thompson WL, Thompson TR: Pulmonary disease, in Psychiatric Care of the Medical Patient. Edited by Stoudemire A, Fogel BS. New York, Oxford University Press, 1993, pp 591–610

Tyrer PJ, Lader MH: Response to propranolol and diazepam in somatic anxiety. BMJ 2:14–16, 1974

Van den Bemt PMLA, Geven LM, Kuitert NA, et al: The potential interaction between oral anticoagulants and acetaminophen in everyday practice. Pharm World Sci 24:201–204, 2002

Viederman M, Perry SW: Use of a psychodynamic life narrative in the treatment of depression in the physically ill. Gen Hosp Psychiatry 3:177–185, 1980

Wald TG, Kathol RG, Noyes R, et al: Rapid relief of anxiety in cancer patients with both alprazolam and placebo. Psychosomatics 34:324–332, 1993

Warr P: A study of psychological well-being. Br J Psychol 69:111–121, 1978

Weinstock L, Cohen LS, Bailey JW, et al: Obstetrical and neonatal outcome following clonazepam use during pregnancy: a case series. Psychother Psychosom 70:158–162, 2001

Wells KB, Golding JM, Burnham MA: Psychiatric disorder in a sample of the population with and without chronic medical conditions. Am J Psychiatry 145:976–981, 1988

Wilson-Barnett J: Psychological reactions to medical procedures. Psychother Psychosom 57:118–127, 1992

Wise TN: The emotional reactions of chronic illness. Prim Care 1:407–415, 1974

Wise TN: The physician–patient relationship, in Behavioral Science. Edited by Wiener J. Media, PA, Harwal, 1990, pp 193–202

Wisocki PA: Worry as a phenomenon relevant to the elderly. Behav Ther 19:369–379, 1988

Wittkowsky AK, Boccuzzi SJ, Wogen J, et al: Frequent of concurrent use of warfarin with potentially interacting drugs. Pharmacotherapy 24:1668–1674, 2004

Wolkowitz OM, Weingartner H, Thompson K, et al: Diazepam-induced amnesia: a neuropharmacological model of an "organic amnestic syndrome." Am J Psychiatry 144:25–29, 1987

Wooley CF: Where are the diseases of yesteryear? DaCosta's syndrome, soldiers heart, the effort syndrome, neurocirculatory asthenia, and the mitral valve prolapse syndrome. Circulation 53:749–751, 1976

World Health Organization: The ICD-10 Classification of Mental and Behavioural Disorders: Clinical Descriptions and Diagnostic Guidelines. Geneva, Switzerland, World Health Organization, 1992

Yellowlees P, Alpers J, Bowden J, et al: Psychiatric morbidity in patients with chronic airflow obstruction. Med J Aust 146:305–307, 1987

Yeragani VK, Pohl R, Berger R, et al: Decreased heart rate variability in panic disorder patients: a study of power-spectral analysis of heart rate. Psychiatry Res 46:89–103, 1993

Yuan Y, Tsoi K, Hunt RH: Selective serotonin reuptake inhibitors and risk of upper GI bleeding: confusion or confounding? Am J Med 119:719–727, 2006

Zinbarg RE, Barlow DH, Leibowitz M, et al: The DSM-IV field trial for mixed anxiety-depression. Am J Psychiatry 151:1153–1162, 1994

Recommended Readings

Colon EA, Popkin MK, Hocking LB, et al: Anxiety and panic anxiety in medically ill older patients: a review and update (review). Int J Psychiatry Med 25:221–238, 1995

Derogatis LR, Wise TN: Anxiety and Depressive Disorders in the Medical Patient. Washington, DC, American Psychiatric Press, 1989

Viederman M, Perry SW: Use of a psychodynamic life narrative in the treatment of depression in the physically ill. Gen Hosp Psychiatry 3:177–185, 1980

Chapter 38

Anxiety and Insomnia

Thomas W. Uhde, M.D.
Bernadette M. Cortese, Ph.D.

The high comorbidity of anxiety and sleep complaints, including insomnia, is widely recognized among clinicians. Among the anxiety disorders, DSM-IV-TR (American Psychiatric Association 2000) lists sleep disturbances as a core feature of generalized anxiety disorder (GAD) and posttraumatic stress disorder (PTSD). The prevalence rates for sleep disturbances range between 70% and 91% (Maher et al. 2006) in PTSD and 70% (for insomnia) in GAD. Moreover, panic disorder (PD) is characterized by a high prevalence of nocturnal panic attacks, that is, fearful sleep arousals, which are conceptualized by some investigators to produce conditioned fear of sleep and resultant avoidance of sleep and the sleep environment (Uhde 2000). This latter constellation of symptoms, probably representing different pathophysiological disturbances, is often collectively described as "insomnia" by patients with nocturnal panic attacks. Interestingly, patients with primary insomnia have also been found to experience coexistent anxiety problems (Benca 2001; Spira et al. 2008), and patients with chronic insomnia may be at greater risk for developing anxiety or anxiety disorders later in life (Breslau et al. 1996; Neckelmann et al. 2007; Weissman et al. 1997). Thus, the high prevalence of comorbid insomnia in primary anxiety disorders and comorbid anxiety symptoms in primary insomnia suggests an important underlying relationship between these clinical entities. The exact nature of this relationship remains unclear, but emerging advances in our knowledge may lead, in the near future, to more targeted or evidence-based interventions in the management of patients who experience comorbid anxiety and insomnia.

The purpose of this chapter is to provide an overview of knowledge regarding the comorbidity, clinical course, neurobiology, and treatment of insomnia in GAD, PTSD, and PD—anxiety disorders that manifest sleep disturbances as core features of their phenomenology. In addition, we conclude this chapter with suggestions for future research.

Comorbidity

Insomnia, as a subjective sleep complaint, is reported by many patients with anxiety disorders. The report of insomnia is so prevalent among patients with anxiety disorders that it is widely assumed among clinicians, and even among most anxiety disorder specialists, that the treatment of core anxiety symptoms in anxiety disorder patients will be associated with parallel improvement in sleep quality. Whether this assumption plays out in reality, however, requires more systematic study under controlled conditions. Some anxiety disorders appear to be more commonly associated with insomnia. Two specific anxiety disorders, PD and GAD, deserve special mention insofar as they appear to share important but different symptom characteristics compared with patients with primary insomnia.

Characterized by chronic and excessive worry, GAD is associated with numerous additional symptoms, including sleep disturbance. Insomnia complaints range between 60% and 70% (Monti and Monti 2000), and Ohayon et al. (1998) reported greater comorbidity for GAD and insomnia than for all other psychiatric disorders assessed. Often, the subjective sleep complaints reported by individuals diagnosed with GAD are nearly identical to those reported by patients with primary insomnia; they include worry about obtaining good quality or sufficient amounts of sleep and problems falling or maintaining sleep. Patients with primary insomnia report almost identical sleep complaints, but for reasons that remain unclear, they experience their complaints within the context of a sleep problem rather than of a mental health problem. Patients with GAD and primary insomnia typically report symptoms of physiological hyperarousal and increased vigilance (feeling "keyed up"), with intermittent fatigue and disturbances in concentration and memory. There are also nearly identical polysomnographic findings; sleep architecture and rapid eye movement (REM) measures are normal, whereas both syndromes have electroencephalogram (EEG) evidence of increased sleep latency and disturbances in maintaining sleep (for reviews, see Papadimitriou and Linkowski 2005; Uhde 2000).

Notably, patients with GAD, when awakened under experimental conditions after several minutes of EEG-documented stage 2 sleep, report not having been asleep or experiencing any drowsiness whatsoever. These observations, combined with our ongoing studies in patients with recurrent sleep paralysis, indicate that some individuals find it nearly impossible to distinguish between awake and sleep states, including REM-stage sleep. We have reported that patients with recurrent sleep paralysis, as well as some patients with GAD and PD (especially those with nocturnal panic attacks), find it difficult to separate at the experiential level the difference between sleep and wakeful states (Uhde et al. 2006).

Objective measures of sleep also demonstrate an association between PD and impaired sleep initiation and maintenance. Specifically, increased sleep latency, decreased sleep time, and decreased sleep efficiency in PD patients have all been confirmed through sleep EEG (Lydiard et al. 1989; Mellman and Uhde 1989; Sloan et al. 1999). Patients with PD, particularly those who experience nocturnal panic, also report a high incidence of insomnia. Singareddy and Uhde (2008) described both individual and interactive effects of nocturnal panic attacks and depression on subjective sleep disturbances in PD patients. In this study, 78.5% of PD patients with nocturnal panic reported difficulty sleeping, whereas an even greater proportion (91%) of PD patients with a history of both nocturnal panic and depression reported sleep problems. In addition, significantly more panic patients with nocturnal panic (9.2%) or nocturnal panic plus depression (20%) reported particularly severe sleep restriction by subjective report (i.e., sleep duration of ≤5 hours per night) compared with pure PD patients (2.5%). Singareddy and Uhde (2008) also identified a subgroup of patients with hypersomnia (i.e., patients sleeping 9 or more hours per sleeping period). Whether hypersomnia in these subjects extends to excessive daytime sleepiness, a diagnostic characteristic of narcolepsy, is unknown. Of interest, however, is an independent finding that cataplexy, another classic feature of narcolepsy, is more prevalent in patients with primary anxiety disorders compared with healthy control subjects (Flosnik et al. 2009).

These observations suggest that GAD and PD patients, particularly PD patients with nocturnal panic attacks, share many symptomatic and sleep EEG characteristics with chronic insomnia sufferers. Preliminary observations also suggest a possible link between PD and hypersomnia and, possibly, even cataplexy. Taken together, these findings suggest that it may be reasonable to conceptualize PD as a condition associated with a broad array of sleep disturbances, which most often involves classic symptoms of insomnia, but may also involve hypersomnia in a subset of individuals. On the other hand, selective anxiety disorders, such as social phobia (Brown et al. 1994), can be easily distinguished from chronic insomnia on a number of clinical and physiological criteria (for review, see Uhde 2000), largely based on the absence of impressive clinical or EEG findings.

Clinical Course

Anxiety and insomnia are, in many cases, both disabling and chronic conditions that putatively place sufferers at increased risk for developing secondary complications. Some research on insomnia and anxiety has assessed the longitudinal course of these illnesses in relation to each other. The findings, however, are limited and inconsistent; important questions remain as to whether insomnia typically precedes anxiety or if insomnia more often develops subsequent to anxiety.

Some findings suggest that anxiety symptoms/disorders can develop from primary insomnia. For example, longitudinal data from the National Institute of Mental Health Epidemiologic Catchment Area study revealed that adults with uncomplicated insomnia (defined as insomnia without the lifetime presence of a psychiatric disorder) at baseline were five times more likely to experience a panic attack than healthy adults with no sleep or psychiatric disorder. In addition, the individuals were at a significant increased risk for developing PD by the time of a follow-up interview 1 year later, compared with those who did not have baseline insomnia or a psychiatric disorder (Weissman et al. 1997). Neckelmann et al. (2007), who utilized a much longer follow-up interval (11 years) in their longitudinal study, reported a significant association between chronic insomnia and the development of anxiety. Individuals who reported chronic insomnia at either time point were more likely to have or develop an anxiety disorder than those who did not report chronic insomnia. Moreover, the relationship to developing anxiety disorders was significantly stronger in the group that reported chronic insomnia at both the baseline and follow-up assessments, compared with the group that reported chronic insomnia at just the follow-up. These finding suggest that in addition to chronic insomnia being a state marker for anxiety disorders, it may also be a trait marker for those at risk of developing anxiety disorders later in life. Breslau et al. (1996) also found that individuals with a history of insomnia were at increased risk for developing anxiety, compared with individuals with no history of insomnia (odds ratio [OR]=1.97, 95% confidence interval [CI] 1.08–3.60).

Other evidence supports the course of illness progression from primary anxiety to secondary insomnia. Ohayon and Roth (2003) retrospectively assessed the temporal relationship between insomnia and anxiety in a large, multinational, European, general population study. In this study, current severe insomnia was the strongest predictor of a past psychiatric history (OR=5.8, 95% CI 2.4–14.0). Further evidence demonstrating an illness progression from anxiety to insomnia included the finding that the onset of anxiety preceded the insomnia in more than 43% of the cases, whereas the onset of insomnia preceded the development of anxiety in only 18% of the cases. In another retrospective analysis of a community-based sample of adolescents ages 13–15 years, Johnson et al. (2006) assessed the directionality of association between insomnia and psychiatric disorders. This study reported a high prevalence rate of insomnia in individuals with a history of anxiety that varied between 24% and 43%, depending on the specific anxiety disorder. Additionally, in 73% of the individuals with comorbid anxiety and insomnia, the anxiety disorder preceded the onset of the insomnia. Risk associated with either anxiety or insomnia by the prior onset of the other disorder was also assessed to evaluate directionality. This analysis revealed that a prior anxiety disorder increased the risk of subsequent insomnia more than three-fold, but that prior insomnia was unrelated to the later development of an anxiety disorder.

Thus, the studies of Ohayon and Roth (2003) and Johnson et al. (2006), in contrast to the research teams of Breslau, Necklemann, and Weissman (Breslau et al. 1996; Neckelmann et al. 2007; Weissman et al. 1997), both reported illness directionality from primary anxiety to secondary insomnia. Critical differences in methodology may in part account for the disparity in directionality-related findings. In contrast to retrospective studies (Johnson et al. 2006; Ohayon and Roth 2003), prospectively designed investigations tend to report the onset of insomnia prior to anxiety in individuals who have comorbid anxiety-insomnia syndromes.

Although additional research is required before conclusions can be drawn regarding the prevalence and distinctions between subgroups of patients with earlier-onset anxiety versus insomnia, the more rigorously designed (i.e., prospective) investigations suggest a more typical progression of illness from primary insomnia to the later development of secondary anxiety.

Neurobiology

Although a single neurobiological/neurotransmitter system clearly does not alone mediate fear, anxiety, and sleep-wake states, several neurotransmitter systems (noradrenergic, γ-aminobutyric acid [GABA]–ergic, serotonergic and, more recently, hypocretinergic) are implicated in the interactive pathophysiology of anxiety and insomnia.

Noradrenergic System

Within the noradrenergic system, the pontine nucleus locus coeruleus (LC) plays a key role in arousal and vigilance in animals, and disturbances in this nucleus or its neuronal projections to the amygdala and related limbic substrates, hypothalamus and nucleus accumbens, have been implicated in PD, GAD, PTSD, and insomnia (Abelson et al. 2007; Alttoa et al. 2007; Aston-Jones et al. 1991; Charney and Redmond 1983; Charney et al. 1990, 1995; DeViva et al. 2004; Sullivan et al. 1999; Uhde and Singareddy 2002). Preclinical studies in rodents and monkeys have demonstrated that noradrenergic effects associated with fear and stress are in part mediated through LC activation and subsequent increase of norepinephrine in the brain regions associated with anxiety (Aston-Jones and Cohen 2005; Korf et al. 1973; Redmond 1981).

The noradrenergic LC system has been strongly implicated in arousal and sleep-wake functions. The LC likely mediates its wakefulness-promoting effects, and, presumably, insomnia, via a number of actions, including direct activation of the cortex and pedunculopontine tegmental nucleus and inhibitory inputs to the ventral lateral preoptic nucleus, a galanin-related structure implicated in insomnia associated with aging (Gaus et al. 2002).

GABAergic System

As the brain's major inhibitory neurotransmitter system, crucial to the regulation of brain excitability, the GABAergic system is the neurotransmitter pathway most widely implicated in both anxiety and insomnia, with the ionotropic $GABA_A$-benzodiazepine-chloride (GBC) receptor complex that regulates chloride channels being particularly relevant for the biological functions of alarm, arousal, and sedation. The role of the GABAergic system in animal fear and anxiety-like behaviors is well established (Zorumski and Isenberg 1991). Alterations in GABAergic receptor function are also linked to arousal states, involving the full range of sedation-drowsiness to alertness-hypervigilance and alarm states in humans. Although there is no known specific or final common pathway disturbance known to be associated with insomnia, anxiety, or any anxiety disorder, it remains possible that disturbances in benzodiazepine receptor distribution, location, or sensitivity, or secondary GABAergic influences, could play a role in the pathophysiology of anxiety or insomnia (Kalueff and Nutt 1997; Kaschka et al. 1995; Malizia et al. 1998; Mohler et al. 2002, 2005). Interestingly, Buhr et al. (2002) reported a mutation in the β_3 subunit of the $GABA_A$ receptor in a person with chronic insomnia from a family with sleep problems. Unfortunately, there was no comprehensive information provided, or available, on the specific qualities of insomnia or anxiety within the individual or family. Nonetheless, these observations, combined with separate lines of evidence in rodents and humans, suggest that the $GABA_A$ receptors, perhaps particularly α_1, α_2, α_3, and β_3 subunits, may play a partial role in the pathophysiology and treatment of insomnia and comorbid anxiety symptoms (Laposky et al. 2001; Mohler et al. 2002, 2005; Rowlett et al. 2005; Rush 1998).

Serotonergic System

With respect to the serotonergic system, the reticular formation has long been associated with functions of wakefulness. Moruzzi and Magoun (1949) conducted studies demonstrating that the transection of the reticular formation above the pons in the face of intact sensory inputs to higher brain regions are associated with behavior and EEG patterns consistent with sleep, whereas lesions of the reticular formation below the pons are associated with a reduction in sleep. These classic studies and subsequent research indicate that different neural networks within and impinging on the reticular formation mediate wakefulness and arousal functions, including serotonergic projections and activation of 5-HT_{2A} receptors at the level of the cerebral cortex and, possibly, the hypothalamus. The serotonergic receptor system is also strongly implicated in fearful animal behaviors and human anxiety disorders, particularly panic and obsessive-compulsive disorders (for review, see Uhde and Singareddy 2002). Knockouts of 5-HT_{1A} receptors are associated with increased fear behaviors in animal models, including, but not limited to, performance on elevated-plus maze and footshock (Heisler et al. 1998), forced-swim (Ramboz et al. 1998), and open-field (Parks et al. 1998) tests.

Hypocretinergic System

Several lines of evidence suggest that hypocretins, neuropeptides synthesized in the hypothalamus, play a role in the full range of arousal-alarm functions including anxiety and sleep regulation, as well as the sleep disorder narcolepsy (Chemelli et al. 1999). Among several other areas of the central nervous system, hypocretin neurons densely project to the LC, where they have been shown to have a direct impact on the noradrenergic system (Horvath et al. 1999). A study in our laboratory assessed the impact of hypocretins on startle behavior in the rat (Singareddy et al. 2006). Intracerebroventricular administration of hypocretin A and B, compared with saline vehicle, produced a significant reduction in noise-alone startle amplitude, a measure of unconditioned fear in the startle-potentiated startle paradigm (Winston et al. 2001). That neither hypocretin A nor hypocretin B had any effect on fear conditioning (i.e., potentiated startle) suggests that the anxiolytic properties of hypocretins might be selectively limited to unconditioned fear states, which is potentially relevant to theorized neurobiological "alarm" systems that must exist and play a role in maintaining vigilance during sleep. Although highly speculative, the possibility exists that the hypocretinergic system emerged during evolution as a specialized system to maintain vigilance during sleep, a period of maximum vulnerability to threats in the wild. Such a system might be particularly relevant to patients with nocturnal panic attacks, individuals who appear to experience an increased vulnerability to sleep-related panic attacks during transitions into greater degrees of relaxation and increasing drowsiness.

Treatment

With the high comorbidity of anxiety and insomnia, and convergence of the underlying neuroanatomical and neurochemical substrates for these disorders, it is not surprising that both disorders often respond favorably to similar pharmacological treatments and nonpharmacological interventions (e.g., cognitive-behavioral therapy). In line with the neurobiological systems previously described, this overview of pharmacological treatments for anxiety and insomnia focuses on the noradrenergic, GABAergic, and serotonergic systems. It should be emphasized that discussions about drugs in this section are intended as a tool for examining evidence for and against a theoretical convergence of anxiety and insomnia from a pharmacodynamic perspective. We would, in fact, like to underscore that many of the drugs mentioned in this section are untested under double-blind, controlled, experimental conditions and do not have a U.S. Food and Drug Administration (FDA) indication for the treatment of either anxiety or insomnia.

Given that the emphasis of this textbook is the treatment of anxiety and the anxiety disorders, we provide two tables: Table 38–1 lists current anxiolytics with their FDA-approved indications, and Table 38–2 describes the best available information regarding the effects of these anxiolytics on sleep.

Pharmacological Treatments

Noradrenergic System

Clonidine, an α_2-adrenergic agonist, has short-term but not long-term anti-anxiety actions in humans (Uhde et al. 1989). Theoretically, this effect parallels the inhibition of, followed by tolerance to, the direct application of clonidine via iontophoresis onto the LC in animals (Aghajanian and VanderMaelen 1982). LC inhibition is likely to mediate the sedating and antianxiety effects of other α_2-adrenergic agonists such as dexmedetomidine and lofexidine. Similarly, the α_1-adrenergic antagonist prazosin has been recently reported to have beneficial effects in the treatment of the hyperarousal, anxiety, and sleep-related problems in PTSD, including insomnia and nightmares (Raskind et al. 2003). Some treatment limitations, however, have been reported by the same group of investigators (Peskind et al. 2003), who found that nightmares strongly reappeared in all subjects once prazosin was discontinued.

GABAergic System

Many drugs with direct or indirect actions at the GABAergic-benzodiazepine-chloride (GBC) receptor complex have short-term sedating, sleep-promoting, and anti-anxiety profiles. Barbiturates, alcohol, benzodiazepines, and anesthetic agents, which act at different sites of the GBC receptor complex, have both sedating and subjective anxiety-reducing effects in humans, although the behavioral effects of barbiturates, alcohol, and anesthetic agents in patients who meet contemporary DSM-IV-TR diagnostic criteria for anxiety or sleep disorders have not been thoroughly examined. Propofol, an anesthetic agent with $GABA_A$ receptor actions, is often reported by subjects undergoing colonoscopy to produce the equivalent of a full night's restful and restorative sleep (author observations).

Traditional hypnotic benzodiazepine drugs such as flurazepam, estazolam, temazepam, triazolam, and quazepam, which have FDA indications for the short-term treatment of insomnia, produce short-term anxiolysis, but are generally considered impractical for such off-label use due to short half-life pharmacokinetics. Benzodiazepine hypnotics administered to patients with insomnia as target symptoms have been shown to improve insomnia as well as reduce comorbid daytime anxiety (Fontaine et al. 1990) and improve a sense of physical well-being (Roth et al. 2005). It is widely appreciated among clinicians that benzodiazepine compounds and so-called Z drugs reduce anxiety and subjective insomnia. These observations are consistent with the notion that anxiety and insomnia share overlapping neuroanatomical substrates, at least in terms of the therapeutic response patterns to drugs acting at the GBC receptor complex. These observations, however, contribute to the possible misperception that a critical, or even requisite, ingredient of drug-mediated anxiolysis, and especially sleep-promotion, is the induction of drowsiness or sedation. Drug properties of drowsiness and sedation may not only be unnecessary for the effective treatment of anxiety, insomnia, or comorbid anxiety-insomnia conditions but may actually increase anxiety in selective patients, such as those with nocturnal panic

TABLE 38–1. List of FDA-approved anxiolytics and indications

Drug and site	Trade name	Indication
GABAergic		
Alprazolam	Xanax	Anxiety disorders, GAD, PD
Chlordiazepoxide	Librium	Anxiety disorders
Clonazepam	Klonopin	PD
Clorazepate dipotassium	Tranxene	Anxiety disorders
Diazepam	Valium	Anxiety disorders
Lorazepam	Ativan	Anxiety disorders
Meprobamate	Equanil	Anxiety disorders
Oxazepam	Serepax	Anxiety disorders
Serotonergic		
Escitalopram	Lexapro	GAD
Fluoxetine	Prozac	OCD, PD
Fluvoxamine maleate	Luvox	OCD
Paroxetine	Paxil	GAD, PD, PTSD, SD, OCD
Paroxetine mesylate	Pexeva	GAD, PD, PTSD, SD, OCD
Sertraline	Zoloft	PD, PTSD, SD, OCD
Noradrenergic/serotonergic		
Buspirone	BuSpar	Anxiety disorders
Duloxetine	Cymbalta	GAD
Venlafaxine	Effexor	GAD, PD, SP
Mixed targets		
Amitriptyline-chlordiazepoxide	Limbitrol	Mixed depression/anxiety
Amitriptyline-perphenazine	Triavil	Mixed depression/anxiety
Amoxapine	Asendin	Mixed depression/anxiety
Clomipramine	Anafranil	OCD
Doxepin	Sinequan	Depression and/or anxiety
Hydroxyzine dihydrochloride	Atarax	Psychoneurotic anxiety
Hydroxyzine pamoate	Vistaril	Psychoneurotic anxiety
Prochlorperazine dimaleate	Compazine	Generalized nonpsychotic anxiety
Trifluoperazine dihydrochloride	Stelazine	Generalized nonpsychotic anxiety

Note. FDA=U.S. Food and Drug Administration; GAD=generalized anxiety disorder; OCD=obsessive-compulsive disorder; PD=panic disorder; PTSD=posttraumatic stress disorder; SP=social phobia.

who may be prone to monitor threat cues during sleep (Singareddy et al. 2006).

Serotonergic System

Selective serotonin reuptake inhibitors (SSRIs) are widely used by clinicians to treat most of the anxiety disorders, whereas trazodone, a tetracylic SSRI with 5-HT_2 antagonist effects, may be the most frequently prescribed medication for the treatment of insomnia by psychiatrists and primary care physicians. There are limited data regarding the secondary improvement in insomnia following the targeted treatment of anxiety (or vice versa). It is known that older patients with anxiety disorders (≥60 years, with mainly GAD) show

TABLE 38–2. FDA-approved anxiolytics: subjective and objective effects on sleep

Drug (trade name) and site	Subjective effects	Objective effects	References
GABAergic			
Alprazolam (Xanax)	Improved sleep quality in PD/reduced insomnia in PTSD	↑ Sleep efficiency in PD	Braun et al. 1990; Saletu-Zyhlarz et al. 2000
Chlordiazepoxide (Librium)			
Clonazepam (Klonopin)	Improved symptoms in chronic insomniacs/no change in PTSD	↓ Total wake time in primary insomnia	Cates et al. 2004; Kales et al. 1991; Schenck et al. 1996
Clorazepate (Tranxene)			
Diazepam (Valium)	Improved sleep soundness/quality in primary insomnia	↓ Total wake time/sleep latency, ↑ stage 2/REM in primary insomnia	Kales et al. 1988
Lorazepam (Ativan)	Improved sleep quality in GAD	↓ Awakenings/time awake in GAD	Saletu et al. 1997b
Meprobamate (Equanil)			
Oxazepam (Serepax)		↑ Sleep duration/↓ awakenings for insomnia	Gallais et al. 1983
Serotonergic			
Escitalopram (Lexapro)	Trend-level improvement in sleep disturbance in PTSD		Robert et al. 2006
Fluoxetine (Prozac)	Some improvement in sleep disturbance in MDD w/insomnia	↓ Sleep efficiency/REM sleep, ↑ awakenings in MDD with insomnia	Gillin et al. 1997
Fluvoxamine (Luvox)	Improved HAM-D sleep items score in MDD/ improved sleep quality in PTSD	↑ REM latency/↓ REM sleep in MDD	Neylan et al. 2001; Wilson et al. 2000
Paroxetine (Paxil)	Improved sleep quality in primary insomnia/ reduced sleep disturbance in PTSD	No significant change in objective measures in primary insomnia	Nowell et al. 1999; Stein et al. 2003
Paroxetine mesylate (Pexeva)			
Sertraline (Zoloft)	No change in sleep in MDD/insomnia most common adverse event in PTSD	↑ Sleep latency/↓ REM sleep in MDD	Davidson et al. 2001; Jindal et al. 2003
Noradrenergic/serotonergic			
Buspirone (BuSpar)	No significant change in sleep in primary insomnia	↑ Time awake in primary insomnia	Manfredi et al. 1991
Duloxetine (Cymbalta)	Gradually improved insomnia symptoms in MDD	↑ REM latency/↓ REM sleep in MDD	Hirschfeld et al. 2005; Kluge et al. 2007
Venlafaxine (Effexor)	Gradually improved insomnia symptoms in GAD		Stahl et al. 2007

TABLE 38–2. FDA-approved anxiolytics: subjective and objective effects on sleep *(continued)*

Drug (trade name) and site	Subjective effects	Objective effects	References
Mixed targets			
Amitriptyline-chlordiazepoxide (Limbitrol)	Improved HAM-D, GAS, POMS, SAS in MDD with insomnia	↑ Sleep efficiency, ↓ awakenings/REM sleep in MDD with insomnia	Scharf et al. 1986
Amitriptyline-perphenazine (Triavil)			
Amoxapine (Asendin)			
Clomipramine (Anafranil)		↓ REM sleep/sleep efficiency/maintenance, ↑ wakefulness in MDD	Kupfer et al. 1989
Doxepin (Sinequan)	Improved sleep quality/working ability in primary insomnia	↑ Sleep efficiency in primary insomnia	Hajak et al. 2001; Roth et al. 2007
Hydroxyzine dihydrochloride (Atarax)			
Hydroxyzine pamoate (Vistaril)			
Prochlorperazine (Compazine)			
Trifluoperazine (Stelazine)			

Note. FDA=U.S. Food and Drug Administration; GAD=generalized anxiety disorder; GAS=Global Assessment Scale; HAM-D=Hamilton Rating Scale for Depression; MDD=major depressive disorder; PD=panic disorder; POMS=Profile of Mood State; PTSD=posttraumatic stress disorder; REM=rapid eye movement; SAS=State Anxiety Scale.

decreased scores on the Pittsburgh Sleep Quality Index, suggesting that quality of sleep improves after the targeted treatment of anxiety in elderly patients (Blank et al. 2006). Not all individuals with anxiety disorders (e.g., PTSD), however, show convergent and parallel improvements in anxiety symptoms and insomnia (or sleep efficiency on polysomnography) when treated with SSRIs. Moreover, responses to some SSRIs may be either ineffective or may actually induce insomnia in people with PTSD, people with primary insomnia, or psychiatrically healthy subjects (Davis et al. 2006; Winokur et al. 2001). Thus, although the SSRIs play a crucial role in the treatment of many anxiety disorders, including those in which sleep problems are a core feature, the effects of these same agents on the treatment of insomnia appear to be less predictable.

Hypocretinergic System

There are no hypocretinergic agonists or antagonists that have FDA approval for the treatment of anxiety or insomnia, or comorbid anxiety-insomnia, although this will be an area for future research.

Nonpharmacological Interventions

Cognitive-behavioral therapy (CBT) is the most commonly used nonpharmacological intervention for both anxiety and insomnia, with numerous studies demonstrating its effectiveness (Foa 2006; Morin et al. 1999; Newman and Borkovec 1995). In patients with comorbid GAD and insomnia, one might predict that CBT specifically designed to target the cognitive distortions of worry would be useful in treating both conditions. In an important preliminary investigation, Belanger et al. (2004) administered group CBT to GAD patients, based on targeting GAD-related worries (Dugas and Ladouceur 2000), in which sleep complaints were not specifically addressed as part of the treatment. In this study, 86.5% of the GAD patients reported that they had never experienced insomnia without worry, and the majority reported difficulties maintaining sleep; indeed, 25% reported suffering from all phases of insomnia (i.e., early, middle, and late). In addition, CBT treatment for GAD was associated with a significant improvement on the Insomnia Severity Index (Morin 1993). The authors concluded that even though sleep dysfunction was not directly addressed, the CBT treatment specific for GAD had a significant positive impact on sleep dysfunction.

CBT has also been assessed for comorbid PTSD and insomnia. Although PTSD, along with some symptoms of sleep disturbance such as nightmares (Cooper and Clum 1989; Keane et al. 1989), improves with treatment, insomnia may not respond well to general CBT treatment for PTSD. Therefore it may be necessary for patients to undergo additional CBT targeting insomnia specifically. In one study, DeViva et al. (2005) administered a 5-session CBT for insomnia to PTSD patients who had previously responded well to CBT for their PTSD symptoms but still reported significant insomnia. In this small sample of treated PTSD patients, additional behavioral treatment targeting insomnia improved self-reported sleep time, sleep-onset latency, wake-time after sleep onset, sleep efficiency, sleep quality, impairment resulting from sleep difficulty, and maladaptive sleep-related cognitions. Residual insomnia symptoms remained after clinical improvement of PTSD in this small sample. However, the study findings suggest that additional CBT targeting PTSD-related insomnia, may be necessary to achieve a more complete response.

A typical component of CBT for insomnia is sleep restriction, with the targeted goal of maximizing sleep efficiency (i.e., the time spent sleeping while in bed; Buysse and Dorsey 2002). Sleep deprivation/restriction has also been used as an acute therapeutic approach in depressed patients, improving scores on both anxiety and mood (Roy-Byrne et al. 1986; Wehr 1990). Although limited data exist concerning the effects of sleep deprivation on anxiety and insomnia, what evidence is available suggests possible opposing effects for these two disorders, demonstrating some success as a treatment for insomnia, but no consistent or sustained benefits in patients with primary anxiety. Specifically, sleep deprivation is associated with an increase in anxiety symptoms in psychiatrically healthy individuals, and has been shown to worsen anxiety in patients with some but not all anxiety disorders. Roy-Byrne et al. (1986) assessed depression and anxiety levels after one night of total sleep deprivation in patients with PD who were not currently depressed. Individual responses of panic patients to sleep deprivation varied, with a subset of panic patients (7/12; 58%) demonstrating a worsening of anxiety and 4 of the 12 panic patients (33%) experiencing a spontaneous panic attack the day following the sleep deprivation procedure. Labbate et al. (1997) also assessed the effects of sleep deprivation on anxiety and reported a worsening of anxiety symptoms after sleep deprivation in a small sample of panic patients. In this study, 3 of the 5 patients with PD experienced at least one panic attack the morning after sleep deprivation, whereas none of the control subjects experienced sleep deprivation-induced panic. With respect to other anxiety subtypes, one night of sleep deprivation revealed inconsistent, and, in some instances, negative effects in patients with primary obsessive-compulsive disorder (OCD) (Joffe and Swinson 1988; Labbate et al. 1997), social phobia, and GAD (Labbate et al. 1998). Smith et al. (2005) reported that their very anxious patients found it difficult to comply with sleep restriction methods due to increased worry and a spiral of anxiety created by having less time in bed.

In contrast to the studies conducted with anxious patients, several studies describe the positive effects of sleep deprivation/restriction on insomnia and suggest its potential utility in treating this disorder. In one study, Stepanski et al. (2000) assessed the effects of one night of total sleep deprivation in primary insomniacs, and found that sleepiness and total sleep time were significantly increased, compared with baseline, during the recovery night following the sleep deprivation night. In addition, postdeprivation sleep measures in the subjects with insomnia were comparable with the age- and sex-matched control subjects with normal sleep function.

These observations suggest that the behavioral (and, possibly, neurobiological) responses to sleep deprivation might serve as a "diagnostic" research tool for investigating the distinctions between primary anxiety versus primary insomnia syndromes. These findings also raise the practical possibility that "natural" circumstances of sleep deprivation (e.g., shift work, military duty in war zones) might have "mixed" effects in individuals who experience comorbid anxiety and insomnia problems. However, it is also theoretically possible that individuals with "insomnia" who respond positively to sleep deprivation largely represent a subgroup of individuals with poor sleeping habits or sleep hygiene. On the other hand, individuals who do not respond to sleep deprivation, including those with primary insomnia or primary anxiety, share a common diathesis (Uhde and Cortese 2008) and are most likely to develop comorbid anxiety and insomnia.

Limitations of the Evidence

The lack of experimental data regarding the long-term impact of drug versus nondrug therapies in the management of patients with comorbid anxiety plus insomnia, or even primary insomnia alone, presents a challenge for clinicians who wish to practice evidence-based medicine. Even more problematic is the lack of information on the course of anxiety and insomnia after treatment discontinuation. In the end, clinicians must rely heavily on the best available research advances combined with specific information that emerges from working in close partnership with patients (e.g., obtaining a comprehensive history with a focus on longitudinal course of illness relationships between anxiety versus insomnia symptoms).

In view of the prevalence of insomnia reported by patients with anxiety disorders (Brown and Uhde 2003; Craske and Tsao 2005; Hoehn-Saric 1981; Mellman and Uhde 1989, 1990; Saletu et al. 1997a, 1997b; Uhde 2000), the portfolio of polysomnography and related sleep research studies in patients with anxiety disorders is fairly modest. The greatest amount of polysomnography and related sleep research has been conducted in PD, PTSD, GAD, and, to a lesser extent, OCD (Dow et al. 1996; Engdahl et al. 2000; Hurwitz et al. 1988; Mellman 1997; Papadimitriou and Linkowski 2005; Ross et al. 1994; Sheikh et al. 2003; Uhde 2000; Uhde et al. 1984). Although sleep disturbances are a "core" and distinguishing feature of PTSD, the anxiety disorders of GAD and PD, especially in those patients with nocturnal panic attacks (Cortese and Uhde 2006; Craske and Tsao 2005; Mellman and Uhde 1989; Singareddy and Uhde 2008), appear to share particularly significant characteristics with primary insomnia patients in terms of symptomatology, comorbidity, pharmacologic treatment response, and sleep-EEG measures. Because symptoms of "psychic distress"—worry, difficulty concentrating, feelings of jitteriness, agitation, and muscle tension—are almost universally reported in part or whole by patients with GAD and primary insomnia, it is not surprising that GAD was found to be the most prevalent comorbid anxiety disorder assessed in a large general population study of individuals with insomnia complaints (Ohayon et al. 1998). We cannot help but speculate that cultural or socioeconomic factors might largely influence whether one self-identifies anxiety-insomnia as a medical (i.e., sleep) problem versus a mental health (i.e., anxiety) problem, which, in the case of GAD and primary insomnia, might lead to the conclusion that major differences in primary insomnia and GAD patients are mainly related to help-seeking strategies.

From a *theoretical* perspective (see Uhde and Cortese 2008), the most rational approach for managing the patient with comorbid anxiety and insomnia, whether these represent different manifestations of a single underlying diathesis or different disorders with secondary complications (i.e., primary anxiety with secondary insomnia or primary insomnia with secondary anxiety), is to select medications that target the presenting cluster of symptoms that heralded the onset of illness. Despite the inherent logic of such an approach, it should be underscored that no controlled study with appropriate methods has been conducted to justify such a strategy. Even if there was proven efficacy for this method of drug selection, we have not yet established reliable methods for obtaining accurate information on anxiety-insomnia relationships using retrospective methods. Moreover, we do not yet understand the impact of self-selection (i.e., why some individuals with apparently identical symptom clusters emphasize "sleep" versus "anxiety" as their core problem) on drug treatment responses. Finally, even if all of these sources of variance were taken into account, it is highly likely that there would be a sizable number of people who failed to achieve a full remission of *both* anxiety and insomnia. From a *practical* perspective, therefore, it will often be necessary to treat the anxiety and insomnia symptoms separately.

Future Research

Both cross-sectional and retrospective (Uhde et al. 1985) life-charting as well as prospective methods should be used to investigate patients with primary insomnia and anxiety disorders. Prospective studies in patients whose initial presentation is anxiety versus insomnia or, in well-defined, at-risk populations, are particularly desirable. Assessment tools must be developed, validated, and employed in a systematic fashion. Conducting these studies will be particularly challenging because of pragmatic considerations, which will necessitate that such investigations be conducted across different institutional sites and specialty clinics (i.e., sleep medicine clinics versus anxiety disorder clinics). Ideally, it is desirable to conduct such studies within departments or institutions that have research expertise in *both* sleep and anxiety disorder research in order to minimize internal and external sources of variation. To investigate the convergent, comorbid relationship between anxiety and insomnia, priority might be given to the study of 1) patients who meet DSM-IV-TR criteria for GAD *plus* seek treatment at anxiety disorder clinics, versus 2) patients meeting *International Statistical Classification of Diseases and Related Health Problems* (ICD-10; World Health Organization 1992) criteria for insomnia *plus* seek treatment from sleep clinics. Other than these entry criteria, we recommend that there be few, if any, exclusion criteria in designing such comparator studies. Specifically, we would not include or exclude on the basis of sleep misperception or, perhaps, even the degree or duration of subjective insomnia. Such differences or similarities across groups seeking treatment for anxiety versus insomnia might themselves be markers that distinguish group differences.

From a genetic or neurophysiological perspective, we know that several neurotransmitter systems have particular relevance to anxiety and insomnia. However, we cannot characterize to any definitive degree the neuroanatomical substrates or functional neurocircuits that mediate primary anxiety versus primary insomnia versus comorbid anxiety-insomnia syndromes, or even whether these syndromes reflect meaningful or fundamentally different neuropathological pathways. Although magnetic resonance imaging, magnetic resonance spectroscopy, and functional magnetic resonance imaging methods have intrinsic limitations (e.g., lack of resolution power), these technologies provide new types of experimental data, which go beyond information that can be obtained with polysomnography or spectral analysis methods (Nofzinger 2004; Nofzinger et al. 1999, 2002).

The use of sleep deprivation and related chemical endocrine challenge techniques, two "older" investigational strategies, remains valuable but underutilized research tools for investigating mixed anxiety-insomnia syndromes. Caffeine is an ideal chemical model for panic attacks (Lin et al. 1997; Uhde 1995) and, not surprisingly, has recently emerged as a tool for the study of insomnia (Drake et al. 2006). Disturbances in hypothalamic-pituitary-adrenal axis function remain a separate focus of research among investigators with an interest in either anxiety (for review, see Uhde and Singareddy 2002) or primary insomnia (Drake et al. 2003; Vgontzas and Chrousos 2002). Yet the specific origin, maintenance, and neuroanatomical impact of putative glucocorticoid disturbances in mixed anxiety-insomnia syndromes have been largely overlooked by the scientific community. We suggest that "older" research techniques (i.e., sleep restriction, chemical-endocrine probes) should not be discarded simply in favor of emergent technologies, but, rather, should be prudently combined with newer imaging and genetic strategies to improve our understanding of the neuropathophysiological processes that mediate the important biological functions of fear, arousal, and sleep. By combining "older" and "newer" strategies, the scientific community will be better positioned to identify meaningful endophenotypes, which will take into account the spectrum of anxiety-insomnia symptoms that characterize most mental illnesses.

Perhaps the most exciting area for future research is the theoretical development of drugs with nonsedating anxiolysis or, even, cognitive enhancing, pro-vigilance, anxiolytic properties. As reviewed elsewhere (Dawson et al. 2005; Mohler et al. 2002, 2005), the development of a compound that binds to α_2 $GABA_A$ and/or α_3 $GABA_A$ sites, which are located primarily in the fear-related substrates (i.e., amygdala) and cortex, but without binding to the sedation-associated α_1 $GABA_A$ binding site, would theoretically have nonsedating anxiolytic properties. Such a drug would be particularly useful for patients who wish to maintain alertness or who experience increased anxiety as a result of increasing relaxation or sedation (e.g., patients with nocturnal panic attacks). Even more speculative, but equally provocative, is the idea that drugs with hypocretin agonist actions might also be useful in the treatment of patients with nocturnal panic attacks or those whose insomnia is related to a fear of sleeping (Singareddy et al. 2006; Uhde 2000).

◀ Key Clinical Points ▶

- The high prevalence of comorbid insomnia in primary anxiety disorders and comorbid anxiety symptoms in primary insomnia suggest an important underlying relationship between these clinical entities.
- Several neurotransmitter systems (noradrenergic, GABAergic, serotonergic and, more recently, hypocretinergic) are implicated in the interactive pathophysiology of anxiety and insomnia.
- Anxiety and insomnia often respond favorably to similar pharmacological treatments (e.g., benzodiazepines, selective serotonin reuptake inhibitors) and nonpharmacological interventions (e.g., cognitive-behavioral therapy).
- Although no controlled study with appropriate methods has been conducted to justify such a strategy, the most rational approach for managing the patient with comorbid anxiety and insomnia is to select medications that target the presenting cluster of symptoms that heralded the onset of illness.
- In all likelihood, a number of comorbid anxiety and insomnia patients will fail to achieve a full remission of both disorders after successful treatment of one of the disorders, making separate treatment for the anxiety and insomnia symptoms necessary.

References

Abelson JL, Khan S, Liberzon I, et al: HPA axis activity in patients with panic disorder: review and synthesis of four studies. Depress Anxiety 24:66–76, 2007

Aghajanian GK, VanderMaelen CP: Alpha 2-adrenoceptor-mediated hyperpolarization of locus coeruleus neurons: intracellular studies in vivo. Science 215:1394–1396, 1982

Alttoa A, Eller M, Herm L, et al: Amphetamine-induced locomotion, behavioral sensitization to amphetamine, and striatal D2 receptor function in rats with high or low spontaneous exploratory activity: differences in the role of locus coeruleus. Brain Res 1131:138–148, 2007

American Psychiatric Association: Diagnostic and Statistical Manual of Mental Disorders, 4th Edition, Text Revision. Washington, DC, American Psychiatric Association, 2000

Aston-Jones G, Cohen JD: Adaptive gain and the role of the locus coeruleus-norepinephrine system in optimal performance. J Comp Neurol 493:99–110, 2005

Aston-Jones G, Chiang C, Alexinsky T: Discharge of noradrenergic locus coeruleus neurons in behaving rats and monkeys suggests a role in vigilance. Prog Brain Res 88:501–520, 1991

Bélanger L, Morin CM, Langlois F, et al: Insomnia and generalized anxiety disorder: effects of cognitive behavior therapy for gad on insomnia symptoms. J Anxiety Disord 18:561–571, 2004

Benca RM: Consequences of insomnia and its therapies. J Clin Psychiatry 62:33–38, 2001

Blank S, Lenze E, Mulsant BH, et al: Outcomes of late-life anxiety disorders during 32 weeks of citalopram treatment. J Clin Psychiatry 67:468–472, 2006

Braun P, Greenberg D, Dasberg H, et al: Core symptoms of posttraumatic stress disorder unimproved by alprazolam treatment. J Clin Psychiatry 51:236–238, 1990

Breslau N, Roth T, Rosenthal L, et al: Sleep disturbance and psychiatric disorders: a longitudinal epidemiological study of young adults. Biol Psychiatry 39:411–418, 1996

Brown T, Uhde TW: Sleep panic attacks: a micro-movement analysis. Depress Anxiety 18:214–220, 2003

Brown T, Black B, Uhde TW: Sleep architecture in social phobia. Biol Psychiatry 35:420, 1994

Buhr A, Bianchi MT, Baur R, et al: Functional characterization of the new human GABAA receptor mutation 3(R192H). Hum Genet 111:154–160, 2002

Buysse DJ, Dorsey CM: Current and experimental therapeutics of insomnia, in Neuropsychopharmacology: The Fifth Generation of Progress. Edited by Davis KL, Charney D, Coyle JT, et al. Nashville, TN, American College of Neuropsychopharmacology, 2002, pp 1931–1943

Cates ME, Bishop MH, Davis LL, et al: Clonazepam for treatment of sleep disturbances associated with combat-related posttraumatic stress disorder. Ann Pharmacother 38:1395–1399, 2004

Charney DS, Redmond DE: Neurobiological mechanisms in human anxiety: evidence supporting central noradrenergic hyperactivity. Neuropharmacology 22:1531–1536, 1983

Charney DS, Woods SW, Nagy LM, et al: Noradrenergic function in panic disorder. J Clin Psychiatry 51:5–11, 1990

Charney DS, Deutch AY, Southwick SM, et al: Neural circuits and mechanisms of post-traumatic stress disorder, in Neurobiological and Clinical Consequences of Stress: From Normal Adaptation to Post Traumatic Stress Disorder. Edited by Friedman MJ, Charney DS, Deutch AY. Philadelphia, PA, Lippincott-Raven, 1995, pp 271–287

Chemelli RM, Willie JT, Sinton CM, et al: Narcolepsy in orexin knockout mice: molecular genetics of sleep regulation. Cell 98:437–451, 1999

Cooper NA, Clum GA: Imaginal flooding as a supplementary treatment for PTSD in combat veterans: a controlled study. Behav Ther 20:381–391, 1989

Cortese BM, Uhde TW: Immobilization panic. Am J Psychiatry 163:1453–1454, 2006

Craske MG, Tsao JC: Assessment and treatment of nocturnal panic attacks. Sleep Med Rev 9:173–184, 2005

Davidson JR, Rothbaum BO, van der Kolk BA, et al: Multicenter, double-blind comparison of sertraline and placebo in the treatment of posttraumatic stress disorder. Arch Gen Psychiatry 58:485–492, 2001

Davis LL, Frazier EC, Williford RB, et al: Long-term pharmacotherapy for post-traumatic stress disorder. CNS Drugs 20:465–476, 2006

Dawson GR, Collinson N, Atack JR: Development of subtype selective GABAA modulators. CNS Spectr 10:21–27, 2005

DeViva JC, Zayfert C, Mellman TA: Factors associated with insomnia among civilians seeking treatment for PTSD: an exploratory study. Behav Sleep Med 2:162–176, 2004

DeViva JC, Zayfert C, Pigeon WR, et al: Treatment of residual insomnia after CBT for PTSD: case studies. J Trauma Stress 18:155–159, 2005

Dow BM, Kelsoe JR Jr, Gillin JC: Sleep and dreams in Vietnam PTSD and depression. Biol Psychiatry 39:42–50, 1996

Drake CL, Roehrs T, Roth T: Insomnia causes, consequences, and therapeutics: an overview. Depress Anxiety 18:163–176, 2003

Drake CL, Jefferson C, Roehrs T, et al: Stress-related sleep disturbance and polysomnographic response to caffeine. Sleep Med 7:567–572, 2006

Dugas MJ, Ladouceur R: Treatment of GAD: targeting intolerance of uncertainty in two types of worry. Behav Modif 24:635–657, 2000

Engdahl BE, Eberly RE, Hurwitz TD, et al: Sleep in a community sample of elderly war veterans with and without posttraumatic stress disorder. Biol Psychiatry 47:520–525, 2000

Flosnik DL, Cortese BM, Uhde TW: Cataplexy in anxious patients: is subclinical narcolepsy underrecognized in anxiety disorders? J Clin Psychiatry (in press)

Foa EB: Psychosocial therapy for posttraumatic stress disorder. J Clin Psychiatry 67:40–45, 2006

Fontaine R, Beaudry P, Le Morvan P, et al: Zopiclone and triazolam in insomnia associated with generalized anxiety disorder: a placebo-controlled evaluation of efficacy and daytime anxiety. Int Clin Psychopharmacol 5:173–183, 1990

Gallais H, Casanova P, Fabregat H: Midazolam and oxazepam in the treatment of insomnia in hospitalized patients. Br J Clin Pharmacol 16:145S–149S, 1983

Gaus SE, Strecker RE, Tate BA, et al: Ventrolateral preoptic nucleus contains sleep-active, galaninergic neurons in multiple mammalian species. Neuroscience 115:285–294, 2002

Gillin JC, Rapaport M, Erman MK, et al: A comparison of nefazodone and fluoxetine on mood and on objective, subjective, and clinician-rated measures of sleep in depressed patients: a double-blind, 8-week clinical trial. J Clin Psychiatry 58:185–192, 1997

Hajak G, Rodenbeck A, Voderholzer U, et al: Doxepin in the treatment of primary insomnia: a placebo-controlled, double-blind, polysomnographic study. J Clin Psychiatry 62:453–463, 2001

Heisler LK, Chu HM, Brennan TJ, et al: Elevated anxiety and antidepressant-like responses in serotonin 5-HT1A receptor mutant mice. Proc Natl Acad Sci USA 95:15049–15054, 1998

Hirschfeld RM, Mallinckrodt C, Lee TC, et al: Time course of depression-symptom improvement during treatment with duloxetine. Depress Anxiety 21:170–177, 2005

Hoehn-Saric R: Characteristics of chronic anxiety patients, in Anxiety: New Research and Changing Concepts. Edited by Klein DF, Rabkin JG. New York, Raven Press, 1981, pp 399–409

Horvath TL, Peyron C, Diano S, et al: Hypocretin (orexin) activation and synaptic innervation of the locus coeruleus noradrenergic system. J Comp Neurol 415:145–159, 1999

Hurwitz TD, Mahowald MS, Kuskowski M, et al: Polysomnographic sleep is not clinically impaired in Vietnam combat veterans with chronic posttraumatic stress disorder. Biol Psychiatry 44:1066–1073, 1988

Jindal RD, Friedman ES, Berman SR, et al: Effects of sertraline on sleep architecture in patients with depression. J Clin Psychopharmacol 23:540–548, 2003

Joffe RT, Swinson RP: Total sleep deprivation in patients with obsessive-compulsive disorder. Acta Psychiatr Scand 77:483–487, 1988

Johnson EO, Roth T, Breslau N: The association of insomnia with anxiety disorders and depression: exploration of the direction of risk. J Psychiatr Res 40:700–708, 2006

Kales A, Soldatos CR, Bixler EO, et al: Diazepam: effects on sleep and withdrawal phenomena. J Clin Psychopharmacol 8:340–346, 1988

Kales A, Manfredi RL, Vgontzas AN, et al: Clonazepam: sleep laboratory study of efficacy and withdrawal. J Clin Psychopharmacol 11:189–193, 1991

Kalueff A, Nutt DJ: Role of GABA in memory and anxiety. Depress Anxiety 4:100–110, 1997

Kaschka W, Feistel H, Ebert D: Reduced benzodiazepine receptor binding in panic disorders measured by iomazenil SPECT. J Psychiatr Res 29:427–434, 1995

Keane TM, Fairbank JA, Caddell JM, et al: Implosive (flooding) therapy reduces symptoms of PTSD in Vietnam combat veterans. Behav Ther 20:245–260, 1989

Kluge M, Schüssler P, Steiger A: Duloxetine increases stage 3 sleep and suppresses rapid eye movement (REM) sleep in patients with major depression. Eur Neuropsychopharmacol 17:527–531, 2007

Korf J, Aghajanian GK, Roth RH: Increased turnover of norepinephrine in the rat cerebral cortex during stress: role of the locus coeruleus. Neuropharmacology 12:933–938, 1973

Kupfer DJ, Ehlers CL, Pollock BG, et al: Clomipramine and EEG sleep in depression. Psychiatry Res 30:165–180, 1989

Labbate LA, Johnson MR, Lydiard RB, et al: Sleep deprivation in panic disorder and obsessive-compulsive disorder. Can J Psychiatry 42:982–983, 1997

Labbate LA, Johnson MR, Lydiard RB, et al: Sleep deprivation in social phobia and generalized anxiety disorder. Biol Psychiatry 43:840–842, 1998

Laposky AD, Homanics GE, Baile A, et al: Deletion of the GABA(A) receptor beta 3 subunit eliminates the hypnotic actions of oleamide in mice. Neuroreport 12:4143–4147, 2001

Lin AS-K, Uhde TW, Slate SO, et al: Effects of intravenous caffeine administered to healthy males during sleep. Depress Anxiety 5:21–28, 1997

Lydiard RB, Zealberg J, Laraia MT, et al: Electroencephalography during sleep of patients with panic disorder. J Neuropsychiatry Clin Neurosci 1:372–376, 1989

Maher MJ, Rego SA, Asnis GM: Sleep disturbances in patients with post-traumatic stress disorder: epidemiology, impact and approaches to management. CNS Drugs 20:567–590, 2006

Malizia AL, Cunningham VJ, Bell CJ, et al: Decreased brain GABA(A)-benzodiazepine receptor binding in panic disorder: preliminary results from a quantitative PET study. Arch Gen Psychiatry 55:715–720, 1998

Manfredi RL, Kales A, Vgontzas AN, et al: Buspirone: sedative or stimulant effect? Am J Psychiatry 148:1213–1217, 1991

Mellman TA: Psychobiology of sleep disturbance in posttraumatic stress disorder. Ann NY Acad Sci 821:142–149, 1997

Mellman TA, Uhde TW: Sleep panic attacks: new clinical findings and theoretical implications. Am J Psychiatry 146:1204–1207, 1989

Mellman TA, Uhde TW: Patients with frequent sleep panic: clinical findings and response to medication treatment. J Clin Psychiatry 51:513–516, 1990

Mohler H, Fritschy JM, Rudolph U: A new benzodiazepine pharmacology. J Pharmacol Exp Ther 300:2–8, 2002

Mohler H, Fritschy JM, Vogt K, et al: Pathophysiology and pharmacology of GABA(A) receptors. Handb Exp Pharmacol 169:225–247, 2005

Monti JM, Monti D: Sleep disturbance in generalized anxiety disorder and its treatment. Sleep Med Rev 4:263–276, 2000

Morin CM: Insomnia: Psychological Assessment and Management. New York, Guilford, 1993

Morin CM, Hauri PJ, Espie CA, et al: Nonpharmacologic treatment of chronic insomnia: an American Academy of Sleep Medicine review. Sleep 22:1134–1156, 1999

Moruzzi G, Magoun HW: Brain stem reticular formation and activation of the EEG. Electroencephalogr Clin Neurophysiol 1:455–473, 1949

Neckelmann D, Mykletun A, Dahl AA: Chronic insomnia as a risk factor for developing anxiety and depression. Sleep 30:873–880, 2007

Newman MG, Borkovec TD: Cognitive-behavioral treatment of generalized anxiety disorder. Clin Psychol 48:5–7, 1995

Neylan TC, Metzler TJ, Schoenfeld FB, et al: Fluvoxamine and sleep disturbances in posttraumatic stress disorder. J Trauma Stress 14:461–467, 2001

Nofzinger EA: What can neuroimaging findings tell us about sleep disorders? Sleep Med 5:S16–S22, 2004

Nofzinger EA, Nichols TE, Meltzer CC, et al: Changes in forebrain function from waking to REM sleep in depression: preliminary analyses of [18F]FDG PET studies. Psychiatry Res 91:59–78, 1999

Nofzinger EA, Buysse DJ, Miewald JM, et al: Human regional cerebral glucose metabolism during non-rapid eye movement sleep in relation to waking. Brain 125:1105–1115, 2002

Nowell PD, Reynolds CF 3rd, Buysse DJ, et al: Paroxetine in the treatment of primary insomnia: preliminary clinical and electroencephalogram sleep data. J Clin Psychiatry 60:89–95, 1999

Ohayon MM, Roth T: Place of chronic insomnia in the course of depressive and anxiety disorders. J Psychiatr Res 37:9–15, 2003

Ohayon MM, Caulet M, Lemoine P: Comorbidity of mental and insomnia disorders in the general population. Compr Psychiatry 39:185–197, 1998

Papadimitriou GN, Linikowski P: Sleep disturbance in anxiety disorders. Int Rev Psychiatry 17:229–236, 2005

Parks CL, Robinson PS, Sibille E, et al: Increased anxiety of mice lacking the serotonin1A receptor. Proc Natl Acad Sci USA 95:10734–10739, 1998

Peskind ER, Bonner LT, Hoff DJ, et al: Prazosin reduces trauma-related nightmares in older men with chronic posttraumatic stress disorder. J Geriatr Psychiatry Neurol 16:165–171, 2003

Ramboz S, Oosting R, Amara DA, et al: Serotonin receptor 1A knockout: an animal model of anxiety-related disorder. Proc Natl Acad Sci USA 95:14476–14481, 1998

Raskind M, Peskind E, Kanter E, et al: Reduction of nightmares and other PTSD symptoms in combat veterans by prazosin: a placebo-controlled study. Am J Psychiatry 160:371–373, 2003

Redmond DE Jr: Clonidine and the primate locus coeruleus: evidence suggesting anxiolytic and anti-withdrawal effects. Prog Clin Biol Res 71:147–163, 1981

Robert S, Hamner MB, Ulmer HG, et al: Open-label trial of escitalopram in the treatment of posttraumatic stress disorder. J Clin Psychiatry 67:1522–1526, 2006

Ross RJ, Ball WA, Dinges DF, et al: Rapid eye movement sleep disturbance in posttraumatic stress disorder. Biol Psychiatry 35:195–202, 1994

Roth T, Walsh JK, Krystal A, et al: An evaluation of the efficacy and safety of eszopiclone over 12 months in patients with chronic primary insomnia. Sleep Med 6:487–495, 2005

Roth T, Rogowski R, Hull S, et al: Efficacy and safety of doxepin 1 mg, 3 mg, and 6 mg in adults with primary insomnia. Sleep 30:1555–1561, 2007

Rowlett JK, Cook JM, Duke AN, et al: Selective antagonism of GABAA receptor subtypes: an in vivo approach to exploring the therapeutic and side effects of benzodiazepine-type drugs. CNS Spectr 10:40–48, 2005

Roy-Byrne PP, Uhde TW, Post RM: Effects of one night's sleep deprivation on mood and behavior in panic disorder: patients with panic disorder compared with depressed patients and normal controls. Arch Gen Psychiatry 43:895–899, 1986

Rush CR: Behavioral pharmacology of zolpidem relative to benzodiazepines: a review. Pharmacol Biochem Behav 61:253–269, 1998

Saletu B, Saletu-Zyhlarz G, Anderer P, et al: Nonorganic insomnia in generalized anxiety disorder: controlled studies on sleep: awakening and daytime vigilance utilizing polysomnography and EEG mapping. Neuropsychobiology 36:117–129, 1997a

Saletu B, Saletu-Zyhlarz G, Anderer P, et al: Nonorganic insomnia in generalized anxiety disorder, 2: comparative studies on sleep, awakening, daytime vigilance and anxiety under lorazepam plus diphenhydramine (Somnium) versus lorazepam alone, utilizing clinical, polysomnographic and EEG mapping methods. Neuropsychobiology 36:130–152, 1997b

Saletu-Zyhlarz GM, Anderer P, Berger P, et al: Nonorganic insomnia in panic disorder: comparative sleep laboratory studies with normal controls and placebo-controlled trials with alprazolam. Hum Psychopharmacol 15:241–254, 2000

Scharf MB, Hirschowitz J, Zemlan FP, et al: Comparative effects of limbitrol and amitriptyline on sleep efficiency and architecture. J Clin Psychiatry 47:587–591, 1986

Schenck CH, Mahowald MW: Long-term, nightly benzodiazepine treatment of injurious parasomnias and other disorders of disrupted nocturnal sleep in 170 adults. Am J Med 100:333–337, 1996

Sheikh JI, Woodward SH, Leskin GA: Sleep in post-traumatic stress disorder: convergence and divergence. Depress Anxiety 18:187–197, 2003

Singareddy R, Uhde TW: Nocturnal sleep panic and depression: relationship to subjective sleep in panic disorder. J Affect Disord 2008 [Epub ahead of print]

Singareddy R, Uhde TW, Commissaris R: Differential effects of hypocretins on noise alone versus potentiated startle responses. Physiol Behav 89:650–655, 2006

Sloan EP, Natarajan M, Baker B, et al: Nocturnal and daytime panic attacks: comparison of sleep architecture, heart rate variability, and response to sodium lactate challenge. Biol Psychiatry 45:1313–1320, 1999

Smith MT, Huang MI, Manber R: Cognitive behavior therapy for chronic insomnia occurring within the context of medical and psychiatric disorders. Clin Psychol Rev 25:559–592, 2005

Spira AP, Friedman L, Aulakh JS, et al: Subclinical anxiety symptoms, sleep, and daytime dysfunction in older adults with primary insomnia. J Geriatr Psychiatry Neurol 21:149–153, 2008

Stahl SM, Ahmed S, Haudiquet V: Analysis of the rate of improvement of specific psychic and somatic symptoms of general anxiety disorder during long-term treatment with venlafaxine ER. CNS Spectr 12:703–711, 2007

Stein DJ, Davidson J, Seedat S, et al: Paroxetine in the treatment of post-traumatic stress disorder: pooled analysis of placebo-controlled studies. Expert Opin Pharmacother 4:1829–1838, 2003

Stepanski E, Zorick F, Roehrs T, et al: Effects of sleep deprivation on daytime sleepiness in primary insomnia. Sleep 23:215–219, 2000

Sullivan GM, Coplan JD, Kent JM, et al: The noradrenergic system in pathological anxiety: a focus on panic with relevance to generalized anxiety and phobias. Biol Psychiatry 46:1205–1218, 1999

Uhde T: Caffeine-induced anxiety: an ideal chemical model of panic disorder. Einstein Monograph Series in Psychiatry. Edited by Asnis GM, van Praag HM. New York, Wiley-Liss, 1995, pp 181–205

Uhde T: The anxiety disorders, in Principles and Practice in Sleep Medicine, 3rd Edition. Edited by Kryger MH, Roth T, Dement W. Philadelphia, PA, WB Saunders, 2000, pp 1123–1139

Uhde T, Cortese BM: Anxiety and insomnia: theoretical relationship and future research, in Anxiety in Health Behaviors and Physical Illness. Edited by Zvolensky MJ, Smits JA. New York, Springer, 2008, pp 105–127

Uhde TW, Singareddy R: Biological research in anxiety disorders, in Psychiatry as a Neuroscience. Edited by Maj M. New York, Wiley, 2002, pp 237–285

Uhde T, Roy-Byrne PP, Gillin JC, et al: The sleep of patients with panic disorder: a preliminary report. Psychiatry Res 12:251–259, 1984

Uhde T, Boulenger J-P, Roy-Byrne PP, et al: Longitudinal course of panic disorder: clinical and biological considerations. Prog Neuropsychopharmacol Biol Psychiatry 9:39–51, 1985

Uhde TW, Stein MB, Siever LJ, et al: Behavioral and physiological effects of short-term and long-term administration of clonidine in panic disorder. Arch Gen Psychiatry 46:170–177, 1989

Uhde T, Merritt-Davis, O, Yaroslavsky Y, et al: Sleep paralysis: overlooked fearful arousal. Presented at the 159th Annual Meeting of the American Psychiatric Association, Toronto, ON, Canada, May 2006

Vgontzas AN, Chrousos GP: Sleep, the hypothalamic-pituitary-adrenal axis, and cytokines: multiple interactions and disturbances in sleep disorders. Endocrin Metab Clin North Am 31:15–36, 2002

Wehr TA: Manipulations of sleep and phototherapy: nonpharmacological alternatives in the treatment of depression. Clin Neuropharmacol 13:S54–S65, 1990

Weissman MM, Greenwald S, Niño-Murcia G, et al: The morbidity of insomnia uncomplicated by psychiatric disorders. Gen Hosp Psychiatry 19:245–250, 1997

Wilson SJ, Bell C, Coupland NJ, et al: Sleep changes during long-term treatment of depression with fluvoxamine: a home-based study. Psychopharmacology (Berl) 149:360–365, 2000

Winokur A, Gary KA, Rodner S, et al: Depression, sleep physiology, and antidepressant drugs. Depress Anxiety 14:19–28, 2001

Winston CR, Leavell BJ, Ardayfio PA, et al: A nonextinction procedure for long-term studies of classically conditioned enhancement of acoustic startle in the rat. Physiol Behav 73:9–17, 2001

World Health Organization: International Statistical Classification of Diseases and Related Health Problems (ICD-10). Geneva, Switzerland, World Health Organization, 1992

Zorumski CF, Isenberg KE: Insights into the structure and function of GABA-benzodiazepine receptors: ion channels and psychiatry. Am J Psychiatry 148:162–173, 1991

Recommended Readings

Dement WC, Vaughn C: Promise of Sleep: A Pioneer in Sleep Medicine Explores the Vital Connection Between Health, Happiness, and a Good Night's Sleep. New York, Dell Trade Paperbacks, 1999

Epstein L, Mardon S: The Harvard Medical School Guide to a Good Night's Sleep (Harvard Medical School Guides). New York, McGraw-Hill, 2007

Hauri P, Linde S: No More Sleepless Nights, Revised Edition. New York, Wiley, 1996

Kryger MH, Roth T, Dement WC (eds): Principles and Practice of Sleep Medicine, 3rd Edition. Philadelphia, PA, WB Saunders, 2000

Pawlyk AC, Morrison AR, Ross RJ, et al: Stress-induced changes in sleep in rodents: models and mechanisms. Neurosci Biobehav Rev 32:99–117, 2008

Roth T: Insomnia: definition, prevalence, etiology, and consequences. Clin Sleep Med 3(suppl):S7–S10, 2007

Spoormaker VI, Montgomery P: Disturbed sleep in post-traumatic stress disorder: secondary symptom or core feature? Sleep Med Rev 12:169–184, 2008

Stewart R, Besset A, Bebbington P, et al: Insomnia comorbidity and impact and hypnotic use by age group in a national survey population aged 16 to 74 years. Sleep 29:1391–1397, 2006

Web Sites of Interest

American Academy of Sleep Medicine: Sleep Education. http://www.sleepeducation.com

Anxiety Disorders Association of America. http://www.adaa.org

Sleep (journal). http://www.journalsleep.org

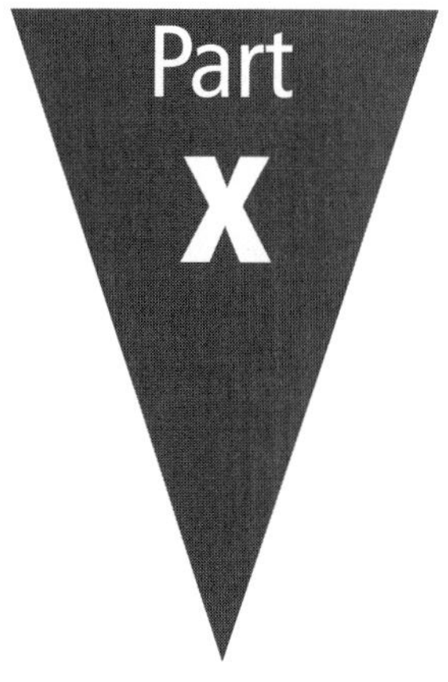

Social Aspects of Anxiety Disorders

Chapter 39

Cultural and Social Aspects of Anxiety Disorders

Dan J. Stein, M.D., Ph.D.
David Williams, Ph.D.

Recent expanding interest in the anxiety disorders has been driven by advances in our understanding of their psychobiological mediators and interventions. At the same time, however, advances in cross-cultural and social psychiatry may have fundamental implications for a comprehensive understanding of these conditions. The work of Kleinman and his colleagues (Good and Good 1982; Kleinman 1988), for example, has played a major role in the development of a "new cross-cultural psychiatry" (Kleinman 1977; Littlewood 1990). This field focuses on psychopathology in non-Western cultures but also emphasizes the potentially significant contribution of anthropological theories and methods to the Western clinical setting.

This chapter focuses on cultural and social aspects of the anxiety disorders. We begin by considering different ways of approaching the intersection between culture and the anxiety disorders. We then consider each of the anxiety disorders in turn from a clinical anthropological perspective. We propose that a number of anxiety disorders do in fact occur universally, but that their experience and expression may differ in crucial ways. In addition, we note that socioeconomic factors may play a crucial role in mediating the pathogenesis of some anxiety disorders.

Culture and Psychiatry

A number of different approaches to the intersection of culture and medicine have been outlined (Hahn and Kleinman 1983). One way of classifying the approaches is to distinguish between a clinical position, an anthropological position, and a clinical anthropological position. These positions reflect different stances on key debates within the philosophy of science and medicine. This section draws extensively on other discussions of the strengths and weaknesses of these positions (D.J. Stein 1993, 2008). It should be emphasized that this division is intended to be a heuristic one and may not reflect the work of any single clinician or anthropologist.

Clinical Position

The clinical position is occupied by clinicians and anthropologists who are primarily interested in applying Western medical and psychiatric nosologies, in post hoc fashion, to diverse populations. The DSM-IV categories and criteria, for example, constructed in a particular (Western) setting, are used to classify psychiatric data obtained in other (non-Western) contexts. Cross-cultural psychiatrists such as Prince and Tcheng-Larouche (1987),

This work is supported by the Medical Research Council Research Unit on Anxiety and Stress Disorders (South Africa).

for example, have argued that relatively minor alterations in the DSM system would result in a truly international classification of diseases.

This position has a long tradition in medical and psychiatric nosology. Kraepelin, for example, the father of contemporary psychiatric nosology, applied his system of classifying psychoses in German patients to data collected in Java. Kraepelin's nosology was predicated on a biological hypothesis—that the major psychoses each had a distinctive underlying neuropathogenesis, which accounted for their particular symptomatology and course. Thus psychotic symptomatology had universal forms, which were biologically determined, but diverse contents, which were colored by cultural factors (Littlewood 1990).

Similarly, a clinical position might argue that anxiety disorders are simply biomedical disorders and that culture can influence only their content rather than their form. For example, the form of obsessive-compulsive disorder (OCD) necessarily comprises obsessions or compulsions, but the content may vary from obsessions about syphilis in one culture to obsessions about AIDS in another culture. Proponents of such a position would argue that OCD has a specific neurobiological basis and that cross-cultural differences in the disorder are therefore likely to be only superficial.

The strength of the clinical approach lies in its willingness to extend a particular theoretical framework to diverse settings. The position highlights the scientific process of constructing nosologies. Indeed, international employment of the DSM system has allowed the work of different clinicians to converge and has contributed to increased knowledge of psychiatric disorders. Furthermore, advances in our understanding of the neurobiology of psychiatric disorders, including the anxiety disorders, would seem to strengthen this position.

Nevertheless, this position has been criticized for committing a "category fallacy"—of reifying the categories and criteria of one ethnocentric classification as universal natural kinds. Indeed, routinized application of one theoretical framework of disease may prevent the nosologist from recognizing the existence, or appreciating the character, of unfamiliar categories and symptoms. The DSM system, particularly prior to DSM-IV, gives short shrift to the so-called culture-bound syndromes and pays little attention to the differences in psychopathology between different cultures. Conversely, this approach downplays the possible contribution that cross-cultural theories and methods make in helping us recognize the particular sociocultural influences on our own nosology.

Anthropological Position

The anthropological approach states that the form and content of medical disorders are crucially determined by culture; our nosologies are themselves cultural artifacts. Such disorders are inevitably culture bound (Yap 1951, 1962): they are expressed and experienced in terms of a particular sociocultural context. Thus clinicians and anthropologists who are proponents of this position are interested, for example, in exploring the relationship between the construction of DSM-IV and its forerunners and their particular sociocultural setting.

Again, this position has a long history. Boas, a pioneering figure in American anthropology, wrote: "If it is our serious purpose to understand the thoughts of a people the whole analysis of experience must be based on their concepts, not ours" (Boas 1943, p. 314). Furthermore, Boas increasingly came to believe that an appreciation of the historical and environmental factors that shaped a culture is required in order to understand these psychological forms (Boas 1943). These ideas have also been applied in medical and psychiatric anthropology, and an extensive literature devoted to the cultural meanings of disease, and to the social construction of disease, has emerged (Conrad and Schneider 1980; Cooper 2004; Wright and Treacher 1982).

Critics of the DSM classification of anxiety disorders might, for example, emphasize that this system is itself a social construction. In their early review of the anxiety disorders, Good and Kleinman (1985) noted the following:

1. That cross-cultural comparisons using Western scales of anxiety (Spielberger and Diaz-Guerrero 1990) have several crucial methodological problems
2. That there is tremendous variation across societies in the experience and expression of symptoms of anxiety, as well as in the experienced source of anxiety
3. That anxiety disorders are not simply the result of culturally influenced interpretations of an underlying disease, but rather that anxiety disorders are also disorders of the interpretive process

Similarly, Young (1980) emphasized the extent to which the concept of stress and diagnoses such as posttraumatic stress disorder (PTSD) are embedded within our particular Western sociocultural context. In particular, he argues that the focus of DSM on the individual and his or her biology reflects the individualistic, technological aspects of Western society. Conversely, a disorder such as koro, an anxiety about penile shrinkage, is not simply a biomedical entity but rather is constructed within certain non-Western cultures.

The anthropological approach has a number of strengths. It emphasizes the relationship between psychiatric nosology and the social forms in which it is produced. It therefore points to the importance of considering the ways in which cultural factors determine the experience and perception of a mental disorder (rather than simply influencing its form). Kleinman (1980), for example, has suggested that the emphasis in DSM on the psychological rather than somatic symptoms of depressive spectrum disorders makes sense only within Western culture and is not universally applicable. Furthermore, this position points to the importance of thinking through the relationship between our nosology and our particular sociocultural setting in a self-reflexive process.

Nevertheless, the anthropological position also falls prey to a number of criticisms. A view of mental disorder as merely a social construction undermines the existence of mental disorders in DSM as real phenomena that are generated by underlying biopsychological mechanisms. A view of nosology as simply a cultural product undermines the importance of scientific explanation as a component of clinical work. Indeed, important strengths of DSM are its inclusion of advances in contemporary psychiatric science (e.g., recognizing panic disorder as a separate entity with a specific phenomenology and pathophysiology) and its explicit attitude that future editions of DSM will need to change to incorporate new findings. Thus, the anthropological position tends to neglect the reality of the entities and processes of mental disorders and the validity of our explanations of their mechanisms. It tends to downplay commonalities in underlying psychobiology across different cultures.

Clinical Anthropological Position

A synthetic or clinical anthropological position attempts to reach a compromise between the clinical and the anthropological positions. This position conceptualizes biomedical disorders as reflecting the operation of real psychobiological mechanisms but acknowledges that disorders are necessarily expressed and experienced within sociocultural contexts. Classifications such as DSM, which are based on scientific knowledge, may be argued to have both intransitive dimensions (they do allow a knowledge of real entities) and transitive dimensions (they are always produced in social forms) (Bhaskar 1978).

An early Greek classification of infectious diseases, for example, divided infectious diseases into those that resolve after the "krisis" and those in which there is deterioration after the turning point. At this point little was known about the underlying mechanisms of infection, and the classification was informed primarily by a wide-ranging theory, which also pertained to other aspects of social life. As knowledge of infectious entities progressed, so classifications have incorporated discoveries about different bacteria, viruses, and, more recently, prions. Knowledge about infectious disease continues to be produced in social forms and may, for example, reflect a Western focus on individual susceptibility to infection rather than on social responsibility for disease prevention (Young 1980). Nevertheless, the structure of classifications of infectious diseases is based on knowledge of real entities and processes.

Similarly, certain psychobiological mechanisms may result in the phenomenon of social anxiety; however, in Western culture, body dysmorphic disorder is common, whereas in Eastern cultures olfactory reference syndrome is seen. Both entities may well involve overlapping serotonergic mechanisms (D.J. Stein et al. 1998), but the experience of each disorder may differ in crucial ways. It is not that "psychotic" disorders are more biological than "neurotic" ones (Leff 1990)—rather, all psychiatric disorders comprise psychopathological phenomena that are generated by underlying neurobiological and psychosocial mechanisms.

The strength of the clinical anthropological approach is that it has a place for both scientific knowledge and meaning construction. Increasingly, the psychobiological mechanisms underlying cross-cultural variations are open to empirical exploration (Han and Northoff 2008). The reality of disease and its biopsychological underpinnings is emphasized, and the construction of disease within a particular sociocultural context is also incorporated. One way to draw on this approach is by employing a differentiation between disease and illness. We discuss this distinction in the subsequent section.

Disease Versus Illness

A central theoretical distinction in modern medical anthropology is that between disease and illness (Fabrega 1987; Good and Good 1982; Kleinman 1977, 1980; Westmeyer 1987). The term *disease* refers to biomedical disorders that are present across cultures (e.g., raised blood pressure, depressed mood), whereas *illness* refers to the subjective perception and experience of such disorders. Medical anthropologists have emphasized a point well known to psychiatrists—that the perception of a disorder can itself affect its course and outcome (D.J. Stein and Rapoport 1996; D.J. Stein et al. 2007). Furthermore, medical anthropologists have emphasized that in order to negotiate clinical interventions with the patient, it is imperative that the physician obtain an understanding of the illness (rather than simply the disease).

For example, the experience of the medical disorder known as *depression* in Chinese culture is informed by explanatory models that highlight the relevance of somatic symptoms and that expect management to involve the family. In this context, patients in fact experience the illness known as *neurasthenia*, in which somatic symptoms are prominent. In order to achieve compliance with an appropriate treatment, an understanding of the patient's explanatory model is needed; this then allows an understanding of the patient's illness and negotiation of a shared model of the disorder and its treatment (Kleinman 1988).

In the next sections, we employ the distinction between *disease* and *illness* to address the intersection between cultural and social studies and the anxiety disorders. From a clinical anthropological perspective, although there do appear to be universal disease processes, cross-cultural factors result in different manifestations of psychopathological phenomena. Thus, although DSM diagnoses are culture bound, this appears to be characteristic of all psychiatric disorders. To define a particular psychiatric disorder as culture bound is to lose sight of the psychosocial factors in all such disorders. Furthermore, although psychiatric nosologies ought to be applied tentatively, with self-reflexive criticism (Kleinman 1988), this should be a feature of all psychological science.

In general, we argue that the anxiety disorders do not in fact represent a category fallacy. From a theoretical perspective, neuroevolutionary approaches to the anxiety disorders suggest that universal psychobiological mechanisms are important in the pathophysiology of these conditions. Empirical epidemiological and neurobiological data provide some support for this argument, and clinical data confirm that patients can experience the onset of anxiety disorders in the absence of exposure to cultural narratives about their symptoms.

Nevertheless, culture may exert important influences on the experience and expression of anxiety disorders (Friedman 1997; Good and Kleinman 1985; Guarnacia and Kirmayer 1997; Neal and Turner 1991). In particular, it is possible that culture influences the course and outcome of these conditions (D.J. Stein and Rapoport 1996; D.J. Stein et al. 2007). Certainly there is strong evidence that the adversity and stress associated with low social status play a causal role in mood and other psychiatric disorders (Dohrenwend et al. 1992; Yu and Williams 1999). Even controlling for sociodemographic variables, stress from marginal minority status may affect rates of anxiety disorders (Brown et al. 1990).

Panic Disorder

Panic Disorder as Disease

A range of evidence indicates that panic disorder is a universal biomedical disorder and that this diagnosis does not represent a category fallacy. First, there is increasing evidence that specific neuroanatomical circuits and neurochemical systems underpin the symptoms of panic disorder. Second, epidemiological studies suggest that the prevalence of the disorder in different settings is similar (although differences between populations do emerge). Third, clinical and epidemiological studies have found that variables such as age at onset, sex ratio, and psychiatric sequelae of panic disorder are similar in a range of different contexts (Gorman et al. 2000).

A neuroevolutionary account of panic disorder would bolster claims that it is a universal biomedical entity. Klein (1993) has made perhaps the most comprehensive attempt to do just this. He proposed that panic attacks occur when a suffocation monitor erroneously signals a lack of oxygen and maladaptively triggers an evolved suffocation alarm system. This hypothesis relies on the argument that the physiological mechanism for detecting potential suffocation depends on increased PCO_2 (partial pressure of carbon dioxide in the blood) and brain lactate levels.

The false suffocation alarm theory seems to account for the prominent symptoms of dyspnea during a panic attack (indicating a specific emergency reaction to suffocation) (Anderson et al. 1984) and for the chronic hyperventilation that predicts lactate-induced panic (indicating an attempt to avoid dyspnea by lowering PCO_2) (Papp et al. 1993). This hypothesis also buttresses the differentiation, which Klein was instrumental in drawing, between episodic spontaneous panic and chronic fearlike anxiety (in which there is hypothalamic-pituitary-adrenal activation) (Klein 1964). The hypothesis also provides an explanation of the lack of panic in patients with absent suffocation alarms (Ondine's curse) and during pregnancy and delivery (when PCO_2 is lowered) (Pine et al. 1994). Conversely, the hypothesis provides an explanation for increased panic during relaxation and sleep, during the premenstrual period, and for the high frequency of panic in patients with respiratory insufficiency (in whom PCO_2 is increased) (Klein 1993).

A possible objection to Klein's hypothesis is the observation that panic attacks have features similar to those of many other kinds of fear responses. Thus, it might be suggested that panic attacks serve as a common adaptation for situations from which fleeing is an appropriate response (Nesse 1987). Various kinds of triggers, including separation anxiety, other kinds of loss, and traumatic suffocation, might then all be expected to increase the threshold for this more general danger response. Indeed, Klein (1981) earlier put forward a hypothesis that panic attacks could be understood as homologous to an evolved separation anxiety response.

Panic Disorder as Illness

If panic disorder is understood as a biomedical disorder involving a false suffocation alarm, how is this condition perceived and experienced by different persons and in different cultures? As is the case with many other anxiety disorders, there are relatively few data on this issue.

Nevertheless, panic attacks and panic disorder have been documented in a range of different cultures. Of course, they may manifest in somewhat different ways. Simons (1985), for example, provided an example of an Inuit person whose agoraphobic avoidance manifested not in the usual Western avoidance of driving but as a fear of kayaking. Liebowitz et al. (1994) noted that *ataque de nervios* in Hispanic Americans can be used to refer to several different patterns of emotional symptoms, including diagnosable anxiety and mood disorders such as panic disorder. Indeed, of their subjects who met diagnostic criteria for both ataque de nervios and panic disorder, 80% seemed to employ the term *ataque* to label their panic attacks.

Is it possible that the perception of panic symptoms itself influences the disorder's course and prognosis? Certainly, panic attacks are commonly misdiagnosed as medical disorders in Western settings. Self-diagnosis of panic attacks as ataque de nervios in Hispanic Americans might similarly lead to ineffective interventions; for example, Salman et al. (1997) noted that many such patients take medications only on an as-needed basis. On the other hand, it is possible that in certain cultures, responses that invoke current cognitive-behavioral principles, such as exposure, are more prevalent. Cultural norms regarding gender roles, for example, have been argued to facilitate increased rates of agoraphobia in women (Starcevic et al. 1998).

Social Anxiety Disorder

Social Anxiety Disorder as Disease

As with panic disorder, there is again some evidence that social anxiety disorder is a universal biomedical disorder and that this diagnosis does not represent a category fallacy. First, although our knowledge of the neurobiology of social anxiety disorder remains in an early stage, there is work indicating that serotonergic and dopaminergic mechanisms as well as particular brain regions are crucial in mediating the disorder. Second, epidemiological studies indicate that the disorder is highly prevalent in almost all countries studied (Weissman et al. 1996). Third, clinical and epidemiological studies have found that variables such as age at onset, sex ratio, and psychiatric sequelae of social anxiety disorder are similar in a range of different countries (M.B. Stein and D.J. Stein 2008).

It has been hypothesized that social anxiety disorder involves pathological triggering of an appeasement display, often characterized by blushing (D.J. Stein and Bouwer 1997). This hypothesis relies on the argument that blushing is a communicative, fixed-action pattern and that there are similarities between blushing in humans and primate appeasement displays that serve to deflect peer aggression (Leary and Meadows 1991). The neurobiology of social anxiety disorder, of blushing, and of appeasement displays is not well understood, so the false appeasement hypothesis currently lacks empirical support. Nevertheless, there is increasing literature that attempts to understand social anxiety disorder in terms of different innate defense systems (M.B. Stein and D.J. Stein 2008; Trower and Gilbert 1989).

Social Anxiety Disorder as Illness

Again the question can be asked: If social anxiety disorder is understood as a biomedical disorder involving a particular kind of false alarm, how is this condition perceived and experienced by different persons and in different cultures? Perhaps the most relevant body of literature here is that on *taijin kyofusho* (TKS) or *anthropophobia*, a condition that has been described in Japanese and other Eastern cultures (Kirmayer 1991). This is a disorder characterized by "the presence of extraordinary intense anxiety and tension in social settings with others, a fear of being looked down upon by others, making others feel unpleasant, and being disliked by others, so that it leads to withdrawal from or avoidance of social relations" (Kashara 1975, as cited in Tseng et al. 1992). Typical fears in TKS include blushing, unpleasant body odor, and stuttering.

TKS overlaps with and differs from social anxiety disorder in interesting ways. Both disorders involve social anxiety and fears of embarrassment. However, while patients with social anxiety disorder typically worry about embarrassing themselves, patients with TKS often worry about offending or embarrassing others (Kleinknecht et al. 1994). This may reflect important cultural differences between the West and East, particularly the value given to the group over the individual in traditional Asian thought. Although there has been relatively little work on the neurobiology of TKS, it is interesting to note that its symptoms, like those of social anxiety disorder, may respond to treatment with serotonin reuptake inhibitors (Kizu et al. 1994; Matsunaga et al. 2001) or to Morita therapy (which has elements in common with cognitive-behavioral therapy) (D.J. Stein and Matsunaga 2001).

An argument that TKS and social anxiety disorder overlap to an important extent is perhaps strengthened by the appearance of cases in the West in which concerns are precisely those that characterize the offensive subtype of TKS (Clarvit et al. 1996) or in which symptoms are those of olfactory reference syndrome (D.J. Stein et al. 1998). Such patients may respond to standard treatments used for social anxiety disorder (Clarvit et al. 1996; D.J. Stein et al. 1998). On the other hand, it should be noted that not all patients who receive a culture-bound diagnosis meet criteria for the overlapping DSM category. Thus, for example, patients with TKS may occasionally be best diagnosed as having a psychotic disorder.

Obsessive-Compulsive Disorder

Obsessive-Compulsive Disorder as Disease

It seems reasonable to assert that OCD, too, is a biomedical disorder mediated by specific neurobiological mechanisms. Certainly, there is increasing evidence that specific neuroanatomical circuits and neurochemical systems underpin the symptoms of OCD. Again, epidemiological studies indicate that the prevalence of the disorder in almost all countries so far studied is similar, in this case affecting approximately 2%–3% of the population (Karno et al. 1988; Weissman et al. 1994). Finally, clinical and epidemiological studies have found that variables such as age at onset, sex ratio, and kinds of obsessions and compulsions are again similar in a range of different countries (Greenberg and Witztum 1994; Weissman et al. 1994).

There are, however, some data indicating that the prevalence and symptomatology of OCD do vary in some respects from country to country. For example, an increased prevalence of religious obsessions may occur in places where religious concerns are dominant (de Bilbao and Giannakopoulos 2005; Okasha et al. 1994). Nevertheless, it may be argued that close examination of symptoms pertaining to religious beliefs reveals remarkable overlap with the content of symptoms in nonreligious patients (Greenberg and Witztum 1994). Thus, religious obsessions and compulsions can be reframed in terms of the physical contamination symptoms seen in OCD in other cultures. Similarly, while some authors have suggested that OCD is uncommon in Africa, this is contradicted by clinical reports of such cases (Gangdev et al. 1996).

A number of authors have suggested that from an evolutionary perspective, OCD may be considered as involving an alarm that erroneously signals the need to groom or to perform other behaviors that are ordinarily useful in responding to perceived danger (Rapoport et al. 1992; D.J. Stein et al. 1992; Swedo 1989). This hypothesis relies on the argument that the basal ganglia, which appear to play a significant role in the pathogenesis of OCD, are a repository of species-specific motoric and cognitive procedural strategies (i.e., learned habits, response sets).

A possible objection to this view of OCD emerges from an early ethological literature that focused on displacement behaviors. Ethologists have, for example, described the elicitation of repetitive incomplete motoric patterns in response to conflicting triggers (e.g., for attack and flight) (Tinbergen 1953). In this account, grooming in animals and OCD in humans might be conceived of as a nonspecific response to stress. It has been suggested that there is a prepotency for rituals at ages 5–8 (Marks 1987), so a stressful environment at that time may be important in reinforcing such behaviors. However, this view does not seem able to explain the specificity of the phenomenology and neurobiology of OCD.

Obsessive-Compulsive Disorder as Illness

The question of how OCD may be experienced and expressed differently in different countries has been considered by D.J. Stein and Rapoport (1996), and this section draws closely on their work. In certain non-Western cultures, it is possible that obsessions are understood in terms of constructs such as intentional witchcraft or ancestor displeasure. Such an understanding would in turn lead the patient to present to a traditional healer. In Africa, for example, Carothers (1953) noted that anxiety was commonly associated with fear of bewitchment and poisoning or fear of having broken some taboo or having neglected a ritual. Similarly, Lambo (1962) noted that morbid fear of bewitchment was the commonest cause of an acute anxiety state in Africans. It is possible, therefore, that African patients with symptoms revolving around bewitchment and other culturally syntonic concerns may in fact have had OCD.

More radically, the question that arises is whether certain kinds of disorders represent culture-bound variations of OCD. Are body dysmorphic disorder and anorexia nervosa Western forms of OCD? Is koro (concern about penile retraction) an Eastern form of OCD? Overall, there seems to be too little confirmatory evidence for this. The alternatives are then to classify the cross-cultural category by using more than one DSM diagnosis or to consider adding the culture-bound category as a separate diagnosis. Body dysmorphic disorder and koro, for example, overlap insofar as a concern with a body defect is present in each (D.J. Stein et al. 1991). Nevertheless, koro is often accompanied by panic, and the concern about penile retraction is often relatively transient. Perhaps koro overlaps with body dysmorphic disorder and/or panic disorder. Alternatively, the constellation of symptoms in koro may be sufficiently distinct to warrant a separate diagnosis.

Another question is whether the perception of OCD symptoms itself influences the disorder's course and prognosis. Okasha et al. (1994) noted that OCD patients seen in psychiatric settings in Egypt have high scores on the Yale-Brown Obsessive Compulsive Scale, suggesting that there is a high tolerance for symptoms before medical, rather than religious, help is sought. Explanations that highlight cultural differences in tolerance for symptoms may also contribute to understanding gender differences in presentation; in Egypt, more males present for treatment, perhaps because tolerance for symptoms is higher in females. Similarly, in Western cultures, nonmedical belief systems may influence treatment-seeking behavior. Thus, religious patients with scrupulosity are perhaps more likely to seek spiritual advice than medical care. It has been argued that in the United States certain groups of OCD patients, such as African Americans, do not present as commonly for psychiatric care and are more likely to voice somatic complaints (Hollander and Cohen 1994).

It is noteworthy that empirical investigation of OCD has demonstrated that modification of patients' reactions to obsessions may result in changes in brain activity and in symptom levels (Baxter et al. 1992). Unfortunately, there are relatively little data on the various health-seeking pathways taken by OCD patients in different settings. Further research along these lines is clearly called for, with additional exploration of the beliefs and circumstances that prevent OCD patients from seeking medical care. Further work on the course and outcome of OCD in different settings would also be of interest.

Posttraumatic Stress Disorder

Posttraumatic Stress Disorder as Disease

In recent years it has become clear that PTSD is characterized not by a normal stress response but rather by pathological sensitization of certain neurochemical systems and changes in functional neuroanatomy (Yehuda and McFarlane 1995). Epidemiological studies in a range of different settings have demonstrated that PTSD is more likely to occur after more severe traumas but that certain individuals appear to be vulnerable to developing the disorder (Yehuda and McFarlane 1995). There is also a good deal of evidence demonstrating that PTSD symptoms are similar in different historical eras and in different cultures (Marsella et al. 1996).

A neuroevolutionary approach to PTSD has not been well defined, but presumably this disorder involves a dissociation of classical conditioned responses from their cortical control mechanisms. Preclinical studies demonstrate that thalamo-amygdaloid pathways play a crucial role in conditioned responses, and clinical studies of PTSD patients demonstrate hyperactivity of the amygdala during symptom provocation. Preclinical studies suggest that slow cortico-amygdaloid pathways can override faster thalamo-amygdaloid pathways; this allows habituation to previously feared stimuli (LeDoux 1996). In PTSD patients, however, it might be hypothesized that thalamo-amygdaloid responses, which ordinarily are activated only in emergency situations, are continuously recruited.

Posttraumatic Stress Disorder as Illness

How is PTSD experienced and expressed differently in different societies? One point that may shed light on this is the question of how PTSD is experienced and expressed differently in men and women in Western culture; similarities and differences have been described between male combat veterans and female rape survivors, for example. This may reflect differences in cultural narratives about the experience of combat and of rape. Similarly, differences may be seen across different cultures in the aftermath of trauma. Marsella et al. (1996), for example, suggest that while the reexperiencing and hyperarousal symptoms of PTSD are universal, the avoidant and numbing symptoms are more likely experienced in those ethnocultural settings where avoiding and numbing behaviors are common expressions of distress. There may also be historical and cross-cultural variations in the extent of different symptoms after trauma (Jones et al. 2002; Lewis-Fernández et al. 2008; Stamm and Friedman 2000; Yeomans et al. 2008). Cultural and social factors may be important determinants of vulnerability to PTSD by shaping concepts of what constitutes a trauma and by affecting known vulnerability factors such as early childhood experiences, comorbidity (e.g., alcohol abuse), and social resources for responding to trauma.

Once again, many of these questions remain open for future rigorous empirical research (Jones et al. 2002). Nevertheless, a strong theoretical argument can be made that particular cultural rituals, performed after exposure to trauma, do play a role in preventing PTSD (Shay 1994). Conversely, it is possible to speculate that the repression of trauma narratives in certain cultures exacerbates posttraumatic suffering. An interesting experiment at a national level took place in South Africa, where a Truth and Reconciliation Commission encouraged public acknowledgment of past gross human rights violations (Kaminer et al. 2001). In the absence of rigorous empirical data, it is not clear whether this exercise had a psychotherapeutic effect; there is, however, a small amount of literature on the therapeutic effect of bearing witness to past human rights violations (Weine et al. 1998).

Given that the psychopathology of PTSD frequently involves not only discrete symptoms but also a broad questioning of the self and of identity, understanding the patient's sociocultural background is particularly important. Several authors have emphasized that inadequate appreciation of the sociocultural context of trauma and of responses to trauma may impede the therapeutic process (Stamm and Friedman 2000). On the other hand, a comprehensive and sensitive assessment of this context may allow appropriate individual and community interventions that promote symptomatic improvement as well as broader healing (D.J. Stein et al. 2007).

Generalized Anxiety Disorder

Generalized Anxiety Disorder as Disease

The question of whether generalized anxiety disorder (GAD) is a universal category is perhaps not as clear as in the case of other anxiety disorders. Early on, Good and Kleinman (1985) concluded that "generalized anxiety disorders exist in nearly all cultures." Nevertheless, the particular overlaps of anxiety, depression, and somatic symptoms may differ substantially from culture to culture. Even using the DSM characterization of GAD, there is significant comorbidity with depression and with somatization symptoms. Furthermore, although there have been advances in the neurobiology of GAD, it is presently unclear whether the underlying mechanisms are specific to this disorder. Finally, it has taken longer for a body of cross-national data on the symptoms and epidemiology of GAD to accumulate.

What has been investigated are various combinations of anxiety, depression, and somatization symptoms in different cultures. Consider, for example, the entity of neurasthenia, which is included in the *International Statistical Classification of Diseases and Related Health Problems,* 10th Revision (ICD-10; World Health Organization 1992). For example, an early study by Good and Kleinman (1985) found that on interviewing 100 patients with neurasthenia using the Schedule for Affective Disorders and Schizophrenia, 93 had depression and 69 had anxiety disorders (including 13 with GAD). A majority of the patients demonstrated major depression along with anxiety disorder, chronic pain, and somatoform disorders. The majority also reported a history of significant stressors. Treatment of patients with neurasthenia who also met diagnostic criteria for depression with tricyclic antidepressants led to decreased symptoms (although not necessarily to decreased social impairment). These agents are of course useful both in treating depression and in treating GAD.

It is possible, then, to argue that in a range of different cultures there is an anxiety-depression-somatization disorder that may respond to treatment with antidepressants. Individual vulnerabilities and various stressors are likely to contribute to the pathogenesis of this syndrome. Certainly, there is growing evidence of an inverse and causal relationship between socioeconomic status and mental health (Dohrenwend et al. 1992; Yu and Williams 1999). In the National Comorbidity Survey, for example, an anxiety disorder was 2.82 times as common in those who had not completed high school as in those with a college education or more (i.e., with

16 or more years of education) and 2.12 times as common in those with yearly income of less than $20,000 as in those with an income of more than $70,000 (Kessler et al. 1994).

Generalized Anxiety Disorder as Illness

In some cultures or groups this anxiety-depression-somatic disorder may be described and experienced in primarily psychological terms (e.g., the sadness of major depression, the worries of GAD). However, in other cultures or groups, somatization may be more central. Certainly, the experience of anxiety and depression in Chinese culture is informed by explanatory models that highlight the relevance of somatic symptoms and that expect that management will involve the family. In this context, patients may experience the illness known as *neurasthenia*. Nevertheless, somatic symptoms have also been shown to be present in many Western patients with anxiety and mood disorders. Different kinds of somatic symptoms of anxiety may be experienced in different cultures; in Nigeria, for example, a core symptom of anxiety appears to be the sensation of an insect crawling through the head or other parts of the body (Awaritefe 1988; Ebigbo 1986).

There are clear clinical implications of such an argument. First, it is important to determine the explanatory model of patients having mixtures of anxiety, depression, and somatic symptoms (Kleinman 1988). A comprehensive clinical interview should include an inquiry into the patient's own causal model of his or her symptoms; this may reveal significant differences from that of the clinician. Careful negotiation around these models may allow the clinician to justify his or her treatment choices in a way that the patient experiences as empathic, which improves compliance.

Second, there needs to be additional research that focuses on whether or not similar psychobiological mechanisms are responsible for the range of anxiety, mood, and somatic symptoms experienced by these patients. The DSM system has encouraged a focus on studies of patients who meet diagnostic criteria for particular disorders. However, even in the West, such a focus runs into difficulties with disorders with high comorbidity. Furthermore, there is a strong rationale for focusing instead on particular symptoms, such as anhedonia, that cut across diagnostic categories and that may be mediated by specific psychobiological mechanisms in all of these categories (van Praag et al. 1990).

Conclusion

Important recent advances in the anxiety disorders have included more reliable nosological criteria, an increased understanding of psychobiology, and more effective treatments. To some extent this work has been so successful that it is possible to argue that our concepts of the anxiety disorders are universal and that this work never entails a category fallacy. From this perspective, the importance of sociocultural factors in the anxiety disorders is limited only to a consideration of ethnic and gender differences in pharmacokinetics and pharmacodynamics when medications are used. Certainly, one of the astonishing things about working in the anxiety disorders field is how media educational campaigns result in "discovery" of these conditions; patients often endure symptoms for years, with no awareness that others have similar symptoms or that specific medical treatments exist.

However, with these important advances we run the risk of failing to address cultural and social contexts. Although DSM-IV-TR (American Psychiatric Association 2000) highlights cultural issues in psychiatric diagnosis, the DSM system arguably remains a Western cultural product that does not entirely come to grips with anxiety entities such as TKS and neurasthenia. Such entities deserve increased phenomenological and neurobiological study. Arguably, a more comprehensive approach to anxiety disorders in different cultures and social groups will ultimately result in a better understanding of their pathogenesis and management.

Even for disorders for which we can posit universal underlying mechanisms, it is crucial to consider the impact of culture and society on the diagnosis and treatment of the disorder, on its expression, and on the patient's experience. The literature on misdiagnosis of psychiatric disorders in American minority groups deserves to be extended to the anxiety disorders. Ethnicity and gender affect important aspects of pharmacological management (ranging from patient compliance to pharmacogenetic variation), psychotherapeutic treatment, and broader interventions (such as the national media campaigns to improve the recognition and treatment of anxiety disorders).

Women are at greater risk of developing anxiety disorders than men; the psychobiological and sociocultural mechanisms underlying this predisposition require much further analysis. There is evidence for an association between low education or income and the diagnosis of an anxiety disorder; investigation of the possible mechanisms whereby low socioeconomic status may play a role in the pathogenesis of anxiety disorders may ultimately lead to new avenues of prevention and management. It is increasingly recognized that specific psychosocial interventions may lead to particular brain changes; it is therefore not implausible that sociocultural variations result in different courses of anxiety disorders. Social anxiety disorder may, for example, be experienced somewhat differently in the West and the East. Similarly, it is possible that different reactions to severe trauma result in changes in the experience and expression of PTSD. Much additional research in this area is required.

◀ Key Clinical Points ▶

- Diagnosis of an anxiety disorder does not appear to be a category fallacy; these conditions are characterized by universal psychobiological mechanisms, and there are therefore important similarities in their symptoms and clinical features across cultures and social groups.
- At the same time, the expression and experience of anxiety disorders can be molded in important ways by sociocultural contexts. It is useful for clinicians to determine the explanatory models that patients have of their disorders. This allows clinician and patient to negotiate a shared understanding of symptoms and an approach to treatment.
- A balance is needed between understanding anxiety disorders from the perspective of their being a disease and from the perspective of their being an illness; for example, in the aftermath of trauma, it is important to encourage an expectation of recovery, but also to be aware that some patients will develop PTSD, which requires intervention.

References

American Psychiatric Association: Diagnostic and Statistical Manual of Mental Disorders, 4th Edition, Text Revision. Washington, DC, American Psychiatric Association, 2000

Anderson DJ, Noyes R, Crowe RR: A comparison of panic disorder and generalized anxiety disorder. Am J Psychiatry 141:572–575, 1984

Awaritefe A: Clinical anxiety in Nigeria. Acta Psychiatr Scand 77:729–735, 1988

Baxter LR, Schwartz JM, Bergman KS, et al: Caudate glucose metabolic rate changes with both drug and behavior therapy for OCD. Arch Gen Psychiatry 49:681–689, 1992

Bhaskar R: A Realist Theory of Science, 2nd Edition. Hassocks, Sussex, UK, Harvester Press, 1978

Boas F: Recent anthropology. Science 98:311–314, 1943

Brown DR, Eaton WW, Sussman L: Racial differences in prevalence of phobic disorders. J Nerv Ment Dis 178:434–441, 1990

Carothers J: The African Mind in Health and Disease: A Study in Ethnopsychiatry. Geneva, World Health Organization, 1953

Clarvit SR, Schneier FR, Liebowitz MR: The offensive subtype of taijin-kyofu-sho in New York City: the phenomenology and treatment of a social anxiety disorder. J Clin Psychiatry 57:523–527, 1996

Conrad P, Schneider J: Deviance and Medicalization: From Badness to Sickness. St Louis, MO, Mosby, 1980

Cooper R: What is wrong with the DSM? Hist Psychiatry 15:5–25, 2004

de Bilbao F, Giannakopoulos P: Effect of religious culture on obsessive compulsive disorder symptomatology: a transcultural study in monotheistic religions [in French]. Rev Med Suisse 30:2818–2821, 2005

Dohrenwend BP, Levav I, Shrout PE, et al: Socioeconomic status and psychiatric disorders: the causation-selection issue. Science 255:946–952, 1992

Ebigbo PO: A cross sectional study of somatic complaints of Nigerian females using the Enugu Somatization Scale. Cult Med Psychiatry 10:167–186, 1986

Fabrega H: Psychiatric diagnosis: a cultural perspective. J Nerv Ment Dis 175:383–394, 1987

Friedman S (ed): Cultural Issues in the Treatment of Anxiety. New York, Guilford, 1997

Gangdev P, Stein DJ, Ruzibiza JB: Obsessive-compulsive disorder in African South Africans. S Afr Med J 86:1592–1598, 1996

Good BJ, Good MD: Towards a meaning-centred analysis of popular illness categories: "fright-illness" and "heart distress" in Iran, in Cultural Conceptions of Mental Health and Therapy. Edited by Marsella AJ, White GM. Boston, MA, Dordrecht, 1982, pp 141–166

Good BJ, Kleinman AM: Culture and anxiety: cross-cultural evidence for the patterning of anxiety disorders, in Anxiety and the Anxiety Disorders. Edited by Tuma AH, Maser J. Hillsdale, NJ, Erlbaum, 1985, pp 297–323

Gorman JM, Kent JM, Sullivan GM, et al: Neuroanatomical hypothesis of panic disorder, revised. Am J Psychiatry 157:493–505, 2000

Greenberg D, Witztum E: Cultural aspects of obsessive compulsive disorder, in Current Insights in Obsessive Compulsive Disorder. Edited by Hollander E, Zohar J, Marazzati D, et al: Chichester, UK, Wiley, 1994, pp 11–21

Guarnaccia PJ, Kirmayer LJ: Culture and the anxiety disorders, in DSM-IV Sourcebook, Vol 3. Edited by Widiger TA, Frances A, Pincus HA, et al. Washington, DC, American Psychiatric Press, 1997, pp 925–932

Hahn RA, Kleinman A: Biomedical practice and anthropological theory. Ann Rev Anthropol 12:305–333, 1983

Han S, Northoff G: Culture-sensitive neural substrates of human cognition: a transcultural neuroimaging approach Nat Rev Neurosci 9:646–654, 2008

Hollander E, Cohen LJ: Obsessive-compulsive disorder, in Anxiety Disorders in African Americans. Edited by Friedman S. New York, Springer, 1994, pp 185–202

Jones E, Hodgins-Vermaas R, McCartney H, et al: Post-combat syndromes from the Boer war to the Gulf war: a cluster analysis of their nature and attribution. Br Med J 324:321–324, 2002

Kaminer D, Stein DJ, Mbanga I, et al: The Truth and Reconciliation Commission in South Africa: relation to psychiatric status and forgiveness among survivors of human rights abuses. Br J Psychiatry 178:373–377, 2001

Karno M, Golding JM, Sorenson SB, et al: The epidemiology of obsessive-compulsive disorder in five US communities. Arch Gen Psychiatry 45:1094–1099, 1988

Kessler RC, McGonagle KA, Zhao S, et al: Lifetime and 12-month prevalence of DSM-III-R psychiatric disorders in the United States. Arch Gen Psychiatry 51:8–19, 1994

Kirmayer L: The place of culture in psychiatric nosology: taijin kyofusho and DSM-III-R. J Nerv Ment Dis 179:19–28, 1991

Kizu A, Miyoshi N, Yoshida Y, et al: A case with fear of emitting body odour resulted in successful treatment with clomipramine. Hokkaido Igaku Zasshi 69:1477–1480, 1994

Klein DF: Delineation of two drug-responsive anxiety syndromes. Psychopharmacologia 5:397–408, 1964

Klein DF: Anxiety reconceptualized, in Anxiety: New Research and Changing Concepts. Edited by Klein DF, Rabkin J. New York, Raven, 1981, pp 235–264

Klein DF: False suffocation alarms, spontaneous panics, and related conditions: an integrative hypothesis. Arch Gen Psychiatry 50:306–317, 1993

Kleinknecht RA, Dinnel DL, Tanouye-Wilson S, et al: Cultural variation in social anxiety and phobia: a study of Taijin Kyofusho. Behav Ther 17:175–178, 1994

Kleinman A: Depression, somatisation, and the new "cross-cultural psychiatry." Soc Sci Med 11:3–10, 1977

Kleinman A: Patients and Healers in the Context of Culture: An Exploration of the Borderland Between Anthropology, Medicine, and Psychiatry. Los Angeles, University of California Press, 1980

Kleinman A: Rethinking Psychiatry: From Cultural Category to Personal Experience. New York, Free Press, 1988

Lambo TA: Malignant anxiety: a syndrome associated with criminal conduct in Africans. J Ment Sci 108:256–264, 1962

Leary MR, Meadows S: Predictors, elicitors, and concomitants of social blushing. J Pers Soc Psychol 60:254–262, 1991

LeDoux JE: The Emotional Brain: The Mysterious Underpinnings of Emotional Life. New York, Simon and Schuster, 1996

Leff J: The "new cross-cultural psychiatry." Br J Psychiatry 157:296–297, 1990

Lewis-Fernández R, Turner JB, Marshall R, et al: Elevated rates of current PTSD among Hispanic veterans in the NVVRS: true prevalence or methodological artifact? J Trauma Stress 21:123–132, 2008

Liebowitz MR, Salman E, Jusino CM, et al: Ataque de nervios and panic disorder. Am J Psychiatry 151:871–875, 1994

Littlewood R: From categories to contexts: a decade of the "new cross-cultural psychiatry." Br J Psychiatry 156:308–327, 1990

Marks IM: Fears, Phobias, and Rituals: Panic, Anxiety, and Their Disorders. Oxford, UK, Oxford University Press, 1987

Marsella AJ, Friedman MJ, Gerrity ET, et al: Ethnocultural aspects of PTSD: some closing thoughts, in Ethnocultural Aspects of Posttraumatic Stress Disorder: Issues, Research, and Clinical Applications. Edited by Marsella AJ, Friedman MJ, Gerrity ET, et al. Washington, DC, American Psychological Association, 1996, pp 529–538

Matsunaga H, Kiriike N, Matsui T, et al: Taijin kyofusho: a form of social anxiety disorder that responds to serotonin reuptake inhibitors? Int J Neuropsychopharmacol 4:231–237, 2001

Neal AM, Turner SM: Anxiety disorders research with African Americans: current status. Psychol Bull 109:400–410, 1991

Nesse RM: An evolutionary perspective on panic disorder and agoraphobia. Ethology and Neurobiology 8(suppl):73S–83S, 1987

Okasha A, Saad A, Khalil AH, et al: Phenomenology of obsessive-compulsive disorder: a transcultural study. Compr Psychiatry 35:191–197, 1994

Papp LA, Klein DF, Gorman JM: Carbon dioxide hypersensitivity, hyperventilation, and panic disorder. Am J Psychiatry 150:1149–1157, 1993

Pine DS, Weese-Mayer DE, Silvestri JM, et al: Anxiety and congenital central hypoventilation syndrome. Am J Psychiatry 151:864–870, 1994

Prince R, Tcheng-Larouche F: Culture-bound syndromes and international disease classifications. Cult Med Psychiatry 11:3–20, 1987

Rapoport JL, Ryland DH, Kriete M: Drug treatment of canine acral lick: an animal model of obsessive-compulsive disorder. Arch Gen Psychiatry 48:517–521, 1992

Salman E, Diamond K, Jusino C, et al: Hispanic Americans, in Cultural Issues in the Treatment of Anxiety. Edited by Friedman S. New York, Guilford, 1997, pp 59–80

Shay J: Achilles in Vietnam: Combat Trauma and the Undoing of Character. New York, Atheneum, 1994

Simons RC: Sorting the culture-bound syndromes, in The Culture-Bound Syndromes: Folk Illnesses of Psychiatric and Anthropological Interest. Edited by Simons RC, Hughes CC. Boston, Dordrecht, 1985, pp 25–38

Spielberger C, Diaz-Guerrero R (eds): Cross-Cultural Anxiety. London, Taylor & Francis, 1990

Stamm BH, Friedman MJ: Cultural diversity in the appraisal and expression of trauma, in International Handbook of Human Response to Trauma. Edited by Shalev AY, Yehuda R, McFarlane AC. New York, Kluwer Academic/Plenum, 2000, pp 69–86

Starcevic V, Djordjevic A, Latas M, et al: Characteristics of agoraphobia in women and men with panic disorder with agoraphobia. Depress Anxiety 8:8–13, 1998

Stein DJ: Cross-cultural psychiatry and the DSM-IV. Compr Psychiatry 34:322–329, 1993

Stein DJ: Philosophy of Psychopharmacology: Happy Pills, Smart Pills, and Pep Pills. Cambridge, UK, Cambridge University Press, 2008

Stein DJ, Bouwer C: Blushing and social phobia: a neuroethological speculation. Med Hypotheses 49:101–108, 1997

Stein DJ, Matsunaga H: Cross-cultural aspects of social anxiety disorder. Psychiatr Clin N Am 24:773–782, 2001

Stein DJ, Rapoport JL: Cross-cultural studies and obsessive-compulsive disorder. CNS Spectr 1:42–46, 1996

Stein DJ, Frenkel M, Hollander E: Classification of koro. Am J Psychiatry 148:1278–1280, 1991

Stein DJ, Shoulberg N, Helton K, et al: The neuroethological model of obsessive-compulsive disorder. Compr Psychiatry 33:274–281, 1992

Stein DJ, Le Roux L, Bouwer C, et al: Is olfactory reference syndrome on the obsessive-compulsive spectrum? Two cases and a discussion. J Neuropsychiatry Clin Neurosci 10:96–99, 1998

Stein DJ, Seedat S, Iversen A, et al: Post-traumatic stress disorder: medicine and politics. Lancet 369:139–144, 2007

Stein MB, Stein DJ: Social anxiety disorder. Lancet 371:1115–1125, 2008

Swedo SE: Rituals and releasers: an ethological model of obsessive-compulsive disorder, in Rapoport JL (ed): Obsessive-Compulsive Disorder in Children and Adolescents. Washington, DC, American Psychiatric Press, 1989, pp 269–288

Tinbergen H: Social Behavior in Animals. London, Chapman & Hall, 1953

Trower P, Gilbert P: New theoretical conceptions of social phobia. Clin Psychol Rev 9:19–35, 1989

Tseng W, Asai M, Kitanishi K, et al: Diagnostic patterns of social phobia: comparison in Tokyo and Hawaii. J Nerv Ment Dis 180:380–386, 1992

van Praag HM, Asnis GM, Kahn RS, et al: Monoamines and abnormal behaviour: a multi-aminergic perspective. Br J Psychiatry 157:723–734, 1990

Weine SM, Kulenovic AD, Pavkovic I, et al: Testimony psychotherapy in Bosnian refugees: a pilot study. Am J Psychiatry 155:1720–1726, 1998

Weissman MM, Bland RC, Canino GJ, et al: The cross-national epidemiology of obsessive compulsive disorder: the Cross National Collaborative Group. J Clin Psychiatry 55(March, suppl):5–10, 1994

Weissman MM, Bland RC, Canino GJ, et al: The cross-national epidemiology of social phobia: a preliminary report. Int Clin Psychopharmacol 11(suppl):9–14, 1996

Westmeyer J: Cultural factors in clinical assessment. J Consult Clin Psychol 55:471–478, 1987

World Health Organization: International Statistical Classification of Diseases and Related Health Problems, 10th Revision. Geneva, World Health Organization, 1992

Wright P, Treacher A (eds): The Problem of Medical Knowledge: Examining the Social Construction of Medicine. Edinburgh, UK, Edinburgh University Press, 1982

Yap PM: Mental diseases peculiar to certain cultures: a survey of comparative psychiatry. J Ment Sci 97:313–327, 1951

Yap PM: Words and things in comparative psychiatry, with special reference to the exotic psychoses. Acta Psychiatr Scand 38:163–169, 1962

Yehuda R, McFarlane AC: Conflict between current knowledge about posttraumatic stress disorder and its original conceptual basis. Am J Psychiatry 152:1705–1713, 1995

Yeomans PD, Herbert JD, Forman EM: Symptom comparison across multiple solicitation methods among Burundians with traumatic event histories. J Trauma Stress 21:231–234, 2008

Young A: The discourse on stress and the reproduction of conventional knowledge. Soc Sci Med 14:133–146, 1980

Yu Y, Williams DR: Socioeconomic status and mental health, in Handbook of the Sociology of Mental Health. Edited by Aneshensel CS, Phelan J. New York, Plenum, 1999, pp 151–166

Recommended Readings

Ballenger JC, Davidson JR, Lecrubier Y, et al: Consensus statement on transcultural issues in depression and anxiety from the International Consensus Group on Depression and Anxiety. J Clin Psychiatry 62 (suppl 13):47–55, 2001

Friedman S (ed): Cultural Issues in the Treatment of Anxiety. New York, Guilford, 1997

Greenberg D, Witztum E: Cultural aspects of obsessive compulsive disorder, in Current Insights in Obsessive Compulsive Disorder. Edited by Hollander E, Zohar J, Marazzati D, et al. Chichester, UK, Wiley, 1994, pp 11–21

Kleinman A: Rethinking Psychiatry: From Cultural Category to Personal Experience. New York, Free Press, 1988

Stein DJ, Matsunaga H: Cross-cultural aspects of social anxiety disorder. Psychiatr Clin N Am 24:773–782, 2001

Stein DJ, Seedat S, Iversen A, et al: Post-traumatic stress disorder: medicine and politics. Lancet 369:139–144, 2007

Chapter 40

The Economic and Social Burden of Anxiety Disorders

David F. Tolin, Ph.D.
Christina M. Gilliam, Ph.D.
Danielle Dufresne, M.A.

In 2007, the United States spent over $2 trillion on health care; by 2016, this figure is expected to rise to $4.2 trillion, or 20% of the gross domestic product (Poisal et al. 2007). Chronic diseases cost over $1 trillion, with mental disorders accounting for 16% of this cost (DeVol and Bedroussian 2007). Globally, mental disorders account for 5 of the top 10 causes of years lived with disability (Murray and Lopez 1996). The aim of this chapter is to describe the burden of anxiety disorders from an economic and quality-of-life perspective. After reviewing research on the prevalence of anxiety disorders, we describe the financial burden of anxiety in terms of its direct and indirect costs, including new analyses showing the impact of anxiety disorders on work impairment and income. We also discuss the effect of anxiety on quality of life at the individual and family level. Finally, we discuss the potential for effective treatment to improve quality of life and reduce the overall burden of illness for those suffering from anxiety disorders.

Prevalence of Anxiety Disorders

The prevalence of mental disorders in the United States was first examined in the Epidemiologic Catchment Area (ECA) study (Regier et al. 1988, 1990), followed by the National Comorbidity Survey (NCS) (Kessler et al. 1994) and the National Comorbidity Survey Replication (NCS-R) (Kessler et al. 2005a, 2005b) (see Table 40–1). Using diagnostic criteria from DSM-III (American Psychiatric Association 1980), DSM-III-R (American Psychiatric Association 1987), and DSM-IV (American Psychiatric Association 1994), respectively, these studies describe the current and lifetime prevalence of a broad range of mental disorders, including anxiety disorders. As shown in Table 40–1, all three epidemiologic surveys showed a high lifetime prevalence of anxiety disorders (ranging from 16% in the ECA to 29% in the NCS-R), with rates equaling or exceeding those of affective disorders and substance use disorders. Similar results have been found in other countries. The World Health Organization (WHO) found 12-month rates of anxiety disorders ranging from 6% to 12% in Europe and from 2% to 5% in Asia; despite these international discrepancies, the rates of anxiety disorders consistently equaled or exceeded those of mood, impulse control, and substance use disorders (WHO World Mental Health Survey Consortium 2004). Examining data across 27 studies of the European Union, Wittchen and Jacobi (2005) estimated

TABLE 40–1. 12-month and lifetime prevalence of anxiety disorders

	ECA study		NCS		NCS-R		Clinical Significance Revision
Disorder	**Current**	**Lifetime**	**Current[b]**	**Lifetime**	**Current[b]**	**Lifetime**	**Current[b]**
Panic disorder	0.8[a]	1.4	2.3	3.5	2.7	4.7	1.4
Phobia	8.5[a]	14.0	—	—	—	—	—
Agoraphobia without panic	—	—	2.8	5.3	0.8	1.4	2.1
Social phobia	—	—	7.9	13.3	6.8	12.1	3.2
Simple (specific) phobia	—	—	8.8	11.3	8.7	12.5	4.3
Generalized anxiety disorder	2.3[b]	—	3.1	5.1	3.1	5.7	2.8
Obsessive-compulsive disorder	1.6[a]	2.5	—	—	1.0	1.6	2.1
Posttraumatic stress disorder	—	1.0	—	7.8	3.5	6.8	3.6
Separation anxiety disorder	—	—	—	—	0.9	5.2	—
Any anxiety	9.8[a]	16.0	17.2	24.9	18.1	28.8	11.8
Any affective	5.7[a]	7.8	11.3	19.3	9.5	20.8	5.1
Any substance use	6.4[a]	16.7	11.3	26.6	3.8	14.6	6.0

[a]6-month prevalence.
[b]12-month prevalence.

Source. Epidemiologic Catchment Area (ECA) study (Blazer et al. 1987; Helzer et al. 1987; Regier et al. 1990; Robins et al. 1984), National Comorbidity Survey (NCS) (Kessler et al. 1994, 1995), National Comorbidity Survey Replication (NCS-R) (Kessler et al. 2005a, 2005b), and Clinical Significance Revision of the ECA and NCS (Narrow et al. 2002).

median 12-month prevalence rates ranging from 0.7% for obsessive-compulsive disorder (OCD) to 6.4% for specific phobia; the prevalence of any anxiety disorder was 12%, higher than those of mood, substance dependence, psychotic, somatoform, or eating disorders.

It is noteworthy that the NCS and NCS-R yielded substantially higher rates of anxiety disorders than did the earlier ECA. To some extent, these discrepancies can be attributed to changes in diagnostic criteria after DSM-III, the absence of older adults (age 55 or above) in the NCS, and subtle differences in the interview questions (Regier et al. 1998). To reconcile the ECA and NCS further, Narrow et al. (2002) applied questions concerning clinical significance (e.g., interference with functioning, service utilization) so that a disorder was considered present only if symptoms were described as causing substantial distress or impairment. As shown in Table 40–1, 1-year prevalence estimates were reduced, although rates of anxiety disorders overall (11.8%) remained higher than those of affective disorders (5.1%) and substance use disorders (6%).

Factors Associated With Increased Risk of Anxiety Disorders

Gender

Women were approximately twice as likely as men to report lifetime anxiety disorder in the ECA (odds ratio [OR]=2.2), NCS (OR=1.8), and NCS-R (OR=1.6). By comparison, "externalizing" disorders (e.g., conduct disorders, substance use disorders) appear more prevalent in men than in women (Kessler et al. 2005b). (A more detailed discussion of the relationship between gender and anxiety disorders can be found in Craske 2003.)

Age

The NCS yielded the highest rates of 12-month and lifetime anxiety disorders in respondents ages 15–24 years, with decreasing rates of illness in older respondents. The NCS-R showed a slightly different pattern, with the greatest prevalence among respondents ages 30–44 (35.1%), followed by ages 45–59 (30.8%), 18–29 (30.2%), and 60 and older (15.3%). This pattern was similar to that obtained in the earlier ECA, in which the highest current prevalence was seen in respondents ages 25–44 (8.3%), followed by ages 18–24 (7.7%), 45–64 (6.6%), and age 65 and older (5.5%). Therefore, all three epidemiologic surveys found the lowest rates of anxiety disorders among their oldest participants, with risk of anxiety disorders peaking at some point between ages 15 and 44. The fact that lifetime rates of anxiety disorders are lowest in the oldest respondent groups suggests one of two possibilities. First, the decreased rates may reflect cohort differences rather than age differences. Second, the structured interviews used in these surveys may systematically underestimate the presence of anxiety-related symptoms among older respondents.

Race/Ethnicity

The NCS found no significant differences in rates of lifetime anxiety disorder between White and Nonwhite respondents. In the NCS-R, however, non-Hispanic black and Hispanic respondents showed significantly lower rates of lifetime anxiety disorder than did white respondents (OR=0.8 and 0.7, respectively). The ECA found higher rates of anxiety disorders among black respondents compared with white and Hispanic respondents, although these differences were no longer significant when controlling for socioeconomic status.

Socioeconomic Status

The ECA yielded the highest rates of anxiety disorders (phobia, panic disorder, and OCD) among participants in the lowest socioeconomic status (SES) group (10.5%), with a linear decline in anxiety rates with increasing SES. The highest SES group showed only a 4.6% rate of current (1 month) anxiety disorders. In the NCS, rates of lifetime and current (12 months) anxiety disorders (and all other disorders) were lowest among respondents with a yearly household income of $70,000 or more (approximately $103,000 in 2007 dollars). A linear increase in risk of anxiety disorders was found with lower income, with the highest rates (OR=2 lifetime, 2.12 current) seen in respondents earning $19,000 or less (approximately $28,000 in 2007 dollars). The lowest rates of anxiety disorders (and all other disorders) also were seen among respondents with 16 or more years of education, with the highest rates (OR=1.86 lifetime, 2.82 current) in those with less than a high school education.

In summary, anxiety disorders are among the most prevalent of all mental disorders according to three large-scale epidemiologic surveys. Women are at increased risk for anxiety disorders, as are individuals with low SES. There is some evidence to suggest that older adults are at lower risk than are their younger counterparts, although cohort effects cannot be ruled out. The impact of race and ethnicity on risk of anxiety disorders is unclear.

Estimating the Economic Burden of Anxiety Disorders

Psychiatric Work Impairment

One way to measure the economic burden of anxiety disorders is to examine the extent of work or role impairment. In the NCS, participants were asked about *psychiatric work loss days* (number of days in the past month that the respondent was unable to work or carry out usual activities due to mental health issues) and *psychiatric work cutback days* (number of days in the past month that the respondent was less effective at work or in activities due to mental health issues) in the past 30 days (Kessler and Frank 1997). *Psychiatric work impairment days* are then calculated from the combination of psychiatric work loss and cutback days. Previous research with the NCS (Kessler and Frank 1997) as well as the Australian National Survey of Mental Health and Well-Being (Lim et al. 2000) has indicated that all of the anxiety disorders assessed in those surveys were associated with a significantly increased number of psychiatric work impairment days, with particularly high rates of work impairment days seen in respondents meeting criteria for panic disorder, generalized anxiety disorder (GAD), posttraumatic stress disorder (PTSD), and agoraphobia.

In this chapter we examine psychiatric work impairment in the Collaborative Psychiatric Epidemiology Surveys (CPES), a compilation of three nationally representative surveys (*N*=20,013), conducted by the Institute for Social Research at the University of Michigan. The core CPES questionnaire was based largely on the World Mental Health Composite International Diagnostic Interview (WMH-CIDI), a standardized psychiatric diagnostic interview developed for administration by lay interviewers. The three surveys comprising the CPES are:

1. NCS-R (Kessler and Merikangas 2004). The NCS-R was administered in two parts. Part 1 included a core diagnostic assessment of all 9,282 respondents. Part 2 included questions about risk factors, consequences, other correlates, and additional disorders. Part 2 was administered to only 5,692 of the 9,282 Part 1 respondents.
2. National Survey of American Life (NSAL) (Jackson et al. 2004). The NSAL was designed to explore racial and ethnic differences in mental disorders and service utilization in African-American (*N*=3,570) and Afro-Caribbean (*N*=1,621) populations of the United States as compared with non-Hispanic white respondents (*N*=891) living in the same communities.
3. National Latino and Asian American Study (NLAAS) (Alegria et al. 2004). The NLAAS examined the prevalence of mental disorders and service utilization by Latinos and Asian Americans in the United States. The NLAAS survey was administered to Latino (*N*=2,554) and Asian-American (*N*=2,095) adults as well as a small sample of non-Latino whites (*N*=215).

All of these surveys consisted of home-based interviews of noninstitutionalized adults ages 18 and older living in the United States. The NCS-R and NSAL were conducted from 2001 to 2003; the NLAAS was conducted from 2002 to 2003.

As was done with previous research (Kessler et al. 2001), for the present analyses the number of psychiatric work impairment days was calculated as the number of psychiatric work loss days plus 50% of the number of psychiatric work cutback days. Although studies have differed in how psychiatric work impairment was calculated, this method is now preferred (R.C. Kessler, personal communication, February 10, 2007).

Information about psychiatric work loss and work cutback days was available from 14,162 CPES respondents, allowing for the calculation of psychiatric work impairment days over the last 30-day period. Table 40–2 shows the average number of psychiatric work impairment days for respondents meeting DSM-IV criteria for anxiety disorders within the past 30 days. For each anxiety disorder, those with and without the condition (even if other mental disorders were present) were compared using independent-sample *t*-tests as well as the effect size estimate *d*, for which values of 0.2, 0.5, and 0.8 are interpreted conventionally to mean small, medium, and large effects, respectively (Cohen 1988). As shown in the table, anxiety disorders overall were associated with a mean 2.2 psychiatric work impairment days per month, with the greatest number of impairment days seen in respondents meeting criteria for agoraphobia, adult separation anxiety disorder, PTSD, panic disorder, and OCD. All anxiety disorders were associated with a significantly higher rate of work impairment, compared to those without the disorder.

Next, we compared respondents with current anxiety disorders (*N*=1,433), those with remitted anxiety disorders (*N*=1,491), and those with no history of anxiety disorders (*N*=2,644). The three groups differed

TABLE 40–2. Psychiatric work impairment days in the past 30 days, according to 30-day anxiety disorder diagnoses

DSM-IV diagnosis	*N*	Mean (SD) impairment days	*t* versus those without disorder	*d* versus those without disorder
Adult separation anxiety disorder	72	4.74 (8.14)	12.49*	0.68
Agoraphobia without panic disorder	99	5.57 (8.70)	19.81*	0.80
Generalized anxiety disorder	105	1.52 (4.24)	4.01*	0.29
Obsessive-compulsive disorder[a]	92	3.23 (6.01)	9.92*	0.60
Panic disorder	146	3.50 (6.03)	14.13*	0.65
Posttraumatic stress disorder	131	3.90 (7.16)	13.84*	0.62
Social phobia	432	2.59 (5.82)	17.12*	0.48
Specific phobia	492	1.97 (5.20)	11.27*	0.37
Any anxiety disorder	1,245	2.23 (5.40)	19.08*	0.47

Note. t=Student's t-test, ; d=Cohen's d (effect size).

*$P<0.001$.

[a]Calculated according to the presence of obsessions or compulsions plus interference attributed to obsessions or compulsions or presence of symptoms for more than 60 minutes per day.

in psychiatric work impairment days ($F_{2,\,5{,}565}$=196.84, $P<0.001$). Tukey honestly significant difference (HSD) post hoc tests revealed significant differences among all three groups ($P<0.05$; see Figure 40–1). Thus, even individuals with remitted anxiety disorders exhibit residual work impairment.

Income

We identified the proportion of respondents in each group whose household income was below the federal poverty line for a family of that size. Chi-square analysis indicated that the three groups differed, $\chi^2(2)=125.971$, $P<0.001$. Respondents with current anxiety disorders were more likely to live below the federal poverty threshold (22.4%) than were those with remitted (10.2%) or no anxiety disorders (11.5%). As shown in Figure 40–2, the highest poverty rates were seen among respondents with OCD. Over one-third of respondents with OCD or agoraphobia were below the federal poverty line; over one-quarter of those with panic disorder, separation anxiety disorder, and social phobia were below the poverty line.

Overall Cost to Society

Psychiatric work impairment is only one of several possible contributors to the economic burden of anxiety. Historically, economic burden of illness has been defined as including *direct costs* and *indirect costs.* Direct costs include psychiatric service costs (e.g., counseling and hospitalizations), nonpsychiatric medical costs (e.g., emergency room treatment), and the costs of medications. Indirect costs include lost productivity resulting from suicide (mortality), excessive absenteeism, or reduced work capacity.

In the first major examination of the overall financial costs of anxiety disorders, DuPont et al. (1996a) reanalyzed data from survey respondents with panic disorder with and without agoraphobia, social phobia, simple phobia, OCD, and GAD (importantly, however, PTSD was not assessed). Similarly, Greenberg et al. (1999) reanalyzed data from the NCS, supplemented by cost data from a health maintenance organization, the U.S. Census Bureau, costs from professional associations and news periodicals, suicide data from the National Center for Health Statistics, and industry sources regarding prescription drugs. Anxiety disorders included in this review were panic disorder, agoraphobia, PTSD, social phobia, simple phobia, and GAD (however, OCD was not assessed).

Overall, these two studies found relatively similar costs of anxiety disorders: Dupont et al. (1996a) estimated the total cost to be $46.6 billion in 1990 (approximately $73.9 billion in 2007 dollars), or 31.5% of the total economic burden of mental illness. Greenberg et al. (1999) estimated this cost to be $42.3 billion in 1990 (approximately $67.1 billion in 2007 dollars). However,

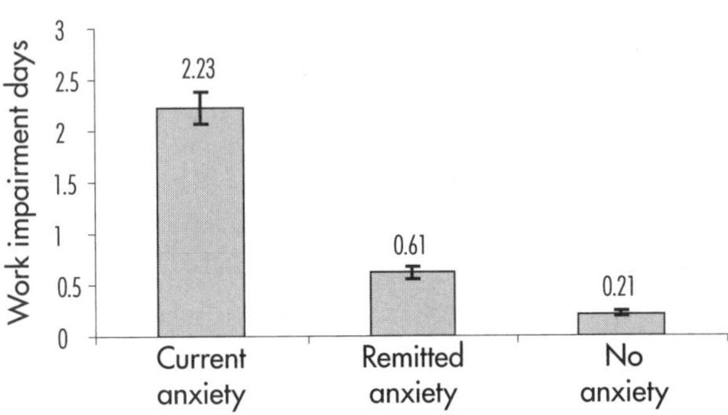

FIGURE 40–1. Psychiatric work impairment in respondents with current, remitted, or no anxiety disorders.

Mean (standard error) psychiatric work impairment days in the past month for respondents with current anxiety disorders, those with remitted (lifetime but not in the past 30 days) anxiety disorders, and those with no history of anxiety disorders.

as shown in Figure 40–3, the distribution of costs was quite different between the two studies. Dupont et al. reported that approximately three-quarters of the total cost of anxiety disorders stemmed from indirect costs, particularly income loss from work ($34.2 billion, or $54.2 billion in 2007 dollars). Mortality costs added $1.3 billion ($2.1 billion in 2007 dollars) to the indirect costs. Direct costs accounted for less than one-quarter of the total cost, $10.7 billion ($17.0 billion in 2007 dollars). Of the direct costs, nursing home costs accounted for the largest percentage ($5.5 billion, or $8.7 billion in 2007 dollars), followed by prescription drug costs ($1.2 billion, or $1.9 billion in 2007 dollars), nonphysician mental health visits ($645 million, or $1.0 billion in 2007 dollars), short-stay hospital care ($388 million, or $615 million in 2007 dollars), and office-based physician visits ($356 million, or $564 million in 2007 dollars).

Conversely, Greenberg et al. (1999) reported that 85% of the total costs were due to direct costs, particularly nonpsychiatric medical treatment ($23 billion, or $36.5 billion in 2007 dollars). Psychiatric treatment costs accounted for $13.3 billion ($21.1 billion in 2007 dollars), and pharmaceutical costs $759 million ($1.20 billion in 2007). Indirect costs, on the other hand, represented a much smaller proportion of the total costs. Total workplace costs accounted for $4.1 billion ($6.5 billion in 2007 dollars), followed by mortality costs ($1.2 billion, or $1.9 billion in 2007 dollars).

Why was the cost distribution so different, with DuPont et al. (1996a) showing mostly indirect costs and Greenberg et al. (1999) showing mostly direct costs? One possible contributor is the difference in patient groups between the two studies. DuPont et al. did not examine individuals with PTSD. In the Greenberg et al. study, individuals with PTSD were among the highest utilizers of health care services and were significantly more likely than those without PTSD to utilize virtu-

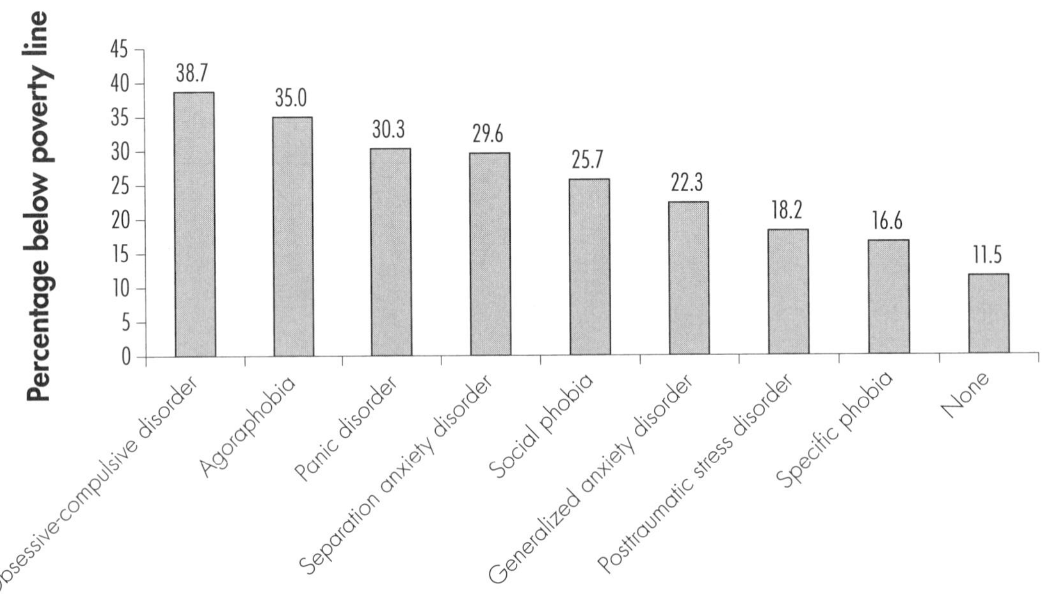

FIGURE 40–2. Proportion of respondents with current anxiety disorders living below the federal poverty line.

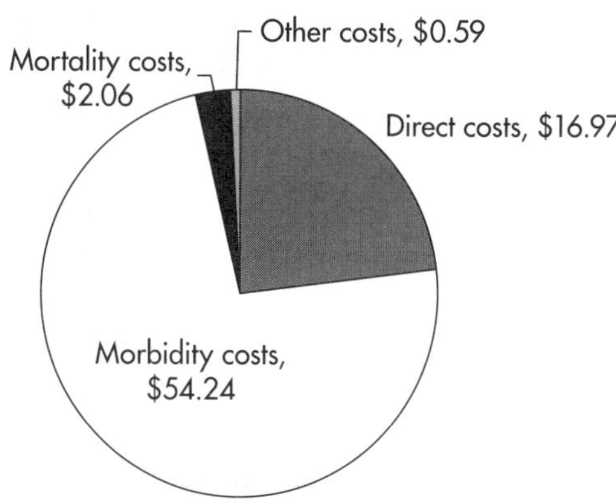

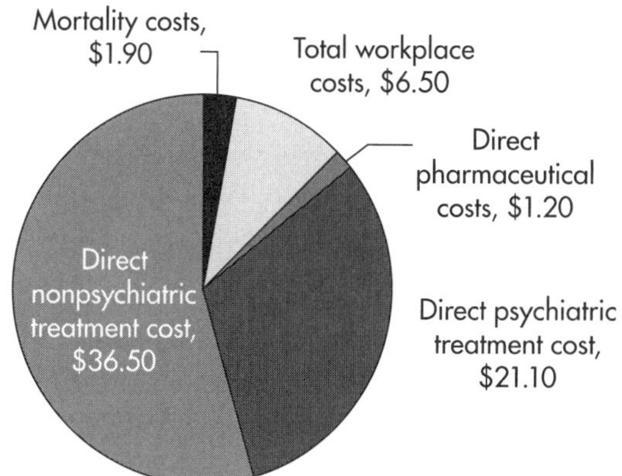

FIGURE 40–3. Economic costs of anxiety disorders.

Adjusted to 2007 dollars, in billions of dollars.

Source. Top: DuPont et al. 1996a, 1996b. Bottom: Greenberg et al. 1999.

ally all levels of mental health treatment, including psychiatric hospitalization. Among veterans seen in a Veteran's Affairs medical center, those suffering from PTSD demonstrated a greater number of medical conditions/complaints than did those without PTSD (Deykin et al. 2001) and were more likely to have received recent inpatient or outpatient medical treatment (Schnurr et al. 2000). PTSD is associated with substantially higher health care costs than are other anxiety disorders (Marciniak et al. 2005). Therefore, the inclusion of individuals with PTSD (as well as attention to the nonpsychiatric medical treatment of such individuals) might well have increased the direct cost estimates in that study. Greenberg et al. (using NCS data) did not examine individuals with OCD. Given the high rates of unemployment and reduced work capacity among individuals with OCD (DuPont et al. 1996b; Murray and Lopez 1996; Steketee et al. 1987), the inclusion of this population might have increased the indirect cost estimate. Another likely contributor to the difference is the expanded inclusion of direct nonpsychiatric medical costs in the Greenberg et al. study. In the DuPont et al. study, medical treatment visits were included only if they were associated with a primary or secondary diagnosis of an anxiety disorder.

Thus, in addition to being the most common forms of mental disorder, anxiety disorders are also among the most costly. All of the anxiety disorders are associated with significant impairment in work and role functioning, and even individuals whose anxiety disorders have remitted continue to report residual functional impairment. Individuals with anxiety disorders are significantly more likely than those without anxiety disorders to live below the poverty threshold, with poverty particularly common in individuals with OCD and agoraphobia. The relationship between anxiety and income might well be bidirectional: low SES may increase the risk of developing anxiety disorders, and the presence of anxiety-related symptoms can add to work impairment and subsequently reduce income from work. The overall economic burden of anxiety disorders is estimated at $67–$74 billion in 2007 dollars. The breakdown of expenditures (e.g., direct vs. indirect costs) is not clear, although direct costs of psychiatric treatment clearly do not account for the majority of the cost. Rather, direct costs of nonpsychiatric medical treatment (e.g., emergency room visits, general practitioner visits) and lost revenue from work appear to be stronger contributors.

Estimating the Social Burden of Anxiety Disorders

Family Burden

Although considerable research has been conducted on the impact of mental illness (e.g., schizophrenia) on the family, anxiety disorders have received considerably less attention in this regard; most of the existing studies examined family burden in relation to OCD and (typically combat-related) PTSD. Overall, family members of patients with OCD and PTSD generally report levels of distress, impairment, and burden comparable to those of patients with severe mental illness, such as schizophrenia (Kalra et al. 2008; Veltro et al. 1994).

Anxiety disorders such as OCD and PTSD appear to have a negative impact on partner relationships, with patients and their partners in both groups reporting high levels of relationship distress (Cook et al. 2004; Cooper 1996; Dekel et al. 2005; Jordan et al. 1992;

Riggs et al. 1998). Among veterans with PTSD, emotional numbing has been identified as a specific symptom associated with greater relationship distress (Cook et al. 2004; Riggs et al. 1998). Further, the presence of combat-related PTSD appears to increase the risk of interpersonal physical and verbal aggression (Beckham et al. 1997; Taft et al. 2007b) including domestic violence (Carroll et al. 1985; Taft et al. 2007a). Not surprisingly, individuals with OCD or PTSD are more likely to be divorced in comparison to individuals without these disorders (Card 1987; Karno et al. 1988).

In addition to partner relationship problems and distress, there is some evidence to suggest that anxiety disorders may negatively affect other aspects of family functioning. Individuals with OCD and veterans with PTSD both report problems with family functioning (Davidson and Mellor 2001; Hollander et al. 1996). Family members also report general family dysfunction (Davidson and Mellor 2001; Van Noppen and Steketee 2003) as well as specific burden in areas such as financial strain, disruption of family activities, and impaired family interactions (Black et al. 1998; Calvocoressi et al. 1995; Chakrabarti et al. 1993; Van Noppen and Steketee 2003; Verbosky and Ryan 1988). Similar to research findings on the potential impact of PTSD on partner relationships among veterans, emotional numbing appears to be particularly related to impairment in the relationship between the child and the veteran parent with PTSD (Ruscio et al. 2002).

Finally, an anxiety disorder in a family member has been associated with psychological distress, poor psychosocial functioning, and reduced quality of life among other members of the family. In some studies, family members of individuals with PTSD or OCD reported impairment in their social and leisure functioning as a result of their family member's illness (Black et al. 1998; Cooper 1996; Magliano et al. 1996; Stengler-Wenzke et al. 2006). In comparison to the general population, family members also reported lower levels of physical and psychological well-being (Stengler-Wenzke et al. 2006) and life satisfaction (Jordan et al. 1992), as well as poorer psychological adjustment such as greater general distress and psychiatric symptoms including depressive, obsessive-compulsive, and anxious symptoms (Calhoun et al. 2002; Dekel et al. 2005; Solomon et al. 1992; Waysman et al. 1993). Among family members of relatives with OCD, severity of family members' depressive and anxious symptoms was found to be related to degree of modifications made in routine activities because of OCD and the patient's reactions when the family member refused to assist in rituals (Amir et al. 2000). Some evidence indicates that children of veterans with PTSD exhibit greater behavioral, academic, and psychiatric problems than do children of veterans without PTSD or children of civilians (Caselli and Motta 1995; Davidson et al. 1989; Harkness 1991; Jordan et al. 1992).

Quality of Life

Quality of life is a multidimensional construct that extends beyond anxiety symptoms to include subjective well-being and life satisfaction (Angermeyer and Kilian 1997; Gladis et al. 1999). Documented quality of life problems in the anxiety disorders have included marital and financial problems in panic disorder (Weissman 1991), impaired relationships in social phobia (Eng et al. 2005; Stein and Kean 2000), high rates of public financial assistance and diminished subjective well-being in PTSD (Warshaw et al. 1993; Zatzick et al. 1997), role limitations in OCD (Hollander et al. 1996; Koran et al. 1996), and high rates of disability in GAD (Wittchen 2002).

Olatunji et al. (2007) have conducted a quantitative review of 32 patient samples from 23 separate studies (N=2,892). Effect size estimates were calculated between anxiety and control samples. Overall, there was a large effect size (d=1.31), indicating poorer quality of life among anxiety patients versus control subjects, with no significant difference seen between studies using epidemiologic versus treatment-seeking clinical samples. No diagnosis was associated with significantly poorer overall quality of life (compared with control samples) than was any other diagnosis. Across anxiety disorders, mental health and social functioning were rated as more impaired than was physical health.

Figure 40–4 shows, for each anxiety disorder, mean effect size estimates for specific quality of life domains (physical health, mental health, work, social, home and family). With few exceptions, each anxiety disorder was associated with large and significant effect sizes versus control samples. For physical health, all disorders except social phobia were associated with significant impairment. For mental health, the effect size for PTSD, GAD, panic disorder, and mixed anxiety was significantly higher than that for social phobia. For work, PTSD was associated with a significantly larger effect size estimate than was panic disorder. For social and home and family, there were no significant differences among the anxiety disorders.

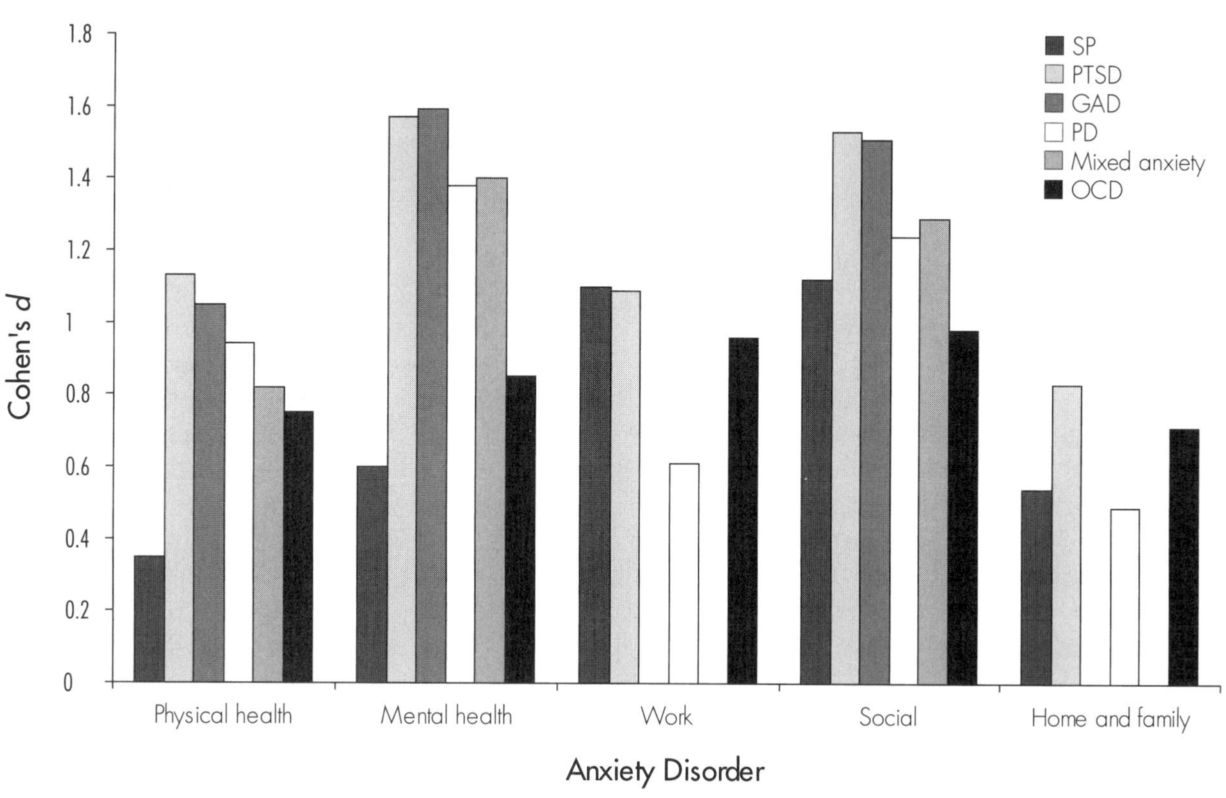

FIGURE 40–4. Effect size estimates for specific domains of quality of life in specific anxiety disorders compared with control samples.

SP=social phobia; PTSD=posttraumatic stress disorder; GAD=generalized anxiety disorder; PD=panic disorder; OCD=obsessive-compulsive disorder.

Source. Adapted from Olatunji et al. 2007.

The Effects of Treatment on Quality of Life Impairment

Pharmacotherapy

There has been considerable research on the impact of pharmacotherapy on quality of life among individuals with anxiety disorders. Patients with panic disorder have reported improvements in quality of life following treatment with different classes of medications, including selective serotonin reuptake inhibitors (SSRIs) (Bandelow et al. 2007; Hoehn-Saric et al. 1993; Michelson et al. 1998; Pohl et al. 1998; Pollack et al. 1998, 2007), serotonin-norepinephrine reuptake inhibitors (SNRIs) (Pollack et al. 2007), tricyclic antidepressants (Mavissakalian et al. 1998), and benzodiazepines (Jacobs et al. 1997). Bandelow et al. (2007) noted that the quality of life of patients with panic disorder fell within the normal range after escitalopram treatment on the Quality of Life Enjoyment and Satisfaction Questionnaire (Endicott et al. 1993), although Jacobs et al. (1997) reported that posttreatment quality of life scores of patients with panic disorder, although improved from pretreatment, ranked at the 17th percentile (indicating poorer quality of life) in comparison with the general population on the Medical Outcomes Study 36-Item Short-Form Health Survey (SF-36) (Ware and Kosinski 1994). Patients with PTSD have reported improvements in quality of life in response to treatment with SSRIs (Brady et al. 2000; Connor et al. 1999; Malik et al. 1999; Marshall et al. 1976; Rabin and de Charro 2001; Rapaport et al. 2002; Tucker et al. 2001) and nefazodone (McRae et al. 2004). For social phobia, there is evidence that quality of life is improved following treatment with mirtazapine (Muehlbacher et al. 2005) as well as SSRIs (M.B. Stein et al. 1998, 1999). Patients with GAD report significant improvements in quality of life following treatment with SSRIs (Pollack et al. 2001; D.J. Stein et al. 2005) as well as an adjunct course of an atypical antipsychotic to antidepressants (Menza et al. 2007). In one study, both an SNRI and

SSRI demonstrated comparable improvements in quality of life among patients with OCD (Tenney et al. 2003). With the exception of a few studies (Mavissakalian et al. 1998; Tenney et al. 2003), a placebo comparison group was employed, demonstrating that changes in quality of life from pre- to posttreatment were not attributable to nonspecific effects such as the passage of time, attention, expectancy, and so on.

Long-term effects of pharmacotherapy on quality of life are mixed. Patients with panic disorder generally report continued improvements in certain aspects of quality of life at follow-up (Lecrubier and Judge 1997; Mavissakalian et al. 1998; Rapaport et al. 2002). In one study, however, patients with panic disorder who discontinued SSRI medication after several months of treatment reported gradual deterioration in some aspects of their quality of life (Rapaport et al. 2002). Carpiniello et al. (2002) found that among patients who received pharmacotherapy in an outpatient clinic approximately 3 years prior, 60% reported a significant level of disability, and 40% reported being dissatisfied with at least 50% of assessed life domains.

Cognitive-Behavioral Therapy

Although research on the impact of cognitive-behavioral therapy (CBT) on quality of life in anxiety disorders has been less extensive compared with research on the impact of pharmacotherapy, the available evidence suggests that CBT is associated with significant improvements in various measures of quality of life. Improvements in quality of life following CBT have been found among patients with OCD (Bystritsky et al. 1999, 2001; Cordioli et al. 2003; Diefenbach et al. 2007; Moritz et al. 2005), panic disorder (Heldt et al. 2006; Telch et al. 1995), PTSD (Rabin and de Charro 2001), GAD (Stanley et al. 2003), and social phobia (Rapee et al. 2007). In studies utilizing a control group (e.g., minimal contact or wait-list control), those who received CBT generally reported significantly greater improvements in quality of life than did the control group, whereas the control group did not show significant changes in quality of life over the same time period (Cordioli et al. 2003; Rapee et al. 2007; Stanley et al. 2003; Telch et al. 1995). Improvements in quality of life following CBT appear to be not only statistically significant but also clinically meaningful. For example, patients with panic disorder who received group CBT fell in the 62nd percentile (indicating average quality of life) on the Social Adjustment Scale (Weissman and Bothwell 1976) in comparison with a community sample, whereas untreated (wait-list control) patients fell in the 89th percentile (suggesting worse quality of life) (Telch et al. 1995).

In general, improvements in quality of life at the end of treatment appear to be maintained at follow-up, with some loss of gains in certain areas compared with posttreatment (Cordioli et al. 2003; Stanley et al. 2003; Telch et al. 1995). For example, gains in quality of life were maintained at follow-up assessments 12 months following CBT for late-life GAD (Stanley et al. 2003). However, even "remitted" patients with panic disorder continued to report significantly worse quality of life compared with healthy control subjects at follow-up (Fava et al. 2001). Patients receiving combined pharmacotherapy and CBT generally appear to maintain improvements in work and social adjustment (O'Sullivan et al. 1991) as well as to demonstrate some mild improvements in social and occupational functioning from pretreatment to long-term follow-up in areas such as relationship and work status (Rufer et al. 2006).

Treatment Attainment

The good news, therefore, is that pharmacotherapy and CBT appear to have a positive impact not only on anxiety symptoms but also on quality of life more broadly. The bad news, however, is that most individuals with anxiety disorders never receive these treatments. In the NCS, for example, only one in four respondents meeting criteria for a psychiatric disorder obtained treatment from a mental health specialist (Kessler et al. 1994). These findings were replicated in the NCS-R: only 22% of respondents meeting diagnostic criteria for an anxiety disorder reported seeking treatment from a mental health professional, and 24% reported seeking mental health services from nonpsychiatric health care providers (e.g., primary care physicians). Among those with anxiety disorders, those with panic disorder (35%) and PTSD (34%) were most likely to seek treatment from a mental health professional, whereas those with specific phobia (19%), social phobia (25%), and GAD (26%) were less likely to seek such treatment. Compared with respondents with affective disorders, those with anxiety disorders were less likely to seek treatment for their condition from either mental health professionals (33% affective disorders vs. 22% anxiety disorders) or from general medical practitioners (33% affective disorders vs. 24% anxiety disorders) (Wang et al. 2005).

Equally concerning is the finding that even when individuals with anxiety disorder seek treatment from a healthcare professional, many do not receive evidenced-based or minimally adequate treatment. Despite accumulating evidence favoring the effectiveness of CBT as a psychosocial treatment for anxiety disorders (Nathan and Gorman 2002), individuals with anxiety disorders in the United States are more likely to receive non-evidence–based psychosocial treatment. In the Harvard/Brown Anxiety Disorders Research Program (*N*=711 adults with panic disorder, agoraphobia, social phobia, or GAD), for example, only a small proportion of participants reported receiving cognitive (9%–14%) or behavioral therapy (9%–14%); the most frequently reported type of psychosocial treatment received was psychodynamic therapy (26%–29%) (Goisman et al. 1999).

Similar results were found in the NCS-R. Wang et al. (2005) defined *minimally adequate* treatment as 2 months or more of pharmacotherapy with an appropriate medication along with greater than four visits with a physician or eight or more sessions of psychotherapy. Approximately 52% of respondents meeting criteria for anxiety disorders received minimally adequate treatment from a mental health professional, with those who sought services from a nonpsychiatrist mental health professional (e.g., psychologist, social worker) being slightly more likely to receive minimally adequate treatment (51%) compared with those who sought treatment from a psychiatrist (46%). Only a small minority of those who sought treatment from a general medical practitioner (13%) received minimally adequate treatment. In the Australian National Survey of Mental Health and Well-Being, the majority (79%) of those who identified anxiety symptoms as a primary complaint reported never seeking any consultations or treatment for their anxiety symptoms. Even among respondents meeting diagnostic criteria for an anxiety disorder, more than half (59%) never sought any treatment for this condition. Of respondents who did seek treatment, only 52% received CBT or pharmacotherapy, resulting in less than one-quarter of individuals with anxiety disorder receiving appropriate treatment (Issakidis and Andrews 2002).

In summary, the burden of anxiety disorders can be measured not only in terms of economic impact but also in terms of quality of life, both for the individual with an anxiety disorder and for his or her family members. Subjective quality of life is significantly reduced for individuals with anxiety disorders. Although no overall differences in quality of life are evident among the different anxiety disorders, PTSD, GAD, and panic disorder appear to affect specific domains of quality of life more than do other anxiety-related conditions. There is considerable evidence to suggest that anxiety disorders (at least OCD and combat-related PTSD) are associated with problems in the partner relationship and family functioning as well as impairments in the individual family members' psychosocial functioning and quality of life. Although this has not been examined directly, it is reasonable to hypothesize that family members of patients with other anxiety disorders also suffer. Panic disorder and agoraphobia, for example, may have significant implications for family members because these patients often rely on family members to serve as safety signals by accompanying them out of the home. The presence of impairment in the family does not necessarily indicate unidirectional causality. Just as an individual's anxiety symptoms might negatively affect family functioning, it is equally possible that family dysfunction contributes to the etiology and/or maintenance of anxiety-related symptoms.

It is encouraging that research on the impact of evidenced-based pharmacotherapy and CBT generally shows a favorable impact on quality of life following an adequate trial of therapy. Although limited by a small number of studies assessing the long-term effect of treatment on quality of life as well as the long-term economic and societal benefits of quality of life improvement over time, the available evidence suggests that evidence-based treatment results in improved (although not necessarily normalized) quality of life. However, the rate of treatment attainment among individuals with anxiety disorders is abysmal, creating a major challenge for researchers and clinicians: although treatments have been developed that quite clearly reduce symptoms, improve quality of life, and decrease the overall burden of anxiety disorders, for the most part these interventions are not being delivered to the patients who need them. Advances in treatment dissemination to both clinicians and the public are clearly needed if the economic and social burden of anxiety is to be diminished.

Key Clinical Points

- Anxiety disorders are the most common category of mental disorder, with lifetime estimates ranging from 16% to 29%.
- Women, younger adults, and individuals of low socioeconomic status report the highest rates of anxiety disorders.
- Anxiety disorders are associated with an average of two psychiatric work impairment days per month, with the greatest number of impairment days seen in individuals with agoraphobia, adult separation anxiety disorder, posttraumatic stress disorder, panic disorder, and obsessive-compulsive disorder.
- Even individuals with remitted anxiety disorders report residual work impairment.
- Individuals with anxiety disorders are more likely to live below the federal poverty threshold than are those without anxiety disorders, with over one-third of respondents with OCD or agoraphobia living below the federal poverty line.
- The overall cost of anxiety disorders is estimated between $67 and $74 billion in 2007 dollars. Direct costs of nonpsychiatric medical treatment and lost revenue from work appear to be major contributors to the overall cost.
- Family members of individuals with anxiety disorders report high levels of distress, impairment, and caregiver burden.
- Anxiety disorders are associated with reduced quality of life, with no clear difference across diagnoses of anxiety disorder.
- Pharmacotherapy and cognitive-behavioral therapy have been demonstrated to improve quality of life, although some degree of long-term impairment is evident.
- Most individuals with anxiety disorders do not receive empirically supported treatments for their condition.

References

Alegria M, Takeuchi D, Canino G, et al: Considering context, place and culture: the National Latino and Asian American Study. Int J Methods Psychiatr Res 13:208–220, 2004

American Psychiatric Association: Diagnostic and Statistical Manual of Mental Disorders, 3rd Edition. Washington, DC, American Psychiatric Association, 1980

American Psychiatric Association: Diagnostic and Statistical Manual of Mental Disorders, 3rd Edition, Revised. Washington, DC, American Psychiatric Association, 1987

American Psychiatric Association: Diagnostic and Statistical Manual of Mental Disorders, 4th Edition. Washington, DC, American Psychiatric Association, 1994

Amir N, Freshman M, Foa EB: Family distress and involvement in relatives of obsessive-compulsive disorder patients. J Anxiety Disord 14:209–217, 2000

Angermeyer MC, Kilian R: Theoretical models of quality of life for mental disorders, in Quality of Life in Mental Disorders. Edited by Sartorius N. New York, Wiley, 1997, pp 19–54

Bandelow B, Stein DJ, Dolberg OT, et al: Improvement of quality of life in panic disorder with escitalopram, citalopram, or placebo. Pharmacopsychiatry 40:152–156, 2007

Beckham JC, Feldman ME, Kirby AC, et al: Interpersonal violence and its correlates in Vietnam veterans with chronic posttraumatic stress disorder. J Clin Psychol 53: 859–869, 1997

Black DW, Gaffney G, Schlosser S, et al: The impact of obsessive-compulsive disorder on the family: preliminary findings. J Nerv Ment Dis 186:440–442, 1998

Blazer D, Hughes D, George LK: Stressful life events and the onset of a generalized anxiety syndrome. Am J Psychiatry 144:1178–1183, 1987

Brady K, Pearlstein T, Asnis GM, et al: Efficacy and safety of sertraline treatment of posttraumatic stress disorder: a randomized controlled trial. JAMA 283:1837–1844, 2000

Bystritsky A, Saxena S, Maidment K, et al: Quality-of-life changes among patients with obsessive-compulsive disorder in a partial hospitalization program. Psychiatr Serv 50:412–414, 1999

Bystritsky A, Liberman RP, Hwang S, et al: Social functioning and quality of life comparisons between obsessive-compulsive and schizophrenic disorders. Depress Anxiety 14:214–218, 2001

Calhoun PS, Beckham JC, Bosworth HB: Caregiver burden and psychological distress in partners of veterans with chronic posttraumatic stress disorder. J Trauma Stress 15:205–212, 2002

Calvocoressi L, Lewis B, Harris M, et al: Family accommodation in obsessive-compulsive disorder. Am J Psychiatry 152:441–443, 1995

Card JJ: Epidemiology of PTSD in a national cohort of Vietnam veterans. J Clin Psychol 43:16–17, 1987

Carpiniello B, Baita A, Carta MG, et al: Clinical and psychosocial outcome of patients affected by panic disorder with or without agoraphobia: results from a naturalistic follow-up study. Eur Psychiatry 17:394–398, 2002

Carroll EM, Rueger DB, Foy DW, et al: Vietnam combat veterans with posttraumatic stress disorder: analysis of marital and cohabitating adjustment. J Abnorm Psychol 94: 329–337, 1985

Caselli LT, Motta RW: The effect of PTSD and combat level on Vietnam veterans' perceptions of child behavior and marital adjustment. J Clin Psychol 51:4–12, 1995

Chakrabarti S, Kulhara P, Verma SK: The pattern of burden in families of neurotic patients. Soc Psychiatry Psychiatr Epidemiol 28:172–177, 1993

Cohen J: Statistical Power Analysis for the Behavioral Sciences, 2nd Edition. Hillsdale, NJ, Lawrence Erlbaum Associates, 1988

Connor KM, Sutherland SM, Tupler LA, et al: Fluoxetine in post-traumatic stress disorder. Randomised, double-blind study. Br J Psychiatry 175:17–22, 1999

Cook JM, Riggs DS, Thompson R, et al: Posttraumatic stress disorder and current relationship functioning among World War II ex-prisoners of war. J Fam Psychol 18:36–45, 2004

Cooper M: Obsessive-compulsive disorder: effects on family members. Am J Orthopsychiatry 66:296–304, 1996

Cordioli AV, Heldt E, Bochi DB, et al: Cognitive-behavioral group therapy in obsessive-compulsive disorder: a randomized clinical trial. Psychother Psychosom 72:211–216, 2003

Craske MG: Origins of Phobias and Anxiety Disorders: Why More Women Than Men? New York, Elsevier, 2003

Davidson AC, Mellor DJ: The adjustment of children of Australian Vietnam veterans: is there evidence for the transgenerational transmission of the effects of war-related trauma? Aust N Z J Psychiatry 35:345–351, 2001

Davidson J, Smith R, Kudler H: Familial psychiatric illness in chronic posttraumatic stress disorder. Compr Psychiatry 30:339–445, 1989

Dekel R, Zahava S, Bleich A: Emotional distress and marital adjustment of caregivers: contribution of level of impairment and appraised burden. Anxiety Stress Coping 18:71–82, 2005

DeVol R, Bedroussian A: An Unhealthy America: The Economic Burden of Chronic Disease. Santa Monica, CA, Milken Institute, 2007

Deykin EY, Keane TM, Kaloupek D, et al: Posttraumatic stress disorder and the use of health services. Psychosom Med 63:835–841, 2001

Diefenbach GJ, Abramowitz JS, Norberg MM, et al: Changes in quality of life following cognitive-behavioral therapy for obsessive-compulsive disorder. Behav Res Ther 45:3060–3068, 2007

DuPont RL, Rice DP, Miller LS, et al: Economic costs of anxiety disorders. Anxiety 2:167–172, 1996a

DuPont RL, Rice DP, Shiraki S, et al: Economic costs of obsessive-compulsive disorder. Med Interface 8:102–109, 1996b

Endicott J, Nee J, Harrison W, et al: Quality of Life Enjoyment and Satisfaction Questionnaire: a new measure. Psychopharmacol Bull 29:321–326, 1993

Eng W, Coles ME, Heimberg RG, et al: Domains of life satisfaction in social anxiety disorder: relation to symptoms and response to cognitive-behavioral therapy. J Anxiety Disord 19:143–156, 2005

Fava GA, Rafanelli C, Ottolini F, et al: Psychological well-being and residual symptoms in remitted patients with panic disorder and agoraphobia. J Affect Disord 65:185–190, 2001

Gladis MM, Gosch EA, Dishuk NM, et al: Quality of life: Expanding the scope of clinical significance. J Consult Clin Psychol 67:320–331, 1999

Goisman RM, Warshaw MG, Keller MB: Psychosocial treatment prescriptions for generalized anxiety disorder, panic disorder, and social phobia, 1991–1996. Am J Psychiatry 156:1819–1821, 1999

Greenberg PE, Sisitsky T, Kessler RC, et al: The economic burden of anxiety disorders in the 1990s. J Clin Psychiatry 60:427–435, 1999

Harkness LL: The effect of combat-related PTSD on children. National Center for PTSD Clinical Newsletter 2:12–13, 1991

Heldt E, Blaya C, Isolan L, et al: Quality of life and treatment outcome in panic disorder: cognitive behavior group therapy effects in patients refractory to medication treatment. Psychother Psychosom 75:183–186, 2006

Helzer JE, Robins LN, McEvoy L: Post-traumatic stress disorder in the general population: findings of the epidemiologic catchment area survey. N Engl J Med 317:1630–1634, 1987

Hoehn-Saric R, McLeod DR, Hipsley PA: Effect of fluvoxamine on panic disorder. J Clin Psychopharmacol 13:321–326, 1993

Hollander E, Kwon JH, Stein DJ, et al: Obsessive-compulsive and spectrum disorders: overview and quality of life issues. J Clin Psychiatry 57 (suppl 8):3–6, 1996

Issakidis C, Andrews G: Service utilisation for anxiety in an Australian community sample. Soc Psychiatry Psychiatr Epidemiol 37:153–163, 2002

Jackson JS, Torres M, Caldwell CH, et al: The National Survey of American Life: a study of racial, ethnic and cultural influences on mental disorders and mental health. Int J Methods Psychiatr Res 13:196–207, 2004

Jacobs RJ, Davidson JR, Gupta S, et al: The effects of clonazepam on quality of life and work productivity in panic disorder. Am J Manag Care 3:1187–1196, 1997

Jordan BK, Marmar CR, Fairbank JA, et al: Problems in families of male Vietnam veterans with posttraumatic stress disorder. J Consult Clin Psychol 60:916–926, 1992

Kalra H, Kamath P, Trivedi JK, et al: Caregiver burden in anxiety disorders. Curr Opin Psychiatry 21:70–73, 2008

Karno MG, Sorensen SB, Burnam A: The epidemiology of OCD in five U.S. communities. Arch Gen Psychiatry 45:1094–1099, 1988

Kessler RC, Frank RG: The impact of psychiatric disorders on work loss days. Psychol Med 27:861–873, 1997

Kessler RC, Merikangas KR: The National Comorbidity Survey Replication (NCS-R): background and aims. Int J Methods Psychiatr Res 13:60–68, 2004

Kessler RC, McGonagle KA, Zhao S, et al: Lifetime and 12-month prevalence of DSM-III-R psychiatric disorders in the United States: results from the National Comorbidity Survey. Arch Gen Psychiatry 51:8–19, 1994

Kessler RC, Sonnega A, Bromet E, et al: Posttraumatic stress disorder in the National Comorbidity Survey. Arch Gen Psychiatry 52:1048–1060, 1995

Kessler RC, Mickelson KD, Barber CB, et al: The effects of chronic medical conditions on work impairment, in Caring and Doing for Others: Social Responsibility in the Domains of the Family, Work, and Community. Edited by Rossi AS. Chicago, IL, University of Chicago Press, 2001, pp 403–426

Kessler RC, Berglund P, Demler O, et al: Lifetime prevalence and age-of-onset distributions of DSM-IV disorders in the National Comorbidity Survey Replication. Arch Gen Psychiatry 62:593–602, 2005a

Kessler RC, Chiu WT, Demler O, et al: Prevalence, severity, and comorbidity of 12-month DSM-IV disorders in the National Comorbidity Survey Replication. Arch Gen Psychiatry 62:617–627, 2005b

Koran LM, Thienemann ML, Davenport R: Quality of life for patients with obsessive-compulsive disorder. Am J Psychiatry 153:783–788, 1996

Lecrubier Y, Judge R: Long-term evaluation of paroxetine, clomipramine and placebo in panic disorder. Collaborative Paroxetine Panic Study Investigators. Acta Psychiatr Scand 95:153–160, 1997

Lim D, Sanderson K, Andrews G: Lost productivity among full-time workers with mental disorders. J Ment Health Policy Econ 3:139–146, 2000

Magliano L, Tosini P, Guarneri M, et al: Burden on families of patients with obsessive-compulsive disorder: a pilot study. Eur Psychiatry 11:192–197, 1996

Malik ML, Connor KM, Sutherland SM, et al: Quality of life and posttraumatic stress disorder: a pilot study assessing changes in SF-36 scores before and after treatment in a placebo-controlled trial of fluoxetine. J Trauma Stress 12:387–393, 1999

Marciniak MD, Lage MJ, Dunayevich E, et al: The cost of treating anxiety: the medical and demographic correlates that impact total medical costs. Depress Anxiety 21:178–184, 2005

Marshall WL, Presse L, Andrews WR: A self-administered program for public speaking anxiety. Behav Res Ther 14:33–39, 1976

Mavissakalian MR, Perel JM, Talbott-Green M, et al: Gauging the effectiveness of extended imipramine treatment for panic disorder with agoraphobia. Biol Psychiatry 43:848–854, 1998

McRae AL, Brady KT, Mellman TA, et al: Comparison of nefazodone and sertraline for the treatment of posttraumatic stress disorder. Depress Anxiety 19:190–196, 2004

Menza MA, Dobkin RD, Marin H: An open-label trial of aripiprazole augmentation for treatment-resistant generalized anxiety disorder. J Clin Psychopharmacol 27:207–210, 2007

Michelson D, Lydiard RB, Pollack MH, et al: Outcome assessment and clinical improvement in panic disorder: evidence from a randomized controlled trial of fluoxetine and placebo. The Fluoxetine Panic Disorder Study Group. Am J Psychiatry 155:1570–1577, 1998

Moritz S, Rufer M, Fricke S, et al: Quality of life in obsessive-compulsive disorder before and after treatment. Compr Psychiatry 46:453–459, 2005

Muehlbacher M, Nickel MK, Nickel C, et al: Mirtazapine treatment of social phobia in women: a randomized, double-blind, placebo-controlled study. J Clin Psychopharmacol 25:580–583, 2005

Murray CJ, Lopez AD (eds): The Global Burden of Disease: A Comprehensive Assessment of Mortality and Disability From Diseases, Injuries, and Risk Factors in 1990 and Projected to 2020. Cambridge, MA, Harvard University Press, 1996

Narrow WE, Rae DS, Robins LN, et al: Revised prevalence estimates of mental disorders in the United States: using a clinical significance criterion to reconcile 2 surveys' estimates. Arch Gen Psychiatry 59:115–123, 2002

Nathan PE, Gorman JM: A Guide to Treatments That Work, 2nd Edition. New York, Oxford University Press, 2002

Olatunji BO, Cisler JM, Tolin DF: Quality of life in the anxiety disorders: a meta-analytic review. Clin Psychol Rev 27:572–581, 2007

O'Sullivan G, Noshirvani H, Marks I, et al: Six-year follow-up after exposure and clomipramine therapy for obsessive compulsive disorder. J Clin Psychiatry 52:150–155, 1991

Pohl RB, Wolkow RM, Clary CM: Sertraline in the treatment of panic disorder: a double-blind multicenter trial. Am J Psychiatry 155:1189–1195, 1998

Poisal JA, Truffer C, Smith S, et al: Health spending projections through 2016: modest changes obscure part D's impact. Health Aff (Millwood) 26:W242–W253, 2007

Pollack MH, Otto MW, Worthington JJ, et al: Sertraline in the treatment of panic disorder: a flexible-dose multicenter trial. Arch Gen Psychiatry 55:1010–1016, 1998

Pollack MH, Zaninelli R, Goddard A, et al: Paroxetine in the treatment of generalized anxiety disorder: results of a placebo-controlled, flexible-dosage trial. J Clin Psychiatry 62:350–357, 2001

Pollack MH, Lepola U, Koponen H, et al: A double-blind study of the efficacy of venlafaxine extended-release, paroxetine, and placebo in the treatment of panic disorder. Depress Anxiety 24:1–14, 2007

Rabin R, de Charro F: EQ-5D: a measure of health status from the EuroQol Group. Ann Med 33:337–343, 2001

Rapaport MH, Endicott J, Clary CM: Posttraumatic stress disorder and quality of life: results across 64 weeks of sertraline treatment. J Clin Psychiatry 63:59–65, 2002

Rapee RM, Abbott MJ, Baillie AJ, et al: Treatment of social phobia through pure self-help and therapist-augmented self-help. Br J Psychiatry 191:246–252, 2007

Regier DA, Boyd JH, Burke JD, et al: One-month prevalence of mental disorders in the United States: based on five Epidemiologic Catchment Area sites. Arch Gen Psychiatry 45:977–986, 1988

Regier DA, Narrow WE, Rae DS: The epidemiology of anxiety disorders: The Epidemiologic Catchment Area (ECA) experience. J Psychiatr Res 24:3–14, 1990

Regier DA, Kaelber CT, Rae DS, et al: Limitations of diagnostic criteria and assessment instruments for mental disorders: implications for research and policy. Arch Gen Psychiatry 55:109–115, 1998

Riggs DS, Byrne CA, Weathers FW, et al: The quality of the intimate relationships of male Vietnam veterans: problems associated with posttraumatic stress disorder. J Trauma Stress 11:87–101, 1998

Robins LN, Helzer JE, Weissman MM, et al: Lifetime prevalence of specific psychiatric disorders in three sites. Arch Gen Psychiatry 41:949–958, 1984

Rufer M, Fricke S, Moritz S, et al: Symptom dimensions in obsessive-compulsive disorder: prediction of cognitive-behavior therapy outcome. Acta Psychiatr Scand 113:440–446, 2006

Ruscio AM, Weathers FW, King LA, et al: Male war-zone veterans' perceived relationships with their children: the importance of emotional numbing. J Trauma Stress 15:351–357, 2002

Schnurr PP, Friedman MJ, Sengupta A, et al: PTSD and utilization of medical treatment services among male Vietnam veterans. J Nerv Ment Dis 188:496–504, 2000

Solomon Z, Waysman M, Levy G, et al: From front line to home front: a study of secondary traumatization. Fam Process 31:289–302, 1992

Stanley MA, Beck JG, Novy DM, et al: Cognitive-behavioral treatment of late-life generalized anxiety disorder. J Consult Clin Psychol 71:309–319, 2003

Stein DJ, Andersen HF, Goodman WK: Escitalopram for the treatment of GAD: efficacy across different subgroups and outcomes. Ann Clin Psychiatry 17:71–75, 2005

Stein MB, Kean YM: Disability and quality of life in social phobia: epidemiologic findings. Am J Psychiatry 157:1606–1613, 2000

Stein MB, Liebowitz MR, Lydiard RB, et al: Paroxetine treatment of generalized social phobia (social anxiety disorder): a randomized controlled trial. JAMA 280:708–713, 1998

Stein MB, Fyer AJ, Davidson JR, et al: Fluvoxamine treatment of social phobia (social anxiety disorder): a double-blind, placebo-controlled study. Am J Psychiatry 156:756–760, 1999

Steketee G, Grayson JB, Foa EB: A comparison of characteristics of obsessive-compulsive disorder and other anxiety disorders. J Anxiety Disord 1:325–335, 1987

Stengler-Wenzke K, Kroll M, Matschinger H, et al: Quality of life of relatives of patients with obsessive-compulsive disorder. Compr Psychiatry 47:523–527, 2006

Taft CT, Street AE, Marshall AD, et al: Posttraumatic stress disorder, anger, and partner abuse among Vietnam combat veterans. J Fam Psychol 21:270–277, 2007a

Taft CT, Vogt DS, Marshall AD, et al: Aggression among combat veterans: relationships with combat exposure and symptoms of posttraumatic stress disorder, dysphoria, and anxiety. J Trauma Stress 20:135–145, 2007b

Telch MJ, Schmidt NB, Jaimez TL, et al: Impact of cognitive-behavioral treatment on quality of life in panic disorder patients. J Consult Clin Psychol 63:823–830, 1995

Tenney NH, Denys DA, van Megen HJ, et al: Effect of a pharmacological intervention on quality of life in patients with obsessive-compulsive disorder. Int Clin Psychopharmacol 18:29–33, 2003

Tucker P, Zaninelli R, Yehuda R, et al: Paroxetine in the treatment of chronic posttraumatic stress disorder: results of a placebo-controlled, flexible-dosage trial. J Clin Psychiatry 62:860–868, 2001

Van Noppen BL, Steketee G: Family responses and multifamily behavioral treatment for obsessive-compulsive disorder. Brief Treat Crisis Interv 3:231–247, 2003

Veltro F, Magliano L, Lobrace S, et al: Burden on key relatives of patients with schizophrenia vs neurotic disorders: a pilot study. Soc Psychiatry Psychiatr Epidemiol 29:66–70, 1994

Verbosky SJ, Ryan DA: Female partners of Vietnam veterans: stress by proximity. Issues Ment Health Nurs 9:95–104, 1988

Wang PS, Lane M, Olfson M, et al: Twelve-month use of mental health services in the United States: results from the National Comorbidity Survey Replication. Arch Gen Psychiatry 62:629–640, 2005

Ware J, Kosinski M: SF-36 Physical and Mental Health Summary Scales: A User's Manual. Boston, MA, The Health Institute, 1994

Warshaw MG, Fierman E, Pratt L, et al: Quality of life and dissociation in anxiety disorder patients with histories of trauma or PTSD. Am J Psychiatry 150:1512–1516, 1993

Waysman M, Mikulincer M, Solomon Z, et al: Secondary traumatization among wives of PTSD combat veterans: a family typology. J Fam Psychol 7:104–118, 1993

Weissman MM: Panic disorder: impact on quality of life. J Clin Psychiatry 52(suppl):6–9, 1991

Weissman MM, Bothwell S: Assessment of social adjustment by patient self-report. Arch Gen Psychiatry 33:1111–1115, 1976

WHO World Mental Health Survey Consortium: Prevalence, severity, and unmet need for treatment of mental disorders in the World Health Organization World Mental Health Surveys. JAMA 291:2581–2590, 2004

Wittchen HU: Generalized anxiety disorder: prevalence, burden, and cost to society. Depress Anxiety 16:162–171, 2002

Wittchen HU, Jacobi F: Size and burden of mental disorders in Europe—a critical review and appraisal of 27 studies. Eur Neuropsychopharmacol 15:357–376, 2005

Zatzick DF, Marmar CR, Weiss DS, et al: Posttraumatic stress disorder and functioning and quality of life outcomes in a nationally representative sample of male Vietnam veterans. Am J Psychiatry 154:1690–1695, 1997

Recommended Readings

DuPont RL, Rice DP, Shiraki S, et al: Economic costs of obsessive-compulsive disorder. Med Interface 8:102–109, 1996

Greenberg PE, Sisitsky T, Kessler RC, et al: The economic burden of anxiety disorders in the 1990s. J Clin Psychiatry 60:427–435, 1999

Kessler RC, Frank RG: The impact of psychiatric disorders on work loss days. Psychol Med 27:861–873, 1997

Murray CJ, Lopez AD (eds): The Global Burden of Disease: A Comprehensive Assessment of Mortality and Disability From Diseases, Injuries, and Risk Factors in 1990 and Projected to 2020. Cambridge, MA, Harvard University Press, 1996

Olatunji BO, Cisler JM, Tolin DF: Quality of Life in the Anxiety Disorders: A Meta-Analytic Review. Clin Psychol Rev 27:572–581, 2007

Chapter 41

Consumer Considerations

Jerilyn Ross, M.A., L.I.C.S.W.

Nam et ipsa scientia potestas est. [Knowledge is power.]

—Francis Bacon, *Meditationes Sacrae* (1597)

In an address delivered at the University of California, Berkeley, on March 23, 1962, John Fitzgerald Kennedy, the 35th president of the United States, said, "In a time of turbulence and change, it is more true than ever that knowledge is power." Truer words could not be uttered today to echo the discrepancy that exists in turbulent health care systems throughout the world; namely, the educated, well-informed consumer has a distinct advantage over his or her uninformed counterpart. As Herzlinger (1997) wrote, "The relationship between education and health seems beyond dispute. People who understand the relationship between their own behavior and their health are better prepared to manage their health."

Education, information, and knowledge appear to be key elements for today's demanding health care consumer. These skills empower individuals to gain mastery over their illnesses and to place realistic demands on the health care marketplace. To paraphrase Sir Francis Bacon, the sixteenth-century English philosopher, and President Kennedy, knowledge is power—especially as it pertains to the health care consumer, supplier, and legislator. In this chapter, I attempt to summarize consumer-relevant information on several key facets of anxiety disorders, including their severity, the consequences if they are not treated or are inadequately treated, the economic burden such disorders impose on society, and barriers to treatment for the consumer.

In recent years, a proliferation of newspaper and magazine articles, Internet resources, television and radio talk shows, and books—both academic and self-help—has been tremendously helpful in raising consciousness about the seriousness and the treatability of anxiety disorders. Yet, as evidenced by the many people who contact the Anxiety Disorders Association of America (ADAA), Mental Health America (formerly known as the National Mental Health Association), the National Alliance on Mental Illness (NAMI), the Obsessive Compulsive Foundation (OCF), and other consumer organizations focused on anxiety and related disorders, people continue to be unable to find and/or afford effective treatment. Further, millions of people remain in the dark about their anxiety-related conditions.

Severity of the Problem

Anxiety disorders are among the most common psychiatric illnesses (Ross 1994). Yet despite the prevalence of anxiety disorders, they have been and continue to be grossly underdiagnosed, misdiagnosed, or inadequately treated. Moreover, the mortality rate is higher in individuals with anxiety disorders, especially panic disorder, than in individuals without anxiety disorders. The data, although controversial, also suggest that premature mortality is increased in persons with anxiety disorders because of an increased suicide rate in both sexes and because of an increased rate of cardiovascular disease in men. Comorbidity with other psychiatric illnesses has been cited extensively and includes comorbid anxiety disorders, major depressive disorder, and personality disorders. The concomitant use of alcohol and illegal drugs is also a complication for individuals with anxiety disorders. In an attempt to self-medicate the dreaded signs and symptoms of anxiety disorders, particularly panic disorder, individuals will often receive temporary relief from the use of alcohol and illicit street drugs. However, they often experience rebound symptoms of anxiety, intensifying their anxiety disorder and laying the groundwork for a concomitant substance abuse problem. In fact, studies show that approximately 10% of the adults with alcoholism meet the criteria for panic disorder.

Millions of persons with anxiety disorders suffer in silence or go from doctor to doctor; many have no idea what is wrong with them (Ross 1994). Simply identifying the correct diagnosis can be a challenge, because the physical symptoms that accompany some anxiety disorders send the patients to medical doctors who often have little or no training in the diagnosis and management of anxiety disorders. This category of mental disorders, therefore, is both underrecognized and underdiagnosed by the medical profession. In response to this problem, the ADAA and other consumer organizations have initiated the following proactive activities:

- Promote the education and training of mental health professionals about effective treatments for anxiety disorders.
- Educate non–mental health specialists, such as medical general practitioners, gynecologists, and cardiologists, in the diagnosis and treatment of anxiety disorders. Provide these health care professionals with referral information and literature for patients with anxiety disorders.
- Help consumers, families, and friends recognize anxiety disorders and get help.

Rosalynn Carter, former first lady of the United States, maintains that discrimination against those with mental disorders and stigmatization of them by society, and particularly by health care professionals, is common in the United States today. She writes:

> We must end discrimination against those with mental disorders. Discrimination has denied those who need care access to appropriate services for far too long, and it continues to limit resources available to pay for care. We must recognize that mental health is an integral part of every person's health. Awareness of mental health problems needs to permeate the health-care system. Primary-care physicians, nurses, physicians' assistants—all must have sufficient knowledge about the interdependency between mind and body to know when intervention is necessary and who is best able to intervene. (Ross 1994, p. xi)

The stigma that comes with mental illness in American society has yet to be dissipated, and it certainly affects those who have an anxiety disorder. Indeed, many persons with agoraphobia, for instance, cite "fear of going crazy" as one of the symptoms of a panic attack. It also was startling to learn that although anxiety disorders are the most common psychiatric illnesses in the population and are among the most treatable of psychiatric illnesses, a subanalysis of data from the National Comorbidity Survey indicates that only about 20% of persons with anxiety disorders perceive the need for treatment, and even fewer seek help (Mojtabai et al. 2002).

Consequences of Untreated Anxiety Disorders

Untreated or inadequately treated anxiety disorders can have significant costs to the patient, to the patient's family, and to society, affecting the use of health care services, the gross domestic product, and other sectors. As Mrs. Carter noted:

> When an anxiety disorder is not recognized or appropriately treated, the toll is great, not only to the individual, but to his or her family and the community at large. Many people with panic disorder, for instance, have markedly constrained lifestyles because of fear of traveling any distance from home, which often leaves

> them unable to fulfill family responsibilities, career functions, and social obligations. Many also have concurrent depression. Treating the underlying disorder will not only decrease a great deal of personal suffering, but will also have a positive effect on families, communities, and the workplace. (Ross 1994)

The ADAA averages between 5 and 6 million hits on its Web site each month from individuals seeking information and help. In addition, ADAA receives thousands of e-mails, letters, and phone calls. Not everyone tells his or her whole story—many of them are simply seeking information or want to find help. Many individuals, however, do give details, and in particular they talk about the consequences of untreated anxiety disorders. Some of the issues that many of these poignant stories have in common include the following:

- Repeated doctor and emergency room visits
- Extensive, expensive, and often unnecessary medical examinations
- Reliance on disability insurance
- Academic underperformance
- Vocational limitations
- Use of alcohol to self-medicate
- Depression
- Suicidal ideation and attempts

These individuals write and talk about disrupted personal lives, aborted careers, substance abuse, and a great deal of despair and discouragement. Sometimes they describe symptoms of outright depression and discuss suicidal ideation and attempts. They describe what it is like to live on disability because they are unable to work. Clearly, this raises issues about their quality of life, which obviously appears to be diminished. In addition, they experience decreased family involvement, increased family burdens on caregivers, decreased career functioning, and decreased social functioning.

Overall Cost of Anxiety Disorders to Society

The overall costs of an illness include not only the direct and indirect costs but also what may be termed intangible costs, including pain and suffering experienced by the patient and his or her family (Andreasen 1991; Martin 1995). It is especially important for the medical profession to embrace the concept of the intangible costs of an illness to society, particularly in this era of constrained health care dollars because of increased managed care penetration. The lost potential of those with an anxiety disorder, excluded from the cultural, economic, or social life of the United States through fear and ignorance, cannot be quantified in dollars, and even the most conservative estimates barely scratch the surface. (For a more detailed discussion of these issues, see Chapter 40 of this volume, "The Economic and Social Burden of Anxiety Disorders.")

Barriers to Diagnosis and Treatment

Anxiety disorders cost the nation more than $42 billion per year, much of it attributable to misdiagnosis and undertreatment. More than half the tab is associated with repeated use of health care services because those with anxiety disorders seek relief from symptoms that mimic physical illnesses. People with an anxiety disorder are three to five times more likely to go to the doctor and 6 times more likely to be hospitalized than people without an anxiety disorder (Greenberg et al. 1999).

In 1996, the National Institute of Mental Health (NIMH) conducted focus groups among patients with anxiety disorders to determine their level of knowledge about the signs and symptoms of anxiety disorders. In addition, they collected data regarding attitudes, motivations, and barriers to both diagnosis and treatment among individuals with anxiety disorders. Unequivocally, the response given most often as the major common barrier to those persons either seeking or receiving treatment for their anxiety disorders was lack of medical coverage in the United States. Of paramount importance was that several focus group participants also cited the receipt of inadequate or poor treatment for their disease, either as a direct result of their uninsured status or because of inadequate coverage by their particular plan.

Other barriers to treatment mentioned in these focus groups included the consumer's concern that medical professionals would not have knowledge about the correct treatment for their particular form of anxiety disorder or that they would not be sympathetic to an individual with an anxiety disorder. Several participants said that they have been reluctant to seek treatment because they did not know what treatment would entail. Furthermore, many participants reported that they saw numerous medical and mental health professionals before they were given the correct diagnosis of an anxiety disorder.

Ignorance about anxiety disorders on the part of both physicians and patients, together with a widespread misunderstanding about the relation of mind and body, has been among the chief barriers to treatment of anxiety disorders for most of those who need it.

These barriers are compounded by a tendency on the part of physicians and other professionals to ignore or belittle many complaints that affect primarily women, as most anxiety disorders do. A wall of ignorance—and to some extent injustice—has separated those who have an anxiety disorder from those who could treat it (Ross 1994).

To be fair, much of the knowledge about these disorders has emerged only in the past three decades, and much remains to be discovered—about genetic predisposition and about emotional and environmental factors that precipitate the disorders. Nevertheless, as mentioned earlier in this chapter, the stigma that comes with mental illness in our society has yet to be dissipated.

Other barriers to treatment of anxiety disorders for today's health care consumer include the role of the gatekeeper physician in many managed care plans or health maintenance organizations. As we read on a daily basis in our newspapers and hear repeatedly on television, the demanding health care consumer is annoyed with the gatekeeper physician concept. Consumers want to go to a specialist without having to obtain permission in advance from the gatekeeper—hence the increasing demand for those managed care plans that allow for some choice and for point-of-service plans—and if they do have to go to a gatekeeper, they want that clinician to be well informed about the signs and symptoms of anxiety disorders. Among legislators, who are crucial in shaping health care policy in the United States, many lack an understanding of the widespread prevalence of anxiety disorders and of their severity and treatment profiles. Education and information, such as that provided by consumer organizations, may help inform these key legislators and enable them to make more prudent health care policy choices for their constituents.

The Consumer Organization as Voice and Resource

The ADAA, founded in 1980 as the Phobia Society of America, targets the elimination of ignorance surrounding anxiety disorders as its first priority. This national group is devoted to relieving the trivialization and stigma of anxiety disorders. In addition, the ADAA is dedicated to the early identification, prevention, and treatment of anxiety disorders, as well as to improving the lives of people who have them (Ross 1997).

Other consumer organizations, such as the Obsessive Compulsive Foundation and Mental Health America, similarly focus on public and professional awareness, on promoting research, on advocacy, and on increasing the availability of cost-effective treatment for the anxiety disorders. Public and professional awareness activities seek to raise awareness, reduce and eliminate stigma, increase understanding about recognition, increase diagnostic skills, and increase knowledge about effective treatments.

Consumer organizations serve as clearinghouses for information related to the anxiety disorders and provide a forum for mental health researchers, clinicians, and consumers. Diverging views about some elements of anxiety disorders are often recognized, debate is encouraged, and input from different disciplines is welcomed.

Such organizations handle tens of thousands of requests for help each year and have become public symbols of reassurance to those with anxiety disorders and their friends and families.

Cooperative efforts with other mental health organizations and government agencies to increase access to treatment and erase the stigma surrounding anxiety disorders are another top priority for many consumer organizations, as is the development of self-help groups. Self-help groups have played an increasingly vital role in providing support to individuals with anxiety disorders, helping patients find treatment, and advocating public policies that help ease the burdens of anxiety disorders.

The news media are also a target of consumer groups because of their ability to home in on the idea that these disorders can affect anybody at any time. Information on anxiety disorders has been provided on the Internet, on dozens of national television and radio programs, and in several hundred newspapers and magazines. Indeed, extensive strategies of public education and policy advocacy can lower treatment barriers and promote the welfare of individuals with anxiety disorders.

Too often, individuals with anxiety disorders have been victimized by ignorance, misdiagnosis, and misunderstanding. In response to these difficulties, consumer organizations can:

- Teach clergy, school counselors, and employee assistance personnel how to recognize anxiety disorders, make referrals, and provide information and guidance
- Extend information outreach to new constituencies, including hospitals and emergency rooms, university networks, and libraries
- Alert national and state legislators to the societal costs of anxiety disorders, including the expense to the health care system of unnecessary tests and repeat examinations because of misdiagnoses

- Persuade government agencies to commit increased funds to anxiety disorders research
- Inform private industry about the economic waste and lost productivity because of untreated anxiety disorders and help them better understand anxiety disorders in the workplace
- Work for increased insurance reimbursement for anxiety disorders treatment
- Conduct joint efforts with other mental health organizations to stimulate more focused attention on anxiety disorders
- Maintain a position as centers of exchange for new information on anxiety disorders
- Conduct broad-based fundraising to support high-quality research either directly or through existing organizations

The mission and activities of many consumer organizations are consistent with the philosophy that knowledge is power. These organizations seek to provide education and information to today's health care consumers, providers, and legislators in an effort to give the individual who has an anxiety disorder a sense of self-empowerment and mastery over the disorder.

Stories From the Front Lines: Consumer Frustrations

In addition to the thousands of e-mails and letters that are received annually by consumer organizations, scores of telephone calls are received daily. Most of those who contact the organizations want reassurance that they have a real and treatable condition, that they are not alone, and that help is available for them. Examples of some of the most common frustrations expressed by individuals who contact the ADAA are:

- "I feel like a hypochondriac."
- "Everyone thinks I act anxious for attention. They think I should just pull myself together."
- "My health insurance paid thousands of dollars for medical tests, but when I was finally given the diagnosis of an anxiety disorder, I was denied coverage for treatment."
- "My community mental health center said they couldn't help me. Isn't an anxiety disorder a mental health problem?"

Most of the participants in the focus groups conducted by the NIMH in 1996, discussed earlier in this chapter, reported the following key statements:

- Anxiety disorder symptoms or behaviors were present for years before help was sought.
- The anxiety or behaviors experienced by patients with an anxiety disorder were different from those of people without an anxiety disorder.
- Patients were seen by many health professionals before receiving a correct diagnosis.
- The worst thing about undiagnosed anxiety disorders was the inability to do what one wanted in life.
- The best thing about receiving an anxiety disorder diagnosis was knowing that one was not "crazy."
- The disorder was seldom discussed with people other than close friends and family.

Other frustrations voiced by today's more demanding health care consumers, some of whom are patients with anxiety disorders, include a direct challenge to the current managed care environment. In particular, many consumers seem dissatisfied with 1) the role of the gatekeeper physician, especially if that clinician is uninformed about the signs and symptoms of the different types of anxiety disorders; 2) the difficulty in getting an appointment with a specialist (e.g., a psychiatrist, a psychopharmacologist, or a psychologist)—in part because of capitation, in which the goal of the health care provider is to reduce the number of referrals to specialists; and 3) the fact that many insurance plans have "carved out" mental health benefits, making it very difficult for persons with anxiety disorders to obtain adequate and appropriate treatment.

In addition, today's educated, well-informed health care consumer is more familiar with the widespread prevalence of anxiety disorders and the ease with which most can be successfully treated. However, many individuals with anxiety disorders feel that their "voices in the government" (i.e., health care policymakers) do not understand the severity of the disease or the ease with which it can be properly treated.

The Human Side: Patient Vignettes

Three letters recently received by the ADAA from people describing what it is like to live with these disorders are illustratively poignant.

36-Year-Old Man From North Carolina

When I get out of bed each morning, I am faced with fighting…to survive…. My body is filled with so much anxiety; many times I actually feel…I am dying. I have gone to all kinds of doctors…even spent some time in the hospital to try to figure out what the symptoms are or what is causing them. The frustrating part...I am told that it is only my nerves. Even worse...my insurance paid for all the doctors and hospitals when no one could help me, but they won't pay for a psychiatrist.

17-Year-Old Girl From California

My fears have taken over my life. I can't leave my house. I was a straight-A student, and now I'm too scared to go to school. I don't know what to do. I would like to be able to do things that normal people do...school...job...ride in a car. It's hard remembering what I used to do...all I have are the memories. I'm at a point where I either get on the right track now or I give up. Your organization is my last hope.

39-Year-Old Woman From Michigan

I am becoming a very unpleasant burden to my family. I'm a failure as a human being. People/friends make me feel that I'm like this on purpose. I treat my husband awful because I'm mad at me. I have given suicide a lot of thought.... I'm scared of everything. Please, can you help me and my family? My life depends on it.

These are truly tragic stories; however, they are not extraordinary. They are typical of what we read and hear about every day at consumer organizations.

Medical Agenda

In today's tightly regulated managed care environment, most patients with symptoms consistent with an anxiety disorder initially are evaluated by a primary care physician in the role of gatekeeper. Primary care physicians see roughly half of the adult population with an anxiety disorder (Harmon et al. 2002). Because of the myriad signs and symptoms associated with anxiety disorders, the differential diagnosis is obviously lengthy and complicated. Therefore, a full battery of standard medical procedures, including history, physical examination, and basic laboratory data, is indicated when working up a patient with a suspected anxiety disorder. However, because the signs and symptoms consistent with anxiety accompany many medical and psychiatric conditions, the differential diagnosis is not always straightforward.

The successful treatment of anxiety disorders often involves collaboration between medical and nonmedical clinicians. However, this can pose a problem in today's competitive health care provider marketplace because turf battles often arise among the various mental health professionals, including psychiatrists, psychologists, and social workers. If each is able to place the needs of the patient over the economic needs of the professional's parent organization (i.e., managed care company/health maintenance organization) or private practice, then the medical and nonmedical clinicians should be able to work in harmony.

Time and reimbursement constraints are placed on psychiatrists who practice in a managed care setting; therefore, the psychiatrist's role in psychotherapy for many psychopathological conditions has markedly diminished (Wilson et al. 1997). Teamwork and a collaborative effort between medical and nonmedical providers have become crucial to the successful management of anxiety disorders. The ability of the nonmedical clinician to share problems and issues that arise in the management of a particular patient with their medical colleagues can only strengthen the team's ability to maintain a comprehensive, adequate treatment plan that best serves the needs of that patient.

The primary care physician plays a vital role in today's managed care organization and often is active in the treatment and management of psychiatric disorders, including anxiety disorders. From a health consumer perspective this may be problematic, because primary care physicians often lack knowledge about anxiety disorders and are not always sympathetic to the plight of the afflicted patients. Limited training in primary care residency programs may affect their treatment decision making. For example, the primary care physician may not be willing to prescribe a benzodiazepine when it is the drug of choice for a particular patient's signs and symptoms, or the physician may taper a patient's medication too rapidly, causing an iatrogenic withdrawal syndrome. In addition, the primary care physician may not be familiar with the evidence-based efficacy of nonmedical therapies, and this may cause difficulties with referrals to nonmedical behavioral health professionals.

Wilson et al. (1997) suggested a list of questions for the health care consumer to ask his or her treating physician or therapist:

1. What training have you received in the treatment of anxiety disorders?
2. What are your views on medication management of this disorder? On cognitive-behavioral therapy?
3. What are your views regarding the origin of anxiety disorders?
4. How do you evaluate treatment progress and outcome?

5. Describe, in general, your treatment protocols for
   - A. Panic disorder
   - B. Agoraphobia
   - C. Social phobia (e.g., public speaking)
   - D. Specific phobia (e.g., fear of flying)
   - E. Generalized anxiety disorder
   - F. Obsessive-compulsive disorder
   - G. Posttraumatic stress disorder

Government's Role

Any comprehensive discussion of the political agenda of health care reform must take into account the fact that even in the United States, 44 million Americans are estimated to be uninsured (Mental Health Liaison Group 2000), and the number continues to rise. Coupled with this fact, it is clear that many legislators who are involved in creating health care policy are not properly informed about the severity and the treatment success of anxiety disorders (Ross 1994).

Those of us involved in anxiety disorders research, treatment, and public and professional education are all too familiar with the gaps and frustrations in our health care system—in particular, the lack of access for people with anxiety disorders to publicly funded mental health facilities and to adequate health insurance to cover private treatment (Ross 1994).

Key goals of the ADAA and other consumer organizations include promoting research on anxiety disorders and the equal treatment of mental and physical illnesses. In 1990, following the NIMH's Consensus Conference on Panic Disorder, consumer organizations were instrumental in encouraging NIMH to launch a major national education campaign to promote awareness of panic disorder. Following the success of that program, NIMH expanded its efforts to embrace all of the anxiety disorders. In a subsequent partnership in 1995, the ADAA and NIMH conducted a survey that found that Americans misunderstand panic disorder and that the most at-risk group (women ages 18–34) is the least likely to recognize the illness and the most likely to incorrectly believe that the condition is a result of a person's difficulty in handling stress. Consumer organizations look forward to their continued involvement in the government's efforts to educate the public and health professionals about the fact that anxiety disorders are real, serious, and treatable.

The progress and the momentum that were generated in the research and treatment of anxiety disorders in the 1990s, dubbed the "Decade of the Brain," are ongoing. Consumer organizations have entered the new millennium with continued determination to provide hope, help, and resources (both governmental and private) for those tormented by anxiety disorders and those dedicated to treating these mental illnesses. The goal is to bring anxiety disorders under control and move them nearer the top of the national health care agenda, with support from an enlightened public, with increased awareness by the health care community, and with firm and steady pressure from those with anxiety disorders (i.e., the consumers) (Ross 1997).

Conclusion

Although the NIMH has reported that about 40 million Americans have an anxiety disorder, the good news is that anxiety disorders are among the most treatable of all psychiatric disorders. In fact, research data compiled during the "Decade of the Brain" suggest that cognitive-behavioral therapy and new medications have mitigated the disturbing signs and symptoms consistent with anxiety disorders in approximately 60%–90% of the afflicted individuals, allowing them to lead normal lives again.

The pervasive problems posed by anxiety disorders have several solutions, which are being addressed on a national level (through the NIMH) and through mental health advocacy groups. The messages concerning anxiety disorders recommended by the NIMH focus groups are consistent with what have found to be most effective in motivating those with anxiety disorders to reach out for help. The following key messages were identified by the NIMH focus groups:

- Anxiety disorders are common, treatable biochemical or genetic disorders.
- Anxiety disorders have a lengthy duration of symptoms and interfere with day-to-day functioning.
- The tone of anxiety disorder education messages should be positive and comforting, not threatening or scary.
- In addition to describing the wide range of behavioral, cognitive, and physical symptoms, education messages should stress the common effects of these symptoms across disorders: 1) feeling a lack of control over one's life, 2) not being able to live the life one wants to live, and 3) wasting time and energy on nonproductive behaviors.

Consumers can advocate for the early recognition and diagnosis of anxiety disorders; access to affordable, effective treatment; and increased funding for research from the government and private sources. The psychiatric community is encouraged to join in efforts to educate health care consumers, other health care providers, and legislators at both the state and the national levels about the severity and treatability of anxiety disorders. It is our responsibility to help those who have anxiety disorders to have access to the care they need and deserve.

Finally, one encouraging letter can be shared to show what can happen when the whole system—the media, physicians, and an advocacy group—works together.

44-Year-Old Woman From Oklahoma

It's been a long ten years—two years on disability, extensive medical tests, thousands of dollars, a broken marriage, lost friendships.... I had no idea what was wrong with me or that help was available. I could go on, but what I want to tell you is that I have returned to a productive life.... I'm now practicing law again ... believe it or not, it was an Ann Landers article on panic disorder that saved my life. I cried for three days after reading it, wrote to you to get the name of a psychiatrist in my city who could help me, and within three months this nearly suicidal recluse returned to work and got back in touch with friends.

◀ Key Clinical Points ▶

Educational efforts directed at the health care consumer, the health care provider (e.g., the primary care physician), and legislators at both national and local levels must emphasize the following messages:

- Anxiety disorders are prevalent, undertreated, disabling, costly, and often comorbid with depression and/or substance abuse.
- Patients and physicians should be aware of the most common signs and symptoms of anxiety disorders.
- Managed correctly, the treatment of anxiety disorders can be highly successful.
- Appropriate treatment can allow patients with anxiety disorders to lead normal, productive lives.
- Successful treatment often involves both medical and nonmedical interventions.
- Knowledge and skill of the health care provider is a major variable affecting treatment outcome.
- Funding for research on anxiety disorders by the NIMH and from pharmaceutical companies in the private sector must be increased.
- Consumer organizations are working on the patient's behalf to improve the lives of people who have anxiety disorders.

References

Andreasen NC: Assessment issues and the cost of schizophrenia. Schizophr Bull 17:475–481, 1991

Greenberg PE, Sisitsky T, Kessler RC, et al: The economic burden of anxiety disorders in the 1990s. J Clin Psychiatry 60:427–435, 1999

Harmon JS, Rollman, BL, Shear MK, et al: Physician office visits of adults for anxiety disorders in the United States, 1987–1998. J Gen Intern Med 17:165–172, 2002

Herzlinger RE: Market-Driven Health Care. Reading, MA, Addison-Wesley, 1997

Martin P: Medical economic impact of schizophrenia. Encephale 3:67–73, 1995

Mental Health Liaison Group: Responding to the Mental Health Needs of America: A Briefing Document for Candidates and Policy Makers. Washington, DC, Mental Health Liaison Group, 2000

Mojtabia R, Olfson M, Mechanic D: Perceived need and help-seeking in adults with mood, anxiety, or substance use disorders. Arch Gen Psychiatry 59:77–84, 2002

Ross J: Triumph Over Fear: A Book of Help and Hope for People With Anxiety, Panic Attacks, and Phobias. New York, Bantam Books, 1994

Ross J: ACNP and the Anxiety Disorders Association of America: sharing an advocacy agenda. ACNP Bulletin, March 2–7, 1997

Wilson JO, Ross J, DuPont RL: Anxiety disorders in managed care. Behavioral Health Management 17:33–38, 1997

Recommended Readings

Anxiety Disorders Association of America: Improving the Diagnosis and Treatment of Generalized Anxiety Disorder: A Dialogue Between Mental Health Professionals and Primary Care Physicians. Silver Spring, MD, Anxiety Disorders Association of America, 2004

Kramer M, Ross J, Davidson J: Brief reports: consumers who call the Anxiety Disorders Association of America: characteristics and satisfaction. J Nerv Ment Dis 189:328–331, 2001

Laden S: Promoting Better Outcomes for Primary Care Patients With Anxiety Disorders. Silver Spring, MD, Anxiety Disorders Association of America, 2006

Web Sites of Interest

Anxiety Disorders Association of America. http://www.adaa.org

Mental Health America. http://www.mentalhealthamerica.net

National Institute of Mental Health, National Anxiety Disorders Program. http://intramural.nimh.nih.gov/mood

Obsessive Compulsive Foundation. http://www.ocfoundation.org

Index

Page numbers printed in **boldface** type refer to tables or figures.